Evidence-Based Gastroenterology and Hepatology
THIRD EDITION

Evidence-Based Gastroenterology and Hepatology

THIRD EDITION

EDITED BY

John WD McDonald

Professor of Medicine
Robarts Clinical Trials, Robarts Research Unit
University of Western Ontario
London, Ontario, Canada

Andrew K Burroughs

Professor of Hepatology and Consultant Physician/Hepatologist
The Royal Free Sheila Sherlock Liver Centre
Royal Free Hospital, and University College London
London, UK

Brian G Feagan

Professor of Medicine
Robarts Clinical Trials, Robarts Research Unit
University of Western Ontario
London, Ontario, Canada

M Brian Fennerty

Professor of Medicine
Oregon Health and Science University
Division of Gastroenterology and Hepatology
Portland, Oregon, USA

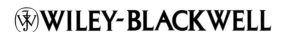
WILEY-BLACKWELL
A John Wiley & Sons, Ltd., Publication

BMJ|Books

This edition first published 2010. © 2010, 2004, 1999 by Blackwell Publishing Ltd

Blackwell Publishing was acquired by John Wiley & Sons in February 2007. Blackwell's publishing program has been merged with Wiley's global Scientific, Technical and Medical business to form Wiley-Blackwell.

Registered office: John Wiley & Sons Ltd, The Atrium, Southern Gate, Chichester, West Sussex, PO19 8SQ, UK
Editorial offices: 9600 Garsington Road, Oxford, OX4 2DQ, UK

The Atrium, Southern Gate, Chichester, West Sussex, PO19 8SQ, UK

111 River Street, Hoboken, NJ 07030-5774, USA

For details of our global editorial offices, for customer services and for information about how to apply for permission to reuse the copyright material in this book please see our website at www.wiley.com/wiley-blackwell

The right of the author to be identified as the author of this work has been asserted in accordance with the Copyright, Designs and Patents Act 1988.

Wiley also publishes its books in a variety of electronic formats. Some content that appears in print may not be available in electronic books.

Designations used by companies to distinguish their products are often claimed as trademarks. All brand names and product names used in this book are trade names, service marks, trademarks or registered trademarks of their respective owners. The publisher is not associated with any product or vendor mentioned in this book. This publication is designed to provide accurate and authoritative information in regard to the subject matter covered. It is sold on the understanding that the publisher is not engaged in rendering professional services. If professional advice or other expert assistance is required, the services of a competent professional should be sought.

The contents of this work are intended to further general scientific research, understanding, and discussion only and are not intended and should not be relied upon as recommending or promoting a specific method, diagnosis, or treatment by physicians for any particular patient. The publisher and the author make no representations or warranties with respect to the accuracy or completeness of the contents of this work and specifically disclaim all warranties, including without limitation any implied warranties of fitness for a particular purpose. In view of ongoing research, equipment modifications, changes in governmental regulations, and the constant flow of information relating to the use of medicines, equipment, and devices, the reader is urged to review and evaluate the information provided in the package insert or instructions for each medicine, equipment, or device for, among other things, any changes in the instructions or indication of usage and for added warnings and precautions. Readers should consult with a specialist where appropriate. The fact that an organization or Website is referred to in this work as a citation and/or a potential source of further information does not mean that the author or the publisher endorses the information the organization or Website may provide or recommendations it may make. Further, readers should be aware that Internet Websites listed in this work may have changed or disappeared between when this work was written and when it is read. No warranty may be created or extended by any promotional statements for this work. Neither the publisher nor the author shall be liable for any damages arising herefrom.

Library of Congress Cataloging-in-Publication Data
Evidence-based gastroenterology and hepatology / edited by John W.D. McDonald . . . [et al.]. – 3rd ed.
    p. ; cm.
  Includes bibliographical references and index.
    ISBN 978-1-4051-8193-8 (alk. paper)
  1. Gastroenterology–Textbooks.   2. Hepatology–Textbooks.   3. Gastrointestinal system–Diseases–Textbooks.   4. Liver–Diseases–Textbooks.   5. Evidence-based medicine–Textbooks.   I. McDonald, John W.D.
    [DNLM: . Gastrointestinal Diseases–diagnosis.   2. Gastrointestinal Diseases–therapy.   3. Evidence-based Medicine–methods.   4. Liver Diseases–diagnosis.   5. Liver Diseases–therapy. WI 140 E928 2010]
  RC801.E95 2010
  616.3'3–dc22

                                                                                                    2010011010

A catalogue record for this book is available from the British Library.

Set in 9.25/12pt Palatino by Toppan Best-set Premedia Limited
Printed and bound in Singapore by Fabulous Printers Pte Ltd

1   2010

Contents

Contents

The colour plate section can be found facing p. 266.

Evidence-Based Medicine Series
Updates and additional resources for the books in this series are available from:
www.evidencebasedseries.com

Contributors

Bincy P Abraham
Section of Gastroenterology and Hepatology, Baylor College of Medicine, Houston, USA

Paul C Adams
London Health Sciences Centre, London, Ontario, Canada

Aftab Ala
Centre for Gastroenterology, Hepatology and Nutrition, Department of Medicine, Frimley Park Hospital NHS Foundation Trust, Surrey, UK

Piero Luigi Almasio
Division of Gastroenterology, Academic Department of Internal Medicine, University of Palermo, Palermo, Italy

Raúl J Andrade
Liver Unit, Gastroenterology Service, "Virgen de la Victoria" University Hospital and School of Medicine, Centro de Investigación Biomédica en Red de Enfermedades Hepáticas y Digestivas (CIBEREHD), Málaga, Spain

Vicente Arroyo
Liver Unit and GI Unit, Hospital Clínic and University of Barcelona, Institut d'Investigacions Biomèdiques August Pi-Sunyer (IDIBAPS), Ciber de Enfermedades Hepáticas y Digestivas (CIBERHED), Barcelona, Spain

Johan Bohr
Department of Gastroenterology, Örebro University Hospital, Örebro, Sweden

Michel Boucher
HTA Development, CADTH, Ottawa, Canada

Marc Bradette
Division of Gastroenterology, Centre Hospitalier Universitaire de Québec, Québec City, Canada

Andrew K Burroughs
The Royal Free Sheila Sherlock Liver Centre, Royal Free Hospital *and* Department of Surgery, University College London, London, UK

James R Burton, Jr
University of Colorado, Denver, Colorado, USA

Stephen Caldwell
Department of Hepatology, University of Virginia, Charlottesville, Virginia, USA

Calogero Cammà
Division of Gastroenterology, Academic Department of Internal Medicine, University of Palermo, Palermo, Italy

Andrés Cárdenas
Liver Unit and GI Unit, Hospital Clínic and University of Barcelona, Institut d'Investigacions Biomèdiques August Pi-Sunyer (IDIBAPS), Ciber de Enfermedades Hepáticas y Digestivas (CIBERHED), Barcelona, Spain

Hélène Castel
Department of Hepatology, Hôpital Claude Huriez, Lille, France

Nishchay Chandra
Gastroenterology Unit, John Radcliffe Hospital, Oxford, UK

Roger W Chapman
Gastroenterology Unit, John Radcliffe Hospital, Oxford, UK

Naoki Chiba
Division of Gastroenterology, McMaster University Medical Centre, Hamilton *and* Guelph General Hospital, Guelph, Canada

Evangelos Cholongitas
The Royal Free Shiila Sherlock Liver Centre, Royal Free Hospital *and* Department of Surgery, University College London, London, UK

Contributors

Nicholas Church
Centre for Liver and Digestive Disorders, Royal Infirmary of
  Edinburgh, Edinburgh, UK

Paul Collins
School of Clinical Sciences, University of Liverpool, Liverpool, UK

Massimo Colombo
Department of Medicine, First Division of Gastroenterology,
  Fondazione IRCCS Cà Granda Ospedale Maggiore Policlinico,
  Università degli Studi di Milano, Milan, Italy

Ann Cranney
Canadian Protective Medical Association *and*
  Clinical Epidemiology, Ottawa Hospital Research Institute *and*
  Faculty of Medicine, University of Ottawa,
  Ottawa, Canada

Antonio Craxì
Division of Gastroenterology, Academic Department of Internal
  Medicine, University of Palermo, Palermo, Italy

Susan N Cullen
Buckinghamshire Hospitals NHS Trust, High Wycombe, UK

Christopher P Day
Institute of Cellular Medicine, Newcastle University, Newcastle
  Upon Tyne, UK

Amar P Dhillon
Histopathology Department, Royal Free Hospital, London, UK

Vito Di Marco
Division of Gastroenterology, Academic Department of Internal
  Medicine, University of Palermo, Palermo, Italy

James S Dooley
Centre for Hepatology, University College London Medical School
  (Royal Free Campus), University College London *and* the Royal
  Free Sheila Sherlock Liver Centre, Royal Free Hampstead NHS
  Trust, London, UK

Catherine Dubé
Division of Gastroenterology, University of Calgary, Calgary,
  Canada

Herbert L DuPont
Center for Infectious Disease, University of Texas Health Science
  Center at Houston, School of Public Health *and* Internal
  Medicine Service, St. Luke's Episcopal Hospital, Department of
  Medicine, Baylor College of Medicine, Houston, USA

Hassan Elberm
Department of Surgery, Southampton University Hospitals,
  Southampton, UK

Elizabeth J Elliott
Discipline of Paediatrics and Child Health, University of Sydney
  and The Children's Hospital of Westminster, Sydney *and* Centre
  for Evidence-Based Paediatrics, Gastroenterology and Nutrition,
  Sydney, Australia

Carlo A Fallone
Division of Gastroenterology, McGill University Health Center,
  Montreal, Canada

Brian G Feagan
Robarts Clinical Trials, Robarts Research Unit, University of
  Western Ontario, London, Ontario, Canada

M Brian Fennerty
Oregon Health and Science University,
  Division of Gastroenterology and Hepatology,
  Portland, Oregon, USA

Peter Ferenci
Division of Gastroenterology and Hepatology, Medical University
  Vienna, Vienna, Austria

Alexander C Ford
Department of Gastroenterology, St James's University Hospital,
  Leeds, UK

Brett E Fortune
University of Colorado, Denver, Colorado, USA

Giacomo Germani
The Royal Free Sheila Sherlock Liver Centre, Royal Free Hospital
  and Department of Surgery, University College London,
  London, UK

Pere Ginès
Liver Unit and GI Unit, Hospital Clínic and University of
  Barcelona, Institut d'Investigacions Biomèdiques August
  Pi-Sunyer (IDIBAPS), Ciber de Enfermedades Hepáticas y
  Digestivas (CIBERHED), Barcelona, Spain

John Goulis
Fourth Department of Medicine, Aristotelian University of
  Thessaloniki, Hippokration General Hospital of Thessaloniki,
  Thessaloniki, Greece

Leah Gramlich
Division of Gastroenterology, Royal Alexandra Hospital
  University of Alberta, Edmonton, Canada

James Gregor
Department of Medicine, University of Western Ontario, London,
  Ontario, Canada

E Jenny Heathcote
Francis Family Liver Centre, Toronto Western Hospital, University
  Health Network *and* Department of Medicine, University of
  Toronto, Toronto, Canada

Gideon M Hirschfield
Francis Family Liver Centre, Toronto Western Hospital, University Health Network *and* Department of Medicine, University of Toronto, Toronto, Canada

Massimo Iavarone
Department of Medicine, First Division of Gastroenterology, Fondazione IRCCS Maggiore Cà Granda Ospedale Maggiore Policlinico, Università degli Studi di Milano, Milan, Italy

Gary P Jeffrey
Western Australia Liver Transplantation Service, Sir Charles Gairdner Hospital, Nedlands, Australia

Derek P Jewell
Experimental Medicine Division, John Radcliffe Hospital, Oxford, UK

Colin D Johnson
Department of Surgery, Southampton University Hospitals, Southampton, UK

Emilie Jolicoeur
Department of Gastroenterology, Montfort Hospital, Ottawa, Canada

Bret A Lashner
Center for Inflammatory Bowel Disease, Cleveland Clinic, Cleveland, USA

Calvin HL Law
Hepatobiliary, Pancreatic and Gastrointestinal Surgery, Department of Health Policy, Management and Evaluation, University of Toronto *and* Institute for Clinical Evaluative Sciences, Toronto, Ontario, Canada

Theodore R Levin
The Permanente Medical Group, Inc., Walnut Creek, California, USA

Robert Löfberg
IBD Unit, HMQ Sophia Hospital, Karolinska Institute, Stockholm, Sweden

M Isabel Lucena
Clinical Pharmacology Service, "Virgen de la Victoria" University Hospital and School of Medicine, Centro de Investigación Biomédica en Red de Enfermedades Hepáticas y Digestivas (CIBEREHD), Málaga, Spain

John WD McDonald
Robarts Clinical Trials, Robarts Research Unit, University of Western Ontario, London, Ontario, Canada

Lynne V McFarland
Department of Medicinal Chemistry, School of Pharmacy, University of Washington, Washington, USA

John G McHutchison
Division of Gastroenterology, Duke Clinical Research Institute *and* Duke University Medical Center, North Carolina, USA

Michael MP Manns
Department of Gastroenterology, Hepatology and Endocrinology, Medical School, Hanover, Germany

Philippe Mathurin
Department of Hepatology, Hôpital Claude Huriez, Lille, France

Paul Moayyedi
Gastroenterology Division, McMaster University Medical Centre, Hamilton, Canada

Rachid Mohamed
Division of Gastroenteology, University of Calgary, Calgary, Canada

Katherine Muir
University of Toronto, Toronto, Canada

Christian Müller
Division of Gastroenterology and Hepatology, Medical University Vienna, Vienna, Austria

Nicholas Murphy
Queen Elizabeth Hospital (Birmingham), Edgbaston, Birmingham, UK

Miquel Navasa
Liver Unit, Institut de Malalties Digestives i Metaboliques, Hospital Clinic, IDIBAPS, CIBEREHD, Barcelona, Spain

James O'Beirne
Royal Free Hospital, London, UK

Kelvin Palmer
Gastroenterology Unit, Western General Hospital, Edinburgh, UK

George V Papatheodoridis
Department of Internal Medicine, Athens University Medical School, Hippokration General Hospital, Athens, Greece

Darrell S Pardi
Inflammatory Bowel Disease Clinic, Division of Gastroenterology and Hepatology, Mayo Clinic, Rochester, USA

David Patch
The Royal Free Sheila Sherlock Liver Centre, Royal Free Hospital *and* Department of Surgery, University College London, London, UK

Keyur Patel
Division of Gastroenterology, Duke Clinical Research Institute *and* Duke University Medical Center, North Carolina, USA

Contributors

Maria Pleguezuelo
The Royal Free Shiila Sherlock Liver Centre, Royal Free Hospital *and* Department of Surgery, University College London, London, UK

Linda Rabeneck
University of Toronto, Toronto, Canada

Joel E Richter
Department of Medicine, Temple University School of Medicine, Philadelphia, USA

Antoni Rimola
Liver Unit, Institut de Malalties Digestives i Metaboliques, Hospital Clinic, IDIBAPS, CIBEREHD, Barcelona, Spain

Jason R Roberts
Division of Gastroenterology and Hepatology, Medical University of South Carolina, South Carolina, USA

Juan Rodés
Liver Unit and GI Unit, Hospital Clínic and University of Barcelona, Institut d'Investigacions Biomèdiques August Pi-Sunyer (IDIBAPS), Ciber de Enfermedades Hepáticas y Digestivas (CIBERHED), Barcelona, Spain

Hugo R Rosen
University of Colorado, Denver, Colorado, USA

Alaa Rostom
Forzani & MacPhail Colon Cancer Screening Centre University of Calgary, Calgary, Canada

Michael Sai Lai Sey
Department of Medicine, University of Western Ontario, London, Ontario, Canada

William J Sandborn
Inflammatory Bowel Disease Clinic, Division of Gastroenterology and Hepatology, Mayo Clinic, Rochester, USA

Michael D Saunders
Digestive Diseases Center, University of Washington School of Medicine, Washington, USA

Joseph H Sellin
Section of Gastroenterology and Hepatology, Baylor College of Medicine, Houston, USA

Neeral Shah
Department of Hepatology, University of Virginia, Charlottesville Virginia, USA

Arya M Sharma
Division of Endocrinology, University of Alberta, Edmonton, Canada

Marco Senzolo
Department of Surgical and Gastroenterological Sciences, University-Hospital of Padua, Padua, Italy

Marika Simon-Rudler
UPMC Service d'Hépato-Gastroentérologie, Assistance Publique-Hôpitaux de Paris, Groupe Hospitalier Pitié-Salpêtrière, Université Pierre et Marie Curie, Paris, France

Constantine A Soulellis
Division of Gastroenterology, McGill University Health Center, Montreal, Canada

Christina M Surawicz
Department of Gastroenterology, Harborview Medical Center, Washington, USA

Lloyd R Sutherland
Department of Community Health Sciences, University of Calgary, Health Sciences Centre, Calgary, Canada

Nicholas J Talley
Department of Medicine, The Mayo Clinic Jacksonville, USA

Véd R Tandan
Department of Surgery, St Joseph's Healthcare Hamilton, McMaster University, Hamilton, Ontario, Canada

Dominique Thabut
UPMC Service d'Hépato-Gastroentérologie, Assistance Publique-Hôpitaux de Paris, Groupe Hospitalier Pitié-Salpêtrière, Université Pierre et Marie Curie, Paris, France

Hans L Tillmann
Division of Gastroenterology, Duke Clinical Research Institute and Duke University Medical Center, North Carolina, USA

Christos Trianto
Division of Gastroenterology, Department of Internal Medicine, University Hospital, Patras, Greece *and* The Royal Free Sheila Sherlock Liver Centre, Royal Free Hospital *and* Department of Surgery, University College London, London, UK

Peter Tugwell
Department of Epidemiology and Community Medicine, University of Ottawa *and* Ottawa Hospital Research Institute, Ottawa, Canada

Curt Tysk
Department of Gastroenterology, Örebro University Hospital, Örebro, Sweden

Laura VanderBeek
McMaster University, Hamilton, Ontario, Canada

Sander Veldhuyzen van Zanten
Division of Gastroenterology, Department of Medicine, University of Alberta, Edmonton, Canada

Marcelo F Vela
Gastroenterology Section, Baylor College of Medicine, Houston, Texas, USA

Arndt Vogel
Department of Gastroenterology, Hepatology and Endocrinology, Medical School, Hanover, Germany

Alastair JM Watson
School of Clinical Sciences, University of Liverpool, Liverpool, UK

George Wells
Department of Epidemiology and Community Medicine and Cardiovascular Research Methods Centre, University of Ottawa, Ottawa, Canada

Julia Wendon
King's College London School of Medicine *and* King's College Hospital, London, UK

Marilyn Zeman
Division of Gastroenterology, Royal Alexandra Hospital University of Alberta, Edmonton, Canada

Introduction

John WD McDonald[1], Andrew K Burroughs[2], Brian G Feagan[1] and M Brian Fennerty[3]

[1] Robarts Clinical Trials, Robarts Research Unit, University of Western Ontario, London, Ontario, Canada
[2] The Royal Free Sheila Sherlock Liver Centre, Royal Free Hospital, *and* University College London, London, UK
[3] Oregon Health and Science University, Division of Gastroenterology and Hepatology, Ontario Oregon, USA

Over the past three decades the emergence of evidence-based medicine (EBM) has had a substantial impact on clinical practice. In the first half of the twentieth century, diagnostic tests or treatments, usually based on a strong scientific rationale and experimental work in animals, were routinely introduced into clinical care without good scientific proof of efficacy in people. Some of these interventions, such as gastric freezing for the treatment of ulcers and penicillamine therapy for primary biliary cirrhosis, were ultimately shown to be ineffective and harmful [1, 2]. There is little doubt that the widespread acceptance by physicians of unproved treatments has been detrimental to the well-being of many patients.

Fortunately, the need for a more critical approach to medical practice was recognized. In 1948 the first randomized controlled trial (RCT) in humans was carried out under the direction of the British Medical Research Council [3]. Epidemiologists and statisticians, notably Sir Richard Doll and Sir Bradford Hill, provided scientific leadership to the medical community, which responded with improvements in the quality of clinical research. The use of randomized allocation to control for confounding variables and to minimize bias was recognized as invaluable for conducting valid studies of treatments. The initiation of these landmark experiments defined a new era in clinical research; the RCT soon became the benchmark for the evaluation of medical and surgical interventions. Gastroenterologists played an important part in these early days. In 1955, Professor Sidney Truelove conducted the first randomized trial in the discipline of gastroenterology [4]. He and his colleagues proved that cortisone was more effective than a placebo for the treatment of ulcerative colitis. As noted in Chapter 12, this treatment has stood the test of time. The ascendancy of the RCT was accompanied by a call for greater scientific rigor in the usual practice of clinical medicine. Strong advocates of the application of epidemiological principles to patient care emerged and found a growing body of support among clinicians.

As the number of randomized trials grew to the point of becoming unmanageable, it was recognized that there was a need to provide summaries of the evidence provided by these trials for the use of practitioners, who frequently lack both time and expertise to consult the primary research. Busy clinicians may consult local experts, with the tacit assumption that they will make recommendations based on evidence. Liberati and colleagues provided evidence that this approach led to inappropriate care for many women with breast cancer [5]. Subsequently, convincing evidence became available through the work of Antman *et al.* and of Mulrow that the conventional review article and the traditional textbook chapter are seldom comprehensive, and are frequently biased [6, 7]. More recently, Jefferson reinforced this conclusion on the basis of a survey concerning recommendations for vaccination for cholera, which appeared in editorials and review articles [8]. He pointed out that authors of editorials and reviews frequently resort to the "desk drawer" technique, pulling out evidence with which they are very familiar, but failing to assemble and review all of the evidence in a systematic way.

In the UK, Archie Cochrane, as early as 1979, made a compelling case that there was a need to prepare and maintain summaries of all randomized trials [9]. Cochrane's challenge to the medical community to use scientific methods to identify, evaluate and systematically summarize the world's medical literature pertaining to all health care interventions is now being met. From its inception in 1993, the electronic database prepared by the volunteer members of the Cochrane Collaboration and published as the *Cochrane Library* has grown exponentially [10]. Systematic reviews and especially Cochrane reviews are now widely used by clinicians in the daily practice of medicine, by researchers and by the public. Accordingly, data from systematic reviews published in the *Cochrane Library*

Evidence-Based Gastroenterology and Hepatology, 3rd edition.
J. McDonald, A.K. Burroughs, B. Feagan, and M.B. Fennerty. © 2010 Blackwell Publishing Ltd

are featured prominently in several chapters in *Evidence-based Gastroenterology and Hepatology*. Unfortunately, coverage in the *Cochrane Library* of topics in gastroenterology and hepatology is still far from complete.

Several other clinical epidemiologists played important roles in the evolution of evidence-based medicine. Beginning in the 1970s, David Sackett encouraged practicing physicians to become familiar with the basic principles of critical appraisal. Criteria developed by Sackett and others for the evaluation of clinical studies assessing therapy, causation, prognosis and other clinical topics were widely published [11, 12]. His text, *Clinical Epidemiology: a Basic Science for Clinical Medicine*, co-authored by colleagues Gordon Guyatt, Brian Haynes and Peter Tugwell, introduced many physicians to the concepts of EBM [13]. In the USA, Alvin Feinstein called attention to the need for increased rigor in the design and interpretation of observational studies and explored the scientific principles of diagnostic testing [14, 15]. Among gastroenterologists, Thomas Chalmers, a strong, early advocate for the RCT [16], was responsible for introducing gastroenterologists and others to the importance of randomized trials in gastroenterology and hepatology and to the concept of systematic reviews and meta-analysis as means of summarizing data from these studies [17, 18].

Despite the opposition of some, the popularity of EBM continues to grow [19]. Although the explanations for this phenomenon are complex, one factor is that many practitioners recognize that ethical patient care should be based on the best possible evidence. For this, and other reasons, the fundamental concept behind EBM – the use of the scientific method in the practice of clinical medicine – has been widely endorsed by medical opinion leaders, patients and governments.

What is evidence-based gastroenterology and hepatology?

Evidence-based gastroenterology and hepatology is the application of the most valid scientific information to the care of patients with gastrointestinal and hepatic diseases. Physicians who treat patients with digestive diseases must provide their patients with the most appropriate diagnostic tests, the most accurate prognosis and the most effective and safe therapy. To meet this high standard individual clinicians must have access to and be able to evaluate scientific evidence. Although many practitioners argue that this has always been the standard of care in clinical medicine, a great deal of evidence exists to the contrary. Wide variations in practice patterns among physicians have been documented for many treatments, despite the presence of good data from widely publicized RCTs and the promotion of practice guidelines by content experts. For example,

Scholefield *et al.* carried out a survey of British surgeons who were questioned regarding the performance of screening colonoscopy for colon cancer [20]. Although this study was done in 1998 (after publication of the results of the RCTs described in Chapter 18 which demonstrated a benefit of this practice), many of these physicians failed to make appropriate recommendations for screening patients at risk. What is the explanation for this finding? One possibility is that many clinicians rely for information on their colleagues, on local experts, or on review articles or textbook chapters that are not based on the principles of EBM.

Two important points about EBM should be emphasized. First, use of the principles of EBM in the management of patients is complementary to traditional clinical skills and will never supersede the recognized virtues of careful observation, sound judgment and compassion for the patient. It is noteworthy that many good doctors have intuitively used the basic principles of EBM; hence the promotion of such well-known clinical aphorisms as "go where the money is" and "do the last test first". Knowledge of EBM enables physicians to understand why these basic rules of clinical medicine are valid through the use of a quantitative approach to decision making. This paradigm can in no way be considered detrimental to the doctor-patient relationship.

Second, although RCTs are the most valuable source of data for evaluating health care interventions, other kinds of evidence must frequently be used. In some instances, most obviously in studies of causation, it is neither possible nor ethical to conduct RCTs. Here, data from methodologically rigorous observational studies are extremely valuable. A dramatic example was the demonstration by several authors (quoted in Chapter 27) that the relative risk of hepatocellular carcinoma in chronic carriers of the hepatitis B virus is dramatically higher than in persons who are not infected. Although these data are observational, the strength of the association is such that it is exceedingly unlikely that a cause other than hepatitis B virus is responsible for the development of cancer in these people. Case-control studies are especially useful for studying rare diseases and for the initial development of scientific hypotheses regarding causation. The etiological role of non-steroidal anti-inflammatory drugs in the development of gastric ulcer was recognized using this methodology [21]. Finally, case series can provide compelling evidence for the adoption of a new therapy in the absence of data from RCTs, if the natural history of the disease is both well characterized and severe. An example is the identification of orthotopic liver transplantation as a dramatically effective intervention for patients with advanced liver disease.

Box 1.1 shows a generally agreed approach to ranking the strength of evidence that arises from various types of studies of health care interventions, and this system is used throughout the book. This ranking of evidence has

Box 1.1 Grading of recommendations and levels of' evidence used in *Evidence-based Gastroenterology and Hepatology*

Grade A

Level 1a
- Evidence from large randomized clinical trials (RCTs) or systematic reviews (including meta-analyses) of multiple randomized trials which collectively have at least as much data as one single well-defined trial.

Level 1b
- Evidence from at least one "All or none" high quality cohort study; in which *all* patients died/failed with conventional therapy and some survived/succeeded with the new therapy (e.g. chemotherapy for tuberculosis, meningitis, or defibrillation for ventricular fibrillation): or in which many died/failed with conventional therapy and *none* died/failed with the new therapy (e.g. penicillin for pneumococcal infections).

Level 1c
- Evidence from at least one moderate sized RCT or a meta-analysis of small trials which collectively only has a moderate number of patients.

Level 1d
- Evidence from at least one RCT.

Grade B

Level 2
- Evidence from at least one high quality study of non-randomized cohorts who did and did not receive the new therapy.

Level 3
- Evidence from at least one high quality case control study.

Level 4
- Evidence from at least one high quality case series.

Grade C

Level 5
- Opinions from experts without reference or access to any of the foregoing (for example, argument from physiology, bench research car first principles)

appeared in a number of publications; we have chosen to reproduce it from *Evidence-based Cardiology*, along with the system used by its editors, Yusuf *et al.*, for making recommendations on the basis of these levels of evidence [22]. As mentioned in Box 1.1, throughout this book recommendation grades appear as **A** or **A1a**.

Clinical decision making in gastroenterology and hepatology

Clinical decision making by gastroenterologists usually falls into one of the following categories:

- Deciding whether to apply a specific diagnostic test in arriving at an explanation of a patient's problem, or determining the status of the patient's disease.
- Offering a prognosis to a patient.
- Deciding among a number of interventions available for managing a patient's problem. In this category, the first question is "Does a given intervention do more good than harm?" The second is "Does it do more good than other effective interventions?" The third is "Is it more or less cost-effective than other interventions?"

A comprehensive approach would incorporate many different types of evidence (e.g. RCTs, non-RCTs, epidemiologic studies and experimental data), and examine the architecture of the information for consistency, coherence and clarity. Occasionally, the evidence does not completely fit into neat compartments. For example, there is strong (A1a) evidence through very large randomized trials that fecal occult blood testing on an annual or semi-annual basis modestly reduces mortality from colon cancer in a population at average risk for this disease. The evidence that direct examination of the colon at intervals of five to ten years results in even greater benefit has been derived only from case control studies (B3). Physicians, patients and policy advisers should have both levels of evidence available to make informed decisions.

Recommendation grades appear either within the text, for example **A** and **A1a** or within a table in the chapter.

The grading system clearly is only applicable to preventative or therapeutic interventions. It is not applicable to many other types of data such as descriptive, genetic or pathophysiologic.

Application of a diagnostic test

Example: A four-year-old child is experiencing diarrhea and has a positive family history of celiac disease. Should a serological test for antiendomysial antibody (EMA) be done?

Chapter 10 includes an extensive treatment of this topic with a summary of studies (see Table 10.1) that included various groups of patients with a greater or lesser probability of having celiac disease (ranging from patients with gastrointestinal symptoms to patients in whom celiac disease was suspected on clinical grounds). Several studies listed in Table 10.1 and the study of Cataldo *et al.* [23] are relevant to this patient.

When evaluating this test the reader may wish to adopt the approach of Kitching *et al.* for deciding on the clinical usefulness of a diagnostic test (Figure 1.1) [24].

The criteria listed in Figure 1.1 for validity of a diagnostic test were clearly met in Cataldo's study. In Chapter 10 Gregor and Say explore the utility of the test and point out that tests with high positive likelihood ratios (LR > 10) and

- **Are the study results valid?**
1 Was there an independent blind comparison (or unbiased comparison) with a reference ("gold") standard of diagnosis?
2 Was the diagnostic test evaluated in an appropriate spectrum of patients (like those seen in the reader's practice)?
3 Was the reference standard applied regardless of the diagnostic test result?

- **What are the results?**
Cataldo F, Ventura A, Lazzari R *et al*. Antiendomysium antibodies and celiac disease: solved and unsolved questions. An Italian multicentre study. *Acta Paediatr* 1995;**84**:1125–31.
A study of IgA endomysium antibodies (EMA) in 1485 children with gastrointestinal disease (688 with celiac disease confirmed by intestinal biopsy)

Results for antiendomysial antibody (EMA) test

| | No. of patients with biopsy proven celiac disease | | |
	Present	Absent	Totals
EMA positive	645	20	665
	a	b	a+b
EMA negative	c	d	c+d
	43	777	810
	a+c	b+d	a+b+c+d
Totals	688	797	1485

Sensitivity = a/(a + c) = 645/688 = 0·94
Specificity = d/(b + d) = 777/797 = 0·97
Likelihood ratio (positive result) = sensitivity/(1–specificity) = 0·94/(1–0·97) = 31
Likelihood ratio (negative result) = (1–sensitivity)/specificity = (1–0·94)/0·97 = 0·06
Positive predictive value = a/(a + b) = 645/665 = 0·97
Negative predictive value = d/c + d = 777/810 = 0·96

Figure 1.1 Approaches to evaluating evidence about diagnosis.

low negative likelihood ratios (LR < 0.1) are generally considered to be clinically useful. The EMA test clearly falls into this category. The authors draws attention to the fact that the probability that a specific patient actually has celiac disease (based on a positive test), or does not have it (based on a negative test), also depends on the pretest odds of the patient having the disease (see Table 1.1).

If the child in question, whose pretest likelihood of celiac disease is estimated to be 8%, has a negative test it may be concluded that the child almost certainly does not have celiac disease; on the other hand, if the child has a positive test, the likelihood of him or her having celiac disease is still only 65%.

As Gregor and Alidina point out, the implications of misdiagnosis must be considered carefully. In the circumstance of a positive test in the child with non-specific symptoms the physician and the child's parents should consider whether it is now reasonable to proceed to intestinal biopsy to confirm the diagnosis, rather than recommending a gluten-free diet, presumably for life. If a search for other clinical or laboratory clues reveals that celiac disease is very likely to be the correct diagnosis, the pretest likelihood may

Table 1.1 The anti-endomysial antibody (EMA) test for celiac disease. Dependence of post-test likelihood of celiac disease on pretest likelihood, assuming positive LR = 31, negative LR = 0.06.

Pretest likelihood of celiac disease	Post-test likelihood with a positive EMA test (%)	Post-test likelihood with a negative EMA test (%)
8% (non-specific symptoms, positive family history)	65	0.5
50% (more specific symptoms)	97	6
0.25% (population screen)	8	0.02

Data from Chapter 10.

be as high as 50%. This would raise the post-test likelihood to 97%. The physician and parents may be comfortable accepting the diagnosis and proceed to a trial of a gluten-free diet, rather than subjecting a young child to intestinal biopsy. This is an excellent example of how a skilled clinician must integrate the principles of evidence-based medicine with traditional clinical skills and judgment.

Offering a prognosis

Example: A 50-year-old woman with recently diagnosed celiac disease. has learned at a meeting of the local celiac society that patients with celiac disease have a substantial increase in the risk of developing a number of cancers and that this cancer risk is reduced by strict adherence to a gluten-free diet.

Chapter 10 describes the types of study which are relevant to determination of prognosis and discusses the strengths and weaknesses of case-control and cohort studies.

Gregor and Alidina point out that certain case-control studies which reported very high mortality and malignancy rates may have been subject to selection bias (inclusion of particularly ill or refractory patients) and measurement bias (patients with abdominal symptoms being more likely to undergo investigations such as small bowel biopsy which may lead to a diagnosis of celiac disease). They refer to a British study in which a cohort of patients with celiac disease was assembled and followed for ten years. This design attempts to minimize the biases that are inherent in the case-control studies. Table 1.2 shows that the risk of certain cancers is increased compared to the risk in the general population. Table 1.3 shows that strict adherence to a gluten-free diet significantly reduced this risk and may have eliminated the excess risk for several of the identified cancers.

On the basis of this evidence it is reasonable to advise the patient that her disease does carry with it an increased risk of certain relatively uncommon cancers and that adherence to a strict gluten-free diet appears to minimize this increased risk.

Recommendations concerning therapy

We have provided examples of how evidence concerning the use of diagnostic tests and prognosis can be analyzed and incorporated into clinical practice. Most chapters in this book deal more extensively with evidence concerning therapy and rely heavily on data from randomized trials and meta-analyses.

Example: Should a 28-year-old woman who has had an uncomplicated resection of the terminal ileum for Crohn's disease receive maintenance therapy with an S-aminosalicylate (ASA) product? Prior to the surgery she had had steroid-dependent disease and had failed treatment with both azathioprine and methotrexate.

A search of the literature for placebo-controlled randomized trials of 5-ASA for maintenance of remission in patients with a surgically induced remission of disease would reveal several trials. The largest published trial is that of McLeod and colleagues, who randomized 163 adult patients to receive either 3 g/day of 5-ASA or a placebo following surgery [26]. The primary outcome of interest was the recurrence of active Crohn's disease as defined by the recurrence of symptoms and the documentation of active disease either radiologically or endoscopically. At

Table 1.2 Cancer mortality in 210 patients with celiac disease at the end of 1985.

Site of cancer	ICD8	O	E	O/E	P
All sites	140–208	31	15.48	2.0	b
Mouth and pharynx	141–147	3	0.31	9.7	a
Esophagus	150	3	0.24	12.3	a
Non-Hodgkin's lymphoma	200, 202	9	0.21	42.7	b
Gastrointestinal tract	151–154	3	3.07	1.0	NS
Remainder		13	11.65	1.1	NS

[a] $p < 0.01$.
[b] $p < 0.001$.
O: observed numbers; E: expected numbers.
Source: Holmes GKT *et al. Gut* 1989; **30**: 333–338 [25].

Table 1.3 Cancer morbidity by diet group.

Site of cancer	Diet group[a]	No.	O	E	O/E	P
All sites	1	108	14	9.06	1.5	
	2	102	17	6.42	2.6	c
Mouth, pharynx,	1	108	1	0.33	3.0	
esophagus	2	102	5	0.22	22.7	c
Non-Hodgkin's	1	108	2	0.12	16.7	b
lymphoma	2	102	7	0.09	77.8	c
Remainder	1	108	11	8.61	1.3	
	2	102	5	6.11	0.8	

[a] Diet group 1, strict adherence to gluten-free diet; group 2, reduced gluten diet or normal diet. Source: Holmes G KT *et al. Gut* 1989; **30**: 333–338 [25].
[b] $p < 0$–01.
[c] $p < 0.001$.

- **Are the results valid?**
1 Was the assignment of patients to treatment really randomized (and the randomization code concealed)?
2 Were all patients who entered the study accounted for at its conclusion?
3 Were the clinical outcomes measured blindly?

- **Is the therapeutic effect important?**
1 Were both statistical and clinical significance considered?
2 Were all clinically important outcomes reported?

- **What are the results?**
  McLeod RS, Wolff BG, Steinhart AH *et al*. Prophylactic mesalamine treatment decreases postoperative recurrence of Crohn's disease. *Gastroenterology* 1995;**109**:404–13.

  Randomized controlled trial in which 163 patients with Crohn's disease who had all visible disease resected were randomized to receive mesalamine (Pentasa) 3 g daily or a placebo for a median period of 34 months. Primary outcome was recurrent Crohn's disease defined by recurrence of symptoms and radiographic or endoscopic documentation of recurrence.

	Recurrent Crohn's disease		Risk (%)	ARR (%)	RRR (%)
	Yes	No			
5-ASA	27	60	31	10	24
Placebo	31	45	41	–	–

  ARR, absolute risk reduction; RRR, relative risk reduction.

- **Are the results relevant to my patient?**
1 Were the study patients recognizably similar to my own?
2 Is the therapeutic maneuver feasible in my practice?

Figure 1.2 Elements of a valid and useful randomized trial.

the end of the follow-up period (maximum duration 72 months, median duration 34 months), 31% of patients who received active treatment remained in remission compared with 41% of those who received a placebo (p = 0.031); 5-ASA was well tolerated. A low proportion of patients developed adverse reactions in the control and active treatment groups. One patient treated with 5-ASA developed pancreatitis that was attributed to the study drug. The results of this study can be evaluated using the guidelines described in Figure 1.2, which is modeled after the approach of Kitching *et al.* [24].

Are the results of this study valid?

A review of the methods section of the article confirms that an appropriate method of randomization was employed (computer-generated in permutated blocks), which insured concealment of the randomization code [26]. Furthermore, inspection of the baseline characteristics of the treatment and control groups shows that they are well balanced with respect to such confounding variables as the time from surgery to randomization. This information further supports the legitimacy of the randomization process. Assessment of the method of randomization is important, because non-randomized designs are especially vulnerable to the effects of bias. Studies which employ "quasi-randomization" schemes such as allocation to treatment according to the day of the week or alphabetically by the patient's surname have been shown to consistently overestimate the treatment effect identified by RCTs that employ a valid randomization scheme [27, 28]. However, it may be noted that 87 patients were randomized to 5-ASA, compared with only 76 patients in the control group. This observation raises the concern that the analysis might not have been done according to the "intent to treat" principle which specifies that patients are analyzed in the group to which they were originally assigned, irrespective of the treatment that was ultimately received. The use of this strategy reduces the possibility of bias, which might occur if investigators selectively withdrew from the analysis patients who had done poorly or experienced toxicity. For this reason, the intent to treat principle yields a conservative estimate of the true benefit of the treatment. However, detailed review shows that in this study the discrepancy in patient numbers occurred because five patients who were randomized to the active treatment group withdrew consent prior to receiving the study medication and were not included. Thus, it appears that the analysis was based on the intent to treat principle.

Approximately 10% of patients in both treatment groups had incomplete follow-up. Methodologically rigorous studies have a very low proportion of patients for whom data are missing. This issue is important, since patients who are lost to follow-up usually have a different prognosis from those for whom complete information is available. If there is incomplete follow-up data for a substantial proportion of patients then the results are uninterpretable [29].

Turning to an assessment of the outcomes in this study, both the patients and investigators were unaware of the treatment allocation. Blinding is used to reduce bias in the interpretation of outcomes. This is especially important when a subjective outcome is evaluated [30]. In this study, objective demonstration of recurrent disease (endoscopy and/or radiology) was required in addition to the more subjective measure of the introduction of treatment for recurrent symptoms. Thus, the reader can be satisfied that the primary outcome measure was both clinically meaningful and objectively assessed.

Finally, the data analysis and results should be examined. A great deal of useful information can be obtained by reviewing the assumptions that were used in the sample size calculation. In this study, which analyzes a difference in proportions, the investigators had to define four variables: the alpha (type 1) error rate, the beta (type 2) error rate, the expected proportion of patients who would be expected to relapse in the placebo group, and the minimum difference in the rate of relapse which the investigator wished to detect. In this publication these parameters are easily identified. The rate of symptomatic recurrence was estimated to be 12.5% per year and it was anticipated that treatment with 5-ASA would reduce this rate by 50% to an absolute value of 6.25% per year. In contrast to the expected 50% relative risk reduction which was anticipated, the three-year actuarial risk of recurrence was 26% in the treatment group compared to 45% in the group that received 5-ASA (p = 0.039). Therefore, the relative risk reduction ((45–26%)/45% = 42%) is slightly lower than the figure which the investigators considered to be clinically meaningful. Furthermore, the probability of a type 1 error is described as a one-tailed value of p = 0.05. This implies that one-tailed statistical testing was used to derive the p value of 0.039. The use of one-sided statistical testing raises legitimate concerns regarding the statistical inferences made in the study [31]. It is inappropriate to hypothesize that 5-ASA therapy could only be beneficial, given that the drug can cause diarrhea and colitis [32]. For these reasons, uncer-

tainty exists regarding both the clinical and statistical interpretation of these data.

Are the results of this valid study important?

To assess the importance of this result it is necessary to quantify the magnitude of the treatment effect. How the evidence is presented may influence both physicians and patients in making choices. The most basic means of expressing the magnitude of a treatment of fact is the absolute risk reduction (ARR), which is defined as the proportion of patients in the experimental group with a treatment success minus the proportion of patients with this outcome in the control group. In this instance the annual rate of relapse in the placebo-treated patients was 15% (success rate of 85%) compared with 8.7% (success rate of 91.3%) in those who received the active treatment. This yields an ARR of 6.3%. The number needed to treat (NNT), the number of patients with Crohn's disease who would have to be treated with 3 g/day of 5-ASA to maintain remission over a year, can be calculated as the reciprocal of this number, and is 16. Alternative ways of describing effectiveness include calculating the observed relative risk reduction (RRR = 63/15) of 42%, or even stating that about 90% of patients respond to maintenance therapy, ignoring the substantial placebo effect which is evident. The evidence presented as the ARR or NNT, rather than the numbers which show the treatment in a more favorable light, may still lead the physician to recommend this form of treatment and cause the patient to choose to accept this strategy over no intervention. However, the expectations of the physician and patients are likely to be more realistic than they may be if the physician accepts and promotes in an uncritical way the information that 90% of patients who receive 5-ASA maintenance therapy will remain in remission over one year [33].

Are these results applicable to my patient?

Following an assessment of the validity of the evidence using the criteria described in the preceding paragraphs, it is necessary to decide whether the conclusions of the study are relevant and important to the individual patient. An initial step is to evaluate the demographic characteristics of the patients in the RCT and compare them to those of the patient in question. If the patient for whom maintenance therapy is being considered is similar to the patients who were evaluated in the trial, it is reasonable to assume that she will experience the same benefit of therapy and is at no greater risk for the development of adverse drug

Study or subgroup	5-ASA Events	5-ASA Total	Placebo Events	Placebo Total	Weight	Risk ratio M-H, fixed, 95% CI	Risk ratio M-H, fixed, 95% CI
Lochs 2000	36	152	50	166	38.7%	0.79 (0.54, 1.14)	
Brignola 1995	7	44	10	43	8.2%	0.68 (0.29, 1.63)	
Mcleod 1995	27	87	31	76	26.8%	0.76 (0.50, 1.15)	
Hanauer 2004	26	44	31	40	26.3%	0.76 (0.57, 1.03)	
Total (95% CI)		327		325	100.0%	0.76 (0.62, 0.94)	
Total events	96		122				

Heterogeneity: Chi^2 = 0.09, df = 3 (p = 0.99); I^2 = 0%
Test for overall effect: Z = 2.51 (p = 0.01)

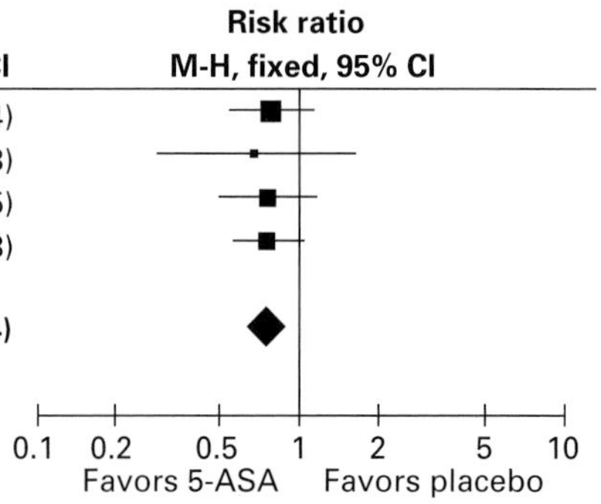

Scale: 0.1 0.2 0.5 1 2 5 10
Favors 5-ASA   Favors placebo

Figure 1.3 Interventions for prevention of post-operative recurrence of Crohn's disease.
Source: Doherty G, Bennett G, Patil S, Cheifetz A, Moss AC. Interventions for prevention of post-operative recurrence of Crohn's disease. In: *Cochrane Database of Systematic Reviews* 2009, Issue 4. Art. No.: CD006873. DOI: 10.1002/14651858.CD006873.pub2.

reactions. Alternatively, this patient may have characteristics that make it unlikely that a benefit from 5-ASA will be realized. For example, if the patient had residual active Crohn's disease it would be difficult to generalize the results of the study of McLeod *et al.*, since the patients in this trial had resection of all visible disease prior to study entry [26].

At this point, if we accept that the results are generalizable to our patient example, the relative risks and benefits of the therapy must be weighed and the patient's preferences should be considered. Evaluation of the data reveals that the trial was methodologically rigorous and evaluated an important outcome. However, it is doubtful whether conventional statistical significance was demonstrated. This raises the question of whether the observed differences between the treatment groups might have occurred by chance. Furthermore, the magnitude of the treatment effect is relatively small. In presenting to the patient the benefit of an annual reduction in the risk of recurrence of 6.3% it is also necessary to consider the cost and inconvenience of taking medication for an asymptomatic condition. One observation in favor of recommending the treatment is that the risk of serious toxicity with 5-ASA appears to be low.

Because there is a degree of uncertainty concerning the true benefit of 5-ASA maintenance therapy based on analysis of this single RCT, it would be prudent to review additional published data. A meta-analysis of 5-ASA therapy has been published [34]. Meta-analysis, the process of combining the results of multiple RCTs using quantitative methods, is an important tool for the practitioner of EBM. Pooling the results of multiple RCTs increases statistical power and thus may resolve the contradictory results of individual studies. Combining data from RCTs statistically also increases the precision of the estimate of a treatment effect. Moreover, the greater statistical power afforded by meta-analysis may allow insight into the benefits of treatment for specific subgroups of patients. These properties are particularly relevant to the case under consideration, given the previously identified concerns.

The meta-analysis summarized data from 15 RCTs which evaluated the efficacy of 5-ASA maintenance therapy in 1371 patients with quiescent Crohn's disease. Patients were randomly assigned to receive either 5-ASA or placebo for treatment periods of 4–48 months. Although 5-ASA was superior to placebo in 13 of the 15 studies, the results of only two trials were statistically significant. Separate analyses were done using data from the four trials that included patients with a surgically induced remission (see Figure 1.3) in distinction to those that evaluated patients after a medically induced remission. Sensitivity analyses assessed the response to therapy in specific subgroups of patients. The overall analysis concluded that 5-ASA has a statistically significant benefit; the risk of symptomatic relapse in patients who received 5-ASA was reduced by 6.3% (95% confidence interval −10.4% to −2.1%, 2 p = 0.0028), which corresponds to an NNT of 16. Importantly, the greatest benefit was observed in the four trials that evaluated patients following a surgical resection. In these studies there was a 13.1% reduction in the risk of a relapse (95% CI: −21.8 − −4.5%, 2 p = 0.0028), which corresponds to an NNT of 8. No statistically significant effect was demonstrable in the analysis, which was restricted to the patients with medically induced remission.

Are the results of this meta-analysis valid and reliable?

Figure 1.4 provides some useful guidelines for the interpretation of overview analyses. It is important that a comprehensive search strategy be adopted since publication bias, the selective publication of studies with positive results, is an important threat to the validity of meta-analysis [35]. This criterion was met. Camma and colleagues' review of the literature was extensive and not limited to English lan-

- Are the results of this overview valid and reliable?
1 Is it an overview of randomized trials of treatments?
2 Does it include a methods section that describes:
   (a) finding and including all the relevant trials?
   (b) assessing their individual validity?
   (c) using valid statistical methods that compare "like with like" stratified by study?

3 Were the results consistent from study to study?
4 Are the conclusions based on sufficiently large amounts of data to exclude a spurious difference (type 1 error) or missing a real difference (type II error).

- Are these applicable to your patient?
Differences between subgroups should only be believed if you can say "yes" to all of the following:
1 Was it hypothesized before the study began (rather than the product of dredging the data), and has it been confirmed in other, independent studies?
2 Was it one of just a few subgroups analyses carried out in this study?
3 Is the difference both clinically (beneficial for some but useless or harmful for others) and statistically significant?
4 Does it really make biologic and clinical sense?

Figure 1.4 Approaches to evaluating evidence concerning overviews.
Reproduced from Yusuf S *et al.*, eds. *Evidence-based Cardiology*. BMJ Books, London, 1998 [22].

guage publications. The investigators also searched review articles, primary studies and abstracts by hand. Quality scores were used to evaluate the validity of the individual studies and a sensitivity analysis was done which assessed the effect of trial quality on the result. No important change in the overall result was noted when studies of lower quality were excluded from consideration. However this type of analysis was not carried out in the analysis of the subgroups of four trials (411 patients) which evaluated 5-ASA after a surgically induced remission.

One of the included studies, that of Caprilli *et al.*, which involved 95 patients, showed a greater benefit for 5-ASA than any other trial, medical or surgical, which has been performed [36]. An important methodological deficiency of this RCT was the failure to conceal the treatment allocation from the investigators. Since these physicians were aware of the treatment assignment, and the definition of relapse used required clinical interpretation, it is possible that the 27% reduction in the risk of relapse identified is an overestimation of the true treatment effect. Accordingly, the inclusion of the results of this study in the subgroup analysis of the surgical studies may overestimate the true benefit of 5-ASA. Furthermore, Camma *et al.* did not include an additional trial by Lochs *et al.*, which was only available as a preliminary report at the time the meta-analysis was done [37]. This study, which is the largest RCT to evaluate 5-ASA following surgery, assigned 318 patients to receive either 4 g of active drug or a placebo for 18 months. Although Camma and colleagues described this study as "confirming" a benefit of 5-ASA after surgery, the results are not impressive. Only a 6.9% reduction in the rate of relapse was observed in patients who received the active treatment (24.5% 5-ASA compared with 31.4% placebo). This difference was *not* statistically significant.

This example underscores the importance of updating systematic reviews as new information becomes available, which is the approach of the Cochrane Collaboration, but not of reviews in conventional publications. When the data provided by Lochs *et al.* were aggregated with those of the other trials, the overall estimate of benefit for 5-ASA was less (ARR 4%, NNT 25) [38]. On the basis of these data it can be concluded that 5-ASA may be an effective maintenance therapy following surgery, but the magnitude of the treatment effect is modest at best.

Chapter 11 includes a meta-analysis performed as part of a Cochrane review that also supports this conclusion (see Figure 1.3).

Are these results applicable to our patient example?

The meta-analysis of surgical trials by Camma *et al.* provides important information to the clinician who must decide whether or not to offer patients 5-ASA for maintenance therapy. The concern regarding statistical significance raised by the critique of the McLeod study has been reduced. It seems likely that the beneficial effect of 5-ASA following surgery is real. However, although the majority of the criteria outlined in Figure 1.4 have been met, the issue of clinical relevance remains. The most optimistic estimate of the size of the treatment effect, derived from the meta-analysis, is an NNT of 8. However, given the possibility of bias in the study of Caprilli *et al.*, a more conservative estimate could be based on the data of Lochs and colleagues from the single large randomized trial which yielded an NNT of 15, or from the revision by Sutherland of Camma's meta-analysis that yielded an ARR of only 4%, and an NNT of 25.

In presenting this information to the patient the following points should be emphasized.
• The existing data suggest that 5-ASA is not effective, or at the most, very marginally effective.
• The annual risk of relapse following surgery is relatively low without treatment.
• 5-ASA therapy is safe.
• The cost of 5-ASA therapy is approximately US$70 per month.
• To derive a benefit from the treatment the medication must be taken on a regular basis. This requires the patient to take six pills each day.

Patients undoubtedly will react in different ways to this information. Our patient chose not to accept this therapy.

Rationale for a book on evidence-based gastroenterology and hepatology

Gastroenterologists, hepatologists and general surgeons are fortunate to have many excellent textbooks that provide a wealth of information regarding digestive diseases. Such traditional textbooks concentrate on the pathophysiology of disease and are comprehensive in their scope. *Evidence-based Gastroenterology and Hepatology* is not intended to replace these texts, since its focus is on clinical evidence.

Excellent electronic databases are available, and many traditional publications contain relevant research evidence and important summaries and reviews to support evidence-based practice. However, Cumbers and Donald have found that physicians in clinical practice find the acquisition of data from these sources time consuming [39]. Their study revealed that even locating relevant articles required on average three days for practitioners with an on-site library and a week for those without such a facility. This book has been written for the purpose of saving valuable time for busy practitioners of gastroenterology and hepatology, and for general internists and general surgeons who deal with substantial numbers of patients with disorders ranging from gastroesophageal reflux disease to liver transplantation.

It has been extensively revised since the second edition was published in 2004, in order to provide more recent evidence that serves as the basis for recommendations. For example, we present data from Cochrane reviews that summarize the strong evidence that anti-TNF agents are effective for both induction and maintenance of remission of Crohn's disease, along with a careful consideration of the adverse effect profile of these agents.

The book cannot claim to be comprehensive. However, the third edition has been expanded significantly, with new chapters on eosinophilic esophagitis, travelers' diarrhea, antibiotic- associated diarrhea, non-invasive markers for the diagnosis of fibrosis, drug-induced liver injury, liver biopsy, and hepatic outflow syndromes and splanchnic thrombosis. In addition, all chapters have been extensively revised and updated to reflect current evidence. A limitation of any textbook is the timeliness of the information that it is possible to provide in print form. New evidence accumulates rapidly in clinical medicine and it is impossible to include the most up-to-date information in a textbook because of the time required for production. To meet the needs of our readers for the most timely information the editors have endeavored to include, where possible, new evidence that became available during the editorial process. It is also planned to produce electronic updates of chapters at regular intervals. These updates will appear on the Evidence-Based Medicine Series website: http://www.evidencebasedseries.com/Summary of updated evidence in the Third Edition.

These summaries highlight the most significant changes to *Evidence-based Gastroenterology and Hepatology* since the second edition, particularly regarding treatment recommendations in specific conditions. The full discussion of the evidence can be found in the relevant chapters.

Part I: Gastrointestinal disorders

Gastroesophageal reflux disease (Chapter 2)

Data support the use of empiric antisecretory therapy for patients presenting with symptoms thought to be caused by GERD, without performing confirmatory diagnostic testing. PPI are significantly better than H_2-RA for healing esophagitis and relieving symptoms. There are insufficient data to support routinely using PPI doses higher than standard doses for healing esophagitis, treating symptomatic GERD or atypical symptoms of GERD, although higher doses may be effective for preventing relapse that occurs at standard doses. The most cost-effective strategies are PPI based "step-down" or PPI "on-demand" approaches. Laparoscopic fundoplication is an effective alternative to medical therapy, particularly for patients whose symptoms responded to medication.

Barrett's esophagus (Chapter 3)

Aggressive anti-reflux therapy with either high-dose PPI or surgery has not been shown to revert Barrett's esophagus to normal squamous mucosa or reduce the risk of developing cancer. Although endoscopic ablative therapy is a reasonable option in the Barrett's patient with high grade dysplasia or superficial adenocarcinoma, these therapies are not recommended for the Barrett's patient without neoplasia, since continued surveillance will still be required, complications are frequent and the risk/benefit ratio is not established. Estimates of the cost effectiveness of surveillance of Barrett's esophagus vary widely, and it is not possible currently to make a recommendation for population screening for Barrett's either in the general population or in those with chronic GERD.

Esophageal motility disorders (Chapter 4)
The costs and cost effectiveness of Botulinum toxin injections and pneumatic dilation for achalasia are lower than the cost of Heller myotomy. In the longer term, pneumatic dilatation appears to be more cost-effective than Botulinum toxin injection therapy.

Eosinophilic esophagitis (Chapter 5)
Conventional oral corticosteroids and swallowed inhaled fluticasone both appear to be effective for this condition. However, the adverse effects of oral steroids are more frequent and severe, and inhaled (swallowed) steroids should be used as initial treatment for uncomplicated EE.

Ulcer disease and *Helicobacter pylori* infection (Chapter 6)
Half of ulcer bleeding may be attributable to NSAIDs, and patients who are also positive for *H. pylori* have a synergistically high risk of re-bleeding. *H. pylori* eradication significantly reduces ulcer re-bleeding rates. Clarithromycin resistance accounts for most treatment failures. When a clarithromycin-based eradication regimen has failed, it is not worthwhile to administer it again. More effective options include PPI/amoxicillin/metronidazole or PPI with amoxicillin and levofloxacin for ten days, as well as more conventional bismuth-based quadruple regimens.

NSAID induced gastroduodenal toxicity (Chapter 7)
H. pylori contributes to an excess ulcer-risk in NSAID naive patients, whereas ulcers occurring in long-term NSAID users are probably largely caused by the NSAIDs, irrespective of *H. pylori* status. It is appropriate to eradicate *H. pylori* in NSAID naive patients prior to starting chronic ASA or NSAID therapy. However, *H. pylori* eradication alone appears to be insufficient for ulcer prophylaxis in chronic non-ASA NSAID users. Misoprostol prophylaxis and substitution of COX-2 inhibitors appear to reduce the risk of developing endoscopically diagnosed gastric ulcers by 80% and the risk of complicated ulcers by 50%.

Functional dyspepsia (Chapter 9)
Patients undergoing endoscopy for dyspeptic symptoms tend to be more satisfied and have improved quality of life and subsequently create significantly lower health care costs than patients initially treated empirically. The practical bottom line for use of PPIs in functional dyspepsia is that it is reasonable to give patients a trial of 4–8 weeks of therapy, with the understanding that heartburn is a predictor of response and that the majority of patients will not respond (NNT = 15). *H. pylori* infection is present in 30–70% of patients, and eradication may lead to long-term symptom improvement in a small proportion of these patients. There is no convincing evidence for the use of prokinetic or antidepressant medications.

Celiac disease (Chapter 10)
Although the human recombinant anti-tissue transglutamase antibody test (tTG) has a sensitivity of 96% and a specificity of 99% for diagnosis of celiac disease in some studies, the sensitivity in other studies is considerable lower. The tTG will likely remain as an adjunct to endoscopy for the diagnosis of celiac disease, rather than a replacement. A substantial amount of evidence demonstrates a lack of toxicity of oats in newly diagnosed patients with celiac disease, and in celiac disease patients in remission.

Crohn's disease (Chapter 11)
Infliximab, adalimumab and certolizumab have all been shown to be effective for induction and maintenance of remission. There is emerging evidence that early combined immunosuppression with infliximab combined with azathioprine and, if necessary, steroids is superior to conventional management with corticosteroids, followed in sequence by azathioprine and infliximab in terms of steroid-free remission and avoidance of surgery at 26 and 52 weeks. Serious adverse events are not significantly more frequent in the early combined immunosuppression group. The combination of infliximab and methotrexate, although safe, has not been shown to be more effective than infliximab alone in Crohn's disease patients who are also receiving treatment with prednisone.

Although an earlier small randomized placebo-controlled trial suggested that omega-3 fatty acids are effective for maintenance of remission in patients at a relatively high risk of relapse of Crohn's disease, two large randomized trials that included 762 patients have now shown that this approach is not effective.

Natalizumab (300 mg or 3 to 4 mg/kg) is effective for induction of clinical response and remission in patients with moderately to severely active Crohn's disease. One patient with Crohn's disease treated with natalizumab in combination with azathioprine developed progressive multifocal leukoencephalopathy (PML). A retrospective investigation suggests that the incidence of PML is approximately 1 case per 1000 patients.

Ulcerative colitis (Chapter 12)
Probiotic preparations of a specific lyophilized *E. coli* strain, or mixtures of several bacteria, when added to conventional therapy, may increase rates of induction and enhance maintenance of remission in mild ulcerative colitis. An

apheretic technique that removes granulocytes from the blood of patients is ineffective. Infliximab is effective for induction of remission in severe refractory disease.

Pouchitis (Chapter 13)
Small controlled trials have demonstrated the efficacy of ciprofloxacin and metronidazole for acute pouchitis, of budesonide enemas for active chronic pouchitis, and of probiotic bacteria for maintaining remission of chronic pouchitis and for prophylaxis.

Microscopic colitis (Chapter 14)
Budesonide is effective for short-term treatment, but the optimal strategy for long-term management needs further study. The long-term prognosis is good, and the risk of complications including colonic cancer is low.

Drug-induced diarrhea: (Chapter 15)
Faced with an aging patient population and an ever increasing population of diabetic patients physicians should be aware that cholinesterase inhibitors, increasingly used in Alzheimer's disease, produce diarrhea in 14% of patients and metformin produces malabsorptive diarrhea in up to 50% of patients.

Metabolic bone disease in gastrointestinal disorders (Chapter 16)
Bisphosphonate therapy reduces the risk of vertebral fractures in IBD patients by 6.3%. The improvement in BMD in IBD patients taking infliximab + a bisphosphonate may be greater than that observed with a bisphosphonate alone.

Chronic PPI users may not have an increase in the risk of hip fracture with PPI use if they have no other identifiable risk factor. If there is a true association (as opposed to an association with confounding variables) between PPI use and decreased bone density, the fracture risk in chronic PPI users is low. The increased risk may be clinically relevant in patients with multiple other risk factors for osteoporosis, especially in patients with long-term, high-dose therapy.

Colorectal cancer in ulcerative colitis: surveillance (Chapter 17)
Chromoendoscopy with targeted biopsies may increase the yield of surveillance colonoscopy. Estimates of sensitivity and specificity are made from an increased number of large surveillance programs.

Colon cancer screening (Chapter 18)
The sensitivity of fecal occult blood testing, when three stools are tested using a sensitive immunochemical technique, approaches 90%. The miss rate for significant lesions at colonoscopy may be as high as 5%. There is consistent evidence that colonoscopy is less effective for reduction in right-sided CRC than it is for left-sided CRC. Colonoscopy may be more cost effective than CT colonography, depending on relative procedural costs.

Prevention and treatment of traveler's diarrhea (Chapter 19)
This new chapter summarizes the evidence for a number of interventions for chemoprohylaxis (with Rifaximin being the recommended agent). Early evidence for the efficacy of immunoprohylaxis is also presented.

Clostridium difficile disease (Chapter 20)
Preventive strategies, including enhanced infection control programs and antibiotic stewardship, are effective in reducing the incidence of CDAD. Complicated cases of CDAD have increased in frequency in some outbreaks, and it is postulated that the emergent hypervirulent BI/NAP10/27 strain is responsible. Evidence still favors metronidazole for treatment of initial episodes, but vancomycin appears to be the more effective treatment for severe disease. Observational studies suggest that tapered and pulsed vancomycin regimens may be effective for recurrent disease.

Irritable bowel syndrome (Chapter 21)
Colonic investigation has a very low yield in patients presenting with symptoms that are highly suggestive of IBS in the absence of alarm features. Screening to exclude celiac disease and thyroid dysfunction appears to be of value, but a panel of blood tests, including ESR and CRP, often performed when patients with suspected IBS are first seen in the outpatient clinic, has a low yield in detecting organic disease. Data to support the role of lactose hydrogen breath testing to exclude lactose intolerance are conflicting. Soluble fibre, antispasmodics (particularly hyoscine) and peppermint oil may be of some benefit in treatment of IBS patients, although the evidence is less than convincing. Both TCADs and SSRIs are effective (NNT = 4). Probiotics may also be used as second-line interventions in individuals with particularly troublesome abdominal pain and bloating. Psychological interventions should be reserved for individuals who are unresponsive to, or intolerant of, more conventional therapies, since they are time-consuming and expensive.

Ogilvie's syndrome (Chapter 22)
Evidence is presented that polyethylene glycol may reduce the frequency of recurrent cecal dilatation in patients who had initial resolution with neostigmine or decompression. Polyethylene glycol may also prevent the development of acute pseudoobstruction in patients with multiple organ failure admitted to an ICU.

Gallstone disease (Chapter 23)
The natural history of asymptomatic cholelithiasis in diabetic patients appears to be similar to that in the general population, and preventative surgery should not be recom-

mended routinely. Laparoscopic cholecystectomy appears to be as safe as open cholecystectomy and may provide short-term improvement in quality of life. Acute cholecystitis should be treated with early laparoscopic cholecystectomy. In patients with gallstone pancreatitis preoperative ERCP may increase overall morbidity compared with the approach of cholecystectomy with intraoperative cholangiography. Patients with acute severe gallstone pancreatitis should undergo cholecystectomy following resolution of the acute episode, but during the initial hospital stay. Patients with mild to moderate pancreatitis can be considered for early laparoscopic cholecystectomy. Three approaches to the management of common duct stones (open common bile duct exploration, ERCP and sphincterotomy, and laparoscopic common bile duct exploration) have been compared, and conflicting data may relate to variation in operator expertise. The approach to CBD stones should be individualized and based on the type of expertise available at each institution.

Acute pancreatitis (Chapter 24)
Several recent, well-planned RCTs provided no evidence for benefit from the early use of prophylactic antibiotics in severe pancreatitis, and it is no longer recommended.

Obesity (Chapter 25)
The risk for co-morbidities, including cardiovascular disease, type 2 diabetes, obstructive sleep apnea and certain cancers, is reduced up to 40% by bariatric surgery.

Part II: Liver disease

Hepatitis C (Chapter 26)
There are concise guidelines for treatment of naive patients, based on genotype and viral load. Re-treatment is reviewed in detail as much more evidence is available from randomized studies. In the main, relapsers are worth re-treating, but genotype 1 non-responders may not yield cost-effective benefit.

Hepatitis B (Chapter 27)
New therapies and new evaluation of interferon have revolutionized the management of these patients. The importance of monitoring for viral resistance, and using the correct combination, or sequential use, of agents is outlined.

Alcoholic related liver disease (Chapter 28)
In alcoholic hepatitis there has been a consolidation of the evidence for the use of steroids and evidence for "stopping rules", and validation of indices of non-response. Trials of agents to help abstention are reviewed.

Non-alcoholic fatty liver disease (Chapter 29)
This disease spectrum is far better characterized, including the association with the other factors which make up the metabolic syndrome. Whilst diagnostic methodology has improved, specific therapeutic agents are not available. What has been tried so far is summarized, with an outline of future prospects.

Hemochromatosis (Chapter 30)
Genetic hemochromatosis is underdiagnosed in the general population, and overdiagnosed in patients with secondary iron overload. A mild elevation in ferritin is very common, and may be related to obesity with NAFLD, regular alcohol consumption, or inflammation.

The hepatic iron index reported on histological examination has limited use with the advent of genetic testing. The C282Y homozygote is the classic genetic pattern in >90% of typical cases. With other genetic variants severe iron overload is usually seen in the setting of a concomitant risk factor (alcoholism, viral hepatitis, NAFLD). Several studies have documented reversal of fibrosis following iron depletion therapy.

Wilson's disease (Chapter 31)
Despite isolation of several genes, the diagnosis remains a clinical one in patients presenting with abnormal liver function. Trientene and zinc therapy have further documentation of their efficacy.

Primary biliary cirrhosis (Chapter 32)
Updated information on the use of ursodeoxycholic acid (UDCA), particularly in early PBC, still leave this drug as the one most frequently used for this disease, but with gaps in robust evidence for its efficacy.

Autoimmune hepatitis (Chapter 33)
Classical autoimmune hepatitis is well recognized, but "difficult to treat" cases not responding to standard immunosuppression, and the occurrence of overlap syndromes make some cases difficult to diagnose and to treat. Good outcomes have now been obtained with budenoside, tacrolimus and mycophenalate. New diagnostic algorithms have helped distinguish true overlap syndromes from disease variants.

Primary sclerosing cholangitis (Chapter 34)
It is important to exclude IgG4 associated sclerosing cholangitis in the differential diagnosis. Use of UDCA is under scrutiny, and the use of high dose UDCA is reviewed.

Non-histological assessment of fibrosis (Chapter 35)
This is a new chapter, which has evaluated both serum markers and transient elastography and the comparison with liver biopsy for the assessment of fibrosis.

Portal hypertensive bleeding (Chapter 36)
Evolution of combined therapies using endoscopic and pharmacological ones, has replaced single mode approaches.

The use of primary prophylaxis with non-selective beta-blockers has been extended to grade Child C patients with cirrhosis even if varices are small. Antibiotics are now mandatory in the treatment of acute variceal bleeding as they improve control of bleeding, and mortality over and above specific endoscopic and pharmacological methods.

Hepatic outflow syndromes and splanchnic thrombosis (Chapter 37)

This is a new chapter, updating current management of hepatic outflow obstruction with a defined algorithm and use of anticoagulation for portal venous thrombosis.

Ascites, hepatorenal syndrome and spontaneous bacterial peritonitis (Chapter 38)

This is an updated review of therapy, particularly for hepatorenal syndrome, for which terlipressin and albumin improve renal function in about 30% of patients. Selection for antibiotic prophylaxis in a primary setting has expanded beyond patients with low concentrations of albumin in ascites.

Hepatic encephalopathy: treatment (Chapter 39)

The diagnosis and management of minimal hepatic encephalopathy are integral to this chapter, as this is an evolving area, which does affect quality of life, ability to drive safely and so on.

Hepatocellular carcinoma (Chapter 40)

Combined clinical and imaging characteristics have allowed a much better clinical staging system, which guides therapy. Indications and use of loco-regional therapy, liver resection and transplantation, as well as new agents such as sorafenib have evolved, and a rationale basis for therapy is presented.

Fulminant hepatic failure (Chapter 41)

Supportive management has greatly improved over the past few years. Current best practice is reviewed by new authors, and referral and indications for liver transplantation are fully discussed. The current status of liver support devices is evaluated on the basis of the few controlled trials and observational studies.

Liver transplantation: prevention and treatment of rejection (Chapter 42)

New data from randomized trials has been incorporated against a background of the method of diagnosis of rejection and long-term complications and outcomes, where these have been documented.

Liver transplantation: prevention and treatment of infection (Chapter 43)

New authors have completely revised this chapter, dealing with the major cause of morbidity and mortality within one year of transplantation. Hepatologists who may not be in transplant centers, but who follow up patients who have had liver transplant, need to be aware of infectious complications, their diagnosis and treatment.

Management of HCV infection and liver transplantation (Chapter 44)

This is a major clinical problem, for which only recently there has been data from randomized studies and careful prospective observational studies to give some evidence-based guidance for therapy.

Management of HBV infection and liver transplantation (Chapter 45)

The new therapies for HBV infection have revolutionized the outcome for HBV infected patients who come to liver transplantation. Treatment algorithms are now simplified and the importance for monitoring for viral resistance fully outlined.

Liver biopsy (Chapter 46)

This is a new chapter reviewing the evidence base for diagnosis of liver disease, and staging/grading for chronic viral hepatitis. A full review of transjugular liver biopsy is given.

Drug induced liver injury (DILI) (Chapter 47)

This is a new chapter, including etiopathogenetic mechanisms and practical algorithms to reach a diagnosis for this problem, which is being seen more frequently.

References

1 Ruffin JM, Grizzle JE, Hightower NC, McHardy G, Shull H, Kirsner JB. A co-operative double blind evaluation of gastric "freezing" in the treatment of duodenal ulcer. *N Engl J Med* 1969; **281**: 16–19.

2 Dickson ER, Fleming TR, Wiesner RH *et al.* Trial of penicillamine in advanced primary biliary cirrhosis. *N Engl J Med* 1985; **312**: 1011–1015.

3 A Medical Research Council Investigation. Streptomycin treatment of pulmonary tuberculosis. *BMJ* 1948; **ii**: 770–782.

4 Truelove SC, Witts LJ. Cortisone in ulcerative colitis. Final report on a therapeutic trial. *BMJ* 1955: 1041–1048.

5 Liberati A, Apolone G, Nicolucci A *et al.* The role of attitudes, beliefs, and personal characteristics of Italian physicians in the surgical treatment of early breast cancer. *Am J Public Health* 1990; **81**: 38–41.

6 Antman EM, Lau J, Kupelnick B, Mosteller F, Chalmers TC. A comparison of results of meta-analyses of randomized control trials and recommendations of clinical experts. Treatments for myocardial infarction. *JAMA* 1992; **268**: 240–248.

7 Mulrow CD. The medical review article: state of the science. *Ann Intern Med* 1987; **106**: 485–488.

8 Jefferson T. What are the benefits of editorials and nonsystematic reviews? *BMJ* 1999; **318**: 135.

9 Cochrane AL. Archie Cochrane in his own words. Selections arranged from his 1972 introduction to "Effectiveness and efficiency: random reflections on the health services" 1972. *Control Clin Trials* 1989; **10**: 428–433.

10 The Cochrane Collaboration. *Cochrane Library* 1999: www.cochrane.org.

11 Sackett DL. Clinical epidemiology. *Am J Epidemiol* 1969; **89**: 125–128.

12 Sackett DL. Interpretation of diagnostic data: 1. How to do it with pictures. *Can Med Assoc J* 1983; **129**: 429–432.

13 Sackett D, Haynes RB, Tugwell P, Guyatt GH. *Clinical Epidemiology: a Basic Science for Clinical Medicine*, 2nd edn. Little, Brown and Company, Boston, MA, 1991.

14 Reid MC, Lachs MS, Feinstein AR. Use of methodological standards in diagnostic test research. getting better but still not good. *JAMA* 1995; **274**: 645–651.

15 Ransohoff DF, Feinstein AR. Problems of spectrum and bias in evaluating the efficacy of diagnostic tests. *N Engl J Med* 1978; **299**: 926–930.

16 Chalmers TC. Randomization of the first patient. *Med Clin North Am* 1975; **59**: 1035–1038.

17 Resnick RH, Iber FL, Ishihara AM, Chalmers TC, Zimmerman H. A controlled study of the therapeutic portacaval shunt. *Gastroenterology* 1974; **67**: 843–587.

18 Sacks HS, Berrier J, Reitman D, Ancona-Berk VA, Chalmers TC. Meta-analyses of randomized controlled trials. *N Engl J Med* 1987; **316**: 450–455.

19 Kernick D. Lies, damned lies, and evidence-based medicine. Jabs and jibes. *Lancet* 1998; **351**: 1824.

20 Scholefield JH, Johnson AG, Shorthouse AJ. Current surgical practice in screening for colorectal cancer based on family history criteria. *Br J Surg* 1998; **85**: 1543–1546.

21 Gabriel SE, Jaakkimainen L, Bombardier C. Risk for serious gastrointestinal complications related to use of nonsteroidal anti-inflammatory drugs. A meta-analysis. *Ann Intern Med* 1991; **115**: 787–796.

22 Yusuf S, Cairns JA, Camm AJ, Fallen EL, Gersh BJ. *Evidence-based Cardiology*, 2nd edn. BMJ Books, London, 2003.

23 Cataldo F, Ventura A, Lazzari R. Anti-endomysium antibodies and celiac disease: solved and unsolved questions. An Italian multicentre study. *Acta Paediatr* 1995; **84**: 1125–1131.

24 Kitching A, Sackett D, Yusuf S. Approaches to evaluating evidence. *Evidence-based Cardiology*. BMJ Books, London, 1998.

25 Holmes GKT, Prior R, Lane MR *et al.* Malignancy in celiac disease: effect of a gluten-free diet. *Gut* 1989; **30**: 333–338.

26 McLeod RS, Wolff BG, Steinhart AH *et al.* Prophylactic mesalamine treatment decreases postoperative recurrence of Crohn's disease. *Gastroenterology* 1995; **109**: 404–413.

27 Chalmers TC, Celano P, Sacks HS, Smith H Jr. Bias in treatment assignment in controlled clinical trials. *N Engl J Med* 1983; **309**: 1358–1361.

28 Schulz KF, Chalmers I, Hayes RJ, Altman DG. Empirical evidence of bias. Dimensions of methodological quality associated with estimates of treatment effects in controlled trials. *JAMA* 1995; **273**: 408–412.

29 ICH Steering Committee. *ICH Harmonised Tripartite Guideline. Statistical Principles for Clinical Trials.* Section 5.3-Missing Values and Outliers. Geneva: International Conference on Harmonisation of Technical Requirements for Registration of Pharmaceuticals for Human Use, 1998.

30 Feagan BG, McDonald JWD, Koval JJ. Therapeutics and inflammatory bowel disease: a guide to the interpretation of randomized controlled trials. *Gastroenterology* 1996; **110**: 275–823.

31 Koch GG. One-sided and two-sided tests and p values. *J Biopharm Stat* 1991; **1**: 161–170.

32 Kapur KC, Williams GT, Allison MC. Mesalazine induced exacerbation of ulcerative colitis. *Gut* 1995; **37**: 838–839.

33 Naylor CD, Chen E, Strauss B. Measured enthusiasm: does the method of reporting trial results alter perceptions of therapeutic effectiveness? *Ann Intern Med* 1992; **117**: 916–921.

34 Camma C, Giunta M, Rosselli M, Cottone M. Mesalamine in the maintenance treatment of Crohn's disease: a meta-analysis adjusted for confounding variables. *Gastroenterology* 1997; **113**: 1465–1473.

35 Oxman AD, Cook DJ, Guyatt GH. User's guides to the medical literature. VI How to use an overview. Evidence-Based Medicine Working Group. *JAMA* 1994; **272**: 1367–1371.

36 Caprilli R, Andreoli A, Capurso L *et al.* Oral mesalazine (5-aminosalicylic acid; asacol) for the prevention of postoperative recurrence of Crohn's disease. *Aliment Pharmacol Ther* 1994; **8**: 35–43.

37 Lochs H, Mayer M, Fleig WE *et al.* Prophylaxis of postoperative relapse in Crohn's disease with mesalazine (Pentasa) in comparison to placebo. *Gastroenterology* 2000; **119**: 264–273.

38 Sutherland LR. Mesalamine for the prevention of postoperative recurrence: is nearly there the same as being there? *Gastroenterology* 2000; **118**: 264–273.

39 Cumbers B, Donald A. Evidence-based practice. Data day. *Health Serv J* 1999; **109**: 30–31.

Gastrointestinal disorders

2 Gastroesophageal reflux disease

Naoki Chiba[1] and M Brian Fennerty[2]

[1] Division of Gastroenterology, McMaster University Medical Centre, Hamilton *and* Guelph General Hospital, Guelph, Canada
[2] Oregan Health and Science University, Division of Gastroenterology and Hepatology, Oregon, USA

Introduction

Heartburn and or regurgitation are very common symptoms encountered in patients seen in a clinical practice. Most patients with gastroesophageal reflux disease (GERD) will have these symptoms of heartburn and/or regurgitation, but many patients with these symptoms do not have GERD. Clinical studies prior to the mid-1990s focused on management of patients with predominant heartburn based on the endoscopic findings of esophagitis, as healing of the esophageal mucosa was an easily measured objective endpoint compared to subjectively assessing a patient's symptom response to a therapy. More recently it has become known that GERD symptom severity does not predict the presence or absence of endoscopic mucosal damage (e.g. esophagitis), and patients with GERD including those with and without esophagitis, experience decrements in quality of life (QoL) associated with their symptoms. In treating GERD patients with esophagitis and those with non-erosive reflux disease (NERD), as well as those patients with symptomatic heartburn that have not undergone endoscopy, proton pump inhibitors (PPIs) offer better healing and symptom relief than less potent acid inhibitors (e.g. histamine-2 receptor antagonists or H2-blockers) or acid neutralizing agents (e.g. antacids). The available PPIs are, for the most part, equally effective as treatment for GERD symptoms and healing esophagitis, although esomeprazole more effectively heals the small minority of GERD patients with more severe grades of esophagitis (Los Angeles Grades C and D). For patients with documented erosive esophagitis and in those with NERD and/or uninvestigated heartburn that relapses quickly upon discontinuing treatment, maintenance therapy with a PPI may be appropriate. For patients with documented NERD, lower doses of PPI therapy are often adequate, and treatment can also be given on demand or prn. The PPIs are very safe and offer excellent long-term control of symptoms, although recent evidence suggests that long-term use may be associated with some adverse outcomes. Anti-reflux surgery is also an effective option for treating GERD symptoms and healing esophagitis, especially since a laparoscopic alternative has now become well established and is widely available. The choice for surgery should be based on patient preference rather than issues of efficacy or cost, as there is ample evidence that neither therapeutic approach is substantially more cost-effective than the other.

Definition of gastroesophageal reflux disease

Gastroesophageal reflux (GER) is a normal physiological process that most commonly occurs during and after meals in an upright position. However, due to acid neutralization by saliva and prompt esophageal clearance of physiologic refluxate, symptoms associated with physiologic GER occur in only a minority of people. Conversely, GERD occurs when reflux is frequent or caustic enough to cause the typical symptoms of heartburn, acid regurgitation and or dysphagia or result in esophageal mucosal injury. GERD also may result in extraesophageal manifestations such as non-cardiac chest pain, asthma, cough or posterior laryngitis and hoarseness [1]. Moreover, patients will often present not only with reflux symptoms but also with epigastric pain and/or discomfort, symptoms associated with "dyspepsia" rather than GERD [1–3]. It is difficult to determine at what point GER transforms a normal physiological state into a disease state, GERD. Many patients and providers regard some degree of heartburn as normal. Moreover only a small proportion of patients with GERD actually seek medical care, as noted in Castell's "GERD iceberg" [4].

Early literature often incorrectly used the terms hiatus hernia and gastroesophageal reflux synonymously, imply-

Evidence-Based Gastroenterology and Hepatology, 3rd edition.
J. McDonald, A.K. Burroughs, B. Feagan, and M.B. Fennerty. © 2010
Blackwell Publishing Ltd

ing that the hernia was the cause of the symptoms of GERD or the root cause of GERD itself. Hiatus hernia is a common structural abnormality, whereas reflux is most often caused by functional or mechanical events. Once the hiatus hernia was dismissed as the root cause of GERD, reflux disease was considered to be present when abnormally prolonged esophageal acid exposure resulted in esophageal damage, either macroscopic (endoscopic esophagitis and/or Barrett's esophagus) or microscopic (histological esophagitis). However, more recently, it has been recognized that symptomatic gastroesophageal reflux without obvious macroscopic or microscopic esophageal injury, otherwise known as "endoscopy negative reflux disease" (ENRD) or "non-erosive reflux disease" (NERD), is an important and large part of the spectrum of reflux disease [5]. Another term, symptomatic GERD, has been used to refer to these patients previously classified as having NERD. However, this term is also imprecise and should be applied only to patients with uninvestigated reflux-like symptoms that adversely impact their normal quality of life (QoL).

It is now generally accepted that GERD is really a spectrum of diseases. Attention has been focused on the typical symptoms of heartburn and acid regurgitation that are often not accompanied by any easily identified pathological findings. Even without endoscopic esophagitis, these patients have reduced health-related QoL comparable with that experienced by patients with esophagitis [6–89]. Awareness of this fact has led some experts to erroneously equate a patient with the predominant symptom of heartburn with a confident diagnosis of GERD [10, 11]. Patients with heartburn alone have only a little better than chance probability of having GERD as defined by an abnormal ambulatory esophageal acid exposure [12]. Most patients with endoscopic esophagitis will complain of heartburn [13], and even if heartburn is not the predominant symptom, endoscopic esophagitis can be identified in up to 36% of patients with suspected GERD [14]. Thus, it is clear that the symptom of heartburn in and of itself is an insufficient criterion to diagnose GERD.

Many authors continue to mix symptoms and mucosal damage in the same definition of GERD. The American College of Gastroenterology definition of GERD is, "chronic symptoms or mucosal damage produced by the abnormal reflux of gastric contents into the esophagus" [15]. Experts from the Genval Workshop further expanded this definition to include the patient-centered perspective that gastroesophageal reflux is defined by the presence of "clinically significant impairment of health-related well-being (quality of life) due to reflux-related symptoms" [11]. These are similar to the 2004 Canadian GERD Consensus Conference definition: "GERD applies to individuals with reflux of gastric contents into the esophagus causing (a) symptoms sufficient to reduce quality of life and/or (b) esophageal injury" [9]. The subsequent 2006 Montreal definition:

"GERD is a condition which develops when the reflux of stomach contents causes troublesome symptoms and/or complications" was similar [1].

In summary, these data indicate that an encompassing, objective and validated definition of GERD is lacking and instead we are relying on imperfect measures to define this disease. Furthermore, the varied phenotypic expression of the disease(s) indicates that a single reproducible measure is unlikely to be an effective tool for the definition of GERD.

Symptoms of gastroesophageal reflux disease

The typical symptoms of GERD include heartburn (usually defined as a rising retrosternal burning discomfort) and acid regurgitation [1, 9]. Many investigators suggest that the diagnosis of GERD should be based primarily on the presence of these typical symptoms, as the specificity of heartburn and acid regurgitation for GERD is approximately 89% and 95% respectively [27]. Indeed, up to 96% of patients with documented erosive esophagitis also have heartburn [13]. An early study reported that when heartburn or regurgitation occurred daily, there was a positive predictive value of 59% and 66% respectively, for the diagnosis of GERD [28]. When an abnormal pH-metry is used as the gold standard, these symptoms have demonstrated 72% sensitivity and 63% specificity for GERD [29]. Many patients also have other upper abdominal symptoms as noted previously, but according to recent concepts, these patients are probably more correctly classified as having dyspepsia rather than GERD [30].

In summary, the only validated symptom measure for GERD at this time is the word description for heartburn (e.g. a burning discomfort arising behind the breastbone towards the neck).

Epidemiology of gastroesophageal reflux disease

Considering the lack of consistency of symptom based definitions and methods of diagnosis of GERD, it is difficult to determine the absolute prevalence of GERD in the general population. For instance, are we measuring the prevalence of the symptoms of heartburn or acid regurgitation, and to what degree, or are we measuring the prevalence of endoscopic esophagitis? The prevalence of GERD also varies between surveys of the general population and studies of symptomatic patients that present to the family practitioner. Heartburn is experienced by 4–7% of the general US population on a daily basis and by 34–44% of the population at least once a month (Table 2.1) [5, 20, 31–33]. Similarly high rates have been observed in New Zealand [34]. Recent data suggest that Asian patients have a lower prevalence of GERD symptoms than Western pop-

Table 2.1 Population-based questionnaire studies of the prevalence of the symptom of heartburn.

Authors	Country	Daily (%)	At least once weekly (%)	At least once a month (%)	Total at least once/month (%)
Nebel *et al.* (1976) [16]	USA	7	14	15	36
Thompson and Heaton (1982) [17]	UK	4	10	21	34
Gallup Organization (1988) [18]	USA	—	—	—	44
Isolauri and Laippala (1995) [19]	Finland	9	15	21	41
Locke *et al.* (1997) [20]	USA	—	18	—	42
Wong *et al.* (2003) [21]	China	—	2.5	8.9	—
Diaz-Rubio *et al.* (2004) [22]	Spain	—	9.8	—	—
Cho *et al.* (2005) [23]	Korea	—	2.0	4.7	—
Bor *et al.* (2005) [24]	Turkey	—	10	—	—
Moraes-Filho *et al.* (2005) [25]	Brazil	—	4.6	—	—
Yamagishi *et al.* (2008) [26]	Japan	—	—	—	20

ulations [21, 35], as well as a much lower prevalence of esophagitis [36].

In contrast, the overall prevalence of reflux esophagitis in Western countries has been estimated to be about 2% [33]. However, this figure likely underestimates the true prevalence. In a group of 27% of adults self-treating with antacids more than twice a month, objective evidence of reflux esophagitis is revealed in 84% during investigation, suggesting that esophagitis is not uncommonly found in those with symptoms of heartburn [37]. Furthermore, some have estimated that the prevalence of GERD is as high as 20% of the adult population and that esophagitis is found in 35–50% of those with GERD. If these data are correct the prevalence of esophagitis in the adult population may be as high as 7–10%. A recent systematic review by El-Serag has shown an overall increase in the prevalence of GERD over the past two decades, particularly for North America and Europe, but not Asia [38].

The incidence of GERD is estimated to be 4.5 per 100,000 with a dramatic increase in persons over the age of 40 years [39]. A Canadian study found that heartburn occurred at least once a week in 19% of persons > 60 years old, compared with 4.8% of persons < 27 years old [17]. A large American retrospective cohort study in VA patients also identified older age along with being a white male as the group associated with the most severe forms of GERD [40].

Nebel *et al.* in 1976 [16] studied the point prevalence and precipitating factors associated with symptomatic gastroesophageal reflux using a questionnaire in 446 hospitalized and 558 outpatients (see Table 2.1). Age, sex or hospitalization did not significantly affect prevalence. In a Finnish study of 1700 adults, only 16% of symptomatic patients reported taking medications and only 5% had sought medical care [19].

In clinical practice, the relevant population is the group of patients that present with symptomatic heartburn. In this population, it has been estimated that about 50–70% of patients have normal endoscopies and the minority of patients (30–50%) have endoscopic esophagitis [41]. However, in a recently reported Canadian study of prompt endoscopy in patients with uninvestigated dyspepsia, the overall prevalence of endoscopic esophagitis was 43%, and in those with dominant heartburn, the prevalence of esophagitis was 55% [14]. Thus in this population, NERD was seen in less than half of the patients (45%).

In summary, the true population prevalence of GERD and esophagitis is unknown but appears to be approximately 10–15% and 3–7% based on current data.

Pathophysiology of gastroesophageal reflux disease

GERD is primarily a motility and/or anatomical disorder of the esophagus, perturbations of which allow an abnormal amount or frequency of injurious gastric contents to reflux into the esophagus. Reflux occurs as a consequence of a defect of the normal anatomic and physiological antireflux barrier that is provided primarily by actions of the lower esophageal sphincter (LES) and crural diaphragm. The two key abnormalities are thought to be abnormal transient lower esophageal sphincter relaxations (TLESRs) [42, 43], precipitated by gastric distension in the postprandial period [44] and poor basal LES tone [42]. The result of these and other less common anatomic and physiological abnormalities is an increased intraesophageal exposure of gastric refluxate and increasing damage as the pH of refluxate falls below 4, which is optimal for pepsin activation [45,

46]. A hiatus hernia may act as a reservoir for acid refluxate that can then re-reflux up the esophagus [47, 48]. GERD patients with hiatus hernia have been found to have greater esophageal acid exposure and more reflux episodes vs GERD patients without a hernia [49].

Pathophysiology in non-erosive reflux disease

Further support for the concept that acid alone can be the pathophysiological basis for reflux disease comes from the observation that in patients that have typical symptoms of reflux with a normal endoscopy, 6–15% with symptomatic reflux had normal 24-hour esophageal pH-metry [50–52]. Additionally, pathological reflux on pH studies has been identified in 21–61% of endoscopy negative patients [53–55]. A recent study identified abnormal acid reflux in 84% of patients with either erosive esophagitis or NERD, a much higher proportion than previously reported. The reason for these variable results is unknown. In contrast, 71–91% of patients with erosive esophagitis at endoscopy have pathological reflux on pH studies. Thus, abnormal intraesophageal acid exposure as measured by pH studies is more frequent but not an optimal gold standard for documenting reflux disease [53–55]. However, despite these limitations the data clearly demonstrate that the proportion of intraesophageal acid exposure increases over the spectrum from NERD to worsening grades of esophagitis and Barrett's esophagus [56].

Another conundrum in reflux disease is the patient with an apparent suprasensitive esophagus. Of 96 patients with normal 24-hour esophageal acid exposure, 12.5% were found to have a statistically significant association between their reflux symptoms and actual reflux episodes, despite having "normal" intraesophageal acid exposure [51]. In these patients, the duration of reflux episodes was shorter and the pH of reflux episodes was often lower than in patients with typical GERD, suggesting that esophageal hypersensitivity was the cause of their symptoms. These and other data have led to the concept of an acid-sensitive esophagus.

An esophageal balloon distension study provided further experimental evidence of esophageal hypersensitivity in patients with normal acid exposure times with a value for a symptom index (SI) > 50% [50]. In general, these patients had significantly lower thresholds for initial perception and discomfort from esophageal balloon distension, compared with both normal controls and patients with confirmed reflux. In contrast, Fass *et al.* studied patients with GERD and controls without GERD and determined that patients showed enhanced perception of acid perfusion but not of esophageal distension [57]. They concluded that chronic acid reflux by itself was not the cause of esophageal hypersensitivity to distension in patients with non-cardiac chest pain, although subsequent data from this group

suggest that the esophagus can be primed to be hypersensitive by repeated reflux events.

Carlsson *et al.* [58] have also demonstrated an impaired esophageal mucosal barrier in symptomatic GERD patients by measuring the transmucosal epithelial potential difference, suggesting a role for alteration in cell barrier function as a cause for reflux symptoms in some individuals.

Another study examined differences in spatiotemporal reflux characteristics between symptomatic and asymptomatic reflux episodes [59]. They used a pH sensor positioned 3, 6, 9, 12 and 15 cm above the LES and found that the duration of acid exposure was longer and the proximal extent was higher in symptomatic than in asymptomatic reflux episodes. A similar study also determined that patients with NERD compared with healthy controls, had a higher, intraesophageal proximal reflux of acid [60]. Even NERD patients with normal acid exposure time seemed to perceive proximal reflux very readily, implying that their proximal esophageal mucosa is more sensitive to short duration refluxes than that of patients with esophagitis.

More recently, there is a suggestion that up to two-thirds of patients with NERD have histological evidence of esophageal injury [61]. The commonest finding is dilation of intercellular spaces irrespective of esophageal acid exposure. Basal cell hyperplasia and papillary elongation were seen more frequently in NERD patients with abnormal acid exposure. However, these findings are not found consistently enough to reliably serve as the basis for the diagnosis of GERD.

Hiatus hernia

The mere presence of a hiatus hernia (HH) bears no relationship to the diagnosis of esophagitis and is frequently seen in those without esophagitis. Moreover, up to half the healthy population has a hiatus hernia [62] and only half of the patients with symptoms of heartburn and regurgitation have a hiatus hernia [63]. However, some studies have suggested that patients with a hiatus hernia have greater esophageal acid exposure and more reflux episodes [49] and more severe reflux esophagitis than patients without, suggesting that a HH does have a role in some patients with reflux disease [64, 65]. A large HH may act as a reservoir for acid that re-refluxes more readily when a swallow is initiated and in this fashion contributes to GERD [47, 48].

Other supporting evidence for the role of HH in GERD comes from a study in patients with pathologic reflux (pH < 4 for more than 5% of a 24-hour intraesophageal pH-metry study) that identified hiatus hernia in 71% of patients with mild esophagitis, compared with 39% of those without esophagitis [66]. Patients with a hiatus hernia also had higher 24-hour intraesophageal acid exposure compared with those without, particularly during the night. However, there were no differences in symptoms of heartburn or regurgitation, whether or not patients had a hiatus hernia or esophagitis.

Another study demonstrated that the presence of hiatus hernia correlated with more severe manifestations of GERD [67]. Hiatus hernia was seen in 29% of symptomatic patients, 71% with erosive esophagitis, and 96% with long segment Barrett's esophagus.

Although transient lower esophageal sphincter relaxations (TLESRs) are thought to be a key mechanism for pathological reflux, van Herwaarden et al. [49] did not find differences in LES pressure, and the incidence of TLESRs, and the proportion of TLESRs associated with acid reflux were comparable in those with and without hiatus hernia. They felt that the excess reflux in GERD patients with hiatus hernia was caused by malfunction of the gastroesophageal barrier during low LES pressure, swallow-associated normal LES relaxations, deep inspiration and straining.

In summary, the pathophysiology of GERD is varied, and the most common mechanism appears to be TLESRs but mechanical defects of the gastroesophageal junction and LES also play a role in many patients with this disorder.

Natural history of gastroesophageal reflux disease

There are few data about this important topic, and existing studies are limited in that they usually include heterogeneous populations. In one such study using a Swedish population-based survey of over a thousand citizens conducted over seven years, the prevalence of GERD remained stable over time at about 17–19% [68]. In a more recent 10-year follow-up Swedish study of 197 respondents out of the original 337 subject cohort, 83% reported no change in their global symptom assessment, indicating relative stability of symptoms over time [69].

A small retrospective study published in 1991 identified patients with symptoms of GERD but with a normal endoscopy and 24-hour pH study [70]. All patients received antacids or prokinetic drugs or both for 3–6 months. Thus, this was not a study of untreated patients but a study that employed treatments now recognized to be relatively ineffective (vs true untreated controls). However, 19 of the 33 patients still had symptoms at the end of six months and of these, five (26%) developed erosive esophagitis. The remainder of the patients remained asymptomatic. There was no difference in baseline pH-metry between those that went on to develop esophagitis and those that did not.

Another study reported data on patients with objectively proven GERD conservatively managed without treatment over a 17–22-year follow-up [71]. The authors reported on 60 patients from an initial cohort of 87 patients. Ten of these patients ultimately had an anti-reflux procedure, but of the remaining "untreated" 50 patients, 36 (72%) were less symptomatic at follow-up. Of this group, only six became symptom "free". The majority no longer used anti-reflux medications. Only five patients remained unchanged and nine became worse. The prevalence of erosive esophagitis fell from 40% at referral to 27% at follow-up endoscopy, and six new cases of Barrett's metaplasia developed. At follow-up, 66% of the patients had objective evidence of GERD with esophagitis, a pathological pH study or newly recognized Barrett's metaplasia. Neither the presence of esophagitis or of hiatal hernia, nor the severity of symptoms at baseline predicted the course of the disease at follow-up. The authors concluded that the severity of reflux symptoms declined in the long term, but pathological reflux persisted in the majority of the conservatively managed patients.

For patients with mild esophagitis, the course of the disease may also be relatively benign from an oesophageal injury perspective, with only 23% progressing to more severe esophagitis, while 31% improved and 46% spontaneously healed with no further episodes. However, from an impact on quality of life GERD does not appear to be a benign disease. In one study, patients with endoscopic esophagitis diagnosed more than 10 years earlier were contacted by postal questionnaire and phone interview [71]. Of the respondents, over 70% continued to have significant symptoms of reflux, and 40–50% were still taking acid suppressive medications regularly and had reduced QoL (lower Short Form (SF)-36, physical and social function domain scores). Thus, GERD is a chronic disease with significant morbidity and it impacts negatively on QoL.

Despite frequent symptoms, even severe reflux disease has little effect on life expectancy, with almost no deaths directly due to GERD reported in long-term follow-up [39, 71, 72]. However, a recent population-based study identified GERD as a strong risk factor for esophageal adenocarcinoma, but not squamous cell carcinoma [73].

In summary, the above data indicate that GERD is a chronic but not static disease; progression and regression may occur, although this is not common. Despite impacting QoL adversely, GERD has little effect on life expectancy.

Esophageal complications of gastroesophageal reflux disease

Complications of GERD include bleeding (< 2%), ulceration (approximately 5%) and strictures (1.2% to 20%) [71, 74, 75]. Patients with strictures are generally older and more frequently have a hiatus hernia [74]. Barrett's esophagus has been identified in 10–20% of GERD patients [76]. Six of 50 patients (12%) developed Barrett's esophagus during approximately 20 years of follow-up, a crude incidence of 0.6% per year [72]. The association of Barrett's esophagus and esophageal adenocarcinoma are covered in Chapter 3.

Effects of gastroesophageal reflux disease on quality of life (QoL)

Increased attention is being paid to patient QoL assessments, as opposed to histology of the esophagus as an outcome measure of importance in patients with GERD. Indeed, as there is no single physical marker for this disease, most experts now include decrements in QoL as part of the definition of GERD [9]. Several general health status and reflux-specific QoL instruments have been developed, validated and used. Examples include: Medical Outcomes Study SF-36 [77], Psychological General wellbeing (PGWB) index [78], the Gastrointestinal Symptom Rating Scale (GSRS) [79–81], the Gastroesophageal Reflux Disease – Health Related Quality of Life (GERD-HRQL) instrument [82], ReQuest [83–85], Reflux Disease Questionnaire [86], REFLUX-QUAL (RQS) [87], the Reflux questionnaire [88] and the Quality of Life in Reflux and Dyspepsia questionnaire (QOLRAD) [89]. Because of the development and availability of QoL instruments, more recent GERD clinical studies have used validated GERD-specific instruments focusing more on assessing patient satisfaction and QoL as primary endpoints [89–96]. Despite the development of more specific health-related QoL questionnaires, a 2008 systematic review identified that existing scales were still somewhat suboptimal [97]. Patients with gastrointestinal disorders have decreased functional status and well-being [98]. Those patients with chronic gastrointestinal disorders, including GERD, and congestive heart failure have the poorest health perceptions. These perceptions are worse than those that characterize some other chronic conditions such as hypertension and arthritis [79, 99, 100]. In patients with heartburn there was a substantial impairment of all aspects of health-related QoL when measured using the GSRS, QOLRAD, SF-36 and the Hospital Anxiety and Depression (HAD) scale [98].

Other studies have shown that successful treatment of GERD results in improvement in QoL. In general, patients with reflux esophagitis are considered to have equally impaired QoL to those with non-erosive disease, but those with very severe reflux esophagitis may have even more impairment [101]. NERD patients do not have objective markers such as endoscopic esophagitis that can be used to define treatment success. Symptom reduction to a level that does not cause significant impairment of health-related QoL is therefore an appropriate outcome by which to measure a therapy. Both the PGWB and GSRS scores show

good discriminative ability to reflect the severity of impairments in quality of life in NERD patients [102]. Improvements in health-related QoL with treatment of NERD and of erosive esophagitis have also been documented [7, 103, 104]. There are also now scales such as the Proton pump inhibitor Acid Suppression test (PASS) [105], the Gastrooesophageal reflux disease impact scale [106] and the Reflux Disease Questionnaire (RDQ) [107] that have been developed as instruments to help guide patient care.

In summary, these data demonstrate that the impact GERD has on QoL is substantial and equivalent to many other diseases considered to be severe and important.

Diagnostic tests for gastroesophageal reflux disease

The diagnosis of GERD depends on the definition of "pathological" in diagnostic tests. Problems in defining GERD have been recognized for more than two decades [62]. Methods of diagnosing GERD are outlined in Table 2.2. These tests evaluate different features of GERD, and none of them measures all aspects of the disease. Tests such as barium studies, scintigraphy and ambulatory oesophageal pH studies demonstrate whether reflux is occurring; endoscopy demonstrates mucosal injury and complications of GERD; ambulatory oesophageal pH studies quantify the amount of oesophageal acid exposure, the number and duration of reflux events and allow the correlation of reflux events with recorded symptoms; oesophageal sensitivity to acid is assessed by the Bernstein test. The correct interpretation of these diagnostic tests for GERD is critically important. For example, a patient with documented endoscopic esophagitis with a negative Bernstein test should not be regarded as having a "false negative" Bernstein test, but rather an acid insensitive esophagus as measured by this test. With variable patient populations, and with differences in definitions, techniques and gold standards, it is impossible to compare sensitivity and specificity values between the various diagnostic tests for GERD [108].

Manometry and lower esophageal pressure measurement

LES pressures alone are not of diagnostic value, as there is considerable variation in the normal LES pressure as well as overlap of pressures in those with and without esophagitis. Furthermore, the most common finding of an LES pressure in patients with GERD is a normal one. In a review of six studies [109], LES pressure < 10 mmHg did correlate with abnormal oesophageal acid exposure but with a sensitivity of only 58% and specificity of 84%. However, there may still be some utility in low LES pressures as a predictor

Table 2.2 Summary of diagnostic tests in gastroesophageal reflux disease.

Test	What does it measure?	Comments
Esophageal manometry	• Measures lower esophageal sphincter pressure • Low (<10 mmHg) LES pressure: 58% sensitivity and 84% specificity for abnormal oesophageal acid exposure [109] • Does not measure risk for reflux or assess for the presence of esophagitis	• Overlap with normal prevents one from using LES pressure as a diagnostic criteria for GERD • Does not detect transient LES relaxation • May be useful in pre/post operative evaluation
Radiology	• Demonstrates some of the morphological findings of GERD, for example strictures and ulcers • Detects gastroesophageal reflux but cannot differentiate pathological reflux of GERD from physiological reflux of normals • Detects hiatus hernia • Poor detection for mild esophagitis 0–53% [111] • Does not assess symptom correlation with reflux event	• In patients with GERD detects reflux in 10–50% [111] • Unclear role in most patients with GERD • Presence of a hiatus hernia does not correlate with GERD [111]
Scintigraphy	• Detects gastroesophageal reflux but cannot differentiate pathological reflux of GERD from physiological reflux of normals	• Sensitivity 14–86% [111] • Requires radioactivity exposure
Endoscopy	• Detects esophagitis, strictures and Barrett's esophagus • Allows biopsy, but esophageal histology has limited utility	• Lacks sensitivity
Bernstein (acid perfusion test)	• Measures esophageal acid sensitivity • Can be positive in patients with normal endoscopy and normal oesophageal pH studies (hypersensitive esophagus) • Determines oesophageal origin of pain	• Sensitivity 42–100%, mean 77% [111] • Specificity 50–100%, mean 86% [111] • May be useful in patients with atypical symptoms and NCCP
Esophageal pH monitoring	• Catheter based • Quantifies gastroesophageal reflux • Allows assessment of whether "pathological reflux" occurs • Allows for determination of a symptom index (correlation between symptoms and reflux events) • Does not detect mucosal damage • Wireless pH testing • Longer duration of measurement possible	• Normal in 14–29% of those with esophagitis • Normal in 6–15% of patients with abnormal SI • Better patient tolerance
SI with oesophageal pH monitoring	• Correlates symptoms with reflux events	• Bimodal predictive value • Can be positive when pH study is normal
PPI test	• Positive test suggests acid reflux as probable cause of symptoms	• Simplicity, reduced cost

GERD: gastroesophageal reflux disease; LES: lower esophageal sphincter; SI: symptom index; NCCP: non-cardiac chest pain; PPI: proton pump inhibitor.

for identifying patients with the most severe reflux or in identifying those at higher risk of complications associated with regurgitation [62]. Manometry prior to surgery has been advocated to document a mechanically defective lower esophageal sphincter [110], but there is no good evidence that this affects outcome. Some experts still advocate for preoperative manometry in GERD patients as it also measures distal esophageal amplitudes, a measure that may affect surgical decision making (type of wrap, whether to perform the surgery, etc.).

Radiological diagnosis

A variety of outcome measures have been used in studies of the use of radiology procedures in GERD. Some of these tests have assessed gastroesophageal reflux (with and without reflux provoking maneuvers) and correlated this with other measures of reflux such as esophageal pH studies. Other studies and tests examined the ability of radiological studies to identify esophagitis.

The radiological diagnosis of esophagitis is generally considered to be unreliable, especially in mild reflux esophagitis. The diagnostic accuracy of barium radiography compared with endoscopy has been demonstrated to be 0–53% for mild, 79–93% for moderate and 95–100% for severe esophagitis [28, 111]. Many of the early studies [112] compared radiological techniques to endoscopy as a gold standard. By 1980, it was recognized that about half the patients with symptomatic reflux did not have endoscopic esophagitis [54, 62]. Thus, many, if not most, patients with GERD would be expected to have normal barium studies. Additionally, from a technical perspective, the gastroesophageal junction (the site most involved by oesophageal inflammation, and fibrosis) is not well visualized in up to a third of patients, due to inadequate distension [112, 113].

Documenting that reflux occurs during a radiological examination does not determine whether patients have GERD, nor does it correlate with patients' symptoms. With provocative tests, reflux is seen in 25–71% of symptomatic patients but also is noted in 20% of controls [114]. Low density contrast medium does not improve the diagnostic accuracy over that observed with the use of regular barium contrast [115]. When taken as a whole, radiological studies are frequently falsely negative in patients in whom endoscopy or esophageal pH-metry studies are abnormal and are not recommended as a diagnostic test for GERD.

Measurement of the internal diameter of the cardiac esophagus was shown to predict 89% of patients with mild endoscopic esophagitis [116]. However, this was not confirmed in a study that found that the gastroesophageal junction could not be adequately visualized in 29% of patients [112].

Free, severe reflux as seen on barium studies may be a highly specific predictor of reflux as defined by esophageal pH monitoring [109, 112, 117, 118]. However, esophagitis is often not diagnosed radiographically in patients with abnormal intraesophageal pH studies [119].

Scintigraphy

Reflux can also be measured following the ingestion of a liquid containing a radiolabeled pharmaceutical such as sulfur colloid or ^{99m}Tc in an acidified liquid suspension. This procedure is similar to the assessment of reflux during radiology, although scintigraphy may be superior in this regard [63]. Graded abdominal compression to induce and detect reflux is unreliable, with variable sensitivity of 14–90% [63, 111, 112, 114, 120]. The biggest problem with this method of testing for reflux appears to be the short duration of the imaging test, as reflux occurs intermittently and therefore can often go undetected in any study of short duration that depends on demonstrating abnormal frequency of reflux as part of the diagnostic criteria. With the availability of endoscopy and intraesophageal pH monitoring, this test also appears to have little value in the diagnosis of GERD.

Upper gastrointestinal endoscopy

Endoscopy provides the most accurate means of assessing mucosal detail of the esophagus, but remains insensitive in diagnosing reflux. Definite endoscopic reflux esophagitis is unequivocal evidence that the patient suffers from GERD. However, patients with an "acid sensitive" esophagus who experience symptoms in the absence of esophagitis (the majority of patients with reflux) cannot be diagnosed by endoscopy. Recent efforts attempting to increase the sensitivity of endoscopic detection of the mucosal changes of GERD using imaging enhancements such as narrow band imaging (NBI) have not been as promising as hoped. The intraesophageal pH study is abnormal in 50% or more of patients with reflux symptoms and normal endoscopy [54, 121]. Thus, using current endoscopic technology, a negative endoscopy does not exclude GERD. Histological diagnosis of reflux may be more sensitive than endoscopy alone in diagnosing reflux, but the sensitivity of this test is problematic due to inadequate size of the biopsy [122], patchy distribution of the histological findings [123] or minimal changes with variable interpretation [124].

Berstad and Hatlebakk [125] prospectively evaluated patients with GERD using their own unique endoscopic grading system. Those with "true" GERD all had endoscopic findings according to their classification, but the presence of whitish exudate in the lesions and the width of the lesions were the only two endoscopic features that correlated with the severity of esophageal acid exposure as measured by pH-metry [126]. Confirmatory data from other investigators using this endoscopic classification are lacking.

Previously, the most widely applied esophagitis grading system had been the Savary-Miller classification in the original and modified forms. A newer classification [127], which measures metaplasia, ulcer, stricture and erosions (known as the MUSE classification), records the degree of severity of each as absent, mild, moderate and severe. This is now adapted as the Los Angeles (LA) classification and is the one that is now most commonly used [118]. The key features are:
• Grade A: one (or more) mucosal break no longer than 5 mm that does not extend between the tops of two mucosal folds
• Grade B: one (or more) mucosal break more than 5 mm long that does not extend between the tops of two mucosal folds
• Grade C: one (or more) mucosal break that is continuous between the tops of two or more mucosal folds but which involves less than 75% of the circumference
• Grade D: one (or more) mucosal break which involves at least 75% of the esophageal circumference [128]

The LA classification has been tested in a study that evaluated the circumferential extent of esophagitis by the criterion of whether mucosal breaks extended between the tops of mucosal folds and gave acceptable agreement (kappa 0.4) among observers [128]. Severity of esophageal acid exposure was significantly ($P < 0.001$) related to the LA severity grade of esophagitis. The pretreatment esophagitis grades A–C were related to heartburn severity ($P < 0.01$), outcomes of omeprazole treatment ($P < 0.01$), and the risk for symptom relapse off therapy ($P < 0–05$).

Bernstein test as a measure of esophageal acid sensitivity

This test was first described in 1958 and used to attempt to distinguish chest pain of esophageal from that of cardiac origin [129]. In an early 1978 prospective, comparative study of upper gastrointestinal endoscopy, upper gastrointestinal barium series, esophageal manometry and the Bernstein test in patients with suspected reflux esophagitis, the Bernstein test had the greatest sensitivity (85%) for diagnosing esophagitis. However, there were many false positives, as half the patients without esophagitis also had a positive Bernstein test. The lack of specificity for esophagitis is not very surprising, since most of these patients are now considered to have an acid sensitive esophagus, consistent with NERD. Another study found the sensitivity of the Bernstein test to be 70% in patients with typical reflux symptoms. However, 97% of patients with a negative test had either endoscopic, histologic or scintigraphy evidence of GERD [130]. In a review of seven studies [131], the overall sensitivity of this test was 77% and specificity 86%. Although the Bernstein test does not establish that there is mucosal damage (esophagitis), and patient acceptance is limited, a positive test result (defined as reproduction of symptoms during acid perfusion and not during saline perfusion) implies that the esophagus is likely to be the origin of the symptoms.

Ambulatory esophageal pH monitoring

Catheter based esophageal pH recordings have been used for over 30 years. Previous versions of this chapter have critically reviewed and covered the standards and thresholds of esophageal acid exposure. Whether an abnormal intraesophageal pH study is the gold standard for diagnosing GERD remains controversial [54]. This test is useful in quantifying the amount and frequency of acid reflux that occurs. However, it can be difficult to separate physiological from low-level pathological reflux, and the threshold levels that separate "normal" from "abnormal" test results are not clear. A cutoff pH of 4 to define pathological reflux has been validated with catheter based systems [108, 132]. Furthermore, this pH threshold makes physiological sense, as proteolytic activity of pepsin is low at a pH above 4, and high below pH 3 [46]. Unfortunately, even this cutoff may mischaracterize up to 50% of reflux episodes [133]. The technique has many limitations, including lack of availability, invasiveness, cost, lack of patient acceptability, debatable reproducibility, and technical problems such as improper placement of the pH probe, probe failures and recording device failures [134].

The technique is now improved with a wireless pH monitoring method [135]. The main advantage is that a patient does not have to walk around with a conspicuous and uncomfortable transnasal catheter. Since patients do not restrict their usual daily activities, the results are considered to be a more reflective and accurate identification of the true intraesophageal acid profile. The Bravo system is an example that transmits esophageal pH data every six seconds. With this new technique, thresholds were re-established and an acceptable discriminating threshold was determined to be 5.3% of 24 hours. The capsule is placed endoscopically and clipped into place 6 cm above the squamocolumnar junction. While a foreign body sensation is felt by the patient, the discomfort is minimal. As the capsule is clipped into place, prolonged pH measurements are possible and this factor may increase the sensitivity for the diagnosis of GERD [136, 137]. However, capsule detachment can occur and esophageal perforation has been reported [135].

These tests may be useful for investigating patients with atypical reflux symptoms or non-cardiac chest pain in whom GERD is suspected to be the cause of symptoms.

Symptom index (SI)

A quantitative method for correlating symptoms and esophageal acid reflux events was developed in 1986 and called the "symptom index". This index is calculated as the number of times the symptom occurred when the pH is < 4, divided by the total number of symptoms, multiplied by 100. Initial validation studies in 100 patients found the SI to be distributed in a bimodal fashion. Of patients with SI above 75%, 97.5% had an abnormal esophageal pH study [138]. If the SI was less than 25%, the proportion of patients with a normal esophageal pH study was 81%, and 90% of this group had a normal endoscopy [139]. Endoscopy was normal in nearly 30% of patients with a high SI. Thus, if endoscopy is found to be normal in the course of evaluating patients suspected of having GERD, an esophageal pH study combined with a measurement of SI may be a useful diagnostic test. There was very poor correlation between results of the Bernstein test and the SI. The negative predictive value of a low SI is useful. A limitation of the SI is that it does not take into account the reflux episodes that were symptom free. The SI was not found to be useful for diagnosing non-cardiac chest pain [140]. The next method to be developed was the symptom sensitivity index (SSI) that failed to take into account the total number of symptom episodes [141].

The symptom association probability (SAP) is another method that has been developed, with the intent to reduce the shortcomings of the SI [142]. This method correlates pH data during both symptomatic and asymptomatic reflux episodes and requires further validation, although some experts have suggested that this index is superior to the SI [135].

All three methods: SI, SSI and SAP were prospectively compared using symptom response to high dose omeprazole. SSI and SAP had better sensitivities of 74% and 65% compared to 35% with SI, but none predicted the response to PPI particularly well [143]. In summary, these data demonstrate that an objective gold-standard diagnostic test for GERD is lacking. Endoscopy has insufficient sensitivity but high PPV. Esophageal ambulatory pH monitoring has the highest diagnostic test sensitivity for GERD.

Symptoms as a diagnostic test for GERD

An important study of patients with reflux-like symptoms was reported by Joelsson and Johnsson [144]. Erosive esophagitis (Savary-Miller grade I or worse) was identified in a third of patients with symptoms of GERD. Whether the patient had erosive disease or not, the frequency of heartburn and acid regurgitation correlated with median esophageal acid exposure time, measured by 24-hour pH monitoring. Although patients with an endoscopically normal esophagus had lower overall median acid exposure, there was a trend towards more acid exposure in those with more severe symptoms. Figure 2.1 shows the relationship between severity of symptoms and acid exposure time. The authors concluded that reflux-like dyspepsia is accompanied by increased esophageal acid exposure, a finding that is supported by others [55, 145]. Unfortunately, severity of symptoms is still a poor predictor of mucosal damage [54, 146, 147].

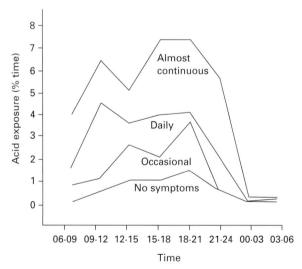

Figure 2.1 Acid exposure of the distal part of the esophagus during eight three-hour periods expressed as median% time spent with pH < 4 in 190 patients with different degrees of heartburn and acid regurgitation and 50 asymptomatic endoscopically normal subjects. Reproduced with permission from Joelsson B *et al. Gut* 1989; **30**: 1523–1525 [144].

Johannessen *et al.* [148] determined that the symptom of heartburn showed the best discrimination for patients with esophagitis. Typical symptoms of GERD, such as heartburn, correlate with abnormal intraesophageal pH exposure in 56–73% of patients [29, 54].

In an effort to improve the diagnostic value of the symptoms of GERD based on the patient's history, investigators have applied structured questionnaires [149–154]. Using the questionnaire developed by Johnsson [149], a positive response to all four questions was required to achieve a high positive predictive value, thus limiting its usefulness. The description of symptoms as opposed to using the term heartburn, may be a factor that improves the predictive value of this questionnaire.

DeMeester reported a retrospective review of 100 consecutive patients with symptoms of GERD [54]. The combination of the presence of grade II or III symptoms on the standardized questionnaire and endoscopic esophagitis, predicted increased acid exposure on 24-hour intraesophageal pH monitoring, with a specificity of 97% and a positive predictive value of 98%.

The Carlsson-Dent questionnaire that is intended to identify responders to PPI therapy has been extensively validated for reflux esophagitis detected at endoscopy and abnormal 24-hour intraesophageal pH-metry [150]. The questionnaire has a maximum score of 18. In the endoscopic comparison, using a threshold score of 4, the questionnaire had 70% sensitivity but only 46% specificity for diagnosis of esophagitis. When used in dyspeptic patients, the questionnaire had a sensitivity of 92% but a specificity of only 19% for diagnosis of GERD when compared with abnormal 24-hour intraesophageal pH monitoring. The mean score of 11 for GERD patients was higher than that observed in the dyspepsia cohort (mean 4.6). Symptom relief during treatment with omeprazole was predicted by the presence of heartburn, described as "a burning feeling rising from the stomach or lower chest up towards the neck" (odds ratio 4) and by "relief from antacids" (odds ratio 2.2). Even in a non-ulcer dyspepsia study from which patients with predominant heartburn were excluded, 42% of the patients indicated that they had a "rising burning feeling", a description that has been validated to define GERD-related heartburn in the Carlsson-Dent questionnaire. Even in this group of presumed non-GERD patients, those patients who answered positively to this key question had the best symptom relief with omeprazole. One prospective validation of this questionnaire in a primary care population did not find that the questionnaire was better than the physician's provisional diagnosis for discriminating omeprazole responders [155]. The utility of this questionnaire as a clinical practice tool appears to be limited, although it remains an important tool for research purposes because it allows for stratification of patients enrolled in GERD studies.

Similar in its goal to the Carlsson-Dent questionnaire, the 12-item "GERD Screener" demonstrated construct, convergent and predictive validity. This instrument was practical, short and easily administered and was intended to serve as a valuable case-finding instrument in primary care and managed care organizations [154].

Locke *et al.* [156] developed a GERD questionnaire in 1994 [152] and used it in a study in which patients underwent open access endoscopy. The study provided evidence that heartburn frequency was associated with esophagitis, that duration of acid regurgitation was associated with Barrett's esophagus and that strictures were associated with dysphagia severity and duration. Unfortunately, despite these somewhat encouraging findings, the questionnaire overall was only able to modestly predict endoscopic findings. This questionnaire has also been adapted to the Spanish population with excellent reproducibility and concurrent validity [157].

Subsequent validated GERD questionnaires focused more on creating instruments for assessing QoL rather than for diagnosis of GERD [89–95]. However, a new, reliable and valid questionnaire to better diagnose GERD was developed [153] and the internal consistency, interobserver reliability, criteria validity using 24-hour esophageal pH monitoring, construct validity and extreme group validation were assessed using patients with pathologic GERD. This questionnaire had sensitivity, specificity and positive predictive values of over 90%, while the negative predictive value was 79% [153]. A new Chinese GERD questionnaire was found to discriminate between controls and GERD patients with a sensitivity of 82% and a specificity of 84% [158].

In summary, these data indicate that at the present, symptom based questionnaires have been demonstrated to be useful research tools but they are of insufficient validity or are too complicated to use to be useful in clinical practice.

Therapeutic trial of acid suppression as a diagnostic test for GERD

All of the diagnostic tests described above are cumbersome or invasive and they detect different aspects of reflux. PPIs are the most effective intervention for all grades of esophagitis and for treatment of symptoms such as heartburn. The therapeutic response to a trial with a PPI was therefore thought possibly to be useful in diagnosing GERD in a variety of patient populations including patients with typical symptoms of GERD (heartburn), patients with GERD-related non-cardiac chest pain, and patients with positive and negative findings for GERD on endoscopy or pH monitoring. The variation of patient populations studied makes direct comparisons between studies impossible.

In a double-blind, placebo-controlled study of patients with reflux symptoms (92% had heartburn) and only minor or no esophagitis at endoscopy, patients were randomized to receive omeprazole 40 mg once daily or a placebo for 14 days [159]. A 75% reduction in heartburn was considered to be a positive diagnostic test. There was a significant (P = 0.04) correlation between response to the PPI and the results of the pH-metry. A response to PPI occurred in 68% of patients with abnormal reflux and in only 37% of patients with a normal pH study. Only 13% of patients responded to placebo.

A randomized trial of omeprazole 20 mg twice daily or placebo for one week tested the efficacy of omeprazole to diagnose reflux disease among dyspeptic patients [160]. A diagnosis of GERD was made on the basis of either grade II–III esophagitis or esophageal reflux with pH < 4 for more than 4% of the esophageal pH monitoring time. Using this definition, 135 of 160 (84%) patients were found to have GERD. Of those patients with presumed NERD, 63% had an abnormal pH study. Twenty percent (18/92) of patients with esophagitis had normal pH studies. Using symptom improvement of at least one grade for the definition of a positive test, the "omeprazole test" had a sensitivity of 71–81% for diagnosing GERD, compared with the sensitivity of placebo of 36–47%. With a more stringent definition for a positive test of total symptom relief, the sensitivity of omeprazole to diagnose reflux was lower at 48–59%, compared with 6–19% for placebo. However, the specificity of the test was also low, and actually was higher with placebo than with omeprazole. Thus, the test in this study was more useful for ruling out the diagnosis than for ruling it in. Even patients who did not have GERD by definition had better symptom relief with omeprazole than with placebo. These may be patients with an acid sensitive esophagus who respond well to acid suppression despite their esophageal pH being within normal limits.

A recent UK study of 90 patients with dyspeptic symptoms suggestive of GERD evaluated the cost-effectiveness of an open course of treatment with omeprazole 40 mg daily for 14 days as a diagnostic test [161]. The cost per correct diagnosis was £47 for omeprazole (95% CI: £40 to £59) compared with £480 for endoscopy (95% CI: £396 to £608). The authors concluded that an empirical trial of omeprazole was cost-effective both for symptom relief and for diagnosing GERD in patients with typical symptoms.

In a small, four-week, randomized placebo-controlled crossover study [162] in patients with normal endoscopy and esophageal pH-metry, but with an SI of > 50, 10 of 12 (83%) of patients with a positive SI showed improvement on omeprazole 20 mg twice daily for decreased symptom frequency, severity and consumption of antacids (P < 0.01). The SF-36, QoL parameters for bodily pain and vitality also significantly improved. In the group with a negative SI only one patient clearly improved.

Thirty-three consecutive patients with symptoms of reflux, abnormal pH studies, but normal endoscopies were sequentially allocated to receive ranitidine 150 mg twice daily, omeprazole 40 mg once daily, or omeprazole 40 mg twice daily for 7–10 days [163]. On the last day of treatment an esophageal pH study was repeated, and the results were correlated with symptoms. Using a 75% reduction in symptoms as a positive test, and the pH test as the gold standard, the sensitivity of the omeprazole test using a dose of 40 mg twice daily was 83.3%, while the sensitivity with omeprazole 40 mg once daily was only 27.2%. The authors concluded that the diagnosis of GERD could be ruled out if a patient failed to respond to a short course of high dose PPI.

Fass *et al.* [164] also used an omeprazole 60 mg daily test versus placebo in GERD positive (35/42, 83%) and GERD negative patients (17%). Twenty-eight GERD-positive and three GERD-negative patients responded to the omeprazole test, providing sensitivity of 80.0% and specificity of 57.1%. Economic analysis revealed that the omeprazole test saved US$348 per average patient evaluated, with 64% reduction in the number of upper endoscopies and a 53% reduction in the use of pH testing.

Most studies have used omeprazole in the "PPI test". However, a study using 60 mg of lansoprazole once daily versus placebo for five days found that 85% tested positive during active treatment compared with 9% with placebo [165]. The PPI test sensitivity was 85% and specificity was 73%.

Esomeprazole is more potent than omeprazole and it also has been evaluated as a diagnostic tool [166]. Patients (n = 440) were randomized to receive esomeprazole 40 mg once daily, esomeprazole 20 mg twice daily or a placebo for 14 days. Endoscopy and 24-hour esophageal pH-monitoring were carried out to determine the presence of gastroesophageal reflux disease (GERD). The esomeprazole treatment test had sensitivity in confirming the diagnosis of GERD of between 79% and 86% (for the two doses of PPI) after five days, while the corresponding value for placebo was 36%.

In a small, eight-week, placebo-controlled study of 36 patients with non-cardiac chest pain and abnormal esophageal 24-hour pH-metry, overall pain improvement was reported by 81% of omeprazole and 6% of placebo-treated patients [167]. Similar results were reported in another small study of 39 patients [168]. The omeprazole test correctly classified 78% of patients considered to be GERD patients by 24-hour esophageal monitoring and/or endoscopy and was positive in only 14% of patients considered not to have GERD by these criteria. Thus, a therapeutic trial may be useful in conditions other than typical GERD such as non-cardiac chest pain, an observation that is further supported by more recent studies [169, 170].

A meta-analysis of studies that used a trial of acid suppression for diagnosing GERD systematically and quantifiably evaluated all published studies prior to 2004 and concluded that "successful short-term treatment with a PPI in patients suspected of having GERD does not confidently establish the diagnosis, when GERD is defined by currently accepted reference standards" [171]. In summary, these data indicate that a therapeutic trial of a PPI for 1–2 weeks may be a reasonably useful clinical tool but it is by no means a gold-standard test for the diagnosis of GERD. The advantages of this approach include simplicity, non-invasiveness, ease of prescription and consumption, tolerability, and savings in terms of direct costs and time lost by the patient, but it does not demonstrate optimal sensitivity or specificity. A positive therapeutic trial may also predict longer term therapeutic response, but data confirming this notion are limited. These studies also support the notion that a symptom-based treatment is reasonable for most patients with reflux disease without a specific diagnosis. Perhaps the greatest value of this test lies in determining that GERD is not likely to be the cause of a given patient's symptoms (high negative predictive value) when no response to high-dose PPI is achieved.

Treatment of gastroesophageal reflux disease

Symptoms of gastroesophageal reflux are common and have a significant adverse impact on QOL. The costs of disease include both drug acquisition costs and indirect costs such as testing, physician visits and time off work. Because of the difficulty in making a definitive diagnosis of GERD through diagnostic investigations, the physician must make a presumptive diagnosis and initiate a management plan. The goals of therapy are to provide adequate symptom relief, heal esophagitis and prevent complications. Since initial studies in GERD have focused on mucosal healing; healing of erosive esophagitis will be discussed first, followed by discussions on NERD, and finally on symptomatic treatments in the uninvestigated patient.

Acid suppression therapy for gastroesophageal reflux disease

While transient relaxations of the LES and defective basal LES tone are thought to be the primary pathophysiological determinants of reflux, symptoms and damage arising from the esophagus are the result of acidic reflux as a consequence of these and other physiological perturbations [43]. Thus, the focus of treatment has been on acid suppression.

Acid secretion and/or gastric pH can be affected by various drugs. Antimuscarinic agents are weak inhibitors of the parietal cell M_3 cholinergic receptors, and their clinical use is limited by their anticholinergic side effects. H_2-receptor antagonists (H_2-RAs) inhibit parietal cell histamine receptors; thus acid inhibition can be largely overcome by stimulation of gastrin and cholinergic receptors, as occurs when food is eaten [172]. Tolerance or tachyphylaxis to H_2-RAs develops rapidly and reduces their efficacy with continued use over time [173]. PPIs provide the most potent acid inhibition through covalent binding to the H^+, K^+-ATPase (acid or proton pump) located in the secretory canaliculus of the parietal cell. Inhibiting the proton pump, which is the final common pathway of acid secretion, diminishes acid secretion to all known stimuli. Despite short serum half-lives, the PPIs have a longer duration of pharmacological action owing to the dependence of acid secretion recovery on the rate of synthesis of new proton pumps by the parietal cell.

Studies of intragastric acidity have been used to assess the degree and duration of acid inhibition with anti-secretary drugs [174, 175]. These studies have confirmed that PPIs are far superior to H_2-RAs in their ability to suppress food stimulated, daytime and total 24-hour acid secretion. Bell *et al.* [174] have shown, by meta-analysis, that the healing rate of erosive esophagitis correlated directly with the duration of gastric acid suppression over a 24-hour period. The primary determinants of healing were the duration of antisecretory treatment, the degree of acid suppression and the duration of acid suppression over the 24-hour period. There was also a highly significant correlation between the time that the pH in the esophagus was above 4 and the ability to heal erosive esophagitis. The authors concluded that if intragastric acidity could be maintained above a mean pH of 4 for 20–22 hours of the day, 90% of patients with erosive esophagitis would be healed by eight weeks. Thus, the superiority of PPIs over H_2-RAs was predicted prior to the performance of clinical trials based on their pharmacologic ability to achieve more effective suppression of acid secretion.

Lifestyle modifications

Although lifestyle modifications as a treatment for GERD are frequently recommended, there is little evidence that these are of benefit (Box 2.1). Changing dietary habits and lifestyle modifications are generally considered useful by physicians [176, 177]. However, when patients were asked about advice they had received from physicians, lifestyle changes were only modestly recommended [178]. If a patient is under the age of 50, and has no serious "alarm symptoms" such as unexplained weight loss, dysphagia or hematemesis, it is reasonable to start empirical therapy [9, 163] as the most cost-effective approach [179].

One study assessed patients with 24-hour esophageal pH testing and found no difference in lifestyle alteration and

BOX 2.1 Recommended lifestyle modifications in gastroesophageal reflux disease

- Avoid precipitating foods and drinks: fat [200, 201] (two studies found no effect of fat [202, 203], another found no effect of caloric density [204]), chocolate [205, 206], peppermint [207], spices [208], raw onions [209], carbonated beverages [198, 210], caffeine [4, 185, 211–213], coffee [185], orange juice and tomato drink [210, 214]
- Avoid alcohol [4, 210, 215–217]
- Avoid cigarette smoking [4, 186, 216–218]
- Avoid large meals and gastric distension [44, 219]
- Avoid lying down within 3–4 hours of a meal [220]
- Aggravating factors to be avoided: posture [220], physical exertion especially running [188, 189], weightlifting and cycling [189, 193]
- Raising the head of the bed may have some efficacy [220–223]
- Sleeping on the left lateral position reduces reflux [195–197]
- Avoid tight clothes [4]
- Obesity may be a risk factor [4, 22, 216–224], weight reduction helps symptoms [225], weight reduction does not help [226, 227], Roux-en-Y gastric bypass may benefit [224]
- Avoid certain drugs if possible: β-blockers, anticholinergics including certain antidepressants, theophylline, calcium antagonists, nitrates

anxiety between those with positive and negative pH profiles [180]. However, the data that white wine (vs red wine) induces reflux is reasonably robust [181, 182]. There are several mechanisms identified, including reduced LES pressure [182], disturbed esophageal clearance due to increased simultaneous contractions and failed peristalsis [183, 184]. The most recently identified mechanism is the occurrence of repeated reflux events into the esophagus when pH is still acidic from a previous reflux episode, the so-called "re-reflux" phenomenon [185]. Although caffeine itself is thought to be associated with reflux, one study has proposed that it is something in coffee other than caffeine that is responsible [186]. Smoking is also often implicated (Box 2.1) but results concerning its role are controversial. One 24-hour pH study has shown an association with smoking [186] while another has not [187]. Vigorous exercise has also been implicated as exacerbating reflux, with emphasis on running [188–193], but with evidence also for weightlifting and cycling [189, 193]. Thus, there is some rationale for "mother's advice" not to exercise right after eating. In one study ranitidine 300 mg, given one hour before running, reduced esophageal acid exposure [192]. While there is some evidence that elevating the head of the bed is beneficial, not all investigators agree as the effectiveness has been studied using esophageal acid exposure (which is improved but not normalized) and not symptoms as an outcome [194]. Lastly, the effect of posture is interesting, as more acid reflux seems to occur in the right lateral position. Thus the left lateral position is recommended for sleeping [195–197]. Meining and Classen reviewed the efficacy of lifestyle modifications as a treatment for GERD in detail and determined that for many of the recommendations, the data are conflicting, weak and, at best, equivocally supportive [198]. A recent systematic review investigating the effect of lifestyle modifications on GERD found that most were not evidence based and had little to recommend their routine use [199].

In summary, these data do not allow one to recommend lifestyle modifications as a therapy for GERD, although some of the modifications are known to positively affect health in other ways (smoking cessation, weight loss, etc.) and can be recommended on that basis alone.

Placebo response rates

Because healing of moderate to severe esophagitis with placebo therapy occurs in about 28% of patients [13, 228], the use of placebo controls has been important, especially for the less effective drugs, such as H_2-RAs and prokinetics. Additionally, the symptomatic placebo response rate ranges from 37–64%, further underscoring the need for placebo controls in less effective therapies for GERD [229]. For PPIs, the therapeutic gain is so large that placebo-controlled trials are less necessary, although they remain useful [13].

Antacids and alginate

A small randomized placebo-controlled trial of Maalox TC at a full dose of 15 ml seven times daily for four weeks in 32 GERD patients showed no significant symptom relief [230]. Other trials have reported marginal if any benefit of antacids and alginates over placebo, and antacids do not heal esophagitis [231–233]. **A1d** However, a recent meta-analysis concluded that compared with the placebo response the relative benefit increase was up to 60% with alginate/antacid combinations, and 11% with antacids [229].

In an uncontrolled study of patients with grade I to III esophagitis healed with either an H_2-RA or omeprazole, patients were given alginate for symptomatic maintenance treatment [234]. At six months, 76% were in remission. Those with more severe baseline esophagitis relapsed more frequently. In a randomized controlled trial, sodium alginate 10 ml four times daily was slightly more effective than cisapride 5 mg four times daily for reducing both symptoms measured on a visual analog scale (0–100) (alginate

29 ± 22, cisapride 35 ± 25, p = 0.01) and the number of reflux episodes in a four-week period (alginate 2 ± 2, cisapride 3±4, p = 0.001) [235]. Conservative symptomatic therapy with alginate may be useful in some patients. **A1d**

Collings et al. [236] recently demonstrated that a calcium carbonate gum decreased heartburn and intraesophageal acidity more than chewable antacids, with effects that lasted for a couple of hours. This observation suggests that such a gum may be useful for intermittent therapy, possibly because of an effect on salivation.

In summary, there are sufficient data supporting a recommendation for antacids as a short-term treatment for symptomatic heartburn; alginate/antacid combinations appear to be superior to antacid use alone.

Prokinetic drugs

In a randomized, placebo-controlled trial, metoclopramide and domperidone did not improve esophageal motility, duration of acid exposure or esophageal clearance, although both agents significantly increased LES pressure [237]. Cisapride is the only prokinetic drug that increases both esophageal clearance and enhances LES tone [238, 239]. However, one study provided evidence that cisapride increased acid reflux in comparison with omeprazole and famotidine [240].

Placebo-controlled trials show marginal benefit for cisapride in healing esophagitis and improving symptoms [239, 241–243]. **A1d** For mild grades of esophagitis, cisapride has been demonstrated to be as effective as H_2-RA for healing and symptom relief with comparable tolerability [243–248]. However, this drug requires prolonged use for up to 12 weeks before clinical benefit is seen [242, 243, 245, 247, 249–251].

In one randomized trial in patients with milder GERD, omeprazole 10 or 20 mg daily was significantly more effective than cisapride 10 mg four times daily for relief of heartburn, regurgitation and epigastric pain [104]. This and other studies suggest that for symptomatic GERD, the degree of acid suppression is a more important determinant of symptom relief than prokinetic activity. **A1d**

In healing grades I and II esophagitis, adding cisapride to omeprazole did not significantly increase efficacy over omeprazole alone [252]. In another study of healing grades II and III esophagitis, cisapride 20 mg twice daily added to pantoprazole 40 mg once daily did not improve healing over pantoprazole alone [253]. Thus, these two studies provide strong evidence that the addition of cisapride does not add any clinical benefit to treating with PPIs alone. **A1d**

Cisapride has demonstrated only modest benefit for maintenance therapy for mild esophagitis [251, 252, 254, 255]. However, in patients with more severe erosive esophagitis initially healed with antisecretory therapy, cisapride was not effective for maintenance treatment [243, 245, 256, 257] and was not more effective than placebo [258]. **A1d**

The recent Cochrane meta-analysis concluded that there was a paucity of evidence on prokinetic therapy, with no substantive evidence that it is superior to placebo [259]. Cisapride has also been associated with the development of serious cardiac arrhythmias including torsades de pointes, when used with other drugs that inhibit cytochrome P450 3A4. These include fluconazole, itraconazole, ketoconazole, erythromycin, clarithromycin, ritonavir, indinavir, nefazodone, tricyclic antidepressants and certain tetracyclic antidepressants, certain antipsychotics, astemizole, terfenadine, and class IA and III anti-arrhythmics [260]. Thus, cisapride is not recommended for the treatment of GERD because its potential for producing significant adverse events is greater than that for other more effective agents, and in many countries the drug has now been withdrawn.

In summary, there are insufficient data to recommend the use of cisapride in the treatment of GERD.

Sucralfate in gastroesophageal reflux disease

For grade I–III GERD, there have been four small, randomized trials of sucralfate 1 g four times daily compared with standard dose H_2-RA, none of which demonstrated any significant differences with respect to symptom resolution and healing [261–264]. However, none of these studies showed very large benefits from either intervention, with low rates of heartburn relief (34–62%) and healing (31–64%). Combining sucralfate and cimetidine was not better than monotherapy with either drug [265, 266]. The meta-analysis of randomized trials for grade II–IV esophagitis performed by Chiba *et al.* yielded a pooled value for healing of 39.2% for sucralfate compared with 28% for placebo [13]. However, the 95% CI was wide (3.6 to 74.8%). **A1c**

In a six-month study of grade I–II GERD, sucralfate was more effective than placebo for preventing relapse (sucralfate 31%, placebo 65%; ARR 34%, NNT 3, p < 0.001) [267]. **A1d**

It is interesting that sucralfate, which does not lower acid output, reduce esophageal acid exposure or improve esophageal transit time [268] has any efficacy given our understanding of the pathophysiology of this condition. The adverse effect of constipation, the need for four times daily dosing and the modest observed benefit make sucralfate a less than optimal GERD treatment choice for most patients.

In summary, there are insufficient data to support a recommendation for the use of sucralfate in the treatment of GERD.

H$_2$-receptor antagonists

H_2-RAs are not optimally effective in the treatment of GERD but still maintain a role in symptomatic therapy and are discussed here somewhat briefly.

Intermittent/on-demand therapy for heartburn relief

Acid suppressive therapy with H_2-RAs has been the mainstay of treatment for acid-related disorders and in many countries these agents are available for over-the-counter (OTC) use [269]. This availability permits intermittent, on demand use by the patient. A blinded crossover trial of famotidine 5, 10 and 20 mg versus placebo showed that all famotidine doses were more effective than placebo for the prevention of meal-induced heartburn and other dyspeptic symptoms [270]. This study established that heartburn severity peaked 1–2 hours after a meal. Thus, a small dose of H_2-RA taken before eating is useful to reduce GERD symptoms induced by meals.

A unique formulation of a readily dissolving famotidine wafer (20 mg) was compared with standard dose (150 mg) ranitidine [271]. With both treatments, about half the patients had some symptom relief within three hours. A similar randomized trial found trivial but statistically significant differences between ranitidine and famotidine for time to adequate symptom relief (ranitidine 15 minutes, famotidine 18.5 minutes, p = 0.005) and for the proportion of patients with symptom relief at one hour (ranitidine 92%, famotidine 84%; p = 0.02) [272].

A recent meta-analysis of OTC medications determined from ten trials, yielded a relative benefit increase of up to 41% with H_2-RAs compared to placebo [229]. Thus, for mild reflux symptoms, use of H_2-RA on an as needed basis remains a useful therapy for GERD.

High dose H$_2$-receptor antagonists

While standard doses of H_2-RAs heal more severe, grade II to IV esophagitis in about 52% of patients [13], higher doses of H_2-RA (150–300 mg four times daily) are more effective, healing 74–80% of patients in 12 weeks, under conditions in which the healing rate with placebo is 40–58% [273, 274]. Silver *et al.* [275] compared regimens of ranitidine 300 mg twice daily and 150 mg four times daily for treatment of erosive esophagitis. At 12 weeks, the healing proportion observed for the four times daily regimen was 77% and for the twice daily regimen, 66% (absolute risk reduction (ARR) 11%, number needed to treat (NNT) 9). Ranitidine 150 mg four times daily was superior to standard dose (150 mg twice daily) ranitidine or cimetidine (800 mg twice daily) in patients with erosive esophagitis [276]. In another randomized trial in patients with erosive esophagitis [277], with ranitidine 150 mg twice daily the proportion of patients healed was 54% at eight weeks compared with 75% with 300 mg four times daily (ARR 21%, NNT 5). **A1d** Famotidine is pharmacologically more potent than ranitidine and a large dose of 40 mg twice daily was superior to standard dose 20 mg twice daily or ranitidine 150 mg twice daily in patients with erosive or worse esophagitis [278]. **A1d** These data suggest that standard dose H_2-RAs can be effective in GERD symptom relief, but higher doses are necessary for healing and maintenance of healing of esophagitis.

More complete data on oesophagitis healing with H_2-RAs is found in the recently updated Cochrane Review [259], where there was a statistically significant benefit of H_2-RAs compared to placebo.

In summary, these data indicate that H_2-RAs have a limited but measurable effect in treating GERD, and symptoms respond better than healing to treatment.

Erosive gastroesophageal reflux disease

Meta-analysis of healing and symptom relief with proton-pump inhibitors and H_2-receptor antagonists

An early meta-analysis of randomized trials of patients with more severe esophagitis (grade II in 61.8%, grade III in 31.7% and grade IV in 6.5%) established the clinical efficacy of PPIs [13]. Subsequent published studies support the conclusions derived from this meta-analysis [259, 279–295]. **A1d**

In the meta-analysis [13], the rate of healing, expressed as "percent healed per week", was significantly superior with PPI therapy compared with H_2-RA, particularly early in the course of treatment (weekly healing rate in first two weeks: PPI 32%, H_2-RA 15%). The rate of healing slowed with increasing duration of treatment as fewer patients remained unhealed, but PPI remained superior to H_2-RA. The overall healing proportions during 12 weeks, using pooled results irrespective of dose and duration were: PPI 84% (95% CI: 79 to 88), H_2-RA 52% (95% CI: 47 to 57), sucralfate 39% (95% CI: 4 to 75) and placebo 28% (95% CI: 19 to 37). These data were used to plot rate of healing against time on a "healing time curve" (Figure 2.2). By the end of the second week, PPI had healed 63.4 ± 6.6% of patients, while H_2-RA required 12 weeks to achieve healing in a similar proportion of patients (60.2 ± 5.9%). Linear regression analysis of individual study results showed that PPI heal at an overall rate of 11.7% per week (95% CI: 10.7 to 12.6), twice as rapidly as H_2-RA (5.9% per week, 95% CI: 5.5 to 6.3) and four times more rapidly than placebo (2.9, 95% CI: 2.4 to 3.4).

Heartburn was present in all but 3.8% (95% CI: 2.1 to 5.5) of patients at baseline. Overall, heartburn relief was seen in 77.4 ± 10.4% of patients treated with PPI and in 47.6 ± 15.5% treated with H_2-RA. Data for heartburn relief were plotted against time to create a "symptom relief time curve" (Figure 2.3). Linear regression analysis of the data yielded an overall heartburn relief rate of 11.5% per week

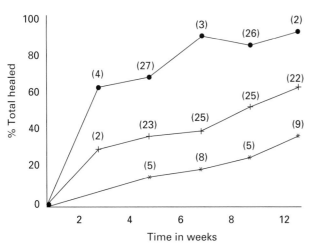

Figure 2.2 Healing-time curve expressed as the mean total healing for each drug class per evaluation time in weeks. By week 4, PPIs (proton pump inhibitors) heal more patients than any other drug class, even after a much longer duration of treatment (12 weeks), implying a substantial therapeutic gain despite the fact that all drug classes achieve higher healing with longer durations of therapy. The number of studies is shown in parentheses. •: PPI; +: H_2-RA, *: placebo. Reproduced with permission from Chiba N *et al. Gastroenterology* 1997; **112**: 1798–1810 [13].

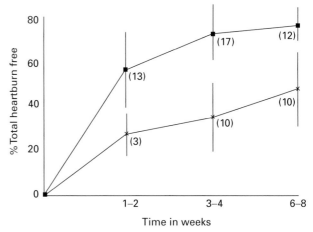

Figure 2.3 Symptom relief-time curve expressed as the mean total heartburn relief for each drug class corrected for patients free of heartburn at baseline at 1–2, 3–4, and 6–8 weeks. By week 2, more patients treated with PPIs (proton pump inhibitors) are asymptomatic compared with H_2-RA (H2-receptor antagonists) even after a much longer duration of treatment (eight weeks), implying a substantial therapeutic gain despite the fact that both drug classes achieve greater symptom relief with longer durations of treatment. The number of studies is shown in parentheses. ■: PPI; x: H_2-RA. Reproduced with permission from Chiba N *et al. Gastroenterology* 1997; **112**: 1798–1810 [13].

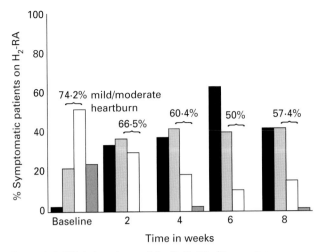

Figure 2.4 Shift in heartburn relief with H₂-RAs (H₂ receptor antagonists). From studies using a symptom scale of none, mild, moderate, or severe, the shift in symptom severity with duration of treatment can be observed. With H₂-RAs, although there is an increase in the number of patients completely heartburn free, at the end of the study, more than half of the patients still have mild to moderate symptoms: none (■); mild (□); moderate (□); severe (▨). Reproduced with permission from Chiba N *et al. Gastroenterology* 1997; **112**: 1798–1810 [13].

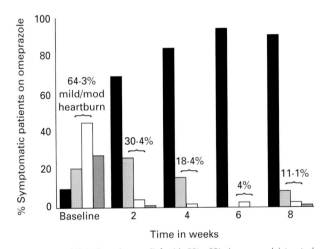

Figure 2.5 Shift in heartburn relief with PPIs. PPIs (omeprazole)-treated patients have a dramatic shift in the number of patients completely symptom free, particularly early in-treatment, and at the end of the study, very few patients have any residual heartburn in contrast to patients treated with H₂-RAs: none (■); mild (□); moderate (□); severe (▨). Reproduced with permission from Chiba N *et al. Gastroenterology* 1997; **112**: 1798–1810 [13].

for PPI (95% CI: 9.9 to 13.0) and 6.4% per week for H₂-RA (95% CI: 5.4 to 7.4).

Some studies measured heartburn in categories of none, mild, moderate or severe and reported the shift in heartburn relief with treatment (Figures 2.4 and 2.5). The proportion of patients with residual mild to moderate symptoms after eight weeks of therapy was 11.1% for PPI and 57.4% for H₂-RAs.

This meta-analysis provided evidence that PPI are significantly better than H₂-RA for both healing esophagitis and relieving symptoms in patients with moderately severe esophagitis. There was also evidence in one RCT that PPI therapy is effective for healing persistent grade II–IV esophagitis after treatment failure with 12 weeks standard dose H₂-RA [296]. **A1d**

Other more recent Cochrane meta-analyses have demonstrated similar findings, with PPIs being superior to H₂-RAs in healing and maintenance of healing of esophagitis [259, 297]. These data support a recommendation for the use of PPIs rather than H₂-RAs for the healing and maintenance of healing of esophagitis, as well as for heartburn relief.

Differences in efficacy between proton pump inhibitors

There are now five proton-pump inhibitors available in North America. These are omeprazole, lansoprazole, pantoprazole, rabeprazole and esomeprazole.

For symptom relief, esomeprazole has been shown to be more rapidly effective than omeprazole [32, 290], lansoprazole [284, 298] and pantoprazole [299]. In other studies, lansoprazole was more rapidly effective than omeprazole [33] and pantoprazole non-inferior to esomeprazole [300]. However, differences in symptom relief were no longer apparent at the end of these studies [279, 287, 301, 302]. In another study, omeprazole and pantoprazole were found to be equivalent with each other but not with lansoprazole regarding rapidity of symptom relief [303]. Similar results were found in a comparison of rabeprazole and omeprazole [294]. Low, half-doses of PPIs compared with standard doses were not found to be as effective for healing esophagitis or for symptom relief [146, 279]. However, for maintenance therapy some data suggest that low dose PPIs are as effective as standard doses [37, 304, 305]. While there were small differences between overall study results, the data from these studies were insufficient to establish the superiority of any one drug over all others [306].

Vakil and Fennerty recently carried out a careful systematic review of randomized controlled trials that directly compared PPIs to determine whether there is a difference in clinical outcomes between any of these agents [306]. They restricted this review to more recent (1998–2002), better quality trials. They found similar healing rates for the following comparisons:

• lansoprazole 30 mg daily compared with omeprazole 20 mg [301] or 40 mg [280], or pantoprazole 40 mg daily [291]

• pantoprazole 40 mg [307] or rabeprazole 20 mg [281, 289] compared with omeprazole 20 mg daily **A1c**

They found that for esophagitis healing, esomeprazole was superior to omeprazole and lansoprazole [32, 284, 290]. Earlier randomized trials comparing two different

PPIs (lansoprazole, omeprazole, pantoprazole and rabeprazole) had also failed to show a difference in healing rates with drugs used at standard recommended doses [27, 31, 279, 280, 287, 301, 307, 308]. **A1d**

Two other meta-analyses also have shown that esomeprazole was superior to omeprazole and that other PPIs did not produce higher healing rates than omeprazole [309–311]. **A1c** Another review concluded that lansoprazole, pantoprazole and rabeprazole were comparable with omeprazole in terms of heartburn control, healing rates and relapse rates [312]. Systematic reviews of data from randomized trials performed up to 2005 that compared esomeprazole to other PPIs showed that esomeprazole was more effective than omeprazole, lansoprazole and pantoprazole for healing esophagitis at four and eight weeks, but there is still no direct comparative trial of esomeprazole against rabeprazole [311, 313]. Esomeprazole 40 mg daily was more effective for healing the more severe LA grades C and D esophagitis in randomized trials in which it was compared with omeprazole 20 mg daily [32, 290, 313], lansoprazole 30 mg [284, 298, 313] or pantoprazole [299, 313, 314]. **A1d** One randomized trial that included only 284 patients but was otherwise similar in design to the trial that included 5241 patients showed no difference between esomeprazole 40 mg and lansoprazole 30 mg for healing of erosive (or more severe) esophagitis in four or eight weeks; the smaller trial may have lacked statistical power [285]. **A1c** Subsequently, another study showed esomeprazole superior to pantoprazole [314].

Esomeprazole is the first PPI shown to be more effective than any other PPI; all other direct comparisons have shown that healing rates are essentially the same for all agents in this class [285]. However, in elderly patients over age 65 there may be some differences [315]. In a relatively small randomized trial, Pilotto and colleagues compared standard dose omeprazole, pantoprazole, rabeprazole and lansoprazole for healing of esophagitis using the outdated Savary-Miller classification [315]. They determined that at eight weeks, pantoprazole and rabeprazole were significantly more effective than omeprazole for healing esophagitis and were also more effective than omeprazole or lansoprazole for relieving symptoms. The authors were unable to provide an adequate explanation for apparent differences in response in the elderly population [315].

Esomeprazole, the (S)-isomer of omeprazole, produces potent acid suppression as a result of increased systemic exposure and less inter-individual variability in response to it. Hatlebakk [316] reviewed available data and concluded that esomeprazole 40 mg daily was significantly more effective at controlling gastric acidity than lansoprazole 30 mg daily, pantoprazole 40 mg daily and rabeprazole 20 mg daily in a mixed population of healthy volunteers and patients with GERD. Comparable results were also reported in patients with GERD symptoms [317]. Similar

results for greater potency of esomeprazole compared to pantoprazole have been reported [318–321]. Esomeprazole 20 mg daily was also significantly more effective than lansoprazole 15 mg daily. Another study reviewing half healing doses concluded that esomeprazole was significantly more effective than rabeprazole, lansoprazole or pantoprazole for control of intragastric acid [322]. Thus, the reports of greater clinical efficacy are consistent with the greater pharmacological potency of this drug.

A study of the Food and Drug Administration database reported very few drug interactions for omeprazole, lansoprazole and pantoprazole [323]. Of the rare interactions, vitamin K antagonist reactions were most common, but even these were seen in only 0.09–0.11 per million packages prescribed. This report concluded that the safety of the drugs was likely to be a class effect, with no significant differences among the PPIs.

In summary, these data indicate that there are statistically significant differences in potency and healing rates observed with the various proton pump inhibitors, with esomeprazole demonstrating the highest healing rates. However, these data do not indicate that the differences in healing or symptom response rates are sufficiently large to conclude that one agent should be used in preference to another.

Is there a rationale for higher dose proton pump inhibitor therapy?

The standard doses of PPI are very effective for healing most cases of esophagitis, and it is clear that there is a correlation between the degree of acid suppression and healing [174]. In clinical practice, patients with persistent or recurrent symptoms are often told to double their dose of PPI, typically to take the doses on a twice daily regimen. This clinical recommendation was based on the 9–12 hour physiological effect these compounds have on gastric acid secretion; the pharmacological data demonstrated that a standard dose taken bid was more effective at prolonging acid control than a double dose taken once daily [324]. Patients with complicated or atypical GERD were randomly assigned to receive lansoprazole or pantoprazole once daily [325]. Esophageal acid exposure was normalized in all lansoprazole patients (in 35% of cases with double dose), whereas 25% of the pantoprazole treated patients did not have lowered or normalized esophageal acid exposure, even with the dose doubled (p = 0.008). A study in patients with stage II or III esophagitis randomized to pantoprazole 40 mg or 80 mg daily healing was observed in 78% and 72% of subjects at four weeks [282]. These data suggest that increasing the dose of pantoprazole beyond the standard dose is not likely to be of any benefit.

Klinkenberg-Knol *et al.* have followed a cohort of GERD patients for many years and reported that doubling the dose of omeprazole to 40 mg daily was effective to treat relapses [326]. A longer term report followed 230 patients for up to 11 years on continuous therapy [327]. Of those followed, a third each had grade II, III and IV disease. It was estimated that there was only one relapse for every nine years of treatment and the median maintenance dose was 20 mg daily. Dose titration (range 20 mg every second day to 120 mg once daily) allowed most patients to remain in remission. Another study showed that titrating the dose of omeprazole to 40–60 mg daily was as effective for maintenance of remission as anti-reflux surgery [328]. **B4**

In a randomized trial in which patients with erosive esophagitis were randomized to receive rabeprazole 20 mg daily or omeprazole 40 mg daily in for 4–8 weeks, there were no significant differences in the rates of symptom relief or healing [294]. **A1d**

Further lack of support for using higher than normal doses of PPIs to treat GERD come from two recent meta-analyses of placebo controlled trials of standard and high doses of PPIs to treat laryngeal symptoms of GERD, providing no evidence for efficacy of these therapies for symptomatic improvement or resolution of laryngo-pharyngeal symptoms [329, 330]. There is also concern about having patients on multiple daily doses of PPIs, a practice that increases cost. Inadomi *et al.* [331] identified and recruited such patients through the use of pharmacy records of PPI prescriptions. Eligible subjects were stepped-down to single dose PPI (lansoprazole 30 mg or omeprazole 20 mg daily), and 80% did not report recurrent symptoms of heartburn or acid regurgitation. These authors concluded that "this intervention can decrease management costs without adversely affecting quality of life" [331]. **B4** Additionally, Lee *et al.* performed a systematic review that also confirmed the over utilisation of both increased and standard dose PPIs in clinical practice [332]. In summary, there are insufficient data to support a recommendation for routinely using PPI doses higher than standard doses for healing esophagitis, treating symptomatic GERD or atypical symptoms of GERD, although higher doses may be effective in preventing relapse that occurs at standard doses of PPIs. Higher doses are appropriate in only a minority of patients.

Maintenance therapy for patients with documented healed esophagitis

For mild forms of esophagitis, as seen at a community level, 46% of patients will heal spontaneously [334]. For moderately severe GERD, healing and symptom relief are more readily obtained with PPI therapy. However, within 6–12 months, irrespective of the initial healing agent, relapses are reported in 36–82% of patients in the absence of maintenance therapy [335–338]. When maintenance therapy is either not commenced after an initial course of

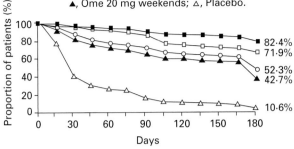

Figure 2.6 Actuarial life-table analysis. Estimated proportion of patients in endoscopic remission at the end of the 6-month follow up period with maintenance treatment. Reproduced with permission from Carlsson *et al. Aliment Pharmacol Ther* 1997; **11**: 473–482 [333].

therapy, or is stopped, symptoms often recur within a day, and erosive esophagitis can recur in many patients within 10 days [339] to one month [340]. Thus, maintenance therapy is required in most patients with esophagitis in order to maintain healing and symptom relief. However, a recent systematic review provided evidence that despite continuous therapy with PPI, 28% of patients suffer a relapse of esophagitis within six months [338].

A meta-analysis of the rate of relapse of erosive esophagitis reported in five omeprazole trials that included 1154 patients in whom erosive GERD was initially healed by omeprazole 20–40 mg was carried out by Carlsson *et al.* [341]. Figure 2.6 shows the effects of various regimens. Omeprazole 20 mg daily, which maintained 82.4% of patients in remission for six months, was significantly better than omeprazole 10 mg daily (p = 0.04). Both of these regimens were significantly better than ranitidine 150 mg twice daily and omeprazole 20 mg on weekends. PPI therapy taken on a regimen of three times in a week is less effective than daily dosing [342, 343]. Two trials have assessed maintenance over 12 months. Omeprazole 20 mg daily was superior to ranitidine 150 mg twice daily (omeprazole 80.2%, ranitidine 39.4%; ARR 40.8%, NNT 2). **A1a** The proportions of patients with asymptomatic endoscopic esophagitis relapse were: omeprazole 20 mg 4.5%, omeprazole 10 mg 12.5%, and ranitidine 14.6%. Regression analysis identified four risk factors for recurrence: pretreatment severity of esophagitis, younger age, non-smoking status and moderate to severe reflux pre-entry. A previous systematic review of continuous maintenance therapy [344] in patients with initial grades II–IV esophagitis was updated in the first and second editions of this book and readers are referred there for details [345, 346]. There are methodological issues in pooling these results. Not all studies provided precise numbers of patients in remission/relapse, and data were analysed on either an intention to treat basis or using data from all the evaluable patients in life-table analysis.

Most trials were of only six months' duration. The esomeprazole studies used the LA classification to grade esophagitis. LA grade A is not directly comparable to either the Hetzel-Dent or Savary-Miller grade I classifications. However, given these shortcomings, 12-month placebo relapse rates ranged from 71 to 91% [346], H$_2$-blockers were not significantly more effective with relapse rates between 51 and 88% [346]. The data supported the concept that the greater degree of acid suppression resulted in better remission rates. PPIs resulted in the highest remission rate, particularly when the dose given was the full healing dose for omeprazole, lansoprazole, pantoprazole, rabeprazole and esomeprazole [346]. These data were also confirmed in a more recent Cochrane Review [297]. PPIs were rarely compared directly, but in one study, lansoprazole and omeprazole were comparable [347].

In trials comparing half doses, esomeprazole 20 mg was more effective than lansoprazole 15 mg once daily [348, 349]. With more severe LA grades of esophagitis, esomeprazole treatment provided a significantly longer time to relapse than was observed in the lansoprazole treated patients [348]. At six months, pantoprazole 20 mg and esomeprazole 20 mg were comparable [350]. Using half doses of these PPIs was less effective for maintenance therapy than full healing doses [346]. In the Cochrane Review of placebo-controlled trials, the observed relative risk of relapse was 0.46 for half doses of PPIs, compared to only 0.26 for full dose PPI therapy [297].

One trial [37] suggested that esomeprazole 20 mg was as effective as 40 mg daily. Another suggested that rabeprazole 10 mg was as effective as 20 mg daily [351], although this observation was not confirmed in two other similar trials [352, 353].

Studies looking specifically at patients aged 65 years and over have not found different esophagitis healing rates [354, 355]. There are no data indicating that the elderly respond any differently from younger patients with esophagitis.

There are limited data from maintenance studies of greater duration than one year. An observational maintenance study with pantoprazole 40 mg once daily in 157 patients with healed stage II or III reflux esophagitis (Savary-Miller classification) showed endoscopic remission in 87% and 76% of patients after one and two years [356]. **B4** Another five-year follow-up study in patients with both peptic ulcer and reflux esophagitis found estimated rates of remission on maintenance treatment with pantoprazole (n = 115) of 82% at one year, 75% at two years, 72% at three years, 70% at four years and 68% at five years [357]. There have been two randomized trials of five years' duration. In the first, patients with initially healed erosive or worse esophagitis were randomized to receive rabeprazole 20 mg once daily, rabeprazole 10 mg once daily or omeprazole 20 mg once daily [351]. Of the initial 243

patients, 123 completed the five-year study. Relapse rates were 11.5%, 9.8% and 13.3%, respectively. In the second study, patients were randomized to rabeprazole 20 mg, 10 mg or placebo with five-year relapse rates of 11%, 23% and 63% respectively [358]. All treatments were safe and well tolerated. These data provide evidence that remission can be effectively maintained over long time periods.

The problem of healing the more severe grades of esophagitis is well known. The proportion of patients who experience acute healing for grade II esophagitis ranges from 76–100%, for grade III from 63–95% and for grade IV from 56–75% [344]. Grade IV disease relapses more frequently than grade II and III disease [340, 359].

In summary, in clinical practice, it is suggested that the dose of PPI can be titrated upwards to maintain healing in most patients [326] or alternatively, the most potent PPI be used. **A1d C5** In some patients, lower doses of PPIs may be effective for maintenance therapy in patients with healed esophagitis. **B4**

On-demand therapy as a strategy for maintenance of healing of mild/moderate esophagitis

Lansoprazole (15 mg daily and 30 mg on alternate days) was studied for maintenance of endoscopic healing and symptom relief over a six-month period after healing of Savary-Miller grades I–III reflux esophagitis [360]. After six months, recurrence of esophagitis was observed in 12% of the 15 mg once daily group and in 19% of the 30 mg alternate day group. This difference was not statistically significant. However, 12.1% of patients who received 15 mg daily and 28.6% of those who received alternate day higher dose therapy (p = 0.007) had heartburn. **A1d**

In another study, patients with esophagitis were initially treated until symptoms had resolved. Thereafter, they took "on-demand" lansoprazole (30 mg) or omeprazole (20 mg) for six months, only when reflux symptoms relapsed [361]. There were no differences observed in the frequency of reflux symptoms or in the number of doses taken by subjects in the lansoprazole (0.73 doses/day) and omeprazole (0.71 doses/day) groups. **A1d**

In a study population of mild LA grades A and B esophagitis, esomeprazole 40 mg was more effective than omeprazole 20 mg once daily, on-demand for symptom relief and fewer tablets were consumed [362]. Another study examined patients with more severe LA grades A–D initially healed with esomeprazole 40 mg daily [363]. On continuous esomeprazole 20 mg once daily, 81% remained in remission at six months compared to 58% with on-demand treatment (ARR 23%, NNT = 4, p < 0.0001). Heartburn was significantly more common in the on-demand group, and continuous therapy more effectively maintained healing of erosive esophagitis [363].

There are relatively few studies that have examined this strategy in patients with more severe initial erosive esophagitis compared to patients with mild esophagitis, uninvestigated heartburn or NERD. An important factor reducing efficacy of an on-demand strategy is obesity [364]. In a recent systematic review on the use of on-demand therapy, Pace and colleagues demonstrated that "on-demand therapy", while effective for the treatment of GERD symptoms, was less effective than continuous PPI maintenance therapy for maintenance of healing of esophagitis [365].

In summary, these data do not support a recommendation for "on-demand" therapy for patients with documented erosive esophagitis, since relapse is more common with this strategy, patients must experience recurrent symptoms before treatment is taken, and these patients are left with unhealed lesions. **C5**

Cost-effectiveness of maintenance therapy

PPIs are the most effective treatments available to treat GERD. PPIs are in general more costly than H_2-RAs, although the availability of multiple generic forms and OTC formulations of PPIs has markedly narrowed this disparity in cost. Therefore, cost-effectiveness analyses can be important in decision making regarding treatment options. Studies differ substantially with respect to methods, assumptions, interventions and outcomes being evaluated, the inclusiveness of cost items and the jurisdiction to which the analyses are applied. No perfect cost-effectiveness study exists, and new advances in therapy and changes in cost over time tend to render the conclusions out of date rather quickly. However, despite these limitations, these modelling studies are useful to put the role of existing interventions into perspective.

Many studies have indicated that PPIs are likely to be more cost-effective than H_2-RAs in the treatment of patients with GERD, despite their higher initial acquisition costs [366–375]. Cost-effectiveness data from Canada [376], Sweden [377] and the USA [378, 379] arrived at similar conclusions. Maintenance PPI over a one-year period is consistently the most effective, but also the most costly intervention [376–379]. Intermittent omeprazole to treat symptomatic relapse was more cost-effective than continuous omeprazole therapy, although there was an increase in the number of symptomatic weeks per year [376]. Maintenance therapy with ranitidine or cisapride was less effective for controlling symptoms, but was of intermediate cost.

High dose H_2-RA was both more costly and less effective than PPI, with more frequent relapses that ultimately led to PPI maintenance therapy [373]. Harris *et al.* [378] reported that treatment with continuous PPI becomes more cost-effective than H_2-RA if patients with active symptoms of GERD experience a 9% decrement in QoL. When considering three different PPI maintenance strategies, starting continuous PPI after the second recurrence was least costly and least effective [379]. Continuous PPI started after the first recurrence added only a small increment of cost per recurrence prevented, compared with continuous PPI from the outset, which was ten times more costly [379]. However, for patients with a 22% decrement in QoL, continuous therapy became cost-effective when compared with maintenance after first relapse. All these strategies are modelled for only one year and may not be generalizable to lifelong treatment. Countering the potentially negative effect of acquisition costs is the fact that PPI unit costs have decreased substantially with the availability of multiple generic forms and OTC forms of this class of drugs.

More recent work has focused on comparisons between PPIs and various dosings. One paper using a Markov model compared low versus standard dose PPI therapy [380]. The standard dose PPI was found to be the more cost-effective strategy on the strength of the highest number of symptom-free patient-years and the quality adjusted life years gained. However, this study did not include estimates based on data from studies of esomeprazole 20 mg or rabeprazole 10 mg daily, two effective lower dosing regimens that may have altered the results. In another study, esomeprazole was found to be more cost-effective than lansoprazole in the maintenance of healing of erosive esophagitis [381]. In a UK study that compared all the PPIs, generic omeprazole and rabeprazole dominated the other PPIs, i.e. they cost less and resulted in more symptom free days [382].

In summary, these data support a recommendation for the use of PPIs as the most cost-effective for maintance therapy for patients with GERD.

Treatment of non-erosive reflux disease (NERD)

NERD or endoscopy-negative reflux disease (ENRD) is defined as GERD in the absence of macroscopic findings at endoscopy. Patients in this category are identified as having GERD, based on characteristic symptoms, occasionally an abnormal ambulatory esophageal pH test, a positive Bernstein test, or a positive symptom index and/or experience improvement with empirical acid suppressive therapy. These are patients with GERD symptoms often without objective abnormalities in other investigations undertaken.

One of the first studies in this group of patients was reported by Bate *et al.* in 1996 [383]. Patients with NERD were randomized in a double blind trial to receive omeprazole 20 mg once daily (n = 98) or placebo (n = 111). At four weeks, omeprazole was more effective than placebo (p < 0.0001) with respect to the proportion of subjects with freedom from heartburn (omeprazole 57%, placebo 19%), or regurgitation (omeprazole 75%, placebo 47%) and complete relief of symptoms (omeprazole 43%, placebo 14%). **A1c** Patients in the omeprazole arm used less antacids and time to first heartburn-free day was more rapid with omeprazole.

Another randomized trial in 495 patients with NERD compared low dose omeprazole 10 mg or a placebo for six months [163]. Placebo-treated patients were nearly twice as likely to discontinue treatment before the end of six months. Life-table estimates for cumulative remission at six months, were 73% for omeprazole and 48% for placebo (ARR 25%, NNT 4, p = 0.0001). QoL assessments showed a more significant deterioration in the GSRS reflux domain for placebo patients (p < 0.05), but no significant differences were noted in PGWB. Thus, a continuous dose of omeprazole 10 mg daily is effective maintenance therapy for the majority of patients with heartburn but no esophagitis (NERD). However, a larger dose of omeprazole may be required for up to a quarter of patients.

A Cochrane Review evaluating short-term treatment in NERD was updated in 2006 [384], and determined that PPIs are more effective than H_2-RA therapy, but the magnitude of benefit was smaller than was observed in patients treated empirically.

A randomized trial compared omeprazole in doses of 20 mg or 10 mg daily and placebo in 509 patients with NERD in whom heartburn was the predominant complaint [80]. Symptomatic remission of heartburn (no more than one day of mild symptoms in the week prior to the final visit) was significantly more frequent after 2–4 weeks of therapy with omeprazole in either dose, and the standard dose of omeprazole was more effective than the lower dose. Symptom relief occurred in most patients by the end of the second week. With four weeks of treatment the proportion of patients indicating sufficient control of heartburn was 66% and 57% for the standard and low doses of omeprazole and only 31% for the placebo group. **A1c** The more abnormal the initial pH study, the better the response to a greater degree of acid suppression. There was a significant correlation of response to therapy with acid reflux, age and the presence of a hiatus hernia. No correlation was identified between body mass index and degree of acid exposure, despite the widely held view that being overweight worsens reflux. A randomized trial of four weeks' duration in NERD patients in the USA [385] found omeprazole 20 mg once daily to be better than omeprazole 10 mg once daily or placebo for increasing the proportion of patients with no heartburn at both day 7 (omeprazole 20 mg 62%, 10 mg 41%, placebo 14%) or day 27 (omeprazole 20 mg 74%, 10 mg 49%, placebo 23%). Omeprazole was also significantly (p = 0.003) more effective than placebo for relief of acid regurgitation, dysphagia, epigastric pain and nausea. **A1c**

Katz *et al.* [386] reported the results of two randomized, double-blind trials with identical methodology that compared esomeprazole 40 mg once daily or 20 mg once daily with placebo for four weeks in 717 NERD patients. Complete resolution of heartburn was achieved in 65% of patients treated with either esomeprazole dose compared with 40% of placebo patients (ARR = 25%, NNT = 4, p < 0.001). **A1a**

Two studies of lansoprazole in NERD patients have been reported by Richter [387, 388]. The first study [387] compared lansoprazole 15 mg, lansoprazole 30 mg or placebo for eight weeks. Lansoprazole patients reported less daytime and night-time heartburn and antacid usage, compared with placebo patients. The second study [388] found lansoprazole to be more effective than ranitidine 150 mg twice daily or placebo. In this study, lansoprazole 15 mg and 30 mg daily were equally effective. **A1c**

A randomized trial compared pantoprazole 20 mg once daily versus omeprazole 20 mg once daily in patients with very mild grade I reflux esophagitis [389]. While these patients are not strictly a NERD population, grade I is considered by some investigators to be almost normal. The rates of symptom relief and healing were comparable at four and eight weeks. Another trial of pantoprazole 20 mg once daily versus ranitidine 150 mg twice daily in a similar patient group with grades 0–I GERD found pantoprazole to be superior to ranitidine [390]. **A1c** In a trial with a similar population of grade 0 and I esophagitis, pantoprazole 20 mg was more effective than placebo with lower numbers of patients showing "unwillingness to continue" or numbers of additional antacids taken [391]. In a similar trial, pantoprazole 20 mg and 40 mg were not significantly different and both were more effective than placebo [392].

A randomized trial comparing rabeprazole (10 mg or 20 mg once daily) with placebo in NERD patients with moderately severe symptoms found that rabeprazole, like other PPIs, rapidly and effectively relieved heartburn [393]. Other symptoms such as regurgitation, belching, bloating, early satiety and nausea were also improved. There was no difference in efficacy between the two rabeprazole doses. A six-month on-demand trial with rabeprazole 20 mg once daily was effective for symptom control in 85% of patients, limited PPI consumption to a mean of 0.3 tablets per day and improved HRQoL [394]. **A1c**

Bytzer [395] has performed a comprehensive review of the studies dealing with symptomatic GERD [80, 146, 383, 385, 387, 388, 393, 396–401]. The studies included patients with mild erosive esophagitis as well as patients with NERD. Bytzer noted that the endpoint in many of these studies was that of complete heartburn relief, a result that most patients probably do not aim for in the long term. For example, in the "on-demand" studies, patients took their PPIs once every 2–3 days, suggesting that patients accept relapse of their symptoms before they took on-demand medication. Also, the lowest response rates were observed in the studies that evaluated complete symptom relief, compared with those studies in which the endpoint was less rigorous and which permitted continued therapy despite lack of complete symptom relief.

In summary, these data support the recommendation for the use of PPIs as being more effective than H$_2$-RAs for the treatment of NERD, but the magnitude of the treatment effect is not as great as that seen in patients with esophagitis [402, 403]. This apparent difference in efficacy may be explained in part by the difficulty of ensuring that patients enrolled in these studies actually have GERD rather than functional heartburn or dyspepsia.

Long-term treatment of non-erosive reflux disease

Another approach in endoscopy negative heartburn patients is the use of patient-controlled, on-demand therapy. The first methodologically sound on-demand randomized trial in 424 NERD patients compared omeprazole 20 mg or 10 mg, with placebo [400] for the outcome of time to discontinuation of treatment (due to unwillingness to continue) over a six-month period. With life-table analysis, the remission rates were: omeprazole 20 mg 83% (95% CI: 77% to 89%) omeprazole 10 mg 69% (61% to 77%) and placebo 56% (46% to 64%) (p < 0–01 for all intergroup differences). **A1c** The mean number of study medications used daily was 0.43–0.47. Treatment failure was associated with more than a doubling of antacid use and deterioration in patient QoL.

The results of several "on-demand" trials with esomeprazole have been published. The first of these compared esomeprazole 20 mg once daily with placebo in 342 NERD patients for six months after initial symptom relief with PPI [401]. The proportion of patients who discontinued treatment due to lack of heartburn relief were esomeprazole 14% and placebo 51% (ARR = 37%, NNT = 3, p < 0.0001). **A1c** Most patients took the study medication for periods of 1–3 consecutive days (esomeprazole) or 4–13 consecutive days (placebo). Use of antacids was more than two-fold higher among placebo recipients. In the second study, patients who had achieved complete heartburn resolution after short-term esomeprazole or omeprazole treatment (n = 721) were randomized to esomeprazole 20 mg (n = 282), 40 mg, n = 293) or placebo (n = 146) on-demand (maximum one dose/day) for six months [404]. Treatment was discontinued (due to unwillingness to continue) less often by esomeprazole treated patients (esomeprazole 20 mg 8%, 40 mg 11%, placebo 42% ARR = 34%, 0.31, NNT = 3). **A1c** Patients took an average of one esomeprazole tablet every three days.

In another trial, patients were randomized to either esomeprazole 20 mg on-demand or to lansoprazole 15 mg

daily continuously for six months [405]. Those in the esomeprazole 20 mg on-demand arm took a pill only 38% of the time as opposed to 100% of the time with lansoprazole, yet still reported greater willingness to continue taking on-demand therapy, and greater satisfaction [405]. This strategy greatly lowers the cost of treatment and the evidence from this trial indicates that not all PPI are the same with respect to maintenance.

In an open study in patients with moderate to severe heartburn but normal endoscopy, rabeprazole at the low dose of 10 mg daily was highly effective, with an 83% complete response rate at four weeks [406]. Responders entered a six-month on-demand phase of rabeprazole 10 mg vs placebo and patients in the PPI arm had significantly lower rates of strategy discontinuation and antacid use [406]. **A1d**

Cost-effectiveness analysis using a Markov model was designed to compare the following three strategies for six months: on-demand esomeprazole 20 mg daily, intermittent four-week acute treatment courses of omeprazole 20 mg daily, and continuous omeprazole 20 mg daily treatment following acute treatment. The expected number of relapses per patient was estimated to be 0.10 for the on-demand esomeprazole strategy, 0.47–0.75 for continuous omeprazole treatment and 0.57–1.12 for the intermittent omeprazole strategy. The on-demand treatment with esomeprazole 20 mg was found to be cost-effective compared with the other strategies [407]. Another study evaluated costs and effectiveness of on-demand maintenance therapy with all available PPIs: omeprazole, esomeprazole, lansoprazole, pantoprazole and rabeprazole. There were no significant differences in outcomes but differences in cost were significant [408].

A meta-analysis has also confirmed the utility of intermittent or "on-demand" therapy for milder forms of GERD. In this study adequate symptom relief and maintenance of QoL was demonstrated for on-demand therapy [365].

In summary, there is evidence that on-demand therapy for maintenance treatment of NERD is clinically effective and cost-effective.

Adverse effects of long-term antisecretory drug use

While the short-term and long-term use of PPIs and H$_2$-RAs has been proven to be remarkably safe and effective, the profound alteration on gastric secretory physiology that occurs with PPI use has been postulated potentially to result in deleterious effects. Even if such effects are rare, the widespread and ubiquitous use of these agents over the last 20 years and the expected continued widespread use increases the probability that even rare adverse effects may become commonly encountered clinical issues. The preponderance of data suggests that potent inhibition of parietal cell secretion can adversely impact cobalamin serum levels, although no discrete adverse clinical outcomes have been reported related to B12 deficiency [409]. There is also concern about the possibility that PPIs raise the risk of community acquired pneumonia [410]. The Canadian Association of Gastroenterology has presented a position statement with the conclusion that an association appears to be present, but this translates into an attributable risk of one case of community acquired pneumonia per 100 years of acid suppressive use [411].

An observed association between prolonged acid suppression with PPIs and an increase in hip fracture [412–414] may not be seen until seven years or more of exposure [415]. A recent matched nested case-control study in patients without major risk factors found no increased risk of hip fracture with PPIs [416]. This result suggests that confounding factors may account for the association found in earlier studies. Additionally, Moayyedi and Cranney critically reviewed the data and found no evidence to support either causation or biological plausibility [417].

Enteric infections, particularly those caused by *Clostridium difficile*, also appear to be more common in patients taking PPIs, even away from the usual hospital based setting for these infections. The adjusted odds ratio for this infection was nearly three for those taking PPIs in a large population based controlled study [418]. A systematic review of acid suppressive drugs and the risk of enteric infections has confirmed this association, but the authors also warned that this result does not prove causation [419]. In summary, these data suggest that the safety record for antisecretory treatment is substantial and enviable, but there are potential concerns with long-term use. Population based studies indicate an association between PPI use and complications such as community acquired pneumonia, hip fracture and *C. difficile* infection but causation has not been proven. Despite the apparent rarity of these events, the recommendation to use the lowest, effective dose of antisecretory medicine needed to control symptoms is justified, given the possibility of cause and effect.

Symptomatic gastroesophageal reflux disease: empirical therapy for uninvestigated patients

At the primary care level, patients often present with predominant reflux symptoms of heartburn or acid regurgitation with no prior diagnostic studies or trials of therapy. If these patients do not have alarm symptoms, especially if they are under the age of 50 years, there is a considerable degree of agreement that they can be treated empirically with antisecretory therapy without prior endoscopy. With this approach in mind there has been an increase in the number of studies in patients with GERD-like symptoms without any initial investigations, i.e studies in which therapy is studied in uninvestigated patients with the predominant symptom of heartburn. These studies obviously include a mixed group of patients, many of whom do not have esophagitis and some in whom GERD is not the cause of their symptoms.

A randomized trial that included 424 patients with a history of proved esophagitis enrolled from general practices in the UK [420] showed that omeprazole 20 mg once daily was more effective for relief of heartburn and regurgitation than ranitidine 150 mg twice daily for four weeks (omeprazole 59%, ranitidine 27%, ARR = 22%, NNT = 5). **Ala** The prior history of esophagitis limits generalizability of this study to all patients in primary care practices, but the good relief of symptoms regardless of initial symptom severity is noteworthy.

In a trial in primary care settings in the USA, 590 patients with moderately severe symptomatic GERD were randomized without endoscopy to receive ranitidine 150 mg twice daily or a placebo [421]. Ranitidine rapidly and significantly improved heartburn severity scores, physician global assessment of the response to treatment, and the SF-36 score for physical functioning, bodily pain and vitality dimensions. **Ala** Using a heartburn specific questionnaire a significant improvement in all dimensions: physical, heartburn pain, sleep, diet, social functioning and mental health was observed for ranitidine-treated patients.

In another trial conducted in the USA, uninvestigated heartburn patients were randomized to receive either ranitidine, lansoprazole or stepped up therapy from ranitidine to lansoprazole or stepped down therapy from lansoprazole to ranitidine [422]. The continuous lansoprazole treatment was more effective than the other strategies in terms of reducing heartburn severity and increasing the number of heartburn-free days, and there appeared to be little rationale to stepping down to ranitidine.

A randomized trial [423] of 307 patients with GERD symptoms in Australian primary care settings showed that even a low dose of pantoprazole (20 mg daily) was significantly more effective than ranitidine 300 mg daily for complete control of symptoms at four weeks (40% vs 19%; $p < 0.001$), eight weeks (55% vs 33%; $p < 0.001$), six months (71% vs 56%; $p = 0007$) and twelve months (77% vs 59%; $p = 0.001$).

In the CADET-HR randomized, double blind trial in Canadian primary care settings, 390 patients with reflux predominant symptoms were randomized to receive ranitidine 150 mg twice daily or omeprazole 20 mg daily [424]. Heartburn relief at four weeks was reported by 55% of omeprazole and 27% of ranitidine-treated patients (ARR = 22%, NNT = 5). **Ala** Greater improvements in GSRS for indigestion, abdominal pain, and reflux ($p < 0.05$) and in the GASTROQoL health-related QoL scales ($p < 0.003$) were also observed in omeprazole patients. After four weeks, patients with inadequate symptom relief were stepped up every 4–8 weeks from ranitidine to omeprazole 20 mg once daily or from omeprazole 20 mg once to twice daily [424]. "Step up" occurred in 100 patients with ranitidine and 57 with omeprazole. With step-up therapy, by 16 weeks, heartburn relief resulted in 88% of patients who started with omeprazole and in 87% of those who started with ranitidine. **Ala** In the first eight weeks, omeprazole provided complete heartburn relief in 53% while it took 16 weeks to achieve a similar degree of relief in the group who were treated initially with ranitidine. Thus, starting with omeprazole therapy produced significantly faster symptom relief. Patient responders then had the medications stopped and 50% of patients experienced symptomatic relapse within nine days [424]. Only 10% of patients had no further relapse over a six-month period of follow-up.

In a Cochrane Review evaluating short-term treatment in symptomatic, non-endoscoped patients updated in 2006 [384], van Pinxteren *et al.* identified 15 empiric treatment trials. The relative risk for heartburn remission in placebo-controlled trials was 0.37 for PPI, 0.77 for H_2-RAs and 0.86 for prokinetics. In direct comparative trials PPIs were significantly more effective than H_2-RAs (seven trials, RR 0.66, 95% CI: 0.60 to 0.73) and prokinetics. Thus, PPIs were superior to H_2-RAs in empirical treatment of typical GERD symptoms. **Ala**

In a large, methodologically sound, double-blind, randomized trial in 3034 patients in 360 sites in the USA, patients with symptomatic, uninvestigated GERD symptoms received lansoprazole 30 mg once daily or esomeprazole 40 mg once daily [425] and heartburn assessments were carried out at days 1, 3, 7 and 14. The study setting was unclear and was unlikely to include only primary care practice. No statistically significant difference in heartburn relief was observed [425]. **Ala** Patients indicated that they were very pleased with their treatment, experienced substantial benefit and would recommend the medication to others. However, nearly 40% of patients still had some degree of day or night heartburn at the end of two weeks.

More studies are now available that compare various PPIs. Furthermore, longer term maintenance studies to assess the effectiveness of PPIs are now available [426–430], In a Norwegian study, patients were initially treated with esomeprazole 40 mg for four weeks. They were then randomized to esomeprazole 20 mg daily continuously or on-demand, or to ranitidine 150 mg twice daily for six months [428]. Either esomeprazole strategy gave better symptom relief and better patient satisfaction than was observed with ranitidine, indicating that on-demand therapy is a viable option.

In a rabeprazole study 331 uninvestigated heartburn-predominant patients, were treated with rabeprazole 20 mg daily for four weeks [427]. Responders were then randomized to receive either rabeprazole 20 mg continuously daily (COT) or on demand (ODT) for six months. Not surprisingly, the continuous therapy arm experienced a greater mean percentage of heartburn-free days (COT 90.3% +/− 14.8%, ODT 64.8% +/− 22.3%, p < 0.0001). Ninety-two percent of COT patients and 79% of ODT patients were either "satisfied" or "very satisfied" with treatment. While COT provides better symptom improvement, both strategies were acceptable [427].

An interesting study evaluated a patient's willingness to pay for complete symptom relief in GERD [431]. The authors found that patients were willing to pay up to US$182 to obtain more complete and faster symptom relief without side effects. Older patients were less willing to pay than younger patients to obtain symptom relief.

In summary, these data support a recommendation for the use of empirical antisecretory therapy for patients presenting with symptoms thought to be caused by GERD, without performing confirmatory diagnostic testing.

Economic evaluation in uninvestigated symptomatic heartburn

The costs and effectiveness of each drug and of each management strategy need to be evaluated. However, there are many subtle variations between studies that render direct comparisons difficult. Furthermore, decision analyses suffer from the inherent weakness of having to rely on estimates of treatment outcomes. Ofman recently reviewed the cost-effectiveness studies in symptomatic GERD [432]. He concluded that the most cost-effective strategies are PPI based step-down or PPI on-demand strategies [432]. He noted that most decision analyses had been constructed around uninvestigated GERD symptoms.

One recent study comparing esomeprazole 20 mg daily or on-demand provided estimates of similar efficacy with either strategy but reduced cost of the on-demand strategy over six months [426]. Similarly, it has been shown that esomeprazole 20 mg daily on-demand is more cost-effective than esomeprazole 20 mg continuously or than ranitidine [429]. In a large trial of 1357 uninvestigated heartburn patients, the esomeprazole 20 mg on-demand strategy was less costly, with comparable efficacy and satisfaction to esomeprazole 40 mg prescribed intermittently by the physician for either two or four weeks [430].

In summary, on-demand therapy requires that a patient becomes symptomatic before self-treating. However, patient satisfaction with this approach is high, and this management strategy is cost-effective and is recommended.

Does symptom improvement predict healing of esophagitis?

There is evidence that relief of symptoms by H_2-RAs does not reliably predict healing of mucosal damage. Patients with heartburn initially treated in a four-week study with omeprazole or cimetidine [433] were randomized to receive maintenance therapy with either omeprazole 10 mg once daily or cimetidine 800 mg qhs for 24 weeks [434]. Symptomatic remission, defined as no more than mild heartburn on one out of the seven previous days, was significantly more frequent with omeprazole (omeprazole 60%, cimetidine 24%; ARR 36%%, NNT 3). Erosive esophagitis was seen in only 10% of patients in symptomatic remission on omeprazole compared with 33% on cimetidine.

One-third of patients with relapse of erosive esophagitis by endoscopy during maintenance therapy with famotidine 40 mg twice daily were completely asymptomatic [435].

A meta-analysis [333] suggested that if heartburn resolved, only 4.5% of patients treated with omeprazole 20 mg once daily, but 14.6% with ranitidine 150 mg twice daily, experienced asymptomatic relapse of erosive esophagitis at endoscopy. **A1c**

The more recent trials show that significantly fewer esomeprazole-treated patients had persistent esophagitis, despite symptom relief, than is the case for omeprazole-treated patients [32, 290]. In patients with heartburn resolution at four weeks, esophagitis remained unhealed in 14.8% [290] to 16.8% [32] of patients receiving esomeprazole 40 mg daily compared with 23.2% [290] to 26.9% [32] of those receiving omeprazole 20 mg daily. **A1a** A similar result was seen in a comparison of esomeprazole 40 mg daily and lansoprazole 30 mg daily, with unhealed esophagitis in spite of heartburn resolution in 17.3% and 20.5% of these patients [284]. In the most severe forms of esophagitis, the healing was 11% more frequent for grade C and 17% for grade D disease in esomeprazole-treated patients. It is unclear why, despite effective symptom resolution, many patients still have esophagitis. The most likely explanation in these studies is that when patients were healed at four weeks, they came out of the studies, and the healing and symptom resolution could not be assessed at eight weeks. In all these studies, esophagitis healing was much more frequent at eight weeks than at four weeks. Therefore, if patients been endoscoped at that interval, the proportion of healed patients among those with heartburn resolution would have probably been higher.

In summary, these data demonstrate that esophagitis relapse is unusual in patients who remain asymptomatic while being treated with PPIs, but relapse is more common in those without symptoms who are being treated with an H$_2$-RA. Thus, continuous PPI therapy is recommended as maintenance therapy in patients with esophagitis, particularly with more severe esophagitis.

Treatment of esophageal peptic stricture

Esophageal peptic stricture, the most severe GERD complication, can be difficult to manage. H$_2$-RA are at best mar-

ginally more effective than a placebo for reducing the need for repeat dilatations [436, 437]. One study found no benefit from ranitidine 300 mg daily compared with placebo [438]. There are three randomized trials comparing standard dose omeprazole 20 mg daily with H$_2$-RA [439–441] and one comparing lansoprazole with high dose ranitidine [442].

In one small study [440], 34 patients with strictures were randomized to receive omeprazole 20 mg once daily, or ranitidine 150 mg or famotidine 20 mg twice daily. After three months, if esophagitis remained unhealed, the dose of medication was doubled and the patient was re-endoscoped at six months. At three months, there was no significant difference between PPI and H$_2$-RA for esophagitis healing or relief of dysphagia, although there was a trend in favor of the PPI. By six months, omeprazole treatment resulted in significantly better healing of esophagitis (omeprazole 100%, H$_2$-RA 53%; ARR 47%, NNT 2; p < 0.01) and relief of dysphagia (omeprazole 94%, H$_2$-RA 40%; ARR 54%, NNT = 2; p < 0.01). **A1d** *Post hoc* analysis also showed a trend toward reduction in the proportions of patients requiring dilatations in omeprazole-treated patients (omeprazole 41%, H$_2$-RA 73%; ARR = 32%, NNT = 3, p = 0.07). The number of dilatations required was significantly less for the omeprazole treated patients (11 vs 31 dilatations, mean of 0.6 vs 2.1 sessions per patient, p < 0.01). Cost-effectiveness analysis for healing and relief of dysphagia, that included costs of drugs, endoscopy and dilatations, and management of perforations, showed that omeprazole was 40–50% more cost-effective than H$_2$-RA.

A second adequately powered trial compared constant doses of omeprazole 20 mg once daily and ranitidine 150 mg twice daily for one year [439]. Endoscopy was done as required and at the end of the study. Repeat dilatation was required less frequently in omeprazole-treated patients (omeprazole 30%, ranitidine 46%; ARR = 16%, NNT = 6). **A1c** Fewer dilatation sessions were required in omeprazole-treated patients (omeprazole 0.48, ranitidine 1.08; p < 0.01). Omeprazole was also superior with respect to the number of patients without stricture at the end of the study, esophagitis healing and improved heartburn and dysphagia.

In a study of 158 patients over six months, lansoprazole 30 mg daily was more effective than ranitidine 300 mg twice daily for relieving dysphagia. There was a trend toward a reduction in the need for repeat dilatations (lansoprazole 30.8%, ranitidine 43.8%; p = 0.09) over 12 months [442]. **A1d**

Omeprazole 20 mg once daily was found to be more effective but more expensive than ranitidine in a cost-utility study [443].

In an observational study 30 of 36 patients with reflux esophagitis and stricture treated with dilatation and omeprazole 20 mg twice daily for 6–8 weeks experienced healing of esophagitis and relief of dysphagia [444]. These 30 patients were then randomized to receive omeprazole 20 mg twice daily, lansoprazole 30 mg twice daily or pantoprazole 40 mg twice daily (n = 10 each arm). After four weeks of treatment, significantly more omeprazole-treated patients remained healed, but no difference was seen with respect to the need to repeat dilatation of strictures. This small study may lack power to demonstrate differences between effects of these strategies. **A1d**

In summary, these data lead to the recommendation for the use of PPI vs an H$_2$-RA in those with peptic strictures as a means of reducing recurrence of the stricture or symptomatic dysphagia following dilatation.

Endoscopic treatments

Several endoscopic techniques for treating GERD have now been investigated and all demonstrated some early promise [445–452]. However, all of these techniques (injection, radiofrequency ablation, endoscopic stapling and or suturing), were either less effective than hoped, produced more adverse effects than anticipated or were too expensive or complex to be incorporated into clinical practice. All have either been withdrawn from the marketplace or remain as investigational tools. A recently published systematic review details the devices, and preclinical and clinical studies published up to the end of 2006, before this field collapsed from a clinical standpoint [453]. However, there continue to be developments in endoscopic anti-reflux therapies, and one or more of these devices may be introduced for clinical use in the foreseeable future.

Anti-reflux surgery

Medical therapy versus surgical anti-reflux therapy

Early randomized trials comparing open anti-reflux surgery (ARS) with medical therapy (H$_2$-receptor antagonists and or prokinetic agents) demonstrated that surgery was more effective than medical therapy in treating patients with esophagitis [454, 455]. However, these studies are no longer relevant, since they did not compare present day medical therapy with PPIs with surgical therapy using laparoscopic techniques. Spechler et al. have provided an update of a cohort of patients from the original study [456]. They were able to account for 97% (239/247) of the original cohort, 79 of whom had died. After a mean of 9–10 years follow-up, of the surviving and measurable patients 92% of the medical treated patients and 62% of the surgically treated patients (p < 0.001) were regularly taking anti-reflux medications. Patients with Barrett's esophagus at

baseline developed esophageal adenocarcinomas at an annual rate of 0.4%, whereas these cancers developed at a lower 0.07% annual rate in patients without Barrett's. This study indicates that anti-reflux surgery should not be recommended, with the expectation that patients with GERD will no longer need to take antisecretory medications or that the procedure prevents esophageal cancer among those with GERD and Barrett metaplasia. **A1c**

There are few direct comparisons of a PPI versus anti-reflux surgery. The first was a study by Lundell et al. with five-year follow-up [328]. Three hundred and ten patients were randomized to receive open surgical fundoplication or continuous omeprazole therapy and followed for up to five years. Only 11 of 155 patients randomized to surgery refused the treatment. Omeprazole-treated patients were allowed dose increases to 40–60 mg daily to control symptoms. No significant differences in efficacy were demonstrated and QoL assessments (PGWB and GSRS) improved in both groups. Thus, surgical therapy was demonstrated to be as effective as continuous omeprazole therapy in this trial. **A1a** However, laparoscopic fundoplication, the technique that is now widely used, was not performed. The seven-year follow up suggested that surgery was more effective than omeprazole but there were specific post-fundoplication complaints that remained problematic [457]. A more recent, short-term observational study compared the efficacy of laparoscopic fundoplication and lansoprazole in normalizing abnormal reflux in patients with GERD [458]. After anti-reflux surgery, all 55 patients were heartburn free, and esophageal pH-monitoring 3–6 months after surgery was normal in 85% of patients. Patients treated with lansoprazole were titrated upwards to 90 mg daily and esophageal acid exposure was normalized in 96% of cases. Patients who became heartburn free did not necessarily normalize their esophageal acid exposure. The results suggest that either approach may be reasonable for any given patient. **B4**

A more recent study has compared outcomes of modern laparoscopic ARS and potent antisecretory therapy using esomeprazole. In this three-year interim analysis of 554 patients with GERD randomized as part of an open-label prospective randomized trial comparing laparoscopic ARS to esomeprazole, the proportion of patients in remission in the two groups was similar (surgically treated 90%, and medically treated 93%) in an intention to treat analysis [459].

These data do not support the contention that either anti-reflux surgery or use of PPIs is a more effective GERD therapy, as both are safe and similarly effective therapies [460]. Surgical proponents often argue that medical therapies do not correct the underlying anatomical abnormalities. However, there are no long-term data to support the view that surgery achieves this result permanently either. One small follow-up observational study of patients after

20 years demonstrated that about 30% of the fundoplications were defective, and abnormal reflux on esophageal pH studies was also seen in about 30% of patients assessed [461]. **B4** Another study of 441 patients after a mean follow-up of 18 years following the Hill procedure for GERD, reported good and excellent subjective results in 80% of patients [462]. **B4** A ten-year follow-up study after laparoscopic anti-reflux surgery suggested that while 89% would select surgery again, 28% were taking acid suppressive drugs [463]. Thus, the long-term results of fundoplication are good but not completely durable. Even after one year, 6% of patients will require PPI therapy [464]. A retrospective questionnaire of 844 patients at a mean of six years after ARS identified that 26% of patients still had abnormal pH despite being on medication and in total, 37% were taking acid suppressive therapy [465]. There is also no credible evidence that surgery prevents progression to Barrett's metaplasia or protects against esophageal cancer, an often claimed benefit of surgery [464].

One randomized trial of open versus laparoscopic fundoplication [466] found no difference between the two approaches and more than 85% of patients were satisfied with their results. The major advantage for laparoscopic fundoplication is a significant reduction in hospital stay from 8–9 days for an open procedure to 2–5 days [467–469], and less time off work for the patient (laparoscopic 21.3 days, open surgery 38.2 days, p = 0.02) [468]. Thus, the procedure of choice is laparoscopic fundoplication; **A1d** however, data on long-term outcomes are lacking.

Surgical results continue to depend on surgical expertise, and the issue of a learning curve remains [468, 470]. An intra-operative complication rate of 8% has been reported [470]. The most frequent adverse effects are dysphagia, inability to belch or vomit, postprandial fullness, bloating, pain and flatus [471]. Also, laparoscopic fundoplication is not without serious complications such as esophageal perforation, paraesopheageal herniations, pneumothorax and splenic damage requiring splenectomy [472].

For some patients, there may be incomplete symptom relief with PPI therapy. In one randomized trial of anti-reflux surgery and omeprazole, those patients who were not improved on omeprazole 40 mg daily were offered anti-reflux surgery and fared well [464]. **B4** Thus, some patients with a partial response to PPIs may improve with anti-reflux surgery. However, it is of concern that 6/178 (3%) of these patients experienced postoperative complications that necessitated reoperation.

The best results with ARS are obtained in the patient with typical reflux symptoms, an abnormal esophageal pH study and good symptomatic response to PPIs [473]. Thus, the best indication for surgery is a patient who responds well to PPI but does not wish to take continuous medications to control their reflux [474, 475]. **B4 C5** With the relative ease and safety of laparoscopic surgery, it has become

a reasonable alternative for selected patients. As with all surgery, patient selection has improved through objective testing with pre-operative esophageal pH-metry and manometry. Even if cost-effectiveness modelling studies favor surgery, a decision to have surgery should not be imposed upon a patient. Ultimately, the final decision should rest on the preferences of an informed patient.

In summary, these data lead to a recommendation that surgery can be offered as an effective alternative to medical therapy in patients with reflux. The patients most likely to benefit from this treatment are patients who have been effectively treated for their symptoms with medication. Neither medical therapy nor surgery has proven more effective than the other in managing GERD symptoms or avoiding the complications of this disorder, and treatment choices should be based on patient preference for treatment.

References

1 Vakil N, van Zanten SV, Kahrilas P, Dent J, Jones R. The Montreal definition and classification of gastroesophageal reflux disease: A global evidence-based consensus. *Am J Gastroenterol* 2006; **101**: 1900–1920.

2 Chiba N. Definitions of dyspepsia: time for a reappraisal. *Eur J Surg Suppl* 1998; **164**: 14–23.

3 Veldhuyzen van Zanten SJ, Flook N, Chiba N *et al.* An evidence-based approach to the management of uninvestigated dyspepsia in the era of *Helicobacter pylori*. Canadian Dyspepsia Working Group. *CMAJ* 2000; **162**(Suppl 12): S3–23.

4 Kitchin LI, Castell DO. Rationale and efficacy of conservative therapy for gastroesophageal reflux disease. *Arch Intern Med* 1991; **151**: 448–454.

5 Fass R, Ofman JJ. Gastroesophageal reflux disease – should we adopt a new conceptual framework? *Am J Gastroenterol* 2002; **97**: 1901–1909.

6 Eloubeidi MA, Provenzale D. Health-related quality of life and severity of symptoms in patients with Barrett's esophagus and gastroesophageal reflux disease patients without Barrett's esophagus. *Am J Gastroenterol* 2000; **95**: 1881–1887.

7 Wiklund I, Bardhan KD, Muller-Lissner S *et al.* Quality of life during acute and intermittent treatment of gastro-oesophageal reflux disease with omeprazole compared with ranitidine. Results from a multicentre clinical trial. The European Study Group. *Ital J Gastroenterol Hepatol* 1998; **30**: 19–27.

8 Glise H. Quality of life and cost of therapy in reflux disease. *Scand J Gastroenterol Suppl* 1995; **210**: 38–42.

9 Armstrong D, Marshall JK, Chiba N *et al.* Canadian Consensus Conference on the management of gastroesophageal reflux disease in adults – update 2004. *Can J Gastroenterol* 2005; **19**: 15–35.

10 Talley NJ, Stanghellini V, Heading RC, Koch KL, Malagelada JR, Tytgat GN. Functional gastroduodenal disorders. *Gut* 1999; **45**(Suppl 2): II37–II42.

11 Dent J, Brun J, Fendrick AM, *et al.* on behalf of the Genval Workshop Group. An evidence-based appraisal of reflux

disease management – the Genval Workshop Report. *Gut* 1999; **44**(Suppl 2): S1–16.

12 Moayyedi P, Axon AT. The usefulness of the likelihood ratio in the diagnosis of dyspepsia and gastroesophageal reflux disease. *Am J Gastroenterol* 1999; **94**: 3122–3125.

13 Chiba N, de Gara CJ, Wilkinson JM, Hunt RH. Speed of healing and symptom relief in grade II to IV gastroesophageal reflux disease: A meta-analysis. *Gastroenterology* 1997; **112**: 1798–1810.

14 Thomson AB, Barkun AN, Armstrong D *et al.* The prevalence of clinically significant endoscopic findings in primary care patients with uninvestigated dyspepsia: The Canadian Adult Dyspepsia Empiric Treatment – Prompt Endoscopy (CADET-PE) study. *Aliment Pharmacol Ther* 2003; **17**: 1481–1491.

15 DeVault KR, Castell DO. Updated guidelines for the diagnosis and treatment of gastroesophageal reflux disease. The Practice Parameters Committee of the American College of Gastroenterology. *Am J Gastroenterol* 1999; **94**: 1434–1442.

16 Nebel OT, Forbes MF, Castell DO. Symptomatic gastroesophageal reflux: incidence and precipitating factors. *Am J Dig Dis* 1976; **21**: 953–956.

17 Thompson WG, Heaton KW. Heartburn and globus in apparently healthy people. *Can Med Assoc J* 1982; **126**: 46–48.

18 Anonymous. *Heartburn across America: A Gallup Organization national survey.* Gallup Organization Princeton, NJ, 1988.

19 Isolauri J, Laippala P. Prevalence of symptoms suggestive of gastroesophageal reflux disease in an adult population. *Ann Med* 1995; **27**: 67–70.

20 Locke GR, Talley NJ, Fett SL, Zinsmeister AR, Melton LJ. Prevalence and clinical spectrum of gastroesophageal reflux: a population-based study in Olmsted County, Minnesota. *Gastroenterology* 1997; **112**: 1448–1456.

21 Wong WM, Lai KC, Lam KF *et al.* Prevalence, clinical spectrum and health care utilization of gastro-oesophageal reflux disease in a Chinese population: a population-based study. *Aliment Pharmacol Ther* 2003; **18**: 595–604.

22 Diaz-Rubio M, Moreno-Elola-Olaso C, Rey E, Locke GR, III, Rodriguez-Artalejo F. Symptoms of gastro-oesophageal reflux: prevalence, severity, duration and associated factors in a Spanish population. *Aliment Pharmacol Ther* 2004; **19**: 95–105.

23 Talley NJ, Locke GR, III, McNally M, Schleck CD, Zinsmeister AR, Melton LJ, III. Impact of gastroesophageal reflux on survival in the community. *Am J Gastroenterol* 2008; **103**: 12–19.

24 Bor S, Mandiracioglu A, Kitapcioglu G, Caymaz-Bor C, Gilbert RJ. Gastroesophageal reflux disease in a low-income region in Turkey. *Am J Gastroenterol* 2005; **100**: 759–765.

25 Moraes-Filho JP, Chinzon D, Eisig JN, Hashimoto CL, Zaterka S. Prevalence of heartburn and gastroesophageal reflux disease in the urban Brazilian population. *Arq Gastroenterol* 2005; **42**: 122–127.

26 Yamagishi H, Koike T, Ohara S *et al.* Prevalence of gastro-esophageal reflux symptoms in a large unselected general population in Japan. *World J Gastroenterol* 2008; **14**: 1358–1364.

27 Vcev A, Stimac D, Vceva A *et al.* Lansoprazole versus omeprazole in the treatment of reflux esophagitis. *Acta Med Croatica* 1997; **51**: 171–174.

28 Johnsson F, Joelsson B, Gudmundsson K, Greiff L. Symptoms and endoscopic findings in the diagnosis of gastroesophageal reflux disease. *Scand J Gastroenterol* 1987; **22**: 714–718.

29 Klauser AG, Heinrich C, Schindlbeck NE, Müller-Lissner SA. Is long-term esophageal pH monitoring of clinical value? *Am J Gastroenterol* 1989; **84**: 362–366.

30 Talley NJ, Colin-Jones D, Koch KL, Koch M, Nyren O, Stanghellini V. Functional dyspepsia: a classification with guidelines for diagnosis and management. *Gastroenterology Intl* 1991; **4**: 145–160.

31 Dekkers CP, Beker JA, Thjodleifsson B, Gabryelewicz A, Bell NE, Humphries TJ. Double-blind comparison correction of Double-blind, placebo-controlled comparison of rabeprazole 20 mg vs omeprazole 20 mg in the treatment of erosive or ulcerative gastro-oesophageal reflux disease. The European Rabeprazole Study Group. *Aliment Pharmacol Ther* 1999; **13**: 49–57.

32 Kahrilas PJ, Falk GW, Johnson DA *et al.* Esomeprazole improves healing and symptom resolution as compared with omeprazole in reflux oesophagitis patients: A randomized controlled trial. The Esomeprazole Study Investigators. *Aliment Pharmacol Ther* 2000; **14**: 1249–1258.

33 Richter JE, Kahrilas PJ, Sontag SJ, Kovacs TO, Huang B, Pencyla JL. Comparing lansoprazole and omeprazole in onset of heartburn relief: results of a randomized, controlled trial in erosive esophagitis patients. *Am J Gastroenterol* 2001; **96**: 3089–3098.

34 Haque M, Wyeth JW, Stace NH, Talley NJ, Green R. Prevalence, severity and associated features of gastro-oesophageal reflux and dyspepsia: A population-based study. *N Z Med J* 2000; **113**: 178–181.

35 Ho KY, Kang JY, Seow A. Prevalence of gastrointestinal symptoms in a multiracial Asian population, with particular reference to reflux-type symptoms. *Am J Gastroenterol* 1998; **93**: 1816–1822.

36 Wong WM, Lam SK, Hui WM *et al.* Long-term prospective follow-up of endoscopic oesophagitis in southern Chinese – prevalence and spectrum of the disease. *Aliment Pharmacol Ther* 2002; **16**: 2037–2042.

37 Johnson DA, Benjamin SB, Vakil NB *et al.* Esomeprazole once daily for 6 months is effective therapy for maintaining healed erosive esophagitis and for controlling gastroesophageal reflux disease symptoms: A randomized, double-blind, placebo-controlled study of efficacy and safety. *Am J Gastroenterol* 2001; **96**: 27–34.

38 El-Serag HB. Time trends of gastroesophageal reflux disease: A systematic review. *Clin Gastroenterol Hepatol* 2007; **5**: 17–26.

39 Brunnen PL, Karmody AM, Needham CD. Severe peptic oesophagitis. *Gut* 1969; **10**: 831–837.

40 el Serag HB, Sonnenberg A. Associations between different forms of gastro-oesophageal reflux disease. *Gut* 1997; **41**: 594–599.

41 Fass R. Epidemiology and pathophysiology of symptomatic gastroesophageal reflux disease. *Am J Gastroenterol* 2003; **98**: S2–S7.

42 Dent J, Holloway RH, Toouli J, Dodds WJ. Mechanisms of lower oesophageal sphincter incompetence in patients with symptomatic gastro-oesophageal reflux. *Gut* 1988; **29**: 120–128.

43 Dent J. Recent views on the pathogenesis of gastro-oesophageal reflux disease. *Baillières Clin Gastroenterol* 1987; **1**: 727–745.

44 Holloway RH, Hongo M, Berger K, McCallum RW. Gastric distension: A mechanism for postprandial gastroesophageal reflux. *Gastroenterol* 1985; **89**: 779–784.

45 Venables CW. Mucus, pepsin and peptic ulcer. *Gut* 1986; **27**: 233–238.

46 Goldberg HI, Dodds WJ, Gee S, Montgomery C, Zboralske FF. Role of acid and pepsin in acute experimental esophagitis. *Gastroenterology* 1969; **56**: 223–230.

47 Mittal RK, Lange RC, McCallum RW. Identification and mechanism of delayed esophageal acid clearance in subjects with hiatus hernia. *Gastroenterol* 1987; **92**: 130–135.

48 Sloan S, Kahrilas PJ. Impairment of esophageal emptying with hiatal hernia. *Gastroenterology* 1991; **100**: 596–605.

49 van Herwaarden MA, Samsom M, Smout AJ. Excess gastro-esophageal reflux in patients with hiatus hernia is caused by mechanisms other than transient LES relaxations. *Gastroenterology* 2000; **119**: 1439–1446.

50 Trimble KC, Pryde A, Heading RC. Lowered oesophageal sensory thresholds in patients with symptomatic but not excess gastro-oesophageal reflux: evidence for a spectrum of visceral sensitivity in GORD. *Gut* 1995; **37**: 7–12.

51 Shi G, Bruley des Varannes S, Scarpignato C, Le Rhun M, Galmiche JP. Reflux related symptoms in patients with normal oesophageal exposure to acid. *Gut* 1995; **37**: 457–464.

52 Eriksen CA, Cullen PT, Sutton D, Kennedy N, Cushieri A. Abnormal esophageal transit in patients with typical reflux symptoms but normal endoscopic and pH profiles. *Am J Surg* 1991; **161**: 657–661.

53 Schlesinger PK, Donahue PE, Schmid B, Layden TJ. Limitations of 24-hour intraesophageal pH monitoring in the hospital setting. *Gastroenterology* 1985; **89**: 797–804.

54 DeMeester TR, Wang CI, Wernly JA *et al.* Technique, indications, and clinical use of 24 hour esophageal pH monitoring. *J Thorac Cardiovasc Surg* 1980; **79**: 656–670.

55 Masclee AAM, De Best ACAM, De Graaf R, Cluysenaer OJJ, Jansen JBMJ. Ambulatory 24-hour pH-metry in the diagnosis of gastroesophageal reflux disease. Determination of criteria and relation to endoscopy. *Scand J Gastroenterol* 1990; **25**: 225–230.

56 Fiorucci S, Santucci L, Chiucchiú S, Morelli A. Gastric acidity and gastroesophageal reflux patterns in patients with esophagitis. *Gastroenterology* 1992; **103**: 855–861.

57 Fass R, Naliboff B, Higa L *et al.* Differential effect of long-term esophageal acid exposure on mechanosensitivity and chemosensitivity in humans. *Gastroenterology* 1998; **115**: 1363–1373.

58 Carlsson R, Fandriks L, Jonsson C, Lundell L, Orlando RC. Is the esophageal squamous epithelial barrier function impaired in patients with gastroesophageal reflux disease? *Scand J Gastroenterol* 1999; **34**: 454–458.

59 Weusten BL, Akkermans LM, vanBerge-Henegouwen GP, Smout AJ. Symptom perception in gastroesophageal reflux disease is dependent on spatiotemporal reflux characteristics. *Gastroenterology* 1995; **108**: 1739–1744.

60 Cicala M, Emerenziani S, Caviglia R *et al.* Intra-oesophageal distribution and perception of acid reflux in patients with non-erosive gastro-oesophageal reflux disease. *Aliment Pharmacol Ther* 2003; **18**: 605–613.

61 Dent J. Microscopic esophageal mucosal injury in nonerosive reflux disease. *Clin Gastroenterol Hepatol* 2007; **5**: 4–16.

62 Breen KJ, Whelan G. The diagnosis of reflux oesophagitis: an evaluation of five investigative procedures. *Aust NZ J Surg* 1978; **48**: 156–161.

63 Kaul B, Petersen H, Grette K, Erichsen H, Myrvold HE. Scintigraphy, pH measurement, and radiography in the evaluation of gastoesophageal reflux. *Scand J Gastroenterol* 1985; **20**: 289–294.

64 Kaul B, Petersen H, Myrvold HE. Hiatus hernia in gastro-esophageal reflux disease. *Scand J Gastroenterol* 1986; **21**: 31–34.

65 Berstad A, Weberg R, Frøyshov Larsen I, Hoel B, Hauer Jensen M. Relationship of hiatus hernia to reflux esophagitis. A prospective study of coincidence, using endoscopy. *Scand J Gastroenterol* 1986; **21**: 55–58.

66 Smout AJPM, Geus WP, Mulder PGH, Stockbrügger RW, Lamers CBHW. Gastro-oesophageal reflux disease in the Netherlands. Results of a multicentre pH study. *Scand J Gastroenterol* 1996; **31**(Suppl 218): 10–15.

67 Cameron AJ. Barrett's esophagus: Prevalence and size of hiatal hernia. *Am J Gastroenterol* 1999; **94**: 2054–2059.

68 Agreus L, Svardsudd K, Talley NJ, Jones MP, Tibblin G. Natural history of gastroesophageal reflux disease and functional abdominal disorders: A population-based study. *Am J Gastroenterol* 2001; **96**: 2905–2914.

69 Ruth M, Finizia C, Lundell L. Occurrence and future history of oesophageal symptoms in an urban Swedish population: results of a questionnaire-based, ten-year follow-up study. *Scand J Gastroenterol* 2005; **40**: 629–635.

70 Pace F, Santalucia F, Bianchi Porro G. Natural history of gastro-esophageal reflux disease without esophagitis. *Gut* 1991; **32**: 845–848.

71 McDougall NI, Johnston BT, Kee F, Collins JSA, McFarland RJ, Love AHG. Natural history of reflux oesophagitis: A 10 year follow up of its effect on patient symptomatology and quality of life. *Gut* 1996; **38**: 481–486.

72 Isolauri J, Luostarinen M, Isolauri E, Reinikainen P, Viljakka M, Keyriläinen O. Natural course of gastroesophageal reflux disease: 17–22 year follow-up of 60 patients. *Am J Gastroenterol* 1997; **92**: 37–41.

73 Lagergren J, Bergstrom R, Lindgren A, Nyren O. Symptomatic gastroesophageal reflux as a risk factor for esophageal adenocarcinoma. *N Engl J Med* 1999; **340**: 825–831.

74 Ben Rejeb M, Bouché O, Zeitoun P. Study of 47 consecutive patients with peptic esophageal stricture compared with 3880 cases of reflux esophagitis. *Dig Dis Sci* 1992; **37**: 733–736.

75 Heading RC. Epidemiology of oesophageal reflux disease. *Scand J Gastroenterol* 1989; **24**: 33–37.

76 Wienbeck M, Barnert J. Epidemiology of reflux disease and reflux esophagitis. *Scand J Gastroenterol* 1989; **24**: 7–13.

77 Ware JEJ, Sherbourne CD. The MOS 36-item short-form health survey (SF-36). I. Conceptual framework and item selection. *Med Care* 1992; **30**: 473–483.

78 Dupuy HJ. (1984) The Psychological General Well-Being (PGWB) index. In: Wenger NK, Mattson ME, Furberg CF, and Elinson J, eds. *Assessment of quality of life in clinical trials of cardiovascular therapies.* Le Jacq Publishing Inc, New York **1984**: 170–183.

79 Dimenas E, Glise H, Hallerback B, Hernqvist H, Svedlund J, Wiklund I. Well-being and gastrointestinal symptoms among patients referred to endoscopy owing to suspected duodenal ulcer. *Scand J Gastroenterol* 1995; **30**: 1046–1052.

80 Lind T, Havelund T, Carlsson R *et al.* Heartburn without oesophagitis: efficacy of omeprazole therapy and features deter-

mining therapeutic response. *Scand J Gastroenterol* 1997; **32**: 974–979.

81 Revicki DA, Wood M, Wiklund I, Crawley J. Reliability and validity of the Gastrointestinal Symptom Rating Scale in patients with gastroesophageal reflux disease. *Qual Life Res* 1998; **7**: 75–83.

82 Velanovich V. The development of the GERD-HRQL symptom severity instrument. *Dis Esophagus* 2007; **20**: 130–134.

83 Stanghellini V. ReQuest– the challenge of quantifying both esophageal and extra-esophageal manifestations of GERD. *Best Pract Res Clin Gastroenterol* 2004; **18**(Suppl): 27–30.

84 Monnikes H, Bardhan KD, Stanghellini V, Berghofer P, Bethke TD, Armstrong D. Evaluation of GERD symptoms during therapy. Part II. Psychometric evaluation and validation of the new questionnaire ReQuest in erosive GERD. *Digestion* 2007; **75**(Suppl 1): 41–47.

85 Rubin G, Uebel P, Brimo-Hayek A, Hey KH, Doerfler H, Heading RC. Validation of a brief symptom questionnaire (ReQuest in Practice) for patients with gastro-oesophageal reflux disease. *Aliment Pharmacol Ther* 2008; **27**: 846–851.

86 Nocon M, Kulig M, Leodolter A, Malfertheiner P, Willich SN. Validation of the Reflux Disease Questionnaire for a German population. *Eur J Gastroenterol Hepatol* 2005; **17**: 229–233.

87 Amouretti M, Nalet B, Robaszkiewicz M *et al.* Validation of the short-form REFLUX-QUAL (RQS), a gastro-esophageal reflux disease (GERD) specific quality of life questionnaire. *Gastroenterol Clin Biol* 2005; **29**: 793–801.

88 Macran S, Wileman S, Barton G, Russell I. The development of a new measure of quality of life in the management of gastro-oesophageal reflux disease: the Reflux questionnaire. *Qual Life Res* 2007; **16**: 331–343.

89 Wiklund IK, Junghard O, Grace E *et al.* Quality of life in reflux and dyspepsia patients. Psychometric documentation of a new disease-specific questionnaire (QOLRAD). *Eur J Surg* 1998; **164**: 41–49.

90 Schunemann HJ, Armstrong D, Degl'innocenti A *et al.* A randomized multicenter trial to evaluate simple utility elicitation techniques in patients with gastroesophageal reflux disease. *Med Care* 2004; **42**: 1132–1142.

91 Rothman M, Farup C, Stewart W, Helbers L, Zeldis J. Symptoms associated with gastroesophageal reflux disease: development of a questionnaire for use in clinical trials. *Dig Dis Sci* 2001; **46**: 1540–1549.

92 Allen CJ, Parameswaran K, Belda J, Anvari M. Reproducibility, validity, and responsiveness of a disease-specific symptom questionnaire for gastroesophageal reflux disease. *Dis Esophagus* 2000; **13**: 265–270.

93 Shaw MJ, Talley NJ, Beebe TJ *et al.* Initial validation of a diagnostic questionnaire for gastroesophageal reflux disease. *Am J Gastroenterol* 2001; **96**: 52–57.

94 Colwell HH, Mathias SD, Pasta DJ, Henning JM, Hunt RH. Development of a health-related quality-of-life questionnaire for individuals with gastroesophageal reflux disease: A validation study. *Dig Dis Sci* 1999; **44**: 1376–1383.

95 Raymond JM, Marquis P, Bechade D *et al.* Assessment of quality of life of patients with gastroesophageal reflux. Elaboration and validation of a specific questionnaire. *Gastroenterol Clin Biol* 1999; **23**: 32–39.

96 Coyne KS, Wiklund I, Schmier J, Halling K, Degl'innocenti A, Revicki D. Development and validation of a disease-specific treatment satisfaction questionnaire for gastro-oesophageal reflux disease. *Aliment Pharmacol Ther* 2003; **18**: 907–915.

97 Chassany O, Holtmann G, Malagelada J, Gebauer U, Doerfler H, DeVault K. Systematic review: health-related quality of life (HRQOL) questionnaires in gastro-oesophageal reflux disease. *Aliment Pharmacol Ther* 2008; **27**: 1053–1070.

98 Madisch A, Kulich KR, Malfertheiner P *et al.* Impact of reflux disease on general and disease-related quality of life – evidence from a recent comparative methodological study in Germany. *Z Gastroenterol* 2003; **41**: 1137–1143.

99 Stewart AL, Greenfield S, Hays RD, *et al.* Functional status and well-being of patients with chronic conditions: results from the medical outcomes study. *JAMA* 1989; **262**: 907–913.

100 Dimenas E. Methodological aspects of evaluation of quality of life in upper gastrointestinal disease. *Scand J Gastroenterol* 1993; **28**: 18–21.

101 Dimenas E, Glise H, Hallerback B, Hernqvist H, Svedlund J, Wiklund I. Quality of life in patients with upper gastrointestinal symptoms: An improved evaluation of treatment regimens? *Scand J Gastroenterol* 1993; **28**: 681–687.

102 Dimenas E, Carlsson R, Glise H, Israelsson B, Wiklund I. Relevance of norm values as part of the documentation of quality of life instruments for use in upper gastrointestinal diseases. *Scand J Gastroenterol* 1996; **31**(Suppl 221): 8–13.

103 Mathias SD, Castell DO, Elkin EP, Matosian ML. Health-related quality of life of patients with acute erosive reflux esophagitis. *Dig Dis Sci* 1996; **41**: 2123–2129.

104 Galmiche JP, Barthelemy P, Hamelin B. Treating the symptoms of gastro-oesophageal reflux disease: a double-blind comparison of omeprazole and ciaspride. *Aliment Pharmacol Ther* 1997; **11**: 765–773.

105 Armstrong D, Veldhuyzen SJ, Chung SA *et al.* Validation of a short questionnaire in English and French for use in patients with persistent upper gastrointestinal symptoms despite proton pump inhibitor therapy: the PASS (Proton pump inhibitor Acid Suppression Symptom) test. *Can J Gastroenterol* 2005; **19**: 350–358.

106 Jones R, Coyne K, Wiklund I. The gastro-oesophageal reflux disease impact scale: A patient management tool for primary care. *Aliment Pharmacol Ther* 2007; **25**: 1451–1459.

107 Shaw M, Dent J, Beebe T *et al.* The Reflux Disease Questionnaire: A measure for assessment of treatment response in clinical trials. *Health Qual Life Outcomes* 2008; **6**: 31.

108 Howard PJ, Maher L, Pryde A, Heading RC. Symptomatic gastro-oesophageal reflux, abnormal oesophageal acid exposure, and mucosal acid sensitivity are three separate, though related, aspects of gastro-oesophageal reflux disease. *Gut* 1991; **32**: 128–132.

109 Richter JE, Castell DO. Gastroesophageal reflux; pathogenesis, diagnosis, and therapy. *Ann Int Med* 1982; **97**: 93–103.

110 Fuchs KH, DeMeester TR, Albertucci M. Specificity and sensitivity of objective diagnosis of gastroesophageal reflux disease. *Surgery* 1987; **102**: 575–580.

111 Wu WC. Ancillary tests in the diagnosis of gastroesophageal reflux disease. *Gastroenterol Clin North Am* 1990; **19**: 671–682.

112 Sellar RJ, De Caestecker JS, Heading RC. Barium radiology: A sensitive test for gastro-oesophageal reflux. *Clin Radiology* 1987; **38**: 303–307.

113 Chen YM, Ott DJ, Gelfand DW, Munitz HA. Multiphasic examination of the esophagogastric region for strictures, rings and hiatal hernia: evaluation of the individual techniques. *Gastrointestinal Radiology* 1985; **10**: 311–316.

114 DeVault KR, Castell DO. Guidelines for the diagnosis and treatment of gastroesophageal reflux disease. *Arch Intern Med* 1995; **155**: 2165–2173.

115 Fransson SG, Sökjer H, Johansson KE, Tibbling L. Radiologic diagnosis of gastro-oesophageal reflux. Comparison of barium and low-density contrast medium. *Acta Radiologica* 1987; **28**: 295–298.

116 Graziani L, De Nigris E, Pesaresi A, Baldelli S, Dini L, Montesi A. Reflux oesophagitis: Radiographic-endoscopic correlation in 39 symptomatic cases. *Gastrointestinal Radiology* 1983; **8**: 1–6.

117 Pope CE. Pathophysiology and diagnosis of reflux esophagitis. *Gastroenterol* 1976; **70**: 445–454.

118 Armstrong D, Bennett JR, Blum AL *et al.* The endoscopic assessment of esophagitis: A progress report on observer agreement. *Gastroenterology* 1996; **111**: 85–92.

119 Chen MY, Ott DJ, Sinclair JW, Wu WC, Gelfand DW. Gastroesophageal reflux disease: correlation of esophageal pH testing and radiographic findings. *Radiology* 1992; **185**: 483–486.

120 Jenkins AF, Cowan RJ, Richter JE. Gastroesophageal scintigraphy: is it a sensitive screening test for gastroesophageal reflux disease? *J Clin Gastroenterol* 1985; **7**: 127–131.

121 Spechler SJ. Epidemiology and natural history of gastro-oesophageal reflux disease. *Digestion* 1992; **51**(Suppl 1): 24–29.

122 Knuff TE, Benjamin SB, Worsham GF, Hancock J, Castell DO. Histologic examination of chronic gastroesophageal relux: An evaluation of biopsy methods and diagnostic criteria. *Dig Dis Sci* 1984; **29**: 194–201.

123 Ismail-Beigi F, Pope CE. Distribution of the histological changes of gastroesophageal reflux in the distal esophagus of man. *Gastroenterol* 1974; **66**: 1109–1113.

124 Schindlbeck NE, Wiebecke B, Klauser AG, Voderholzer WA, Müller-Lissner SA. Diagnostic value of histology in non-erosive gastro-oesophageal reflux disease. *Gut* 1996; **39**: 151–154.

125 Berstad A, Hatlebakk JG. The predictive value of symptoms in gastro-oesophageal reflux disease. *Scand J Gastroenterol* 1995; **30**(Suppl 211): 1–4.

126 Hatlebakk JG, Berstad A. Endoscopic grading of reflux oesophagitis: What observations corelate with gastro-oesophageal reflux? *Scand J Gastroenterol* 1997; **32**: 760–765.

127 Armstrong D, Emde C, Inauen W, Blum AL. Diagnostic assessment of gastroesophageal reflux disease: What is possible vs what is practical? *Hepato-gastroenterol* 1992; **39**(Suppl 1): 3–13.

128 Lundell LR, Dent J, Bennett JR *et al.* Endoscopic assessment of oesophagitis: clinical and functional correlates and further validation of the Los Angeles classification. *Gut* 1999; **45**: 172–180.

129 Bernstein LM, Baker LA. A clinical test for esophagitis. *Gastroenterol* 1958; **34**: 760–781.

130 Kaul B, Petersen H, Grette K, Myrvold HE, Halvorsen T. The acid perfusion test in gastroesophageal reflux disease. *Scand J Gastroenterol* 1986; **21**: 93–96.

131 Richter JE. (1985) Acid perfusion (Bernstein) test. In: Castell DO, Wu WC, and Ott DJ, eds. *Gastroesophageal Reflux Disease: Pathogenesis, Diagnosis and Therapy.* Futura Publishing Co Inc, London, 1985: 139–148.

132 Johnsson F, Joelsson B, Isberg PE. Ambulatory 24 hour intraesophgeal pH-monitoring in the diagnosis of gastro-esophageal reflux disease. *Gut* 1987; **28**: 1145–1150.

133 Wyman JB, Dent J, Holloway RH. Changes in oesophageal pH associated with gastro-oesophageal reflux. Are traditional criteria sensitive for detection of reflux? *Scand J Gastroenterol* 1993; **28**: 827–832.

134 Rosen SN, Pope CE. Extended esophageal pH monitoring. An analysis of the lterature and assessment of its role in the diagnosis and management of gastroesophageal reflux. *J Clin Gastroenterol* 1989; **11**: 260–270.

135 Hirano I, Richter JE. ACG practice guidelines: Esophageal reflux testing. *Am J Gastroenterol* 2007; **102**: 668–685.

136 Gillies RS, Stratford JM, Booth MI, Dehn TC. Oesophageal pH monitoring using the Bravo catheter-free radio capsule. *Eur J Gastroenterol Hepatol* 2007; **19**: 57–63.

137 Pandolfino JE, Kwiatek MA. Use and utility of the Bravo pH capsule. *J Clin Gastroenterol* 2008; **42**: 571–578.

138 Ward BW, Wu WC, Richter JE, Lui KW, Castell DO. Ambulatory 24-hour esophageal pH monitoring: technology seaching for a clinical application. *J Clin Gastroenterol* 1986; **8**(Suppl 1): 59–67.

139 Wiener GJ, Richter JE, Copper JB, Wu WC, Castell DO. The symptom index: A clinically important parameter of ambulatory 24-hour esophageal pH monitoring. *Am J Gastroenterol* 1988; **83**: 358–361.

140 Dekel R, Martinez-Hawthorne SD, Guillen RJ, Fass R. Evaluation of symptom index in identifying gastroesophageal reflux disease-related noncardiac chest pain. *J Clin Gastroenterol* 2004; **38**: 24–29.

141 Breumelhof R, Smout AJPM. The symptom sensitivity index: A valuable additional parameter in 24-hour esophageal pH recording. *Am J Gastroenterol* 1991; **86**: 160–164.

142 Weusten BL, Roelofs JM, Akkermans LM, Berge-Henegouwen GP, Smout AJ. The symptom-association probability: An improved method for symptom analysis of 24-hour esophageal pH data. *Gastroenterology* 1994; **107**: 1741–1745.

143 Taghavi SA, Ghasedi M, Saberi-Firoozi M *et al.* Symptom association probability and symptom sensitivity index: Preferable but still suboptimal predictors of response to high dose omeprazole. *Gut* 2005; **54**: 1067–1071.

144 Joelsson B, Johnsson F. Heartburn – the acid test. *Gut* 1989; **30**: 1523–1525.

145 Vitale GC, Cheadle WG, Sadek S, Michel ME, Cushieri A. Computerized 24-hour ambulatory esophageal pH monitoring and esophagogastroduodenoscopy in the reflux patient. *Ann Surg* 1984; **200**: 724–728.

146 Venables TL, Newland RD, Patel AC, Hole J, Wilcock C, Turbitt ML. Omeprazole 10 milligrams once daily, omeprazole 20 milligrams once daily, or ranitidine 150 milligrams twice daily, evaluated as initial therapy for the relief of symptoms of gastro-oesophageal reflux disease in general practice. *Scand J Gastroenterol* 1997; **32**: 965–973.

147 Galmiche JP, Bruley des Varannes S. Symptoms and disease severity in gastro-oesophageal reflux disease. *Scand J Gastroenterol* 1994; **29**(Suppl 201): 62–68.

148 Johannessen T, Petersen H, Kleveland PM *et al.* The predictive value of history in dyspepsia. *Scand J Gastroenterol* 1990; **25**: 689–697.

149 Johnsson F, Roth Y, Damgaard Pedersen NE, Joelsson B. Cimetidine improves GERD symptoms in patients selected by a validated GERD questionnaire. *Aliment Pharmacol Ther* 1993; **7**: 81–86.

150 Carlsson R, Dent J, Bolling-Sternevald E *et al.* The usefulness of a structured questionnaire in the assessment of symptomatic gastroesophageal reflux disease. *Scand J Gastroenterol* 1998; **33**: 1023–1029.

151 Tefera L, Fein M, Ritter MP *et al.* Can the combination of symptoms and endoscopy confirm the presence of gastroesophageal reflux disease? *The American Surgeon* 1997; **63**: 933–936.

152 Locke GR, Talley NJ, Weaver AL, Zinsmeister AR. A new questionnaire for gastroesophageal reflux disease. *Mayo Clin Proc* 1994; **69**: 539–547.

153 Manterola C, Munoz S, Grande L, Bustos L. Initial validation of a questionnaire for detecting gastroesophageal reflux disease in epidemiological settings. *J Clin Epidemiol* 2002; **55**: 1041–1045.

154 Ofman JJ, Shaw M, Sadik K *et al.* Identifying patients with gastroesophageal reflux disease: validation of a practical screening tool. *Dig Dis Sci* 2002; **47**: 1863–1869.

155 Numans ME, de Wit NJ. Reflux symptoms in general practice: diagnostic evaluation of the Carlsson-Dent gastro-oesophageal reflux disease questionnaire. *Aliment Pharmacol Ther* 2003; **17**: 1049–1055.

156 Locke GR, Zinsmeister AR, Talley NJ. Can symptoms predict endoscopic findings in GERD? *Gastrointest Endosc* 2003; **58**: 661–670.

157 Moreno Elola-Olaso C, Rey E, Rodriguez-Artalejo F, Locke GR, III, Diaz-Rubio M. Adaptation and validation of a gastroesophageal reflux questionnaire for use on a Spanish population. *Rev Esp Enferm Dig* 2002; **94**: 745–758.

158 Wong WM, Lam KF, Lai KC *et al.* A validated symptoms questionnaire (Chinese GERDQ) for the diagnosis of gastro-oesophageal reflux disease in the Chinese population. *Aliment Pharmacol Ther* 2003; **17**: 1407–1413.

159 Schenk BE, Kuipers EJ, Klinkenberg-Knol EC *et al.* Omeprazole as a diagnostic tool in gastroesophageal reflux disease. *Am J Gastroenterol* 1997; **92**: 1997–2000.

160 Johnsson F, Weywadt L, Solhaug JH, Hernqvist H, Bengtsson L. One-week omeprazole treatment in the diagnosis of gastro-oesophageal reflux disease. *Scand J Gastroenterol* 1998; **33**: 15–20.

161 Bate CM, Riley SA, Chapman RW, Durnin AT, Taylor MD. Evaluation of omeprazole as a cost-effective diagnostic test for gastro-oesophageal reflux disease. *Aliment Pharmacol Ther* 1999; **13**: 59–66.

162 Watson RG, Tham TC, Johnston BT, McDougall NI. Double blind cross-over placebo controlled study of omeprazole in the treatment of patients with reflux symptoms and physiological levels of acid reflux – the "sensitive oesophagus". *Gut* 1997; **40**: 587–590.

163 Schindlbeck NE, Klauser AG, Voderholzer WA, Müller-Lissner SA. Empiric therapy for gastroesophageal reflux disease. *Arch Intern Med* 1995; **155**: 1808–1812.

164 Fass R, Ofman JJ, Gralnek IM, Johnson C, Camargo E, Sampliner RE, Fennerty MB. Clinical and economic assessment of the ome-

prazole test in patients with symptoms suggestive of gastro-esophageal reflux disease. *Arch Intern Med* 1999; **159**: 2161–2168.

165 Juul-Hansen P, Rydning A, Jacobsen CD, Hansen T. High-dose proton-pump inhibitors as a diagnostic test of gastro-oesophageal reflux disease in endoscopic-negative patients. *Scand J Gastroenterol* 2001; **36**: 806–810.

166 Johnsson F, Hatlebakk JG, Klintenberg AC *et al.* One-week esomeprazole treatment: an effective confirmatory test in patients with suspected gastroesophageal reflux disease. *Scand J Gastroenterol* 2003; **38**: 354–359.

167 Achem SR, Kolts BE, MacMath T, Richter J, Mohr D, Burton L, Castell DO. Effects of omeprazole versus placebo in treatment of noncardiac chest pain and gastroesophageal reflux. *Dig Dis Sci* 1997; **42**: 2138–2145.

168 Fass R, Fennerty MB, Ofman JJ, Gralnek IM, Johnson C, Camargo E, Sampliner RE. The clinical and economic value of a short course of omeprazole in patients with noncardiac chest pain. *Gastroenterology* 1998; **115**: 42–49.

169 Fass R, Fennerty MB, Johnson C, Camargo L, Sampliner RE. Correlation of ambulatory 24-hour esophageal pH monitoring results with symptom improvement in patients with noncardiac chest pain due to gastroesophageal reflux disease. *J Clin Gastroenterol* 1999; **28**: 36–39.

170 Pandak WM, Arezo S, Everett S *et al.* Short course of omeprazole: a better first diagnostic approach to noncardiac chest pain than endoscopy, manometry, or 24-hour esophageal pH monitoring. *J Clin Gastroenterol* 2002; **35**: 307–314.

171 Numans ME, Lau J, de Wit NJ, Bonis PA. Short-term treatment with proton-pump inhibitors as a test for gastroesophageal reflux disease: a meta-analysis of diagnostic test characteristics. *Ann Intern Med* 2004; **140**: 518–527.

172 Hunt RH. The relationship between the control of pH and healing and symptom relief in gastro-oesophageal reflux disease. *Aliment Pharmacol Ther* 1995; **9**: 3–7.

173 Hatlebakk JG, Berstad A. Gastro-oesophageal reflux during 3 months of therapy with ranitidine in reflux oesophagitis. *Scand J Gastroenterol* 1996; **31**: 954–958.

174 Bell NJV, Burget D, Howden CW, Wilkinson J, Hunt RH. Appropriate acid suppression for the management of gastro-oesophageal reflux disase. *Digestion* 1992; **51**: 59–67.

175 Bell NJV, Hunt RH. Role of gastric acid suppression in the treatment of gastro-oesophageal reflux disease. *Gut* 1992; **33**: 118–124.

176 Chiba N, Bernard L, O'Brien BJ, Goeree R, Hunt RH. A Canadian physician survey of dyspepsia management. *Can J Gastroenterol* 1998; **12**: 83–90.

177 Meining A, Driesnack U, Classen M, Rosch T. Management of gastroesophageal reflux disease in primary care: results of a survey in 2 areas in Germany. *Z Gastroenterol* 2002; **40**: 15–20.

178 Blair DI, Kaplan B, Spiegler J. Patient characteristics and life-style recommendations in the treatment of gastroesophageal reflux disease. *J Fam Pract* 1997; **44**: 266–272.

179 Sonnenberg A, Delco F, el Serag HB. Empirical therapy versus diagnostic tests in gastroesophageal reflux disease: a medical decision analysis. *Dig Dis Sci* 1998; **43**: 1001–1008.

180 Lim PL, Gibbons MJ, Crawford EJ, Watson RG, Johnston BT. The effect of lifestyle changes on results of 24-h ambulatory

oesophageal pH monitoring. *Eur J Gastroenterol Hepatol* 2000; **12**: 655–656.

181 Pehl C, Wendl B, Pfeiffer A, Schmidt T, Kaess H. Low-proof alcoholic beverages and gastroesophageal reflux. *Dig Dis Sci* 1993; **38**: 93–96.

182 Pehl C, Pfeiffer A, Wendl B, Kaess H. Different effects of white and red wine on lower esophageal sphincter pressure and gastroesophageal reflux. *Scand J Gastroenterol* 1998; **33**: 118–122.

183 Pehl C, Frommherz M, Wendl B, Schmidt T, Pfeiffer A. Effect of white wine on esophageal peristalsis and acid clearance. *Scand J Gastroenterol* 2000; **35**: 1255–1259.

184 Pehl C, Frommherz M, Wendl B, Pfeiffer A. Gastroesophageal reflux induced by white wine: the role of acid clearance and "rereflux". *Am J Gastroenterol* 2002; **97**: 561–567.

185 Wendl B, Pfeiffer A, Pehl C, Schmidt T, Kaess H. Effect of decaffeination of coffee or tea on gastro-oesophageal reflux. *Aliment Pharmacol Ther* 1994; **8**: 283–287.

186 Kadakia SC, Kikendall JW, Maydonovitch C, Johnson LF. Effect of cigarette smoking on gastroesophageal reflux measured by 24-h ambulatory esophageal pH monitoring. *Am J Gastroenterol* 1995; **90**: 1785–1790.

187 Pehl C, Pfeiffer A, Wendl B, Nagy I, Kaess H. Effect of smoking on the results of esophageal pH measurement in clinical routine. *J Clin Gastroenterol* 1997; **25**: 503–506.

188 Van Nieuwenhoven MA, Brouns F, Brummer RJ. Gastrointestinal profile of symptomatic athletes at rest and during physical exercise. *Eur J Appl Physiol* 2004; **91**(4): 429–34.

189 Collings KL, Pierce PF, Rodriguez-Stanley S, Bemben M, Miner PB. Esophageal reflux in conditioned runners, cyclists, and weightlifters. *Med Sci Sports Exerc* 2003; **35**: 730–735.

190 Choi SC, Yoo KH, Kim TH, Kim SH, Choi SJ, Nah YH. Effect of graded running on esophageal motility and gastroesophageal reflux in fed volunteers. *J Korean Med Sci* 2001; **16**: 183–187.

191 Yazaki E, Shawdon A, Beasley I, Evans DF. The effect of different types of exercise on gastro-oesophageal reflux. *Aust J Sci Med Sport* 1996; **28**: 93–96.

192 Kraus BB, Sinclair JW, Castell DO. Gastroesophageal reflux in runners. Characteristics and treatment. *Ann Intern Med* 1990; **112**: 429–433.

193 Clark CS, Kraus BB, Sinclair J, Castell DO. Gastroesophageal reflux induced by exercise in healthy volunteers. *JAMA* 1989; **261**: 3599–3601.

194 Pollmann H, Zillessen E, Pohl J, Rosemeyer D, Abucar A, Armbrecht U, Bornhofen B, Herz R. Effect of elevated head position in bed in therapy of gastroesophageal reflux. *Z Gastroenterol* 1996; **34**(Suppl 2): 93–99.

195 Shay SS, Conwell DL, Mehindru V, Hertz B. The effect of posture on gastroesophageal reflux event frequency and composition during fasting. *Am J Gastroenterol* 1996; **91**: 54–60.

196 Tobin JM, McCloud P, Cameron DJ. Posture and gastro-oesophageal reflux: a case for left lateral positioning. *Arch Dis Child* 1997; **76**: 254–258.

197 Katz LC, Just R, Castell DO. Body position affects recumbent postprandial reflux. *J Clin Gastroenterol* 1994; **18**: 280–283.

198 Meining A, Classen M. The role of diet and lifestyle measures in the pathogenesis and treatment of gastroesophageal reflux disease. *Am J Gastroenterol* 2000; **95**: 2692–2697.

199 Kaltenbach T, Crockett S, Gerson LB. Are lifestyle measures effective in patients with gastroesophageal reflux disease? An evidence-based approach. *Arch Intern Med* 2006; **166**: 965–971.

200 Becker DJ, Sinclair J, Castell DO, Wu WC. A comparison of high and low fat meals on postprandial esophageal acid exposure. *Am J Gastroenterol* 1989; **84**: 782–786.

201 Nebel OT, Castell DO. Lower esophageal sphincter pressure changes after food ingestion. *Gastroenterology* 1972; **63**: 778–783.

202 Pehl C, Waizenhoefer A, Wendl B, Schmidt T, Schepp W, Pfeiffer A. Effect of low and high fat meals on lower esophageal sphincter motility and gastroesophageal reflux in healthy subjects. *Am J Gastroenterol* 1999; **94**: 1192–1196.

203 Penagini R, Mangano M, Bianchi PA. Effect of increasing the fat content but not the energy load of a meal on gastro-oesophageal reflux and lower oesophageal sphincter motor function. *Gut* 1998; **42**: 330–333.

204 Pehl C, Pfeiffer A, Waizenhoefer A, Wendl B, Schepp W. Effect of caloric density of a meal on lower oesophageal sphincter motility and gastro-oesophageal reflux in healthy subjects. *Aliment Pharmacol Ther* 2001; **15**: 233–239.

205 Wright LE, Castell DO. The adverse effect of chocolate on lower esophageal sphincter pressure. *Am J Dig Dis* 1975; **20**: 703–707.

206 Murphy DW, Castell DO. Chocolate and heartburn: Evidence of increased esophageal acid exposure after chocolate ingestion. *Am J Gastroenterol* 1988; **93**: 633–636.

207 Sigmund CJ, McNally EF. The action of a carminative on the lower esophageal sphincter. *Gastroenterol* 1969; **56**: 13–18.

208 Babka JC, Castell DO. On the genesis of heartburn. The effects of specific foods on the lower esophageal sphincter. *Am J Dig Dis* 1973; **18**: 391–397.

209 Allen ML, Mellow MH, Robinson MG, Orr WC. The effect of raw onions on acid reflux and reflux symptoms. *Am J Gastroenterol* 1990; **85**: 377–380.

210 Feldman M, Barnett C. Relationships between the acidity and osmolality of popular beverages and reported postprandial heartburn. *Gastroenterology* 1995; **108**: 125–131.

211 Thomas FB, Steinbaugh JT, Fromkes JJ, Mekhjian HS, Caldwell JH. Inhibitory effect of coffee on lower esophageal sphincter pressure. *Gastroenterology* 1980; **79**: 1262–1266.

212 McArthur K, Hogan D, Isenberg JI. Relative stimulatory effects of commonly ingested beverages on gastric acid secretion in humans. *Gastroenterology* 1982; **83**: 199–203.

213 Pehl C, Pfeiffer A, Wendl B, Kaess H. The effect of decaffeination of coffee on gastro-oesophageal reflux in patients with reflux disease. *Aliment Pharmacol Ther* 1997; **11**: 483–486.

214 Price SF, Smithson KW, Castell DO. Food sensitivity in reflux esophagitis. *Gastroenterology* 1978; **75**: 240–243.

215 Vitale GC, Cheadle WG, Patel B, Sadek SA, Michel ME, Cushieri A. The effect of alcohol on nocturnal gastroesophageal reflux. *JAMA* 1987; **258**: 2077–2079.

216 Locke GR, III, Talley NJ, Fett SL, Zinsmeister AR, Melton LJ, III. Risk factors associated with symptoms of gastroesophageal reflux. *Am J Med* 1999; **106**: 642–649.

217 Watanabe Y, Fujiwara Y, Shiba M *et al.* Cigarette smoking and alcohol consumption associated with gastro-oesophageal reflux disease in Japanese men. *Scand J Gastroenterol* 2003; **38**: 807–811.

218 Waring JP, Eastwood TF, Austin JM, Sanowski RA. The immediate efects of cessation of cigarette smoking on gastroesophageal reflux. *Am J Gastroenterol* 1989; **84**: 1076–1078.

219 Dodds WJ, Dent J, Hogan WJ, Helm JF, Hauser R, Patel GK, Egide MS. Mechanisms of gastroesophageal reflux in patients with reflux esophagitis. *N Engl J Med* 1982; **307**: 1547–1552.

220 Stanciu C, Bennett JR. Effects of posture on gastro-oesophageal reflux. *Digestion* 1977; **15**: 104–109.

221 Harvey RF, Gordon PC, Hadley N *et al.* Effects of sleeping with the bed-head raised and of ranitidine in patients with severe peptic oesophagitis. *Lancet* 1987; **ii**: 1200–1203.

222 Johnson LF, DeMeester TR. Evaluation of elevation of the head of the bed, bethanecol, and antacid foam tablets on gastroesophageal reflux. *Dig Dis Sci* 1981; **26**: 673–680.

223 Hamilton JW, Boisen RJ, Yamamoto DT, Wagner JL, Reichelderfer M. Sleeping on a wedge diminishes exposure of the esophagus to refluxed acid. *Dig Dis Sci* 1988; **33**: 518–522.

224 Friedenberg FK, Xanthopoulos M, Foster GD, Richter JE. The association between gastroesophageal reflux disease and obesity. *Am J Gastroenterol* 2008; **103**: 2111–2122.

225 Fraser-Moodie CA, Norton B, Gornall C, Magnago S, Weale AR, Holmes GK. Weight loss has an independent beneficial effect on symptoms of gastro-oesophageal reflux in patients who are overweight. *Scand J Gastroenterol* 1999; **34**: 337–340.

226 Kjellin A, Ramel S, Rossner S, Thor K. Gastroesophageal reflux in obese patients is not reduced by weight reduction. *Scand J Gastroenterol* 1996; **31**: 1047–1051.

227 Mathus-Vliegen LM, Tytgat GN. Twenty-four-hour pH measurements in morbid obesity: Effects of massive overweight, weight loss and gastric distension. *Eur J Gastroenterol Hepatol* 1996; **8**: 635–640.

228 Pace F, Maconi G, Molteni P, Minguzzi M, Bianchi Porro G. Meta-analysis of the effect of placebo on the outcome of medically treated reflux esophagitis. *Scand J Gastroenterol* 1995; **30**: 101–105.

229 Tran T, Lowry AM, El-Serag HB. Meta-analysis: The efficacy of over-the-counter gastro-oesophageal reflux disease therapies. *Aliment Pharmacol Ther* 2007; **25**: 143–153.

230 Graham DY, Patterson DJ. Double-blind comparison of liquid antacid and placebo in the treatment of symptomatic reflux esophagitis. *Dig Dis Sci* 1983; **28**: 559–563.

231 Farup PG, Weberg R, Berstad A *et al.* Low-dose antacids versus 400 mg cimetidine twice daily for reflux oesophagitis. A comparative, placebo-controlled, multicentre study. *Scand J Gastroenterol* 1990; **25**: 315–320.

232 Grove O, Bekker C, Jeppe-Hansen MG *et al.* Ranitidine and high-dose antacid in reflux oesophagitis. A randomized, placebo-controlled trial. *Scand J Gastroenterol* 1985; **20**: 457–461.

233 Koelz HR. Treatment of reflux esophagitis with H_2-Blockers, antacids and prokinetic drugs. An analysis of randomized clinical trials. *Scand J Gastroenterol* 1989; **24**(Suppl 156): 25–36.

234 Poynard T, A French Co-operative Study Group. Relapse rate of patients after healing of esophagitis – a prospective study of alginate as self-care treatment for 6 months. *Aliment Pharmacol Ther* 1993; **7**: 385–392.

235 Poynard T, Vernisse B, Agostini H, for a multicentre group. Randomized, multicentre comparison of sodium alginate and cisapride in the symptomatic treatment of uncomplicated gastro-oesophageal reflux. *Aliment Pharmacol Ther* 1998; **12**: 159–165.

236 Collings KL, Rodriguez-Stanley S, Proskin HM, Robinson M, Miner PB, Jr. Clinical effectiveness of a new antacid chewing gum on heartburn and oesophageal pH control. *Aliment Pharmacol Ther* 2002; **16**: 2029–2035.

237 Grande L, Lacima G, Ros E *et al.* Lack of effect of metoclopramide and domperidone on esophageal peristalsis and esophageal acid clearance in reflux esophagitis. A randomized, double-blind study. *Dig Dis Sci* 1992; **37**: 583–588.

238 Collins BJ, Spence RAJ, Ferguson R, Laird J, Love AHG. Cisapride: Influence on oesophageal and gastric emptying and gastro-oesoghageal reflux in patients with reflux oesophagitis. *Hepato gastroenterol* 1987; **34**: 113–116.

239 Robertson CS, Evans DF, Ledingham SJ, Atkinson M. Cisapride in the treatment of gastro-oesophageal reflux disease. *Aliment Pharmacol Ther* 1993; **7**: 181–190.

240 Sekiguchi T, Nishioka T, Matsuzaki T *et al.* Comparative efficacy of acid inhibition by drug therapy in reflux esophagitis. *Gastroenterologia* 1991; **26**: 137–144.

241 Castell DO, Sigmund C Jr, Patterson D, Lambert R, Hasner D, Clyde C, Zeldis JB, and the CIS-USA-52 investigator group. Cisapride 20 mg b.i.d. provides symptomatic relief of heartburn and related symptoms of chronic mild to moderate gastro-esophageal reflux disease. *Am J Gastroenterol* 1998; **93**: 547–552.

242 Richter JE, Long JF. Cisapride for gastroesophageal reflux disease: a placebo-controlled, double-blind study. *Am J Gastroenterol* 1995; **90**: 423–430.

243 Geldof H, Hazelhoff B, Otten MH. Two different dose regimens of cisapride in the treatment of reflux oesophagitis: A double-blind comparison with ranitidine. *Aliment Pharmacol Ther* 1993; **7**: 409–415.

244 Dakkak M, Jones BP, Scott MG, Tooley PJ, Bennett JR. Comparing the efficacy of cisapride and ranitidine in oesophagitis: a double-blind, parallel group study in general practice. *Br J Clin Pract* 1994; **48**: 10–14.

245 Galmiche JP, Fraitag B, Filoche B *et al.* Double-blind comparison of cisapride and cimetidine in treatment of reflux esophagitis. *Dig Dis Sci* 1990; **35**: 649–655.

246 Janisch HD, Hüttemann W, Bouzo MH. Cisapride versus ranitidine in the treatment of reflux esophagitis. *Hepatogastroenterology* 1988; **35**: 125–127.

247 Maleev A, Mendizova A, Popov P *et al.* Cisapride and cimetidine in the treatment of erosive esophagitis. *Hepatogastroenterology* 1990; **37**: 403–407.

248 Arvanitakis C, Nikopoulos A, Theoharidis A *et al.* Cisapride and ranitidine in the treatment of gastro-oesophageal reflux disease – a comparative andomized double-blind trial. *Aliment Pharmacol Ther* 1993; **7**: 635–641.

249 Baldi F, Bianchi PG, Dobrilla G *et al.* Cisapride versus placebo in reflux esophagitis. A multicenter double-blind trial. *J Clin Gastroenterol* 1988; **10**: 614–618.

250 Lepoutre L, VanDerSpek P, Vanderlinden I, Bollen J, Laukens P, Van der Spek P. Healing of grade-II and III oesophagitis through motility stimulation with cisapride. *Digestion* 1990; **45**: 109–114.

251 Toussaint J, Gossuin A, Deruyttere M, Huble F, Devis G. Healing and prevention of relapse of reflux oesophagitis by cisapride. *Gut* 1991; **32**: 1280–1285.

252 Kimmig JM. Treatment and prevention of relapse of mild oesophagitis with omeprazole and cisapride: a comparison of two strategies. *Aliment Pharmacol Ther* 1995; **9**: 281–286.

253 van Rensburg CJ, Bardhan KD. No clinical benefit of adding cisapride to pantoprazole for treatment of gastro-oesophageal reflux disease. *Eur J Gastroenterol Hepatol* 2001; **13**: 909–914.

254 Blum AL, Adami B, Bouzo MH *et al.* Effect of cisapride on relapse of esophagitis. A multinational, placebo-controlled trial in patients healed with an antisecretory drug. The Italian Eurocis Trialists. *Dig Dis Sci* 1993; **38**: 551–560.

255 Vigneri S, Termini R, Leandro G *et al.* A comparison of five maintenance therapies for reflux esophagitis. *N Engl J Med* 1995; **333**: 1106–1110.

256 Tytgat GN, Anker-Hansen O, Carling L *et al.* Effect of cisapride on relapse of reflux oesophagitis, healed with antisecretory drugs. *Scand J Gastroenterol* 1992; **27**: 175–183.

257 McDougall NI, Watson RGP, Collins JSA, McFarland RJ, Love AHG. Maintenance therapy with cisapride after healing of erosive oesophagitis: a double-blind placebo-controlled trial. *Aliment Pharmacol Ther* 1997; **11**: 487–495.

258 Hatlebakk JG, Johnsson F, Vilien M, Carling L, Wetterhus S, Thøgersen T. The effect of cisapride in maintaining symptomatic remission in patients with gastro-oesophageal reflux disease. *Scand J Gastroenterol* 1997; **32**: 1100–1106.

259 Moayyedi P, Santana J, Khan M, Preston C, Donnellan C. Medical treatments in the short term management of reflux oesophagitis. *Cochrane Database of Systematic Reviews* 2007; Issue 2. Art. No.: CD003244. DOI: 10.1002/14651858.CD003244.pub2.

260 Wysowski DE, Bacsanyi J. Cisapride and fatal arrhythmia. *N Engl J Med* 1996; **335**: 290–291.

261 Hameeteman W, v.d.Boomgaard DM, Dekker W, Schrijver M, Wesdorp ICE, Tytgat GNJ. Sucralfate versus cimetidine in reflux esophagitis. A single-blind multicentre study. *J Clin Gastroenterol* 1987; **9**: 390–394.

262 Chopra BK, Kazal HL, Mittal PK, Sibia SS. A comparison of the clinical efficacy of ranitidine and sucralfate in reflux esophagitis. *J Assoc Physicians India* 1992; **40**: 439–441.

263 Bremner CG, Marks IN, Segal I, Simjee A. Reflux esophagitis therapy: Sucralfate versus ranitidine in a double blind multi-center trial. *The American Journal of Medicine* 1991; **91**: 119S–122S.

264 Simon B, Mueller P. Comparison of the effect of sucralfate and ranitidine in reflux esophagitis. *The American Journal of Medicine* 1987; **83**: 43–47.

265 Schotborgh RH, Hameeteman W, Dekker W *et al.* Combination therapy of sucralfate and cimetidine, compared with sucralfate monotherapy, in patients with peptic reflux esophagitis. *The American Journal of Medicine* 1989; **86**: 77–80.

266 Herrera JL, Shay SS, McCabe M, Peura DA, Johnson LF. Sucralfate used as adjunctive therapy in patients with severe erosive peptic esophagitis resulting from gastroesophageal reflux. *Am J Gastroenterol* 1990; **85**: 1335–1338.

267 Tytgat GNJ, Koelz HR, Vosmaer GDC, and the Sucralfate Investigational Working Team. Sucralfate maintenance therapy in reflux esophagitis. *Am J Gastroenterol* 1995; **90**: 1233–1237.

268 Jorgensen F, Elsborg L. Sucralfate versus cimetidine in the treatment of reflux esophagitis, with special reference to the esophageal motor function. *Am J Med* 1991; **91**: 114S–118S.

269 Hunt RH. Habit, prejudice, power and politics: issues in the conversion of H2-receptor antagonists to over-the-counter use, editorial. *Can Med Assoc J* 1996; **154**: 49–53.

270 Gottlieb S, Decktor DL, Eckert JM, Simon TJ, Stauffer L, Ciccone PE. Efficacy and tolerability of famotidine in preventing heart-burn and related symptoms of upper gastrointestinal discomfort. *Am J Therapeutics* 1995; **2**: 314–319.

271 Johannessen T, Kristensen P. On-demand therapy in gastro-esophageal relux disease: a comparison of the early effects of single doses of fast-dissolving famotidine wafers and ranitidine tablets. *Clin Ther* 1997; **19**: 73–81.

272 Engzelius JM, Solhaug JH, Knapstad LJ, Kjærsgaard P. Ranitidine effervescent and famotidine wafer in the relief of episodic symptoms of gastro-oesophageal reflux disease. *Scand J Gastroenterol* 1997; **32**: 513–518.

273 Euler AR, Murdock RH, Jr., Wilson TH, Silver MT, Parker SE, Powers L. Ranitidine is effective therapy for erosive esophagitis. *Am J Gastroenterol* 1993; **88**: 520–524.

274 Roufail W, Belsito A, Robinson M, Barish C, Rubin A. Ranitidine for erosive oesophagitis: a double-blind, placebo- controlled study. Glaxo Erosive Esophagitis Study Group. *Aliment Pharmacol Ther* 1992; **6**: 597–607.

275 Silver MT, Murdock RH, Jr., Morrill BB, Sue SO. Ranitidine 300mg twice daily and 150mg four-times daily are efffective in healing erosive esophagitis. *Aliment Pharmacol Ther* 1996; **10**: 373–380.

276 McCarty-Dawson D, Sue SO, Morrill B, Murdock RH, Jr. Ranitidine versus cimetidine in the healing of erosive esophagitis. *Clin Ther* 1996; **18**: 1150–1160.

277 Johnson NJ, Boyd EJS, Mills JG, Wood JR. Acute treatment of reflux oesophagitis: a multi-centre trial to compare 150mg ranitidine b.d. with 300mg ranitidine q.d.s. *Aliment Pharmacol Ther* 1989; **3**: 259–266.

278 Simon TJ, Berlin RG, Tipping R, Gilde L. Efficacy of twice daily doses of 40 or 20 milligrams famotidine or 150 milligrams ranitidine for treatment of patients with moderate to severe erosive esophagitis. Famotidine Erosive Esophagitis Study Group. *Scand J Gastroenterol* 1993; **28**: 375–380.

279 Castell DO, Richter JE, Robinson M, Sontag S, Haber MM, and the Lansoprazole Group. Efficacy and safety of lansoprazole in the treatment of erosive reflux esophagitis. *Am J Gastroenterol* 1996; **91**: 1749–1757.

280 Mulder CJ, Dekker W, Gerretsen M. Lansoprazole 30mg versus omeprazole 40mg in the treatment of reflux oesophagitis grade II, III and IVa (a Dutch multicentre trial). Dutch Study Group. *Eur J Gastroenterol Hepatol* 1996; **8**: 1101–1106.

281 Dekkers CP, Beker JA, Thjodleifsson B, Gabryelewicz A, Bell NE, Humphries TJ. Double-blind comparison of rabeprazole 20mg vs omeprazole 20mg in the treatment of erosive or ulcerative gastro-oesophageal reflux disease. The European Rabeprazole Study Group. *Aliment Pharmacol Ther* 1999; **13**: 49–57.

282 van Rensburg CJ, Honiball PJ, Grundling HD *et al.* Efficacy and tolerability of pantoprazole 40mg versus 80mg in patients with reflux oesophagitis. *Aliment Pharmacol Ther* 1996; **10**: 397–401.

283 Earnest DL, Dorsch E, Jones J, Jennings DE, Greski-Rose PA. A placebo-controlled dose-ranging study of lansoprazole in the management of reflux esophagitis. *Am J Gastroenterol* 1998; **93**: 238–243.

284 Castell DO, Kahrilas PJ, Richter JE *et al.* Esomeprazole (40 mg) compared with lansoprazole (30 mg) in the treatment of erosive esophagitis. *Am J Gastroenterol* 2002; **97**: 575–583.

285 Howden CW, Ballard EDII, Robieson W. Evidence for therapeutic equivalence of lansoprazole 30 mg and esomeprazole 40 mg in the treatment of erosive oesophagitis. *Clin Drug Invest* 2002; **22**: 99–109.

286 Vcev A, Stimac D, Vceva A *et al.* Pantoprazole versus omeprazole in the treatment of reflux esophagitis. *Acta Med Croatica* 1999; **53**: 79–82.

287 Mee AS, Rowley JL & the Lansoprazole clinical research goup. Rapid symptom relief in reflux oesophagitis: a comparison of lansoprazole and omeprazole. *Aliment Pharmacol Ther* 1996; **10**: 757–763.

288 Farley A, Wruble LD, Humphries TJ. Rabeprazole versus ranitidine for the treatment of erosive gastroesophageal reflux disease: a double-blind, randomized clinical trial. Rabeprazole Study Group. *Am J Gastroenterol* 2000; **95**: 1894–1899.

289 Delchier JC, Cohen G, Humphries TJ. Rabeprazole, 20 mg once daily or 10 mg twice daily, is equivalent to omeprazole, 20 mg once daily, in the healing of erosive gastrooesophageal reflux disease. *Scand J Gastroenterol* 2000; **35**: 1245–1250.

290 Richter JE, Kahrilas PJ, Johanson J *et al.* Efficacy and safety of esomeprazole compared with omeprazole in GERD patients with erosive esophagitis: a randomized controlled trial. *Am J Gastroenterol* 2001; **96**: 656–665.

291 Dupas JL, Houcke P, Samoyeau R. Pantoprazole versus lansoprazole in French patients with reflux esophagitis. *Gastroenterol Clin Biol* 2001; **25**: 245–250.

292 Korner T, Schutze K, Van Leendert RJ *et al.* Comparable efficacy of pantoprazole and omeprazole in patients with moderate to severe reflux esophagitis. Results of a multinational study. *Digestion* 2003; **67**: 6–13.

293 Meneghelli UG, Boaventura S, Moraes-Filho JP *et al.* Efficacy and tolerability of pantoprazole versus ranitidine in the treatment of reflux esophagitis and the influence of *Helicobacter pylori* infection on healing rate. *Dis Esophagus* 2002; **15**: 50–56.

294 Holtmann G, Bytzer P, Metz M, Loeffler V, Blum AL. A randomized, double-blind, comparative study of standard-dose rabeprazole and high-dose omeprazole in gastro-oesophageal reflux disease. *Aliment Pharmacol Ther* 2002; **16**: 479–485.

295 Richter JE, Bochenek W. Oral pantoprazole for erosive esophagitis: a placebo-controlled, randomized clinical trial. Pantoprazole US GERD Study Group. *Am J Gastroenterol* 2000; **95**: 3071–3080.

296 Sontag SJ, Kogut DG, Fleischmann R *et al.* Lansoprazole heals erosive reflux esophagitis resistant to histamine H2-receptor antagonist therapy. *Am J Gastroenterol* 1997; **92**: 429–437.

297 Donnellan C, Preston C, Moayyedi P, Sharma N. Medical treatments for the maintenance therapy of reflux oesophagitis and endoscopic negative reflux disease. *Cochrane Database of Systematic Reviews* 2004, Issue 4. Art. No.: CD003245. DOI: 10.1002/14651858.CD003245.pub2.

298 Fennerty MB, Johanson JF, Hwang C, Sostek M. Efficacy of esomeprazole 40 mg vs lansoprazole 30 mg for healing moderate to severe erosive oesophagitis. *Aliment Pharmacol Ther* 2005; **21**: 455–463.

299 Labenz J, Armstrong D, Lauritsen K *et al.* A randomized comparative study of esomeprazole 40 mg versus pantoprazole 40 mg for healing erosive oesophagitis: the EXPO study. *Aliment Pharmacol Ther* 2005; **21**: 739–746.

300 Glatzel D, Abdel-Qader M, Gatz G, Pfaffenberger B. Pantoprazole 40 mg is as effective as esomeprazole 40 mg to relieve symptoms of gastroesophageal reflux disease after 4 weeks of treatment and superior regarding the prevention of symptomatic relapse. *Digestion* 2007; **75** Suppl 1: 69–78.

301 Furuta T, Kaneko E, Baba S, Arai H, Futami H. Percentage changes in serum pepsinogens are useful as indices of eradication of Helicobacter pylori. *Am J Gastroenterol* 1997; **92**: 84–88.

302 Gillessen A, Beil W, Modlin IM, Gatz G, Hole U. 40 mg pantoprazole and 40 mg esomeprazole are equivalent in the healing of esophageal lesions and relief from gastroesophageal reflux disease-related symptoms. *J Clin Gastroenterol* 2004; **38**: 332–340.

303 Mulder CJ, Westerveld BD, Smit JM *et al.* A double-blind, randomized comparison of omeprazole Multiple Unit Pellet System (MUPS) 20 mg, lansoprazole 30 mg and pantoprazole 40 mg in symptomatic reflux oesophagitis followed by 3 months of omeprazole MUPS maintenance treatment: a Dutch multicentre trial. *Eur J Gastroenterol Hepatol* 2002; **14**: 649–656.

304 Thjodleifsson B, Beker JA, Dekkers C, Bjaaland T, Finnegan V, Humphries TJ. Rabeprazole versus omeprazole in preventing relapse of erosive or ulcerative gastroesophageal reflux disease: a double-blind, multicenter, European trial. The European Rabeprazole Study Group. *Dig Dis Sci* 2000; **45**: 845–853.

305 Vakil NB, Shaker R, Johnson DA *et al.* The new proton pump inhibitor esomeprazole is effective as a maintenance therapy in GERD patients with healed erosive oesophagitis: a 6-month, randomized, double-blind, placebo-controlled study of efficacy and safety. *Aliment Pharmacol Ther* 2001; **15**: 927–935.

306 Vakil N, Fennerty MB. Direct comparative trials of the efficacy of proton pump inhibitors in the management of gastro-oesophageal reflux disease and peptic ulcer disease. *Aliment Pharmacol Ther* 2003; **18**: 559–568.

307 Mossner J, Holscher AH, Herz R, Schneider A. A double-blind study of pantoprazole and omeprazole in the treatment of reflux oesophagitis: a multicentre trial. *Aliment Pharmacol Ther* 1995; **9**: 321–326.

308 Corinaldesi R, Valentini M, Belaiche J, Colin R, Geldof H, Maier C, The European Pantoprazole Study Group. Pantoprazole and omeprazole in the treatment of reflux oesophagitis: a European multicentre study. *Aliment Pharmacol Ther* 1995; **9**: 667–671.

309 Edwards SJ, Lind T, Lundell L. Systematic review of proton pump inhibitors for the acute treatment of reflux oesophagitis. *Aliment Pharmacol Ther* 2001; **15**: 1729–1736.

310 Klok RM, Postma MJ, van Hout BA, Brouwers JR. Meta-analysis: comparing the efficacy of proton pump inhibitors in short-term use. *Aliment Pharmacol Ther* 2003; **17**: 1237–1245.

311 Gralnek IM, Dulai GS, Fennerty MB, Spiegel BM. Esomeprazole versus other proton pump inhibitors in erosive esophagitis: a meta-analysis of randomized clinical trials. *Clin Gastroenterol Hepatol* 2006; **4**: 1452–1458.

312 Caro JJ, Salas M, Ward A. Healing and relapse rates in gastroesophageal reflux disease treated with the newer proton-pump inhibitors lansoprazole, rabeprazole, and pantoprazole compared with omeprazole, ranitidine, and placebo: evidence from randomized clinical trials. *Clin Ther* 2001; **23**: 998–1017.

313 Edwards SJ, Lind T, Lundell L. Systematic review: proton pump inhibitors (PPIs) for the healing of reflux oesophagitis – a comparison of esomeprazole with other PPIs. *Aliment Pharmacol Ther* 2006; **24**: 743–750.

314 Vcev A, Begic I, Ostojic R *et al.* Esomeprazole versus pantoprazole for healing erosive oesophagitis. *Coll Antropol* 2006; **30**: 519–522.

315 Pilotto A, Franceschi M, Leandro G *et al.* Comparison of four proton pump inhibitors for the short-term treatment of esophagitis in elderly patients. *World J Gastroenterol* 2007; **13**: 4467–4472.

316 Hatlebakk JG. Review article: gastric acidity–comparison of esomeprazole with other proton pump inhibitors. *Aliment Pharmacol Ther* 2003; **17**(Suppl 1): 10–15.

317 ROhss K, Lind T, Wilder-Smith C. Esomeprazole 40 mg provides more effective intragastric acid control than lansoprazole 30 mg, omeprazole 20 mg, pantoprazole 40 mg and rabeprazole 20 mg in patients with gastro-oesophageal reflux symptoms. *Eur J Clin Pharmacol* 2004; **60**: 531–539.

318 Wilder-Smith C, Backlund A, Eckerwall G, Lind T, Fjellman M, ROhss K. Effect of increasing esomeprazole and pantoprazole doses on acid control in patients with symptoms of gastro-oesophageal reflux disease: a randomized, dose-response study. *Clin Drug Investig* 2008; **28**: 333–343.

319 Piccoli F, Ory G, Hadengue A, Beglinger C, Degen L. Effect of intravenous esomeprazole 40 mg and pantoprazole 40 mg on intragastric pH in healthy subjects. A prospective, open, randomised, two-way cross-over comparative study. *Arzneimittelforschung* 2007; **57**: 654–658.

320 Hartmann D, Eickhoff A, Damian U, Riemann JF, Schilling D. Effect of intravenous application of esomeprazole 40 mg versus pantoprazole 40 mg on 24-hour intragastric pH in healthy adults. *Eur J Gastroenterol Hepatol* 2007; **19**: 133–137.

321 Miner PB, Jr., Tutuian R, Castell DO, Liu S, Sostek MB. Intragastric acidity after switching from 5-day treatment with intravenous pantoprazole 40 mg/d to 5-day treatment with oral esomeprazole 40 mg/d or pantoprazole 40 mg/d: an open-label crossover study in healthy adult volunteers. *Clin Ther* 2006; **28**: 725–733.

322 ROhss K, Wilder-Smith C, Naucler E, Jansson L. Esomeprazole 20 mg provides more effective intragastric Acid control than maintenance-dose rabeprazole, lansoprazole or pantoprazole in healthy volunteers. *Clin Drug Investig* 2004; **24**: 1–7.

323 Labenz J, Petersen KU, Rosch W, Koelz HR. A summary of Food and Drug Administration-reported adverse events and drug interactions occurring during therapy with omeprazole, lansoprazole and pantoprazole. *Aliment Pharmacol Ther* 2003; **17**: 1015–1019.

324 Shimatani T, Inoue M, Kuroiwa T, Horikawa Y. Rabeprazole 10 mg twice daily is superior to 20 mg once daily for night-time gastric acid suppression. *Aliment Pharmacol Ther* 2004; **19**: 113–122.

325 Frazzoni M, De Micheli E, Grisendi A, Savarino V. Effective intra-oesophageal acid suppression in patients with gastro-oesophageal reflux disease: lansoprazole vs pantoprazole. *Aliment Pharmacol Ther* 2003; **17**: 235–241.

326 Klinkenberg-Knol EC, Festen HPM, Jansen JBMJ *et al.* Long-term treatment with omeprazole for refractory reflux esophagitis: efficacy and safety. *Ann Int Med* 1994; **121**: 161–167.

327 Klinkenberg-Knol EC, Nelis F, Dent J *et al.* Long-term omeprazole treatment in resistant gastroesophageal reflux disease: efficacy, safety, and influence on gastric mucosa. *Gastroenterology* 2000; **118**: 661–669.

328 Lundell L, Miettinen P, Myrvold HE *et al.* Continued (5-year) followup of a randomized clinical study comparing antireflux surgery and omeprazole in gastroesophageal reflux disease. *J Am Coll Surg* 2001; **192**: 172–179.

329 Gatta L, Vaira D, Sorrenti G, Zucchini S, Sama C, Vakil N. Meta-analysis: the efficacy of proton pump inhibitors for laryngeal symptoms attributed to gastro-oesophageal reflux disease. *Aliment Pharmacol Ther* 2007; **25**: 385–392.

330 Qadeer MA, Phillips CO, Lopez AR *et al.* Proton pump inhibitor therapy for suspected GERD-related chronic laryngitis: a meta-analysis of randomized controlled trials. *Am J Gastroenterol* 2006; **101**: 2646–2654.

331 Inadomi JM, McIntyre L, Bernard L, Fendrick AM. Step-down from multiple- to single-dose proton pump inhibitors (PPIs): a prospective study of patients with heartburn or acid regurgitation completely relieved with PPIs. *Am J Gastroenterol* 2003; **98**: 1940–1944.

332 Lee TJ, Fennerty MB, Howden CW. Systematic review: Is there excessive use of proton pump inhibitors in gastro-oesophageal reflux disease? *Aliment Pharmacol Ther* 2004; **20**: 1241–1251.

333 Carlsson R, Galmiche JP, Dent J, Lundell L, Frison L. Prognostic factors influencing relapse of oesophagitis during maintenance therapy with antisecretory drugs: a meta-analysis of long-term omeprazole trials. *Aliment Pharmacol Ther* 1997; **11**: 473–482.

334 Ollyo JB, Monnier P, Fontolliet C, Savary M. The natural history, prevalence and incidence of reflux oesophagitis. *Gullet* 1993; **3**(Suppl 3): 3–10.

335 Koelz HR, Birchler R, Bretholz A *et al.* Healing and relapse of reflux esophagitis during treatment with ranitidine. *Gastroenterology* 1986; **91**: 1198–1205.

336 Hetzel DJ, Dent J, Reed WD *et al.* Healing and relapse of severe peptic esophagitis after treatment with omeprazole. *Gastroenterology* 1988; **95**: 903–912.

337 Olbe L, Lundell L. Medical treatment of reflux esophagitis. *Hepatogastroenterology* 1992; **39**: 322–324.

338 Armstrong D. Systematic review: persistence and severity in gastro-oesophageal reflux disease. *Aliment Pharmacol Ther* 2008; **28**: 841–853.

339 Klinkenberg-Knol EC, Jansen JBMJ, Lamers CBHW, Nelis F, Meuwissen SGM. Temporary cessation of long-term maintenance treatment with omeprazole in patients with H₂-receptor-antagonist-resistant reflux oesophagitis. Effects on symptoms, endoscopy, serum gastrin, and gastric acid output. *Scand J Gastroenterol* 1990; **25**: 1144–1150.

340 Sontag SJ, Kogut DG, Fleischmann R, Campbell DR, Richter J, Haber M. Lansoprazole prevents recurrence of erosive reflux esophagitis previously resistant to H2-RA therapy. The Lansoprazole Maintenance Study Group. *Am J Gastroenterol* 1996; **91**: 1758–1765.

341 Carlsson R, Galmiche JP, Dent J, Lundell L, Frison L. Prognostic factors influencing relapse of oesophagitis during maintenance therapy with antisecretory drugs: a meta-analysis of long-term omeprazole trials. *Aliment Pharmacol Ther* 1997; **11**: 473–482.

342 Dent J, Yeomans ND, MacKinnon M *et al.* Omeprazole v ranitidine for prevention of relapse in reflux oesophagitis. A control-

led double blind trial of their efficacy and safety. *Gut* 1994; **35**: 590–598.

343 Sontag SJ, Robinson M, Roufail W *et al.* Daily omeprazole surpasses intermittent dosing in preventing relapse of oesophagitis: a US multi-centre double-blind study. *Aliment Pharmacol Ther* 1997; **11**: 373–380.

344 Chiba N. Proton pump inhibitors in acute healing and maintenance of erosive or worse esophagitis: a systematic overview. *Can J Gastroenterol* 1997; **11** Suppl B: 66B–73B.

345 Chiba N, Hunt RH. (1999) Gastroesophageal reflux disease. In: McDonald J, Burroughs A, and Feagan B, eds. *Evidence Based Gastroenterology and Hepatology*. BMJ Books, London, 1999: 16–65.

346 Chiba N (2004). Gastroesophageal reflux disease. In: McDonald JWD, Burroughs AK, and Feagan BG, eds. *Evidence-based gastroenterology and hepatology*. 2nd ed. Blackwell Publishing Ltd, New Delhi, 2004: 13–54.

347 Carling L, Axelsson CK, Forssell H *et al.* Lansoprazole and omeprazole in the prevention of relapse of reflux oesophagitis: a long-term comparative study. *Aliment Pharmacol Ther* 1998; **12**: 985–990.

348 Lauritsen K, Deviere J, Bigard MA *et al.* Esomeprazole 20 mg and lansoprazole 15 mg in maintaining healed reflux oesophagitis: Metropole study results. *Aliment Pharmacol Ther* 2003; **17**(Suppl 1): 24.

349 DeVault KR, Johanson JF, Johnson DA, Liu S, Sostek MB. Maintenance of healed erosive esophagitis: a randomized six-month comparison of esomeprazole twenty milligrams with lansoprazole fifteen milligrams. *Clin Gastroenterol Hepatol* 2006; **4**: 852–859.

350 Goh KL, Benamouzig R, Sander P, Schwan T. Efficacy of pantoprazole 20 mg daily compared with esomeprazole 20 mg daily in the maintenance of healed gastroesophageal reflux disease: a randomized, double-blind comparative trial – the EMANCIPATE study. *Eur J Gastroenterol Hepatol* 2007; **19**: 205–211.

351 Thjodleifsson B, Rindi G, Fiocca R, Humphries TJ, Morocutti A, Miller N, Bardhan KD. A randomized, double-blind trial of the efficacy and safety of 10 or 20 mg rabeprazole compared with 20 mg omeprazole in the maintenance of gastro-oesophageal reflux disease over 5 years. *Aliment Pharmacol Ther* 2003; **17**: 343–351.

352 Caos A, Moskovitz M, Dayal Y, Perdomo C, Niecestro R, Barth J. Rabeprazole for the prevention of pathologic and symptomatic relapse of erosive or ulcerative gastroesophageal reflux disease. Rebeprazole Study Group. *Am J Gastroenterol* 2000; **95**: 3081–3088.

353 Birbara C, Breiter J, Perdomo C, Hahne W. Rabeprazole for the prevention of recurrent erosive or ulcerative gastro-oesophageal reflux disease. Rabeprazole Study Group. *Eur J Gastroenterol Hepatol* 2000; **12**: 889–897.

354 Pilotto A, Leandro G, Franceschi M. Short- and long-term therapy for reflux oesophagitis in the elderly: a multi-centre, placebo-controlled study with pantoprazole. *Aliment Pharmacol Ther* 2003; **17**: 1399–1406.

355 DeVault KR, Morgenstern DM, Lynn RB, Metz DC. Effect of pantoprazole in older patients with erosive esophagitis. *Dis Esophagus* 2007; **20**: 411–415.

356 van Rensburg CJ, Honiball PJ, van Zyl JH *et al.* Safety and efficacy of pantoprazole 40 mg daily as relapse prophylaxis in patients with healed reflux oesophagitis-a 2-year follow-up. *Aliment Pharmacol Ther* 1999; **13**: 1023–1028.

357 Bardhan KD, Bishop AE, Polak JM *et al.* Pantoprazole in severe acid-peptic disease: the effectiveness and safety of 5 years' continuous treatment. *Dig Liver Dis* 2005; **37**: 10–22.

358 Caos A, Breiter J, Perdomo C, Barth J. Long-term prevention of erosive or ulcerative gastro-oesophageal reflux disease relapse with rabeprazole 10 or 20 mg vs placebo: results of a 5-year study in the United States. *Aliment Pharmacol Ther* 2005; **22**: 193–202.

359 Robinson M, Lanza F, Avner D, Haber M. Effective maintenance treatment of reflux esophagitis with low-dose lansoprazole. A randomized, double-blind, placebo-controlled trial. *Ann Intern Med* 1996; **124**: 859–867.

360 Baldi F, Morselli-Labate AM, Cappiello R, Ghersi S. Daily low-dose versus alternate day full-dose lansoprazole in the maintenance treatment of reflux esophagitis. *Am J Gastroenterol* 2002; **97**: 1357–1364.

361 Johnsson F, Moum B, Vilien M, Grove O, Simren M, Thoring M. On-demand treatment in patients with oesophagitis and reflux symptoms: comparison of lansoprazole and omeprazole. *Scand J Gastroenterol* 2002; **37**: 642–647.

362 Kao AW, Sheu BS, Sheu MJ *et al.* On-demand therapy for Los Angeles grade A and B reflux esophagitis: esomeprazole versus omeprazole. *J Formos Med Assoc* 2003; **102**: 607–612.

363 Sjostedt S, Befrits R, Sylvan A *et al.* Daily treatment with esomeprazole is superior to that taken on-demand for maintenance of healed erosive oesophagitis. *Aliment Pharmacol Ther* 2005; **22**: 183–191.

364 Sheu BS, Cheng HC, Chang WL, Chen WY, Kao AW. The impact of body mass index on the application of on-demand therapy for Los Angeles grades A and B reflux esophagitis. *Am J Gastroenterol* 2007; **102**: 2387–2394.

365 Pace F, Tonini M, Pallotta S, Molteni P, Porro GB. Systematic review: maintenance treatment of gastro-oesophageal reflux disease with proton pump inhibitors taken "on-demand". *Aliment Pharmacol Ther* 2007; **26**: 195–204.

366 Sridhar S, Huang JQ, O'Brien BJ, Hunt RH. Clinical economics review: cost-effectiveness of treatment alternatives for gasto-oesophageal reflux disease. *Aliment Pharmacol Ther* 1996; **10**: 865–873.

367 Sadowski D, Champion M, Goeree R *et al.* Health economics of gastroesophageal reflux disease. *Can J Gastroenterol* 1997; **11**(Suppl B): 108B–112B.

368 Bate CM. Cost-effectiveness of omeprazole in the treatment of reflux oesophagitis. *British Journal of Medical Economics* 1991; **1**: 53–61.

369 Bate CM, Richardson PDI. A one year model for the cost-effectiveness of treating reflux oesophagitis. *Br J Med Econ* 1992; **2**: 5–11.

370 Bate CM, Richardson PDI. Symptomatic assessment and cost effectiveness of treatments for reflux oesophagitis: comparisons of omperazole and histamine H_2-receptor antagonists. *Br J Med Econ* 1992; **2**: 37–48.

371 Bate CM. Omeprazole vs Ranitidine and cimetidine in reflux oesophagitis: The British perspective. *PharmacoEconomics* 1994; **5**: 35–43.

372 Hillman AL, Bloom BS, Fendrick AM, Schwartz JS. Cost and quality effects of alternative treatments for persistent gastro-

esophageal reflux disease. *Arch Intern Med* 1992; **152**: 1467–1472.

373 Bloom BS. Cost and quality effects of treating erosive esophagitis: a re-evaluation. *PharmacoEconomics* 1995; **8**: 139–146.

374 Jones RH, Bosanquet N, Johnson NJ, Chong SL. Cost-effective management strategies for acid-peptic disorders. *Br J Med Econ* 1994; **7**: 99–114.

375 Zagari M, Villa KF, Freston JW. Proton pump inhibitors versus H₂-receptor antagonists for the treatment of erosive gastro-esophageal reflux disease: a cost-comparative study. *Am J Man Care* 1995; **1**: 247–255.

376 O'Brien BJ, Goeree R, Hunt R, Wilkinson J, Levine M, Willan A. *Economic evaluation of alternative therapies in the long term management of peptic ulcer disease and gastroesophageal relux disease.* McMaster University, Canada, 1996.

377 Jonsson B, Stalhammar N-O. The cost-effectiveness of omeprazole in intermittent and maintenance treatment of reflux oesophagitis – the case of Sweden. *British Journal of Medical Economics* 1993; **6**: 111–126.

378 Harris RA, Kuppermann M, Richter JE. Proton pump inhibitors or histamine-2 receptor antagonists for the prevention of recurrences of erosive reflux esophagitis: a cost-effectiveness analysis. *Am J Gastroenterol* 1997; **92**: 2179–2187.

379 Harris RA, Kuppermann M, Richter JE. Prevention of recurrences of erosive reflux esophagitis: a cost-effectiveness analysis of maintenance proton pump inhibition. *Am J Med* 1997; **102**: 78–88.

380 You JH, Lee AC, Wong SC, Chan FK. Low-dose or standard-dose proton pump inhibitors for maintenance therapy of gastro-oesophageal reflux disease: a cost-effectiveness analysis. *Aliment Pharmacol Ther* 2003; **17**: 785–792.

381 Raghunath AS, Green JR, Edwards SJ. A review of the clinical and economic impact of using esomeprazole or lansoprazole for the treatment of erosive esophagitis. *Clin Ther* 2003; **25**: 2088–2101.

382 Remak E, Brown RE, Yuen C, Robinson A. Cost-effectiveness comparison of current proton-pump inhibitors to treat gastro-oesophageal reflux disease in the UK. *Curr Med Res Opin* 2005; **21**: 1505–1517.

383 Bate CM, Griffin SM, Keeling PW *et al.* Reflux symptom relief with omeprazole in patients without unequivocal oesophagitis. *Aliment Pharmacol Ther* 1996; **10**: 547–555.

384 van Pinxteren B, Numans MME, Bonis P, Lau J. Short-term treatment with proton pump inhibitors, H2-receptor antagonists and prokinetics for gastro-oesophageal reflux disease-like symptoms and endoscopy negative reflux disease. *Cochrane Database of Systematic Reviews* 2006, Issue 3. Art. No.: CD002095. DOI: 10.1002/14651858.CD002095.pub3.

385 Richter JE, Peura D, Benjamin SB, Joelsson B, Whipple J. Efficacy of omeprazole for the treatment of symptomatic acid reflux disease without esophagitis. *Arch Intern Med* 2000; **160**: 1810–1816.

386 Katz PO, Castell DO, Levine D. Esomeprazole resolves chronic heartburn in patients without erosive oesophagitis. *Aliment Pharmacol Ther* 2003; **18**: 875–882.

387 Richter JE, Kovacs TO, Greski-Rose PA, Huang B, Fisher R. Lansoprazole in the treatment of heartburn in patients without erosive oesophagitis. *Aliment Pharmacol Ther* 1999; **13**: 795–804.

388 Richter JE, Campbell DR, Kahrilas PJ, Huang B, Fludas C. Lansoprazole compared with ranitidine for the treatment of nonerosive gastroesophageal reflux disease. *Arch Intern Med* 2000; **160**: 1803–1809.

389 Bardhan KD, van Rensburg C. Comparable clinical efficacy and tolerability of 20 mg pantoprazole and 20 mg omeprazole in patients with grade I reflux oesophagitis. *Aliment Pharmacol Ther* 2001; **15**: 1585–1591.

390 Kaspari S, Biedermann A, Mey J. Comparison of pantoprazole 20 mg to ranitidine 150 mg b.i.d. in the treatment of mild gastroesophageal reflux disease. *Digestion* 2001; **63**: 163–170.

391 Kaspari S, Kupcinskas L, Heinze H, Berghofer P. Pantoprazole 20 mg on demand is effective in the long-term management of patients with mild gastro-oesophageal reflux disease. *Eur J Gastroenterol Hepatol* 2005; **17**: 935–941.

392 Scholten T, Dekkers CP, Schutze K, Korner T, Bohuschke M, Gatz G. On-demand therapy with pantoprazole 20 mg as effective long-term management of reflux disease in patients with mild GERD: the ORION trial. *Digestion* 2005; **72**: 76–85.

393 Miner P, Jr., Orr W, Filippone J, Jokubaitis L, Sloan S. Rabeprazole in nonerosive gastroesophageal reflux disease: a randomized placebo-controlled trial. *Am J Gastroenterol* 2002; **97**: 1332–1339.

394 Ponce J, Arguello L, Bastida G, Ponce M, Ortiz V, Garrigues V. On-demand therapy with rabeprazole in nonerosive and erosive gastroesophageal reflux disease in clinical practice: effectiveness, health-related quality of life, and patient satisfaction. *Dig Dis Sci* 2004; **49**: 931–936.

395 Bytzer P. Goals of therapy and guidelines for treatment success in symptomatic gastroesophageal reflux disease patients. *Am J Gastroenterol* 2003; **98**: S31–S39.

396 Venables TL, Newland RD, Patel AC, Hole J, Copeman MB, Turbitt ML. Maintenance treatment for gastro-oesophageal reflux disease. A placebo-controlled evaluation of 10 milligrams omeprazole once daily in general practice. *Scand J Gastroenterol* 1997; **32**: 627–632.

397 Hatlebakk JG, Hyggen A, Madsen PH, Walle PO, Schulz T, Mowinckel P, Bernklev T, Berstad A. Heartburn treatment in primary care: randomised, double blind study for 8 weeks. *BMJ* 1999; **319**: 550–553.

398 Carlsson R, Dent J, Watts R *et al.* Gastro-oesophageal reflux disease in primary care: an international study of different treatment strategies with omeprazole. International GORD Study Group. *Eur J Gastroenterol Hepatol* 1998; **10**: 119–124.

399 Havelund T, Aalykke C. The efficacy of a pectin-based raft-forming anti-reflux agent in endoscopy-negative reflux disease. *Scand J Gastroenterol* 1997; **32**: 773–777.

400 Lind T, Havelund T, Lundell L *et al.* On demand therapy with omeprazole for the long-term management of patients with heartburn without oesophagitis–a placebo-controlled randomized trial. *Aliment Pharmacol Ther* 1999; **13**: 907–914.

401 Talley NJ, Lauritsen K, Tunturi-Hihnala H *et al.* Esomeprazole 20 mg maintains symptom control in endoscopy-negative gastro-oesophageal reflux disease: a controlled trial of "on-demand" therapy for 6 months. *Aliment Pharmacol Ther* 2001; **15**: 347–354.

402 Long JD, Orlando RC. Nonerosive reflux disease. *Minerva Gastroenterol Dietol* 2007; **53**: 127–141.

403 Fass R. Erosive esophagitis and nonerosive reflux disease (NERD): comparison of epidemiologic, physiologic, and therapeutic characteristics. *J Clin Gastroenterol* 2007; **41**: 131–137.

404 Talley NJ, Venables TL, Green JR *et al.* Esomeprazole 40 mg and 20 mg is efficacious in the long-term management of patients with endoscopy-negative gastro-oesophageal reflux disease: a placebo-controlled trial of on-demand therapy for 6 months. *Eur J Gastroenterol Hepatol* 2002; **14**: 857–863.

405 Tsai HH, Chapman R, Shepherd A *et al.* Esomeprazole 20 mg on-demand is more acceptable to patients than continuous lansoprazole 15 mg in the long-term maintenance of endoscopy-negative gastro-oesophageal reflux patients: the COMMAND Study. *Aliment Pharmacol Ther* 2004; **20**: 657–665.

406 Bytzer P, Blum A, De HD, Dubois D. Six-month trial of on-demand rabeprazole 10 mg maintains symptom relief in patients with non-erosive reflux disease. *Aliment Pharmacol Ther* 2004; **20**: 181–188.

407 Wahlqvist P, Junghard O, Higgins A, Green J. Cost effectiveness of proton pump inhibitors in gastro-oesophageal reflux disease without oesophagitis: comparison of on-demand esomeprazole with conventional omeprazole strategies. *PharmacoEconomics* 2002; **20**: 267–277.

408 Hughes DA, Bodger K, Bytzer P, De HD, Dubois D. Economic analysis of on-demand maintenance therapy with proton pump inhibitors in patients with non-erosive reflux disease. *Pharmacoeconomics* 2005; **23**: 1031–1041.

409 Marcuard SP, Albernaz L, Khazanie PG. Omeprazole therapy causes malabsorption of cyanocobalamin (vitamin B12). *Ann Intern Med* 1994; **120**: 211–215.

410 Laheij RJ, Sturkenboom MC, Hassing RJ, Dieleman J, Stricker BH, Jansen JB. Risk of community-acquired pneumonia and use of gastric acid-suppressive drugs. *JAMA* 2004; **292**: 1955–1960.

411 CAG Clinical Affairs Committee. Community-acquired pneumonia and acid-suppressive drugs: position statement. *Can J Gastroenterol* 2006; **20**: 119–125.

412 Yang YX, Lewis JD, Epstein S, Metz DC. Long-term proton pump inhibitor therapy and risk of hip fracture. *JAMA* 2006; **296**: 2947–2953.

413 Vestergaard P, Rejnmark L, Mosekilde L. Proton pump inhibitors, histamine H2 receptor antagonists, and other antacid medications and the risk of fracture. *Calcif Tissue Int* 2006; **79**: 76–83.

414 Yu EW, Blackwell T, Ensrud KE, Hillier TA, Lane NE, Orwoll E, Bauer DC. Acid-suppressive medications and risk of bone loss and fracture in older adults. *Calcif Tissue Int* 2008; **83**: 251–259.

415 Targownik LE, Lix LM, Metge CJ, Prior HJ, Leung S, Leslie WD. Use of proton pump inhibitors and risk of osteoporosis-related fractures. *CMAJ* 2008; **179**: 319–326.

416 Kaye JA, Jick H. Proton pump inhibitor use and risk of hip fractures in patients without major risk factors. *Pharmacotherapy* 2008; **28**: 951–959.

417 Moayyedi P, Cranney A. Hip fracture and proton pump inhibitor therapy: balancing the evidence for benefit and harm. *Am J Gastroenterol* 2008; **103**: 2428–2431.

418 Dial S, Delaney JA, Barkun AN, Suissa S. Use of gastric acid-suppressive agents and the risk of community-acquired Clostridium difficile-associated disease. *JAMA* 2005; **294**: 2989–2995.

419 Leonard J, Marshall JK, Moayyedi P. Systematic review of the risk of enteric infection in patients taking acid suppression. *Am J Gastroenterol* 2007; **102**: 2047–2056.

420 Hungin APS, Gunn SD, Bate CM, Turbitt ML, Wilcock C, Richardson PDI. A comparison of the efficacy of omeprazole 20 mg once daily with ranitidine 150 mg bd in the relief of symptomatic gastro-oesophageal reflux disease in general practice. *Br J Clin Res* 1993; **4**: 73–88.

421 Rush DR, Stelmach WJ, Young TL *et al.* Clinical effectiveness and quality of life with ranitidine vs placebo in gastroesophageal reflux disease patients: a clinical experience network (CEN) study. *The Journal of Family Practice* 1995; **41**: 126–136.

422 Howden CW, Henning JM, Huang B, Lukasik N, Freston JW. Management of heartburn in a large, randomized, community-based study: comparison of four therapeutic strategies. *Am J Gastroenterol* 2001; **96**: 1704–1710.

423 Talley NJ, Moore MG, Sprogis A, Katelaris P. Randomised controlled trial of pantoprazole versus ranitidine for the treatment of uninvestigated heartburn in primary care. *Med J Aust* 2002; **177**: 423–427.

424 Armstrong D, Veldhuyzen van Zanten SJ *et al.* Heartburn-dominant, uninvestigated dyspepsia: a comparison of "PPI-start" and "H2-RA-start" management strategies in primary care—the CADET-HR Study. *Aliment Pharmacol Ther* 2005; **21**: 1189–1202.

425 Chey W, Huang B, Jackson RL. Lansoprazole and esomeprazole in symptomatic GERD: A double-blind, randomised, multicentre trial in 3000 patients confirms comparable symptom relief. *Clin Drug Invest* 2003; **23**: 69–84.

426 Szucs T, Thalmann C, Michetti P, Beglinger C. Cost analysis of long-term treatment of patients with symptomatic gastroesophageal Reflux Disease (GERD) with esomeprazole on-demand treatment or esomeprazole continuous treatment: an open, randomized, multicenter study in Switzerland. *Value Health* 2008; **12**(2): 273–281.

427 Morgan DG, O'Mahony MF, O'Mahony WF *et al.* Maintenance treatment of gastroesophageal reflux disease: an evaluation of continuous and on-demand therapy with rabeprazole 20 mg. *Can J Gastroenterol* 2007; **21**: 820–826.

428 Norman HA, Bergheim R, Fagertun H, Lund H, Moum B. A randomised prospective study comparing the effectiveness of esomeprazole treatment strategies in clinical practice for 6 months in the management of patients with symptoms of gastroesophageal reflux disease. *Int J Clin Pract* 2005; **59**: 665–671.

429 Hansen AN, Wahlqvist P, Jorgensen E *et al.* Six-month management of patients following treatment for gastroesophageal reflux disease symptoms – a Norwegian randomized, prospective study comparing the costs and effectiveness of esomeprazole and ranitidine treatment strategies in a general medical practitioners setting. *Int J Clin Pract* 2005; **59**: 655–664.

430 Meineche-Schmidt V, Juhl HH, ostergaard JE, Luckow A, Hvenegaard A. Costs and efficacy of three different esomeprazole treatment strategies for long-term management of gastro-oesophageal reflux symptoms in primary care. *Aliment Pharmacol Ther* 2004; **19**: 907–915.

431 Kleinman L, McIntosh E, Ryan M *et al.* Willingness to pay for complete symptom relief of gastroesophageal reflux disease. *Arch Intern Med* 2002; **162**: 1361–1366.

432 Ofman JJ. The economic and quality-of-life impact of symptomatic gastroesophageal reflux disease. *Am J Gastroenterol* 2003; **98**: S8–S14.

433 Bate CM, Green JR, Axon AT *et al.* Omeprazole is more effective than cimetidine for the relief of all grades of gastro-oesophageal reflux disease-associated heartburn, irrespective of the presence or absence of endoscopic oesophagitis. *Aliment Pharmacol Ther* 1997; **11**: 755–763.

434 Bate CM, Green JR, Axon AT *et al.* Omeprazole is more effective than cimetidine in the prevention of recurrence of GERD-associated heartburn and the occurrence of underlying oesophagitis. *Aliment Pharmacol Ther* 1998; **12**: 41–47.

435 Bianchi Porro G, Pace F, Sangaletti O *et al.* High-dose famotidine in the maintenance treatment of refractory esophagitis: results of a medium-term open study. *Am J Gastroenterol* 1991; **86**: 1585–1587.

436 Starlinger M, Appel WH, Schemper M, Schiessel R. Long-term treatment of peptic esophageal stenosis with dilation and cimetidine: factors influencing clinical results. *Eur Surg Res* 1985; **17**: 207–214.

437 Ferguson R, Dronfield MW, Atkinson M. Cimetidine in treatment of reflux esophagitis with peptic stricture. *BMJ* 1979; **2**: 472–474.

438 Farup PG, Modalsli B, Tholfsen JK. Long-term treatment with 300 mg ranitidine once daily after dilatation of peptic oesophageal strictures. *Scand J Gastroenterol* 1992; **27**: 594–598.

439 Smith PM, Kerr GD, Cockel R *et al.* A comparison of omeprazole and ranitidine in the prevention of recurrence of benign esophageal stricture. The RESTORE Investigator Group. *Gastroenterology* 1994; **107**: 1312–1318.

440 Marks RD, Richter JE, Rizzo J, Koehler RE, Spenney JG, Mills TP, Champion G. Omeprazole versus H2-receptor antagonists in treating patients with peptic stricture and esophagitis. *Gastroenterology* 1994; **106**: 907–915.

441 Silvis SE, Farahmand M, Johnson JA, Ansel HJ, Ho SB. A randomized blinded comparison of omeprazole and ranitidine in the treatment of chronic esophageal stricture secondary to acid peptic esophagitis. *Gastrointest Endosc* 1996; **43**: 216–221.

442 Swarbrick ET, Gough AL, Foster CS, Christian J, Garrett AD, Langworthy CH. Prevention of recurrence of oesophageal stricture, a comparison of lansoprazole and high-dose ranitidine. *Eur J Gastroenterol Hepatol* 1996; **8**: 431–438.

443 Stal JM, Gregor JC, Preiksaitis HG, Reynolds RP. A cost-utility analysis comparing omeprazole with ranitidine in the maintenance therapy of peptic esophageal stricture. *Can J Gastroenterol* 1998; **12**: 43–49.

444 Jaspersen D, Diehl KL, Schoeppner H, Geyer P, Martens E. A comparison of omeprazole, lansoprazole and pantoprazole in the maintenance treatment of severe reflux oesophagitis. *Aliment Pharmacol Ther* 1998; **12**: 49–52.

445 Galmiche JP, Bruley d, V. Endoluminal therapies for gastro-oesophageal reflux disease. *Lancet* 2003; **361**: 1119–1121.

446 Vakil N, Sharma P. Review article: endoscopic treatments for gastro-oesophageal reflux disease. *Aliment Pharmacol Ther* 2003; **17**: 1427–1434.

447 Filipi CJ, Lehman GA, Rothstein RI *et al.* Transoral, flexible endoscopic suturing for treatment of GERD: a multicenter trial. *Gastrointest Endosc* 2001; **53**: 416–422.

448 Mahmood Z, McMahon BP, Arfin Q *et al.* Endocinch therapy for gastro-oesophageal reflux disease: a one year prospective follow up. *Gut* 2003; **52**: 34–39.

449 Rothstein RI, Filipi CJ. Endoscopic suturing for gastroesophageal reflux disease: clinical outcome with the Bard EndoCinch. *Gastrointest Endosc Clin N Am* 2003; **13**: 89–101.

450 Triadafilopoulos G, DiBaise JK, Nostrant TT *et al.* Radiofrequency energy delivery to the gastroesophageal junction for the treatment of GERD. *Gastrointest Endosc* 2001; **53**: 407–415.

451 Triadafilopoulos G, DiBaise JK, Nostrant TT *et al.* The Stretta procedure for the treatment of GERD: 6 and 12 month follow-up of the U.S. open label trial. *Gastrointest Endosc* 2002; **55**: 149–156.

452 Johnson DA, Ganz R, Aisenberg J *et al.* Endoscopic implantation of enteryx for treatment of GERD: 12-month results of a prospective, multicenter trial. *Am J Gastroenterol* 2003; **98**: 1921–1930.

453 Falk GW, Fennerty MB, Rothstein RI. AGA Institute technical review on the use of endoscopic therapy for gastroesophageal reflux disease. *Gastroenterology* 2006; **131**: 1315–1336.

454 Behar J, Sheahan DG, Biancani P, Spiro HM, Storer EH. Medical and surgical management of reflux esophagitis. A 38-month report of a prospective clinical trial. *N Engl J Med* 1975; **293**: 263–268.

455 Spechler SJ. Comparison of medical and surgical therapy for complicated gastroesophageal reflux disease in veterans. The Department of Veterans Affairs Gastroesophageal Reflux Disease Study Group. *N Engl J Med* 1992; **326**: 786–792.

456 Spechler SJ, Lee E, Ahnen D *et al.* Long-term outcome of medical and surgical therapies for gastroesophageal reflux disease: follow-up of a randomized controlled trial. *JAMA* 2001; **285**: 2331–2338.

457 Lundell L, Miettinen P, Myrvold HE *et al.* Seven-year follow-up of a randomized clinical trial comparing proton-pump inhibition with surgical therapy for reflux oesophagitis. *Br J Surg* 2007; **94**: 198–203.

458 Frazzoni M, Grisendi A, Lanzani A, Melotti G, De Micheli E. Laparoscopic fundoplication versus lansoprazole for gastro-oesophageal reflux disease. A pH-metric comparison. *Dig Liver Dis* 2002; **34**: 99–104.

459 Lundell L, Attwood S, Ell C *et al.* Comparing laparoscopic antireflux surgery with esomeprazole in the management of patients with chronic gastro-oesophageal reflux disease: a 3-year interim analysis of the LOTUS trial. *Gut* 2008; **57**: 1207–1213.

460 Moss SF, Armstrong D, Arnold R *et al.* GERD 2003 – a consensus on the way ahead. *Digestion* 2003; **67**: 111–117.

461 Luostarinen M, Isolauri J, Laitinen J *et al.* Fate of Nissen fundoplication after 20 years. A clinical, endoscopical, and functional analysis. *Gut* 1993; **34**: 1015–1020.

462 Low DE, Anderson RP, Ilves R, Ricciardelli E, Hill LD. Fifteen- to twenty-year results after the Hill antireflux operation. *J Thorac Cardiovasc Surg* 1989; **98**: 444–449.

463 Fein M, Bueter M, Thalheimer A, Pachmayr V, Heimbucher J, Freys SM, Fuchs KH. Ten-year outcome of laparoscopic antireflux surgery. *J Gastrointest Surg* 2008; **12**: 1893–1899.

464 Lundell L, Dalenback J, Hattlebakk J *et al.* Outcome of open antireflux surgery as assessed in a Nordic multicentre prospec-

tive clinical trial. Nordic GORD-Study Group. *Eur J Surg* 1998; **164**: 751–757.

465 Wijnhoven BP, Lally CJ, Kelly JJ, Myers JC, Watson DI. Use of antireflux medication after antireflux surgery. *J Gastrointest Surg* 2008; **12**: 510–517.

466 Laine S, Rantala A, Gullichsen R, Ovaska J. Laparoscopic vs conventional Nissen fundoplication. A prospective randomized study. *Surg Endosc* 1997; **11**: 441–444.

467 Blomqvist AM, Lönroth H, Dalenbäck J, Lundell L. Laparoscopic or open fundoplication? A complete cost analysis. *Surg Endosc* 1998; **12**: 1209–1212.

468 Champault G, Volter F, Rizk N, Boutelier P. Gastroesophageal reflux: conventional surgical treatment versus laparoscopy. A prospective study of 61 cases. *Surg Laparosc Endosc* 1996; **6**: 434–440.

469 Peters JH, Heimbucher J, Kauer WK, Incarbone R, Bremner CG, DeMeester TR. Clinical and physiologic comparison of laparoscopic and open Nissen fundoplication. *J Am Coll Surg* 1995; **180**: 385–393.

470 Eshraghi N, Farahmand M, Soot SJ, Rand LL, Deveney CW, Sheppard BC. Comparison of outcomes of open versus laparoscopic Nissen fundoplication performed in a single practice. *Am J Surg* 1998; **175**: 371–374.

471 Lundell L. Laparoscopic fundoplication is the treatment of choice for gastro-oesophageal reflux disease. Protagonist. *Gut* 2002; **51**: 468–471.

472 Watson DI, Jamieson GG. Antireflux surgery in the laparoscopic era. *Br J Surg* 1998; **85**: 1173–1184.

473 Quigley EM. Factors that influence therapeutic outcomes in symptomatic gastroesophageal reflux disease. *Am J Gastroenterol* 2003; **98**: S24–S30.

474 Galmiche JP, Zerbib F. Laparoscopic fundoplication is the treatment of choice for gastro-oesophageal reflux disease. *Antagonist Gut* 2002; **51**: 472–474.

475 Anvari M, Allen CJ. Prospective evaluation of dysphagia before and after laparoscopic Nissen fundoplication without routine division of short gastrics. *Surg Laparosc Endosc* 1996; **6**: 424–429.

3 Barrett's esophagus

*Constantine A Soulellis[1], Marc Bradette[2], Naoki Chiba[3], M Brian Fennerty[4]
and Carlo A Fallone[1]*

[1]Division of Gastroenterology, McGill University Health Center, Montreal, Canada
[2]Division of Gastroenterology, Centre Hospitalier Universitaire de Québec, Québec City, Canada
[3]Division of Gastroenterology, McMaster University Medical Centre, Hamilton *and* Guelph General Hospital,
Guelph, Canada
[4]Oregon Health and Science University, Division of Gastroenterology and Hepatology, Oregon, USA

Introduction

Barrett's esophagus was first described by Norman Barrett
in 1957 [1]. It is a condition in which the normally squamous mucosa of the esophagus is replaced by metaplastic
columnar epithelium due to injury from gastroesophageal
reflux. Barrett's esophagus is thus one of the complications
of gastroesophageal reflux disease (GERD). Its importance
is derived entirely from its association with esophageal
adenocarcinoma, the latter of which develops in approximately 0.5% of patients with Barrett's esophagus per year
[2].

Definition

The definition of Barrett's esophagus has changed over the
last several years. From its original description as a columnar-lined lower esophagus [1, 3], to one requiring at least
3 cm of circumferential columnar lining or intestinal metaplasia [4], it has evolved most recently to the presence of
any length of columnar epithelium in the tubular esophagus that is characterized histologically as intestinal metaplasia [5, 6]. In keeping with this evolution in diagnostic
criteria the Practice Parameters Committee of the American
College of Gastroenterology has most recently defined this
entity as "a change in the distal esophageal epithelium of
any length that can be recognized as columnar-type mucosa
at endoscopy and is confirmed to have intestinal metaplasia by biopsy of the tubular esophagus" [7].

There are three important components to this definition
that are worth highlighting. First, intestinal metaplasia
must be present. It has been argued, however, that, even if
not present initially, intestinal metaplasia could be subsequently identified in endoscopically characteristic columnar mucosa. This has led to proposals from the British
Society of Gastroenterology to exclude the requirement of
intestinal metaplasia from the definition of Barrett's
esophagus [8]. However, the clinical significance of changing the definition is unclear, since it is the intestinal specialized epithelium that is associated with adenocarcinoma [6,
9, 10].

Second, this definition encompasses not only the classical Barrett's esophagus (≥3 cm of columnar-lined mucosa
of the distal esophagus with intestinal metaplasia) but also
short segment Barrett's esophagus (SSBE) defined as specialized columnar epithelium lining less than 3 cm of the
distal esophagus [11]. Although the risk for developing
dysplasia and esophageal cancer with SSBE is lower than
with classical longer-segment Barrett's esophagus (LSBE)
(OR 0.55), it is not statistically significantly less. Moreover,
as SSBE is much more common than LSBE, most adenocarcinomas arising from Barrett's likely arise in SSBE not LSBE
even if the incidence in LSBE is higher [12–18].

Finally, intestinal metaplasia must be present in the
tubular esophagus (not just the gastric cardia) for a diagnosis of Barrett's esophagus, as the latter does not have the
same implications as intestinal metaplasia of the tubular
esophagus and may actually be a variant of a normal histological finding of the cardia.

Epidemiology

Incidence and prevalence

The estimates of prevalence of Barrett's vary according
to the population studied and the definition used.
Approximately 6–12% of patients undergoing endoscopy
for symptoms of GERD have documented the presence of
Barrett's esophagus, with the majority having SSBE (≈
6–10% versus 5% LSBE) [12, 19–21]. In patients with mod-

Evidence-Based Gastroenterology and Hepatology, 3rd edition.
J. McDonald, A.K. Burroughs, B. Feagan, and M.B. Fennerty. © 2010
Blackwell Publishing Ltd

erate to severe erosive esophagitis, rates of underlying Barrett's esophagus may be as high as 27% [22]. For patients with dyspeptic symptoms as opposed to only GERD symptoms, the prevalence was 2.4% [23]. Another study of dyspeptic patients obtained a rate of only 0.3%, but this estimate excluded patients with alarm symptoms and those over 45 years [24]. Others have also obtained an estimate of ≤1% in unselected patient populations undergoing endoscopy [12, 25, 26]. Autopsy studies, on the other hand, suggest that the prevalence of Barrett's esophagus is about 21 times higher than that detected endoscopically, and these data suggest that the vast majority of patients with Barrett's esophagus remain unrecognized [27].

The incidence of Barrett's esophagus has continued to increase since the 1970s, and has now reached approximately 10 new cases per 100,000/year [28–30]. The median age of development of the condition has been estimated at 40 years and the mean age at diagnosis at 63 years of age [25]. Although this increase in incidence parallels the increasing use of endoscopy, this is probably not the only explanation, and the true incidence has probably increased as well.

Risk factors

Barrett's esophagus appears to occur predominately in male Caucasians [6, 19]. Although the prevalence of Barrett's esophagus in black, Asian and Hispanic populations has been occasionally found to be higher than expected [31–33], most observational data suggest that the prevalence of Barrett's oesophagus is significantly lower (OR 0.35) for these groups compared to white populations [34, 35]. One might expect that as lifestyle and dietary habits change in developing regions, the prevalence will approximate that of the Western World. The decreasing prevalence of *Helicobacter pylori* infection has also been suggested to play a role in the increased incidence, but this association, although plausible, is controversial [36–38].

In addition to age, gender and race, longer duration of GERD is also a risk factor for Barrett's esophagus [19, 38, 39]. Compared to patients with reflux symptoms of less than one year, Barrett's esophagus was three times more common if reflux symptoms were present for one to five years, five times more common for symptoms present for five to ten years, or more than six times more common if reflux symptoms were present longer than ten years [39]. Increased severity of nocturnal reflux symptoms [38–40] and increased complications of GERD such as esophagitis, ulceration, and bleeding are also associated with an increased prevalence [38] but the evidence regarding association with peptic strictures is conflicting [38, 41, 42]. There is also an association of hiatal hernia with Barrett's esophagus [43, 44]. Although these findings are associated with a higher prevalence of Barrett's esophagus, many patients with this condition have reflux symptoms no different than those experienced by other GERD patients [27, 45].

Within the last ten years, some controversy in the literature has emerged concerning the suggestion that obesity is a risk factor for reflux and, by extension, Barrett's esophagus and esophageal adenocarcinoma. Recently, it has been shown that visceral fat deposition that is associated with an increased abdominal circumference (greater than 80 cm) appears to confer perhaps the greatest risk association, potentially explaining the male predominance of Barrett's esophagus [46]. The reasons for this are not entirely clear, but it has been hypothesized that the metabolic activity of visceral fat interferes with the production of cytokines that protect against carcinogenesis [47].

Recently, some data have emerged implicating diet in the relationship between GERD, Barrett's and cancer. In a case-control study, the odds ratio of Barrett's was significantly less in the highest quartile of fruit/vegetable consumers (OR 0.25–0.56) compared with the lowest quartile. Supplemental antioxidants (Vitamin C, E and beta carotene) did not appear to affect the odds ratios [48]. Another recent study examining the effect of "Western" diet (fast-food and meat-based) versus "health-conscious" diet (fruits, vegetables, and non-fried fish) demonstrated a clear advantage for the latter in the association with Barrett's (OR 0.35) [49]. Although no randomized trials have been conducted as of yet, such findings suggest a possible benefit to a diet rich in fruits and vegetables with minimal meat or fast-food consumption in decreasing the incidence of Barrett's and its associated complication of esophageal adenocarcinoma.

Natural history

The survival of a patient with Barrett's esophagus is very similar to that of patients with benign esophageal disorders such as achalasia or Schatzki's ring [50]. The overwhelming majority of patients with Barrett's esophagus will never develop esophageal adenocarcinoma. Yet, if it were not for this association, Barrett's esophagus would not have much clinical importance.

Early studies estimated the incidence of esophageal adenocarcinoma in Barrett's esophagus at 1–2% per annum. More recent analyses of epidemiologic studies have suggested an incidence ranging from 0.5 to 0.6% per annum, in part due to publication bias of the more positive results with initial studies [50]. This incidence is also probably an overestimate as it likely reflects a higher risk population, with men progressing twice as quickly as women [51–56].

Nevertheless, Barrett's esophagus is definitely associated with the occurrence of esophageal adenocarcinoma (EAC), and this cancer is on a dramatic rise in Western societies.

Since the mid-1970s, the incidence of EAC in Caucasian men from the USA rose from 0.7/100,000 person-years to an estimated 5.69/100,000 person-years by 2004 [12, 30]. This rise is not thought to be due to the previous misclassification of gastroesophageal junction esophageal carcinomas as gastric cancer, since there has not been a concomitant decrease of gastric cardia cancers [12]. The proportion of esophageal cancer due to adenocarcinoma has also increased substantially in the same period, but the absolute number of all esophageal cancers is still quite low in comparison to colorectal cancer, for example, which is ten times more common [12, 57]. Indeed, EAC remains a relatively uncommon cancer, ranked fourteenth for males and eighteenth for females in estimated new cancer cases in Canada in 2008 [58].

The length (extent) of Barrett's esophagus is a risk factor for esophageal adenocarcinoma. A landmark study published in 2000 showed that a 5 cm difference in segment length was associated with a 1.7-fold (95% CI: 0.8–3.8) increase in cancer risk [17]. Although this difference is not statistically significant, a similar association has been repeatedly demonstrated. A meta-analysis published in 2007 demonstrated a statistically significant increase in adenocarcinoma with longer segments of Barrett's esophagus [18]. Other reported risk factors for esophageal adenocarcinoma include severity, frequency and duration of reflux symptoms [59–61], size of hiatal hernia [62], obesity [63], smoking [64] and a diet low in raw fruit content [65]. The use of medications that reduce the lower esophageal sphincter pressure has also been found to be associated with esophageal cancer, in some but not in all studies [66, 67]. Also controversial is the possibility that *H. pylori* protects against GERD and esophageal cancer. A meta-analysis of twenty studies demonstrated a lower prevalence of *H. pylori* in patients with GERD (OR 0.6) [68]. A beneficial effect of *H. pylori* on reducing the risk of development of esophageal adenocarcinoma (OR 0.37 in patients under 50 years of age) has also been suggested by a case-control study [69]. It appears that infection with *cagA + H. pylori* is particularly protective [70, 71]. One study found the prevalence of *H. pylori* infection with *cagA* + strains to be inversely associated with GERD complications (non-erosive GERD 41% *cagA* +, erosive GERD 31%, Barrett's esophagus 13% and Barrett's with dysplasia or adenocarcinoma 0%) [70]. These apparent *associations*, however, still remain controversial and are *not necessarily causal (or protective)*.

The presence and degree of dysplasia associated with Barrett's esophagus is also a risk factor for the subsequent development of esophageal adenocarcinoma. Dysplasia is a histological diagnosis primarily considered as absent, indefinite, low grade, or high grade. There is significant interobserver variability (less than 50% agreement) in the interpretation of low grade dysplasia and there are few prospective studies related to risk [72, 73]. Estimates of

progression from normal, indefinite or low-grade dysplasia to high-grade dysplasia or adenocarcinoma are highly variable but there appears to be a low risk [73]. Patients with high-grade dysplasia, however, have been shown to have a substantially increased risk of cancer. Reid *et al.* [74] found that cancer developed in 33 of 76 patients (43%) with high grade dysplasia, compared to 9 of 251 (4%) with negative, indefinite or low-grade dysplasia by five years. The results from different studies, however, vary substantially with five to seven-year cumulative cancer incidence estimates of 16% to 59%. This variation largely appears to be related to prevalent cancers (those found within a year of diagnosis of cancer) suggesting that the lower rate is the more accurate [72, 75, 76]. Other studies have suggested that flow cytometry can also be used to predict outcome [74].

Pathogenesis

Barrett's esophagus is felt to result from a perturbation in the repair of mucosal injury of the esophagus in an abnormal milieu of gastroesophageal reflux (abnormally acidic and/or acid- and bile-exposed esophageal environment) in a genetically predisposed individual. This hypothesis is based, in part, on animal studies, that demonstrated that excision of the esophageal mucosa results in re-epithelialization of the esophagus with columnar epithelium only if performed in an environment of acid reflux or acid and bile reflux [77, 78]. Although there is no direct human experimental evidence that reflux causes Barrett's esophagus, this theory is supported by human ambulatory esophageal pH monitoring studies, which demonstrate a greater esophageal acid exposure in patients with Barrett's esophagus compared to GERD patients without Barrett's esophagus [79, 80]. In addition, the duration of esophageal acid exposure correlates with the length of Barrett's esophagus [81]. The increase in esophageal acid exposure does not appear to be due to increased acid production, as no difference is present in gastric acid outputs [82].

The most widely accepted conceptual approach to GERD is that it represents a spectrum of disease that ranges from non-endoscopic reflux disease (NERD) to esophagitis, Barrett's esophagus, dysplasia and esophageal adenocarcinoma (Figure 3.1a). Acid reflux is felt to contribute to esophagitis and Barrett's, but the cause of development of dysplasia in Barrett's patients is unknown. Patients with NERD, however, uncommonly develop erosive esophagitis [83] and Barrett's esophagus is almost always diagnosed on first endoscopy [84]. It is for this reason that Fass *et al.* [85] have suggested a new conceptual model that divides GERD into three distinct groups of patients: NERD, erosive esophagitis and Barrett's esophagus (Figure 3.1b). They suggested that patients do not usually move into a differ-

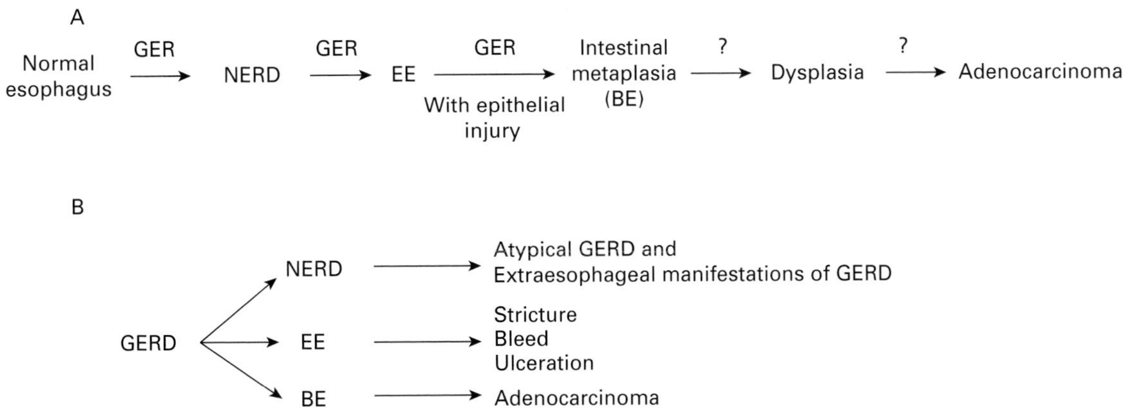

A

Normal esophagus $\xrightarrow{\text{GER}}$ NERD $\xrightarrow{\text{GER}}$ EE $\xrightarrow[\substack{\text{With epithelial} \\ \text{injury}}]{\text{GER}}$ Intestinal metaplasia (BE) $\xrightarrow{?}$ Dysplasia $\xrightarrow{?}$ Adenocarcinoma

B

GERD
- NERD → Atypical GERD and Extraesophageal manifestations of GERD
- EE → Stricture / Bleed / Ulceration
- BE → Adenocarcinoma

Figure 3.1 (a) Conventional concept for GERD.
(b) New concept of GERD as three distinct entities and complications associated with each, Fass *et al.* [85].
Abbreviations: GER: gastroesophageal reflux; NERD: nonendoscopic reflux disease; EE: erosive esophagitis; BE: Barrett's esophagus.

ent group, but each group has its own potential complications (noted in Figure 3.1b).

Diagnosis

As noted previously, the diagnosis of Barrett's esophagus requires the demonstration of intestinal metaplasia on targeted biopsy sampling of endoscopically abnormal appearing esophageal mucosa [7]. The definition and diagnosis of Barrett's is difficult for several reasons. First, there are no symptoms specific for this condition. For the most part, the symptoms are essentially identical to those of GERD and most patients are asymptomatic [27]. In addition, accurate identification of the location of the gastroesophageal junction is required in order to determine if the squamo-columnar junction is displaced proximal to this location, since this displacement is what alerts the endoscopist to the possibility of the diagnosis of Barrett's and thus leads to biopsy of the mucosa. The former junction can at times be very difficult to determine endoscopically because of the presence of a hiatal hernia, esophagitis, and the constant movement of the area. This is highlighted by a multicenter study in which only 72% of the endoscopists correctly recorded endoscopic landmarks in the diagnosis of Barrett's esophagus [86]. SSBE can thus be particularly difficult to identify and distinguish from an irregular Z line (a normal anatomical finding). This is very important because intestinal metaplasia in the gastric cardia does not seem to have the same implications as intestinal metaplasia of the esophagus and, indeed, may be a normal histological finding in this location. Erythema or erosive esophagitis can also impair the visual recognition of Barrett's esophagus, and repeat endoscopy after treatment with acid suppression may be necessary to make the diagnosis of Barrett's in this situation [87].

Currently, intestinal metaplasia is a prerequisite in order to make the diagnosis of Barrett's esophagus. This fact, however, seems not to be fully understood as some pathologists continue to classify patients without intestinal metaplasia as Barrett's esophagus. In one study, correct identification of intestinal metaplasia without dysplasia occurred in only 35% of 20 community-based pathologists [88]. The hematoxylin and eosin stain combined with alcian blue at pH 2.5 can be used to facilitate the recognition of the acid mucin-containing goblet cells characteristic of intestinal metaplasia [5].

A further difficulty with diagnosis is sampling error. When obtaining biopsies for Barrett's esophagus, samples may miss the area with metaplasia and hence fail to lead to the diagnosis. This addresses the important issue of the number of biopsies required; intuitively, the more endoscopic biopsies taken, the more accurate the diagnosis of Barrett's. It has also been suggested that endoscopic adjuncts such as chromoendoscopy and/or narrow band imaging (NBI) may help in targeting biopsies and thus increase the diagnostic yield. Methylene blue, toluene blue, indigo carmine, and Lugol's iodine have all been used as chromoendoscopic agents to identify specialized intestinal metaplasia as well as the characteristic surface patterns suggestive of neoplasia [89–92]. These contrast agents are sprayed over the esophageal mucosa at the time of endoscopy, with areas of intestinal metaplasia and dysplasia demonstrating a variety of characteristic staining patterns. However, interpretation of the staining process may be tedious, and the results are not necessarily reproducible [93]. More recently, the pairing of magnification endoscopy [94] with narrow-band imaging (NBI) has emerged as a new modality that may obviate the need for staining altogether.

Dysplasia is only detectable histologically. Dysplasia, the next step in the neoplastic process, represents a change in architecture of the metaplastic glands and is associated with individual cellular nuclear abnormalities. Dysplasia is felt to progress along a continuum from no dysplasia to low-grade dysplasia, high-grade dysplasia and finally adenocarcinoma, although the time course of this progression is highly variable and not inevitable. Furthermore, it is likely reversible in the stages leading up to adenocarcinoma. Dysplasia is often focal and not easily detectable endoscopically without the aid of stains, magnification and narrow-band imaging, rendering the targeting of biopsy sampling difficult. It has been established that random biopsies taken every 2cm detect 50% fewer cancers than four-quadrant biopsies taken every 1cm [95]. The latter approach has yet to be recommended in formal guidelines because of the effort involved in following such an intensive biopsy protocol. In addition, there is significant interobserver variation in the diagnosis and grading of dysplasia by both academic and non-academic pathologists [12]. Reactive change due to esophagitis is difficult to distinguish from dysplasia and further compounds the problem. However, recent data from a randomized controlled trial demonstrated that roughly half the biopsies are required to detect dysplasia with methylene blue-targeting compared with four-quadrant biopsies every 2cm within Barrett's metaplasia [96]. Furthermore, the combination of NBI and high-magnification endoscopy reportedly identifies microstructural changes suggestive of dysplasia with a sensitivity and specificity of 90% and 100% respectively [97]. Although not formally recommended yet, such advances in endoscopic imaging are likely to be incorporated into endoscopic practice if confirmed and reproducible.

Although the diagnosis of Barrett's esophagus can be difficult, if the endoscopist suspects that the level of the squamo-columnar junction is above the esophagogastric junction (the proximal margin of the gastric folds), biopsies are required. If intestinal metaplasia is present, then the diagnosis of Barrett's esophagus has been established.

Treatment

The goals of treatment for Barrett's esophagus are the same as for GERD; the control of symptoms and maintenance of healed mucosa [6].

Acid suppression

Lifestyle modifications (including dietary adjustment) may help control GERD symptoms somewhat, but these measures are unlikely to have an effect on the regression of Barrett's metaplasia. In fact, some individuals with Barrett's esophagus are asymptomatic, possibly due to the replacement of the normal squamous epithelium with the acid insensitive Barrett's epithelium. Nevertheless, these patients may still benefit from acid suppression given the potential regression of Barrett's metaplasia as discussed below [6].

Histamine H_2-receptor antagonists (H_2-RA) often improve GERD symptoms but they do not effect regression of Barrett's metaplasia [98, 99]. Proton pump inhibitors (PPI) are the most potent antisecretory agents, superior to H_2-RA in the treatment of symptoms and the healing of esophagitis [100]. In Barrett's esophagus, these same endpoints are effectively achieved with PPIs [101–103]. Some studies have also suggested a modest endoscopic regression of Barrett's esophagus with use of PPIs, although these usually utilized a high dose PPI [99, 101, 104–106]. In a randomized controlled trial, Peters *et al.* [99] demonstrated that omeprazole 40mg bid resulted in an 8% reduction of surface area of Barrett's esophagus and a 6% decrease in length, superior to the comparator, ranitidine 150mg bid (Table 3.1). There is also evidence that normalization of intra-esophageal acid exposure decreases cellular proliferation rates and use of PPIs has been associated with a decreased incidence of dysplasia [107, 108]. It is noteworthy that, despite adequate symptom control, even high dose PPI therapy often does not normalize esophageal acid exposure in patients with Barrett's metaplasia [109–112]. However, there is no evidence that normalization of pH leads to a decreased incidence of adenocarcinoma and, therefore, it is not rational to routinely perform pH-metry to determine the level of acid suppression. What is often seen with acid suppression is an increase in islands of squamous epithelium within the Barrett's segment. Biopsies of such islands have often shown underlying intestinal metaplasia, indicating that complete regression of Barrett's does not occur with pharmacological acid inhibition [113]. At this point, no study has shown a reduction of esophageal adenocarcinoma or mortality, although a large randomized control trial examining PPIs and/or aspirin as a chemopreventive agent is underway [114]. Nevertheless, PPIs remain the best pharmacological treatment for Barrett's presently available. **B2**

Given that even high dose PPI may fail to normalize esophageal pH [109–112, 115–117], some have considered anti-reflux surgery as an alternative to decreasing cancer risk with the consideration that continued reflux is the promoting agent. Surgery does provide excellent control of symptoms, and the development of squamous islands after surgery suggests possible regression. One randomized trial comparing medical therapy with anti-reflux surgery with follow up for one to eleven years (Table 3.1) demonstrated a 25% rate of some regression in the surgically treated group (9% progression, 3/32) compared to 7% regression (41% progression, 11/27) in the medical group [118]. However, complete regression of Barrett's metaplasia with surgery is very uncommon and may, in fact, reflect "pseu-

Table 3.1 Summary of randomized controlled trials for the treatment of Barrett's esophagus discussed in this chapter[a].

Therapy	Treatments compared (n)	Outcome	Reference
Acid suppression	Omeprazole 40 mg bid (26) Ranitidine 150 mg bid (27)	• Regression in Barrett's length (p = 0.06) and area (p = 0.02) with omeprazole compared to ranitidine	Peters *et al.* [99]
Surgery	Medical (ranitidine or omeprazole) (27) Anti-reflux surgery (32)	• Length of Barrett's esophagus decreased in 8/27, (increased in 3) in the surgical group compared to 2/32 (increased in 11) in the medical group (p < 0.01). • Dysplasia appeared in 6 medically treated patients (mild in 5, severe in 1) versus 1 surgically treated patient (which was severe)	Ortiz *et al.* [118]
Surgery	Medical (ranitidine 150 mg bid) (91)[b] Surgical therapy (38)[b]	• No difference in incidence of adenocarcinoma between groups, but insufficient power to detect such a difference	Spechler *et al.* [124]
Ablation	PDT with photophrin and omeprazole (138) Omeprazole 20 mg bid (70)	• Ablation of all high grade dysplasia in 77% of PDT group versus 39% in omeprazole group (p < 0.0001) • Cancer in 15% versus 29% respectively (p = 0.027)	Overholt *et al.* [141]
Ablation	PDT + 5 Aminolevulinic acid (ALA) (18) placebo + ALA (16)	• 16/18 of the PDT group had some response compared to 2/18 of the placebo group (p < 0.001)	Ackroyd *et al.* [142]

[a]This list is not meant to be an exhaustive list of all randomized clinical trials in the literature.
[b]This includes all GERD patients, not just those with Barrett's esophagus.
Abbreviations: PDT: Photodynamic therapy.

doregression" due to surgical repositioning of the esophagus [12]. Some studies have also reported a reduced risk of progression of low grade dysplasia [119]. However, both dysplasia and cancer continue to occur after surgery [120–124]. Csendes *et al.* [123] found that dysplasia developed in 17 (10.5%) and adenocarcinoma in 4 (2.5%) of 161 patients who had undergone surgery at late (7–21 years) follow-up. In a small randomized controlled trial comparing medical to surgical anti-reflux therapy, there was no significant difference between groups in incidence of esophageal cancer (Table 3.1) [124], although this study probably lacked power to demonstrate a true difference should one exist. A more recent retrospective observational study of Barrett's patients who underwent Rosetti-Nissen fundoplication for medically-refractory reflux demonstrated regression of LGD to nondysplastic Barrett's esophagus in six of eight patients, and complete regression of metaplasia to normal mucosa in eight of fifty-seven patients (14%). However, six of fifty-seven (11%) demonstrated an increase in length of involvement with Barrett's postoperatively, and two patients went on to develop adenocarcinoma after surgery [125]. Hence, surgery does not reliably prevent dysplasia or cancer and, therefore, does not obviate the need for surveillance and should not be promoted as a cancer prevention therapy.

Chemoprevention of esophageal adenocarcinoma with anti-inflammatory agents

The use of aspirin (ASA) or nonsteroidal anti-inflammatory drugs (NSAID) has been demonstrated to be associated with a significantly reduced risk of developing esophageal adenocarcinoma [126, 127]. Cycooxygenase-2 (COX-2) expression is increased in Barrett's epithelium [128] and COX-2 inhibition has been shown to reduce cell growth in esophageal adenocarcinoma cell lines, as well as inhibit cancer formation in animal models of Barrett's [129, 130]. Modeling the use of aspirin in patients with HGD suggests that this may be a very cost-effective intervention [131]. As such, it has been suggested that using NSAIDs and ASA as chemoprevention agents in Barrett's esophagus may be a viable management option. In a randomized controlled trial reported in 2007 in which 100 patients with low or high-grade dysplasia were randomized to receive celecoxib 200 mg twice daily or placebo, no significant differences were demonstrated in progression of either extent of Barrett's, dysplasia, or cancer at 48 weeks [132]. The possibility of a type II error exists in this study. Despite significant biological plausibility and epidemiological evidence of an ASA/NSAID chemoprevention effect in Barrett's, at this time no recommendation for the use of

NSAIDs as chemopreventive agents in patients with Barrett's can be made. Studies involving larger populations and follow-up periods are in progress and may provide a definitive answer in the future [12, 133, 134].

Ablative therapies

Given the theory that Barrett's esophagus develops in the predisposed individual as a consequence of a perturbation in healing of the injured esophageal epithelium in an abnormal esophageal acidic environment, it was further hypothesized that reversal of Barrett's would require re-injuring of the metaplastic epithelium with ablative therapy in an acid normalized esophageal environment, resulting in re-epithelialization with a native normal squamous epithelium. This effect could eliminate or decrease the risk for dysplasia and esophageal adenocarcinoma. Endoscopic injury or ablation of Barrett's has been demonstrated with a variety of endoscopic techniques, including thermal techniques (radiofrequency energy, electrocoagulation, heater probe, argon plasma coagulation, or laser), cryotherapy, chemical induced injury with photodynamic therapy, or resection via endoscopic mucosal resection.

Reports using a wide variety of different thermal techniques have suggested both complete and incomplete histological regression in Barrett's esophagus, but complications are not uncommon [12]. Multipolar electrocoagulation (MPEC) has resulted in a fibrotic and friable esophagus with adhesions to the pleura in one patient [135]. Argon plasma coagulation (APC) has had significant complications including chest pain and odynophagia (58%), fever and pleural effusion (15%), strictures (9%), pneumomediastinum (3%) and perforation [136, 137]. In addition, one study using heater probe reported buried islands of intestinal metaplasia in 23% of patients [138].

Photodynamic therapy (PDT) is a process in which a light-sensitive agent, which concentrates in neoplastic tissue, is administered and subsequently activated by light of an appropriate wavelength. This results in selective damage of the neoplastic tissue. The sensitizing agents used include porfimer sodium, a hematoporphyrin derivative, or 5-aminolaevulinic acid (5-ALA). Reports describe elimination and regression of dysplasia and early cancers, but complete regression of Barrett's was not achieved in the majority of patients [139]. A randomized trial compared PDT using sodium porfimer to medical therapy with omeprazole in 208 patients (Table 3.1) with high grade dysplasia [140]. At 12-month follow-up, 9% of the PDT group developed cancer compared to 19% of the omeprazole group (NS), but strictures developed in 38% of the patients who underwent PDT. The same authors reported five-year follow-up data on an incomplete subset of these patients in 2007. They demonstrated twice the rate of HGD elimination (77% versus 39%) and nearly half the progres-

sion to cancer (15% versus 29%) for the PDT group. The reported strictures were limited to the first phase of the trial in the PDT group, and all had resolved at five-year follow-up [141]. Another randomized study compared PDT with 5-ALA to placebo in low-grade dysplasia patients and achieved regression of dysplasia in 89% (16/18) versus 11% (2/18) of patients in the placebo group (Table 3.1), but only 30% of the surface area was eliminated in the 5-ALA group [142]. Hence, some risk of progression for residual neoplastic and non-neoplastic tissue still remains with this intervention. In fact, a case of adenocarcinoma developing underneath new squamous epithelium after treatment for high grade dysplasia with PDT using sodium porfimer has been reported [12]. **A1d**

Radiofrequency ablation (RFA) is a relatively new technique that involves the application of high-frequency energy through an endoscopic balloon probe or contact device. The device, comprised of a radiofrequency energy generator and ablation catheter, is usually mounted on a balloon to ensure circumferential ablation. Early uncontrolled trials demonstrate considerable success with this technique. Sharma *et al.* demonstrated elimination of Barrett's with RFA of 70% at one year of follow-up, in addition to a complete absence of buried IM (or squamous overgrowth) [143]. Recent studies have also examined the use of RFA for the treatment of low-grade and high-grade dysplasia, demonstrating elimination rates for both non-dysplastic IM and dysplasia in excess of 90% after one to two years of follow-up [144, 145]. Furthermore, stricturing and buried islands of IM rarely (if ever) occurred in these studies, suggesting potential for this Barrett's ablation modality as a safer (versus PDT) and/or more efficacious (versus MPE or APC) therapy. **B4**

Endoscopic mucosal resection (EMR) has also been performed in patients with and without visible lesions within Barrett's esophagus. In one study, EMR resulted in complete local remission of 97% (34/35) of patients with low-risk lesions characterized by diameter of less than 20mm, well or moderately differentiated histology, lesions limited to mucosa, or non-ulcerated lesions, compared to 59% (13/22) of patients with high-risk lesions characterized by diameter of greater than 20mm, poorly differentiated histology, lesions extending into submucosa, or ulcerated lesions [146]. However, metachronous lesions or recurrent high-grade dysplasia or cancer were detected in the subsequent year in 17% of the low risk and 14% of the high risk group. Larger studies with longer follow-up are required, but EMR also appears to be relatively safe and promising as an effective non-surgical alternative for management of neoplastic Barrett's metaplasia. **B4**

With all endoscopic Barrett's ablative therapies, even if all of the Barrett's epithelium is thought to be eliminated, some residual intestinal metaplasia may be present underneath the neosquamous epithelium, along with the continued risk of cancer development. Thus, these patients have a continued need for surveillance which may be more difficult given that the endoscopic landmarks may be less easily identifiable after ablative therapy [12]. In addition, most of these techniques are associated with a small but significant risk of stricture and perforation. They are (for the most part) costly, the methods have not yet been standardized, and the results are likely very operator dependent. At this time, endoscopic ablative therapy is a reasonable option in the Barrett's patient with high grade dysplasia or superficial adenocarcinoma. **A1d** There are no data allowing one to recommend these therapies in the Barrett's patient without neoplasia, since continued surveillance will still be required, and the risk/benefit ratio is not firmly established.

Screening and surveillance

Screening for the detection of Barrett's esophagus is currently recommended in patients with chronic GERD symptoms, especially in those over age 50 [7, 147]. This recommendation is based in part on the observation that patients with a longer duration of symptoms have a higher prevalence of Barrett's esophagus [39, 60]. GERD patients who are white, male or have more severe acid reflux also have a higher prevalence of Barrett's esophagus [6, 79, 80]; hence the emphasis on screening this population. Most authors have recommended that a "once in a lifetime" endoscopy should be performed in all GERD patients (based on the premise that Barrett's occurs early on in a GERD patient and thus repeat screening endoscopy is not required), although the optimal timing and utility of such a recommendation is unknown [148]. This approach seems to be favored by Canadian gastroenterologists, of whom 76% agreed that all patients with chronic GERD should have a "once in a lifetime" endoscopy [149]. Although the asymptomatic Barrett's esophagus patient would not be picked up with this screening method, a generalized screening endoscopy in the general population is not recommended.

The aim of the "once in a lifetime" gastroscopy in GERD patients is to detect Barrett's esophagus, as this entity increases the risk of developing esophageal adenocarcinoma. Some have argued that cancer surveillance once non-neoplastic Barrett's is discovered is too costly and/or may be ineffective in improving outcomes. In Barrett's patients with dysplasia there is little controversy that either heightened surveillance or an intervention should be recommended, as it is the only method currently available to identify the high risk patients with dysplasia who may benefit from treatment, including new ablative therapies.

Arguments in support of a screening and surveillance strategy

The rationale for screening for and carrying out surveillance of patients with Barrett's esophagus is based on the fact that GERD is a risk factor for esophageal adenocarcinoma (EAC) [60], that Barrett's esophagus represents an intermediate step between esophagitis and adenocarcinoma (and is also the only known precursor of esophageal adenocarcinoma) [6], that the rate of esophageal adenocarcinoma is steadily increasing in Western societies [150] and the prognosis for esophageal adenocarcinoma is very poor unless detected early [151]. Over 50% of all esophageal tumors on the National Cancer database for 1988 were stage III or IV at the time of detection with five-year disease specific survivals of 15% and 3% respectively [152]. It is argued that surveillance programs will detect dysplasia or cancers at an earlier stage when the prognosis is much better. In stage I or II EAC cases the five-year disease specific survival rates were 42% and 29% respectively [152]. In addition, small retrospective observational studies suggest that Barrett's surveillance improves survival. A comparison was made between patients who initially presented with esophageal adenocarcinoma (n = 54) versus those in whom the cancer had been detected during surveillance (n = 16) of Barrett's esophagus [153]. Surveyed patients had significantly earlier stages than non-surveyed patients (75% had stage 0 or I, 25% stage II, and 0% stage III compared to 26%, 25% and 56% respectively, for non-surveyed patients). Survival was also significantly better in the surveyed group, with a two-year survival of 86% versus 43%. Similar results were also demonstrated in an earlier retrospective study comparing 17 adenocarcinoma patients found from surveillance programs versus 35 patients who had not been in a program [154]. Again, the cancers were at an earlier stage and survival was significantly greater in the surveyed group than in the non-surveyed group prior to diagnosis. A third study obtained similar results, with a five-year survival of 62% in those who underwent surveillance, compared to 20% in those that did not [155]. In addition, a prospective study from the UK reported on the results of a surveillance program involving 126 patients and spanning more than nine years; although there was no non-surveillance comparator group, 4% of all patients with Barrett's developed adenocarcinoma, half of which were cured by esophagectomy [156]. These data lead to the recommendation by many experts to advocate for a Barrett's screening and surveillance program in higher risk GERD patients. **B3**

Arguments against a surveillance strategy

Although the incidence of esophageal adenocarcinoma is on the rise, the absolute prevalence of this condition remains relatively low in comparison to other malignancies such as colon cancer. In addition, the benefits of screening and surveying patients with Barrett's esophagus are not as clear as they are with colonic polyps and colon cancer. Decision makers may believe that it is more appropriate to spend health care resources on proven cancer preventive strategies. Furthermore, 93–98% of esophageal adenocarcinomas occur in patients without prior diagnosis of Barrett's esophagus [28, 157–159]. Most patients with Barrett's esophagus do not die from esophageal cancer [160–162]. GERD is very common and approximately 90% of these patients do not have Barrett's esophagus [21]. Surveillance is expensive, time consuming (prevents endoscopists from carrying out other tasks) and not error free; sampling error is a problem, as is interobserver variation in endoscopic and histological diagnosis. In addition, many patients with Barrett's esophagus are asymptomatic. The prevalence of Barrett's esophagus at autopsy was 20 times higher than the estimate from endoscopic diagnosis [27]. Thus, for each case of Barrett's, up to another 20 cases go unrecognized. Considering that the true prevalence of Barrett's esophagus in the community is much higher than previously thought, the observed incidence of adenocarcinoma of the esophagus is very small in relation to the community prevalence of Barrett's epithelium [163].

A group of 166 patients with Barrett's esophagus who chose not to undergo surveillance were re-examined a mean of 9.3 years later [162]. They determined that the incidence of esophageal cancer was one in 180 patient years; a 40-fold increased risk compared to an age and gender-matched group from the general population. All eight patients with cancer were symptomatic and the cancer was detected at diagnostic endoscopy. Only two of these patients died because of their esophageal cancer; one of postoperative complications and the other four years postoperatively with liver metastases. Three had successful surgery, and three died of unrelated illness (pancreatitis, myocardial infarction and asthma). During the follow-up period, there were 77 other unrelated deaths at a mean age of 75 years. The authors concluded that an endoscopic surveillance program in this population of patients with Barrett's would have had marginal benefit, as so few actually died of esophageal cancer. A Danish study found that only 1.3% of patients had a diagnosis of Barrett's esophagus more than one year before cancer was identified [157]. Thus, most cancers were detected in patients who would not have entered into a surveillance program, suggesting that such a strategy would be unlikely to reduce the death rate from esophageal cancer in the general population.

Cost-effectiveness

Unfortunately, there are no randomized controlled trials of surveillance strategies. A cost-effectiveness study examining screening assumed that GERD patients underwent a one-time gastroscopy at age 60 [164]. The calculated screening cost of $24,700 per life-year saved, is considered to be reasonable for a cancer screening program. However, the results were based on a relatively high prevalence of Barrett's esophagus, high-grade dysplasia, and adenocarcinoma, a high sensitivity and specificity of endoscopy, and a minor reduction in quality of life after esophagectomy. Any variation in these parameters altered the cost effectiveness of the strategy.

Another report estimated the cost of detecting one esophageal cancer at $23,000 for male and $65,000 for female patients with Barrett's esophagus [165]. Another found that the cost was lower than the cost of surveillance mammography [166]. Sonnenberg *et al.* [167] found that the incremental cost-effectiveness of surveillance every other year was approximately $16,700 per year of life saved. Provenzale *et al.* [51] evaluated surveillance strategies with a Markov model, and concluded that surveillance every five years was the preferred strategy, with a cost of $98,000 per quality-adjusted life-year gained.

Conclusions regarding screening and surveillance of Barrett's metaplasia

Applying the World Health Organization's 10 principles of early disease detection helps determine whether screening for Barrett's esophagus is beneficial [168, 169]. Although some of these criteria are met, many are not (Table 3.2), and thus one cannot make a recommendation for screening for Barrett's either in the general population or in those with chronic GERD. Furthermore, at this time a recommendation as to whether surveillance should be undertaken once non-neoplastic Barrett's is discovered cannot be made. In the absence of a definitive study, there are arguments to support both sides of the controversy. However, recognizing that Barrett's mucosa is a risk factor for esophageal adenocarcinoma, it may be difficult to disregard present recommendations for surveillance endoscopy until evidence to the contrary is available.

How to perform surveillance

Screening is currently recommended for patients with chronic GERD symptoms [6]. Some are certainly more at risk of Barrett's, and perhaps screening should be focused on those at higher risk (such as white males over age 50 with greater than 10 years of GERD symptoms). Once Barrett's is established, the patient should have the pros and cons of a surveillance program discussed with them. Patients who have co-morbid illness which would not allow them to be candidates for esophagectomy or ablative therapy are unlikely to receive much benefit from surveillance.

Table 3.2 World Health Organization principles for early disease detection.

Principles	Are principles met in Barrett's esophagus?
1 The target health problem is important	Yes (esophageal cancer)
2 There should be an accepted treatment for the target problem	Yes (endoscopic ablation, surgery, or intensive endoscopic surveillance)
3 Facilities for diagnosis and treatment should be available	Yes
4 There should be a recognized latent or early symptomatic stage	Yes (dysplasia)
5 There should exist a suitable screening test or examination	Yes
6 The test should be acceptable to the population to be screened	Yes
7 The natural history and development of the condition should be adequately understood	Possibly
8 There should be an agreed policy on who to treat	No
9 The process of case finding should be cost effective	No
10 Case finding should be a continuing process	Possibly

Updated and modified from references 168 and 169.

During surveillance gastroscopy, four-quadrant biopsy specimens should be obtained at least every 1–2 cm along the entire length of Barrett's epithelium. The endoscopy should be performed in patients receiving acid suppressive therapy so that esophagitis and reactive changes do not confound the diagnosis. In addition, any mucosal abnormalities detected at endoscopy should be targeted for biopsy [12]. It has been suggested that 1 cm intervals with jumbo biopsy forceps is more accurate [95, 170], but this is more labor intensive and also requires endoscopy with a therapeutic gastroscope. Hence, this form of intensive surveillance may not be practical in community practice, despite appearing to be the optimal endoscopic surveillance method.

Summary of practice guidelines

Guidelines for the diagnosis, surveillance and treatment of Barrett's esophagus have been established and updated [7,

171–173]. Table 3.3 summarizes the most recent recommendations. Essentially, the guidelines provided by several groups are very similar. The American Society of Gastrointestinal Endoscopy (ASGE) guidelines (which were generated together with the Society for Surgery of the Alimentary Tract and the American Gastroenterological Association) are similar to those of the American College of Gastroenterology (ACG) and the Canadian Association of Gastroenterology (CAG). For patients without dysplasia, surveillance endoscopy should be repeated within one year, and can then be performed every two to five years, depending upon the guideline followed (Table 3.3). For patients with low-grade dysplasia, confirmation should be sought by a second expert pathologist and a repeat surveillance endoscopy should be performed at six to twelve months. Endoscopies should continue annually until there is no low-grade dysplasia on two successive occasions, at which point a normal surveillance protocol may resume. Finally, for patients with high-grade dysplasia, management should be individualized. The ACG guidelines stipulate that high-grade dysplasia requires expert pathologist confirmation, followed by a repeat endoscopy at three months to rule out esophageal adenocarcinoma. At this point, surgery or endoscopic ablative therapy should be offered to candidates. Those who are unfit for such procedures (or refuse) should be followed with surveillance endoscopy every three months. The recommendations of the French Society of Digestive Endoscopy (FSED) differ slightly from the other guidelines as is demonstrated in Table 3.3. [172].

Conclusion

Barrett's esophagus is likely a complication of chronic gastroesophageal reflux and a risk factor for esophageal adenocarcinoma. It should, however, be realized that esophageal cancer is uncommon and most patients with esophageal cancer do not have clinically recognized Barrett's esophagus before cancer is diagnosed. Also, no randomized controlled trials or large cohort studies have convincingly demonstrated that an endoscopic screening or surveillance strategy prolongs survival or improves quality of life for these patients. However, for some patients, surveillance of Barrett's esophagus may permit detection of cancer at an earlier stage, and therefore improve survival. Therefore, endoscopic screening for Barrett's esophagus can be considered for patients with chronic symptoms of gastroesophageal reflux disease and, particularly, in certain high risk patients such as Caucasian males over the age of 50.

At this time, there is insufficient scientific evidence that aggressive anti-reflux therapy with either high-dose PPI or surgery will revert Barrett's esophagus to normal squa-

Table 3.3 Current practice guidelines for surveillance of Barrett's esophagus.

Source	Date published	No Dysplasia	Surveillance Intervals[a]		
			Low-grade dysplasia	High-grade dysplasia[b]	Biopsy sampling[c]
ACG [7]	2008	3 years after 2 normal EGD (1 year apart) with biopsy	Confirmatory endoscopy in 6 months, then every year until no dysplasia	Continued 3-month surveillance or individualized intervention (ablative therapy, EMR, or surgery)	4 quadrants every 2 cm and mucosal abnormalities
SFED [172]	2007	SSBE – 5 years CBE 3–6 cm – 3 years, >6 cm – 2 years	6 months – 1 year, then annually	Surgery or alternative therapy if still present at 1 month after high dose PPI	4 quadrant CBE – every 2 cm SSBE – every 1 cm
ASGE [173]	2000	Periodic (interval not specified)	More frequent than if no dysplasia	Consider surgery	4 quadrants every 1–2 cm
CAG [171]	2005	2–5 years	Confirmatory endoscopy in 12 months, then annually	Confirmatory in 3 months, then surgery or esophageal mucosal ablation for poor risk patients	4 quadrants every 2 cm

[a] Interval at which surveillance endoscopy should be performed;
[b] requires confirmation;
[c] protocol to be followed for biopsy sampling.
Abbreviations:
ACG: American College of Gastroenterology
ASGE: American Society for Gastrointestinal Endoscopy
EGD: Esophagogastroduodenoscopy
CBE: Classical Barrett's esophagus (length > 3 cm)

SFED: French Society of Digestive Endoscopy
CAG: Canadian Association of Gastroenterology
EMR: Endoscopic mucosal resection
SSBE: Short segment Barrett's esophagus (length < 3 cm)

mous mucosa or reduce the risk of developing cancer. Likewise, there are insufficient data to support the routine use of the various ablative therapies in patients with non-neoplastic Barrett's esophagus. These modalities remain experimental until proven to be effective in randomized trials.

At present, patients with clinically recognized Barrett's esophagus can be offered participation in a surveillance program, with surveillance every 2–3 years for patients without dysplasia (after two normal examinations) and every 6–12 months for patients with low-grade dysplasia. For patients with high-grade dysplasia, surgical intervention or endoscopic therapy should be considered once this change is confirmed by an expert gastrointestinal pathologist, preferably in a center performing a high volume of these procedures.

References

1 Barrett NR. The lower esophagus lined by columnar epithelium. *Surgery* 1957; **41**: 881–894.

2 Shaheen NJ, Crosby MA, Bozymski EM, Sandler RS. Is there publication bias in the reporting of cancer risk in Barrett's esophagus? *Gastroenterology* 2000; **119**: 333–338.

3 Naef AP, Savary M, Ozzello L. Columnar-lined lower esophagus: an acquired lesion with malignant predisposition. Report on 140 cases of Barrett's esophagus with 12 adenocarcinomas. *J Thorac Cardiovasc Surg* 1975; **70**: 826–835.

4 Spechler SJ. Comparison of medical and surgical therapy for complicated gastroesophageal reflux disease in veterans. The Department of Veterans Affairs Gastroesophageal Reflux Disease Study Group. *N Engl J Med* 1992; **326**: 786–792.

5 Sampliner RE. The Practice Parameters Committee of the American College of Gastroenterology. Practice guidelines on the diagnosis, surveillance, and therapy of Barrett's esophagus. *Am J Gastroenterol* 1998; **93**: 1028–1032.

6 Sampliner RE. The Practice Parameters Committee of the American College of Gastroenterology. Updated guidelines for the diagnosis, surveillance, and therapy of Barrett's esophagus. *Am J Gastroenterol* 2002; **97**: 1888–1895.

7 Wang KK and Sampliner RE: Practice Parameters Committee of the American College of Gastroenterology. Updated guidelines 2008 for the diagnosis, surveillance, and therapy of Barrett's esophagus. *Am J Gastroenterol* 2008; **103**: 788–797.

8 Watson A, Heading RC, Shepherd NA. Guidelines for the diagnosis and management of Barrett's columnar-lined oesophagus. *A Report of the Working Party of the British Society of Gastroenterology* 2005. Published online at http://www.bsg.org.uk.

9 Hamilton SR, Smith RR. The relationship between columnar epithelial dysplasia and invasive adenocarcinoma arising in Barrett's esophagus. *Am J Clin Pathol* 1987; **87**: 301–312.

10 Chandrasoma P, Wickramasinghe K, Ma Y, DeMeester T. Is intestinal metaplasia a necessary precursor lesion for adenocarcinomas of the distal esophagus, gastroesophageal junction and gastric cardia? *Dis Esophagus* 2007; **20**: 36–41.

11 Sharma P, Morales TG, Sampliner RE. Short segment Barrett's esophagus – the need for standardization of the definition and of endoscopic criteria. *Am J Gastroenterol* 1998; **93**: 1033–1036.

12 Falk GW. Barrett's esophagus. *Gastroenterology* 2002; **122**: 1569–1591.

13 Sharma P, Morales TG, Bhattacharyya A *et al.* Dysplasia in short-segment Barrett's esophagus: A prospective 3-year follow-up. *Am J Gastroenterol* 1997; **92**: 2012–2016.

14 Schnell TG, Sontag SJ, Chejfec G. Adenocarcinomas arising in tongues or short segments of Barrett's esophagus. *Dig Dis Sci* 1992; **37**: 137–143.

15 Nandurkar S, Martin CJ, Talley NJ, Wyatt JM. Curable cancer in a short segment Barrett's esophagus. *Dis Esophagus* 1998; **11**: 284–287.

16 Weston AP, Krmpotich PT, Cherian R *et al.* Prospective long-term endoscopic and histological follow-up of short segment Barrett's esophagus: Comparison with traditional long segment Barrett's esophagus. *Am J Gastroenterol* 1997; **92**: 407–413.

17 Rudolph RE, Vaughan TL, Storer BE *et al.* Effect of segment length on risk for neoplastic progression in patients with Barrett esophagus. *Ann Intern Med* 2002; **132**: 612–620.

18 Thomas T, Abrams KR, De Caestecker JS, Robinson RJ. Meta analysis: Cancer risk in Barrett's oesophagus. *Aliment Pharmacol Ther* 2007; **26**: 1465–1477.

19 Hirota WK, Loughney TM, Lazas DJ *et al.* Specialized intestinal metaplasia, dysplasia, and cancer of the esophagus and esophagogastric junction: Prevalence and clinical data. *Gastroenterology* 1999; **116**: 277–285.

20 Johnston MH, Hammond AS, Laskin W, Jones DM. The prevalence and clinical characteristics of short segments of specialized intestinal metaplasia in the distal esophagus on routine endoscopy. *Am J Gastroenterol* 1996; **91**: 1507–1511.

21 Winters C Jr, Spurling TJ, Chobanian SJ *et al.* Barrett's esophagus. A prevalent, occult complication of gastroesophageal reflux disease. *Gastroenterology* 1987; **92**: 118–124.

22 Gilani N, Gerkin RD, Ramirez FC *et al.* Prevalence of Barrett's esophagus in patients with moderate to severe erosive esophagitis. *World J Gastroenterol* 2008; **14**: 3518–3522.

23 Thompson AB, Barkun AN, Armstrong D *et al.* The prevalence of clinically significant endoscopic findings in primary care patients with uninvestigated dyspepsia: The Canadian Adult Dyspepsia Empiric Treatment – Prompt Endoscopy (CADET – PE) study. *Aliment Pharmacol Ther* 2003; **17**: 1481–1491.

24 Breslin NP, Thomson ABR, Bailey RJ *et al.* Gastric cancer and other endoscopic diagnoses in patients with benign dyspepsia. *Gut* 2000; **46**, 93–97.

25 Cameron AJ, Lomboy CT. Barrett's esophagus: Age, prevalence, and extent of columnar epithelium. *Gastroenterology* 1992; **103**: 1241–1245.

26 Gruppo Operativo per lo Studio delle Precancerosi dell Esofago (GOSPE). Barrett's esophagus: Epidemiological and clinical results of a multicentric survey. *Int J Cancer* 1991; **48**: 364–368.

27 Cameron AJ, Zinsmeister AR, Ballard DJ, Carney JA. Prevalence of columnar- lined (Barrett's) esophagus. Comparison of population-based clinical and autopsy findings. *Gastroenterology* 1990; **99**: 918–922.

28 Conio M, Cameron AJ, Romero Y *et al.* Secular trends in the epidemiology and outcome of Barrett's oesophagus in Olmsted County, Minnesota. *Gut* 2001; **48**: 304–309.

29 Lagergren J. Adenocarcinoma of the oesophagus: What exactly is the size of the problem and who is at risk? *Gut* 2005; **54**(Suppl 1): i1–5.

30 Brown LM, Devesa SS, Chow WH. Incidence of adenocarcinoma of the esophagus among white Americans by sex, stage, and age. *J Natl Cancer Inst* 2008; **100**: 1184–1187.

31 Bersentes K, Fass R, Padda S *et al.* Prevalence of Barrett's esophagus in Hispanics is similar to Caucasians. *Dig Dis Sci* 1998; **43**: 1038–1041.

32 Fass R. Barrett's esophagus: Are Caucasians the only ethnic group at risk? *Cancer Detect Prev* 1999; **23**: 177–178.

33 Yeh C, Hsu CT, Ho AS *et al.* Erosive esophagitis and Barrett's esophagus in Taiwan: A higher frequency than expected. *Dig Dis Sci* 1997; **42**: 702–706.

34 Abrams JA, Fields S, Lightdale CJ, Neugut AI. Racial and ethnic disparities in the prevalence of Barrett's esophagus among patients who undergo upper endoscopy. *Clin Gastroenterol Hepatol* 2008; **6**: 30–34.

35 Lam KD, Phan JT, Garcia RT *et al.* Low proportion of Barrett's esophagus in Asian Americans. *Am J Gastroenterol* 2008; **103**: 1625–1630.

36 El-Serag HB, Sonnenberg A. Opposing time trends of peptic ulcer and reflux disease. *Gut* 1998; **43**: 327–333.

37 Fallone CA, Barkun AN, Friedman G *et al.* Is *Helicobacter pylori* eradication associated with gastroesophageal reflux disease? *Am J Gastroenterol* 2000; **95**: 914–920.

38 Eisen GM, Sandler RS, Murray S, Gottfried M. The relationship between gastroesophageal reflux disease and its complications with Barrett's esophagus. *Am J Gastroenterol* 1997; **92**: 27–31.

39 Leiberman DA, Oehlke M, Helfand M. Risk factors for Barrett's esophagus in community-based practice. GORGE consortium. Gastroenterology Outcomes Research Group in Endoscopy. *Am J Gastroenterol* 1997; **92**: 1293–1297.

40 Avidan B, Sonnenberg A, Schnell TG, Sontag SJ. There are no reliable symptoms for erosive oesphagitis and Barrett's oesophagus: endoscopic diagnosis is still essential. *Aliment Pharmacol Ther* 2002; **16**: 735–742.

41 Spechler SJ, Sperber H, Doos WG, Schimmel EM. The prevalence of Barrett's esophagus in patients with chronic peptic esophageal strictures. *Dig Dis Sci* 1983; **28**: 769–774.

42 Kim SL, Wo JM, Hunter JG *et al.* The prevalence of intestinal metaplasia in patients with and without peptic strictures. *Am J Gastroenterol* 1998; **93**: 53–55.

43 Avidan B, Sonnenberg A, Schnell TG, Sontag SJ. Hiatal hernia and acid reflux frequency predict presence and length of Barrett's esophagus. *Dig Dis Sci* 2002; **47**: 256–264.

44 Cameron AJ. Barrett's esophagus: prevalence and size of hiatal hernia. *Am J Gastroenterol* 1999; **94**: 2054–2059.

45 Johnson DA, Winters C, Spruling TJ *et al.* Esophageal acid sensitivity in Barrett's esophagus. *J Clin Gastroenterol* 1987; **9**: 23–27.

46 Corley DA, Kobu A, Levin TR *et al.* Abdominal obesity and body mass index as risk factors for Barrett's esophagus. *Gastroenterology* 2007; **133**: 34–41.

47 Konturek PC, Burnat G, Rau T *et al.* Effect of adiponectin and ghrelin on apoptosis of Barrett adenocarcinoma cell line. *Dig Dis Sci* 2008; **53**: 597–605.

48 Kubo A, Levin TR, Block G *et al*. Dietary antioxidants, fruits, and vegetables and the risk of Barrett's esophagus. *Am J Gastroenterol* 2008; **103**: 1614–1623.

49 Kubo A, Levin TR, Block G *et al*. Dietary patterns and the risk of Barrett's esophagus. *Am J Epidemiol* 2008; **167**: 839–846.

50 Katzka DA, Rustgi AK. Gastroesophageal reflux disease and Barrett's esophagus. *Med Clin North Am* 2000; **84**: 1137–1161.

51 Eckardt VF, Kanzler G, Bernhard G. Life expectancy and cancer risk in patients with Barrett's esophagus: A prospective controlled investigation. *Am J Med* 2001; **111**: 33–37.

52 Provenzale D, Schmitt C, Wong JB. Barrett's esophagus: a new look at surveillance based on emerging estimates of cancer risk. *Am J Gastroenterol* 1999; **94**: 2043–2053.

53 Katz D, Rothstein R, Schned A *et al*. The development of dysplasia and adenocarcinoma during endoscopic surveillance of Barrett's esophagus. *Am J Gastroenterol* 1998; **93**: 536–541.

54 O'Conner JB, Falk GW, Richter JE. The incidence of adenocarcinoma and dysplasia in Barrett's esophagus: Report on the Cleveland Clinic Barrett's Esophagus Registry. *Am J Gastroenterol* 1999; **94**: 2037–2042.

55 Drewitz DJ, Sampliner RE, Garewal HS. The incidence of adenocarcinoma in Barrett's esophagus: A prospective study of 170 patients followed 4.8 years. *Am J Gastroenterol* 1997; **92**: 212–215.

56 Yousef F, Cardwell C, Cantwell MM *et al*. The incidence of esophageal cancer and high-grade dysplasia in Barrett's esophagus: A systematic review and meta-analysis. *Am J Epidemiol* 2008; **168**: 237–249.

57 *Cancer Facts and Figures* 2001. American Cancer Society, Atlanta.

58 *Canadian Cancer Statistics* 2008. National Cancer Institute of Canada, Toronto, Canada.

59 Shaheen N, Ransohoff DF. Gastroesophageal reflux, Barrett's esophagus and esophageal cancer: Scientific review. *JAMA* 2002; **287**: 1972–1981.

60 Lagergren J, Bergstrom R, Lindgren A, Nyren O. Symptomatic gastroesophageal reflux as a risk factor for esophageal adenocarcinoma. *N Engl J Med* 1999; **340**: 825–31.

61 Farrow DC, Vaughan TL, Sweeney C *et al*. Gastroesophageal reflux disease, use of H2 receptor antagonists, and risk of esophageal and gastric cancer. *Cancer Causes Control* 2000; **11**: 231–238.

62 Avidan B, Sonnenberg A, Schnell TG *et al*. Hiatal hernia size, Barrett's length, and severity of acid reflux are all risk factors for esophageal adenocarcinoma. *Am J Gastroenterol* 2002; **97**: 1930–1936.

63 Lagergren J, Bergstrom R, Nyren O. Association between body mass and adenocarcinoma of the esophagus and gastric cardia. *Ann Intern Med* 1999; **130**: 883–890.

64 Gammon MD, Schoenberg JB, Ahsan H *et al*. Tobacco, alcohol, and socioeconomic status and adenocarcinomas of the esophagus and gastric cardia. *J Natl Cancer Inst* 1997; **89**: 1277–1284.

65 Brown LM, Swanson CA, Gridley G *et al*. Adenocarcinoma of the esophagus: Role of obesity and diet. *J Natl Cancer Inst* 1995; **87**: 104–109.

66 Lagergren J, Bergstrom R, Adami HO, Nyren O. Association between medications that relax the lower esophageal sphincter and risk for esophageal adenocarcinoma. *Ann Intern Med* 2000; **133**: 165–175.

67 Vaughan TL, Farrow DC, Hansten PD *et al*. Risk of esophageal and gastric adenocarcinomas in relation to use of calcium channel blockers, asthma drugs, and other medications that promote gastroesophageal reflux. *Cancer Epidemiol Biomarkers Prev* 1998; **7**: 749–756.

68 Raghunath A, Hungin AP, Wooff D, Childs S. Prevalence of *Helicobacter pylori* in patients with gastro-oesophageal reflux disease: Systematic review. *BMJ* 2003; **326**: 737.

69 de Martel C, Llosa AE, Farr SM *et al*. *Helicobacter pylori* infection and the risk of development of esophageal adenocarcinoma. *J Infect Dis* 2005; **191**: 761–767.

70 Vicari JJ, Peek RM, Falk GW *et al*. The seroprevalence of cagA-positive *Helicobacter pylori* strains in the spectrum of gastroesophageal reflux disease. *Gastroenterology* 1998; **115**: 50–57.

71 Chow WH, Blaser MJ, Blot WJ *et al*. An inverse relation between cagA+ strains of *Helicobacter pylori* infection and risk of esophageal and gastric cardia adenocarcinoma. *Cancer Res* 1998; **58**: 588–590.

72 Peterson WL, American Gastroenterological Association Consensus Development Panel. Improving the management of GERD; evidence-based therapeutic strategies. *AGA press* 2001; 1–21.

73 Spechler SJ. Clinical practice. Barrett's Esophagus. *N Engl J Med* 2002; **346**: 836–842.

74 Reid BJ, Levine DS, Longton G *et al*. Predictors of progression to cancer in Barrett's esophagus: baseline histology and flow cytometry identify low- and high-risk patient subsets. *Am J Gastroenterol* 2000; **95**: 1669–1676.

75 Buttar NS, Wang KK, Sebo TJ *et al*. Extent of high-grade dysplasia in Barrett's esophagus correlates with risk of adenocarcinoma. *Gastroenterology* 2001; **120**: 1630–1639.

76 Schnell TG, Sontag SJ, Chejfec G *et al*. Long-term nonsurgical management of Barrett's esophagus with high-grade dysplasia. *Gastroenterology* 2001; **120**: 1607–1619.

77 Bremner CG, Lynch VP, Ellis FH Jr. Barrett's esophagus: Congenital or acquired? An experimental study of esophageal mucosal regeneration in the dog. *Surgery* 2008; **68**: 209–216.

78 Gillen P, Keeling P, Byrne PJ *et al*. Experimental columnar metaplasia in the canine oesophagus. *Br J Surg* 1988; **75**: 113–115.

79 Singh P, Taylor RH, Colin-Jones DG. Esophageal motor dysfunction and acid exposure in reflux esophagitis are more severe if Barrett's metaplasia is present. *Am J Gastroenterol* 1994; **89**: 349–356.

80 Oberg S, DeMeester TR, Peters JH *et al*. The extent of Barrett's esophagus depends on the status of the lower esophageal sphincter and the degree of esophageal acid exposure. *J Thorac Cardiovasc Surg* 1999; **117**: 572–580.

81 Fass R, Hell RW, Garewal HS *et al*. Correlation of oesophageal acid exposure with Barrett's oesophagus length. *Gut* 2001; **48**: 310–313.

82 Hirschowitz BI. Gastric acid and pepsin secretion in patients with Barrett's esophagus and appropriate controls. *Dig Dis Sci* 1996; **41**: 1384–1391.

83 Pace F, Santalucia F, Bianchi Porro G. Natural history of gastro-oesophageal reflux disease without oesophagitis. *Gut* 1991; **32**: 845–848.

84 Freston JW, Malagelada JR, Petersen H, McCloy RF. Critical issues in the management of gastroesophageal reflux disease. *Eur J Gastroenterol Hepatol* 1995; **7**: 577–586.

85 Fass R, Ofman JJ. Gastroesophageal reflux disease – should we adopt a new conceptual framework? *Am J Gastroenterol* 2002; **97**: 1901–1909.

86 Ofman JJ, Shaheen NJ, Desai AA *et al.* The quality of care in Barrett's esophagus: Endoscopist and pathologist practices. *Am J Gastroenterol* 2001; **96**: 876–881.

87 Weinstein WM, Lee S, Lewin K *et al.* Erosive esophagitis impairs accurate detection of Barrett's esophagus: A prospective randomized double blind study. *Gastroentrology* 1999; **116**: A 352 (G1538).

88 Alikhan M, Rex D, Khan A *et al.* Variable pathologic interpretation of columnar lined esophagus by general pathologists in community practice. *Gastrointest Endosc* 1999; **50**: 23–26.

89 Canto MI, Setrakian S, Willis J *et al.* Methylene blue-directed biopsies improve detection of intestinal metaplasia and dysplasia in Barrett's esophagus. *Gastrointest Endosc* 2000; **51**: 560–568.

90 Chobanian SJ, Cattau EL Jr, Winters C, Jr *et al.* In vivo staining with toluidine blue as an adjunct to the endoscopic detection of Barrett's esophagus. *Gastrointest Endosc* 1987; **33**: 99–101.

91 Stevens PD, Lightdale CJ, Green PH *et al.* Combined magnification endoscopy with chromoendoscopy for the evaluation of Barrett's esophagus. *Gastrointest Endosc* 1994; **40**: 747–749.

92 Woolf GM, Riddell RH, Irvine EJ, Hunt RH. A study to examine agreement between endoscopy and histology for the diagnosis of columnar lined (Barrett's) esophagus. *Gastrointest Endosc* 1989; **35**: 541–544.

93 Wo JM, Ray MB, Mayfield-Stokes S *et al.* Comparison of methylene blue-directed biopsies and conventional biopsies in the detection of intestinal metaplasia and dysplasia in Barrett's esophagus: A preliminary study. *Gastrointest Endosc* 2001; **54**: 294–301.

94 Guelrud M, Herrera I, Essenfeld H, Castro J. Enhanced magnification endoscopy: A new technique to identify specialized intestinal metaplasia in Barrett's esophagus. *Gastrointest Endosc* 2001; **53**: 559–565.

95 Reid BJ, Blount PL, Feng Z, Levine DS. Optimizing endoscopic biopsy detection of early cancers in Barrett's high-grade dysplasia. *Am J Gastroenterol* 2000; **95**: 3089–3096.

96 Horwhat JD, Maydonovitch CL, Ramos F *et al.* A randomized comparison of methylene blue-directed biopsy versus conventional four-quadrant biopsy for the detection of intestinal metaplasia and dysplasia in patients with long-segment Barrett's esophagus. *Am J Gastroenterol* 2008; **103**: 546–554.

97 Anagnostopoulos GK, Yao K, Kaye P *et al.* Novel endoscopic observation in Barrett's esophagus using high resolution magnification endoscopy and narrow band imaging. *Aliment Pharmacol Ther* 2007; **26**: 501–507.

98 Sampliner RE, Garewal HS, Fennerty MB, Aickin M. Lack of impact of therapy on extent of Barrett's esophagus in 67 patients. *Dig Dis Sci* 1990; **35**: 93–96.

99 Peters FT, Ganesh S, Kuipers EJ *et al.* Endoscopic regression of Barrett's oesophagus during omeprazole treatment; A randomised double blind study. *Gut* 1999; **45**: 489–494.

100 Chiba N, De Gara CJ, Wilkinson JM, Hunt RH. Speed of healing and symptom relief in grade II to IV gastroesophageal reflux disease: A meta-analysis. *Gastroenterology* 1997; **112**: 1798–1810.

101 Sampliner RE. Effect of up to 3 years of high-dose lansoprazole on Barrett's esophagus. *Am J Gastroenterol* 1994; **89**: 1844–1848.

102 Neumann CS, Iqbal TH, Cooper BT. Long term continuous omeprazole treatment of patients with Barrett's oesophagus. *Aliment Pharmacol Ther* 1995; **9**: 451–454.

103 Cooper BT, Neumann CS, Cox MA, Iqbal TH. Continuous treatment with omeprazole 20 mg daily for up to 6 years in Barrett's oesophagus. *Aliment Pharmacol Ther* 1998; **12**: 893–897.

104 Gore S, Healey CJ, Sutton R *et al.* Regression of columnar lined (Barrett's) oesophagus with continuous omeprazole therapy. *Aliment Pharmacol Ther* 1993; **7**: 623–628.

105 Malesci A, Savarino V, Zentilin P *et al.* Partial regression of Barrett's oesophagus by long-term therapy with high-dose omeprazole. *Gastrointest Endosc* 1996; **44**: 700–705.

106 Wilkinson SP, Biddlestone L, Gore S, Shepherd NA. Regression of columnar-lined (Barrett's) oesophagus with omeprazole 40 mg daily: Results of 5 years of continuous therapy. *Aliment Pharmacol Ther* 1999; **13**: 1205–1209.

107 Ouatu-Lascar R, Fitzgerald RC, Triadafilopoulos G. Differentiation and proliferation in Barrett's esophagus and the effects of acid suppression. *Gastroenterology* 1999; **117**: 327–335.

108 El-Serag HB, Aguirre TV, Davis S *et al.* Proton pump inhibitors are associated with reduced incidence of dysplasia in Barrett's esophagus. *Am J Gastroenterol* 2004; **99**: 877–883.

109 Ouatu-Lascar R, Triadafilopoulos G. Complete elimination of reflux symptoms does not guarantee normalization of intraesophageal acid reflux in patients with Barrett's esophagus. *Am J Gastroenterol* 1998; **93**: 711–716.

110 Fass R, Sampliner RE, Malagon IB *et al.* Failure of oesophageal acid control in candidates for Barrett's oesophagus reversal on a very high dose of proton pump inhibitor. *Aliment Pharmacol Ther* 2000; **14**: 597–602.

111 Ortiz A, Martinez de Haro LF, Parrilla P *et al.* 24-h pH monitoring is necessary to assess acid reflux suppression in patients with Barrett's oesophagus undergoing treatment with proton pump inhibitors. *Br J Surg* 1999; **86**: 1472–1474.

112 Katzka DA, Castell DO. Successful elimination of reflux symptoms does not insure adequate control of acid reflux in patients with Barrett's esophagus. *Am J Gastroenterol* 1994; **89**: 989–991.

113 Sharma P, Morales TG, Bhattacharyya A *et al.* Squamous islands in Barrett's esophagus: What lies underneath? *Am J Gastroenterol* 1998; **93**: 332–335.

114 Leedham S and Jankowski J. The evidence base of proton pump inhibitor chemopreventative agents in Barrett's esophagus – the good, the bad, and the flawed! *Am J Gastroenterol* 2007; **102**: 21–23.

115 Fiorucci S, Santucci L, Farroni F *et al.* Effect of omeprazole on gastroesophageal reflux in Barrett's esophagus. *Am J Gastroenterol* 1989; **84**: 1263–1267.

116 Kovacs BJ, Chen YK, Lewis TD *et al.* Successful reversal of Barrett's esophagus with multipolar electrocoagulation despite inadequate acid suppression. *Gastrointest Endosc* 1999; **49**: 547–553.

117 Katz PO, Anderson C, Khoury R, Castell DO. Gastro-oesophageal reflux associated with nocturnal gastric acid breakthrough on proton pump inhibitors. *Aliment Pharmacol Ther* 1998; **12**: 1231–1234.

118 Ortiz A, Martinez de Haro LF, Parrilla P *et al.* Conservative treatment versus antireflux surgery in Barrett's oesophagus:

Long term results of a prospective study. *Br J Surg* 1996; **83**: 274–278.

119 Low DE, Levine DS, Dail DH, Kozarek RA. Histological and anatomic changes in Barrett's esophagus after antireflux surgery. *Am J Gastroenterol* 1999; **94**: 80-85.

120 McDonald ML, Trastek VF, Allen MS *et al.* Barretts's esophagus: does an antireflux procedure reduce the need for endoscopic surveillance? *J Thorac Cardiovasc Surg* 1996; **111**: 1135–1138.

121 Yau P, Watson DI, Devitt PG *et al.* Laparoscopic antireflux surgery in the treatment of gastroesophageal reflux in patients with Barrett esophagus. *Arch Surg* 2000; **135**: 801–805.

122 Csendes A, Braghetto I, Burdiles P *et al.* Long-term results of classic antireflux surgery in 152 patients with Barrett's esophagus: Clinical, radiologic, endoscopic, manometric, and acid reflux test analysis before and late after operation. *Surgery* 1998; **123**: 645–657.

123 Csendes A, Burdiles P, Braghetto I *et al.* Dysplasia and adenocarcinoma after classic antireflux surgery in patients with Barrett's esophagus: The need for long-term subjective and objective follow-up. *Ann Surg* 2002; **235**: 178–185.

124 Spechler SJ, Lee E, Ahnen D *et al.* Long-term outcome of medical and surgical therapies for gastroesophageal reflux disease: Follow-up of a randomized controlled trial. *JAMA* 2001; **285**: 2331–2338.

125 O'Riordan JM, Byrne PJ, Ravi N *et al.* Long-term clinical and pathologic response of Barrett's esophagus after antireflux surgery. *Am J Surg* 2004; **188**: 27–33.

126 Farrow DC, Vaughan TL, Hansten PD *et al.* Use of aspirin and other nonsteroidal anti-inflammatory drugs and risk of esophageal and gastric cancer. *Cancer Epidemiol Biomarkers Prev* 1998; **7**: 97–102.

127 Langman MJ, Cheng KK, Gilman EA, Lancashire RJ. Effect of anti-inflammatory drugs on overall risk of common cancer: Case-control study in general practice research database. *BMJ* 2000; **320**: 1642–1646.

128 Shirvani VN, Ouatu-Lascar R, Kaur BS *et al.* Cyclooxygenase 2 expression in Barrett's esophagus and adenocarcinoma: *Ex vivo* induction by bile salts and acid exposure. *Gastroenterology* 2000; **118**: 487–496.

129 Buttar NS, Wang KK, Leontovich O *et al.* Chemoprevention of esophageal adenocarcinoma by COX-2 inhibitors in an animal model of Barrett's esophagus. *Gastroenterology* 2002; **122**: 1101–1112.

130 Souza RF, Shewmake K, Beer DG *et al.* Selective inhibition of cyclooxygenase-2 suppresses growth and induces apoptosis in human esophageal adenocarcinoma cells. *Cancer Res* 2002; **60**: 5767–5772.

131 Sonnenberg A, Fennerty M. Medical decision analysis of chemoprevention against esophageal adenocarcinoma. *Gastroenterology* 2003; **124**: 1758–1766.

132 Heath EI, Canto MI, Piantadosi S *et al.* Chemoprevention for Barrett's Esophagus Trial Research Group. Secondary chemoprevention of Barrett's esophagus with celecoxib: Results of a randomized trial. *J Natl Cancer Inst* 2007; **99**: 545–557.

133 Fennerty MB, Triadafilopoulos G. Barrett's-related esophageal adenocarcinoma: Is chemoprevention a potential option? *Am J Gastroenterol* 2001; **96**: 2302–2035.

134 Jankowsi J, Barr H. Improving surveillance for Barrett's oesophagus: AspECT and BOSS trials provide an evidence base. *BMJ* 2006; **322**: 1512.

135 Fennerty MB, Coreless CL, Sheppard B *et al.* Pathological documentation of complete elimination of Barrett's metaplasia following endoscopic multipolar electrocoagulation therapy. *Gut* 2001; **49**: 142–144.

136 Pereira-Lima JC, Busnello JV, Saul C *et al.* High power setting argon plasma coagulation for the eradication of Barrett's esophagus. *Am J Gastroenterol* 2000; **95**: 1661–1668.

137 Byrne JP, Armstrong GR, Attwood SE. Restoration of the normal squamous lining in Barrett's esophagus by argon beam plasma coagulation. *Am J Gastroenterol* 1998; **93**: 1810–1815.

138 Michopoulos S, Tsibouris P, Bouzakis H *et al.* Complete regression of Barrett's esophagus with heat probe thermocoagulation: Mid-term results. *Gastrointest Endosc* 1999; **50**: 165–172.

139 Overholt BF, Panjehpour M, Haydek JM. Photodynamic therapy for Barrett's esophagus: Follow-up in 100 patients. *Gastrointest Endosc* 1999; **49**: 1–7.

140 Overholt BF, Lightdale CJ, Wang KK *et al.* International Photodynamic Group for High-Grade Dysplasia in Barrett's Esophagus. Photodynamic therapy with porfimer sodium for ablation of high-grade dysplasia in Barrett's esophagus: International, partially blinded, randomized phase III trial. *Gastrointest Endosc* 2005; **62**: 488–498.

141 Overholt BF, Wang KK, Burdick JS *et al.* International Photodynamic Group for High-Grade Dysplasia in Barrett's Esophagus. . Five-year efficacy and safety of photodynamic therapy with Photofrin in Barrett's high-grade dysplasia. *Gastrointest Endosc* 2007; **66**: 460–468.

142 Ackroyd R, Brown NJ, Davis MF *et al.* Photodynamic therapy for dysplastic Barrett's oesophagus: A prospective, double blind, randomised, placebo controlled trial. *Gut* 2000; **47**: 612–617.

143 Sharma VK, Wang KK, Overholt BF *et al.* Balloon-based, circumferential, endoscopic radiofrequency ablation of Barrett's esophagus: 1-year follow-up of 100 patients. *Gastrointest Endosc* 2007; **65**: 185–195.

144 Sharma VK, Kim HJ, Das A *et al.* A prospective pilot trial of ablation of Barrett's esophagus with low-grade dysplasia using stepwise circumferential and focal ablation (HALO system). *Endoscopy* 2008; **40**: 380–387.

145 Gondrie JJ, Pouw RE, Sondermeijer CM *et al.* Stepwise circumferential and focal ablation of Barrett's esophagus with high-grade dysplasia: Results of the first prospective series of 11 patients. *Endoscopy* 2008; **40**: 359–369.

146 Ell C, May A, Gossner L *et al.* Endoscopic mucosal resection of early cancer and high-grade dysplasia in Barrett's esophagus. *Gastroenterology* 2000; **118**: 670–677.

147 Sharma P, McQuaid K, Dent J *et al.* AGA Chicago Workshop. A critical review of the diagnosis and management of Barrett's esophagus: The AGA Chicago Workshop. *Gastroenterology* 2004; **127**: 310–330.

148 Armstrong D. Motion – All patients with GERD should be offered once in a lifetime endoscopy: Arguments for the motion. *Can J Gastroenterol* 2002; **16**: 549–551.

149 MacNeil-Covin L, Casson AG, Malatjalian D, Veldhuyzen van Zanten S. A survey of Canadian gastroenterologists about man-

agement of Barrett's esophagus. *Can J Gastroenterol* 2003; **17**: 313–317.

150 Devesa SS, Blot WJ, Fraumeni JF, Jr. Changing patterns in the incidence of esophageal and gastric carcinoma in the United States. *Cancer* 1998; **83**: 2049–2053.

151 Farrow DC, Vaughan TL. Determinants of survival following the diagnosis of esophageal adenocarcinoma (United States). *Cancer Causes Control* 1996; **7**: 322–327.

152 Daly JM, Karnell LH, Menck HR. National Cancer Data Base report on esophageal carcinoma. *Cancer* 1996; **78**: 1820–1828.

153 van Sandick JW, van Lanschot JJB, Kuiken BW *et al.* Impact of endoscopic biopsy surveillance of Barrett's oesophagus on pathological stage and clinical outcome of Barrett's carcinoma. *Gut* 1998; **43**: 216–222.

154 Peters JH, Clark GWB, Ireland AP *et al.* Outcome of adenocarcinoma arising in Barrett's esophagus in endoscopically surveyed and nonsurveyed patients. *J Thorac Cardiovasc Surg* 1994; **108**: 813–821.

155 Streitz JM Jr, Andrews CW Jr, Ellis FH, Jr. Endoscopic surveillance of Barrett's esophagus: Does it help? *J Thorac Cardiovasc Surg* 1993; **105**: 383–388.

156 Aldulaimi DM, Cox M, Nwokolo CU, Loft DE. Barrett's surveillance is worthwhile and detects curable cancers. A prospective cohort study addressing cancer incidence, treatment outcome, and survival. *Eur J Gastroenterol Hepatol* 2005; **17**: 943–950.

157 Bytzer P, Christensen PB, Damkier P *et al.* Adenocarcinoma of the esophagus and Barrett's esophagus: A population-based study. *Am J Gastroenterol* 1999; **94**: 86–91.

158 Brown CM, Jones R, Shirazi T *et al.* Prior diagnosis of Barrett's esophagus is rare in patients with esophageal adenocarcinoma. *Gut* 1996; **381**(suppl. 1): A23.

159 Menke-Pluymers MB, Schoute NW, Mulder AH *et al.* Outcome of surgical treatment of adenocarcinoma in Barrett's oesophagus. *Gut* 1992; **33**: 1454–1458.

160 Van der Veen AH, Dees J, Blankensteijn JD, Van Blankenstein M. Adenocarcinoma in Barrett's oesophagus: An overrated risk. *Gut* 1980; **30**: 14–18.

161 Macdonald CE, Wicks AC, Playford RJ. Final results from 10 year cohort of patients undergoing surveillance for Barrett's oesophagus: Observational study. *BMJ* 2000; **321**: 1252–1255.

162 van der Burgh A, Dees J, Hop WC, van Blankenstein M. Oesophageal cancer is an uncommon cause of death in patients with Barrett's oesophagus. *Gut* 1996; **39**: 5–8.

163 Nandurkar S, Talley NJ. Barrett's esophagus: The long and the short of it. *Am J Gastroenterol* 1999; **94**: 30–40.

164 Soni A, Sampliner RE, Sonnenberg A. Screening for high-grade dyplasia in gastroesophageal reflux disease: Is it cost-effective? *Am J Gastroenterol* 2000; **95**: 2086–2093.

165 Wright TA, Gray MR, Morris AI *et al.* Cost effectiveness of detecting Barrett's cancer. *Gut* 1996; **39**: 574–579.

166 Streitz JM Jr, Ellis FH Jr, Tilden RL, Erickson RV. Endoscopic surveillance of Barrett's esophagus: A cost-effectiveness comparison with mammographic surveillance for breast cancer. *Am J Gastroenterol* 1998; **93**: 911–915.

167 Sonnenberg A, Soni A, Sampliner RE. Medical decision analysis of endoscopic surveillance of Barrett's oesophagus to prevent oesophageal adenocarcinoma. *Aliment Pharacol Ther* 2002; **16**: 41–50.

168 Gudlaugsdottir S, van Blankenstein M, Dees J, Wilson JHP. A majority of patients with Barrett's oesophagus are unlikely to benefit from endoscopic cancer surveillance. *Eur J Gastroenterol Hepatol* 2001; **13**: 639–645.

169 Chiba N. Motion – Screening and surveillance of Barrett's epithelium is practical and cost effective: Arguments against the motion. *Can J Gastroenterol* 2002; **16**: 541–545.

170 Levine DS, Haggitt RC, Blount PL *et al.* An endoscopic biopsy protocol can differentiate high-grade dysplasia from early adenocarcinoma in Barrett's esophagus. *Gastroenterology* 1993; **105**: 40–50.

171 Armstrong D, Marshall JK, Chiba N *et al.* Canadian Association of Gastroenterology GERD Consensus Group. Canadian Consensus Conference on the management of gastroesophageal reflux in adults – update 2004. *Can J Gastroenterol* 2005; **19**: 15–35.

172 Boyer J, Laugier R, Chemali M. French Society of Digestive Endoscopy SFED. French Society of Digestive Endoscopy SFED guideline: Monitoring of patients with Barrett's esophagus. *Endoscopy* 2007; **39**: 840–842.

173 SSAT, AGA, ASGE Consensus Panel. Management of Barrett's esophagus. *J Gastrointest Surg* 2000; **4**: 115–116.

4 Esophageal motility disorders: Achalasia and spastic motor disorders

Jason R Roberts[1], Marcelo F Vela[2] and Joel E Richter[3]

[1] Division of Gastroenterology and Hepatology, Medical University of South Carolina, South Carolina, USA
[2] Gastroenterology Section, Baylor College of Medicine, Houston, Texas, USA
[3] Department of Medicine, Temple University School of Medicine, Philadelphia, USA

Esophageal motility disorders present with dysphagia and chest pain as the main symptoms, accompanied by abnormalities on manometric studies. The best characterized esophageal motility disorders are achalasia and diffuse esophageal spasm. The treatment options for these disorders, which range from non-invasive medical therapy to surgery, are presented in this chapter.

Achalasia

Achalasia is a primary esophageal motor disorder characterized by abnormal relaxation of the lower esophageal sphincter (LES) and absent esophageal peristalsis. With an estimated incidence of approximately 1/100 000 and a prevalence of close to 10/100 000 [1], this uncommon disease stands out among the esophageal motility disorders as the most clearly defined (clinically, manometrically and radiographically) and the most successfully treated.

The exact etiology of achalasia remains unknown, but autoimmune, infectious, degenerative and hereditary processes, whether alone or in combination, lead to a chronic inflammatory response in the myenteric plexus that results in selective loss of inhibitory neurons [2]. Manometrically this is manifested by high LES pressure, abnormal LES relaxation and aperistalsis [3]. The combination of an atonic esophageal body with a functional obstruction at the gastroesophageal junction produce esophageal dilatation that can, over a prolonged period of time, lead to the development of a megaesophagus.

The most common symptoms of achalasia are dysphagia for solids and liquids in over 90% of patients, and regurgitation of undigested food and saliva in approximately 75%. Chest pain is present in 40–50% of patients, weight loss in nearly 60%, and heartburn in approximately 40% of sub-

jects [4, 5]. The presence of the disease is strongly supported by a barium esophagram showing a dilated esophagus that tapers into a "bird-beak" at the gastroesophageal junction with fluoroscopy revealing lack of normal peristalsis, usually with to-and-fro disordered bolus movement. The manometric features described above, the most important of which is abnormal LES relaxation, confirm the diagnosis.

Treatment of achalasia

Overview
Currently, there is no available treatment that can correct the underlying neuropathology of achalasia; LES function and peristalsis cannot be restored. Therefore, therapy is based on reduction of the resting LES pressure to allow esophageal emptying by gravity. The goals of treatment are three-fold: relieve symptoms, improve esophageal emptying and prevent the development of megaesophagus. In assessing response to a therapeutic intervention, useful endpoints are symptom relief and physiologic evaluation, the latter through manometric determination of LES pressure and measurement of esophageal emptying by barium examination or nuclear scintigraphy.

Reduction of the LES pressure can be achieved through different therapeutic modalities, including pharmacologic therapy, endoscopic injection of botulinum toxin, pneumatic dilatation and surgical myotomy [6]; the last two being the most effective treatments [4, 7]. "Endstage" cases presenting with a markedly dilated and sometimes sigmoid esophagus may require esophagectomy [8]. The choice of therapy depends on patient characteristics (age, co-morbid illnesses and disease stage), patient's preference, degree of expertise and available modalities in the medical center, and a careful balance between risks and benefits.

Pharmacologic treatment
Pharmacological reduction of the LES basal pressure through smooth muscle relaxants has been attempted with

Evidence-Based Gastroenterology and Hepatology, 3rd edition.
J. McDonald, A.K. Burroughs, B. Feagan, and M.B. Fennerty. © 2010
Blackwell Publishing Ltd

Table 4.1 Nitrates and calcium channel blockers in the treatment of achalasia.

Authors	No. of patients	Treatment	% symptom improvement
Bortolotti and Labo [16]	20	Nifedipine	70
Traube et al. [15]	10	Nifedipine	53
Coccia et al. [17]	14	Nifedipine	77
Gelfond et al. [12]	15	Nifedipine	53
Gelfond et al. [12]	15	ISDN	87
Gelfond et al. [13]	24	ISDN	83
Rozen et al. [14]	15	ISDN	58
Eherer et al. [19]	3	Sildenafil	0

ISDN isosorbide dinitrate.
Modified from Vaezi M, Richter JE. *J Clin Gastroenterol* 1998; **27**: 21–35.

several medications. The most studied classes include nitrates, calcium channel blockers and, more recently, sildenafil (Table 4.1).

Nitrates activate guanylate cyclase, leading to production of a protein kinase that inhibits smooth muscle contraction through dephosphorylation of the myosin light chain. Additionally, nitrates liberate nitric oxide (NO), an inhibitory neurotransmitter mediated by cyclic guanosine monophosphate (cGMP). Significant reduction of LES pressure has been demonstrated 10 minutes after sublingual administration of a 5 mg dose of isosorbide dinitrate [9]. Very few randomized controlled trials have evaluated the effect of nitrates on achalasia. Wong *et al.* [10] found a significant decrease in LES pressure and significant improvement in esophageal emptying 30 minutes after a single dose (0.4 mg) of sublingual nitroglycerin in a randomized crossover study. In several other small studies [11–14], nitrates have decreased LES pressure by 30–65%, with symptom improvement in 58–87% of patients (Table 4.1), but these were uncontrolled studies that traditionally tend to overemphasize the benefits of interventions. Calcium channel blockers produce smooth muscle relaxation by decreasing entry of calcium, necessary for contraction, into smooth muscle cells. In a double-blind randomized controlled trial in 10 achalasia patients [15], sublingual nifedipine (10–30 mg dose, titrated according to patient tolerance) given before meals achieved a significant reduction in LES pressures 30 minutes after administration. However, despite this reduction, LES pressures were still substantial after treatment (mean LES pressure of 30 mmHg). These investigators also reported a modest improvement of dysphagia with nifedipine, with a reduction in the average number of meals per day with dysphagia from 1.9 to 0.9. **A1d** Other uncontrolled studies suggest that calcium

channel blockers decrease LES pressure by 13–49% and improve symptoms in 53–77% of patients [11, 12, 15–17]. **B4**

In a small randomized controlled trial comparing calcium channel blockers and nitrates in 15 patients, 12 found sublingual isosorbide dinitrate (5 mg) to be superior to sublingual nifedipine (20 mg) for the treatment of achalasia. **A1d** In comparison to nifedipine, isosorbide dinitrate achieved a more pronounced reduction in basal LES pressure (47% vs 64%). Additionally, more patients receiving isosorbide dinitrate experienced complete radionuclide meal clearance at 10 minutes (53% vs 15%) and relief of dysphagia (87% vs 53%).

Sildenafil (Viagra) inhibits smooth muscle contraction by promoting accumulation of NO stimulated cGMP (NO-cGMP) through inhibition of NO phosphodiesterase type 5, an enzyme that degrades NO-cGMP. Recently, in a placebo-controlled randomized trial of sildenafil (50 mg) in 14 achalasia patients, Bortolotti *et al.* [18] showed that sildenafil by direct intragastric infusion significantly reduced basal LES pressure, post-deglutitive LES residual pressure and esophageal body contraction amplitude. Peak effect was reached 15–20 minutes after infusion and lasted less than one hour. Eherer *et al.* [19] administered sildenafil orally (50 mg) to 11 patients with esophageal motor disorders, three of whom had a diagnosis of achalasia. LES pressure decreased in two of these patients, but none had relief of symptoms.

Overall, nitrates and calcium channel blockers can reduce LES pressure. The effect on symptoms is variable, short-lived, and usually suboptimal. **A1d** Additionally, adverse effects such as headache, hypotension, and pedal edema that are frequent may limit their use [11]. Therefore, these agents should be reserved for the short-term relief of achalasia symptoms, either as a temporizing measure while awaiting more definitive therapy, or in patients who are too sick or unwilling to undergo other treatments. Sildenafil merits further study in randomized controlled trials.

Botulinum toxin

Endoscopic injection of botulinum toxin into the LES is a relatively recent addition to the treatment options for achalasia. It produces reduction in LES pressure by inhibiting acetylcholine release from nerve endings, thereby counterbalancing the effect of the selective loss of inhibitory neurotransmitters (nitrous oxide and vasoactive intestinal peptide) in achalasia. It is safe, easy to administer and provides symptom relief initially in approximately 85% of patients; however, the effect of a single injection is usually limited to six months or less in over 50% of patients [3]. **B4**

In a six-month randomized controlled trial of 21 patients, the administration of botulinum toxin (100 units) resulted in significant symptom score improvement (from 7.1 ± 1.2 to 1.6 ± 2.2), compared to placebo (from 5.9 ± 1.6 to 5.4 ± 2.0)

Table 4.2 Botulinum toxin injection for the treatment of achalasia: symptomatic improvement after one injection.

Authors	No. of patients	<1 mo	6 mo	12 mo	24 mo	Responding to repeat injections
Pasricha et al. [20, 21]	31	90	55	—	—	27
Cuillere et al. [23]	55	75	50	—	—	33
Rollan et al. [24]	3	100	66	—	—	—
Fishman et al. [25]	60	70	—	36	—	86
Annese et al. [26]	8	100	13	—	—	100
Gordon and Eaker [27]	16	75	44	—	—	—
Muehldorfer et al. [28]	12	75	50	25	10	—
Vaezi et al. [29]	22	63	36	32	—	—
Annese et al. [30]	118	82	—	64	—	100
Kolbasnik et al. [31]	30	77	57	39	25	100
Mikaeli et al. [32]	20	65	25	15	—	60
Allescher et al. [33]	23	74	—	45	30	—
Neubrand et al. [34]	25	65	—	—	36	0

mo: months.

Modified from Hoogerwerf WA et al. Gastrointest. Endosc Clin North Am 2001; **11**: 311–323 [22].

(p = 0.001) at one week. By six months the proportion of patients in remission had declined from 82% to 66% [20]. **A1d** A subsequent study by the same group [21] evaluated the efficacy of botulinum toxin over a 2–3-year period and found that 65% (20/31) of patients had good symptom improvement at six months. However, 19 of these 20 responders eventually relapsed, requiring repeat injections, and two-thirds of the patients eventually chose a more definitive form of therapy. In the analysis of subgoups in this small study the response rate appeared to be higher for patients over the age of 50 years and those with the "vigorous" form of achalasia. Subsequent studies [20–34] have confirmed that botulinum toxin is initially effective, but the benefit of a single injection lasts less than one year in the majority of patients, with all patients requiring repeat injections or other forms of therapy for their achalasia (Table 4.2). **A1d, B4** Botulinum toxin is extremely safe, with 25% of patients presenting with transient, mild, post-procedural chest pain, and 5% developing symptomatic gastroesophageal reflux disease (GERD) [6].

Botulinum toxin is an effective and safe option for the short-term treatment of achalasia. Symptoms are relieved on average for six months with repeat treatments being required to keep patients in long-term remission. Botulinum toxin is inferior to pneumatic dilatation or surgery (see comparative studies below), but it can be particularly useful in the elderly, who may have a higher response rate than younger patients (under age 50 years) and who may have a life expectancy of ≤2 years. Clouse et al. showed the survival analysis curve did not differ significantly for repeated botulinum toxin injections compared to pneumatic dilation at year 1 and year 2 (p = 0.5 and p = 0.4 respectively) [35].

Pneumatic dilatation

Disruption of the muscle fibers of the LES through forceful dilatation has been used as treatment of achalasia for many years. The first description of dilatation dates from 1674 when a patient with achalasia was treated by passing a piece of carved whalebone with a sponge affixed to the distal end down the esophagus into the stomach [7]. The first pneumatic (i.e. air filled) dilators were introduced in the late 1930s, and both the equipment and technique have evolved over the years. Not only are the dilators and techniques varied, but the definitions of success differ across studies. However, there is sufficient experience with the currently used balloon dilators to comment on their efficacy and safety.

Kadakia and Wong calculated the pooled effect of the older dilators (Brown-McHardy Mosher and Hurst-Tucker balloons) among a total of 235 patients studied in five prospective studies. Symptomatic response was excellent or good in 61–100% of patients who were followed for a mean of 2.7 years [36]. **B4** Currently, the most widely used dilator in the USA is the Rigiflex polyethylene balloon (Boston Scientific, Boston), which is available in three different diameters (30, 35 and 40 mm) [11]. The current technique consists of endoscopy to determine landmarks, followed by placement of a balloon across the LES, usually under fluoroscopic guidance. The balloon is then inflated to sufficient pressure (usually 7–12 psi; 48.3–82.7 kPa) for up to 60 seconds to disrupt the muscle fibers of the LES.

There are no clinical trials that compare pneumatic dilatation to placebo (i.e. sham dilatation). In recent randomized controlled trials comparing pneumatic dilatation to Botulinum toxin injection, symptom improvement rates for dilatation at 12 months ranged between 53% and 70% [28,

Table 4.3 Rigiflex balloon dilatation for the treatment of achalasia.

Authors	No. of patients	Study design	% with exc/good response	Follow-up in months (mean)	Perforation rate (%)
Cox et al. [38]	7	P	86	9	0
Gelfand and Kozarek [39]	24	P	93	NR	0
Barkin et al. [40]	50	P	90	20	2
Stark et al. [41]	10	P	74	6	0
Makela et al. [42]	17	R	75	6	5.9
Levine et al. [43]	62	R	85	NR	0
Kim et al. [44]	14	P	75	4	0
Lee et al. [45]	28	P	87	N R	0
Abid et al. [46]	36	P	88	27	6.6
Wehrmann et al. [47]	40	R	87	NR	2.5
Lambroza and Schuman [48]	27	P	89	21	0
Muehldorfer et al. [49]	12	R	83	18	8.3
Bhatnager et al. [50]	15	R	84	14	0
Gideon et al. [51]	24	R	NR	6	4
Khan et al. [52]	9	P	85	NR	0
Kadakia and Wong [37, 53]	56	P	88	59	0
Vela and Richter [5][a]	100	P	82	24	2
Chan et al. [54]	66	R	62	55	4.5
Dobrucali et al. [55]	43	P	54	29	2.3
Kostic et al. [56]	26	P	87	12	NR
Vela et al. [57][a]	106	R	44	36	1.9
Mikaeli et al. [58]	200	P	65	36	00
Ghoshal et al. [59]	126	R	78	15	0.8
Guardino et al. [60][a]	96	R	74	7	1.7
Guardino et al. [60][a,b]	12	R	50	11	0
Boztas et al. [61]	50	R	67	38	0

P: prospective; R: retrospective; NR: not reported.

[a] Patients in these studies overlap.

[b] Patients S/P Heller myotomy.

Modified and updated from Vaezi M F, Richter JE. *J Clin Gastroenterol* 1998; 27: 21–35 [11] and Gelfand MD and Kozarek RA. *Am J Gastroenterol* 1989; 84: 924–927 [39].

29, 32]. **AId** Table 4.3 summarizes the results of 26 uncontrolled studies of Rigiflex pneumatic dilatation for the treatment of achalasia with <5 years follow-up [5, 37–61], the degree of heterogeneity of these studies is not known. The pooled results of 1256 patients followed for a mean of 20 months yield an excellent to good response in 77% of patients. **B4** However, it should be emphasized that uncontrolled studies tend to exaggerate the benefits of interventions, and the criteria used to determine the response to treatment varies among studies. Furthermore, while a graded approach to pneumatic dilation using repeat treatment with a larger balloon size is considered standard, in some studies a repeat procedure within a graded dilation protocol is considered a failure. Zerbib et al. [62] used an iterative approach with pneumatic dilation based on recurrence of patient symptoms. In their protocol, graded dilations were performed every 2–3 weeks until remission

occurred. Patients were considered treatment failures with persistent symptoms after four or five procedures and only 11 of 150 failed with this approach. **B4**

Another important issue is the relative paucity of long-term outcome studies of pneumatic dilatation. There have been few randomized controlled trials evaluating pneumatic dilation performed with the currently available balloons. In the most recent trial by Kostic et al. that included 26 patients treated with pneumatic dilation and followed for 12 months, 77% of patients improved with treatment [56]. In an older randomized controlled trial with follow-up extending beyond 12 months, 50% of patients treated with pneumatic dilatation had relapse of dysphagia at 30 months [28]. **AId** West et al. [63] reported on the success of pneumatic dilatation in patients followed for more than five years. Although this study was characterized by serious methodological limitations, including the use of

Table 4.4 Rigiflex balloon dilatation for the treatment of achalasia: long-term results.

Authors	No. of patients	Study design	% with exc/good response	Follow-up in months (mean)	Perforation rate (%)
Karamanolis et al. [64]	153	R	51	192	0.46
Katsinelos et al. [65]	39	R	58	108	5.4
Mikaeli et al. [58]	62	P	55	71	3.7

P: prospective; R: retrospective.

Modified and updated from Vaezi M F, Richter JE. *J Clin Gastroenterol* 1998; 27: 21–35 [11] and Gelfand MD and Kozarek RA. *Am J Gastroenterol* 1989; 84: 924–7 [39].

different types of balloons and the use of a symptom questionnaire to define therapeutic success, it was the first study with extended follow-up. The overall therapeutic success rate was 50% in 81 patients followed for more than five years, and the mean number of dilatations per patient was four. Success rate decreased in patients with longer follow-up: 60% in patients followed between 5 and 9 years, 50% for those followed between 10 and 14 years, and 40% in the group followed for more than 15 years. **B4** There have been three subsequent studies with extended follow-up beyond five years. The success rate in 254 pooled patients reached 55% after a mean follow-up period of ten years (Table 4.4) [58, 64, 65].

The overall perforation rate associated with pneumatic dilatation is approximately 2% (this varies across different studies, from as low as 0%, to as high as 8%) [11]. Mortality from the procedure is estimated to be 0.2% [6]. Gastroesophageal reflux after pneumatic dilatation occurs in 15–33% of patients [5, 35]. **A1d B4** Overall, pneumatic dilatation results in good to excellent symptom relief in approximately 80% of patients based upon follow-up of one or two years. However, the limited long-term follow-up data suggest that the remission rates decline with time and the few studies with extended follow-up periods beyond five years indicate a 57% success rate [58, 64, 65]. That said, pneumatic dilatation is the most effective non-surgical treatment available for achalasia and has a success rate comparable with that of surgery (see comparative studies below). It should be considered an acceptable alternative to surgery for treatment of achalasia.

Heller myotomy

Surgical myotomy was originally described by Ernest Heller in 1914 and involved cutting the anterior and posterior aspects of the LES through a thoracotomy [66].The surgical technique has evolved first with a laparotomy approach and again with the advent of minimally invasive surgery in the 1990s. While a thoracoscopic approach has been used, laparoscopic myotomy has become the preferred method, as it is associated with less morbidity and

quicker recovery times [67]. Whether an anti-reflux procedure should be performed (to prevent reflux) or not (to avoid postoperative dysphagia) has been a matter of controversy [3, 7]. Recent studies by Rice et al. and Richards et al. determined that the addition of anterior fundoplication (Dor) does reduce the amount of acid reflux following Heller myotomy [68, 69]. In the study conducted by Rice et al., the esophageal acid exposure time in the upright position varied from 0.4% with anterior fundoplication to 2.9% without (p = 0.005). The same study compared the incidence of reflux, resting LESP, and esophageal emptying. The addition of a Dor fundoplication resulted in significantly less reflux (0.4% vs 2.9% p = 0.005), a higher LESP (18 mmHg vs 13 mmHg p = 0.002), and no difference in the esophageal emptying (p = 0.6) [68]. Similar results were demonstrated by Richards et al., who observed that the addition of anterior fundoplication decreased the amount of reflux (p = 0.005), without increasing dysphagia scores [69]. These limited data indicate that anti-reflux procedures may decrease post-esophagomyotomy reflux without impairing emptying, but the long-term effect on this balance is still unknown.

Minimally invasive surgery and especially laparoscopy, has become the standard approach to perform myotomy. Uncontrolled studies of the thoracoscopic [11, 70–75] and laparoscopic [11, 56, 57, 75–100] techniques are summarized in Tables 4.5 and 4.6 respectively. Pooled results of 103 patients in five studies of thoracoscopy yield good to excellent symptom response in 82% of patients with a mean follow-up of 16 months, although GERD developed in 42% of patients. The pooled symptom response rate was 84% in 1420 patients undergoing laparoscopic or open Heller myotomy in 30 uncontrolled trials; 37% of these patients developed GERD [11, 56, 57, 75–100]. **B4**

As with pneumatic dilation, the efficacy of Heller myotomy decreases with longer follow-up periods. In a series of 73 patients treated with Heller myotomy, excellent/good responses were reported in 89% and 57% of patients at six months and six years' follow-up [57]. Csendes et al. observed 80% of patients with good/excellent results

Table 4.5 Thoracoscopic myotomy for the treatment of achalasia.

Authors	No. of patients	Anti-reflux procedure	% symptom good/ excellent	Follow-up months (mean)	% somplication GERD
Patti *et al.* [71]	30	No	87	NR	NR
Cade and Martin [72]	12	No	92	3	18
Raiser *et al.* [73]	10	Yes	62	15	57
Pellegrini *et al.* [74]	35	No	87	12	60
Ramacciato *et al.* [75]	16	No	63	35	31

Modified and updated from Vaezi MF, Richter JE. *J Clin Gastroenterol* 1998; **27**: 21–35 [11].
NR: not reported; GERD: gastroesophageal reflux disease.

Table 4.6 Laparoscopic myotomy for the treatment of achalasia.

Author	No. of patients	Anti-reflux procedure	% symptom improvement good/excellent	Follow-up in months (mean)	% complication GERD
Rosati *et al.* [76]	25	Yes	96	12	N R
Ancona *et al.* [77]	17	Yes (D[a])	100	8	6
Mitchell *et al.* [78]	14	Yes (D)	86	NR	7
Swanstrom and Pennings [76]	12	Yes (T[b])	100	16	16
Raiser *et al.* [73]	39	Yes (D/T)	63	26	27
Morino *et al.* [80]	18	Yes (D)	100	8	6
Robertson *et al.* [81]	10	No	88	14	13
Bonovina *et al.* [82]	33	Yes (D)	97	12	NR
Delgado *et al.* [83]	12	Yes (D)	83	4	NR
Hunter *et al.* [84]	40	Yes (D/T)	90	13	18
Kjellin *et al.* [85]	21	No	52	22	38
Ackroyd *et al.* [86]	82	Yes (D)	87	24	5
Yamamura *et al.* [87]	24	Yes (D)	88	17	0
Patti *et al.* [88]	102	Yes (D)	89	25	NR
Pechlivanides *et al.* [89]	29	Yes (D)	90	12	10
Sharp *et al.* [90]	100	No	87	10	14
Donahue *et al.* [91]	81	Yes (D)	84	45	26
Zaninotto *et al.* [92]	113	Yes (D)	92	12	5
Ramacciato *et al.* [75]	17	Yes (D)	94	18	6
Luketich *et al.* [93]	62	Yes (T/D)	92	19	9
Decker *et al.* [94]	73	Yes (T/D)	83	31	11
Mineo *et al.* [95]	14	Yes (D)	NR	85	14
Gockel *et al.* [96]	108	Yes (D)	97	55	22
Wright *et al.* [97]	52	Yes (D)	83	46	19
Wright *et al.* [97]	63	Yes (T)	95	45	50
Khajanchee *et al.* [98]	121	Yes (T)	84	9	33
Kostic *et al.* [56]	25	Yes (T)	96	12	NR
Zaninotto *et al.* [99]	40	Yes (D/F)	88	38	3
Vela *et al.* [57]	73	Yes (D/T)	57	72	56
Csendes *et al.* [100]	67	Yes (D)	73	190	33

[a] D, Dor.
[b] T, Toupet.
[c] F, Floppy Nissen.
P: prospective; R: retrospective; NR: not reported.
Modified from Vaezi MF, Richter JE. *J Clin Gastroenterol* 1998; **27**: 21–35 [11].

at 7–10 years, 74% at 10–20 years and 65% at >20 years [100].

As stated earlier, the degree of benefit may be overestimated in uncontrolled studies. Heller myotomy, preferably through the laparoscopic approach, should be considered as effective as pneumatic dilatation and should be offered to patients who present an acceptable surgical risk. It can also be offered to those who have failed pneumatic dilatation.

Comparisons of different treatment modalities

Pneumatic dilatation versus botulinum toxin   These two therapeutic approaches have been compared in three randomized controlled trials (Table 4.7). **A1d** Vaezi *et al.* [29] randomized 42 patients to receive botulinum toxin injection or graded pneumatic dilatation with 30 and 35 mm Rigiflex balloons and reported success at 12 months (defined as improvement in symptom score greater than 50%) to be 70% for dilatation and 32% for botulinum toxin. Using a similar design and criteria for symptom response, Mikaeli *et al.* [32] reported response rates at 12 months of 53% with single pneumatic dilatation and 15% with a single botulinum toxin injection. Success after repeat dilation or repeat injection was observed, respectively, in 100% and 60% of patients at 12 months. Muehldorfer *et al.* [28] randomized 24 patients to botulinum toxin or dilatation with a 40 mm latex balloon; symptomatic response was superior with pneumatic dilatation compared with botulinum toxin at 12 months (67% vs 25%) and at 30 months (50% vs 0%). Identification of predictors of response was not possible in any of these three small randomized trials. Although randomization codes were concealed, patients and investigators were not blinded as to the treatments received.

Two studies have compared the costs of Heller myotomy, pneumatic dilation and botox injection. The costs per symptomatic cure over a ten-year horizon were $10,792 for Heller myotomy, $3723 for BoTox injection, and $3111 for pneumatic dilation [101]. A cost-effectiveness study that accounted for quality of life over a five-year horizon determined the costs of BoTox injection, pneumatic dilation and

Heller myotomy to be $7011, $7069, and $21,407 respectively. While the cost of BoTox was slightly lower, PD was more cost-effective, with an incremental cost-effectiveness of $1348 per QALY (quality adjusted life year) [102].

Heller myotomy versus botulinum toxin   There is only one prospective randomized controlled trial comparing the effectiveness of laparoscopic myotomy and botulinum toxin injection. A total of 80 patients were randomized to either treatment group. The lower esophageal resting and relaxation pressures, esophageal body dilation, and dysphagia/regurgitation scores were all measured before and after treatment. After six months there was a greater symptom reduction (82% vs 66%) in the myotomy group compared to the BoTox group. The two-year probability of remaining symptom free was 87% after myotomy and 34% after BoTox. Median LESP was significantly lower in the surgery group (27 mmHg vs 36 mmHg p < 0.05). The esophageal body diameter was not significantly different 4.1 cm vs 3.5 cm [99]. Two cost minimization studies compared Heller myotomy, pneumatic dilation and botox injection. Heller myotomy was associated with greater costs compared to BoTox injection in both studies (US$10,792 vs 3723 and US$21,407 vs 7011) [103].

Pneumatic dilatation versus Heller myotomy   The first randomized controlled trial that compared pneumatic dilatation to myotomy [70, 100] found that myotomy via laparotomy had a success rate of 95% compared with 65% for pneumatic dilatation with the Mosher bag. **A1d** Neither of these techniques are widely used today, and the results may not be generalizable to other techniques. Spiess and Kahrilas [7] pooled all uncontrolled series of ten or more patients undergoing pneumatic dilatation or surgery with follow-up greater than a year performed between 1966 and 1997. They reported response rates as weighted means and found good to excellent symptom response in 80 ± 42% of participants with pneumatic dilatation. Response rates for surgery were 84 ± 20% with thoracotomy, 85 ± 42% with laparotomy, and 92 ± 18% with laparoscopy. However, criteria for including or excluding reports were not stated, and these uncontrolled studies may tend to overestimate

Table 4.7 Randomized trials comparing symptomatic response 12 months after pneumatic dilatation or botulinum toxin injection for treatment of achalasia. No. (%) of patients with symptomatic remission.

Authors	No. of patients	Pneumatic dilatation	Botulinum toxin injection	P value
Vaezi *et al.* [29]	42	14/20(70)	7/22(32)	0.017
Mikaeli *et al.* [32]	39	10/19(53)	3/20(15)	<0.01
Muehldorfer *et al.* [28]	24	8/12(67)	3/12(25)	<0.05

the benefits of treatment. **B4** Kostic *et al.* [56] were the first to conduct a randomized controlled trial comparing patients treated with current techniques, laparoscopic Heller myotomy and pneumatic dilation with the Rigiflex balloon. The results of this trial showed 96% success in the myotomy group versus 87% in the dilation group during a 12-month follow-up period compared to the data reported by Csendes (95% vs 65%). The duration of treatment response for either intervention is not clear, as most studies include follow-up periods <5 years. Vela *et al.* [57] demonstrated the effectiveness of myotomy and dilation declines over time. In 106 patients undergoing pneumatic dilation and 73 treated with Heller myotomy, there were similar results at six months (90% vs 89%), but after six years only 44% and 57% of patients continued to have a good/excellent response. The only variables associated with patient outcomes in the dilation group were sex and age. Women more frequently required a single dilation, and younger patients, especially men, were more likely to have early failure requiring more than one dilation within the first six months. The frequency of post-treatment GER varies among studies for both PD and HM. In a retrospective study comparing PD to HM, the use of PPIs for heartburn was more common in the myotomy patients (56% vs 26%, p < 0.01). Gastroesophageal reflux was a cause for symptom recurrence in only 4% of patients that were dilated, compared to 36% of those who received myotomies. An antireflux procedure was performed in 33% of the patients treated with myotomy. However, reflux still occurred in 39% of them compared to 65% of those who did not receive an anti-reflux procedure [57].

From these data and the uncontrolled studies summarized in Tables 4.5 and 4.6 we conclude that Heller myotomy and pneumatic dilatation have similar success rates. **B4** The success rates for both of these treatments decline over time, and repeat intervention may be required. Pharmacologic acid suppression may be needed in either

case, but it should be strongly considered, and perhaps mandatory, for patients who are treated with Heller myotomy since GER is a cause of late treatment failure [57].

Only one study has compared the costs of pneumatic dilation and Heller myotomy. At a seven-year follow-up period, pneumatic dilation cost US$8474 compared to US$20,064 for myotomy. A limitation of these data is that the myotomy was done through an open approach, and Ancona *et al.* found that a Heller myotomy done through a laparoscopic approach costs less than an open approach (US$2699 vs US$3082) [103].

Esophagectomy

A small number of patients develop "endstage" achalasia, characterized by progressive dilatation and tortuosity of the esophagus [8]. This complication may be seen in cases that are refractory to treatment and in patients with long-standing untreated disease. If these patients do not respond to Heller myotomy, esophageal resection is frequently required. Esophagectomy is associated with a greater morbidity/mortality than laparoscopic Heller myotomy, and should be a "last resort" for patients who have failed pneumatic dilation and/or Heller myotomy. Patti *et al.* [104] demonstrated the technical feasibility of a laparoscopic Heller myotomy in patients with a dilated (>6cm) sigmoid esophagus. There was not an increased complication rate in this group, and success rates (91%) were similar to those observed in patients with less dilated and tortuous organs.

There are few studies that assess the effectiveness of the two approaches to resection of the esophagus, i.e. the use of colonic interposition or a gastric pull-up. No randomized controlled trials have been carried out in this area. The available uncontrolled data show symptom improvement in over 80% of endstage cases of achalasia with mortality rates between 0% and 5.4%, and development of GERD in 8–36% of patients (Table 4.8) [8, 105–112]. The studies per-

Table 4.8 Esophagectomy in the treatment of refractory achalasia.

Authors	No. of patients	% symptom improvement	Follow-up in months (mean)	GERD	% complication postop dilation	Mortality
Pinotti *et al.* [106]	122	83	93	36	17	4.1
Watson *et al.* [107]	104	98	NR	20	30	2
Orringer and Stirling [108]	26	100	30	15	39	3.9
Cecconello *et al.* [109]	64	94	81	16	NR	NR
Miller *et al.* [110]	37	91	76	8	14	5.4
Banbury *et al.* [8]	32	87	43	31	60	0
Peters *et al.* [111]	19	80	72	NR	28	0
Devaney *et al.* [112]	93	95	38	NR	46	2.1

P: prospective; R: retrospective; NR: not reported.

Modified and updated from Khazanchi A, Katz PO. *Gastrointest Endosc Clin North Am* 2001; 111: 325–345 [105].

formed do not provide sufficient evidence to determine whether there are advantages of colonic interposition compared with gastric pull-through. **B4**

Summary

Several options are available for the treatment of achalasia, ranging from medications to esophagectomy. Unfortunately, there have been very few controlled trials with long-term follow-up to guide our approach to these patients. Techniques and outcome measures vary over time and between studies. The outcomes of symptom resolution and objective improvement in esophageal emptying are not always correlated. This problem was demonstrated in a study by Vaezi *et al.* [113] who performed timed studies of barium emptying (measuring the column of barium in the esophagus one and five minutes after a bolus) in patients treated with pneumatic dilatation. They found that 31% of patients who reported near complete symptom resolution had less than 50% improvement in barium emptying after treatment. Studies with at least five years of follow-up indicate the response to treatment decreases over time for myotomy and pneumatic dilation [57, 70]. With these limitations in mind, the available evidence is sufficient to make the following recommendations.

• Pharmacologic therapy has variable and limited response and is hindered by adverse effects.

• Calcium channel blockers and nitrates should be used in patients who cannot tolerate or are unwilling to receive other treatments.

• The use of sildenafil should be restricted to research protocols.

• Botulinum toxin is safe and effective but benefit generally lasts less than six months to one year. It should be used in elderly or frail individuals in whom more aggressive treatments pose a high risk.

• Pneumatic dilatation and laparoscopic Heller myotomy have similar efficacy and should be offered as first-line treatments to all patients who can tolerate these procedures. Pneumatic dilatation appears to be the more cost-effective therapeutic approach over a five-year horizon, but whether this holds true with longer follow-up is not known [114, 115]. Although some patient characteristics such as age and sex and patients' preferences should be taken into consideration, we currently have no way of predicting which patient will respond better to pneumatic dilatation or surgery. The risks and benefits of the intervention need to be carefully weighed in each case.

• Esophagectomy may be necessary in patients with end-stage achalasia.

The algorithm in Figure 4.1 depicts a general approach to the treatment of achalasia supported by a guideline paper by the American College of Gastroenterology [4]. A randomized controlled trial of pneumatic dilatation versus laparoscopic Heller myotomy to compare efficacy, cost and safety over an extended follow-up period, and to identify predictors of response is greatly needed. One such study is currently being conducted in Europe.

Complicated patients, including those who are refractory to initial treatment, may benefit from evaluation and

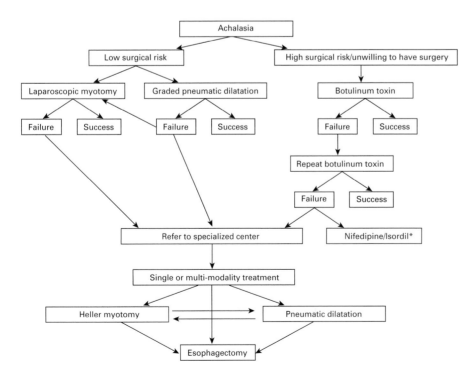

Figure 4.1 Algorithm for the treatment of achalasia. Isosorbide dinitrate (modified from reference 4).

treatment at a tertiary center that can offer expertise in all the treatments available for this disorder. A multi-modality approach is often necessary in this group.

Spastic motility disorders

Spastic motor abnormalities of the esophagus include diffuse esophageal spasm (DES), the nutcracker esophagus (NE), and hypertensive lower esophageal sphincter. These abnormal manometric patterns have been described in association with chest pain and dysphagia. However, whether these abnormal motility patterns represent true diseases, as opposed to manometric findings present in but not responsible for dysphagia and chest pain, remains controversial. Therefore, in contrast to achalasia, the clinical importance of these abnormalities is less clear.

Diffuse esophageal spasm is characterized by normal peristalsis with intermittent simultaneous contractions that can lead to chest pain and dysphagia. The manometric description requires 20% or more simultaneous contractions during water swallows. Adhering to these criteria DES is rare, with an estimated incidence of 0.2/100 000 [116]. This motility disorder is seen in 3–5% of patients who undergo manometry for non-cardiac chest pain or dysphagia [117]. NE, which may be considered a variant of DES, is a manometric abnormality characterized by an average distal esophageal contraction amplitude of 180 mmHg or greater during swallows. Symptoms, i.e. dysphagia and chest pain, are similar for DES and NE. Furthermore, manometric findings may show fluctuation across these disorders, with periods of return to normal peristalsis and, rarely, progression to achalasia.

The etiology of DES and its spastic variants remains unknown. Proposed theories include a dysfunction in endogenous NO synthesis and degradation [118] and defects in cholinergic mechanisms [116]. Other studies suggest that DES can be caused by gastroesophageal reflux [119] and stressful events [120].

The most common presenting symptoms are chest pain, which can occur in association with swallowing or spontaneously, and dysphagia. The chest pain may be clinically indistinguishable from angina of cardiac origin. Dysphagia occurs with both solids and liquids and is transitory and non-progressive.

The diagnosis of a spastic motility disorder is based on the presence of dysphagia or chest pain, accompanied by an abnormal manometry. Chest pain may be stimulated during provocative testing with edrophonium [3]. The diagnosis should only be made after cardiac causes have been thoroughly ruled out. It is important to determine whether gastroesophageal reflux is present by 24-hour pH monitoring, because acid reflux can be a cause of chest pain. If GERD is found, it should be aggressively treated with acid suppression.

Treatment of spastic motility disorders

Overview
Therapeutic trials for spastic motility disorders are scarce, and most of them are uncontrolled studies with small numbers of patients. The unknown etiology and pathophysiology, the controversies surrounding the clinical importance of DES and NE, which make development of therapies challenging, and the rarity of these disorders, have interfered with design and performance of large randomized trials. Furthermore, a high association with psychiatric diseases (depression, anxiety, panic disorder) and issues of heightened visceral sensation pose additional problems [120, 121]. The main goal of therapy is symptomatic relief. An important component in the treatment of DES and NE consists of educating and reassuring the patient about the non-progressive and benign nature of the disease. Many of the treatments used for achalasia have also been used in spastic motility disorders; these include medications such as calcium channel blockers and nitrates, endoscopic botulinum toxin injection, pneumatic dilatation and surgical myotomy.

Additionally, psychotropic agents have been shown to be useful in patients with chest pain of esophageal origin. Observational studies of a number of interventions for these disorders have been carried out [19, 122–132] and the results of a small number of randomized trials are summarized in Table 4.9.

Medications
Treatment aimed at reducing muscle contractility has been attempted with nitrates or calcium channel blockers. Intravenous nitroglycerin (100–200 mg/kg) was shown to decrease the duration of contractions and relieve symptoms in five patients with DES [118]. **B4** There are no randomized controlled trials evaluating the efficacy of nitrates in the treatment of esophageal spasm. In a randomized controlled trial of diltiazem 60 mg three times daily for two weeks, chest pain and dysphagia were not improved [122]. **A1d** In another randomized controlled trial of 14 patients with chest pain, nine of them with manometric diagnosis of NE, diltiazem 60 mg PO four times daily for eight weeks resulted in a significant decrease in mean chest pain scores [123]. **A1d** However, the symptomatic improvement occurred regardless of whether manometry showed NE. In uncontrolled studies, nifedipine resulted in relief of dysphagia in five of six patients with DES [124] and improved chest pain in four of six patients with DES or NE[125]. However, in a 14-week, double-blind crossover study of patients with non-cardiac chest pain and NE, nifedipine 10–30 mg PO three times daily for 14 weeks decreased the

Table 4.9 Randomized controlled trials of treatment for spastic disorders of esophageal motility.

Authors	No. of patients	Treatment	Design	Duration	% symptom improvement
Drenth et al. [122]	8	Diltiazem 60 mg three times daily	Crossover	4 weeks	0
Richter et al. [126]	20	Nifedipine 10–30 mg three times daily	Crossover	6 weeks	10
Clouse et al. [127]	29	Trazadone 100–150 mg/day	Double-blind Parallel	6 weeks	Trazadone 50 Placebo 10 (p = 0.02)
Cannon et al. [121]	49	Imipramine 50 mg at bed time	Double-blind Parallel	3 weeks	Imipramine 52 ± 25 Placebo 1 ± 86 (p = 0.03)

distal esophageal contraction amplitude but did not reduce the frequency or severity of chest pain compared to placebo [126]. **A1d** Although other small studies or anecdotal reports described manometric improvement with nitrates or calcium channel blockers, these were not always accompanied by a good clinical response, and adverse effects such as headache, hypotension or lower extremity edema were frequent. More recently, a small uncontrolled study of sildenafil (50 mg PO every day) for the treatment of four patients with NE and one patient with DES, found a symptom relief rate of 60% [19]. **C5**

The use of psychotropic drugs for DES is aimed at altering visceral sensation and targeting stress as a potential cause of spasm. In a randomized controlled trial of 29 patients with chest pain treated with the serotonin reuptake inhibitor trazodone (100–150 mg/day for six weeks), distress over esophageal symptoms was significantly reduced, with no effect on the manometric abnormalities [127]. In a second randomized controlled trial, the tricyclic antidepressant imipramine (50 mg at bedtime) in patients with chest pain and normal cardiac evaluation achieved a 52 ± 25% reduction in episodes of chest pain compared with only 1 ± 86% reduction in placebo-treated patients (p = 0.03) [121]. **A1d** Abnormal manometry was present in only half of the patients and did not predict the response to treatment.

In summary, there are no good data showing improvement of chest pain or dysphagia with nitrates or calcium channel blockers. However, given the lack of established treatments, and since symptoms may be alleviated in some subjects, a therapeutic trial with these agents is reasonable. Therapeutic trials with trazodone or imipramine are recommended for treating chest pain of esophageal origin, although their effect on dysphagia has not been studied. As in the treatment of achalasia, controlled trials with sildenafil are needed.

Botulinum toxin

Inhibition of esophageal contraction after botulinum toxin injection has been recently introduced as a treatment of spastic motility disorders. Miller et al. [128] used botulinum toxin to treat chest pain in patients with a diagnosis of non-reflux, non-cardiac, non-achalasia spastic esophageal motility disorder (including DES, hypertensive LES or NE). This uncontrolled study of 29 patients receiving botulinum toxin injection at the esophagogastric junction into the LES muscle (the esophageal body was not injected), found 50% or greater reduction in chest pain in 70% of patients and complete relief in 48%. Mean duration of symptom relief was seven months. **B4** Storrs et al. [129] injected botulinum toxin in 1.5 cm intervals into the esophageal body of nine patients with DES, finding 50% or greater improvement in dysphagia and chest pain in 89% of patients at six months. There are no randomized controlled trials evaluating the use of botulinum toxin for the treatment of DES or NE. Uncontrolled studies tend to overestimate the benefits of treatment. However, this agent has a remarkable safety profile and can be tried in patients who fail medical therapy. **B4**

Pneumatic dilatation and Heller myotomy

In an uncontrolled study, Ebert et al. [130] found that pneumatic dilatation improved symptoms in eight of nine (89%) patients with DES and manometry showing high LES pressure in addition to spasm. The procedure, however, did not result in correction of the abnormal esophageal body contractions. Irving et al. [131] used dilatation with Rigiflex balloon to treat 20 DES patients with severe symptoms that were refractory to conservative management; symptom response was reported to be good in 70% of patients. **B4**

Patti et al. [132], using thoracoscopic myotomy in ten patients with DES and NE, found that this minimally invasive approach improved symptoms in 80% of patients. Ellis et al. [133] reported an overall symptomatic improvement rate of 70% in 42 patients with esophageal motor disorders (32 had a diagnosis of esophageal spasm) treated with long esophagomyotomy performed through a thoracotomy. In contrast, a more recent study by Patti et al. [134] compared the symptom scores in patients with primary motility disorders pre and post-intervention with either thoracoscopic or laparoscopic Heller myotomy. In patients with DES, myotomy relieved dysphagia and chest pain in more than 80%; however, patients with nutcracker esophagus had a less predictable response, and surgery most often failed to relieve the symptoms.

There are no randomized controlled trials evaluating pneumatic dilatation or esophageal myotomy as treatment of DES. The uncontrolled studies may overestimate the benefit of these treatments. Given the morbidity associated with these invasive procedures, they should be reserved for patients with severe symptoms who are refractory to other forms of treatment. These procedures should only be carried out after careful discussion of risks and benefits with the patient. **B4**

Summary

Diffuse esophageal spasm and its spastic variants are rare disorders. It is critical that a cardiac etiology is ruled out before making the diagnosis of a spastic motility disorder as a cause of chest pain. Gastroesophageal reflux should be investigated and treated when present. Randomized controlled trials in large populations evaluating treatment for these disorders are lacking. The available data suggest that therapeutic trials of muscle relaxants, such as nitrates and calcium channel blockers, may be warranted in some patients. Psychotropic medications, like trazodone or imipramine, are recommended as symptomatic treatment for chest pain associated with a motility disorder but have no proven role in the treatment of dysphagia. Botulinum toxin has resulted in symptom improvement in uncontrolled trials; this agent warrants further study in randomized controlled trials and is attractive because of its excellent adverse effect profile. Finally, pneumatic dilatation and myotomy should be reserved for patients with severe, refractory symptoms after careful consideration of the risks associated with these procedures.

References

1 Mayberry JF. Epidemiology and demographics of achalasia. *Gastrointest Endosc Clin North Am* 2001; **11**: 235–247.

2 Wong RKH, Maydonovitch CL. Achalasia. In: Castell DO, Richter JE, eds. *The Esophagus*, 3rd edn. Lippincott Williams & Wilkins, Philadelphia 1999: 185–213.

3 Richter JE. Oesophageal motility disorders. *Lancet* 2001; **358**: 823–828.

4 Vaezi MF, Richter JE. Diagnosis and management of achalasia. *Am J Gastroenterol* 1999; **94**: 3406–3412.

5 Vela MF, Richter JE. Management of achalasia at a tertiary center – a complicated disease. *Gastroenterology* 2003; **124**: A236.

6 Spechler SJ. AGA technical review on treatment of patients with dysphagia caused by benign disorders of the distal esophagus. *Gastroenterology* 1999; **117**: 223–254.

7 Spiess AE, Kahrilas PJ. Treating achalasia: From whalebone to laparoscope. *JAMA* 1998; **280**: 638–642.

8 Banbury MK, Rice TW, Goldblum JR *et al.* Esophagectomy with gastric reconstruction for achalasia. *J Thorac Cardiovasc Surg* 1999; **117**: 1077–1085.

9 Gelfond M, Rozen P, Gilat T. Effect of nitrates on LOS pressure in achalasia: a potential therapeutic aid. *Gut* 1981; **22**: 312–138.

10 Wong RK, Maydonovitch C, Garcia JE, Johnson LF, Castell DO. The effect of terbutaline sulfate, nitroglycerin, and aminophylline on lower esophageal sphincter pressure and radionuclide esophageal emptying in patients with achalasia. *J Clin Gastroenterol* 1987; **9**: 386–389.

11 Vaezi MF, Richter JE. Current therapies for achalasia: Comparison and efficacy. *J Clin Gastroenterol* 1998; **27**: 21–35.

12 Gelfond M, Rozen P, Gilat T. Isosorbide dinitrate and nifedipine treatment of achalasia: Clinical, manometric and radionuclide evaluation. *Gastroenterology* 1982; **83**: 963–969.

13 Gelfond M, Rozen P, Keren S, Gilat T. Effect of nitrates on LOS pressure in achalasia: A potential therapeutic aid. *Gut* 1981; **22**: 312–318.

14 Rozen P, Gelfond M, Salzman S *et al.* Radionuclide confirmation of the therapeutic value of isosorbide dinitrate in relieving the dysphasia in achalasia. *J Clin Gastroenterol* 1982; **4**: 17–22.

15 Traube M, Dubovik S, Lange RC, McCallum RW. The role of nifedipine therapy in achalasia: Results of a randomized, double-blind, placebo-controlled study. *Am J Gastroenterol* 1989; **84**: 1259–1262.

16 Bortolotti M, Labo G. Clinical and manometric effects of nifedipine in patients with esophageal achalasia. *Gastroenterology* 1981; **80**: 39–44.

17 Coccia G, Bortolotti M, Michetti P, Dodero M. Prospective clinical and manometric comparing pneumatic dilation and sublingual nifedipine in the treatment of esophageal achalasia. *Gut* 1991; **32**: 604–606.

18 Bortolotti M, Mari C, Lopilato C *et al.* Effects of sildenafil on esophageal motility of patients with idiopathic achalasia. *Gastroenterology* 2000; **118**: 253–257.

19 Eherer AJ, Schwetz I, Hammer HF *et al.* Effect of sildenafil on oesophageal motor function in healthy subjects and patients with oesophageal motor disorders. *Gut* 2002; **50**: 758–764.

20 Pasricha PJ, Ravich WJ, Hendrix TR *et al.* Intrasphincteric botulinum toxin for the treatment of achalasia. *N Engl J Med* 1995; **332**: 774–778.

21 Pasricha PJ, Rudra R, Ravich WJ *et al.* Botulinum toxin for achalasia: Long-term outcome and predictors of response. *Gastroenterology* 1996; **110**: 1410–1415.

22 Hoogerwerf WA, Pasricha PJ. Pharmacologic therapy in treating achalasia. *Gastrointest Endosc Clin North Am* 2001; **11**: 311–323.

23 Cuilliere C, Ducrotte P, Zerbib F *et al.* Achalasia: outcome of patients treated with intrasphincteric injection of botulinum toxin. *Gut* 1997; **41**: 87–92.

24 Rollan A, Gonzales R, Carvajal S *et al.* Endoscopic intrasphincteric injection of botulinum toxin for the treatment of achalasia. *J Clin Gastroenterol* 1995; **20**: 189–191.

25 Fishman VM, Parkman HP, Schiano TD *et al.* Symptomatic improvement in achalasia after botulinum toxin injection of the lower esophageal sphincter. *Am J Gastroenterol* 1996; **91**: 1724–1730.

26 Annese V, Basciani M, Perri F *et al.* Controlled trial of botulinum toxin injection versus placebo and pneumatic dilation in achalasia. *Gastroenterology* 1996; **111**: 1418–1424.

27 Gordon JM, Eaker EY. Prospective study of esophageal botulinum toxin injection in high-risk achalasia patients. *Am J Gastroenterol* 1997; **92**: 1812–1816.

28 Muehldorfer SM, Schneider TH, Hochberger J *et al.* Esophageal achalasia: Intrasphincteric injection of botulinum toxin versus balloon dilation. *Endoscopy* 1999; **31**: 517–521.

29 Vaezi MJ, Richter JE, Wilcox CM *et al.* Botulinum toxin versus pneumatic dilation in the treatment of achalasia: A randomized trial. *Gut* 1999; **44**: 231–239.

30 Annese V, Bassotti G, Coccia G *et al.* A multicenter randomized study of intrasphincteric botulinum toxin in patients with oesophageal achalasia. *Gut* 2000; **46**: 597–600.

31 Kolbasnik J, Waterfall WE, Fachnie B *et al.* Long-term efficacy of botulinum toxin in classical achalasia; A prospective study. *Am J Gastroenterol* 1999; **94**: 3434–3439.

32 Mikaeli J, Fazel A, Montazeri G *et al.* Randomized controlled trial comparing botulinum toxin injection to pneumatic dilatation for the treatment of achalasia. *Aliment Pharmacol Ther* 2001; **15**: 1389–1396.

33 Allescher HD, Storr M, Seige M *et al.* Treatment of achalasia: Botulinum toxin injection vs pneumatic balloon dilation. A prospective study with long-term follow-up. *Endoscopy* 2001; **33**: 1007–1017.

34 Neubrand M, Scheurlen C, Schepke M, Sauerbach T. Long-term results and prognostic factors in the treatment of achalasia with botulinum toxin. *Endoscopy* 2002; **34**: 519–523.

35 Prakash C, Freedland KE, Chan MF, Clouse RE. Botulinum toxin injections for achalasia symptoms can approximate the short term efficacy of a single pneumatic dilation: A survival analysis approach. *Am J Gastroenterol* 1999; **94**: 328–333.

36 Kadakia SC, Wong RKH. Pneumatic balloon dilation for esophageal achalasia. *Gastrointest Endosc Clin North Am* 2001; **11**: 325–345.

37 Wong RKH, Maydonovitch C. Utility of parameters measured during pneumatic dilation as predictors of successful dilation. *Am J Gastroenterol* 1996; **91**: 1126–1129.

38 Cox J, Buckton GK, Bennett JR. Balloon dilatation in achalasia: A new dilator. *Gut* 1986; **27**: 986–989.

39 Gelfand MD, Kozarek RA. An experience with polyethylene balloon for pneumatic dilation for achalasia. *Am J Gastroenterol* 1989; **84**: 924–927.

40 Barkin JS, Guelrud M, Reiner DK *et al.* Forceful balloon dilation: An outpatient procedure for achalasia. *Gastrointest Endosc* 1990; **36**: 123–125.

41 Stark GA, Castell DO, Richter JE *et al.* Prospective randomized comparison of Browne-McHardy and Microvasive balloon dilator in the treatment of achalasia. *Am J Gastroenterol* 1990; **85**: 1322–1326.

42 Makela J, Kiviniemi H, Laitinen S. Heller's cardiomyotomy compared with pneumatic dilation for the treatment of oesophageal achalasia. *Eur J Surg* 1991; **157**: 411–414.

43 Levine ML, Moskowitz GW, Dorf BS *et al.* Pneumatic dilation in patients with achalasia with a modified Gruntzig dilator (Levine) under direct endoscopic control. Results after 5 years. *Am J Gastroenterol* 1991; **86**: 1581–1584.

44 Kim CH, Cameron AJ, Hsu JJ *et al.* Achalasia: Prospective evaluation of relationship between lower esophageal sphincter pressure, esophageal transit, and esophageal diameter and symptoms in response to pneumatic dilation. *Mayo Clin Proc* 1993; **68**: 1067–1073.

45 Lee JD, Cecil BD, Brown PE *et al.* The Cohen test does not predict outcome in achalasia after pneumatic dilation. *Gastrointest Endosc* 1992; **39**: 157–160.

46 Abid S, Champion G, Richter JE *et al.* Treatment of achalasia: The best of both worlds. *Am J Gastroenterol* 1993; **89**: 979–985.

47 Wehrmann T, Jacobi V, Jung M *et al.* Pneumatic dilation in achalasia with a low-compliance balloon. Results of a 5-year prospective evaluation. *Gastrointest Endosc* 1995; **42**: 31–36.

48 Lambroza A, Schuman RW. Pneumatic dilation for achalasia without fluoroscopic guidance: Safety and efficacy. *Am J Gastroenterol* 1995; **90**: 1226–1229.

49 Muehldorfer SM, Hahn EG, Eli C. High- and low-compliance balloon dilators in patients with achalasia: A randomized prospective comparison trial. *Gastrointest Endosc* 1996; **44**: 398–403.

50 Bhatnager MS, Nanivadekar SA, Sawant P *et al.* Achalasia cardia dilation using polyethylene balloon (Rigiflex) dilator. *Indian J Gastroenterol* 1996; **15**: 49–51.

51 Gideon RM, Castell DO, Yarze J. Prospective randomized comparison of pneumatic dilation techniques in patients with idiopathic achalasia. *Dig Dis Sci* 1999; **44**: 1853–1857.

52 Khan AA, Shah WH, Alam A *et al.* Massively dilated esophagus in achalasia: response to pneumatic balloon dilation. *Am J Gastroenterol* 1999; **94**: 2363–2366.

53 Kadakia SC, Wong RKH. Graded pneumatic dilation using Rigiflex achalasia dilators in patients with primary esophageal achalasia. *Am J Gastroenterol* 1993; **88**: 34–38.

54 Chan Wong SKH, Lee DWH *et al.* Short-term and long-term results of endoscopic balloon dilation for achalasia: 12 years' experience. *Endoscopy* 2004; **36**(8): 690–694.

55 Dobrucali A, Erzin Y, Tuncer M, Dirican A. Long-term results of graded pneumatic dilation under endoscopic guidance in patients with primary esophageal achalasia. *World J Gastroenterology* 2004; **10**(22): 3322–3327.

56 Kostic S, Kjellin A, Ruth M, Lonroth H, Johnsson E, Andersson M, Lundell L. Pneumatic Dilation or Laparoscopic Cardiomyotomy in the Management of Newly Diagnosed Idiopathic Achalasia. *World J Surgery* 2007; **31**: 470–478.

57 Vela M, Richter J, Khandwala F, Blackstone E, Wachsberger D, Baker M, Rice T. The long-term efficacy of pneumatic dilatation and Heller myotomy for the treatment of achalasia. *Clinical Gastroenterology and Hepatology* 2006; **4**: 580–587.

58 Mikaeli J, Bishehsari F, Montazeri G, Yaghoobi M, Malekzadeh R. Pneumatic balloon dilation in achalasia: A prospective comparison of safety and efficacy with different balloon diameters. *Aliment Pharmacol Ther* 2004; **20**: 431–436.

59 Ghoshal UC, Kumar S, Saraswat VA, Aggarwal R, Misra A, Choudhuri G. Long-term follow-up after pneumatic dilation for achalasia cardia: Factors associated with treatment failure and recurrence. *Am J Gastroenterol* 2004; **99**: 2304–2310.

60 Guardino J, Vela M, Connor J, Richter J. Pneumatic dilation for the treatment of achalasia in untreated patients and patients with failed Heller Myotomy. *J Clin Gastroenterol* 2004; **38**: 855–860.

61 Boztas G, Mungan Z, Ozdil S *et al.* Pneumatic balloon dilatation in primary achalasia: The long-term follow-up results. *Hepato-Gastroenterology* 2005; **52**: 475–480.

62 Zerbib F, Thetiot V, Richy F, Benajah DA, Message L, Lamouliatte H. Repeated pneumatic dilations as long-term maintencance therapy for esophageal achalasia. *Am J Gastroenterol* 2006; **101**: 692–697.

63 West RL, Hirsch DP, Batelsman JFWM *et al.* Long term results of pneumatic dilatation in achalasia followed for more than 5 years. *Am J Gastroenterol* 2002; **97**: 1346–1351.

64 Karamanolis G, Sgouros S, Karatzias G, Papadopoulou E, Vasiliadis K, Stefanidis G, Mantides A. Long-term outcome of pneumatic dilation in the treatment of achalasia. *Am J Gastroenterol* 2005; **100**: 270–274.

65 Katsinelos P, Kountouras J, Paroutoglou G *et al.* Long-term results of pneumatic dilation for achalasia: A 15 years' experience. *World J Gastroenterol* 2005; **11**(36): 5701–5705.

66 Amjad A, Pellegrini CA. Laparoscopic myotomy: Technique and efficacy in treating achalasia. *Gastrointest Endosc Clin North Am* 2001; **11**: 347–357.

67 Richter JE. Update on the management of achalasia: balloons, surgery, and drugs. *Gastroenterol Hepatol* 2008; **2**(3): 435–445.

68 Rice T, McKelvey A, Richter J *et al.* A physiologic clinical study of achalasia: Should Dor fundoplication be added to Heller myotomy? *J of Thoracic and Cardiovascular Surgery* 2005; **130**: 1593–1600.

69 Richards W, Torquati A, Holzman M *et al.* Heller myotomy versus Heller myotomy with Dor fundoplication for achalasia: A prospective randomized double-blind clinical trial. *Annals of Surgery* 2004; **240**: 405–415.

70 Csendes A, Braghetto I, Heriquez A *et al.* Late results of a prospective randomized study comparing forceful dilatation and esophagomyotomy in patients with achalasia. *Gut* 1989; **30**: 299–304.

71 Patti MG, Pelligrini CA, Arcerito M *et al.* Comparison of medical and minimally invasive surgical therapy for achalasia. *Arch Surg* 1997; **132**: 233–240.

72 Cade RJ, Martin CJ. Thoracoscopic cardiomyotomy for achalasia. *Aust NZ J Surg* 1996; **66**: 107–109.

73 Raiser F, Perdikis G, Hinder RA *et al.* Heller myotomy via minimal access surgery: An evaluation of anti-reflux procedure. *Am J Surg* 1995; **169**: 424–427.

74 Pellegrini CA, Leichter R, Patti M *et al.* Thoracoscopic esophageal myotomy in the treatment of achalasia. *Ann Thorac Surg* 1993; **56**: 680–682.

75 Ramacciato G, Mercantini P, Amodio PM *et al.* The laparoscopic approach with antireflux surgery is superior to the thoracoscopic approach for the treatment of esophageal achalasia. *Surg Endosc* 2002; **16**: 1431–1437.

76 Rosati R, Fumagalli U, Bonavina L *et al.* Laparoscopic approach to esophageal achalasia. *Am J Surg* 1995; **169**: 424–427.

77 Ancona E, Anselmino M, Zaninotto G *et al.* Esophageal achalasia: laparoscopic vs conventional open Heller-Dor operation. *Am J Surg* 1995; **170**: 265–270.

78 Mitchell PC, Watson DI, Devitt PG *et al.* Laparoscopic cardiomyotomy with a Dor patch for achalasia. *J Am Coll Cardiol* 1995; **38**: 445–449.

79 Swanstrom LL, Pennings J. Laparoscopic esophagomyotomy for achalasia. *Surg Endosc* 1995; **9**: 286–272.

80 Morino M, Rebecchi F, Festa V, Garrone C. Laparoscopic Heller cardiomyotomy with intraoperative manometry in the management of oesophageal achalasia. *Int Surg* 1995; **80**: 332–335.

81 Robertson GSM, Lloyd DM, Wicks ACB *et al.* Laparoscopic Heller's cardiomyotomy without an antireflux procedure. *Br J Surg* 1995; **82**: 957–959.

82 Bonovina L, Rosati P, Segalin A, Peracchia A. Laparoscopic Heller-Dor operation for the treatment of oesophageal achalasia: Technique and early results. *Ann Chir Gynaecol* 1995; **84**: 165–168.

83 Delgado F, Bolufer JM, Martinex-Abad M *et al.* Laparoscopic treatment of esophageal achalasia. *Surg Laparosc Endosc* 1996; **2**: 83–90.

84 Hunter JG, Trus TL, Branum GD, Waring JP. Laparoscopic Heller myotomy and fundoplication for achalasia. *Ann Surg* 1997; **225**: 655–665.

85 Kjellin AP, Granquist S, Ramel S, Thor KBA. Laparoscopic myotomy without fundoplication in patients with achalasia. *Eur J Surg* 1999; **165**: 1162–1166.

86 Ackroyd R, Watson DI, Devitt PG, Jamieson GG. Laparoscopic cardiomyotomy and anterior partial fundoplication for achalasia. *Surg Endosc* 2001; **15**: 683–686.

87 Yamamura MS, Gilster JC, Myers BS *et al.* Laparoscopic Heller myotomy and anterior fundoplication for achalasia results in a high degree of patient satisfaction. *Arch Surg* 2000; **135**: 902–906.

88 Patti MG, Molena D, Fisichella PM *et al.* Laparoscopic Heller myotomy and Dor fundoplication for achalasia. Analysis of successes and failures. *Arch Surg* 2001; **136**: 870–877.

89 Pechlivanides G, Chryos E, Athanasakis E *et al.* Laparoscopic Heller cardiomyotomy and Dor fundoplication for esophageal achalasia. *Arch Surg* 2001; **136**: 1240–1243.

90 Sharp KW, Khaitan L, Scholz S *et al.* 100 consecutive minimally invasive Heller myotomies: Lessons learned. *Ann Surg* 2002; **235**: 631–639.

91 Donahue PE, Horgan S, Liu KJM, Madura JA. Floppy Dor fundoplication after esophagocardiomyotomy for achalasia. *Surgery* 2002; **132**: 716–722.

92 Zaninotto G, Costantini M, Portale G *et al.* Etiology, diagnosis and treatment of failures after laparoscopic Heller myotomy for achalasia. *Ann Surg* 2002; **235**: 186–192.

93 Luketich JD, Fernando HC, Christie NA *et al.* Outcome after minimally invasive esophagomyotomy. *Ann Thorac Surg* 2001; **72**: 1909–1913.

94 Decker G, Borie F, Bouamirrene D *et al.* Gastrointestinal quality of life before and after laparoscopic Heller myotomy with partial posterior fundoplication. *Surgery* 2002; **236**: 750–758.

95 Mineo T, Pompeo E. Long-term outcome of Heller myotomy in achalasia sigmoid esophagus. *J of Thoracic and Cardiovascular Surgery* 2004; **128**: 402–407.

96 Gockel I, Junginger T, Eckardt V. Long-term results of conventional myotomy in patients with achalasia: A prospective 20-year analysis. *The Society for Surgery of the Alimentary Tract* 2006; **10**: 1400–1408.

97 Wright AS, Williams CW, Pellegrini CA, Oelschlager BK. Long-term outcomes confirm the superior efficacy of extended Heller myotomy with toupet fundoplication for achalasia. *Surgical Endoscopy* 2007; **21**: 713–718.

98 Khajanchee Y, Kanneganti S, Leatherwood A, Hansen P, Swanstrom L. Laparoscopic Heller myotomy with Toupet fundoplication. *Arch Surg* 2005; **140**: 827–834.

99 Zaninotto G, Annese V, Costantini M *et al.* Randomized controlled trial of botulinum toxin versus laparoscopic Heller myotomy for esophageal achalasia. *Ann Surg* 2004; **239**: 364–370.

100 Csendes A, Braghetto I, Burdiles P, Korn O, Csendes P, Henriquez A. Very late results of esophagomyotomy for patients with achalasia. *Ann Surg* 2006; **243**: 196–203.

101 Imperiale TF, O'Connor JB, Vaezi MF, *et al.* A cost-minimization analysis of alternative treatment strategies for achalasia. *Am J Gastronterol* 2000; **85**: 2737–2745.

102 O'Connor JB, Singer ME, Imperiale TF, Vaezi MF, Richter JE. The cost-effectiveness of treatment strategies for achalasia. *Dig Dis Sci* 2002; **47**(7): 1516–1525.

103 Vela MF, Vaezi MF. Cost-assessment of alternative management strategies for achalasia. *Expert Opin Pharmacother* 2003: **4**(11); 2019–2025.

104 Sweet MP, Nipomnick I, Gasper WJ *et al.* The outcome of laparoscopic Heller myotomy for achalasia is not influenced by the degree of esophageal dilatation. *J Gastrointest Surg* 2008; **12**; 159–165.

105 Khazanchi A, Katz PO. Strategies for treating severe refractory dysphagia. *Gastrointest Endosc Clin North Am* 2001; **11**: 325–345.

106 Pinotti HW, Cecconcello I, Da Rocha JM *et al.* Resection for achalasia of the esophagus. *Hepatogastroenterology* 1991; **38**: 470–473.

107 Watson TJ, DeMeester TR, Kauer WKH *et al.* Esophageal replacement for end-stage benign esophageal disease. *J Thorac Cardiovasc Surg* 1998; **115**: 1241–1247.

108 Orringer MB, Stirling MC. Esophageal resection for achalasia: Indications and results. *Ann Thorac Surg* 1989; **47**: 340–345.

109 Cecconcello I, Da Rocha JM, Pollara W *et al.* Long-term evaluation of gastroplasty in achalasia. In: Siewert JR, Holscher AH (eds). *Diseases of the Esophagus.* Springer Verlag, Berlin, 1998: 975.

110 Miller DL, Allen MS, Trastek VF *et al.* Esophageal resection for recurrent achalasia. *Ann Thorac Surg* 1995; **60**: 922–925.

111 Peters JH, Kauer WKH, Crookes PF *et al.* Esophageal resection with colon interposition for end-stage achalasia. *Arch Surg* 1995; **130**: 632–636.

112 Devaney EJ, Lannettoni MD, Orringer MB, Marshall B. Esophagectomy for achalasia: Patient selection and clinical experience. *Ann Thorac Surg* 2001; **72**: 854–858.

113 Vaezi MF, Baker ME, Richter JE. Assessment of esophageal emptying post-pneumatic dilation: Use of the timed barium esophagram. *Am J Gastroenterol* 1999; **94**: 1802–1807.

114 Imperiale TF, O'Connor JB, Vaezi MF *et al.* A cost analysis of alternative treatment strategies for achalasia. *Am J Gastroenterol* 2000; **85**: 2737–2745.

115 O'Connor JB, Singer ME, Imperiale TF, Vaezi MF, Richter JE. *Dig Dis Sci* 2002; **47**: 1516–1525.

116 Storr M, Allescher HD, Classen M. Current concepts on pathophysiology, diagnosis and treatment of diffuse oesophageal spasm. *Drugs* 2001; **61**: 579–591.

117 Katz PO, Dalton CB, Richter JE. Esophageal testing of patients with non-cardiac chest pain or dysphagia. *Ann Intern Med* 1987; **106**: 593–597.

118 Konturec JW, Gillesen A, Domschke W. Diffuse esophageal spasm: A malfunction that involves nitric oxide? *Scand J Gastroenterol* 1995; **30**: 1041–1045.

119 Peters LJ, Maas LC, Petti D *et al.* Spontaneous non-cardiac chest pain: Evaluation by 24-hour ambulatory esophageal motility and pH monitoring. *Gastroenterology* 1988; **94**: 878–876.

120 Anderson KO, Dalton CB, Bradley LA *et al.* Stress induces alterations of esophageal pressures in healthy volunteers and non-cardiac chest pain patients. *Dig Dis Sci* 1989; **34**: 83–91.

121 Cannon RO, Quyyumi AA, Mincemoyer R *et al.* Imipramine in patients with chest pain despite normal coronary angiograms. *N Engl J Med* 1994; **330**: 1411–1417.

122 Drenth JPH, Bos LP, Engels LGJ. Efficacy of diltiazem in the treatment of diffuse oesophageal spasm. *Aliment Pharmacol Ther* 1990; **4**: 411–416.

123 Cattau EL, Castell DO, Johnson DA *et al.* Diltiazem therapy for symptoms associated with nutcracker esophagus. *Am J Gastroenterol* 1991; **86**: 272–276.

124 Thomas E, Witt P, Willis M, Morse J. Nifedipine therapy for diffuse esophageal spasm. *South Med J* 1986; **79**: 847–849.

125 Nasrallah SM, Tommaso CL, Singleton RT, Backhaus EA. Primary esophageal motor disorders: Clinical response to nifedipine. *South Med J* 1985; **78**: 312–315.

126 Richter JE, Dalton CB, Bradley L, Castell DO. Oral nifedipine in the treatment of noncardiac chest pain in patients with the nutcracker esophagus. *Gastroenterology* 1987; **93**: 21–28.

127 Clouse RE, Lustman PJ, Eckert TC *et al.* Low-dose trazodone for symptomatic patients with esophageal contraction abnormalities. A double-blind, placebocontrolled trial. *Gastroenterology* 1987; **92**: 1027–1036.

128 Miller LS, Pullela SV, Parkman HP *et al.* Treatment of chest pain in patients with noncardiac, nonreflux, nonachalasia spastic esophageal motor disorders using botulinum toxin injection into the gastroesophageal junction. *Am J Gastroenterol* 2002; **97**: 1640–1646.

129 Storr M, Allescher HD, Rosch T *et al.* Treatment of symptomatic diffuse esophageal spasm by endoscopic injections of botulinum toxin: a prospective study with long-term follow-up. *Gastrointest Endosc* 2001; **54**: 754–759.

130 Ebert EC, Ouyang E, Wright SH *et al.* Pneumatic dilatation in patients with symptomatic diffuse esophageal spasm and lower esophageal sphincter dysfunction. *Dig Dis Sci* 1983; **28**: 481–485.

131 Irving JD, Owen WJ, Linsell J, Mc Cullagh M *et al.* Management of diffuse esophageal spasm with balloon dilatation. *Gastrointest Radio* 1992; **17**: 189–192.

132 Patti MG, Pellegrini CA, Arcerito M *et al.* Comparison of medical and minimally invasive surgical therapy for primary esophageal disorders. *Arch Surg* 1995; **130**: 615–616.

133 Ellis FH. Esophagomyotomy for noncardiac chest pain resulting from diffuse esophageal spasm and related disorders. *Am J Med* 1992; **5A**: 129S–131S.

134 Patti MG, Gorodner MV, Galvani C, Tedesco P, Fisichella PM, Ostroff JW, Bagatelos KC, Way LW. Spectrum of esophageal motility disorders. *Arch Surg* 2005; **140**: 442–449.

5 Eosinophilic esophagitis

Elizabeth J Elliott

Discipline of Paediatrics and Child Health, University of Sydney, *and*
The Children's Hospital of Westminster, Sydney, *and*
Centre for Evidence-Based Paediatrics, Gastroenterology and Nutrition, Sydney, Australia

Introduction

Eosinophilic esophagitis (EE) is a relatively "new" disorder, first described in the late 1970s in adult patients who presented with symptoms of esophagitis, often suffered from atopic disease and were noted to have high numbers of eosinophils on esophageal (and sometimes duodenal and gastric) biopsy. Although their symptoms resembled those of gastroesophageal reflux disease (GERD), these patients frequently had no evidence of acid reflux and almost invariably failed to respond to therapy with acid blockers. The putative causes of the disease resulted in the terms idiopathic EE, allergic EE and primary EE being used synonymously with the term EE, which will be used throughout this chapter.

Increasingly, EE is recognised worldwide as an emerging and significant cause of upper gastrointestinal disease in all age groups. Clinicians should be aware of its clinical and pathological features and will need to keep abreast of the literature regarding its management in order to provide optimal patient care.

The 2007 American Gastroenterology Association (AGA) guideline on EE in children and adults, which is based on a systematic review of the literature, highlights our lack of understanding about the pathophysiology of EE and the ways in which eosinophils contribute to tissue damage, and the lack of universally accepted criteria for diagnosis [1]. Above all, they identify the paucity of high level evidence available from randomised controlled trials (RCTs) to inform clinical management, and our current reliance on

evidence from uncontrolled studies, expert opinion and anecdote.

Searching for the evidence

To inform this chapter, the medical literature contained in electronic databases (Cochrane Library, Medline, Embase, Clinical Evidence) was searched (to October 2008) for articles relevant to the etiology, epidemiology, diagnosis, prognosis and management of EE in adults and children. Emphasis was placed on identifying and reporting in this chapter, summary information from well-conducted systematic reviews of the literature on the diagnosis, management and prognosis of EE. With regard to treatment, the aim was to identify high-level evidence (from meta-analyses of RCTs, RCTs and quasi-RCTs) that compared pharmacological, dietary or surgical interventions for the management of established EE with a placebo or an alternative intervention. Interventions of interest included oral and inhaled corticosteroids, sodium cromoglycate, leukotriene-receptor antagonists (e.g. montelukast), immune modulators (e.g. anti-IL-5 and anti-IgE), dietary interventions (e.g. elemental formulae and food exclusion diets) and surgical interventions (e.g. esophageal dilation). The primary outcomes of interest were improvement in clinical symptoms and histological abnormalities. Harms of interest included adverse effects of medications and dietary or surgical interventions and relapse of symptoms and/or histological abnormalities on cessation of treatment. Several systematic reviews (including the AGA guideline [1], a Cochrane Review on the non-surgical management of EE [2], and reviews on the diagnosis [3] and management [4, 5] of EE) were identified, none of which contained a meta-analysis. Recent non-systematic reviews were also useful information sources [6–8]. Three RCTs [9–11] of therapies for EE were identified. The grading of evidence used in this

Evidence-Based Gastroenterology and Hepatology, 3rd edition.
J. McDonald, A.K. Burroughs, B. Feagan, and M.B. Fennerty. © 2010
Blackwell Publishing Ltd

chapter to support treatment is based on the levels proposed in Box 1.1 in Chapter 1.

Definition

Eosinophilic esophagitis (EE) is an inflammatory disorder of the oesophagus characterised clinically by upper gastrointestinal symptoms, histologically by esophageal infiltration with intraepithelial eosinophils (IEE), and endoscopically by a range of abnormalities which vary according to disease severity and chronicity. EE is part of a spectrum of disorders that, while clinically distinct, are characterised by eosinophilic infiltration of different parts of the gastrointestinal tract and include eosinophilic esophagitis, eosinophilic gastroenteritis and eosinophilic proctocolitis.

Etiology

Our understanding of the pathophysiology of EE is incomplete and the exact role of eosinophils in damaging the oesophagus is not known, limiting our ability to develop rational, safe and effective therapies. The most often proposed etiology for EE is intolerance to ingested (food) or inhaled allergens, mediated through IgE (a type I hypersensitivity response) and/or type 2 T-helper cells (Th2) – a type IV immune response. Mast cell numbers are increased in EE and correlate with eosinophil numbers [6] and the presence of activated mucosal mast cells may help distinguish EE from GERD [12]. In support of an allergic etiololgy, many patients with EE have a family or personal history of allergic disease, including eczema, allergic rhinitis, asthma and food allergy, the latter being common in young children [13]. It is estimated that up to 75% of patients with EE are atopic and many have measurable food allergen-specific IgE [6]. Some patients respond clinically and histologically to an elemental or a restricted diet, with recurrence of disease after resumption of a normal diet. Furthermore, there is evidence at the cellular level that the pattern of inflammation seen in EE (including activation of eosinophils, mast cells, and type 2 T-helper cells (Th2) and production of Th2-like cytokines (IL-4, IL-5 and IL-13) and eotaxin chemokines) is consistent with the pattern seen in other allergic diseases [6]. It is proposed that inflammation in the esophagus is driven by Th-2 cytokines, e.g. IL-5, which promote Th2 differentiation, regulate IgE expression and promote the production of eosinophils, their release from the bone marrow, and their movement to and survival in other sites. In further support of an allergic basis for EE, most patients respond positively to treatment with corticosteroids. Of interest, cytokine and microarray profiles are similar in both "allergic" and "non-

allergic" patients with EE, suggesting a common etiological pathway to esophageal inflammation [6]. The importance of eotaxins has been demonstrated in one cohort study, in which children with EE expressed the gene for eotaxin-3 (a substance that attracts circulating eosinophils to disease sites) at levels of more than 100 times the levels found in disease-free controls [14]. The study authors went on to demonstrate that this was due to single nucleotide polymorphisms in the eotaxin-3 gene of affected individuals. Furthermore, they showed that mice lacking eotaxin receptors were protected against developing EE.

It is acknowledged that GERD and EE may coexist: some patients with features typical of EE have abnormal pH studies and respond to PPIs [15]. Indeed, an alternate etiological theory for EE is that acid damage in patients with GERD results in increased esophageal permeability and that the resultant antigen entry results in eosinophilic infiltration and a subsequent inflammatory response that induces fibrotic change in the esophagus. Also, products released by eosinophils may lower esophageal sphincter pressure and alter esophageal motility, predisposing to acid reflux [8]. It is likely that the etiology of EE will prove to be multi-factorial. Nevertheless, future studies of disease pathogenesis and genetics will be crucial to guide rational development and use of new therapies.

Epidemiology

The AGA's guideline, which provides pooled data from epidemiological studies including over 1000 patients, suggest that EE occurs worldwide in most ethnic backgrounds; that adult men are more commonly affected than women; and that the mean age of onset is 38 (range 14–89) years in adults and 8.6 (range 0.5–21.1) years in children and young adults [1]. Familial disease clusters have been reported but it is not clear whether these reflect genetic predisposition or exposure to common environmental triggers. Variations in reported incidence and prevalence rates may simply reflect study selection bias and use of different diagnostic criteria. In the only published population-based study of a random sample of 1000 adults in Sweden, four individuals (0.4%; 95% CI: 0.2–1.2%) had eosinophilic esophagitis on biopsy, using a cutoff of ≥ 20 per HPF and the diagnosis was associated with dysphagia (2/66 vs 2/926; p = 0.025). According to the study definition, an additional seven individuals (0.7%) had "probable" EE (15–19 eosinophils per HPF), which was associated with esophageal narrowing (2/15 vs 5/978; p = 0.005) [16]. Using the AGA definition [1], this study suggests a prevalence of EE of ~1%. Increased clinician awareness of EE may account for the reported increase in disease prevalence in some settings, although the increase may be real [1].

Diagnosis

Criteria for the definitive diagnosis of EE are not internationally agreed upon or uniformly accepted. The diagnosis may be suspected in patients of any age who present with symptoms of oesophageal disease, including symptoms of GERD (e.g. regurgitation, vomiting, heartburn, or epigastric, chest or abdominal pain), which occur in both children and adults. In young children, symptoms may be accompanied by food intolerance or refusal and failure to thrive. Dysphagia with solid food or recurrent food impaction occurs more often in adults, commonly males, with longstanding symptoms. Many patients have a strong family or personal history of atopic diseases. Common clinical, endoscopic and histologic features and positive investigations at diagnosis are shown in Table 5.1, although their frequency varies considerably between studies.

The "gold standard" for the diagnosis of EE is a histological abnormality. However, varying cutoffs are used in the literature for the number of eosinophils required per high power field (HPF) to make the diagnosis of EE and distinguish it from conditions such as GERD [1, 8]. This is demonstrated in a systematic review of the literature [3]. In 318 publications identified, 35% of authors did not state the diagnostic criteria they used: 10 different histological definitions were used, and the criterion for the diagnosis of EE ranged from 5 to 30 eosonophils per HPF. There was also variation in the area of the HPF used in these studies [3]. Another difficulty in making the diagnosis is the patchy nature of EE (hence the patchy distribution of IEE), which influences the number of biopsies necessary and the esophageal sites (distal and proximal) that should be biopsied.

Diagnostic test sensitivity increases with the number of biopsies obtained: in one study sensitivity increased from 55% with one biopsy to 100% with five biopsies [17]. However, the choice of the biopsy site can also be difficult. In one study the appearance of the esophagus was normal at endoscopy in 30% of children with EE [18], suggesting that multiple biopsies should be taken from the length of the esophagus when the diagnosis is suspected, regardless of the endoscopic appearance. In the systematic review, only 39% of authors reported using specific biopsy protocols [3]. In addition, different investigators have used different histological grading systems, including a score that included both eosinophil numbers and thickness of the basal cell layer [9]. The lack of consistency in diagnostic methods makes comparison between epidemiological and intervention studies impossible. Acceptance of a universal, standardised histological definition for EE, such as that proposed in the AGA guideline (≥15 IEE per HPF in one or more biopsy specimens) [1] and of a standardised biopsy protocol and fixing technique (e.g. using formalin or paraformaldehyde), is imperative. Many clinicians biopsy the stomach and duodenum to exclude eosinophilic gastritis and duodenitis and some studies exclude patients in whom eosinophils are identified outside the esophagus and an accepted universal standard must also be reached in this regard.

To complicate matters, it has been suggested that eosinophilic infiltration may be a non-specific response to any injury of the esophageal epithelium [19]. Eosinophilic infiltration of the esophagus has been documented in other conditions including Crohn's disease, drug reactions, parasitic infection and hypereosinophilic syndrome, which should be excluded when considering a diagnosis of EE [1]. Although the AGA guideline suggest that, in order to make

Table 5.1 Clinical, endoscopic and histological features of eosinophilic esophagitis.

Common clinical features	Endoscopic features	Histological features	Laboratory investigations
GERD symptoms: regurgitation vomiting, heartburn, epigastric, chest or abdominal pain	Normal appearing esophagus	≥15 eosinophils per high power field in one or more esophageal biopsy	Skin prick tests for food and environmental allergens
Dysphagia, choking, food impaction (increase with age, usually occur in adults)	Erythema	specimens	Patch tests to food allergens
Food refusal or intolerance, poor weight gain/failure to thrive, fussy eater (in infants and young children)	Edema	Squamous epithelial hyperplasia	Peripheral eosinophil count (~2 fold elevation seen, more commonly in children)
Early satiety	Exudates or micro-abscesses appearing as raised white dots, plaques or nodules (representing eosinophilic microabscesses)	Eosinophilic microabscesses	Distal esophageal pH studies if diagnosis of GERD considered
Hematemesis	Longitudinal furrowing	Degranulation of eosinophils	
Unresponsive to PPI	Esophageal rings or corrugation	Basal zone hyperplasia	
Personal or family history of atopic disease (food allergy, positive skin prick tests, asthma, eczema)	Stricture	Papilliary lengthening	
	Small-calibre esophagus	Normal duodenal, gastric histology	
	Longitudinal shearing or friability (crepe paper mucosa) at endoscopy[a]		

[a] Characteristic of EE.

the diagnosis of EE, GERD should have been excluded by a normal lower oesophageal pH study and partial or complete lack of response to high dose protein pump inhibitor (PPI) therapy [1], this diagnostic criterion is not universally accepted, particularly in children in whom pH studies may be difficult to perform [10]. As discussed above, there is overlap between the clinical and histological features of EE and GERD and the two conditions may coexist with a complex inter-relationship [15]. Nevertheless, a pH study may be helpful to exclude GERD as a cause for esophagitis when the endoscopy and biopsy findings are equivocal.

Endoscopy findings in EE are extremely variable (Table 5.1) and may reflect disease severity and chronicity; at one end of the spectrum the esophagus may appear normal and at the other end luminal narrowing and strictures (usually in adults with long-standing symptoms) may be evident [20]. Furuta suggests that apart from the findings of longitudinal shearing and "crepe paper" mucosa, endoscopic features described in EE are not unique to this condition [1]. Nevertheless, identification of more than one of the typical features (including exudates or micro-abscesses appearing as raised white dots or nodules, esophageal narrowing, ringed (or feline) esophagus, longitudinal furrows or longitudinal shearing and friability) in the context of consistent clinical symptoms should raise the index of suspicion for EE [1]. Barium studies are not routinely recommended but may be useful to define the site and extent of esophageal narrowing found at endoscopy and to exclude other diagnoses.

In accordance with the current AGA guideline [1] diagnostic criteria include:

• Clinical symptoms of esophageal disease *and*
• Histological abnormality: (≥15 IEE in one or more HPF on a biopsy specimen) *and*
• Exclusion of differential diagnoses including GERD (by normal pH study or lack of response to high dose PPI) *and*
• Consistent endoscopic findings

Prognosis

Due to the relative rarity and recent recognition of this disorder, there are few prospective longitudinal cohort studies that provide good evidence about the long-term prognosis of EE. Three follow-up studies in adults were identified in the AGA guideline [1]. In summary, most patients had significant prior symptoms of refractory GERD, dysphagia, or impaction at study entry and up to 86% went on to develop oesophageal narrowing, strictures, or corrugation. Strictures were proximal in over half of the patients and dilation commonly caused longitudinal tears. The diagnosis of EE had frequently been missed and treatment delayed. Symptoms were chronic and in one study, symptoms worsened during the follow-up period (up to 11.5 years) in about one-quarter of patients and remained

stable in about one-third but were not life-threatening [21]. In some patients there was histological evidence of increasing subepithelial fibrosis or thickening of the esophagus over time in the absence of macroscopic change at endoscopy. There is no evidence in these cohorts with relatively short-term follow-up that EE is associated with development of esophageal neoplasia.

Outcomes in children are also poorly studied. Liacouras reported on nearly 400 children with EE who had presented with refractory GERD at less than 10 years of age and were followed for up to 10 years [18]. About 6% developed esophageal narrowing but only one child required dilation. Clinical and histological response to oral steroids was almost universal and response to inhaled fluticasone was about 50%, but most children relapsed when either treatment was ceased. The majority of children subjected to dietary manipulation (with a restriction diet or elemental diet) went into disease remission, which included improvement in esophageal calibre. A recent retrospective review of 89 children with EE supports the observation that EE is both chronic and relapsing; 79% of the 66% who initially responded to treatment had relapsed within the eight-year follow-up period [22].

Management

A range of pharmacological therapies has been used to treat EE, including oral and inhaled (swallowed) corticosteroids, sodium chromoglycate, PPIs, montelukast (a leukotriene inhibiter) and mepolizumab (an IL-5 monoclonal antibody). Dietary interventions include restricted or elemental diets and surgical interventions include esophageal dilation. However, there is a dearth of high-level evidence to support use of any of these interventions. Only three RCTs (two placebo-controlled trials and one comparing two current therapies) have been performed in EE [9–11]. All had methodological limitations, including small sample size, inconclusive results, and potential confounding from simultaneous use of co-therapy. Two of the RCTs were conducted in children and evaluated the role of steroids [9, 10] but used different criteria for the diagnosis of EE, for inclusion of trial participants and for determining histological response. Neither evaluated long-term maintenance therapy (Table 5.2). There is only one small RCT (n = 11) evaluating a novel therapy in adults with EE [11].

Pharmacological therapies

Corticosteroids

Steroids have been widely used in the treatment of EE and several uncontrolled studies, previously summarised [1, 8]

Table 5.2 Randomised controlled trials in patients with eosinophilic esophagitis.

Author date setting	Participants	Intervention	Comparison	Outcome measures	Evidence level; study quality	Results and comments
Schaefer, 2006. Children's Hospital, Indiana, USA	Included: 80 children (age range 1–16 years) with EE (≥15 eosinophils per HPF and negative pH probe study. 58% of children tested positive for food allergies at entry and were asked to eliminate relevant food. Excluded: other esophageal condition, *H. pylori* infection, CIBD, current treatment with corticosteroids.	Oral prednisone (1 mg/kg/dose twice daily (maximum of 30 mg bd) for 4 weeks then weaned for 8 weeks (n = 32).	Topical (swallowed) fluticasone via metered dose inhaler (110 µg per puff (age 1–10 years) and 22 µg per puff (≥11 years of age) (n = 36).	Histological improvement (to <15 eosinophils per HPF) at 4 weeks; symptom remission; adverse drug effects; symptom relapse.	Grade A evidence. Randomisation: yes, random number assignment. Allocation concealment: yes. Blinding: no, open-label. Baseline characteristics: similar. ITT analysis: no. Adequate sample, power. Follow-up: 6 months.	Benefits: histological improvement in majority at 4 weeks (no difference between groups). Majority symptom free at 4 weeks (no difference between groups). Harms: prednisone group: 40% adverse effects and 3 withdrew <4 weeks with severe adverse effects (hyperphagia, weight gain, cushingoid features). Fluticasone group: 15% esophageal candidiasis. Symptom relapse 45% at week 24.
Konikoff, 2006. Children's Hospitals, Cincinnati, San Diego, USA	Included: 36 children (age range 3–18 years with EE (≥24 eosinophils per HPF in ≥1 biopsy from distal/ proximal esophagus *and* epithelial hyperplasia); *not failed PPI.* Excluded: patients with food allergy on SPT who responded to exclusion diet; recent steroid use; pregnant.	Fluticasone propionate (400 µg bd for 3 months) via metered dose inhaler and swallowed (n = 20). Normal diet and PPI (if taken) continued in both groups.	Placebo (bd) for 3 months via metered dose inhaler (n = 11).	Histological remission (<1 eosinophil per hpf); adverse effects	Grade A evidence. Randomisation: yes, computer generated. Allocation concealment: yes. Blinding: yes (participants, clinicians, histologists). Baseline characteristics: similar (participants, clinicians, histologists). Small sample, adequate power. Follow-up at 3 months: 100%. Analysis: ITT. Compliance monitored: yes.	Benefits: fluticasone vs placebo: Histological remission 50% vs 9%; RR 5.5 (95% CI: p = 0.05). Disappearance of distal esophageal furrowing, decreased. Epithelial hyperplasia Response better in non-allergic, young children. Vomiting decrease in responders. Harms: candidiasis in 1 patient receiving fluticasone

HPF: high power field (400x); PPI: proton pump inhibitor.

suggest that both oral and topical steroids may improve histological abnormalities and clinical symptoms. Historically, oral steroids were reserved for patients with EE with severe dyspagia, strictures and weight loss because of concerns of adverse effects. The more recent use of topical steroids (fluticasone propionate or beclomethasone), administered by a metered-dose inhaler and swallowed, has been documented in uncontrolled studies with variable effectiveness for the initial treatment for EE [1, 8] and few adverse effects. There is limited evidence about the long-term use of either topical or oral steroids, although available studies suggest that discontinuation of steroid therapy frequently results in relapse.

Since publication of the AGA guideline [1] two RCTs have been published (summarised in Table 5.2), which provide the only reliable evidence for steroid therapy for EE. The first was a well-designed and adequately powered, open-label RCT that recruited 80 children (16 years or under) with EE (defined as ≥15 IEE per HPF and negative pH studies) [9]. Children were randomised to receive four weeks' initial treatment with either oral prednisone or topical fluticasone and were weaned off treatment over the next eight weeks. A histological grading score incorporating both eosinophil count and thickness of the basal cell zone was used to assess therapeutic response. Although most of the 68 children who completed the study had symptomatic improvement and showed histological improvement within one month, there was no significant advantage for one medication over the other. Importantly, 40% of the prednisone group experienced adverse effects of treatment and three children withdrew from the trial within four weeks of commencing therapy because of severe adverse effects. Of the fluticasone group, the majority (34/36) showed histologic improvement, 35/36 improved clinically and 15% experienced esophageal candidiasis, which was sometimes asymptomatic and responded to anti-fungal treatment.

Symptom relapse usually occurred within six weeks of stopping therapy and had occurred in 45% of all trial participants at six-month follow-up (although endoscopy and biopsy were not performed at this time) with no difference between treatment groups in the rate or timing of relapse. A potential confounder in this study is that 58% of all children tested positive for food allergies prior to commencing steroids and were asked to eliminate the relevant food. Although the proportion receiving a special diet was similar in each group it is possible that benefits of the diet resulted in an overestimation of the beneficial effect of both medications. In view of the similar effectiveness of the two steroid preparations and the potential adverse effects of oral steroids documented in this RCT, inhaled (swallowed) steroids should be used in preference to oral steroids as initial treatment for uncomplicated EE. **A1c** Patients should

be advised to use the medication without a spacer and, after spraying the medication into their pharynx, to swallow rather than inhale. Patients should be asked not to eat or drink or wash out their mouths for half an hour after medicating. **B4** In view of the high relapse rate of EE after treatment is stopped, the long-term use of fluticasone requires evaluation both for efficacy and for adverse effects. Systemic effects from long-term fluticasone use have not been evaluated in EE. It has been suggested that oral therapy should be reserved for short-term use in patients with acute or severe dysphagia or stricture requiring dilation [1], although RCT evidence in this group is lacking.

The second RCT (placebo-controlled and blinded) included 36 patients aged 18 years or under with EE (defined as ≥24 IEE/HPF in ≥1 biopsy specimen from either the proximal or distal esophagus and epithelial hyperplasia) [10]. Patients were randomised to receive either fluticasone propionate or placebo for three months. The primary outcome was histological remission, complete remission being defined as an eosinophil count of ≤1 per HPF. In contrast to Schaefer's study [9], failure to respond to PPI was not a criterion for inclusion in Konikoff's study and children who were receiving PPI continued to take them during the trial, a potential confounder. In contrast to Schaefer's trial, children with food allergy who had responded to an exclusion diet were excluded from Konikoff's trial; children who refused or failed to respond to dietary manipulation were included. Half of the children who received fluticasone responded histologically. Histological remission (the primary outcome of interest) was higher in the treatment group compared with the placebo group (50% vs 9%; p = 0.047) with a RR of 5.5 (95% CI: 0.81–37.49; p = 0.05), which may reflect the small sample size.

The study thus identifies both a considerable proportion of non-responders to fluticasone and the potential for spontaneous remission of EE and highlights the need for placebo-controlled trials. In this trial, distal esophageal furrowing was less frequently seen following treatment with fluticasone than placebo (50% vs 90%) and reduction in epithelial hyperplasia was greater with fluticasone. With fluticasone there was an improvement in vomiting (in 67% compared with 27% in the placebo group) but not in dysphagia, suggesting that caution should be employed in generalizing these findings to adults with EE, who more often have dysphagia. Young children who were found to be non-allergic using skin-prick testing were more likely to respond to fluticasone therapy. Side effects (namely candidiasis) from fluticasone were uncommon. This study supports the use of fluticasone for EE in children: **A1d** the dose recommended in the AGA guideline based on the literature and consensus is 440 to 880 micrograms per day for children in a divided (bd) dose and 880 to1760 micrograms per day for adolescents or adults [1] although there are not RCTs in adults.

Mast cell stabilizers

In one small, uncontrolled cohort there was no clinical or histological benefit from oral sodium cromoglycate given to children with EE at dose of 100mg four times daily for one month [18]. **B** There is no RCT evidence to support use of this medication which is not currently recommended for EE.

Anti IL-5 medications

The finding, in a mouse model, that IL-5 can induce EE and that blocking IL-5 can ameliorate disease [23] led to the successful treatment of a young adult with EE and chronic symptoms with mepolizumab (an anti-IL-5 medication) and supported trial of this intravenous preparation in four adults with chronic EE and dysphagia who had failed to respond to a range of other therapies [24]. In this small, uncontrolled trial in a heterogeneous group, the clinical and histological response was positive but variable (adverse events were not reported). **B4** Similarly, responses to treatment with reslizumab in four patients with EE were variable [25]. **B4** One recent placebo-controlled RCT evaluated use of up to four doses of mepolizumab in 11 adults with EE and confirmed a greater reduction in esophageal eosinophils in the treatment compared with the placebo group (67% vs 25%), but no difference in symptom response. [11] Mepolizumab was given at a dose of 750mg at 0 and 7 days and if the response was incomplete two doses of 1500mg were given at four-weekly intervals up to a maximum of four doses. **A1d** Larger RCTs are required to assess the benefits and harms of these treatments.

Leukotrioene-receptor antagonists

In a small, uncontrolled study (n = 8) in adults with EE, high dose montelukast (Singulair) resulted in symptom resolution in the majority but caused minor adverse effects (nausea and myalgia) and did not result in histological improvement [26]. Recurrence occurred with cessation of or decrease in the dose of the medication. Currently, there is insufficient evidence to recommend use of this medication. **B4**

Proton pump inhibitors

A number of small uncontrolled studies, summarised in recent reviews [1, 8], report variable clinical and histological improvement in patients with EE when PPIs were used alone or in conjunction with dilation in patients with strictures. **B4** RCT evaluation of PPIs for use in EE is required before their routine use can be recommended.

Dietary interventions

Clinical studies suggest that food allergies may be present in up to 50% of cases of EE in children, and the most common foods implicated are peanuts, milk products, eggs, soy, wheat and seafood [13]. Food allergies are more prevalent in children than in adults and in a subset of patients they play an important role in initiating and maintaining esophageal inflammation. The predictive value of food-specific IgE radioallergosorbent testing (RAST) for diagnosing IgE-mediated food allergy in EE is unknown and skin prick tests are recommended [1]. Type IV Th2 delayed hypersensitivity reactions can be diagnosed by skin patch testing. Although elemental diets (consisting of free amino acids, medium-chain triglycerides and corn syrup solids) and diets restricting specific foods (based on food allergy testing) or excluding the six most common food allergens have been used to treat EE [1, 8], there is little high level evidence to support their use.

Bohm [8] identified eight uncontrolled studies which showed a good clinical and histological response to dietary intervention in between 74% and 100% of children. In the largest study, 172 children were treated with an elemental diet (administered by nasogastric tube because children could not tolerate its taste), with a clinical and histological response in 100% [18]. A similar response was observed in 76% of 146 children treated with a restrictive diet based on skin prick and patch testing [27]. Thirty nine of the 40 children who failed to respond initially subsequently went into remission with an elemental diet. Limitations of these studies include the lack of controls, failure to monitor adherence to diet and, in Spergel's study, concomitant use of steroids in more than half the children and lack of standardisation of diagnostic allergy tests. Long-term use of elemental diets may be regarded as impractical: they are poorly tolerated orally, administration by nasogastric tube is invasive, and they are expensive and do not help identify the offending food. Thus, although there is some evidence to support the use of dietary interventions in EE, **B4** and the AGA guideline recommends they be "considered as an effective therapy in all children diagnosed with EE" [1], there remains the need for placebo-controlled and comparative RCTs to adequately assess the effectiveness, tolerability and cost-effectiveness of elemental and restrictive diets in both children and adults.

Endoscopic dilation

Although dilation of esophageal strictures is often used in adult (and occasionally paediatric) patients with EE and has been reported in several uncontrolled studies [1, 8], the procedure has not been adequately evaluated and has been questioned following reports of perforation, esophageal tearing and other complications. In a recent, small, retrospective case series, in 10 patients treated at two tertiary referral centres in Germany, the use of gentle (3 mm) dilation was reviewed in patients with esophageal strictures (of varying number, length and location) and dyspagia (mean 11 years duration) that were secondary to EE and resistant to at least eight weeks of topical treatment with corticosteroids [28]. Patients had had between one and five dilations; mucosal tears and pain on swallowing for a few days following the procedure were common but there were no perforations. All patients had an immediate improvement in dysphagia score, and their response to treatment (almost complete disappearance of dysphagia) was sustained for an average of 6 (range 2–11) months following the procedure. These findings are consistent with previous, heterogeneous, uncontrolled case series in adults [20, 21, 29, 30] and children [31] in which the majority of patients show clinical improvement. **B4** However, lack of consistency in diagnostic criteria, prior treatment and outcome measures makes comparison between studies difficult. Although it is important to relieve symptoms dilation is not curative, it is associated with significant adverse effects and recurrence occurs in up to 50% cases [1]. It is not clear whether this treatment should be reserved only for patients resistant to medical (steroid) treatment (the current recommendation), or whether prior use of steroids increases the risk of adverse outcomes or improves dilation outcomes. There is an urgent need for larger scale, prospective studies examining the safety and long-term efficacy of dilation in well characterized groups of patients.

Future therapies

Based on our increasing understanding of the pathogenesis of EE, a number of novel therapies have been proposed for potential use, but not yet adequately trialled in EE, and these are summarised by Stone [6]. Known immune modulators, Azathiaprine and 6-mercaptopurine, have been used only in a limited number of cases of EE to induce and maintain remission [32]. Omalizumab, the only clinically available monoclonal antibody against IgE, which prevents activation of mast cells, has been used effectively in a small number of patients with eosinophilic gastroenteritis but may increase esophageal eosinophil numbers and its role in EE is unclear [33]. It has been proposed that calcineurin inhibitors (e.g. tacrolimus), which decrease expression of Th2 and mast cell cytokines, may have a role in treating EE. However, the potential for this medication to induce eosinophilic gastrointestinal disease has been noted in some patients after liver transplantation [34]. Other potential therapies include anti-IL-5 receptor monoclonal antibodies (as an alternative to neutralizing IL-5) and monoclonal antibodies to CD25 and TNF-α [6]. Because epithelial TNF-α levels are increased in EE, infliximab, an anti-TNF therapy, has been used in small numbers of adults with severe, refractory EE with equivocal clinical and negligible histological effect [35]. Antagonists to IL-4 and IL-13, which increase eotaxin expression, and to the eotaxin receptor, to eotaxin and to α4β7 (which are involved in recruiting eosinophils to the gastrointestinal tract) may also have a role in therapy [6].

It will be important that putative therapies are carefully selected, based on our knowledge of pathogenesis and rigorously tested by RCT to confirm their safety and efficacy. Although there are now three published RCTs evaluating treatments for EE, it is discouraging that the study authors used different diagnostic and inclusion criteria for patients with EE and different outcome measures, and that the studies had methodological limitations including small sample size. In view of the variable clinical characteristics of EE and the possibly different etiologies of paediatric and adult EE, it will be important that participants recruited to trials are well characterised and that trials are either restricted to subgroups of EE or adequately powered to enable subgroup analysis. Diagnostic criteria and outcome measures must also be standardised. Although symptom relief is the aim in established disease, it will also be important to evaluate long-term therapy to prevent disease complications and to consider possible therapies to prevent development of EE.

Acknowledgements

Elizabeth Elliott is supported by the National Health and Research Council of Australia (Practitioner Fellowship No. 457084 and Enabling Grant No. 402784). The assistance of Dr Diana Thomas from the Centre for Evidence-Based Paediatrics, Gastroenterology and Nutrition in the preparation of this chapter is acknowledged.

References

1 Furuta GT, Liacouras CA, Collins MH *et al.* and members of the First International Gastrointestinal Eosinophil Research Symposium (FIGERS) Subcommittees. *Gastroenterology* 2007; **133**: 1342–1363.

2 Kukurusovic RH, Elliott EJ, O'Loughlin EV, Markowitz JE. (2004) Non-surgical interventions for eosinophilic oesophagitis. Cochrane Database of Systematic Reviews, Issue 3. Art. No.: CD004065. DOI: 10.1002/14651858.CD004065.pub2 (Updated February 2005 and 2006).

3 Dellon ES, Aderoju A, Woolsley JT, Sandler RS, Shaheen NJ. Variability in diagnostic criteria for eosinophilic esophagitis: A systematic review. *Am J Gastroenterol* 2007; **102**: 2300–2313.

4 Sgouros SN, Bergele C, Mantides A. Eosinophilic esophagitis in adults: A systematic review. *Eur J Gastroenterol Hepatol* 2006; **18**(2): 211–217.

5 Spergel JM, Andrew T, Brown-Whiteorn TF *et al.* Treatment of eosinophilic esophagitis in children and adults: A systematic review and consensus recommendations for diagnosis and treatment. *Gastroenterology* 2005; **133**: 1342–1363.

6 Stone KD, Prussin C. Immunomodulatory therapy of eosinophil-associated gastrointestinal diseases. *Clin Exp Allergy* 2008; **38**: 1858–1865.

7 Liacouras CA. Pharmacologic treatment of eosinophilic esophagitis. *Gastrointest Endoscopy Clin N Am* 2008; **18**: 169–178.

8 Bohm M, Richter JE. Treatment of eosinophilic esophagitis: overview, current limitations, and future direction. *Am J Gastroenterol* 2008; **103**: 2635–2644.

9 Schaefer ET, Fitzgerald JF, Molleston JP *et al.* Comparison of oral prednisone and topical fluticsone in the treatment of eosinophilic esophagitis: A randomized trial in children. *Clin Gastroenterol Hepatol* 2008; **6**: 165–173.

10 Konikoff MR, Noel RJ, Blanchard C *et al.* A randomized, double-blind, placebo-controlled trial of fluticasone propionate for pediatric eosinophilic esophagitis. *Gastroenterology* 2006; **131**: 1381–1391.

11 Straumann A, Conus S, Kita H *et al.* Mepolizumab, a humanized monoclonal antibody to IL-5, for severe eosinophilic esophagitis in adults: A randomized, placebo-controlled double-blind trial. *J Allergy Clin Immunol* 2008; **121**: S44.

12 Kirsch R, Bokhary R, Marcon MA, Cutz E. Activated mucosal mast cells differentiate eosinophilic (allergic) esophagitis from gastroesophageal reflux disease. *J Pediatr Gastroenterol Nutr* 2007; **44**: 20–26.

13 Spergel JM, Beausoleil JL, Mascarenhas M, Liacouras CA. The use of skin prick tests and patch tests to identify causative foods in eosinophilic esophagitis. *J Allergy Clin Immunol* 2002; **109**: 363–368.

14 Blanchard C, Wang N, Stringer KF *et al.* Eotaxin-3 and a uniquely conserved gene expression profile in eosinophilic esophagitis. *J Clin Invest* 2006; **116**: 536–547.

15 Spechler SJ, Gneta RM, Souza RF. Thoughts on the complex relationship between gastroesophageal reflux disease and eosinophilic esophagitis. *Am J Gastroenterol* 2007; **102**: 1301–1306.

16 Ronkainen J, Talley NJ, Aro P *et al.* Prevalence of oesophageal eosinophils and eosinophilic oesophagitis in adults: The population-based Kalixanda study. *Gut* 2007; **56**: 615–620.

17 Gonsalves N, Policarpio-Nicolas M, Zhang Q *et al.* Histopathologic variability and endoscopic correlates in adults with eosinophilic esophagitis. *Gastrointest Endosc* 2006; **64**: 313–319.

18 Liacouras CA, Spergel JM, Ruchelli E *et al.* Eosinophilic esophagitis: A 10-year experience in 381 children. *Clin Gastroenterol Hepatol* 2005; **3**: 1198–1206.

19 Rodrigo S, Abboud G, Oh D. High intraepithelial eosinophil counts in esophageal squamous epithelium are not specific for eosinophilic esophagitis in adults. *Am J Gastroenterol* 2008; **103**: 435–442.

20 Croese J, Fairley SK, Masson JW *et al.* Clinical and endoscopic features of eosinophilic esophagitis in adults. *Gastrointest Endosc* 2003; **58**: 516–522.

21 Straumann A, Spichtin HP, Grize L *et al.* Natural history of primary eosinophilic esophagitis: a follow-up of 30 adult patients for up to 11.5 years. *Gastroenterology* 2003; **125**: 1660–1669.

22 Assa'ad AH, Putnam PE, Collins MH *et al.* Pediatric patients with eosinophilic esophagitis: An 8-year follow-up. *J Allergy Clin Immunol* 2007; **119**: 731–738.

23 Mishra A, Rothenberg ME. Intratracheal IL-13 induces eosinophilic esophagitis by an IL-5, eotaxin-1, and STAT6-dependent mechanism. *Gastroenterology* 2003; **125**: 1419–1427.

24 Stein ML, Collins MH, Villanueva JM *et al.* Anti-IL-5 (mepolizumab) therapy for eosinophilic esophatgitis. *J Allergy Clin Immunol* 2006; **118**: 1312–1319.

25 Prussin C, James SP, Huber MM, Klion AD, Metcalfe DD. Pilot study of anti-IL-5 in eosinophilic gastroenteritis. *J Allergy Clin Immunol* 2004; **111**: S275.

26 Attwood SE, Lewis CJ, Bronder CS *et al.* Eosinophilic esophagitis: A novel treatment using montelukast. *Gut* 2003; **52**: 181–185.

27 Spergel JM, Andrew T, Brown-Whiteorn TF *et al.* Treatment of eosinophilic esophagitis with specific food elimination diet directed by a combination of skin prick and patch tests. *Ann Allergy Asthma Immunol* 2005; **95**: 336–343.

28 Schoepfer AM, Gschossmann J, Scheurer U, Selbold F, Straumann A. Esophageal strictures in adult eosinophilic esophagitis: Dilation is an effective and safe alternative after failure of topical steroids. *Endoscopy* 2008; **40**: 161–164.

29 Vasilopoulos S, Murphy P, Auerbach A *et al.* The small-caliber esophagus: An unappreciated cause of dyspagia for solids in patients with eosinophilic esophagitis. *Gastrointest Endosc* 2002; **55**: 99–106.

30 Cantu P, Velio P, Prada A *et al.* Ringed oesophagus and idiopathic eosinophilic oesophagitis in adults: An association in two cases. *Dig Liver Dis* 2005; **37**: 129–134.

31 Nurko S, Teitelbaum JE, Husain K *et al.* Association of Schatzki ring with eosinophilic esophagitis in children. *J Pediatr Gastroenterol Nurt* 2004; **38**: 436–441.

32 Netzer P, Gschossmann JM, Straumann A, Sendensky A, Weimann R, Schoepfer AM. Corticosteroid-dependent eosinophilic oesophagitis: azathioprine and 6-mercaptopurine can induce and maintain long-term remission. *Eur J Gastroenterol Hepatol* 2007; **19**: 865–869.

33 Foroughi S, Foster B, Kim N *et al.* Anti-IgE treatment of eosinophil-associated gastrointestinal disorders. *J Allergy Clin Immunol* 2007; **120**: 594–601.

34 Saeed SA, Integlia MJ, Pleskow RG *et al.* Tacrolimus-associated eosinophilic gastroenterocolitis in pediatric liver transplant recipients: role of potential food lallergies in pathogenesis. *Pediatr Transplant* 2006; **10**: 730–735.

35 Straumann A, Bussmann C, Conus S, Beglinger C, Simon HU. Anti-TNF-alpha (infliximab) therapy for severe adult eosinophilic esophagitis. *J Allergy Clin Immunol* 2008; **122**: 425–427.

6

Ulcer disease and *Helicobacter pylori* infection: Etiology and treatment

Naoki Chiba

Division of Gastroenterology, McMaster University Medical Centre, Hamilton, *and* Guelph General Hospital, Guelph, Canada

Introduction

Peptic ulcer disease, particularly duodenal ulcer disease, was thought to result from gastric acid hypersecretion and pepsin damage. Indeed Schwarz's dictum [1], "no acid, no ulcer" is still relevant, as acid is a prerequisite for most ulcer formation. Peptic ulcers were also thought to be caused by a variety of other cofactors such as smoking, stress and non-steroidal anti-inflammatory drugs (NSAIDs) including aspirin. Therapy was directed primarily against lowering acid production in the stomach to permit healing of ulceration. However, the discovery and characterization of gastric infection with *Helicobacter pylori* has revolutionized our concepts of ulcer pathogenesis and therapy. As duodenal ulcer has long been thought to result from an imbalance between protective and aggressive factors in the mucosa, *H. pylori* can be considered an "aggressive" factor which may tip the balance toward mucosal damage and result in ulceration. Thus, the assignment of an etiologic role to *H. pylori* does not contradict the traditional concepts of ulcer pathogenesis, but rather extends them.

Warren and Marshall's seminal paper in 1983 first identified the spiral bacterium that is now known as *Helicobacter pylori*, associated with active chronic gastritis [2]. Their subsequent paper [3] determined an association between the gastric infection and peptic ulcer, particularly duodenal ulcer, where *H. pylori* was present in all antral biopsies. For their discovery, Doctors Barry Marshall and Robin Warren were awarded the 2005 Nobel Prize in Physiology and Medicine.

Indisputable evidence has dispelled initial skepticism of the role of this infection as an important gastroduodenal pathogen. This chapter reviews and presents the evidence for the etiological role of *H. pylori* in peptic ulcer disease. Causes of ulcers other than *H. pylori* will also be discussed. Last, treatment of ulcer disease with an emphasis on *H. pylori* eradication will be reviewed.

What is the evidence for the role of *H. pylori* in peptic ulcer disease?

One approach would be to determine whether "Koch's postulates" which link an infectious agent with disease(s) are fulfilled. The postulates state that the "agent (1) must be found in patients with the disease only, (2) must be grown outside of the body, (3) when inoculated into a susceptible animal, must cause the same disease, and (4) must be grown from the lesions observed" [4]. Many of the organisms currently accepted as disease causing pathogens do not necessarily fit all of Koch's postulates. Furthermore, there is limited applicability to chronic disease such as that caused by *H. pylori* infection [5]. A more applicable approach is [5] to use the criteria for assessing epidemiological evidence, as outlined by Hill [6].

There is sufficient evidence to establish *H. pylori* as a cause of duodenal ulcer and this evidence is summarized in Box 6.1.

Association of *H. pylori* with ulcer disease (strength, consistency and specificity)

In this section, the prevalence of *H. pylori* in both duodenal and gastric ulcer patients is considered.

Duodenal ulcer

The prevalence of *H. pylori* in ulcer disease had been well reviewed by Kuipers *et al.* [9], who identified relevant studies published since the discovery of *H. pylori* in 1983.

Evidence-Based Gastroenterology and Hepatology, 3rd edition.
J. McDonald, A.K. Burroughs, B. Feagan, and M.B. Fennerty. © 2010 Blackwell Publishing Ltd

---

BOX 6.1 Evidence for role of *H. pylori* in peptic ulcer disease (PUD) according to Hill's criteria

Association (strength, consistency, specificity) of *H. pylori* with PUD

Prevalence of *H. pylori* in DU ~ 90%, GU ~ 80%:
- *strength* and *consistency* of association is high
- *specificity* is low as *H. pylori* seen in many without ulcers
- *overall, data is supportive*

Temporal relationship: does *H. pylori* infection precede PUD?
- self-administration of *H. pylori* shown to cause active chronic gastritis – fulfils one of Koch's postulates
- but, no direct evidence that PUD is caused
- case control study (Nomura [7]) shows preceding *H. pylori* infection increases risk of DU, GU and gastric cancer
- cohort study (Sipponen [8]), >10% *H. pylori* positives developed DU over 10 years but <1% if *H. pylori* negative
- *thus, data is supportive*

Biological gradient: no consistent data to support higher levels of bacterial load correlate with PUD

Biological plausibility: numerous plausible pathophysiological alterations (see text) that include:
- vacA causing epithelial cell damage – not consistent
- cagA associations with disease states such as DU, gastric cancer and MALTomas – not consistent or universally seen
- elevated gastrin and acid secretion that revert to normal after *H. pylori* eradication
- numerous alterations in mucosal cytokines
- *thus, data are supportive*

Effects of interventions: outcomes following *H. pylori* eradication. Alterations in natural history of PUD with *H. pylori* eradication provides strongest evidence that *H. pylori* is a true pathogen. RCT data of *H. pylori* eradication shows:
- DU and GU relapse markedly decreased
- DU heal with eradication of *H. pylori* infection alone without ulcer healing drugs
- DU heal faster when *H. pylori* eradicated than with ulcer healing drugs alone
- DU refractory to ulcer healing drugs can heal if *H. pylori* eradicated
- Re-bleeding from ulcers can be prevented if *H. pylori* eradicated
- *thus, data are strongly supportive*

Coherence of *H. pylori* data with previous epidemiological data:
- consistent historical correlations between presumed *H. pylori* prevalence, ulcer disease prevalences, death rates and perforations from ulcer disease
- improvements in hygiene and sanitation in industrialized nations have resulted in declining prevalence of both *H. pylori* and ulcer disease
- prevalence of *H. pylori* infection and ulcer disease have become the same in males/females
- *thus, data are supportive*

In the decade to 1993 they found that infection with *H. pylori* was present in 94.9% (95% CI: 94–96%) of 1695 duodenal ulcer patients studied. Borody *et al.* found *H. pylori* in 94% of 302 duodenal ulcer patients in Australia [10]. Of the 14 patients who were negative for *H. pylori* at the time of endoscopy, four had taken antibiotics shortly before endoscopy and may have had false negative results, and eight had NSAID induced ulcers. Overall, only one of 302 patients had no cause for duodenal ulcer identified. Thus, almost all duodenal ulcers which were not caused by NSAIDs were associated with infection with *H. pylori*.

A strong association by itself, does not prove causality [4, 5]. While the association of *H. pylori* with duodenal ulcer is strong and consistent, it is not specific since *H. pylori* is also found in many patients without ulcer disease. The reasons why *H. pylori* infection cause disease in a minority of patients infected with the organism are not yet known. This question remains the subject of ongoing research.

The prevalence of *H. pylori* associated DU appears to be getting lower. In Italy, the prevalence of DU in 2001 was 6.5%, declining to 3.1% in 2004 [11]. Also, from another Italian study, over a 10-year period in two different regions,

there was a decline in DU to about 5% [12]. In South Korea, the prevalence of DU had decreased to 39% in 2004/5 compared to 45% a decade before, with an increase in *H. pylori* negative ulcers to 68% from 79% [13]. A Hong Kong study also showed a decline in duodenal ulcer disease between 1997 and 2003 [14].

In summary, there is a reduction in ulcer disease, mostly duodenal ulcer disease associated with the decline in *H. pylori* infection.

Duodenal ulcers not related to *H. pylori* and NSAIDs

The new millennium has seen an increase in *H. pylori* negative duodenal ulcers, perhaps related to successful treatment of *H. pylori* [15]. Quan and Talley [15] concluded that it was difficult to determine the true prevalence of *H. pylori* negative ulcers accurately because of the cross-sectional nature of the studies. Patients could be misclassified as being *H. pylori* negative if there has been recent antibiotic or bismuth use and also if PPI use had not been stopped at least two weeks prior to testing, especially if testing was done by the urea breath test. Also, as the presence of *H. pylori* in the gastric mucosa could be patchy, mucosal biopsy methods required adequate biopsy sampling and preferably, the use of multiple methods of *H. pylori* determination. Retrospective series suffer from the inability to accurately determine surreptitious NSAID use.

A meta-analysis of seven rigorously designed North American duodenal ulcer studies identified that 20% of patients in these studies had ulcer recurrence within six months, despite successful cure of infection and no reported use of NSAIDs [16]. In a review of similar studies, Ciociola *et al.* [17] estimated the prevalence of *H. pylori* and NSAID negative duodenal ulcers was 22%. One American study identified *H. pylori* infection in only 62% of DU and 44% of GU patients [18]. No reason for these lower *H. pylori* prevalence rates in ulcer patients was offered. A similarly high proportion of 29% *H. pylori* and NSAID negative ulcers was recently reported from Pakistan [19]. There may be ethnic differences in the proportion of ulcers related to *H. pylori*. For example, in Japan, the *H. pylori* negative peptic ulcer prevalence appears to be less than 5% [15]. Despite these reports of nearly 20% or more non-*H. pylori*, non-NSAID ulcers, a report from Italy suggested that of their patients, after careful review of *H. pylori* status, NSAID ingestion and recent antibiotic use, only 0.8% (6/774) could be truly considered idiopathic [20].

In an interesting, prospective population survey of 2416 Danish subjects that assessed risk factors for peptic ulcer disease, the *H. pylori* negative duodenal ulcer prevalence was 13% [21]. The causes of these ulcers could not be adequately ascertained as there were so few ulcers, but there were suggestions that smoking, minor tranquilizer use and tea consumption were possibly associated.

In Singapore, a carefully designed study that assessed thromboxane B2 levels as a surrogate for possible NSAID use, determined a corrected non-*H. pylori* and non-NSAID peptic ulcer proportion of about 8% [22].

In the Swedish Kalixandra study, the prevalence of peptic ulcer was 4.1% [23]. Of these 19% were *H. pylori* and NSAID negative duodenal ulcers.

A Spanish study of 754 peptic ulcer patients found only 1.6% of all duodenal ulcers were non-*H. pylori* and non-NSAID associated [24]. A similarly low prevalence of 2% was found in Finland [25] and 1.3–1.5% in Japan [26, 27]. Thus, these reports of varying prevalences of duodenal ulcers unrelated to *H. pylori* or NSAIDs suggests ethnic variability.

Most duodenal ulcer recurrences after eradication of *H. pylori* are related to NSAIDs [28] and the role of pentagastrin-stimulated peak acid output is unclear [29, 30]. Smoking has been implicated as an important additional risk factor to *H. pylori* and NSAIDs [23, 31]. Stress may be a factor [32, 33] as may other co-morbid illness and alcohol abuse [33]. One study suggested that poor socioeconomic status was an important risk factor for PUD independent of *H. pylori* status [34]. A Japanese study suggested that persistent inflammation in the lamina propria may be an important factor for ulcer recurrence [35].

Overall, the proportion of duodenal ulcers that is both *H. pylori* and NSAID negative is between 1 and 20%. There are not a lot of recent data supporting a change in prevalence of these types of ulcer.

Gastric ulcer

There are fewer studies on the role of *H. pylori* in gastric ulcer, and NSAIDS play an important role in their etiology. *H. pylori* infection is diagnosed in 60–100% of gastric ulcer patients (mean about 70%) [9, 36]. As Thijs *et al.* point out [21, 36], many of the earlier studies suffered methodological problems that probably led to an underestimate of the prevalence of *H. pylori* in gastric ulcer disease. Most gastric ulcers are associated with *H. pylori*-related active chronic gastritis whether or not NSAIDs are involved [36–38]. However, from 4 to 11% may have no identifiable cause [24, 37]. The study by Nomura *et al.* [7] also showed that prior infection with *H. pylori* increased the risk that the patient may develop gastric ulcer subsequently.

Other newer drugs such as bisphosphonates [39, 40] have been found to cause gastric ulcers and there may be a synergistic effect with naprosyn [41]. Potassium supplements and chemotherapeutic drugs such as floxuridine have also been identified as causative agents [15].

Thus, *H. pylori* remains an important cause of duodenal (DU) and gastric ulcers (GU) [42]. *H. pylori* negative ulcers are commonly caused by NSAIDs [36]. Furthermore, the proportion of *H. pylori* negative ulcers increases as the overall prevalence of *H. pylori* infection falls [18, 43].

Temporal relationship

Whether *H. pylori* infection precedes the development of ulcer disease cannot be assessed by point prevalence studies, since it is impossible to assess retrospectively when these patients were infected [5].

Marshall [44] described three "self-administration" experiments in humans. In these cases active chronic gastritis ensued, fulfilling one of Koch's postulates for at least the first step in the development of peptic ulceration, although actual ulcer disease did not develop.

The temporal relationship between infection with *H. pylori* and the development of duodenal ulcer has been best demonstrated in a cohort study reported by Sipponen *et al.* [8]. Of the 321 patients with *H. pylori* at study entry, 34 developed a duodenal ulcer over the next 10 years, while only 1 of 133 *H. pylori* negative patients developed an ulcer.

An IgG serological nested case-control study of a group of 5443 Japanese-American men with stored sera obtained between 1967 to 1970 demonstrated that pre-existing *H. pylori* infection increased the subsequent risk of developing either duodenal or gastric ulcer disease over a surveillance period of greater than 20 years [7]. The odds ratio (OR) for development of ulcer was 4.0 (95% CI: 1.1–14.2) for duodenal ulcer and 3.2 (1.6 to 6.5) for gastric ulcer. The relationship was statistically significant even when the ulcer diagnosis was first made 10 or more years after the serum sample had been obtained. A further analysis of this Hawaiian cohort [45] identified that *H. pylori* infected men of higher birth order had an increased risk of gastric (OR 1.64) but not duodenal ulcer. These data are consistent with the hypothesis that early infection with *H. pylori* increases the risk of developing gastric ulcer.

Biological gradient

If there were a higher bacterial load in the stomach of patients with ulcers vs those without an ulcer this would be additional evidence supporting a causative role [4]. In biopsy studies, there has been insufficient gastric mucosal sampling to assess whether there was a biologic gradient present [5]. It is problematic to rely on biopsy specimens due to sampling error. A test such as a urea breath test (UBT) may be more useful in this regard. Ingested urea is digested by bacterial urease activity with the labeled CO_2 breakdown product being excreted in the breath. Significant correlation has been observed between labeled CO_2 excretion in the breath and intragastric bacterial load [46, 47] and mucosal inflammation [46–48]. However, there has not been consistent correlation with endoscopic findings [46]. Most of the available literature did not find a correlation of endoscopic findings with higher urea breath test values, and authors did not report whether the finding of higher test results predicted the finding of a duodenal ulcer [49–51]. Thus, data supporting a relationship between a greater innoculum of *H. pylori* and ulcer development are limited.

Biological plausibility

H. pylori is a unique bacterium that has evolved ecologically to survive and persist in the harsh acidic environment of the stomach. Bacterial urease, flagellar motility and surface adhesins appear necessary for colonization and persistence [52]. Despite the high prevalence of infection, not all infected persons develop ulcer disease, and most remain asymptomatic. Are there more virulent strains that predispose to ulcer disease? The vacuolating cytotoxin (*vacA*) which causes surface epithelial cell damage and vacuolation of epithelial cells, has not been found consistently to correlate with ulcer disease [52]. The *cagA* protein is a marker of the *cag* pathogenicity island of *H. pylori* and several studies have determined that in developed countries, duodenal ulcers, intestinal metaplasia, gastric carcinoma and mucosa-associated lymphoid tissue (MALT) lymphoma are more commonly seen in patients infected with a *cagA* positive strains [52]. However, this relationship is not universally seen in all ethnic origins. The newest potential virulence marker has been the duodenal ulcer promoting gene (dupA). Although there has been a statistically significant association of dupA with DU, it was identified in only 37% of North Indian patients [53]. In another study dupA was not associated with DU disease [54].

If *H. pylori* is primarily an *intragastric* infection, how does it cause ulcers in the duodenal bulb? Observations prior to and after the discovery of *H. pylori* identified that patients with duodenal ulcers had gastric metaplasia and associated *H. pylori* colonization in the duodenal bulb [55–60]. This change is thought to arise as a result of hypersecretion of acid as observed in duodenal ulcer patients. The gastric metaplasia may [61–63] or may not [64] improve after *H. pylori* eradication. Patients infected with *H. pylori* have increased basal and stimulated gastrin release irrespective of whether they have duodenal ulcer disease or not [65–67]. The elevated gastric acid secretion also results in increased postprandial duodenal acid load [68]. Furthermore, *H. pylori* eradication [69, 70] or suppression [71] results in normalization of these gastrin levels in most subjects, with lowering of acid secretion [65, 69]. However, a subset of patients with recurrent duodenal ulcer have persistently high acid secretion despite *H. pylori* eradication [72]. *H. pylori* can colonize islands of gastric metaplasia in the duodenum. Numerous toxigenic factors have been identified by which *H. pylori* might cause mucosal damage, although there is no one pathophysiological factor accepted as being pathognomonic. Adhesion of *H. pylori* to epithelial cells results in elevated levels of mucosal cytokines such as interleukin (IL)-8 which is increased in the mucosa of *H. pylori* infected patients [73]. *CagA* positive strains have higher levels of tumor necrosis factor (TNF)-α, IL-1β, IL-6, IL-8 and are associated with more severe inflammation (active chronic gastritis) in the gastric mucosa [74]. This T-helper subtype 1 (Th1) proinflammatory cytokine response may predominate in ulcer disease whereas a mixed Th1/Th2 pattern predominates in those with chronic gastritis but no ulcer [75]. There may be a link between increased IL-8 and gastrin release that is potentiated by *H. pylori* sonicates [76]. Thus, there are plausible mutifactorial mechanisms by which *H. pylori* may cause pathogenic effects resulting in peptic ulcer.

Effects of interventions: outcomes following *H. pylori* eradication

In the days before recognition of *H. pylori*, ulcers could be healed but inevitably relapsed over the next year [77–82]. The most clinically relevant evidence for the role of *H. pylori* comes from intervention trials in which *H. pylori* was eradicated and recurrence of ulcer disease markedly reduced [83].

The first reported randomized trial in 1987 [84] showed that the risk of recurrent duodenal ulcer could be reduced to virtually zero when *H. pylori* eradication therapy was given. In 1988, Marshall *et al.* [85] reported a randomized double-blind trial in duodenal ulcer patients in which more ulcers healed and fewer ulcers recurred over 12 months with *H. pylori* eradication therapy. Other important early contributions supported these observations [86–90]. **A1c**

Reviews of studies from 1987 to 1994 demonstrated that the recurrence rate for duodenal ulcer at one year ranges from 0 to 9% when *H. pylori* infection is successfully eradicated [36, 91, 92]. There are fewer data on ulcer recurrence after periods longer than one year after *H. pylori* eradication, but reported recurrence rates range from 0 to 18% [92]. Labenz reported that at one year, infection with *H. pylori* and duodenal ulcer recurred in 2.4% and 0.8% of patients, respectively [93]. Longer follow-up showed no further *H. pylori* or ulcer recurrence at three and four years [93]. Another study reported that 92% of patients remained free of *H. pylori* after seven years of follow-up, while those who were *H. pylori* positive remained persistently positive [94]. **B4** In 15 randomized trials in which *H. pylori* eradication was compared with no eradication, the ulcer recurrence rate was 7% in those in whom *H. pylori* was eradicated vs 67% in those who remained infected [92]. A systematic review [95] has shown that the median 12-month duodenal ulcer recurrence rate is 67% if *H. pylori* infection persists, but is reduced to 6% if *H. pylori* is eradicated. **A1a** Comparable results for gastric ulcer recurrence are 59% and 4%, respectively. A more recent meta-analysis examined studies that directly compared gastric and duodenal ulcers and identified that for DU the one-year ulcer recurrence rate was 2% and for GU 3% if *H. pylori* was eradicated, but if the infection persisted, the ulcer relapse rate was 42% for DU and 39% for GU [96]. **A1a** Thus, regardless of whether the patient suffers from DU or GU, successful eradication results in cure for most patients.

Other strongly supportive data include the observations that DU healed without ulcer healing drugs if *H. pylori* was eradicated and that the rate of healing was faster with *H. pylori* eradication. Eradication of *H. pylori* has been shown to prevent re-bleeding from ulcers as well. These important data will be further discussed in the sections below.

Coherence of the data with earlier epidemiological information

The prevalence of *H. pylori* infection parallels data showing that there was a peak in the incidence of ulcer disease at the end of the nineteenth century [4]. This is consistent with epidemiological data that show that the death rate of duodenal ulcer patients was highest in those born around 1890 [97]. The highest risk for ulcer perforation was identified in a cohort of men born between 1900 and 1920 [98]. This is also the generation with the highest *H. pylori* prevalence in an *H. pylori* seropositivity study carried out in the UK [99]. This relationship is consistent with the hypothesis that *H. pylori* plays an important role in ulcer complications.

Improvements in hygiene and sanitation are associated with a declining risk of infection, as is the case today in industrialized nations compared with less developed countries, which still endure a poor socioeconomic status. The number of admissions for ulcer disease has steadily declined since the middle of this century which infers a declining severity and prevalence of duodenal ulcer [100]. This decline parallels a declining prevalence of *H. pylori* infection. However, more recent data suggest that the overall prevalence of peptic ulcer and its complications has not changed much in the USA, likely because of the ulcerogenic effects of increasing NSAID use [101].

While duodenal ulcer disease has long been thought to be a disease of men, data since 1979 have shown that the prevalence of duodenal ulcer and the death rate for men and women have become similar [102]. This is consistent with the effect of *H. pylori* infection of which the prevalence is the same in both sexes [103].

Treatment of duodenal ulcer

Healing of duodenal ulcer with acid suppressive therapy

A meta-analysis [104] has shown a close linear relationship between the degree of suppression of intragastric acidity and duodenal ulcer healing. A more complex meta-analysis of this relationship between the duration of acid suppression and healing led to the definition of three primary determinants of the benefits of antisecretory drugs: (1) the degree of suppression of acidity; (2) the duration of suppression of acidity over the 24-hour period; and (3) the duration of the treatment [105]. For duodenal ulcer, the duration of time the intragastric acidity can be maintained at or above pH 3.0 is the most important factor. This model identified that maintaining intragastric pH at or above the threshold pH of 3.0 for 18–20 hours of the day predicts a 100% healing of duodenal ulcer [105]. Lesser degrees of acid suppression were found to prolong the duration of time needed to achieve optimal healing. Thus, these models of degree of acid suppression help explain the results of controlled trials of agents for healing ulcers.

Treatment of duodenal ulcer in the pre-*H. pylori* era was revolutionized by H_2-receptor antagonists (H_2-RAs), and subsequently PPIs, whose effects were proven in placebo-controlled trials. Numerous methodologically sound, double-blind, randomized controlled trials using comparative healing rates of endoscopically proven ulcers as the outcome measure, have established that PPIs heal ulcers faster than H_2-RAs and also provide more rapid symptom relief [78, 106–111]. In the chapter in the second edition of this textbook [112], the literature of 28 such randomized controlled trials was reviewed and summarized [18, 77–79, 106–111, 113–130]. **A1a** As the data were robust, this evidence was not updated in this present chapter.

There is no proven difference in ulcer healing rates and safety between different PPIs [127, 131, 132]. There are direct comparative trials of lansoprazole vs omeprazole [125, 126], pantoprazole vs omeprazole [127] and rabeprazole vs omeprazole [128] which showed equivalent duodenal ulcer healing. **A1c**

Maintenance therapy for prevention of duodenal ulcer recurrence

Although ulcers were healed effectively by acid suppressive therapy, ulcer recurrence was almost inevitable, with about 80% recurrence at one year once treatment was stopped [77–82]. Thus, in an effort to prevent recurrent ulcer, patients were given maintenance therapy with H_2-RAs. In a large (n = 399) two-year maintenance study of ranitidine 150 mg daily vs placebo, ulcer symptoms remained controlled in only about half the patients but ulcer recurrence was prevented in 83% of patients [133]. This study also identified significantly (p < 0.002) more complications such as bleeding in the placebo arm. **A1a** After a long-term follow up of 464 patients on maintenance ranitidine, 81% remained free of symptomatic DU recurrence over nine years [81]. A one-year relapse rate of between 20 to 30% has been identified consistently through meta-analyses [134, 135] and reviews [80]. Most of the maintenance studies used suboptimal half doses of the H_2-RAs, as full ulcer healing doses are more effective in preventing relapse [80, 136, 137]. **A1c** Ulcers treated with tripotassium dicitrato bismuthate appeared to have a more prolonged remission beyond that seen with H_2-RAs. It has since been suggested that this effect is, in part, due to the suppressive effects of bismuth on *H. pylori* infection and its ability as a single agent to eradicate *H. pylori* in around 20% of patients [138].

For duodenal ulcers resistant to healing with H_2RAs, lansoprazole was more effective than placebo in maintain-ing healing over one year when used in doses of 15 mg (70% remission) and 30 mg (85% remission) [139]. **A1d** The sample size was inadequate to determine whether the larger dose was more effective.

Influence of *H. pylori* eradication on healing of duodenal ulcer

The interval between *H. pylori* eradication therapy and reassessment may influence ulcer healing data. In a cohort study of patients given *H. pylori* eradication therapy it was observed that at one month, 22/212 (10.4%) had persistent DU. These patients were followed for another two months without additional ulcer healing treatment, and ultimately only three ulcers remained unhealed for a total healing success rate of 98.1% [140].

Furthermore, duodenal ulcers heal faster when *H. pylori* infection is eradicated than with acid suppressive therapy alone using either H_2-RAs [85, 88, 90] or omeprazole [141]. Ulcers refractory to healing with conventional acid suppressive therapy may heal with *H. pylori* eradication therapy [86, 142–145] **A1c** and remain healed over a four-year follow-up period [93]. **B4** In the pre-*H. pylori* era, it was shown that ulcers could be healed with antibiotics alone [146–148]. Similar results have been shown in subsequent studies that aimed to heal ulcers with anti-*H. pylori* antibiotic treatment alone, without the need for additional ulcer healing drugs [25, 149–153]. These findings further support the role of *H. pylori* as a bacterial pathogen for ulcer disease.

Acid suppressive therapy need not be continued beyond the duration of eradication treatment

There is good evidence [25, 150, 154–157] that uncomplicated, active duodenal ulcers heal without the need to continue ulcer healing drugs beyond the duration of eradication therapy. **A1c**

There are several methodologically sound trials in which patients all received eradication therapy and were randomized to either placebo or an ulcer healing drug for a further 2–3 weeks to test the hypothesis that continued ulcer healing drugs were not required after the eradication period [154, 158–162]. In all these studies, the ulcer healing proportions at four weeks were the same, regardless of whether an antisecretory drug was continued or not. In one study, the trend towards ulcer healing at two weeks was higher in patients who continued antisecretory therapy (continued therapy 91%, placebo 76%; p = 0.14), but at four weeks all ulcers had healed in both treatment groups [154]. In another study, by three weeks the healing rates were 89% in the continued omeprazole arm and 81% in the placebo arm and by eight weeks, the healing rates were the same [160].

Duodenal ulcer complications and effects of *H. pylori*

Gastroduodenal ulcer disease causes serious complications, such as bleeding, in 15–20% of patients, perforation in about 5% and obstruction in up to 2% of affected patients [163].

Bleeding

A natural history study of duodenal ulcer before the *H. pylori* era provided interesting data from 2119 patients [164]. Of these patients, 13.5% presented with hemorrhage as the first indication of ulcer disease. The overall mortality was 4.5% in those patients who bled and only 1% in those without bleeding. Most deaths not due to bleeding were due to perforation. The re-bleeding rate was 13% overall versus 2% for patients who continued on therapy. **B4** Even in a report to 2006, the mortality rate remained high at 5.4% after ulcer bleeding [165].

As the rate of recurrent bleeding in the past was high, strategies for prevention of re-bleeding were necessary. Two randomized, placebo controlled trials have evaluated the effect of a maintenance dose of ranitidine 150 mg on ulcer bleeding. One trial did not show that ranitidine reduced re-bleeding. However, the study lacked statistical power [166]. The other trial [167] showed a significantly reduced risk of re-bleeding, (ranitidine 9%, placebo 36%, absolute risk reduction (ARR) 27%, number needed to treat (NNT) 4). **A1d** However, the maintenance H_2-blocker arm still carried a re-bleeding risk of nearly 10% and half the episodes were not proceeded by symptoms alerting one to the presence of a recurrent ulcer. The risk of re-bleeding did not diminish over time, as those patients on placebo were at continuous risk of re-bleeding over the three-year follow-up period. Surprisingly, long-term randomized controlled maintenance trials with more potent acid suppressive drugs (proton pump inhibitors) have not been reported [168]. There is one non-randomized report from 1996 where patients were allocated to either eradication therapy or to long-term antisecretory therapy with either omeprazole or ranitidine [169]. Overall, 12% of the patients (5 of 41) had a re-bleed in the 20-week follow-up, compared to only 2.3% in the antibiotic group [169]. One anecdotal report from Japan in a heterogenous population of both gastric and duodenal ulcers showed that in those with persistent *H. pylori*, ulcer re-bleeding occurred in 12% of patients on H2-blockers and 10% of cases on PPIs [170]. The data are insufficient to allow any conclusion of the benefit of the PPIs.

Currently, it is accepted that eradication of *H. pylori* leads to a reduction in peptic ulcer recurrence, and hence prevents recurrent bleeding of both duodenal and gastric ulcers [170–173]. This has been well summarized by Gisbert *et al.* in a 2004 Cochrane Review and their subsequent observational trial [171, 173]. In the Cochrane Review, the mean re-bleeding rate after *H. pylori* eradication therapy compared with continued antisecretory therapy was 1.6% and 5.6% (OR 0.25;, 95% CI: 0.08 to 0.76) respectively [171]. In the studies comparing *H. pylori* eradication to no eradication and no continued antisecretory therapy, the re-bleeding rate was 2.9% and 20% respectively (OR 0.17; 95% CI: 0.10 to 0.32). Levels of evidence included observational studies and randomized controlled trials. Thus, *H. pylori* infection should be looked for in all patients with bleeding ulcers and eradication therapy should be standard of care for those who are infected. In some patients it may not be possible to eradicate *H. pylori*, and in these patients, PPI maintenance therapy is then recommended.

Despite the success of eradicating *H. pylori* and curing the traditional peptic ulcer, the problem of bleeding ulcers has not gone away. As half of ulcer bleeding may be attributable to NSAIDs, this is a substantial problem [174]. Those positive for both *H. pylori* and NSAIDs have a synergistically high risk of re-bleeding [175, 176].

In a Hong Kong study, there was an increasing proportion of bleeding idiopathic (non-*H. pylori* and non-NSAID related with no other cause) ulcers compared to *H. pylori* related ones [177]. Those with idiopathic ulcers seemed to have a worse prognosis with greater recurrent complications compared to *H. pylori*-associated ulcers that were treated with eradication therapy [177]. Another report found that those with idiopathic ulcers had a higher mortality rate and longer hospital stay than those with an *H. pylori* related ulcer [165]. There are no randomized management trials for preventing re-bleeding in these idiopathic ulcers which appear more serious than *H. pylori* related ulcers. It is recommended that these high-risk patients be treated with the most potent acid-suppressive therapy available, that is, with a PPI. As H_2-blockers exhibit tachyphyaxis and heal ulcers less effectively than PPI, there is little rationale to recommend them.

Summary The results of all studies are in agreement that *H. pylori* eradication significantly reduces ulcer re-bleeding rates and hence *H. pylori* should be looked for and eradicated if identified.

Perforation

There are few data available concerning the role of *H. pylori* infection in other complications such as ulcer perforation. A controlled trial involving 60 patients undergoing simple closure of perforated duodenal ulcer demonstrated a significant ($p < 0.05$) benefit for decreasing complications of peptic ulcer disease with postoperative cimetidine treatment [178]. **A1d** This study did not consider the role of *H. pylori* infection. NSAID use increases the risk of ulcer perforation by a factor of 5 to 8 [179] and in one series, 71% of the perforated DU patients had been using NSAIDs

[180]. Separate relative risks for duodenal and gastric ulcers are not known. In 80 patients presenting with acute perforated duodenal ulcer, the prevalence of *H. pylori* infection by serology was only about 50%, approximately equal to that in a control group, and NSAIDs were frequently the cause of the perforation [181]. More recent studies using biopsy based methods of *H. pylori* detection have shown *H. pylori* prevalence of 50% [180], 73% [182, 183] to 80% or more in perforated duodenal ulcer patients [184–186].

A case series of *H. pylori* positive patients with perforated peptic ulcer demonstrated that after *H. pylori* eradication, there was no need for re-operation and no mortality after a median 44-month follow-up [183]. **B4**

There are two randomized trials of *H. pylori* eradication in patients with perforated peptic ulcer [182, 187]. In a Hong Kong study, patients with perforated DU were initially treated with simple closure [187]. The *H. pylori* prevalence was 81% and these 99 patients were randomized to receive eradication therapy or four weeks of PPI alone. After one year, the rate of ulcer relapse was 38% in patients treated with omeprazole alone and 5% in those who received anti-*Helicobacter* therapy [187]. **A1d** Kate *et al.* followed 202 patients for two years after simple closure of a perforated duodenal ulcer and also retrospectively reviewed the records of an additional 60 patients [182]. In the prospective arm, patients were randomized to ranitidine alone or ranitidine quadruple eradication therapy. In patients in whom *H. pylori* was eradicated, the risk of recurrent ulcer was between 4 and 28% and the authors did not report any subsequent perforations. **B4** Thus, there is reasonably strong evidence to support a recommendation for *H. pylori* eradication in infected patients with a perforated ulcer.

Obstruction

The prevalence of this complication may be as low as 0.5%, and the strength of evidence for this rare complication is restricted to case reports [188, 189] and observational studies [190, 191]. The prevalence of *H. pylori* with pyloric obstruction ranges from 45% to 90% [191], with a mean value of 69% reported in one review [192]. Gastric outlet obstruction seems to improve following *H. pylori* eradication in most reports [188, 189, 191, 193] **B4** and in combination with balloon dilatation of the pylorus in some reports [190, 193].

Treatment of gastric ulcer

Healing of gastric ulcer with acid suppressive therapy

Gastric ulcer healing rates with H_2-RAs in the pre-*H. pylori* era were 3–43% at two weeks, 54–70% at four weeks, 82–

92% at eight weeks and 89–94% at 12 weeks [194]. Thus, gastric ulcers take four to eight weeks longer to heal than duodenal ulcers. There are no important differences in healing rate between various H_2-RAs. However, PPIs have been shown to produce higher healing rates than H_2-RAs in several randomized trials [194–197]. An early meta-analysis [194] demonstrated that the most important determinant of healing was duration of treatment. A later meta-analysis, comparing omeprazole and ranitidine in healing gastric ulcers demonstrated more rapid and complete healing with more potent acid suppression [195]. **A1c** Another meta-analysis in which the rates of gastric ulcer healing were expressed as ulcers healed per week, showed that PPI (represented by omeprazole) healed gastric ulcers 24% faster than other agents [198]. **A1c** A more recent update suggested that rabeprazole, pantoprazole, or lansoprazole showed better improvement in the clinical symptoms when compared with omeprazole [199]. **A1c** However, healing of gastric ulcer with pantoprazole [200] and rabeprazole [201] was comparable to that with omeprazole.

Maintenance therapy for prevention of recurrence of gastric ulcer

Maintenance therapy with H_2-RAs (cimetidine, ranitidine, famotidine, nizatidine) in half standard dose at night, has been shown to reduce the risk of symptomatic recurrence in one year to 6.7–36% compared with a rate of 49–76% without therapy [80]. A PPI (omeprazole, lansoprazole, pantoprazole) in standard dose once daily reduced the recurrence of gastric ulcers to only 4.5% over six months [202].

A randomized trial demonstrated that lansoprazole in doses of 15 mg and 30 mg prevented recurrence of healed gastric ulcer in 83% and 93% of patients over a 12-month period (p < 0.001) [203]. **A1c**

H. pylori eradication influence on healing and recurrence of gastric ulcer

Eradication of *H. pylori* speeds gastric ulcer healing in six weeks to 84.9% compared with a rate of 60% in patients with persistent *H. pylori* infection (p = 0.0148) [204]. A larger study has shown that almost all GU can be healed if *H. pylori* is eradicated compared to 60–70% healing if the infection persists [205].

Curing *H. pylori* infection has been shown in randomized controlled trials to reduce the recurrence rate of gastric ulcers, although there are fewer data than is the case for duodenal ulcer [36, 89, 92, 206–210]. **A1c** Gastric ulcers can be healed by *H. pylori* eradication therapy alone, without the need for continued administration of an antisecretory drug for ulcer healing [208, 211–214]. A recent study compared *H. pylori* eradication alone, eradication therapy with continued PPI and PPI without eradication therapy [214]. In this study, *H. pylori* eradication alone resulted in partial gastric ulcer healing, but healing was better if esomeprazole was continued. A corollary of this is that longer duration of treatment is needed to heal gastric ulcers. The accompanying editorial recommended that PPI be continued after eradication therapy to ensure ulcer healing [215].

H. pylori eradication almost eliminates gastric ulcer recurrence, while persistently infected patients have a relapse rate up to 50% [91, 92, 214, 216]. **A1c** Labenz and Börsch reported that at one year, *H. pylori* recurred in 3.4% of patients, while gastric ulcer recurrence was not observed [93]. Longer follow-up showed no *H. pylori* infection or ulcer recurrence at three and four years [93]. **B4** In studies with higher relapse rates, NSAIDs are an important cause of the recurrent ulcers [217].

H. pylori eradication therapy

Antibiotic regimens

The evolution of *H. pylori* eradication treatment has been rapid. It was determined early on that this infection was easy to suppress but difficult to cure. Thus, if the patient were tested too early following completion of a course of an eradication treatment, the organism would be "cleared" but be falsely identified as having been eradicated. A time interval of at least four weeks after the end of eradication treatment was identified as the minimum necessary to define eradication [138, 218].

The first meta-analysis of *H. pylori* eradication regimens [138] established that single antimicrobial agents were insufficient to eradicate *H. pylori*. A later review identified clarithromycin as a drug that can eradicate *H. pylori* infection in up to 54% of patients when given alone. However, as resistance rapidly develops, its use as a single agent is not recommended [219]. Combinations of two antimicrobials were found to result in improved eradication rates, but the best regimens were "bismuth triple therapies" [138]. The best regimen in 1992 was triple therapy with bismuth, metronidazole and tetracycline (BMT) which was superior to triple therapy with bismuth, metronidazole and amoxicillin [92, 138, 220]. However, this combination was felt to be too cumbersome and hence, more "user friendly" PPI based therapies emerged.

Because the literature is extensive, background materials and reviews will be summarized and only recent data about effects of new therapies and treatment of eradication failures will be discussed. Ranitidine bismuth citrate is an effective drug in combination therapy for *H. pylori* eradication. However, since it is no longer available in most parts of the world, it will not be discussed. The previous chapter on *H. pylori* in the second edition of this book contains details of these previously discussed therapies [221].

PPI based combination therapies

The PPIs are potent acid suppressing agents that effectively heal duodenal and gastric ulcers and provide prompt symptom relief. They may have a synergistic effect with antimicrobials by providing an optimal intragastric pH milieu [222, 223]. They also have some direct suppressive effects on *H. pylori* [224]. In an interesting Japanese study patients were treated with lansoprazole, amoxicillin and clarithromycin and 24-hour intragastric pH was measured on day 6 of treatment [225]. Patients with successful eradication had a higher median intragastric pH of 6.4 compared to those who were eradication failures, where the median pH was 5.2 [225]. **B2** Thus, there is good rationale to use these agents as part of an *H. pylori* eradication regimen.

PPI dual therapy
PPI plus amoxicillin Dual therapy with PPI and amoxicillin (PPI-A) enjoyed a brief period of popularity. Overall efficacy in several reviews and meta-analyses was in the order of 60%, and results were not consistent. Therefore this regimen is not recommended for standard therapy [92, 219, 220, 226–230]. However, one potential advantage with an amoxicillin regimen is that *H. pylori* rarely ever becomes resistant to amoxicillin. Thus, this dual regimen could be given more than once. More potent acid inhibition with higher PPI doses [231, 232] are not more effective.

PPI plus clarithromycin With the identification of clarithromycin as the most effective single therapy [233], it came to be used as dual therapy with omeprazole. This combination gave more consistent and reliable results than PPI-A dual therapy, with eradication rates as high as 70% [220, 226, 229, 234]. Two weeks of therapy with relatively high doses of clarithromycin 500 mg bid to tid and hence higher cost [220] were required. More importantly, the high development of clarithromycin resistance in treatment failures would then preclude its use again as part of an H. pylori eradication regimen [235]. Thus, any regimen that uses clarithromycin should be one that has the best possible eradication success to prevent development of secondary clarithromycin resistance [235].

Other PPI dual therapies One study used rabeprazole with levofloxacin for either 5, 7 or 10 days and found low eradication rates of 50–70% while a triple therapy with rabeprazole, amoxicillin and levofloxacin was 90% effective [236]. These data suggest that dual therapy with a PPI and one antibiotic are unlikely to be of clinical utility.

PPI, clarithromycin and amoxicillin or nitroimidazole triple therapies

Better eradication rates were achieved with regimens that combined a PPI with two antimicrobials. The first regimen, known as the Bazzoli regimen [237], used omeprazole 20 mg od, clarithromycin 250 mg bid and tinidazole 500 mg bid for one week and achieved 100% efficacy. A meta-analysis of such treatments suggested that this was the most effective therapy overall [220]. Many subsequent trials using omeprazole, lansoprazole or pantoprazole have demonstrated that the PPI-based triple therapies are consistently superior to dual therapies [220].

The first large randomized placebo controlled eradicaton trial was the MACH 1 study [238]. While this study was criticized for having only one test of *H. pylori* eradication after treatment, the regimens identified as being the most effective have stood the test of time and remain recommended by most consensus conferences as first-line therapy [239–243].

The most effective one week, twice daily regimens in the MACH 1 study were: (1) omeprazole 20 mg, clarithromycin 500 mg and amoxicillin 1 g or (2) omeprazole 20 mg, clarithromycin 250 mg and metronidazole 400 mg [238]. Studies with similar efficacy for analogous regimens have subsequently been reported using lansoprazole [244–252], pantoprazole [220, 253–255], rabeprazole [256–258] and esomeprazole [234, 259–261] based triple therapies. Meta-analyses have shown the same results [262, 263]. **A1a**

Some studies have shown some slight benefit of one PPI over another, but the significance of such observations is unclear. For example, a direct comparative study of rabeprazole or lansoprazole with clarithromycin and amoxicillin found that the rabeprazole triple therapy was significantly more effective (88% ITT) than the lansoprazole triple (78% ITT), and eradication success with clarithromycin resistant strains was poor for both therapies [264]. Whether there are genetic differences to account for this is unclear. A Taiwanese study compared esomeprazole to pantoprazole with clarithromycin and amoxicillin for one week with ITT eradication rates of 94% and 82% (p = 0.009) respectively [265]. The authors speculated that the greater acid inhibition and anti-*H. pylori* effects of esomeprazole may explain this result.

Most experts recommend that the PPI, clarithromycin and amoxicillin be considered first-line over PPI, clarithromycin and a nitroimidazole triple therapy because of the higher prevalence of resistance of *H. pylori* to imidazole compared to clarithromycin. However, in comprehensive meta-analyses, no difference in efficacy between these two regimens was found [266, 267]. **A1a** Also, one study found that the PPI-CA regimen gave slightly lower eradication with more frequent adverse effects (38%) compared to PPI-CM (20%, p < 0.05) [268].

These twice daily, one-week regimens are well tolerated, with few drop-outs due to drug intolerance. A meta-analysis did not show any difference in efficacy between a lower dose of clarithromycin (250 mg bid) vs the conventional 500 mg bid dose in combination with a PPI and metronidazole [269]. Patients treated with the lower dose had only half the incidence of adverse effects [270]. While the smaller dose of clarithromycin may be adequate for many patients, consensus groups have advocated the 500 mg bid dose for consistency and to avoid possible confusion and prescribing errors. For PPI-CA combinations, the larger clarithromycin dose of 500 mg bid was found to be superior to the 250 mg bid dose [269].

Another triple therapy with PPI, amoxicillin and metronidazole is generally less effective than the PPI, clarithromycin and amoxicillin (PPI-CA) and PPI, clarithromycin and metronidazole (PPI-CM) triple therapies in head-to-head trials [205, 238, 252]. However, as empiric second-line therapy, there may be some advantage, as this is not a clarithromycin containing regimen, and efficacy may be reasonable in some populations [271–273]. It seems particularly effective in Japan [274], even after eradication failure with standard triple therapy [275].

Some declining efficacy

Recent data suggest that these PPI based triple therapies may not be quite as effective as was observed some years ago. For example, a randomized Canadian study published in 2003 compared esomeprazole vs omeprazole with metronidazole and clarithromycin for seven days and found that ITT eradication rates were now less than 80% at 76% and 72% [276], whereas in the 1996 MACH-1 study, the eradication rate for the same regimen was 90% [277]. Unfortunately, this study did not assess *H. pylori* antibiotic resistance.

However, other studies published more recently [278–281] demonstrate continued high eradication success, with ITT eradication rates remaining above 80%. Results are indeed variable in various publications, and the true efficacy is unclear. In areas of high clarithromycin and metronidazole resistance, gold standard triple therapy may be less effective.

Optimum duration of PPI triple therapy

Original recommendations were for a one-week treatment course. Laine reviewed triple therapy with esomeprazole, clarithromycin and amoxicillin and demonstrated that a seven-day regimen gave 86–90% ITT eradication rates in DU patients from Europe and Canada but in the USA, even 10 days seemed slightly less successful, with 77–78% success [260]. Thus, this suggested that in America, longer 10–14 day therapy was necessary. However, a recent US study [282] and a Spanish study [283] using rabeprazole, amoxicillin and clarithromycin found comparable eradication rates with 7 and 10-day treatment. More recently, with the apparent decline in treatment success, even the Maastricht II consensus guidelines nebulousy state that treatment should be given for a minimum of seven days [284] and the Maastricht III consensus indicates that 14 days is more effective than seven days [243]. One study that used lansoprazole, clarithromycin and amoxicillin to eradiate *H. pylori* found that one week of treatment eradicated 75% and two weeks eradicated 86%, a difference that was not statistically significant [285].

Calvet *et al.* [286] performed a meta-analysis of 13 randomized studies to 1999 that directly compared different durations of treatment to determine the optimal treatment duration for triple therapy. They found that pooled data suggested that 10–14 day regimens were better than seven-day regimens and in direct head-to-head comparisons, 14-day regimens were more effective than seven-day regimens, with a therapeutic gain of 7–9%. **A1a** These authors performed a cost-effectiveness analysis of the different durations of treatment in relation to two basic strategies; UBT post treatment for all patients or UBT only if symptoms relapsed [287]. They studied the economic costs in Spain (low cost model) and USA (high cost). For either follow-up strategy, the shortest, seven-day duration produced the lowest costs. In sensitivity analyses, the 10-day regimen would have to be 10–12% more effective than seven-day therapy and the 14-day therapy 25–35% more effective than seven days for the longer duration therapies to become cost effective in Spain. For the USA, the corresponding figures were 3–5% and 8–11% respectively. Thus, even though the longer duration regimens are more effective, in terms of economic evaluation, the shorter duration approaches may be cost effective overall. Indeed, a more recent meta-analysis suggests that extending the duration of PPI triple therapy beyond seven days may not be a clinically useful strategy [288].

Influence of antibiotic resistance on PPI triple therapies

Resistance to nitroimidazole (i.e. metronidazole, tinidazole) A meta-analysis of studies performed prior to 1997 evaluated *H. pylori* eradication rates with a variety of regimens in nitroimidazole resistant and sensitive strains [289]. Pooled data from studies using PPI with nitroimidazole and amoxicillin or clarithromycin, showed that eradication was achieved in 93% of sensitive strains and only 69% in resistant strains. PPI, nitroimidazole and amoxicillin was a less effective regimen (64%) than the corresponding regimen that included clarithromycin (76%) for nitroimidazole resistant stains. For sensitive strains, both regimens were very effective, with pooled eradication rates of 92–93%, and the duration of therapy (7, 10 or 14 days) did not influence eradication success.

The MACH-2 study published after this meta-analysis, carefully evaluated antibiotic resistance and determined that baseline metronidazole resistance reduced the efficacy of the OCM triple therapy from 95% to 76% [290, 291]. A similar reduction in efficacy of about 15% was reported in a lansoprazole study [252]. Importantly, the MACH-2 study also showed that the addition of omeprazole, with its potent acid suppression, helped partially to overcome metronidazole resistance. When baseline metronidazole resistance was present, clarithromycin and metronidazole alone was a successful combination in only 43% of cases, but with the addition of omeprazole the efficacy was improved to 76%. For metronidazole sensitive strains, the eradication rate with the antibiotics alone was 86% and the addition of omeprazole improved the eradication rate only slightly to 95% [290]. In the MACH studies, the dosage of metronidazole was 400 mg bid, slightly lower than the 500 mg bid available in Canada. However, a meta-analysis has shown these two doses to be similarly effective [292]. The higher metronidazole dose may be better on theoretical grounds, since higher doses may be more effective against resistant *H. pylori* strains [293].

Amoxicillin allergy is common and this is a contraindication to use of the PCA regimen. Since this regimen does not contain metronidazole, there is rationale for using it in patients with suspected or documented metronidazole resistant strains [294].

Resistance to clarithromycin

There is no doubt that the primary determinant of treatment failure is resistance to clarithromycin (macrolides). Laine *et al.* summarized the data with esomprazole, amoxicillin and clarithromycin and determined that in clarithromycin sensitive strains, the eradication rate was 89% but in those with clarithromycin resistant *H. pylori*, the eradication rate was much reduced to 45% [295]. After treatment with this triple therapy, clarithromycin resistance developed in 33% (2/6) compared to 85% (23/27) after treatment with esomeprazole and clarithromycin dual therapy. Even worse eradication success with clarithromycin resistance was reported by Murakami *et al.* [264]. In patients treated with rabeprazole or lansoprazole combined with amoxicillin and clarithromycin, the eradication success with clarithromycin sensitive strains was 98% and 89% but in clarithromycin resistant strains, the eradication rates were 8.1% and 0% [264]. Other studies have also shown that PPI triple therapies containing clarithromycin are ineffective in the presence of clarithromycin resistance [296].

For patients treated with PPI, clarithromycin and amoxicillin triple therapy, the primary determinant of treatment failure has been found to be clarithromycin resistance with minor if any influence of CPY-2C19 genetic polymorphisms [297, 298]. For clarithromycin sensitive strains, the eradication rate was 97% vs 6% (1/16) for resistant strains [297] in one study, and in another, corresponding rates were 86% vs 24% [298].

The rate of acquired clarithromycin resistance was found to be 88.9% (8/9) in patients treated with PPI-C dual therapy, while with PPI, clarithromycin and amoxycillin or PPI, clarithromycin and metronidazole triple therapies these rates were 38.7% (12/31) and 90.0% (9/10) respectively (p < 0.01) [299]. Murakami *et al.* suggested that amoxicillin containing regimens may help prevent acquired clarithromycin resistance [299].

Other factors affecting eradication success

Wermeille *et al.* [300] treated 78 patients with one week LCA and overall ITT eradication success was only 65.4% (95% CI: 54.8–76.0%). The eradication rate in "good compliers" was 69.6% (95% CI: 58.7–80.5%). **B4** These authors found that presence of an ulcer, age, gender and smoking habit did not differ significantly between the eradicated and non-eradicated groups. They concluded that while poor compliance and bacterial resistance were important in determining treatment success, these factors only explained 40% of failures.

Broutet and colleagues reported a retrospective analysis using individual patient data from triple therapy eradication studies performed prior to 1999 in France in order to identify risk factors for *H. pylori* eradication failure [301]. The key finding was that eradication failure occurred more frequently if the patient diagnosis was functional dyspepsia compared to duodenal ulcer (34% vs 22% failure, p < 0.000001). This result is consistent with another literature review [302]. However, in another review, the use of PPI, clarithromycin and amoxicillin triple therapy, resulted in the same eradication rates in patients with peptic ulcer or functional dyspepsia [303]. With the decline in prevalence of ulcer disease, deciding on treatment choice based on diagnosis is not a practical alternative. Broutet found that for DU patients, eradication failure occurred more often in smokers, while 10-day therapy was better than seven days [301]. For all patients, age over 60 gave better eradication rates. Smoking was also found to impair eradication success in Japan, particularly in functional dyspepsia patients [304].

A very comprehensive meta-analysis by Fischbach identified that there were differences in eradication success according to differences in ethnic origin [305]. She found the highest eradication rates in north-eastern Asia. Populations characterized by a high prevalence of childhood *H. pylori* infection and high levels of drug resistance exhibited lower treatment success.

PPI is an essential component of PPI-triple eradication regimens

There is good evidence to support the view that the PPI is a necessary component of PPI triple therapies, as eradication rates are higher when a PPI is used with the antibiotics than when the antibiotics are given alone [291, 306–308]. In one such study, all patients were given one week clarithromycin 250 mg and tinidazole 500 mg bid and were randomized to receive either no omeprazole, omeprazole 20 mg once daily or omeprazole 20 mg bid. The eradication rates were higher in the omeprazole groups (omeprazole once daily 88%, twice daily 89%, placebo 64%, ARR for twice daily omeprazole vs antibiotics alone = 0.25, NNT = 4) [306]. **A1c** In the omeprazole groups, 22 patients who harboured metronidazole-resistant strains of *H. pylori* were cured by the omeprazole regimen, providing further evidence that the addition of the PPI may help overcome metronidazole resistance. Another study treated ulcer patients with once daily clarithromycin 500 mg, tinidazole 1 g and either placebo or lansoprazole 60 mg and found that the antibiotics alone eradicated *H. pylori* in 39% of patients, but the addition of the PPI increased the eradication success to 72% [153]. Laine pooled results from three American studies treating duodenal ulcer patients with amoxicillin and clarithromycin and either placebo or omeprazole and determined that pooled eradication with antibiotics alone was 39%, but if omeprazole was added, the eradication rate was improved to 84% [152]. **A1c** In another study, the cure rate by ITT was significantly higher for omeprazole, clarithromycin and amoxicillin (82%) than for clarithromycin and amoxicillin alone (18%), while for omeprazole, clarithromycin and metronidazole the cure rate was 67%, only slightly better than the 59% cure observed with clarithromycin and metronidazole alone [309]. This study showed that the impact of the PPI was much more significant in improving the eradication efficiency of the PPI with clarithromycin and amoxicillin triple therapy. **A1a**

A meta-analysis has shown that pretreatment with a PPI prior to triple and quadruple therapies did not influence *H. pylori* eradication [310].

Comparison of H₂-RA vs PPI in triple therapies

Graham *et al.* conducted a meta-analysis of studies that directly compared an H_2-RA with a PPI and two antibiotics [311]. They identified a total of 12 studies with 1415 patients. The overall pooled efficacy was similar in ITT analysis: 78% (549/701) with H_2-RAs vs 81% (575/714) with PPIs (odds ratio, 0.86; 95% CI: 0.66–1.12). **A1c** Thus, they concluded that the PPI and H_2-RA were similarly effective adjuvants for *H. pylori* triple eradication therapy [311]. However, another meta-analysis was published that concluded that PPI based triple therapies were more effective than H$_2$-RA based regimens [312]. This overview included more studies (20) and the population was 2374 patients. The pooled efficacy was 74% (95% CI: 71–76%) for the PPIs and 69% (95% CI: 66–71%) for the H$_2$-RA triples (odds ratio, 1.31; 95% CI: 1.09–1.58). Based on these data, the PPI component remains an important part of combination eradication therapies. **A1a**

Greater acid suppression: PPI twice daily dosing recommended

A meta-analysis found that the eradication rates with double doses of PPI were higher than single doses of PPI in ITT analysis (83.9% vs 77.7%; Peto odds ratio, 1.51; 95% CI: 1.23–1.85; p < 0.01) [313]. **A1c** An earlier study that compared once daily omeprazole 80 mg, metronidazole and amoxicillin (35% success), omeprazole, metronidazole and azithromycin (65%) and omeprazole, metronidazole and clarithromycin found that 78% could be eradicated with the latter regimen [314]. A more recent study using lansoprazole, clarithromycin and tinidazole either as standard doses twice daily or double doses once daily, found that the once daily dosing was less effective [153]. Thus, there is little evidence to suggest that PPI triple therapy should be given less than twice daily.

There is additional evidence that increased levels of acid suppression lead to better eradication efficacy. In a comparison of PPI triple regimens in which rabeprazole 10 mg or 20 mg were used twice daily with amoxicillin and clarithromycin, the higher dose was more effective (eradication proportions: rabeprazole 10 mg, 85%, 20 mg 96%, p < 0.05) [315]. **A1c** Another study used amoxicillin with clarithromycin with a variety of PPI doses designed to produce a range of acid suppression. In increasing order of acid suppression, patients were given one week of omeprazole 20 mg bid, esomeprazole 40 mg once daily and esomeprazole 40 mg bid, and the observed eradication rates were 71%, 81% and 96% respectively [316]. However, there may be a plateau effect, as one study used omeprazole either 20 mg or 40 mg bid with clarithromycin and tinidazole and found no difference in eradication rates. In patients with resistant strains, the eradication rate was lower and was no better with greater acid suppression [317]. With esomeprazole, which is considered to be one of the most potent acid inhibitors, there may be little difference whether a 40 mg dose is used once or twice daily [318, 319]. Overall, a recent meta-analysis showed that high dose PPI was more effective than standard doses for eradicating *H. pylori* with seven-day PPI triple therapy [320]. **A1a**

Triple and quadruple bismuth based therapies

In the first meta-analysis published in 1992, the best regimen was triple therapy with bismuth, metronidazole and tetracycline (BMT), which was superior to triple therapy with bismuth, metronidazole and amoxicillin [92, 138, 220]. However, the large number of pills required and relatively long two-week duration of treatment affected compliance adversely. Poor compliance (<60% of pills) led to only 69% eradication success compared to 96% in patients who take >60% of pills [321]. Later meta-analyses demonstrated that one week was as effective as two weeks of therapy [92, 220, 229]. The greater number of adverse effects suffered with bismuth triple therapies leads to more treatment discontinuation than is observed with PPI triple therapies [220] or PPI-BMT quadruple therapy [322]. In patients who harbour a metronidazole resistant *H. pylori* infection, eradication efficacy was reduced to 58–64% compared to 86–89% for metronidazole sensitive strains [220, 289]. **A1c**

Proton pump inhibitors (PPIs) have been used in combination with the traditional bismuth triple therapy. This quadruple regimen resulted in high eradication rates (80–90%) with one week of treatment [220, 229, 323, 324] and was superior to bismuth triple therapy without a PPI. **A1c** There have been studies using omeprazole [296, 325–328], lansoprazole [329, 330], pantoprazole [322, 331–333] and rabeprazole [334, 335] as the PPI in these quadruple therapies. Most of the regimens were given four times daily. Importantly, using a PPI with bismuth, nitroimidazole and tetracycline (BMT) helps to overcome metronidazole resistance, with higher eradication rates than if the BMT is used without a PPI [336].

PPI-BMT vs PPI-CA

Published studies that have directly compared these regimens were summarized in the previous edition of this book [221]. A variety of different PPIs have been used, and the studies indicate that the PPI-BMT regimens were as effective or slightly more effective [337] than the PPI-CA triple therapies, with no significant differences between study treatments observed in any of the direct, head-to-head comparisons [296, 322, 327, 328, 330]. There appeared to be no real difference in rates of adverse effects with the PPI-BMT quadruple therapy compared to the gold-standard PPI-triple therapies. The proportion of patients who discontinued drugs due to side effects was very small and was comparable with all regimens. Thus, PPI-BMT should be considered an alternative first-line therapy.

Attempts to improve compliance

New triple BMT capsule

The major drawback of this quadruple regimen is that it generally requires four times daily dosing with at least 18 pills. One recent study using a three times daily regimen appeared to be very effective [327]. Adverse events are generally mild, but frequent enough that they may impair compliance. Most patients can complete the treatment if counselled about possible adverse effects, and treatment discontinuation is infrequent.

Recognizing the difficulty of taking large numbers of pills, a unique capsule has been developed that contains bismuth biskalcitrate 140 mg (as 40 mg Bi_2O_3 equivalent), metronidazole 125 mg and tetracycline 125 mg (Helizide or Pylera™, Axcan Pharma, Mont Saint-Hilaire, Quebec, Canada). In an open study, three of these capsules qid with omeprazole 20 mg bid for 10 days eradicated 93% by ITT and 97% by per protocol analysis [338]. **B4** Eradication rates were 93% and 95% in metronidazole-resistant and metronidazole-sensitive strains, by ITT analysis. This capsule was also evaluated in a quadruple therapy regimen and compared to the gold standard PPI-CA triple therapy in a randomized controlled trial. This therapy was well tolerated with an adverse event rate comparable to PPI-CA, and eradication results were equal [296]. **A1c**

Is twice daily dosing with PPI-BMT effective?

Another attempt to improve compliance and tolerability has been to use the PPI-BMT regimen twice daily. Earlier pilot studies reported modest ITT eradication rates of 71–78% using one week of OBMT bid [339, 340] and 70% with 10 days of LBMT [341]. The latter study showed that this LBMT regimen was more effective in metronidazole sensitive strains (90% eradication) than in resistant strains (41% eradication) [341]. These three studies all used bismuth subsalicylate as the bismuth compound.

More recently, two Italian studies reported by Dore revealed excellent rates of eradication [342, 343] with a regimen that included omeprazole 20 mg, tetracycline 500 mg, metronidazole 500 mg and colloidal bismuth subcitrate caplets 240 mg, all twice daily with noon and evening meals for 14 days. This regimen differs from those described above in terms of the bismuth compound used, the dosing at lunch and supper and the longer 14-day duration. In the first study, of 118 dyspeptic patients, of whom 76 were treatment naïve and 42 had experienced two or more previous treatment failures, the regimen was well tolerated, with 95% compliance and 3% drop-out rate due to medication-associated adverse effects. The overall eradication rate was 95% (ITT) or 98% (per-protocol analysis) [342]. There was no difference in eradication rates between naïve and "salvage" patients. **B4** The second study using the same drug regimen updated the data on the 42 patients from the first report and also included data on a total of 71 patients that had failed at least two prior attempts at eradication using a PPI triple regimen [343]. In this study, the observed eradication rate was 93% (ITT) or 97% (per-protocol analysis) [343]. **B4** The regimen was well tolerated, with only trivial adverse effects. In a second study by Dore, in treatment naïve elderly subjects using essentially the same regimen except for the substitution of

esomeprazole as the PPI, for a 10-day duration, the eradication rate was 91% (ITT) and compliance was excellent [344]. **B4**

An American study used similar twice daily dosing at midday and the evening but used rabeprazole 20 mg, two Pepto-bismol tablets (bismuth subsalicylate – formulation of bismuth available in North America), metronidazole 500 mg and tetracycline 500 mg for 14 days [345]. In 37 patients treated, the eradication rate was 92.3%, 96% in metronidazole sensitive and 83% in metronidazole resistant *H. pylori* strains. **B4** Overall, one patient stopped medication because of adverse effects, but all the remaining patients exhibited 100% compliance, despite five patients having moderate to severe side effects. These data suggest that twice daily quadruple therapy may be very effective, and alternative forms of bismuth may be used.

A slightly different quadruple therapy was also evaluated in a twice daily regimen in 43 patients [346]. Treatment with omeprazole 20 mg, amoxicillin 1 g, tinidazole 500 mg and bismuth subcitrate 240 mg all bid (OATinB) for seven days was slightly less effective than the PPI-ACM regimen described below with eradication observed in 84% (ITT) or 86% (PP) of patients. **B4**

Quadruple (PPI-BMT) therapy effective even with nitroimidazole resistance

PPI-BMT may be an effective regimen for treatment failures, and even metronidazole-resistant strains may be successfully eradicated [296, 322, 347]. In van der Wouden's meta-analysis, the only regimen that was not affected by metronidazole resistance was PPI, bismuth, nitromidazole and tetracycline for at least seven days [289]. Adding a PPI is responsible for this effectiveness in patients with metronidazole resistant strains. In the study by Katelaris *et al.* [322], patients were treated with pantoprazole with BMT (PBMT quadruple) for seven days, compared to BMT triple without a PPI for 14 days. In this study, PBMT eradicated 81% of metronidazole resistant strains while the BMT regimen was successful in only 55% (p < 0.02). **A1c** Furthermore, the BMT regimen for 14 days resulted in 9% of patients discontinuing the drugs, compared to 3% observed with PBMT seven-day therapy.

As clarithromycin resistance significantly reduces the efficacy of clarithromycin containing triple therapies, it is noteworthy that OBMT eradication rates were not significantly different between clarithromycin sensitive and resistant strains [296].

PPI-BMT in treatment failures

Observational studies Patients in whom triple therapy with PPI, clarithromycin and amoxicillin had failed were treated with pantoprazole 40 mg twice daily, CBS 120 mg qid, tetracycline 500 mg qid and metronidazole 500 mg tid for seven days [331]. *H. pylori* eradication rate was 82% (95%

CI: 75–88%); treatment was well tolerated and major adverse effects were not observed. No differences in eradication success were observed in relation to underlying disease, i.e. whether the patient had peptic ulcer or functional dyspepsia [331]. **B4**

Patients in whom RBC-based regimens had failed were treated with OCA for a week, and eradication was successful in 68% of patients [348]. Those who failed to respond to OCA were given quadruple therapy (omeprazole 20 mg bid, bismuth subcitrate 120 mg, tetracycline 500 mg and metronidazole 400 mg qid) with 71% (5/7) success. Of those treated previously with clarithromycin containing regimens, OCA was successful in 11 of 19 patients, while quadruple therapy was successful in five of six. **B4** The numbers are too small to permit definite conclusions, but it appears that quadruple therapy maintains some efficacy despite repeated failures of clarithromycin-based therapies.

Direct comparative trials/systematic reviews The study by Peitz [349] compared second-line therapy with OCA and OBMT. While neither regimen was particulary effective, OBMT was superior (68% eradication) to OCA (43%) as second-line therapy. Failures of the second-line treatment were treated with the alternative regiment, and OBMT produced eradication in 50% of these patients, compared to only 16% observed with with OCA. Thus, while overall treatment success was not very good, OBMT had limited efficacy.

Two systematic reviews concluded that PPI-BMT was superior to an alternative PPI based triple therapy for second-line therapy and thus remained the treatment regimen of choice [350, 351]. **A1c**

Treatments for prior eradication failures

In patients who have failed initial therapy, successive therapies are usually less effective than when they are used as primary therapy. A number of regimens that have been studied are discussed below and summarized in Table 6.1. The most studied and consistently effective regimen is quadruple therapy with a PPI, bismuth compound, nitroimidazole and tetracycline for 7–14 days as discussed above. One drawback is that in some countries bismuth compounds are not available. Such is the case in Japan; however, rabeprazole, amoxicillin and metronidazole triple therapies may be an effective rescue regimen in that country [352, 353].

There are two basic approaches to treating an initial treatment failure, the first is to pick an empiric regimen based on the drugs used in the intial attempt, and the second is to perform *H. pylori* anti-microbial sensitivity testing and select antibiotic combinations based on the resistance pattern. The major drawback to this latter

Table 6.1 Promising "new" regimens for treatment failures.

Triple therapies
    PPI, amoxicillin and metronidazole for seven days – observed to be effective in Japan
    PPI, amoxicillin and rifabutin for 10–14 days
    PPI, moxifloxacin, rifabutin for seven days
    PPI, levofloxacin, rifabutin for seven days
    PPI, amoxicillin, levofloxacin for 10 days
    PPI, tinidazole, levofloxacin for 10 days
Quadruple therapies
    PPI, bismuth, metronidazole, tetracycline bid at lunch and supper x 14 days
    PPI, bismuth, tetracycline, furazolidone for seven days (limited availability of furazolidone)

approach is the general lack of availability of *H. pylori* culture and sensitivity testing.

One report of such a second-line approach described the treatment of patients with omeprazole, amoxicillin and clarithromycin (OAC) for 7 to 14 days or omeprazole, amoxicillin and metronidazole (OAM) for 14 days [271]. Re-treating empirically with clarithromycin-based regimens was largely ineffective, with eradication being achieved in 80% and 16% of clarithromycin sensitive and resistant strains respectively. Using the OAM regimen, metronidazole sensitive and resistant strains were eradicated in 81% and 59% of patients respectively. These data suggest that once clarithromycin has been used and the treatment fails, it is not worthwhile to administer it again. Also, while anti-microbial sensitivity testing may be helpful in some cases, this does not guarantee eradication success. **B4**

Rifabutin regimens Rifabutin containing regimens have emerged as an option for treating eradication failures. The regimen was originally studied in Italy, and a randomized trial has shown that rifabutin is more effective in a dose of 300 mg daily than 150 mg daily, when used in combination with pantoprazole and amoxicillin for 10 days [332]. This triple regimen was more effective (87%) than pantoprazole-BMT quadruple therapy (67%), the most commonly recommended salvage therapy. **A1c** The 87% eradication rate observed in this study was better than the 71% eradication rate observed in 41 patients treated in the pilot study [354]. In another small pilot study assessing a regimen that included rifabutin 150 mg, amoxicillin 1 g, and lansoprazole 30 mg all bid for one week the observed eradication rate was 72% (ITT) and 86% (per-protocol analysis) [355]. A regimen that included esomeprazole, amoxicillin and rifabutin produced similar results [356]. In a trial that compared omeprazole, amoxicillin and rifabutin 150 mg bid for seven days to OBMT the rates of eradication were respectively, only 44% and 70% [357]. These data suggest that one week of treatment may not be sufficient.

In a small group of patients who failed two courses of therapy, the first with PPI-CA and the second with either PPI or RBC-BMT, third-line therapy with omeprazole, amoxicillin and rifabutin 150 mg bid for 14 days was successful in 11 of 14 patients [358]. **B4** In treating strains resistant to both metronidazole and clarithromycin, esomeprazole, rifabutin and amoxicillin triple therapy resulted in an eradication rate of 74% (ITT) in a German population [356]. Also in a German population with *H. pylori* strains resistant to both metronidazole and clarithromycin, triple therapy with esomeprazole 40 mg, moxifloxacin 400 mg and rifabutin 300 mg daily for one week was effective in 78% of patients [359]. **B4** Some of these patients had failed four previous treatments. Considering that these dually resistant *H. pylori* strains are difficult to eradicate, these observational data are promising, particularly for amoxicillin allergic patients.

A drawback to rifabutin is that it is an expensive drug and is not readily available in some jurisdictions. In summary, the results of therapy in which a PPI is combined with amoxicillin and rifabutin, have been inconsistent.

A Chinese study compared the combination of rifabutin 300 mg od, levofloxacin 500 mg od and rabeprazole 20 mg bid with rabeprazole-BMT quadruple therapy, each for seven days [335]. This triple therapy regimen is very simple, as both the levofloxacin and the rifabutin are given only once daily. In this study the eradication rate was very high (91%) with both regimens. Even in patients resistant to both metronidazole and clarithromycin, the eradication rates were 85% (17/20) in the triple therapy and 87% (13/15) in the quadruple therapy arm [335]. Thus, these are both promising regimens for treatment failure. **A1d**

Levofloxacin regimens   Analogous to the first-line PPI triple therapies, regimens substituting clarithromycin with levofloxacin have been studied.

PPI (rabeprazole 20 mg bid), amoxicillin 1 g bid and levofloxacin 500 mg od and PPI, tinidazole 500 mg bid and levofloxacin 500 mg od triple therapies were both very effective in treatment failures, with eradication rates of 90% or more with 10 days of treatment, when compared to the present gold standard for treatment failures, a PPI-quadruple therapy (rabeprazole-BMT) regimen for either 7 or 14 days [334]. **A1c** The quadruple therapies in this study produced disappointing eradication rates of 63–69% [334]. Not only were the triple therapies more effective, the adverse effects were significantly less frequent than were observed in the RBMT, 14-day group. In another study, even after patients had failed two or more previous standard regimens, the rabeprazole, amoxicillin and levo-

floxacin triple therapy for 10 days was effective in 83% of patients [360]. **B4** In a similar study in which pantoprazole was used instead of rabeprazole with amoxicillin and levofloxacin for one week the observed eradication rate was 63% [333] **B4**. In Perri's study, the PPI-BMT regimen appeared to be the more effective, with an 83% eradication rate. Another similar study with pantoprazole, amoxicillin and levofloxacin all twice daily for 10 days resulted in an eradication rate of 70% compared to a 37% observed with PPI-BMT [361]. **A1d**

As the results were not all consistent, a meta-analysis by Gisbert *et al.* has been reported where levofloxacin triple therapies were compared against bismuth quadruple therapy [362]. Overall, the levofloxacin triple therapy regimens appeared to be significantly more effective and better tolerated than the quadruple regimens, and highest eradication rates were observed when therapy was given for 10 days [362]. **A1c** The most commonly used regimen was a PPI with amoxicillin and levofloxacin. Another meta-analysis that restricted its scope to PPI, amoxicillin and levofloxacin also indicated that 10 days of this levofloxacin-based triple therapy was more effective and better tolerated that seven days' bismuth based quadruple therapy [363]. **A1c** One study observed that the eradication rate was the same whether levofloxacin was used 500 mg once or twice daily [364]. In an Italian study, primary levofloxacin resistance was found in 30% of patients, and this was associated with a lower eradication rate of 33% compared to 75% in susceptible strains [365].

Levofloxacin has also been used as part of a quadruple therapy regimen in patients who had failed a course of PPI triple therapy [366]. When used with esomeprazole, bismuth and amoxicillin, the eradication rate was 73%, lower than the 88% rate observed with the usual gold standard quadruple therapy of esomeprazole, bismuth, metronidazole and tetracycline [366]. For patients who had failed more than one course of previous eradication therapy, the success of the levofloxacin quadruple regimen was even lower, with an observed eradication rate of 56% compared to 90%, observed with the EBMTregimen (p = 0.013). **A1c**

Moxifloxacin regimens   After a failure of PPI triple therapy, a Korean study compared one week of triple therapy with moxifloxacin, esomeprazole and amoxicillin against the gold standard esomeprazole, bismuth, metronidazole and tetracycline quadruple therapy [367]. The eradication rate with the moxifloxacin triple therapy was 76% and with the quadruple therapy, 55% (p = 0.042). **A1c** In a different Korean population, a study of the same drugs administered for longer durations, 10 days of triple therapy and 14 days of EBMT quadruple therapy resulted in both regimens obtaining eradication rates of 72% [368]. **A1c** The moxifloxacin triple regimen had significantly fewer adverse effects in both studies.

Gatifloxacin regimens In a small open-label study with one-week gatifloxacin 400 mg od, amoxicillin and rabeprazole in patients who had failed one or more clarithromycin containing regimens, the eradication rate was 84%, without significant adverse effects [369]. **B4** Of the seven treatment failures, secondary resistance to gatifloxacin did not develop. There are only limited data on acquired resistance to quinolones.

A Japanese study suggests that culturing *H. pylori* may be useful, in that strains resistant to clarithromycin and metronidazole could be eradicated with a gatifloxacin regimen if the strains were sensitive to gatifloxacin [370].

Furazolidone regimens A triple therapy regimen with omeprazole, amoxicillin and furazolidone was rather ineffective (52% eradication); however, if antibiotic sensitivity testing can be done, this regimen was shown to be 88% effective against strains that are still sensitive to metronidazole and clarithromycin [371]. In clinical practice, antibiotic sensitivity testing as a requirement after the first failure is impractical. Also, the chance that *H. pylori* would still be susceptible to both antibiotics after treatment failure is fairly small. However, another small study with furazolidone quadruple therapy did show some promise. Patients failing an initial regimen that included clarithromycin, metronidazole, and acid suppression with or without amoxicillin were treated with a quadruple therapy of lansoprazole, bismuth, metronidazole and tetracycline with only 39% success [372]. These treatment failures were subsequently treated with lansoprazole 30 mg bid, colloidal bismuth subcitrate 240 mg bid, tetracycline 1 g bid and furazolidone 200 mg bid for one week and eradication was seen in 9 of 10 patients.

A small RCT in patients with metronidazole resistant *H. pylori* by agar dilution [373] compared one-week bismuth, tetracycline and furazolidone 200 mg bid (BTF) with OBMT and the observed eradication rates were 86% and 74% (p = NS). The BTF regimen resulted in fewer adverse effects than were observed with OBMT (31 vs 60%, p = 0.03). Thus, furazolidone may be an excellent substitute for metronidazole.

Faropenem After initial *H. pylori* eradication failure with lansoprazole, amoxicillin and clarithromycin, 52% of patients had *H. pylori* that was resistant to clarithromycin [374]. These Japanese patients who failed therapy were then re-treated with rabeprazole, amoxicillin and faropenem 200 mg tid for seven days, and eradication was achieved in 91% (21/23) of patients, with no serious adverse events. However, another study in treatment naive patients found much lower eradication rates, with 46.5% with seven-day therapy and 62.5% with 14-day therapy, despite the fact that all strains were highly sensitive *in vitro* [375].

In treatment failures resistant to metronidazole, rabeprazole, minocycline and faropenem triple therapy was only 10% effective [376]. Substituting minocycline for amoxicillin is thus ineffective. These data suggest that faropenem needs further study, and faropenem is not widely available outside of Japan.

Minocycline In a Japanese study, first-line therapy with rabeprazole, amoxicillin and minocycline was ineffective [376]. However, after initial therapy, if strains were metronidazole sensitive, rabeprazole, minocycline and metronidazole was 85% effective. Data for this regimen as first-line therapy are lacking; however, minocycline resitance is rare and this may be a useful regimen for penicillin allergic patients.

Third-line and multiple failures

An uncontrolled study in patients with two consecutive eradication failures was reported by Gisbert *et al.* [377]. A wide variety of regimens were used in the first and second attempts that failed, and the investigators decided on one of four different regimens for the third eradication attempt, avoiding duplicating a previously used regimen in any given patient. Overall, in 48 patients, they gave empirical treatments without antibiotic sensitivity testing and achieved eradication success in 71%. This study has limitations because of the heterogeneity of regimens used but it does provide some clinical evidence that in community practice, where sensitivity testing is not available, even two previous eradication failures can be successfully eradicated with careful choosing of a third regimen.

Gisbert reported another study in patients who failed a first attempt with PPI, clarithromycin and amoxicillin, then a second attempt with bismuth based quadruple therapy [378]. These treatment failures were then treated with levofloxacin, amoxicillin and omeprazole for 10 days and the eradication rate was 60%. This modest rate of success is reasonable, considering that patients had failed two prior attempts. Gisbert also reported that this 10-day levofloxacin, amoxicillin and omeprazole triple therapy was more effective than rifabutin, amoxicillin and omeprazole, with eradication rates of 85% and 45% respectively [379]. Rifabutin appears to be not very effective and can cause leucopenia. Therefore it is not readily recommended.

Newer drugs and regimens

Several newer regimens have been explored (see Table 6.1), and a partial summary appears in Table 6.2.

Table 6.2 "Newer" *H. pylori* eradication regimens.

PPI triple therapies
  Lansoprazole, furazolidone and tetracycline or clarithromycin for
    seven days
  PPI, levofloxacin and amoxicillin or nitroimidazole or clarithromycin
    for seven days
  PPI, moxifloxacin and amoxicillin or nitroimidazole or clarithromycin
    for seven days
PPI, gatifloxacin and amoxicillin for seven days
  PPI quadruple therapies
  PPI, amoxicillin, clarithromycin and nitroimidazole for five days
  PPI, amoxicillin, bismuth and furazolidone or clarithromycin for 14
    days
Sequential therapy
  PPI + amoxicillin for five days then PPI, clarithromyin and
    nitroimidazole for five days

Penicillin allergic patients Penicillin allergy is fairly common, and in these patients, PPI-CM or PPI-BMT can be given first line. In a small study of 20 patients treated with esomeprazole 40 mg, tetracycline 500 mg and metronidazole 500 mg all given four times daily, the eradication rate for the 17 patients undergoing first time treatment was 85% and the three patients who had failed prior eradication therapy were successfully eradicated [380]. The regimen was well tolerated, and confirmation in a second study of the efficacy of this promising regimen would be desirable.

Furazolidone Furazolidone is an older, inexpensive antibiotic that may be effective in areas of high metronidazole resistance, although it may not be available in all markets. A large scale Chinese trial has shown that when furazolidone 100 mg bid was used in triple therapy with omeprazole and amoxicillin, an eradication rate of 86% was achieved [381]. In another Chinese study in DU patients, the observed eradication rate was 66% compared to a rate of 91% with the alternative regimen of omeprazole, furazolidone and clarithromycin (OFC). In this trial the eradication rates observed with standard triple therapy with omeprazole, amoxicillin and clarithromycin (OAC) and omeprazole, metronidazole and clarithromycin (OMC) were 90% and 71% respectively [382]. The furazolidone regimens were well tolerated with only minor side effects [382].

An interesting regimen using drugs with very low rates of *H. pylori* resistance was found to be very effective. In this Brazilian study, lansoprazole 30 mg od, tetracycline 500 mg qid and furazolidone 200 mg tid for seven days achieved 88% success [383]. Adverse events were frequent but minor, with only 1 of 52 patients stopping therapy because of

nausea. This regimen deserves further study. For re-treatment the authors use the same regimen for 10 days (personal communication).

In Iran, where baseline metronidazole resistance is said to be high, two-week quadruple therapy with omeprazole, amoxicillin, bismuth subcitrate and either furazolidone or clarithromycin also resulted in high eradication rates of 84% and 85% [384]. A similar quadruple regimen with omeprazole, amoxicillin, bismuth and either furazolidone or metronidazole resulted in eradication rates of 87% and 75% respectively [385]. It appears that the furazolidone quadruple regimens are more effective than a metronidazole-based regimen in areas of high nitroimidazole resistance. Another Iranian study found lower eradication rates of approximately 70%, with no improvement with two weeks compared to one week of treatment [386]. In a study in which relatives of patients with gastric cancer were screened and offered treatment for *H. pylori* (if found) [387], patients were randomized to receive lansoprazole 30 mg, clarithromycin 500 mg and furazolidone either 200 mg or 400 mg for one week. The triple therapy with the 400 mg dose resulted in an eradication rate of 87%. This regimen is interesting as the drugs are given once daily, are well tolerated and relatively inexpensive.

Fluoroquinolones

Levofloxacin Levofloxacin combination regimens continue to look promising. Levofloxacin has been mostly used in place of clarithromycin. The first paper by Cammarota identified that levofloxacin, amoxicillin and rabeprazole and levofloxacin, tinidazole and rabeprazole triple therapies were both very effective with observed eradication rates greater than 90% [388]. A subsequent RCT confirmed that levofloxacin, amoxicillin and rabeprazole triple therapy for one week resulted in a 90% eradication rate [236]. The rabeprazole, levofloxacin and tinidazole regimen, also administered to an Italian population resulted in eradication rates of approximately 95% when used for four to seven days in treatment naive patients [389].

A slightly different regimen in which levofloxacin was used in place of amoxicillin (rather than clarithromycin), compared esomeprazole 20 mg bid, levofloxacin 500 mg od and clarithromycin 500 mg bid for one week and resulted in an eradication rate of 87%, significantly higher than was observed with standard PPI triple therapies that were only 72–75% effective [390]. Cammarota *et al.* [391] also studied the effect of rabeprazole and levofloxacin once daily with clarithromycin in one of two doses, 250 mg or 500 mg twice daily for one week. The higher clarithromycin dose was more effective (94% vs 84%). Furthermore, all patients who failed eradication therapy developed clarithromycin resistance when the smaller dose of clarithromycin was used, compared to 33% who developed resistance with the larger dose of clarithromycin [391].

Moxifloxacin Another new fluoroquinolone, moxifloxacin appears promising. Used by itself or with lansoprazole, it was not effective, but used for one week in a regimen that included lansoprazole 30 mg od, clarithromycin 500 mg bid and moxifloxacin 400 mg od, the eradication rate in 40 Italian patients was 90% [392]. A larger four-arm study of 320 patients compared four different regimens in treatment naïve patients: two standard one-week PPI triple therapies (esomeprazole with clarithromycin and amoxicillin (ECA) or tinidazole (ECT)) and two moxifloxacin triple therapies (esomeprazole with moxifloxacin and amoxicillin (EMA) or tinidazole (EMT)) [393]. Observed eradication rates with standard triple therapies were 73% for ECA and 75% for ECT and the rates in the regimens with moxifloxacin in place of clarithromycin, were 88% with EMA and 90% with EMT. Adverse effects were also less frequent when moxifloxacin was used.

Another four-arm study of 277 patients also compared one week moxifloxacin with clarithromycin [394]. Patients were randomized to receive one of the following regimens: lansoprazole 30 mg bid, metronidazole 400 mg bid and moxifloxacin 400 mg od (LMM), lansoprazole, amoxicillin and moxifloxacin (LAM), or lansoprazole, metronidazole, clarithromycin (LMC), or lansoprazole, amoxicillin and clarithromycin (LAC). Eradication rates were 93.5%, 86.4%, 70.4% and 78.2% respectively [394]. **A1c** In this study, primary resistance to clarithromycin was seen in 10.8% and to moxifloxacin in 5.9% of strains. Moxifloxacin sensitive strains were significantly better eradicated with both LMM and LAM (98% and 91% respectively), while for resistant strains, the corresponding eradication rates were 75% and 67%. Thus, moxifloxacin based therapies were more effective than clarithromycin based regimens. **A1c**

Gatifloxacin Gatifloxacin 400 mg od and amoxicillin 1g bid was used with rabeprazole 20 mg once daily or twice daily for seven days, in patients who were mainly treatment naïve [395]. The eradication rate in the rabeprazole twice daily arm was higher than in the once daily arm, 92% compared to 83%. All seven patients that had failed previous eradication treatment were cured in the twice daily rabeprazole arm. One caveat in this study is that in about half the patients, sensitivity testing was done, and all tested strains were sensitive to gatifloxacin. This may partially account for the high eradication success rate. This gatifloxacin triple regimen with PPI given twice daily was very effective and well tolerated and should be studied further. **A1d**

A twice daily ofloxacin, rabeprazole and amoxicillin triple therapy was given for either seven days or 14 days with a observed eradication rates of 62% and 92% (p = 0.004) [396]. **A1d** As this regimen does not contain clarithromycin or metronidazole, this approach may be useful for patients who have failed treatment regimens with these drugs in the past.

Nitazoxanide This antibiotic has microbiological similarities to the nitroimidazoles without as much problem with resistance. It is ineffective as a single agent [397].

Sequential therapy

An interesting study in 1049 dyspeptic Italian patients was reported by Zullo [398]. In this RCT, sequential therapy was given to an experimental group for a total of 10 days: during which patients were first treated for five days with rabeprazole 40 mg od and amoxicillin 1g bid and then received rabeprazole 20 mg, clarithromycin 500 mg and tinidazole 500 mg twice daily for another five days. The control group received triple therapy with rabeprazole 20 mg, clarithromycin 500 mg and amoxicillin 1g bid for one week. Sequential therapy was significantly more effective (sequential therapy 92%, standard therapy 74%, p < 0.0001). **A1c** Zullo also examined this strategy in patients 65 years of age and over and observed comparable results, indicating that eradication efficacy is not necessarily affected by age [399]. A subsequent trial of this sequential therapy regimen compared two different doses of clarithromycin, 250 mg (low dose) vs 500 mg (high dose). Both doses were very effective, with eradication rates of 92–95% [400]. **A1c** Using pantoprazole as the PPI, Vaira reported that this 10-day sequential therapy was more effective than 10-day PPI triple therapy [401]. An additional observation in this study was that in clarithromycin resistant *H. pylori*, the sequential therapy was 89% effective, compared to only 29% observed with the triple therapy. Further data in resistant strains are awaited as an 89% eradication rate is unheard of in clarithromycin resistant strains. Further evidence showing sequential therapy to be more effective than standard triple therapy with esomeprazole, clarithromycin and amoxicillin for either 7 or 10 days has also been reported [402].

A systematic review also provides evidence that this 10-day sequential regimen has been consistently highly effective, with an eradication rate of approximately 90% and is more effective than the standard triple therapy [403]. Another meta-analysis reported data from 10 RCTs. The observed crude eradication rate with sequential therapy was 93.4% (95% CI: 91.3% to 95.5%) compared to 76.9% (95%CI: 71% to 82.8%) with standard triple therapy [404]. **A1a** The authors noted that the majority of data were from Italy, and data from other populations would be very desirable.

It has repeatedly been observed to be difficult to eradicate *H. pylori* in Turkey. Uygun *et al.* used an alternative sequential therapy, starting with one week pantoprazole and amoxicillin followed by pantoprazole, tetracycline and metronidazole for a second week [405]. This regimen resulted in an eradication rate of 72.6%, compared to the rate of 58% observed with the gold standard pantoprazole, amoxicillin and clarithromycin triple therapy for two weeks (p = 0.01). **A1d**

PPI or RBC with amoxicillin, clarithromycin and metronidazole for five days A short five-day therapy with rabeprazole 20 mg, amoxicillin 750 mg, clarithromycin 200 mg and metronidazole 250 mg (RACM) all twice daily achieved an eradication rate of 93% in 80 Japanese patients compared with rate of 81% with the standard RCA, one-week triple therapy [406]. Serious adverse events were not seen, and compliance was excellent. An earlier study by the same group used the same regimens but each for five days and found an eradication rate of 94% for RACM and 80% for RAC [407].

A similar regimen used for a short duration was also reported from Germany [408]. This was a three-arm study comparing quadruple therapy with lansoprazole 30 mg bid, amoxicillin 1 g bid, clarithromycin 250 mg bid and metronidazole 400 mg bid for five days (LACM5), with ranitidine 300 mg bid with the same antibiotics (RanACM), and with lansoprazole for all five days combined with the antibiotics for three days, from the third to the fifth day (LACM3). The eradication rates were excellent at 89%, 89% and 81% respectively. The rates were not significantly different, but the three-day therapy may be slightly less effective. These results are similar to those reported in the original description of this regimen in 1998. In that study omeprazole with the same antibiotics (OACM) for five days was compared to OCM for seven days, and the observed eradication rate was 90% for each group [409].

Earlier trials of similar regimens have yielded remarkably consistent results. Neville used lansoprazole as the PPI (LACM) with an eradication rate of 88%, better than was observed with the first-line recommended LCM (81%) or LCA (59%) triple therapy regimens [410]. In this study, the baseline metronidazole resistance rate was 52%. Catalano *et al.* compared either omeprazole or RBC as the antisecretory drug for five days combined with ACM for only three days from days 3 to 5 with standard triple therapies of OCA and RBC-CA [411]. The eradication rates were 89% with OACM, 82% with OAC, 95% with RBC-ACM and 78% with RBC-CA. A similar regimen using omeprazole, amoxicillin, clarithromycin and tinidazole all bid for four days resulted in an eradication rate of 88% [412]. One study in 169 patients in which roxithromycin was used in place of clarithromycin for seven days yielded an eradication rate of 92% [413]. **B4**

What is remarkable is that this PPI-ACM regimen for five days has consistently shown eradication rates of 89–95%, compared to rates of 59–90% (mainly approximately 80%) observed with one-week triple therapies in these studies. Considering these results, further study of this approach, especially as a treatment failure regimen, is clearly warranted.

Less promising regimens

Azithromycin

Azithromycin does not appear to be a very useful drug for *H. pylori* eradication. When used in place of clarithromycin as part of a quadruple therapy, a lower eradication rate was observed [414]. Azithromycin is usually administered for five days even when the other drugs are given for seven days. A potentially attractive regimen is that of a PPI with levofloxacin and azithromycin as each drug can be given once daily. In one study using this regimen for one week, the eradication rate was comparable to that observed with standard PPI, clarithromycin and amoxicillin but the success was only 65% [415]. In a study conducted in France the combination of omeprazole, amoxicillin and azithromycin yielded an eradication rate of only 38%, substantially less than the rates of 72% and 61% observed with OCA or OCM [416]. In other studies where azithromycin was used for only three days, eradication success was suboptimal [383, 417–419]. Used in place of clarithromycin in a once daily, six-day regimen with tinidazole and lansoprazole provided eradication in only 67% of patients [420].

Rifaximin is a poorly absorbed antibiotic and when used as triple therapy with rifaximin, esomeprazole and clarithromycin or levofloxacin it was ineffective [421].

Mucosal protective agents

Cetraxate is an anti-ulcer drug with mucosal protective effects and it can inhibit the growth of *H. pylori* [422]. In triple therapy with clarithromycin and amoxicillin, an eradication rate of 70% was observed compared to a rate of 94% observed with standard pantoprazole, clarithromycin and amoxicillin triple therapy, suggesting that cetraxate is less effective than PPI for this purpose [422].

Sofalcone and polaprezinc are mucoprotective agents with anti-*Helicobacter* activity. In a Japanese trial, patients were randomized to receive one of three regimens: rabeprazole, amoxicillin and clarithromycin triple therapy, sofacolone plus triple therapy, or polaprezinc plus triple therapy and the observed eradication rates were 78%, 87% and 80% respectively [423]. The difference between the sofacolone and rabeprozole regimens was statistically significant.

Table 6.3 *H. pylori* eradication treatment recommendations 2009.

Recommended first-line therapies

PPI triples

    PPI bid + clarithromycin 500 mg bid + amoxicillin 1 g bid for seven days

    PPI bid + clarithromycin 500 mg bid + metronidazole 500 mg bid for seven days

PPI-BMT

    PPI bid + colloidal bismuth citrate 240 mg or bismuth subsalicylate two tabs qid, metronidazole 250–500 mg qid, tetracycline 500 mg qid for seven days

PPI-BMT bid

    PPI bid + colloidal bismuth subcitrate 240 mg or bismuth subsalicylate two tabs bid, metronidazole 500 mg bid and tetracycline 500 mg bid, at noon and supper with the meal for 14 days

Promising first-line therapies

Levofloxacin triple therapy

    PPI od or bid, levofloxacin 500 mg od, amoxicillin 1 g bid for seven days

    PPI od or bid, levofloxacin 500 mg od, nitroimidazole 500 mg bid for seven days

    PPI od or bid, levofloxacin 500 mg od, clarithromycin 500 mg bid for seven days

Moxifloxacin triple therapy

    PPI od or bid, moxifloxacin 400 mg od, amoxicillin 1 g bid for seven days

    PPI od or bid, moxifloxacin 400 mg od, nitroimidazole 500 mg bid for seven days

    PPI od or bid, moxifloxacin 400 mg od, clarithromycin 500 mg bid for seven days

Sequential therapy

    PPI bid and amoxicillin 1 g bid for first five days, then PPI, clarithromycin 500 mg and nitroimidazole 500 mg twice daily for five more days (total 10 days)

PPI-ACM for five days

    PPI bid, amoxicillin 750 mg to 1 g bid, clarithromycin 250 mg bid and metronidazole 500 mg bid

Furazolidone regimens

    PPI od, furazolidone 200 mg tid, tetracycline 500 mg qid for seven days

    PPI od, furazolidone 400 mg od, clarithromycin 500 mg od for seven days

    PPI, amoxicillin 1 g, CBS 240 mg, furazolidone 200 mg all bid for 14 days

Recommended for treatment failures

PPI-BMT

    PPI bid + colloidal bismuth citrate 240 mg or bismuth subsalicylate two tabs qid, metronidazole 250–500 mg qid, tetracycline 500 mg qid for 14 days

Promising quadruple therapies

    PPI-BMT bid: PPI bid + colloidal bismuth subcitrate 240 mg or bismuth subsalicylate two tabs bid, metronidazole 500 mg bid and tetracycline 500 mg bid, at noon and supper with the meal for 14 days PPI bid, CBS 240 mg bid. tetracycline 1000 mg bid, furazolidone 200 mg bid for seven days

PPI triple therapy

    PPI, amoxicillin 750–1000 mg, metronidazole 250 mg bid for seven days (best in Japan)

Rifabutin regimens

    PPI bid, amoxicillin 1 g bid, rifabutin 150 mg bid for 10–14 days

    PPI od, moxifloxacin 400 mg od, rifabutin 300 mg od for seven days

    PPI od, levofloxacin 500 mg od, rifabutin 300 mg od for seven days

Levofloxacin regimens

    PPI bid, levofloxacin 500 mg od, amoxicillin 1 g bid for 10 days

    PPI bid, levofloxacin 500 mg od, nitroimidazole 500 mg bid for 10 days

PPI = omeprazole 20 mg, lansoprazole 30 mg, pantoprazole 40 mg, esomprazole 40 mg or rabeprazole 20 mg.

CBS = colloidal bismuth subcitrate.

Nitroimidazole = metronidazole or tinidazole.

Ecabet sodium when added to standard triple therapy did not improve ITT eradication rates in a Korean study [424].

Probiotics in *H. pylori* eradication

An increasing number of studies have evaluated the effects of probiotics such as *Lactobacillus* GG [425, 426], *Lactobacillus reuteri* ATCC 55730 [427], *Saccharomyces boulardii* [426, 428, 429], a combination of *Lactobacillus* and *Bifidobacteria* [426, 430], a combination of *Bacillus subtilis* and *Streptococcus faecium* [431] or *Bacillus clausii* [432] as adjuvant therapies for *H. pylori* treatment. One study used a combination of *Lactobacillus rhamnosus* GG and C705, *Bifidobacterium breve* Bb99 and *Propionibacterium freundenreichii* ssp. *shermnii* JS [433]. Most studies [425, 426, 429, 432] showed no improvement in *H. pylori* eradication rates with the probiotic, but adverse effects of eradication therapy such as diarrhea and taste disturbances were reduced, and this approach may help some patients complete their treatment course [428, 433, 434].

Some probiotic studies have actually shown an improvement in eradication rates [430, 431, 434–436]. In one study, four weeks' pre-treatment with *Lactobacillus* and *Bifidobacterium*-containing yogurt (AB-yogurt) significantly improved eradication of one-week quadruple therapy with omeprazole, bismuth, amoxicillin and metronidazole [437].

Tong *et al.* [438] conducted a meta-analysis of 14 randomized trials of the effects of probiotic supplementation on *H. pylori* eradication. They concluded that probiotics increased eradication rates and reduced adverse effects, particularly diarrhea. **A1c**

Alternative agents

Fish oil (eicosapen) contains ϖ-3-fatty acids which have been shown to have anti-*H. pylori* bacteriostatic effects. However, replacing metronidazole with eicosapen is ineffective [439]. **C5**

Pronase, a mucolytic agent with no antibacterial effect on *H. pylori*, added to lansoprazole, amoxicillin and metronidazole significantly improved eradication success to 94% compared with 77% (p = 0.004) observed with the LAM triple therapy alone [440]. **A1d** Regimens adding pronase deserve further study.

Lactoferrin is a multifunctional protein found in milk and when added to standard esomeprazole, clarithromycin and amoxicillin triple therapy it did not improve the eradication rate [441]. In an Italian study, lactoferrin significantly reduced the rate of adverse effects from 29.41% 17.64% (p < 0.05) [442]. When used with rabeprazole, clarithromycin and tinidazole, the addition of lactoferrin resulted in an eradication rate of 72%, not significantly different from the rate of 68% observed with the alternative triple therapy regimen containing rabeprazole, levofloxacin and amoxycillin [443]. **A1d**

Summary

H. pylori remains an important cause of ulcer disease, with acceptance as a definite pathogen that fulfills almost all of Hill's criteria for causation. In the new millennium, ulcers not caused by *H. pylori* or non-steroidal anti-inflammatory drugs appear to be on the increase. The older data from the pre-*H. pylori* era has become important again as in these patients there may be little else to offer for ulcer healing and prevention of recurrence other than continuous acid-suppressive therapy. For those with *H. pylori* infection, eradication remains important to facilitate ulcer healing, reduce ulcer relapse and prevent complications such as recurrent hemorrhage. Eradication of *H. pylori* heals ulcers without the need to continue ulcer healing drugs, heals refractory ulcers and also results in faster ulcer healing than occurs with traditional acid-suppressive therapy.

The present recommended first-line therapies include triple therapy with either PPI or RBC with clarithromycin and amoxicillin or metronidazole or a quadruple therapy with a PPI, bismuth compound, metronidazole and tetracycline (Table 6.3). First-line therapy should be administered for 7–10 days and for treatment failures, 10–14 days of treatment is recommended.

With emerging antimicrobial resistance, first-line therapies may not be quite as effective as in the recent past. There is evidence to support the use of a number of regimens for these eradication failures (see Table 6.3).

References

1 Schwarz K. Uber penetrierende Magen- und Jejunalgeschwure. *Beiträge Zur Klinische Chirurgie* 1910; **67**: 96–128.

2 Warren JR, Marshall BJ. Unidentified curved bacillus on gastric epithelium in active chronic gastritis. *Lancet* 1983; **1**: 1273–1275.

3 Marshall BJ, Warren JR. Unidentified curved bacilli in the stomach of patients with gastritis and peptic ulceration. *Lancet* 1984; **1**(16 June): 1311–1315.

4 Mégraud F, Lamouliatte H. *Helicobacter pylori* and duodenal ulcer. Evidence suggesting causation. *Dig Dis Sci* 1992; **37**: 769–772.

5 Rabeneck L, Ransohoff DF. Is *Helicobacter pylori* a cause of duodenal ulcer? A methodologic critique of current evidence. *Am J Med* 1991; **91**: 566–572.

6 Hill BA. The environment and disease: Association or causation? *Proc R Soc Med* 1965; **58**: 295–300.

7 Nomura A, Stemmerman GN, Chyou P-H, Perez-Perez GI, Blaser MJ. *Helicobacter pylori* infection and the risk for duodenal and gastric ulceration. *Annals of Internal Med* 1994; **120**: 977–981.

8 Sipponen P, Varis K, Fraki O, Korri UM, Seppala K, Siurala M. Cumulative 10-year risk of symptomatic duodenal and gastric ulcer disease in people with or without chronic gastritis: A clinical follow-up study of 454 outpatients. *Scand J Gastroenterol* 1990; **25**: 966–973.

9 Kuipers EJ, Thijs JC, Festen HPM. The prevalence of *Helicobacter pylori* in peptic ulcer disease. *Aliment Pharmacol Ther* 1995; **9**(Suppl 2): 59–69.

10 Borody TJ, George LL, Brandl S, *et al. Helicobacter pylori* negative duodenal ulcer. *Am J Gastroenterol* 1991; **86**: 1154–1157.

11 Talamini G, Tommasi M, Amadei V *et al.* Risk factors of peptic ulcer in 4943 inpatients. *J Clin Gastroenterol* 2008; **42**: 373–380.

12 Nervi G, Liatopoulou S, Cavallaro LG *et al.* Does *Helicobacter pylori* infection eradication modify peptic ulcer prevalence? A 10 years' endoscopical survey. *World J Gastroenterol* 2006; **12**: 2398–2401.

13 Jang HJ, Choi MH, Shin WG *et al.* Has peptic ulcer disease changed during the past ten years in Korea? A prospective multi-center study. *Dig Dis Sci* 2008; **53**: 1527–1531.

14 Xia B, Xia HH, Ma CW *et al.* Trends in the prevalence of peptic ulcer disease and *Helicobacter pylori* infection in family physician-referred uninvestigated dyspeptic patients in Hong Kong. *Aliment Pharmacol Ther* 2005; **22**: 243–249.

15 Quan C, Talley NJ. Management of peptic ulcer disease not related to *Helicobacter pylori* or NSAIDs. *Am J Gastroenterol* 2002; **97**: 2950–2961.

16 Laine L, Hopkins RJ, Girardi LS. Has the impact of *Helicobacter pylori* therapy on ulcer recurrence in the United States been overstated? A meta- analysis of rigorously designed trials. *Am J Gastroenterol* 1998; **93**: 1409–1415.

17 Ciociola AA, McSorley DJ, Turner K, Sykes D, Palmer JB. *Helicobacter pylori* infection rates in duodenal ulcer patients in the United States may be lower than previously estimated. *Am J Gastroenterol* 1999; **94**: 1834–1840.

18 Cloud ML, Enas N, Humphries TJ, Bassion S. Rabeprazole in treatment of acid peptic diseases: Results of three placebo-controlled dose-response clinical trials in duodenal ulcer, gastric ulcer, and gastroesophageal reflux disease (GERD). The Rabeprazole Study Group. *Dig Dis Sci* 1998; **43**: 993–1000.

19 Yakoob J, Jafri W, Jafri N, Islam M, Abid S, Hamid S, AliShah H, Shaikh H. Prevalence of non-*Helicobacter pylori* duodenal ulcer in Karachi, Pakistan. *World J Gastroenterol* 2005; **11**: 3562–3565.

20 Gisbert JP, Blanco M, Mateos JM *et al. pylori*-negative duodenal ulcer prevalence and causes in 774 patients. *Dig Dis Sci* 1999; **44**: 2295–2302.

21 Rosenstock S, Jorgensen T, Bonnevie O, Andersen L. Risk factors for peptic ulcer disease: A population based prospective cohort study comprising 2416 Danish adults. *Gut* 2003; **52**: 186–193.

22 Ong TZ, Hawkey CJ, Ho KY. Nonsteroidal anti-inflammatory drug use is a significant cause of peptic ulcer disease in a tertiary hospital in Singapore: A prospective study. *J Clin Gastroenterol* 2006; **40**: 795–800.

23 Aro P, Storskrubb T, Ronkainen J *et al.* Peptic ulcer disease in a general adult population: The Kalixanda study: A random population-based study. *Am J Epidemiol* 2006; **163**: 1025–1034.

24 Arroyo MT, Forne M, de Argila CM *et al.* The prevalence of peptic ulcer not related to *Helicobacter pylori* or non-steroidal anti-inflammatory drug use is negligible in southern Europe. *Helicobacter* 2004; **9**: 249–254.

25 Arkkila PE, Seppala K, Kosunen Tu *et al. Helicobacter pylori* eradication as the sole treatment for gastric and duodenal ulcers. *Eur J Gastroenterol Hepatol* 2005; **17**: 93–101.

26 Nishikawa K, Sugiyama T, Kato M *et al.* Non-*Helicobacter pylori* and non-NSAID peptic ulcer disease in the Japanese population. *Eur J Gastroenterol Hepatol* 2000; **12**: 635–640.

27 Miwa H, Sakaki N, Sugano K *et al.* Recurrent peptic ulcers in patients following successful *Helicobacter pylori* eradication: A multicenter study of 4940 patients. *Helicobacter* 2004; **9**: 9–16.

28 Hyvärinen H, Salmenkylä S, Sipponen P. *Helicobacter pylori*-negative duodenal and pyloric ulcer: Role of NSAIDs. *Digestion* 1996; **57**: 305–309.

29 Harris AW, Gummett PA, Phull PS, Jacyna MR, Misiewicz JJ, Baron JH. Recurrence of duodenal ulcer after *Helicobacter pylori* eradication is related to high acid output. *Aliment Pharmacol Ther* 1997; **11**: 331–334.

30 McColl KEL, El-Nujumi AM, Chittajallu RS *et al.* A study of the pathogenesis of *Helicobacter pylori* negative chronic duodenal ulceration. *Gut* 1993; **34**: 762–768.

31 Kurata JH, Nogawa AN. Meta-analysis of risk factors for peptic ulcer. Nonsteroidal antiinflammatory drugs, *Helicobacter pylori*, and smoking. *J Clin Gastroenterol* 1997; **24**: 2–17.

32 Choung RS, Talley NJ. Epidemiology and clinical presentation of stress-related peptic damage and chronic peptic ulcer. *Curr Mol Med* 2008; **8**: 253–257.

33 Chen TS, Chang FY. Clinical characteristics of *Helicobacter pylori*-negative duodenal ulcer disease. *Hepatogastroenterology* 2008; **55**: 1615–1618.

34 Rosenstock SJ, Jorgensen T, Bonnevie O, Andersen LP. Does *Helicobacter pylori* infection explain all socio-economic differences in peptic ulcer incidence? Genetic and psychosocial markers for incident peptic ulcer disease in a large cohort of Danish adults. *Scand J Gastroenterol* 2004; **39**: 823–829.

35 Ohara T, Morishita T, Suzuki H, Masaoka T, Ishii H. Usefulness of proton pump inhibitor (PPI) maintenance therapy for patients with *H. pylori*-negative recurrent peptic ulcer after eradication therapy for H. pylori: pathophysiological characteristics of *H. pylori*-negative recurrent ulcer scars and beyond acid suppression by PPI. *Hepatogastroenterology* 2004; **51**: 338–342.

36 Thijs JC, Kuipers EJ, van Zwet AA, Pena AS, de Graaff J. Treatment of *Helicobacter pylori* infections. *QJM* 1995; **88**: 369–389.

37 Borody TJ, Brandl S, Andrews P, Jankiewicz E, Ostapowicz N. *Helicobacter pylori* negative gastric ulcer. *Am J Gastroenterol* 1992; **87**: 1403–1406.

38 Rauws EAJ, Langenberg W, Houthoff HJ, Zanen HC, Tytgat GNJ. *Campylobacter pyloridis*-associated chronic active antral gastritis. *Gastroenterology* 1988; **94**: 33–40.

39 Graham DY, Malaty HM. Alendronate gastric ulcers. *Aliment Pharmacol Ther* 1999; **13**: 515–519.

40 Thomson AB, Marshall JK, Hunt RH *et al.* 14 day endoscopy study comparing risedronate and alendronate in postmenopausal women stratified by *Helicobacter pylori* status. *J Rheumatol* 2002; **29**: 1965–1974.

41 Graham DY, Malaty HM. Alendronate and naproxen are synergistic for development of gastric ulcers. *Arch Intern Med* 2001; **161**: 107–110.

42 Walsh JH, Peterson WL. The treatment of *Helicobacter pylori* infection in the management of peptic ulcer disease. *N Engl J Med* 1995; **333**: 984–991.

43 Jyotheeswaran S, Shah AN, Jin HO, Potter GD, Ona FV, Chey WY. Prevalence of *Helicobacter pylori* in peptic ulcer patients in greater Rochester, NY: Is empirical triple therapy justified? *Am J Gastroenterol* 1998; **93**: 574–578.

44 Marshall BJ. *Helicobacter pylori* in peptic ulcer: Have Koch's postulates been fulfilled? *Ann Med* 1995; **27**: 565–568.

45 Blaser MJ, Chyou P-H, Nomura A. Age at establishment of *Helicobacter pylori* infection and gastric carcinoma, gstric ulcer, and duodenal ulcer risk. *Cancer Research* 1995; **55**: 562–565.

46 Perri F, Clemente R, Pastore M *et al.* The 13C-urea breath test as a predictor of intragastric bacterial load and severity of *Helicobacter pylori* gastritis. *Scand J Clin Lab Invest* 1998; **58**: 19–27.

47 Labenz J, Börsch G, Peitz U, Aygen S, Hennemann O, Tillenburg B, Becker T, Stolte M. Validity of a novel biopsy urease test (HUT) and a simplified 13C-urea breath test for diagnosis of *Helicobacter pylori* infection and estimation of the severity of gastritis. *Digestion* 1996; **57**: 391–397.

48 Hilker E, Domschke W, Stoll R. 13C-urea breath test for detection of *Helicobacter pylori* and its correlation with endoscopic and histologic findings. *J Physiol Pharmacol* 1996; **47**: 79–90.

49 Moshkowitz M, Konikoff FM, Peled Y *et al.* High *Helicobacter pylori* numbers are associated with low eradication rate after triple therapy. *Gut* 1995; **36**: 845–847.

50 Sharma TK, Prasad VM, Cutler AF. Quantitative noninvasive testing for *Helicobacter pylori* does not predict gastroduodenal ulcer disease. *Gastrointest Endosc* 1996; **44**: 679–682.

51 Lewis JD, Kroser J, Bevan J, Furth EE, Metz DC. Urease-based tests for *Helicobacter pylori* gastritis. Accurate for diagnosis but poor correlation with disease severity. *J Clin Gastroenterol* 1997; **25**: 415–420.

52 Moran AP, Wadström T. Pathogenesis of *Helicobacter pylori*. *Curr Opin Gastroenterol* 1998; **14**(Suppl 1): S9–S14.

53 Arachchi HS, Kalra V, Lal B *et al.* Prevalence of duodenal ulcer-promoting gene (dupA) of *Helicobacter pylori* in patients with duodenal ulcer in North Indian population. *Helicobacter* 2007; **12**: 591–597.

54 Argent RH, Burette A, Miendje Deyi VY, Atherton JC. The presence of dupA in *Helicobacter pylori* is not significantly associated with duodenal ulceration in Belgium, South Africa, China, or North America. *Clin Infect Dis* 2007; **45**: 1204–1206.

55 Yang H, Dixon MF, Zuo J, Fong F, Zhou D, Corthésy I, Blum A. *Helicobacter pylori* infection and gastric metaplasia in the duodenum in China. *J Clin Gastroenterol* 1995; **20**: 110–112.

56 Harris AW, Gummett PA, Walker MM, Misiewicz JJ, Baron JH. Relation between gastric acid output, *Helicobacter pylori*, and gastric metaplasia in the duodenal bulb. *Gut* 1996; **39**: 513–520.

57 Walker MM, Dixon MF. Gastric metaplasia: Its role in duodenal ulceration. *Aliment Pharmacol Ther* 1996; **10** Suppl 1: 119–128.

58 Madsen JE, Vetvik K, Aase S. *Helicobacter*-associated duodenitis and gastric metaplasia in duodenal ulcer patients. *APMIS* 1991; **99**: 997–1000.

59 Steer HW. Surface morphology of the gastroduodenal mucosa in duodenal ulceration. *Gut* 1984; **25**: 1203–1210.

60 Carrick J, Lee A, Hazell S, Ralston M, Daskalopoulos G. *Campylobacter pylori*, duodenal ulcer, and gastric metaplasia: Possible role of functional heterotopic tissue in ulcerogenesis. *Gut* 1989; **30**: 790–797.

61 Khulusi S, Mendall MA, Badve S, Patel P, Finlayson C, Northfield TC. Effect of *Helicobacter pylori* eradication on gastric metaplasia of the duodenum. *Gut* 1995; **36**: 193–197.

62 Rudnicka L, Bobrzynski A, Stachura J. Short-term eradication therapy for *Helicobacter pylori* does not reduce the incidence of gastric metaplasia in duodenal ulcer patients. *Pol J Pathol* 1997; **48**: 103–106.

63 Khulusi S, Badve S, Patel P *et al.* Pathogenesis of gastric metaplasia of the human duodenum: role of *Helicobacter pylori*, gastric acid, and ulceration. *Gastroenterology* 1996; **110**: 452–458.

64 Urakami Y, Kimura M, Seki H. Gastric metaplasia and *Helicobacter pylori*. *Am J Gastroenterol* 1997; **92**: 795–799.

65 el-Omar E, Penman I, Dorrian CA, Ardill JE, McColl KE. Eradicating *Helicobacter pylori* infection lowers gastrin mediated acid secretion by two thirds in patients with duodenal ulcer. *Gut* 1993; **34**: 1060–1065.

66 Gillen D, el-Omar EM, Wirz AA, Ardill JES, McColl KEL. The acid response to gastrin distinguishes duodenal ulcer patients from *Helicobacter pylori*-infected healthy subjects. *Gastroenterol* 1998; **114**: 50–57.

67 Graham DY, Opekun A, Lew GM, Klein PD, Walsh JH. *Helicobacter pylori*-associated exaggerated gastrin release in duodenal ulcer patients. The effect of bombesin infusion and urea ingestion. *Gastroenterol* 1991; **100**: 1571–1575.

68 Hamlet A, Olbe L. The influence of *Helicobacter pylori* infection on postprandial duodenal acid load and duodenal bulb pH in humans. *Gastroenterol* 1996; **111**: 391–400.

69 el Omar EM, Penman ID, Ardill JE, Chittajallu RS, Howie C, McColl KE. *Helicobacter pylori* infection and abnormalities of acid secretion in patients with duodenal ulcer disease. *Gastroenterology* 1995; **109**: 681–691.

70 Harris AW, Gummett PA, Misiewicz JJ, Baron JH. Eradication of *Helicobacter pylori* in patients with duodenal ulcers lowers basal and peak acid outputs in response to gastrin releasing peptide and pentagastrin. *Gut* 1996; **38**: 663–667.

71 Beardshall K, Moss S, Gill J, Levi S, Ghosh P, Playford RJ, Calam J. Suppression of *Helicobacter pylori* reduces gastrin releasing peptide stimulated gastrin release in duodenal ulcer patients. *Gut* 1992; **33**: 601–603.

72 Harris AW, Gummett PA, Phull PS, Jacyna MR, Misiewicz JJ, Baron JH. Recurrence of duodenal ulcer after *Helicobacter pylori* eradication is related to high acid output. *Aliment Pharmacol Ther* 1997; **11**: 331–334.

73 Rieder G, Hatz RA, Moran AP, Walz A, Stolte M, Enders G. Role of adherence in interleukin-8 induction induction in *Helicobacter pylori*-associated gastritis. *Infect Immun* 1997; **65**: 3622–3630.

74 Yamaoka Y, Kita M, Kodama T, Sawi N, Kashima K, Imanishi J. Induction of various cytokines and development of severe mucosal inflammation by *cagA* gene positive *Helicobacter pylori* strains. *Gut* 1997; **41**: 442–451.

75 D'Elios MM, Manghetti M, Almerigogna F, Amedei A, Costa F, Burroni D, *et al.* Different cytokine profile and antigen-specificity repertoire in *Helicobacter pylori*-specific T cell clones from

the antrum of chronic gastritis patients with or without peptic ulcer. *Eur J Immunol* 1997; **27**: 1751–1755.

76 Beales I, Blaser MJ, Srinivasan S *et al.* Effect of *Helicobacter pylori* products and recombinant cytokines on gastrin release from cultured canine G cells. *Gastroenterol* 1997; **113**: 465–471.

77 Londong W, Barth H, Dammann HG *et al.* Dose-related healing of duodenal ulcer with the proton pump inhibitor lansoprazole. *Aliment Pharmacol Ther* 1991; **5**: 245–254.

78 Bardhan KD, Bianchi Porro G, Bose K *et al.* A comparison of two different doses of omeprazole versus ranitidine in treatment of duodenal ulcers. *J Clin Gastroenterol* 1986; **8**: 408–413.

79 Misra SC, Dasarathy S, Sharma MP. Omeprazole versus famotidine in the healing and relapse of duodenal ulcer. *Aliment Pharmacol Ther* 1993; **7**: 443–449.

80 Dammann HG, Walter TA. Efficacy of continuous therapy for peptic ulcer in controlled clinical trials. *Aliment Pharmacol Ther* 1993; **7**(Suppl 2): 17–25.

81 Penston JG, Wormsley KG. Nine years of maintenance treatment with ranitidine for patients with duodenal ulcer disease. *Aliment Pharmacol Ther* 1992; **6**: 629–645.

82 O'Brien BJ, Goeree R, Hunt R, Wilkinson J, Levine M, Willan A. *Economic Evaluation of Alternative Therapies in the Long Term Management of Peptic Ulcer Disease and Gastroesophageal Reflux Disease.* Report to CCOHTA 1996; RFP no.9503-OMEP: 1–130. McMaster University: 1996.

83 Veldhuyzen van Zanten SJO, Bradette M, Farley A *et al.* The DU-MACH study: Eradication of *Helicobacter pylori* and ulcer healing in patients with acute duodenal ulcer using omeprazole based triple therapy. *Aliment Pharmacol Ther* 1999; **13**: 289–295.

84 Coghlan JG, Humphries H, Dooley C, *et al. Campylobacter pylori* and recurrence of duodenal ulcer – a 12 month follow up study. *Lancet* 1987; **2**: 1109–1111.

85 Marshall BJ, Goodwin CS, Warren JR *et al.* Prospective double-blind trial of duodenal ulcer relapse after eradication of *Campylobacter pylori*. *Lancet* 1988; **ii**: 1437–1442.

86 Rauws EAJ, Tytgat GNJ. Cure of duodenal ulcer associated with eradication of *Helicobacter pylori*. *Lancet* 1990; **335**: 1233–1235.

87 George LL, Borody TJ, Andrews P, Devine M, Moore-Jones D, Walton M, Brandl S. Cure of duodenal ulcer after eradication of *Helicobacter pylori*. *Med J Aust* 1990; **153**: 145–149.

88 Graham DY, Lem GM, Evans DG, Evans DJ, Jr, Klein PD. Effect of triple therapy (antibiotics plus bismuth) on duodenal ulcer healing. A randomized controlled trial. *Ann Intern Med* 1991; **115**: 266–269.

89 Graham DY, Lew GM, Klein PD *et al.* Effect of treatment of *Helicobacter pylori* infection on the long-term recurrence of gastric or duodenal ulcer. A randomized, controlled study. *Ann Intern Med* 1992; **116**: 705–708.

90 Hentschel E, Brandstatter G, Dragosics B *et al.* Effect of ranitidine and amoxicillin plus metronidazole on the eradication of *Helicobacter pylori* and the recurrence of duodenal ulcer. *N Engl J Med* 1993; **328**: 308–312.

91 Tytgat GNJ. Review article: treatments that impact favourably upon the eradication of *Helicobacter pylori* and ulcer recurrence. *Aliment Pharmacol Ther* 1994; **8**: 359–368.

92 Penston JG. *Helicobacter pylori* eradication – understandable caution but no excuse for inertia. *Aliment Pharmacol Ther* 1994; **8**: 369–389.

93 Labenz J, Börsch G. Highly significant change of the clinical course of relapsing and complicated peptic ulcer disease after cure of *Helicobacter pylori* infection. *Am J Gastroenterol* 1994; **89**: 1785–1788.

94 Forbes GM, Glaser ME, Cullen DJE, Warren JR, Christiansen KJ, Marshall BJ, Collins BJ. Duodenal ulcer treated with *Helicobacter pylori* eradication: Seven year follow-up. *Lancet* 1994; **343**: 258–260.

95 Hopkins RJ, Girardi LS, Turney EA. Relationship between *Helicobacter pylori* eradication and reduced duodenal and gastric ulcer recurrence: A review. *Gastroenterology* 1997; **110**: 1244–1252.

96 Leodolter A, Kulig M, Brasch H, Meyer-Sabellek W, Willich SN, Malfertheiner P. A meta-analysis comparing eradication, healing and relapse rates in patients with *Helicobacter pylori*-associated gastric or duodenal ulcer. *Aliment Pharmacol Ther* 2001; **15**: 1949–1958.

97 Susser M. Civilization and peptic ulcer. *Lancet* 1962; **1**: 115–119.

98 Svanes C, Lie RT, Kvåle G, Svanes K, Søreide O. Incidence of perforated ulcer in Western Norway 1935–1990: Cohort or period dependent time trends? *Am J Epidemiol* 1995; **141**: 836–844.

99 Banatvala N, Mayo K, Mégraud F, Jennings R, Deeks JJ, Feldman RA. The cohort effect and *Helicobacter pylori*. *J Infect Dis* 1993; **168**: 219–221.

100 Coggon D, Lambert P, Langman MJS. 20 years of hospital admissions for peptic ulcer in England and Wales. *Lancet* 1981; **1**: 1302–1304.

101 Manuel D, Cutler A, Goldstein J, Fennerty MB, Brown K. Decreasing prevalence combined with increasing eradication of *Helicobacter pylori* infection in the United States has not resulted in fewer hospital admissions for peptic ulcer disease-related complications. *Aliment Pharmacol Ther* 2007; **25**: 1423–1427.

102 Kurata JH. Ulcer epidemiology: An overview and proposed research framework. *Gastroenterology* 1989; **96**: 569–580.

103 Mégraud F, Brassens-Rabbé MP, Denis F, Belbouri A, Hoa DQ. Seroepidemiology of *Campylobacter pylori* in various populations. *J Clin Microbiol* 1989; **27**: 1870–1873.

104 Jones DB, Howden CW, Burget DW, Kerr GD, Hunt RH. Acid suppression in duodenal ulcer: A meta-analysis to define optimal dosing with antisecretory drugs. *Gut* 1987; **28**: 1120–1127.

105 Burget DW, Chiverton SG, Hunt RH. Is there an optimal degree of acid suppression for healing of duodenal ulcers? A model of the relationship between ulcer healing and acid suppression. *Gastroenterology* 1990; **99**: 345–351.

106 Wilairatana S, Kurathong S, Atthapaisalsarudee C, Saowaros V, Leethochawalit M. Omeprazole or cimetidine once daily for the treatment of duodenal ulcers? *J Gastroenterol Hepatol* 1989; **4**: 45–52.

107 Archambault AP, Pare P, Bailey RJ *et al.* Omeprazole (20 mg daily) versus cimetidine (1200 mg daily) in duodenal ulcer healing and pain relief. *Gastroenterol* 1988; **94**: 1130–1134.

108 Hawkey CJ, Long RG, Bardhan KD *et al.* Improved symptom relief and duodenal ulcer healing with lansoprazole, a new proton pump inhibitor, compared with ranitidine. *Gut* 1993; **34**: 1458–1462.

109 Judmaier G, Koelz HR, & Pantopazole-duodenal ulcer-study group. Comparison of pantoprazole and ranitidine in the treatment of acute duodenal ulcer. *Aliment Pharmacol Ther* 1994; **8**: 81–86.

110 McFarland RJ, Bateson MC, Green JRB, O'Donogue DP, Dronfield MW. Omeprazole provides quicker symptom relief and duodenal ulcer healing than ranitidine. *Gastroenterology* 1990; **98**: 278–283.

111 van Rensburg CJ, van Eeden PJ, Marks IN *et al*. Improved duodenal ulcer healing with pantoprazole compared with ranitidine: A multicentre study. *Eur J Gastroenterol Hepatol* 1994; **6**: 739–743.

112 Chiba N. (2004) Ulcer disease and *Helicobacter pylori*. In: McDonald JWD, Burroughs AK and Feagan BG, eds. *Evidence-based Gastroenterology and Hepatology*. 2nd ed. Blackwell Publishing Ltd, New Delhi, **2004**: 83–116.

113 Arber N, Avni Y, Eliakim R, Swissa A, Melzer E, Rachmilewitz D, Konikoff F. A multicenter, double-blind, randomized controlled study of omeprazole versus ranitidine in the treatment of duodenal ulcer in Israel. *Isr J Med Sci* 1994; **30**: 757–761.

114 Barbara L, Blasi A, Cheli R *et al*. Omeprazole vs. ranitidine in the short-term treatment of duodenal ulcer: an Italian Multicenter study. *Hepato-gastroenterol* 1987; **34**: 229–232.

115 Classen M, Dammann HG, Domschke W *et al*. Omeprazole heals duodenal, but not gastric ulcers more rapidly than ranitidine. Results of two German multicentre trials. *Hepato-gastroenterol* 1985; **32**: 243–245.

116 Cremer M, Lambert R, Lamers CBHW, Delle Fave G, Maier C, and the European Pantoprazole study group. A double-blind study of pantoprazole and ranitidine in treatment of acute duodenal ulcer. A multicentre study. *Dig Dis Sci* 1995; **40**: 1360–1364.

117 Crowe JP, Wilkinson SP, Bate CM, Willoughby CP, Peers EM, Richardson PDI, & the OPUS (Omeprazole Peptic Ulcer Study) Research Group. Symptom relief and duodenal ulcer healing with omeprazole or cimetidine. *Aliment Pharmacol Ther* 1989; **3**: 83–91.

118 Hui WM, Lam SK, Lau WY *et al*. Omeprazole and ranitidine in duodenal ulcer healing and subsequent relapse: A randomized double-blind study with weekly endoscopic assessment. *J Gastroenterol Hepatol* 1989; **4**: 35–43.

119 Hotz J, Kleiner R, Grymbowski T, Hennig U, Schwarz JA. Lansoprazole versus famotidine: efficacy and tolerance in the acute management of duodenal ulceration. *Aliment Pharmacol Ther* 1992; **6**: 87–95.

120 Lanza F, Goff J, Scowcroft C, Jennings D, Greski RP. Double-blind comparison of lansoprazole, ranitidine, and placebo in the treatment of acute duodenal ulcer. Lansoprazole Study Group. *Am J Gastroenterol* 1994; **89**: 1191–1200.

121 Mulder CJJ, Tijtgat GNJ, Cluysenaer OJJ *et al*. Omeprazole (20 mg o.m.) versus ranitidine (150 mg b.d.) in duodenal ulcer healing and pain relief. *Aliment Pharmacol Ther* 1989; **3**: 445–451.

122 Schepp W, Classen M. Pantoprazole and ranitidine in the treatment of acute duodenal ulce. A multicentre study. *Scand J Gastroenterol* 1995; **30**: 511–514.

123 Wang CY, Wang TH, Lai KH *et al*. Alimentary tract and pancreas. Double-blind comparison of omeprazole 20 mg OM and ranitidine 300 mg NOCTE in duodenal ulcer: A Taiwan multicentre study. *J Gastroenterol Hepatol* 1992; **7**: 572–576.

124 Valenzuela JE, Berlin RG, Snape WJ *et al*. U.S. experience with omeprazole in duodenal ulcer. Multicenter double-blind comparative study with ranitidine. *Dig Dis Sci* 1991; **36**: 761–768.

125 Ekstrom P, Carling L, Unge P, Anker-Hansen O, Sjostedt S, Sellstrom H. Lansoprazole versus omeprazole in active duodenal ulcer. A double-blind, randomized, comparative study. *Scand J Gastroenterol* 1995; **30**: 210–215.

126 Dobrilla G, Piazzi L, Fiocca R. Lansoprazole versus omeprazole for duodenal ulcer healing and prevention of relapse: A randomized, multicenter, double-masked trial. *Clin Ther* 1999; **21**: 1321–1332.

127 Rehner M, Rohner HG, Schepp W. Comparison of pantoprazole versus omeprazole in the treatment of acute duodenal ulceration – a multicentre study. *Aliment Pharmacol Ther* 1995; **9**: 411–416.

128 Dekkers CP, Beker JA, Thjodleifsson B, Gabryelewicz A, Bell NE, Humphries TJ. Comparison of rabeprazole 20 mg versus omeprazole 20 mg in the treatment of active duodenal ulcer: A European multicentre study. *Aliment Pharmacol Ther* 1999; **13**: 179–186.

129 Meneghelli UG, Zaterka S, de Paula CL, Malafaia O, Lyra LG. Pantoprazole versus ranitidine in the treatment of duodenal ulcer: A multicenter study in Brazil. *Am J Gastroenterol* 2000; **95**: 62–66.

130 Breiter JR, Riff D, Humphries TJ. Rabeprazole is superior to ranitidine in the management of active duodenal ulcer disease: results of a double-blind, randomized North American study. *Am J Gastroenterol* 2000; **95**: 936–942.

131 Ekstrom P, Carling L, Unge P, Anker-Hansen O, Sjostedt S, Sellstrom H. Lansoprazole versus omeprazole in active duodenal ulcer. A double-blind, randomized, comparative study. *Scand J Gastroenterol* 1995; **30**: 210–215.

132 Beker J, Bianchi Porro G, Bigard M *et al*. Double-blind comparison of pantoprazole and omeprazole for the treatment of acute duodenal ulcer. *Eur J Gastroenterol Hepatol* 1995; **7**: 407–410.

133 Ruszniewski Ph, Slama A, Pappo M, Mignon M, GEMUD. Two year maintenance treatment of duodenal ulcer disease with ranitidine 150 mg: a prospective multicentre randomised study. *Gut* 1993; **34**: 1662–1665.

134 Palmer RH, Frank WO, Karlstadt R. Maintenance therapy of duodenal ulcer with H$_2$-receptor antagonists – a meta-analysis. *Aliment Pharmacol Ther* 1990; **4**: 283–294.

135 Kurata JH, Koch GG, Nogawa AN. Comparison of ranitidine and cimetidine ulcer maintenace therapy. *J Clin Gastroenterol* 1987; **9**: 644–650.

136 Penston JG, Wormsley KG. Review article: maintenance treatment with H$_2$-receptor antagonists for peptic ulcer disease. *Aliment Pharmacol Ther* 1992; **6**: 3–29.

137 Lee FI, Hardman M, Jaderberg ME. Maintenance treatment of duodenal ulceration: ranitidine 300 mg at night is better than 150 mg in cigarette smokers. *Gut* 1991; **32**: 151–153.

138 Chiba N, Rao BV, Rademaker JW, Hunt RH. Meta-analysis of the efficacy of antibiotic therapy in eradicating *Helicobacter pylori*. *Am J Gastroenterol* 1992; **87**: 1716–1727.

139 Kovacs TO, Campbell D, Richter J, Haber M, Jennings DE, Rose P. Double-blind comparison of lansoprazole 15 mg, lansoprazole 30 mg and placebo as maintenance therapy in patients with

healed duodenal ulcers resistant to H2-receptor antagonists. *Aliment Pharmacol Ther* 1999; **13**: 959–967.

140 Gisbert JP, Boixeda D, Martín De Argila C, Álvarez Baleriola I, Abraira V, García Plaza A. Unhealed duodenal ulcers despite *Helicobacter pylori* eradication. *Scand J Gastroenterol* 1997; **32**: 643–650.

141 Hosking SW, Ling TK, Yung MY *et al.* Randomised controlled trial of short term treatment to eradicate *Helicobacter pylori* in patients with duodenal ulcer. *BMJ* 1992; **305**: 502–504.

142 Avsar E, Kalayci C, Tözün N *et al.* Refractory duodenal ulcer healing and relapse: comparison of omeprazole with *Helicobacter pylori* eradication. *Eur J Gastroenterol Hepatol* 1996; **8**: 449–452.

143 Bianchi Porro G, Parente F, Lazzaroni M. Short and long term outcome of *Helicobacter pylori* positive resistant duodenal ulcers treated with colloidal bismuth subcitrate plus antibiotics or sucralphate alone. *Gut* 1993; **34**: 466–469.

144 Mantzaris GJ, Hatzis A, Tamvakologos G, Petraki K, Spiliadis C, Triadaphyllou G. Prospective, randomized, investigator-blind trial of *Helicobacter pylori* infection treatment in patients with refractory duodenal ulcers. Healing and long-term relapse rates. *Dig Dis Sci* 1993; **38**: 1132–1136.

145 Wagner S, Gebel M, Haruma K *et al.* Bismuth subsalicylate in the treatment of H2-blocker resistant duodenal ulcers: Role of *Helicbacter pylori*. *Gut* 1992; **33**: 179–183.

146 Zheng ZT, Wang ZY, Chu YX *et al.* Double-blind short-term trial of furazolidone in peptic ulcer. *Lancet* 1985; **i**: 1048–1049.

147 Zhao HY, Li G, Guo J *et al.* Furazolidone in peptic ulcer. *Lancet* 1985; **ii**: 276–277.

148 Quintero Diaz M, Sotto Eschobar A. Metronidazole versus cimetidine in the treatment of gastroduodenal ulcer. *Lancet* 1986; **i**: 907.

149 Lam SK, Ching CK, Lai KC *et al.* Does treatment of *Helicobacter pylori* with antibiotics alone heal duodenal ulcer? A randomised double blind placebo controlled study. *Gut* 1997; **41**: 43–48.

150 Hosking SW, Ling TKW, Chung SCS *et al.* Duodenal ulcer healing by eradication of *Helicobacter pylori* without anti-acid treatment: Randomized controlled trial. *Lancet* 1994; **343**: 508–510.

151 Logan RPH, Gummett PA, Misiewicz JJ, Karim QN, Walker MM, Baron JH. One week's anti-*Helicobacter pylori* treatment for duodenal ulcer. *Gut* 1994; **35**: 15–18.

152 Laine L, Suchower L, Frantz J, Connors A, Neil G. Twice-daily, 10-day triple therapy with omeprazole, amoxicillin, and clarithromycin for *Helicobacter pylori* eradication in duodenal ulcer disease: Results of three multicenter, double-blind, United States trials. *Am J Gastroenterol* 1998; **93**: 2106–2112.

153 Wheeldon TU, Hoang TT, Phung DC, Bjorkman A, Granstrom M, Sorberg M. *Helicobacter pylori* eradication and peptic ulcer healing: The impact of deleting the proton pump inhibitor and using a once-daily treatment. *Aliment Pharmacol Ther* 2003; **18**: 93–100.

154 Labenz J, Idstrom JP, Tillenburg B, Peitz U, Adamek RJ, Borsch G. One-week lowdose triple therapy for *Helicobacter pylori* is sufficient for relief from symptoms and healing of duodenal ulcers. *Aliment Pharmacol Ther* 1997; **11**: 89–93.

155 Goh KL, Navaratnam P, Peh SC *et al.* *Helicobacter pylori* eradication with short-term therapy leads to duodenal ulcer healing

without the need for continued acid suppression therapy. *Eur J Gastroenterol Hepatol* 1996; **8**: 421–423.

156 Gisbert JP, Boixeda D, Martín DA *et al.* New one-week triple therapies with metronidazole for the eradication of *Helicobacter pylori*: clarithromycin or amoxycillin as the second antibiotic. *Med Clin (Barc)* 1998; **110**: 1–5.

157 Harris AW, Misiewicz JJ, Bardhan KD *et al.* Incidence of duodenal ulcer healing after 1 week of proton pump inhibitor triple therapy for eradication of *Helicobacter pylori*. The Lansoprazole Helicobacter Study Group. *Aliment Pharmacol Ther* 1998; **12**: 741–745.

158 Tulassay Z, Kryszewski A, Dite P *et al.* One week of treatment with esomeprazole-based triple therapy eradicates *Helicobacter pylori* and heals patients with duodenal ulcer disease. *Eur J Gastroenterol Hepatol* 2001; **13**: 1457–1465.

159 Marchi S, Costa F, Bellini M *et al.* Ranitidine bismuth citrate-based triple therapy for seven days, with or without further anti-secretory therapy, is highly effective in patients with duodenal ulcer and *Helicobacter pylori* infection. *Eur J Gastroenterol Hepatol* 2001; **13**: 547–550.

160 Tepes B, Krizman I, Gorensek M, Gubina M, Orel I. Is a one-week course of triple anti-*Helicobacter pylori* therapy sufficient to control active duodenal ulcer? *Aliment Pharmacol Ther* 2001; **15**: 1037–1045.

161 Colin R. Duodenal ulcer healing with 1-week eradication triple therapy followed, or not, by anti-secretory treatment: a multi-centre double-blind placebo-controlled trial. *Aliment Pharmacol Ther* 2002; **16**: 1157–1162.

162 Marzio L, Cellini L, Angelucci D. Triple therapy for 7 days vs. triple therapy for 7 days plus omeprazole for 21 days in treatment of active duodenal ulcer with *Helicobacter pylori* infection. A double blind placebo controlled trial. *Dig Liver Dis* 2003; **35**: 20–23.

163 Laine L. *Helicobacter pylori* and complicated ulcer disease. *Am J Med* 1996; **100**: 52S–59S.

164 Bardhan KD, Nayyar AK, Royston C. The outcome of bleeding duodenal ulcer in the era of H2 receptor antagonist therapy. *Q J Med* 1998; **91**: 231–237.

165 Liu NJ, Lee CS, Tang JH *et al.* Outcomes of bleeding peptic ulcers: A prospective study. *J Gastroenterol Hepatol* 2008; **23**: e340–e347.

166 Murray WR, Cooper G, Laferla G, Rogers P, Archibald M. Maintenance ranitidine treatment after haemorrhage from a duodenal ulcer: A 3 year follow up study. *Scand J Gastroenterol* 1988; **23**: 183–187.

167 Jensen DM, Cheng S, Kovacs TOG *et al.* A controlled study of ranitidine for the prevention of recurrent hemorrhage from duodenal ulcer. *N Engl J Med* 1994; **330**: 382–386.

168 Leontiadis GI, Sreedharan A, Dorward S *et al.* Systematic reviews of the clinical effectiveness and cost-effectiveness of proton pump inhibitors in acute upper gastrointestinal bleeding. *Health Technol Assess* 2007; **11**: iii–164.

169 Santander C, Grávalos RG, Gómez-Cedenilla A, Cantero J, Pajares JM. Antimicrobial therapy for *Helicobacter pylori* infection versus long-term maintenance antisecretion treatment in the prevention of recurrent hemorrhage from peptic ulcer: prospective nonrandomized trial on 125 patients. *Am J Gastroenterol* 1996; **91**: 1549–1552.

170 Kikkawa A, Iwakiri R, Ootani H *et al*. Prevention of the rehaemorrhage of bleeding peptic ulcers: Effects of *Helicobacter pylori* eradication and acid suppression. *Aliment Pharmacol Ther* 2005; **21** Suppl 2: 79–84.

171 Gisbert JP, Khorrami S, Carballo F, Calvet X, Gené E, Dominguez-Muñoz E. *H. pylori* eradication therapy vs. antisecretory non-eradication therapy (with or without long-term maintenance antisecretory therapy) for the prevention of recurrent bleeding from peptic ulcer. *Cochrane Database of Systematic Reviews* 2004, Issue 2. Art. No.: CD004062. DOI: 10.1002/14651858.CD004062. pub2.

172 Horvat D, Vcev A, Soldo I *et al*. The results of *Helicobacter pylori* eradication on repeated bleeding in patients with stomach ulcer. *Coll Antropol* 2005; **29**: 139–142.

173 Gisbert JP, Calvet X, Feu F *et al*. Eradication of *Helicobacter pylori* for the prevention of peptic ulcer rebleeding. *Helicobacter* 2007; **12**: 279–286.

174 Ramsoekh D, van Leerdam ME, Rauws EA, Tytgat GN. Outcome of peptic ulcer bleeding, nonsteroidal anti-inflammatory drug use, and *Helicobacter pylori* infection. *Clin Gastroenterol Hepatol* 2005; **3**: 859–864.

175 Huang JQ, Sridhar S, Hunt RH. Role of *Helicobacter pylori* infection and non-steroidal anti-inflammatory drugs in peptic-ulcer disease: a meta-analysis. *Lancet* 2002; **359**: 14–22.

176 Papatheodoridis GV, Sougioultzis S, Archimandritis AJ. Effects of *Helicobacter pylori* and nonsteroidal anti-inflammatory drugs on peptic ulcer disease: A systematic review. *Clin Gastroenterol Hepatol* 2006; **4**: 130–142.

177 Hung LC, Ching JY, Sung JJ *et al*. Long-term outcome of *Helicobacter pylori*-negative idiopathic bleeding ulcers: A prospective cohort study. *Gastroenterology* 2005; **128**: 1845–1850.

178 Simpson CJ, Lamont G, Macdonald I, Smith IS. Effect of cimetidine on prognosis after simple closure of perforated duodenal ulcer. *Br J Surg* 1987; **74**: 104–105.

179 Svanes C, Øvrebø K, Søreide O. Ulcer bleeding and perforation: non-steroidal anti-inflammatory drugs or *Helicobacter pylori*. *Scand J Gastroenterol* 1996; **31**(Suppl 220): 128–131.

180 Kumar S, Mittal GS, Gupta S, Kaur I, Aggarwal S. Prevalence of Helicobactor pylori in patients with perforated duodenal ulcer. *Trop Gastroenterol* 2004; **25**: 121–124.

181 Reinbach DH, Cruickshank G, McColl KE. Acute perforated duodenal ulcer is not associated with *Helicobacter pylori* infection. *Gut* 1993; **34**: 1344–1347.

182 Kate V, Ananthakrishnan N, Badrinath S. Effect of *Helicobacter pylori* eradication on the ulcer recurrence rate after simple closure of perforated duodenal ulcer: Retrospective and prospective randomized controlled studies. *Br J Surg* 2001; **88**: 1054–1058.

183 Metzger J, Styger S, Sieber C, von Flue M, Vogelbach P, Harder F. Prevalence of *Helicobacter pylori* infection in peptic ulcer perforations. *Swiss Med Wkly* 2001; **131**: 99–103.

184 Sebastian M, Chandran VP, Elashaal YI, Sim AJ. *Helicobacter pylori* infection in perforated peptic ulcer disease. *Br J Surg* 1995; **82**: 360–362.

185 Ng EK, Chung SC, Sung JJ *et al*. High prevalence of *Helicobacter pylori* infection in duodenal ulcer perforations not caused by non-steroidal anti-inflammatory drugs. *Br J Surg* 1996; **83**: 1779–1781.

186 Matsukura N, Onda M, Tokunaga A *et al*. Role of *Helicobacter pylori* infection in perforation of peptic ulcer: an age- and gender-matched case-control study. *J Clin Gastroenterol* 1997; **25** Suppl 1: S235–S239.

187 Ng EK, Lam YH, Sung JJ *et al*. Eradication of *Helicobacter pylori* prevents recurrence of ulcer after simple closure of duodenal ulcer perforation: randomized controlled trial. *Ann Surg* 2000; **231**: 153–158.

188 De Boer WA, Driessen WM. Resolution of gastric outlet obstruction after eradication of *Helicobacter pylori*. *J Clin Gastroenterol* 1995; **21**: 329–330.

189 Annibale B, Marignani M, Luzzi I, Delle FG. Peptic ulcer and duodenal stenosis: Role of *Helicobacter pylori* infection. *Ital J Gastroenterol* 1995; **27**: 26–28.

190 Lam Y, Lau JY, Law KB, Sung JJ, Chung SS. Endoscopic balloon dilation and *Helicobacter pylori* eradication in the treatment of gastric outlet obstruction. *Gastrointest Endosc* 1997; **46**: 379–380.

191 Taskin V, Gurer I, Ozyilkan E, Sare M, Hilmioglu F. Effect of *Helicobacter pylori* eradication on peptic ulcer disease complicated with outlet obstruction. *Helicobacter* 2000; **5**: 38–40.

192 Gisbert JP, Pajares JM. Review article: *Helicobacter pylori* infection and gastric outlet obstruction – prevalence of the infection and role of antimicrobial treatment. *Aliment Pharmacol Ther* 2002; **16**: 1203–1208.

193 Cherian PT, Cherian S, Singh P. Long-term follow-up of patients with gastric outlet obstruction related to peptic ulcer disease treated with endoscopic balloon dilatation and drug therapy. *Gastrointest Endosc* 2007; **66**: 491–497.

194 Howden CW, Jones DB, Peace KE, Burget DW, Hunt RH. The treatment of gastric ulcer with antisecretory drugs. Relationship of pharmacological effect to healing rates. *Dig Dis Sci* 1988; **33**: 619–624.

195 Holt S, Howden CW. Omeprazole: overview and opinion. *Dig Dis Sci* 1991; **36**: 385–393.

196 Howden CW, Hunt RH. The relationship between suppression of acidity and gastric ulcer healing rates. *Aliment Pharmacol Ther* 1990; **4**: 25–33.

197 Howden CW, Burget DW, Hunt RH. A meta-analysis to predict gastric ulcer healing from acid suppression. *Gastroenterology* 1991; **100**: A13.

198 Howden CW, Burget DW, Hunt RH. A comparison of different drug classes with respect to rapidity of healing of gastric ulcer (GU). *Gastrolenterology* 1993; **104**: A105.

199 Salas M, Ward A, Caro J. Are proton pump inhibitors the first choice for acute treatment of gastric ulcers? A meta analysis of randomized clinical trials. *BMC Gastroenterol* 2002; **2**: 17.

200 Witzel L, Gutz H, Huttemann W, Schepp W. Pantoprazole versus omeprazole in the treatment of acute gastric ulcers. *Aliment Pharmacol Ther* 1995; **9**: 19–24.

201 Dekkers CP, Beker JA, Thjodleifsson B, Gabryelewicz A, Bell NE, Humphries TJ. Comparison of rabeprazole 20 mg vs. omeprazole 20 mg in the treatment of active gastric ulcer–a European multicentre study. The European Rabeprazole Study Group. *Aliment Pharmacol Ther* 1998; **12**: 789–795.

202 Pilotto A, Di Mario F, Battaglia G *et al*. The efficacy of two doses of omeprazole for short-and long-term peptic ulcer treatment in the elderly. *Clin Ther* 1994; **16**: 935–941.

203 Kovacs TO, Campbell D, Haber M, Rose P, Jennings DE, Richter J. Double-blind comparison of lansoprazole 15 mg, lansoprazole 30 mg, and placebo in the maintenance of healed gastric ulcer. *Dig Dis Sci* 1998; **43**: 779–785.

204 Labenz J, Börsch G. Evidence for the essential role of *Helicobacter pylori* in gastric ulcer disease. *Gut* 1994; **35**: 19–22.

205 Malfertheiner P, Kirchner T, Kist M *et al*. *Helicobacter pylori* eradication and gastric ulcer healing–comparison of three pantoprazole-based triple therapies. *Aliment Pharmacol Ther* 2003; **17**: 1125–1135.

206 Tatsuta M, Ishikawa H, Iishi H, Okuda S, Yokota Y. Reduction of gastric ulcer recurrence after suppression of *Helicobacter pylori* by cefixime. *Gut* 1990; **31**: 973–976.

207 Asaka M, Ohtaki T, Kato M *et al*. Causal role of *Helicobacter pylori* in peptic ulcer relapse. *J Gastroenterol* 1994; **29**(Suppl 7): 134–138.

208 Sung JJY, Chung SCS, Ling TKW *et al*. Antibacterial treatment of gastric ulcers associated with *Helicobacter pylori*. *N Engl J Med* 1995; **332**: 139–142.

209 Bayerdörffer E, Miehlke S, Lehn N *et al*. Cure of gastric ulcer disease after cure of *Helicobacter pylori* infection–German Gastric Ulcer Study. *Eur J Gastroenterol Hepatol* 1996; **8**: 343–349.

210 Malfertheiner P, Bayerdorffer E, Diete U *et al*. The GU-MACH study: the effect of 1-week omeprazole triple therapy on *Helicobacter pylori* infection in patients with gastric ulcer. *Aliment Pharmacol Ther* 1999; **13**: 703–712.

211 Higuchi K, Fujiwara Y, Tominaga K, Watanabe T, Shiba M, Nakamura S, Oshitani N, Matsumoto T, Arakawa T. Is eradication sufficient to heal gastric ulcers in patients infected with *Helicobacter pylori*? A randomized, controlled, prospective study. *Aliment Pharmacol Ther* 2003; **17**: 111–117.

212 Hsu CC, Lu SN, Changchien CS. One-week low-dose triple therapy without anti-acid treatment has sufficient efficacy on *Helicobacter pylori* eradication and ulcer healing. *Hepatogastroenterology* 2003; **50**: 1731–1734.

213 Gisbert JP, Pajares JM. Systematic review and meta-analysis: is 1-week proton pump inhibitor-based triple therapy sufficient to heal peptic ulcer? *Aliment Pharmacol Ther* 2005; **21**: 795–804.

214 Tulassay Z, Stolte M, Sjolund M *et al*. Effect of esomeprazole triple therapy on eradication rates of *Helicobacter pylori*, gastric ulcer healing and prevention of relapse in gastric ulcer patients. *Eur J Gastroenterol Hepatol* 2008; **20**: 526–536.

215 Veldhuyzen van Zanten SV, van der Knoop B. Gastric ulcer treatment: Cure of *Helicobacter pylori* infection without subsequent acid-suppressive therapy: Is it effective? *Eur J Gastroenterol Hepatol* 2008; **20**: 489–491.

216 Leodolter A, Kulig M, Brasch H, Meyer-Sabellek W, Willich SN, Malfertheiner P. A meta-analysis comparing eradication, healing and relapse rates in patients with *Helicobacter pylori*-associated gastric or duodenal ulcer. *Aliment Pharmacol Ther* 2001; **15**: 1949–1958.

217 Befrits R, Sjostedt S, Tour R, Leijonmarck CE, Hedenborg L, Backman M. Long-term effects of eradication of *Helicobacter pylori* on relapse and histology in gastric ulcer patients: A two-year follow-up study. *Scand J Gastroenterol* 2004; **39**: 1066–1072.

218 Hopkins RJ, Girardi LS, Turney EA. *Helicobacter pylori* eradication as a surrogate for reduced peptic ulcer recurrence: A literature-based meta-analysis. *Gut* 1995; **37**(suppl 1): A46(181).

219 Huang JQ, Hunt RH. Review: Eradication of *Helicobacter pylori*. Problems and recommendations. *J Gastroenterol Hepatol* 1997; **12**: 590–598.

220 Penston JG, McColl KEL. Eradication of *Helicobacter pylori*: An objective assessment of current therapies. *Br J Clin Pharmacol* 1997; **43**: 223–243.

221 Chiba N. (2004) Ulcer disease and *Helicobacter pylori*. In: McDonald JWD, Burroughs AK, and Feagan BG, eds. *Evidence-based Gastroenterology and Hepatology*. 2nd ed. Blackwell Publishing Ltd, New Dehli, **2004**: 83–116.

222 Hunt RH. Hp and pH: Implications for the eradication of *Helicobacter pylori*. *Scand J Gastroenterol Suppl* 1993; **196**: 12–16.

223 Hunt RH. pH and Hp–gastric acid secretion and *Helicobacter pylori*: implications for ulcer healing and eradication of the organism. *Am J Gastroenterol* 1993; **88**: 481–483.

224 Gatta L, Perna F, Figura N *et al*. Antimicrobial activity of esomeprazole versus omeprazole against *Helicobacter pylori*. *J Antimicrob Chemother* 2003; **51**: 439–442.

225 Sugimoto M, Furuta T, Shirai N *et al*. Evidence that the degree and duration of acid suppression are related to *Helicobacter pylori* eradication by triple therapy. *Helicobacter* 2007; **12**: 317–323.

226 Chiba N, Wilkinson JM, Hunt RH. Clarithromycin (C) or amoxicillin (A) dual and triple therapies in *H. pylori* (Hp) eradication: A meta-analysis. *Gut* 1995; **37**: A31(T124).

227 Unge P, Berstad A. Pooled analysis of anti-*Helicobacter pylori* treatment regimens. *Scand J Gastroenterol* 1996; **31**: 27–40.

228 Unge P. What other regimens are under investigation to treat *Helicobacter pylori* infection? *Gastroenterology* 1997; **113**: S131–S148.

229 Chiba N, Hunt RH. (1999) Drug therapy of *H. pylori* infection: A meta-analysis. In: Bianchi Porro G and Scarpignato C, eds. *Clinical Pharmacology and Therapy of H. pylori Infection*. Karger, Basel 1999, vol. **11**, pp. 227–268

230 Gisbert JP, Khorrami S, Calvet X, Pajares JM. Systematic review: Rabeprazole-based therapies in *Helicobacter pylori* eradication. *Aliment Pharmacol Ther* 2003; **17**: 751–764.

231 Malaty HM, El-Zimaity HMT, Genta RM, Cole RA, Graham DY. High-dose proton pump inhibitor plus amoxycillin for the treatment or retreatment of *Helicobacter pylori* infection. *Aliment Pharmacol Ther* 1996; **10**: 1001–1004.

232 van der Hulst RW, Weel JF, Verheul SB *et al*. Treatment of *Helicobacter pylori* infection with low or high dose omeprazole combined with amoxycillin and the effect of early retreatment. *Aliment Pharmacol Ther* 1996; **10**: 165–171.

233 Peterson WL, Graham DY, Marshall BJ *et al*. Clarithromycin as monotherapy for eradication of *Helicobacter pylori*: A randomized, double-blind trial. *Am J Gastroenterol* 1993; **88**: 1860–1864.

234 Gisbert JP, Pajares JM. Esomeprazole-based therapy in *Helicobacter pylori* eradication: A meta-analysis. *Dig Liver Dis* 2004; **36**: 253–259.

235 Hoshiya S, Watanabe K, Tokunaga K *et al*. Relationship between eradication therapy and clarithromycin-resistant *Helicobacter pylori* in Japan. *J Gastroenterol* 2000; **35**: 10–14.

236 Di Caro S, Assunta ZM, Cremonini F *et al*. Levofloxacin based regimens for the eradication of *Helicobacter pylori*. *Eur J Gastroenterol Hepatol* 2002; **14**: 1309–1312.

237 Bazzoli F, Zagari RM, Fossi S, Pozzato P, Roda A, Roda E. Efficacy and tolerability of a short term, low dose triple therapy for eradication of *Helicobacter pylori*. *Gastroenterology* 1993; **104**(4): A40.

238 Lind T, Veldhuyzen van Zanten SJO, Unge P *et al*. Eradication of *Helicobacter pylori* using one week triple therapies combining omeprazole with two antimicrobials – the MACH 1 study. *Helicobacter* 1996; **1**: 138–144.

239 Hunt RH, Fallone C, Veldhuyzen van Zanten SJO, Sherman P, Smaill F, Thomson ABR, Canadian Helicobacter Study Group. Risks and benefits of *Helicobacter pylori* eradication: Current status. *Can J Gastroenterol* 2002; **16**: 57–62.

240 Peura DA. The Report of the Digestive Health Initiative^SM International Update Conference on *Helicobacter pylori*. *Gastroenterology* 1997; **113**: S4–S8.

241 Lam SK, Talley NJ. Report of the 1997 Asia Pacific Consensus Conference on the management of *Helicobacter pylori* infection. *J Gastroenterol Hepatol* 1998; **13**: 1–12.

242 Chey WD, Wong BC. American College of Gastroenterology guideline on the management of *Helicobacter pylori* infection. *Am J Gastroenterol* 2007; **102**: 1808–1825.

243 Malfertheiner P, Megraud F, O'Morain C *et al*. Current concepts in the management of *Helicobacter pylori* infection: the Maastricht III Consensus Report. *Gut* 2007; **56**: 772–781.

244 Schwartz H, Krause R, Sahba B *et al*. Triple versus dual therapy for eradicating *Helicobacter pylori* and preventing ulcer recurrence: A randomized, double- blind, multicenter study of lansoprazole, clarithromycin, and/or amoxicillin in different dosing regimens. *Am J Gastroenterol* 1998; **93**: 584–590.

245 Lamouliatte H, Cayla R, Zerbib F *et al*. Dual therapy using a double dose of lansoprazole with amoxicillin versus triple therapy using a double dose of lansoprazole, amoxicillin, and clarithromycin to eradicate *Helicobacter pylori* infection: Results of a prospective randomized open study. *Am J Gastroenterol* 1998; **93**: 1531–1534.

246 Spinzi GC, Bierti L, Bortoli A *et al*. Comparison of omeprazole and lansoprazole in short-term triple therapy for *Helicobacter pylori* infection. *Aliment Pharmacol Ther* 1998; **12**: 433–438.

247 Fennerty MB, Kovacs TO, Krause R *et al*. A comparison of 10 and 14 days of lansoprazole triple therapy for eradication of *Helicobacter pylori*. *Arch Intern Med* 1998; **158**: 1651–1656.

248 Cammarota G, Tursi A, Papa A *et al*. *Helicobacter pylori* eradication using one-week low-dose lansoprazole plus amoxicillin and either clarithromycin or azithromycin. *Aliment Pharmacol Ther* 1996; **10**: 997–1000.

249 Takimoto T, Satoh K, Taniguchi Y *et al*. The efficacy and safety of one-week triple therapy with lansoprazole, clarithromycin, and metronidazole for the treatment of *Helicobacter pylori* infection in Japanese patients. *Helicobacter* 1997; **2**: 86–91.

250 Lazzaroni M, Bargiggia S, Porro GB. Triple therapy with ranitidine or lansoprazole in the treatment of *Helicobacter pylori*-associated duodenal ulcer. *Am J Gastroenterol* 1997; **92**: 649–652.

251 Chey WD, Fisher L, Elta GH *et al*. Bismuth subsalicylate instead of metronidazole with lansoprazole and clarithromycin for *Helicobacter pylori* infection: A randomized trial. *Am J Gastroenterol* 1997; **92**: 1483–1486.

252 Misiewicz JJ, Harris AW, Bardhan KD *et al*. One week triple therapy for *Helicobacter pylori*: a multicentre comparative study.

Lansoprazole Helicobacter Study Group. *Gut* 1997; **41**: 735–739.

253 Adamek RJ, Szymanski C, Pfaffenbach B. Pantoprazole vs omeprazole in one-week low-dose triple therapy for cure of *H. pylori* infection. *Gastroenterology* 1997; **112**: A53.

254 Labenz J, Tillenburg B, Weismüller J, Lütke A, Stolte M. Efficacy and tolerability of a one-week triple therapy consisting of pantoprazole, clarithromycin and amoxycillin for cure of *Helicobacter pylori* infection in patients with duodenal ulcer. *Aliment Pharmacol Ther* 1997; **11**: 95–100.

255 Frevel M, Daake H, Janisch HD *et al*. Eradication of *Helicobacter pylori* with pantoprazole and two antibiotics: A comparison of two short-term regimens. *Aliment Pharmacol Ther* 2000; **14**: 1151–1157.

256 Catalano F, Terminella C, Branciforte G, Bentivegna C, Brogna A, Scalia A. Eradication Therapy with rabeprazole versus omeprazole in the treatment of active duodenal ulcer. *Digestion* 2002; **66**: 154–159.

257 Hawkey CJ, Atherton JC, Treichel HC, Thjodleifsson B, Ravic M. Safety and efficacy of 7-day rabeprazole- and omeprazole-based triple therapy regimens for the eradication of *Helicobacter pylori* in patients with documented peptic ulcer disease. *Aliment Pharmacol Ther* 2003; **17**: 1065–1074.

258 Gisbert JP, Khorrami S, Calvet X, Pajares JM. Systematic review: Rabeprazole-based therapies in *Helicobacter pylori* eradication. *Aliment Pharmacol Ther* 2003; **17**: 751–764.

259 Miehlke S, Schneider-Brachert W, Bastlein E *et al*. Esomeprazole-based one-week triple therapy with clarithromycin and metronidazole is effective in eradicating *Helicobacter pylori* in the absence of antimicrobial resistance. *Aliment Pharmacol Ther* 2003; **18**: 799–804.

260 Laine L. Review article: esomeprazole in the treatment of *Helicobacter pylori*. *Aliment Pharmacol Ther* 2002; **16** (Suppl 4): 115–118.

261 Sheu BS, Kao AW, Cheng HC *et al*. Esomeprazole 40 mg twice daily in triple therapy and the efficacy of *Helicobacter pylori* eradication related to CYP2C19 metabolism. *Aliment Pharmacol Ther* 2005; **21**: 283–288.

262 Vergara M, Vallve M, Gisbert JP, Calvet X. Meta-analysis: Comparative efficacy of different proton-pump inhibitors in triple therapy for *Helicobacter pylori* eradication. *Aliment Pharmacol Ther* 2003; **18**: 647–654.

263 Ulmer HJ, Beckerling A, Gatz G. Recent Use of Proton Pump Inhibitor-Based Triple Therapies for the Eradication of H. pylori: A Broad Data Review. *Helicobacter* 2003; **8**: 95–104.

264 Murakami K, Sato R, Okimoto T *et al*. Eradication rates of clarithromycin-resistant *Helicobacter pylori* using either rabeprazole or lansoprazole plus amoxicillin and clarithromycin. *Aliment Pharmacol Ther* 2002; **16**: 1933–1938.

265 Hsu PI, Lai KH, Lin CK *et al*. A prospective randomized trial of esomeprazole- versus pantoprazole-based triple therapy for *Helicobacter pylori* eradication. *Am J Gastroenterol* 2005; **100**: 2387–2392.

266 Gisbert JP, Gonzalez L, Calvet X *et al*. Proton pump inhibitor, clarithromycin and either amoxycillin or nitroimidazole: a meta-analysis of eradication of *Helicobacter pylori*. *Aliment Pharmacol Ther* 2000; **14**: 1319–1328.

267 Janssen MJ, Van Oijen AH, Verbeek AL, Jansen JB, De Boer WA. A systematic comparison of triple therapies for treatment of

Helicobacter pylori infection with proton pump inhibitor/ranitidine bismuth citrate plus clarithromycin and either amoxicillin or a nitroimidazole. *Aliment Pharmacol Ther* 2001; **15**: 613–624.

268 Bazzoli F, Zagari RM, Pozzato P *et al*. Low-dose lansoprazole and clarithromycin plus metronidazole vs. full-dose lansoprazole and clarithromycin plus amoxicillin for eradication of *Helicobacter pylori* infection. *Aliment Pharmacol Ther* 2002; **16**: 153–158.

269 Huang JQ, Hunt RH. The importance of clarithromycin dose in the management of *Helicobacter pylori* infection: A meta-analysis of triple therapies with a proton pump inhibitor, clarithromycin and amoxycillin or metronidazole. *Aliment Pharmacol Ther* 1999; **13**: 719–729.

270 Ellenrieder V, Fensterer H, Waurick M, Adler G, Glasbrenner B. Influence of clarithromycin dosage on pantoprazole combined triple therapy for eradication of *Helicobacter pylori*. *Aliment Pharmacol Ther* 1998; **12**: 613–618.

271 Lamouliatte H, Megraud F, Delchier JC *et al*. Second-line treatment for failure to eradicate *Helicobacter pylori*: A randomized trial comparing four treatment strategies. *Aliment Pharmacol Ther* 2003; **18**: 791–797.

272 Wong WM, Huang J, Xia HH *et al*. Low-dose rabeprazole, amoxicillin and metronidazole triple therapy for the treatment of *Helicobacter pylori* infection in Chinese patients. *J Gastroenterol Hepatol* 2005; **20**: 935–940.

273 Matsuhisa T, Kawai T, Masaoka T *et al*. Efficacy of metronidazole as second-line drug for the treatment of *Helicobacter pylori* Infection in the Japanese population: A multicenter study in the Tokyo Metropolitan Area. *Helicobacter* 2006; **11**: 152–158.

274 Murakami K, Okimoto T, Kodama M, Sato R, Watanabe K, Fujioka T. Evaluation of three different proton pump inhibitors with amoxicillin and metronidazole in retreatment for *Helicobacter pylori* infection. *J Clin Gastroenterol* 2008; **42**: 139–142.

275 Shirai N, Sugimoto M, Kodaira C *et al*. Dual therapy with high doses of rabeprazole and amoxicillin versus triple therapy with rabeprazole, amoxicillin, and metronidazole as a rescue regimen for *Helicobacter pylori* infection after the standard triple therapy. *Eur J Clin Pharmacol* 2007; **63**: 743–749.

276 Veldhuyzen van Zanten SJO, Machado S, Lee J. One-week triple therapy with esomeprazole, clarithromycin and metronidazole provides effective eradication of *Helicobacter pylori* infection. *Aliment Pharmacol Ther* 2003; **17**: 1381–1387.

277 Lind T, Veldhuyzen van Zanten SJO, Unge P *et al*. Eradication of *Helicobacter pylori* using one-week triple therapies combining omeprazole with two antimicrobials: the MACH I Study. *Helicobacter* 1996; **1**: 138–144.

278 Koivisto TT, Rautelin HI, Voutilainen ME, Heikkinen MT, Koskenpato JP, Farkkila MA. First-line eradication therapy for *Helicobacter pylori* in primary health care based on antibiotic resistance: results of three eradication regimens. *Aliment Pharmacol Ther* 2005; **21**: 773–782.

279 Sun WH, Ou XL, Cao DZ *et al*. Efficacy of omeprazole and amoxicillin with either clarithromycin or metronidazole on eradication of *Helicobacter pylori* in Chinese peptic ulcer patients. *World J Gastroenterol* 2005; **11**: 2477–2481.

280 Zagari RM, Bianchi-Porro G, Fiocca R, Gasbarrini G, Roda E, Bazzoli F. Comparison of 1 and 2 weeks of omeprazole, amoxicillin and clarithromycin treatment for *Helicobacter pylori* eradication: the HYPER Study. *Gut* 2007; **56**: 475–479.

281 Wu IC, Wu DC, Hsu PI *et al*. Rabeprazole- versus esomeprazole-based eradication regimens for H. pylori infection. *Helicobacter* 2007; **12**: 633–637.

282 Vakil N, Lanza F, Schwartz H, Barth J. Seven-day therapy for *Helicobacter pylori* in the United States. *Aliment Pharmacol Ther* 2004; **20**: 99–107.

283 Calvet X, Ducons J, Bujanda L, Bory F, Montserrat A, Gisbert JP. Seven versus ten days of rabeprazole triple therapy for *Helicobacter pylori* eradication: A multicenter randomized trial. *Am J Gastroenterol* 2005; **100**: 1696–1701.

284 Malfertheiner P, Megraud F, O'Morain C *et al*. Current concepts in the management of *Helicobacter pylori* infection–the Maastricht 2–2000 Consensus Report. *Aliment Pharmacol Ther* 2002; **16**: 167–180.

285 Maconi G, Parente F, Russo A, Vago L, Imbesi V, Porro GB. Do some patients with *Helicobacter pylori* infection benefit from an extension to 2 weeks of a proton pump inhibitor-based triple eradication therapy? *Am J Gastroenterol* 2001; **96**: 359–366.

286 Calvet X, Garcia N, Lopez T, Gisbert JP, Gene E, Roque M. A meta-analysis of short versus long therapy with a proton pump inhibitor, clarithromycin and either metronidazole or amoxycillin for treating *Helicobacter pylori* infection. *Aliment Pharmacol Ther* 2000; **14**: 603–609.

287 Calvet X, Gene E, Lopez T, Gisbert JP. What is the optimal length of proton pump inhibitor-based triple therapies for H. pylori? A cost-effectiveness analysis. *Aliment Pharmacol Ther* 2001; **15**: 1067–1076.

288 Fuccio L, Minardi ME, Zagari RM, Grilli D, Magrini N, Bazzoli F. Meta-analysis: duration of first-line proton-pump inhibitor based triple therapy for *Helicobacter pylori* eradication. *Ann Intern Med* 2007; **147**: 553–562.

289 van der Wouden EJ, Thijs JC, Van Zwet AA, Sluiter WJ, Kleibeuker JH. The influence of in vitro nitroimidazole resistance on the efficacy of nitroimidazole-containing anti-*Helicobacter pylori* regimens: A meta- analysis. *Am J Gastroenterol* 1999; **94**: 1751–1759.

290 Lind T, Mégraud F, Unge P *et al*. The MACH2 study: role of omeprazole in eradication of *Helicobacter pylori* with 1-week triple therapies. *Gastroenterology* 1999; **116**: 248–253.

291 Megraud F, Lehn N, Lind T, Bayerdorffer E, O'Morain C, Spiller R, Unge P, van Zanten SV, Wrangstadh M, Burman CF. Antimicrobial susceptibility testing of *Helicobacter pylori* in a large multicenter trial: the MACH 2 study. *Antimicrob Agents Chemother* 1999; **43**: 2747–2752.

292 Chiba N, Sinclair P. Metronidazole 500 mg is as effective as metronidazole 400 mg in the MACH 1 regimen for H. pylori eradication: A meta-analysis. *Gastroenterology* 1998; **12**: 91A.

293 Bardhan K, Bayerdorffer E, Veldhuyzen van Zanten SJ *et al*. The HOMER Study: the effect of increasing the dose of metronidazole when given with omeprazole and amoxicillin to cure *Helicobacter pylori* infection. *Helicobacter* 2000; **5**: 196–201.

294 Lerang F, Moum B, Haug JB, Berge T. Highly effective triple therapy with omeprazole, amoxicillin and clarithromycin in previous H. pylori treatment failures. *Gut* 1996; **39**(Suppl 2): A36 (4A: 25).

295 Laine L, Fennerty MB, Osato M, Sugg J, Suchower L, Probst P, Levine JG. Esomeprazole-based *Helicobacter pylori* eradication

therapy and the effect of antibiotic resistance: results of three US multicenter, double-blind trials. *Am J Gastroenterol* 2000; **95**: 3393–3398.

296 Laine L, Hunt R, El Zimaity H, Nguyen B, Osato M, Spenard J, on behalf of the other 45 investigators. Bismuth-based quadruple therapy using a single capsule of bismuth biskalcitrate, metronidazole, and tetracycline given with omeprazole versus omeprazole, amoxicillin, and clarithromycin for eradication of *Helicobacter pylori* in duodenal ulcer patients: a prospective, randomized, multicenter, North American trial. *Am J Gastroenterol* 2003; **98**: 562–567.

297 Miki I, Aoyama N, Sakai T *et al.* Impact of clarithromycin resistance and CYP2C19 genetic polymorphism on treatment efficacy of *Helicobacter pylori* infection with lansoprazole- or rabeprazole-based triple therapy in Japan. *Eur J Gastroenterol Hepatol* 2003; **15**: 27–33.

298 Kawabata H, Habu Y, Tomioka H *et al.* Effect of different proton pump inhibitors, differences in CYP2C19 genotype and antibiotic resistance on the eradication rate of *Helicobacter pylori* infection by a 1-week regimen of proton pump inhibitor, amoxicillin and clarithromycin. *Aliment Pharmacol Ther* 2003; **17**: 259–264.

299 Murakami K, Fujioka T, Okimoto T, Sato R, Kodama M, Nasu M. Drug combinations with amoxycillin reduce selection of clarithromycin resistance during *Helicobacter pylori* eradication therapy. *Int J Antimicrob Agents* 2002; **19**: 67–70.

300 Wermeille J, Cunningham M, Dederding JP *et al.* Failure of *Helicobacter pylori* eradication: Is poor compliance the main cause? *Gastroenterol Clin Biol* 2002; **26**: 216–219.

301 Broutet N, Tchamgoue S, Pereira E, Lamouliatte H, Salamon R, Megraud F. Risk factors for failure of *Helicobacter pylori* therapy–results of an individual data analysis of 2751 patients. *Aliment Pharmacol Ther* 2003; **17**: 99–109.

302 De Boer WA. Eradication therapy should be different for dyspeptic patients than for ulcer patients. *Can J Gastroenterol* 2003; **17** Suppl B: 41B–45B.

303 Boixeda D, Martin dA, Bermejo F, Lopez SA, Hernandez RF, Garcia PA. Seven-day proton pump inhibitor, amoxicillin and clarithromycin triple therapy. factors that influence *Helicobacter pylori* eradications success. *Rev Esp Enferm Dig* 2003; **95**: 206–9, 202.

304 Suzuki T, Matsuo K, Ito H *et al.* Smoking increases the treatment failure for *Helicobacter pylori* eradication. *Am J Med* 2006; **119**: 217–224.

305 Fischbach LA, Goodman KJ, Feldman M, Aragaki C. Sources of variation of *Helicobacter pylori* treatment success in adults worldwide: A meta-analysis. *Int J Epidemiol* 2002; **31**: 128–139.

306 Moayyedi P, Sahay P, Tompkins DS, Axon AT. Efficacy and optimum dose of omeprazole in a new 1-week triple therapy regimen to eradicate *Helicobacter pylori*. *Eur J Gastroenterol Hepatol* 1995; **7**: 835–840.

307 Bazzoli F, Zagari M, Pozzato P *et al.* Evaluation of short-term low-dose triple therapy for the eradication of *Helicobacter pylori* by factorial design in a randomized, double-blind, controlled study. *Aliment Pharmacol Ther* 1998; **12**: 439–445.

308 Bochenek WJ, Peters S, Fraga PD, Wang W, Mack ME, Osato MS, El-Zimaity HM, Davis KD, Graham DY. Eradication of *Helicobacter pylori* by 7-day triple-therapy regimens combining pantoprazole with clarithromycin, metronidazole, or amoxi-cillin in patients with peptic ulcer disease: Results of two double-blind, randomized studies. *Helicobacter* 2003; **8**: 626–642.

309 Laine L, Frantz JE, Baker A, Neil GA. A United States multicentre trial of dual and proton pump inhibitor-based triple therapies for *Helicobacter pylori*. *Aliment Pharmacol Ther* 1997; **11**: 913–917.

310 Janssen MJ, Laheij RJ, De Boer WA, Jansen JB. Meta-analysis: The influence of pre-treatment with a proton pump inhibitor on *Helicobacter pylori* eradication. *Aliment Pharmacol Ther* 2005; **21**: 341–345.

311 Graham DY, Hammoud F, el Zimaity HM, Kim JG, Osato MS, el Serag HB. Meta-analysis: Proton pump inhibitor or H2-receptor antagonist for *Helicobacter pylori* eradication. *Aliment Pharmacol Ther* 2003; **17**: 1229–1236.

312 Gisbert JP, Khorrami S, Calvet X, Gabriel R, Carballo F, Pajares JM. Meta-analysis: proton pump inhibitors vs. H2-receptor antagonists–their efficacy with antibiotics in *Helicobacter pylori* eradication. *Aliment Pharmacol Ther* 2003; **18**: 757–766.

313 Vallve M, Vergara M, Gisbert JP, Calvet X. Single vs. double dose of a proton pump inhibitor in triple therapy for *Helicobacter pylori* eradication: a meta-analysis. *Aliment Pharmacol Ther* 2002; **16**: 1149–1156.

314 Laine L, Estrada R, Trujillo M *et al.* Once-daily therapy for H. pylori infection: A randomized comparison of four regimens. *Am J Gastroenterol* 1999; **94**: 962–966.

315 Kositchaiwat C, Ovartlarnporn B, Kachintorn U, Atisook K. Low and high doses of rabeprazole vs. omeprazole for cure of *Helicobacter pylori* infection. *Aliment Pharmacol Ther* 2003; **18**: 1017–1021.

316 Anagnostopoulos GK, Tsiakos S, Margantinis G, Kostopoulos P, Arvanitidis D. Esomeprazole versus omeprazole for the eradication of *Helicobacter pylori* infection: Results of a randomized controlled study. *J Clin Gastroenterol* 2004; **38**: 503–506.

317 Manes G, Pieramico O, Perri F *et al.* Twice-daily standard dose of omeprazole achieves the necessary level of acid inhibition for *Helicobacter pylori* eradication. A randomized controlled trial using standard and double doses of omeprazole in triple therapy. *Dig Dis Sci* 2005; **50**: 443–448.

318 Gisbert JP, Dominguez-Munoz A, Dominguez-Martin A, Gisbert JL, Marcos S. Esomeprazole-based therapy in *Helicobacter pylori* eradication: Any effect by increasing the dose of esomeprazole or prolonging the treatment? *Am J Gastroenterol* 2005; **100**: 1935–1940.

319 Hsu PI, Lai KH, Wu CJ *et al.* High-dose versus low-dose esomeprazole-based triple therapy for *Helicobacter pylori* infection. *Eur J Clin Invest* 2007; **37**: 724–730.

320 Villoria A, Garcia P, Calvet X, Gisbert JP, Vergara M. Meta-analysis: High-dose proton pump inhibitors vs. standard dose in triple therapy for *Helicobacter pylori* eradication. *Aliment Pharmacol Ther* 2008; **28**: 868–877.

321 Graham DY, Lew GM, Malaty HM *et al.* Factors influencing the eradication of *Helicobacter pylori* with triple therapy. *Gastroenterology* 1992; **102**: 493–496.

322 Katelaris PH, Forbes GM, Talley NJ, Crotty B. A randomized comparison of quadruple and triple therapies for *Helicobacter pylori* eradication: The QUADRATE Study. *Gastroenterology* 2002; **123**: 1763–1769.

323 Chiba N, Hunt RH. Bismuth, metronidazole and tetracycline (BMT) +/− acid suppression in H. pylori eradication: A meta-analysis. *Gut* 1996; **39**: A36(4A:27).

324 Huang JQ, Chiba N, Wilkinson J, Hunt RH. Attempt by meta-analysis to define the optimal treatment regimen for eradicating *Helicobacter pylori* (*H. pylori*) infection. *Can J Gastroenterology* 1997; **11**(Suppl A): 44A(S14).

325 de Boer W, Driessen W, Jansz A, Tytgat G. Effect of acid suppression on efficacy of treatment for *Helicobacter pylori* infection. *Lancet* 1995; **345**: 817–820.

326 De Boer WA, Driessen WMM, Potters HVPJ, Tytgat GNJ. Randomized study comparing 1 with 2 weeks of quadruple therapy for eradicating *Helicobacter pylori*. *Am J Gastroenterol* 1994; **89**: 1993–1997.

327 Calvet X, Ducons J, Guardiola J et al. One-week triple vs. quadruple therapy for *Helicobacter pylori* infection – a randomized trial. *Aliment Pharmacol Ther* 2002; **16**: 1261–1267.

328 Mantzaris GJ, Petraki K, Archavlis E et al. Omeprazole triple therapy versus omeprazole quadruple therapy for healing duodenal ulcer and eradication of *Helicobacter pylori* infection: a 24-month follow-up study. *Eur J Gastroenterol Hepatol* 2002; **14**: 1237–1243.

329 De Boer WA, van Etten RJXM, Lai JYL, Schneeberger PM, van de Wouw BAM, Driessen WMM. Effectiveness of quadruple therapy using lansoprazole, instead of omeprazole, in curing *Helicobacter pylori* infection. *Helicobacter* 1996; **1**: 145–150.

330 Pai CG, Thomas CP, Biswas A, Rao S, Ramnarayan K. Quadruple therapy for initial eradication of *Helicobacter pylori* in peptic ulcer: comparison with triple therapy. *Indian J Gastroenterol* 2003; **22**: 85–87.

331 Boixeda D, Bermejo F, Martin-de-Argila C et al. Efficacy of quadruple therapy with pantoprazole, bismuth, tetracycline and metronidazole as rescue treatment for *Helicobacter pylori* infection. *Aliment Pharmacol Ther* 2002; **16**: 1457–1460.

332 Perri F, Festa V, Clemente R et al. Randomized study of two "rescue" therapies for *Helicobacter pylori*-infected patients after failure of standard triple therapies. *Am J Gastroenterol* 2001; **96**: 58–62.

333 Perri F, Festa V, Merla A, Barberani F, Pilotto A, Andriulli A. Randomized study of different "second-line" therapies for *Helicobacter pylori* infection after failure of the standard "Maastricht triple therapy". *Aliment Pharmacol Ther* 2003; **18**: 815–820.

334 Nista EC, Candelli M, Cremonini F et al. Levofloxacin-based triple therapy vs. quadruple therapy in second-line *Helicobacter pylori* treatment: A randomized trial. *Aliment Pharmacol Ther* 2003; **18**: 627–633.

335 Wong WM, Gu Q, Lam SK et al. Randomized controlled study of rabeprazole, levofloxacin and rifabutin triple therapy vs. quadruple therapy as second-line treatment for *Helicobacter pylori* infection. *Aliment Pharmacol Ther* 2003; **17**: 553–560.

336 Fischbach L, Evans EL. Meta-analysis: the effect of antibiotic resistance status on the efficacy of triple and quadruple first-line therapies for *Helicobacter pylori*. *Aliment Pharmacol Ther* 2007; **26**: 343–357.

337 Uygun A, Kadayifci A, Safali M, Ilgan S, Bagci S. The efficacy of bismuth containing quadruple therapy as a first-line treatment option for *Helicobacter pylori*. *J Dig Dis* 2007; **8**: 211–215.

338 O'Morain C, Borody T, Farley A et al. Efficacy and safety of single-triple capsules of bismuth biskalcitrate, metronidazole and tetracycline, given with omeprazole, for the eradication of *Helicobacter pylori*: an international multicentre study. *Aliment Pharmacol Ther* 2003; **17**: 415–420.

339 Lahaie RG, Chiba N, Farley A. Efficacy of OBMT, in a twice daily (bid) dosage, for the eradication of *H. pylori*: A preliminary study. *Can J Gastroenterology* 1998; **12**(Suppl A): 134A(S162).

340 Chiba N, Marshall C. Omeprazole, bismuth, metronidazole and tetracycline (OBMT) quadruple therapy given twice daily for *H. pylori* eradication in a community gastroenterology practice. *Gastroenterology* 1998; **114**(4): A91.

341 Graham DY, Hoffman J, el Zimaity HM, Graham DP, Osato M. Twice a day quadruple therapy (bismuth subsalicylate, tetracycline, metronidazole plus lansoprazole) for treatment of *Helicobacter pylori* infection. *Aliment Pharmacol Ther* 1997; **11**: 935–938.

342 Dore MP, Graham DY, Mele R, Marras L, Nieddu S, Manca A, Realdi G. Colloidal bismuth subcitrate-based twice-a-day quadruple therapy as primary or salvage therapy for *Helicobacter pylori* infection. *Am J Gastroenterol* 2002; **97**: 857–860.

343 Dore MP, Marras L, Maragkoudakis E, Nieddu S, Manca A, Graham DY, Realdi G. Salvage therapy after two or more prior *Helicobacter pylori* treatment failures: The super salvage regimen. *Helicobacter* 2003; **8**: 307–309.

344 Dore MP, Maragkoudakis E, Pironti A, Tadeu V, Tedde R, Realdi G, Delitala G. Twice-a-day quadruple therapy for eradication of *Helicobacter pylori* in the elderly. *Helicobacter* 2006; **11**: 52–55.

345 Graham DY, Belson G, Abudayyeh S, Osato MS, Dore MP, El-Zimaity HM. Twice daily (mid-day and evening) quadruple therapy for H. pylori infection in the United States. *Dig Liver Dis* 2004; **36**: 384–387.

346 Garcia N, Calvet X, Gene E, Campo R, Brullet E. Limited usefulness of a seven-day twice-a-day quadruple therapy. *Eur J Gastroenterol Hepatol* 2000; **12**: 1315–1318.

347 Tytgat GNJ. (1996) Aspects of anti-*Helicobacter pylori* eradication therapy. In: Hunt RH and Tytgat GNJ, eds. *Helicobacter pylori: Basic Mechanisms to Clinical Cure.* Kluwer Academic Publishers, Lancaster, UK. **1996**: 340–347.

348 Chan FK, Sung JJ, Suen R, Wu JC, Ling TK, Chung SC. Salvage therapies after failure of *Helicobacter pylori* eradication with ranitidine bismuth citrate-based therapies. *Aliment Pharmacol Ther* 2000; **14**: 91–95.

349 Peitz U, Sulliga M, Wolle K et al. High rate of post-therapeutic resistance after failure of macrolide-nitroimidazole triple therapy to cure *Helicobacter pylori* infection: impact of two second-line therapies in a randomized study. *Aliment Pharmacol Ther* 2002; **16**: 315–324.

350 Hojo M, Miwa H, Nagahara A, Sato N. Pooled analysis on the efficacy of the second-line treatment regimens for *Helicobacter pylori* infection. *Scand J Gastroenterol* 2001; **36**: 690–700.

351 Nash C, Fischbach L, Veldhuyzen van Zanten SJO. What are the global response rates to *Helicobacter pylori* eradication therapy? *Can J Gastroenterol* 2003; **17** Suppl B: 25B–29B.

352 Isomoto H, Inoue K, Furusu H et al. High-dose rabeprazole-amoxicillin versus rabeprazole-amoxicillin-metronidazole as second-line treatment after failure of the Japanese standard

regimen for *Helicobacter pylori* infection. *Aliment Pharmacol Ther* 2003; **18**: 101–107.

353 Murakami K, Sato R, Okimoto T *et al.* Efficacy of triple therapy comprising rabeprazole, amoxicillin and metronidazole for second-line *Helicobacter pylori* eradication in Japan, and the influence of metronidazole resistance. *Aliment Pharmacol Ther* 2003; **17**: 119–123.

354 Perri F, Festa V, Clemente R, Quitadamo M, Andriulli A. Rifabutin-based "rescue therapy" for *Helicobacter pylori* infected patients after failure of standard regimens. *Aliment Pharmacol Ther* 2000; **14**: 311–316.

355 Bock H, Koop H, Lehn N, Heep M. Rifabutin-based triple therapy after failure of *Helicobacter pylori* eradication treatment: preliminary experience. *J Clin Gastroenterol* 2000; **31**: 222–225.

356 Miehlke S, Hansky K, Schneider-Brachert W *et al.* Randomized trial of rifabutin-based triple therapy and high-dose dual therapy for rescue treatment of *Helicobacter pylori* resistant to both metronidazole and clarithromycin. *Aliment Pharmacol Ther* 2006; **24**: 395–403.

357 Navarro-Jarabo JM, Fernandez N, Sousa FL *et al.* Efficacy of rifabutin-based triple therapy as second-line treatment to eradicate *Helicobacter pylori* infection. *BMC Gastroenterol* 2007; **7**: 31.

358 Gisbert JP, Calvet X, Bujanda L, Marcos S, Gisbert JL, Pajares JM. "Rescue" therapy with rifabutin after multiple *Helicobacter pylori* treatment failures. *Helicobacter* 2003; **8**: 90–94.

359 Miehlke S, Schneider-Brachert W, Kirsch C *et al.* One-week once-daily triple therapy with esomeprazole, moxifloxacin, and rifabutin for eradication of persistent *Helicobacter pylori* resistant to both metronidazole and clarithromycin. *Helicobacter* 2008; **13**: 69–74.

360 Zullo A, Hassan C, de Francesco V *et al.* A third-line levofloxacin-based rescue therapy for *Helicobacter pylori* eradication. *Dig Liver Dis* 2003; **35**: 232–236.

361 Bilardi C, Dulbecco P, Zentilin P *et al.* A 10-day levofloxacin-based therapy in patients with resistant *Helicobacter pylori* infection: a controlled trial. *Clin Gastroenterol Hepatol* 2004; **2**: 997–1002.

362 Gisbert JP, Morena F. Systematic review and meta-analysis: Levofloxacin-based rescue regimens after *Helicobacter pylori* treatment failure. *Aliment Pharmacol Ther* 2006; **23**: 35–44.

363 Saad RJ, Schoenfeld P, Kim HM, Chey WD. Levofloxacin-based triple therapy versus bismuth-based quadruple therapy for persistent *Helicobacter pylori* infection: a meta-analysis. *Am J Gastroenterol* 2006; **101**: 488–496.

364 Cheng HC, Chang WL, Chen WY, Yang HB, Wu JJ, Sheu BS. Levofloxacin-containing triple therapy to eradicate the persistent *H. pylori* after a failed conventional triple therapy. *Helicobacter* 2007; **12**: 359–363.

365 Perna F, Zullo A, Ricci C, Hassan C, Morini S, Vaira D. Levofloxacin-based triple therapy for *Helicobacter pylori* re-treatment: role of bacterial resistance. *Dig Liver Dis* 2007; **39**: 1001–1005.

366 Yee YK, Cheung TK, Chu KM *et al.* Clinical trial: Levofloxacin-based quadruple therapy was inferior to traditional quadruple therapy in the treatment of resistant *Helicobacter pylori* infection. *Aliment Pharmacol Ther* 2007; **26**: 1063–1067.

367 Cheon JH, Kim N, Lee DH *et al.* Efficacy of moxifloxacin-based triple therapy as second-line treatment for *Helicobacter pylori* infection. *Helicobacter* 2006; **11**: 46–51.

368 Kang JM, Kim N, Lee DH *et al.* Second-line treatment for *Helicobacter pylori* infection: 10-day moxifloxacin-based triple therapy versus 2-week quadruple therapy. *Helicobacter* 2007; **12**: 623–628.

369 Sharara AI, Chaar HF, Aoun E, Abdul-Baki H, Araj GF, Kanj SS. Efficacy and safety of rabeprazole, amoxicillin, and gatifloxacin after treatment failure of initial *Helicobacter pylori* eradication. *Helicobacter* 2006; **11**: 231–236.

370 Nishizawa T, Suzuki H, Nakagawa I, Iwasaki E, Masaoka T, Hibi T. Gatifloxacin-based triple therapy as a third-line regimen for *Helicobacter pylori* eradication. *J Gastroenterol Hepatol* 2008; **23** (Suppl 2): S167–S170.

371 Wong WM, Wong BC, Lu H *et al.* One-week omeprazole, furazolidone and amoxicillin rescue therapy after failure of *Helicobacter pylori* eradication with standard triple therapies. *Aliment Pharmacol Ther* 2002; **16**: 793–798.

372 Treiber G, Ammon S, Malfertheiner P, Klotz U. Impact of furazolidone-based quadruple therapy for eradication of *Helicobacter pylori* after previous treatment failures. *Helicobacter* 2002; **7**: 225–231.

373 Isakov V, Domareva I, Koudryavtseva L, Maev I, Ganskaya Z. Furazolidone-based triple "rescue therapy" vs. quadruple "rescue therapy" for the eradication of *Helicobacter pylori* resistant to metronidazole. *Aliment Pharmacol Ther* 2002; **16**: 1277–1282.

374 Togawa J, Inamori M, Fujisawa N *et al.* Efficacy of a triple therapy with rabeprazole, amoxicillin, and faropenem as second-line treatment after failure of initial *Helicobacter pylori* eradication therapy. *Hepatogastroenterology* 2005; **52**: 645–648.

375 Ogura K, Mitsuno Y, Maeda S *et al.* Efficacy and safety of faropenem in eradication therapy of *Helicobacter pylori*. *Helicobacter* 2007; **12**: 618–622.

376 Murakami K, Sato R, Okimoto T *et al.* Effectiveness of minocycline-based triple therapy for eradication of *Helicobacter pylori* infection. *J Gastroenterol Hepatol* 2006; **21**: 262–267.

377 Gisbert JP, Gisbert JL, Marcos S, Pajares JM. Empirical *Helicobacter pylori* "rescue" therapy after failure of two eradication treatments. *Dig Liver Dis* 2004; **36**: 7–12.

378 Gisbert JP, Castro-Fernandez M, Bermejo F *et al.* Third-line rescue therapy with levofloxacin after two H. pylori treatment failures. *Am J Gastroenterol* 2006; **101**: 243–247.

379 Gisbert JP, Gisbert JL, Marcos S, Moreno-Otero R, Pajares JM. Third-line rescue therapy with levofloxacin is more effective than rifabutin rescue regimen after two *Helicobacter pylori* treatment failures. *Aliment Pharmacol Ther* 2006; **24**: 1469–1474.

380 Rodriguez-Torres M, Salgado-Mercado R, Rios-Bedoya CF *et al.* High eradication rates of *Helicobacter pylori* infection with first- and second-line combination of esomeprazole, tetracycline, and metronidazole in patients allergic to penicillin. *Dig Dis Sci* 2005; **50**: 634–639.

381 Xiao SD, Liu WZ, Hu PJ *et al.* A multicentre study on eradication of *Helicobacter pylori* using four 1-week triple therapies in China. *Aliment Pharmacol Ther* 2001; **15**: 81–86.

382 Guo CY, Wu YB, Liu HL, Wu JY, Zhong MZ. Clinical evaluation of four one-week triple therapy regimens in eradicating *Helicobacter pylori* infection. *World J Gastroenterol* 2004; **10**: 747–749.

383 Frota LC, da Cunha MP, Luz CR, de Araujo-Filho AH, Frota LA, Braga LL. *Helicobacter pylori* eradication using tetracycline

and furazolidone versus amoxicillin and azithromycin in lansoprazole based triple therapy: an open randomized clinical trial.
Arq Gastroenterol 2005; **42**: 111–115.

384 Fakheri H, Malekzadeh R, Merat S *et al*. Clarithromycin vs.
furazolidone in quadruple therapy regimens for the treatment
of *Helicobacter pylori* in a population with a high metronidazole
resistance rate. *Aliment Pharmacol Ther* 2001; **15**: 411–416.

385 Khatibian M, Ajvadi Y, Nasseri-Moghaddam S *et al*.
Furazolidone-based, metronidazole-based, or a combination
regimen for eradication of *Helicobacter pylori* in peptic ulcer
disease. *Arch Iran Med* 2007; **10**: 161–167.

386 Daghaghzadeh H, Emami MH, Karimi S, Raeisi M. One-week
versus two-week furazolidone-based quadruple therapy as the
first-line treatment for *Helicobacter pylori* infection in Iran.
J Gastroenterol Hepatol 2007; **22**: 1399–1403.

387 Coelho LG, Martins GM, Passos MC *et al*. Once-daily, low-cost,
highly effective *Helicobacter pylori* treatment to family members
of gastric cancer patients. *Aliment Pharmacol Ther* 2003; **17**:
131–136.

388 Cammarota G, Cianci R, Cannizzaro O *et al*. Efficacy of two
one-week rabeprazole/levofloxacin-based triple therapies for
Helicobacter pylori infection. *Aliment Pharmacol Ther* 2000; **14**:
1339–1343.

389 Giannini EG, Bilardi C, Dulbecco P, Mamone M, Santi ML, Testa
R, Mansi C, Savarino V. Can *Helicobacter pylori* eradication regimens be shortened in clinical practice? An open-label, randomized, pilot study of 4 and 7-day triple therapy with
rabeprazole, high-dose levofloxacin, and tinidazole. *J Clin
Gastroenterol* 2006; **40**: 515–520.

390 Nista EC, Candelli M, Zocco MA *et al*. Levofloxacin-based triple
therapy in first-line treatment for *Helicobacter pylori* eradication.
Am J Gastroenterol 2006; **101**: 1985–1990.

391 Cammarota G, Cianci R, Cannizzaro O *et al*. High-dose versus
low-dose clarithromycin in 1-week triple therapy, including
rabeprazole and levofloxacin, for *Helicobacter pylori* eradication.
J Clin Gastroenterol 2004; **38**: 110–114.

392 Di Caro S, Ojetti V, Zocco MA *et al*. Mono, dual and triple
moxifloxacin-based therapies for *Helicobacter pylori* eradication.
Aliment Pharmacol Ther 2002; **16**: 527–532.

393 Nista EC, Candelli M, Zocco MA *et al*. Moxifloxacin-based strategies for first-line treatment of *Helicobacter pylori* infection.
Aliment Pharmacol Ther 2005; **21**: 1241–1247.

394 Bago P, Vcev A, Tomic M, Rozankovic M, Marusic M, Bago J.
High eradication rate of H. pylori with moxifloxacin-based
treatment: A randomized controlled trial. *Wien Klin Wochenschr*
2007; **119**: 372–378.

395 Sharara AI, Chaar HF, Racoubian E *et al*. Efficacy of two rabe-
prazole/gatifloxacin-based triple therapies for *Helicobacter
pylori* infection. *Helicobacter* 2004; **9**: 255–261.

396 Bosques-Padilla FJ, Garza-Gonzalez E, Calderon-Lozano IE
et al. Open, randomized multicenter comparative trial of rabeprazole, ofloxacin and amoxicillin therapy for *Helicobacter pylori*
eradication: 7 vs. 14 day treatment. *Helicobacter* 2004; **9**:
417–421.

397 Guttner Y, Windsor HM, Viiala CH, Dusci L, Marshall BJ.
Nitazoxanide in treatment of *Helicobacter pylori*: A clinical and
in vitro study. *Antimicrob Agents Chemother* 2003; **47**:
3780–3783.

398 Zullo A, Vaira D, Vakil N *et al*. High eradication rates of
Helicobacter pylori with a new sequential treatment. *Aliment
Pharmacol Ther* 2003; **17**: 719–726.

399 Zullo A, Gatta L, de Francesco V *et al*. High rate of *Helicobacter
pylori* eradication with sequential therapy in elderly patients
with peptic ulcer: A prospective controlled study. *Aliment
Pharmacol Ther* 2005; **21**: 1419–1424.

400 Hassan C, de Francesco V, Zullo A, Scaccianoce G, Piglionica
D, Ierardi E, Panella C, Morini S. Sequential treatment for
Helicobacter pylori eradication in duodenal ulcer patients:
Improving the cost of pharmacotherapy. *Aliment Pharmacol Ther*
2003; **18**: 641–646.

401 Vaira D, Zullo A, Vakil N *et al*. Sequential therapy versus standard triple-drug therapy for *Helicobacter pylori* eradication: A
randomized trial. *Ann Intern Med* 2007; **146**: 556–563.

402 Scaccianoce G, Hassan C, Panarese A, Piglionica D, Morini S,
Zullo A. *Helicobacter pylori* eradication with either 7-day or 10-
day triple therapies, and with a 10-day sequential regimen. *Can
J Gastroenterol* 2006; **20**: 113–117.

403 Zullo A, de Francesco V, Hassan C, Morini S, Vaira D. The
sequential therapy regimen for *Helicobacter pylori* eradication: A
pooled-data analysis. *Gut* 2007; **56**: 1353–1357.

404 Jafri NS, Hornung CA, Howden CW. Meta-analysis: Sequential
therapy appears superior to standard therapy for *Helicobacter
pylori* infection in patients naive to treatment. *Ann Intern Med*
2008; **148**: 923–931.

405 Uygun A, Kadayifci A, Yesilova Z, Safali M, Ilgan S, Karaeren
N. Comparison of sequential and standard triple-drug regimen
for *Helicobacter pylori* eradication: A 14-day, open-label, randomized, prospective, parallel-arm study in adult patients with
nonulcer dyspepsia. *Clin Ther* 2008; **30**: 528–534.

406 Nagahara A, Miwa H, Yamada T, Kurosawa A, Ohkura R, Sato
N. Five-day proton pump inhibitor-based quadruple therapy
regimen is more effective than 7-day triple therapy regimen for
Helicobacter pylori infection. *Aliment Pharmacol Ther* 2001; **15**:
417–421.

407 Nagahara A, Miwa H, Ogawa K *et al*. Addition of metronidazole
to rabeprazole-amoxicillin-clarithromycin regimen for
Helicobacter pylori infection provides an excellent cure rate with
five-day therapy. *Helicobacter* 2000; **5**: 88–93.

408 Treiber G, Wittig J, Ammon S, Walker S, van Doorn LJ, Klotz
U. Clinical outcome and influencing factors of a new short-term
quadruple therapy for *Helicobacter pylori* eradication: A randomized controlled trial (MACLOR study). *Arch Intern Med* 2002;
162: 153–160.

409 Treiber G, Ammon S, Schneider E, Klotz U. Amoxicillin/met-
ronidazole/omeprazole/clarithromycin: A new, short quadruple therapy for *Helicobacter pylori* eradication. *Helicobacter* 1998;
3: 54–58.

410 Neville PM, Everett S, Langworthy H *et al*. The optimal antibiotic combination in a 5-day *Helicobacter pylori* eradication
regimen. *Aliment Pharmacol Ther* 1999; **13**: 497–501.

411 Catalano F, Branciforte G, Catanzaro R, Cipolla R, Bentivegna
C, Brogna A. *Helicobacter pylori*-positive duodenal ulcer: Three-
day antibiotic eradication regimen. *Aliment Pharmacol Ther* 2000;
14: 1329–1334.

412 Calvet X, Tito L, Comet R, Garcia N, Campo R, Brullet E. Four-
day, twice daily, quadruple therapy with amoxicillin, clarithro-

mycin, tinidazole and omeprazole to cure *Helicobacter pylori* infection: A pilot study. *Helicobacter* 2000; **5**: 52–56.

413 Okada M, Nishimura H, Kawashima M *et al.* A new quadruple therapy for *Helicobacter pylori*: influence of resistant strains on treatment outcome. *Aliment Pharmacol Ther* 1999; **13**: 769–774.

414 Sullivan B, Coyle W, Nemec R, Dunteman T. Comparison of azithromycin and clarithromycin in triple therapy regimens for the eradication of *Helicobacter pylori*. *Am J Gastroenterol* 2002; **97**: 2536–2539.

415 Iacopini F, Crispino P, Paoluzi OA *et al.* One-week once-daily triple therapy with esomeprazole, levofloxacin and azithromycin compared to a standard therapy for *Helicobacter pylori* eradication. *Dig Liver Dis* 2005; **37**: 571–576.

416 Laurent J, Megraud F, Flejou JF, Caekaert A, Barthelemy P. A randomized comparison of four omeprazole-based triple therapy regimens for the eradication of *Helicobacter pylori* in patients with non-ulcer dyspepsia. *Aliment Pharmacol Ther* 2001; **15**: 1787–1793.

417 Anagnostopoulos GK, Kostopoulos P, Margantinis G, Tsiakos S, Arvanitidis D. Omeprazole plus azithromycin and either amoxicillin or tinidazole for eradication of *Helicobacter pylori* infection. *J Clin Gastroenterol* 2003; **36**: 325–328.

418 Silva FM, Eisig JN, Chehter EZ, da Silva JJ, Laudanna AA. Low efficacy of an ultra-short term, once-daily dose triple therapy with omeprazole, azithromycin, and secnidazole for *Helicobacter pylori* eradication in peptic ulcer. *Rev Hosp Clin Fac Med Sao Paulo* 2002; **57**: 9–14.

419 Ivashkin VT, Lapina TL, Bondarenko OY *et al.* Azithromycin in a triple therapy for H. pylori eradication in active duodenal ulcer. *World J Gastroenterol* 2002; **8**: 879–882.

420 Tindberg Y, Casswall TH, Blennow M, Bengtsson C, Granstrom M, Sorberg M. *Helicobacter pylori* eradication in children and adolescents by a once daily 6-day treatment with or without a proton pump inhibitor in a double-blind randomized trial. *Aliment Pharmacol Ther* 2004; **20**: 295–302.

421 Gasbarrini A, Lauritano EC, Nista EC *et al.* Rifaximin-based regimens for eradication of *Helicobacter pylori*: a pilot study. *Dig Dis* 2006; **24**: 195–200.

422 Wu CJ, Hsu PI, Lo GH *et al.* Comparison of cetraxate-based and pantoprazole-based triple therapies in the treatment of *Helicobacter pylori* infection. *J Chin Med Assoc* 2004; **67**: 161–167.

423 Isomoto H, Furusu H, Ohnita K, Wen CY, Inoue K, Kohno S. Sofalcone, a mucoprotective agent, increases the cure rate of *Helicobacter pylori* infection when combined with rabeprazole, amoxicillin and clarithromycin. *World J Gastroenterol* 2005; **11**: 1629–1633.

424 Kim HW, Kim GH, Cheong JY *et al.* H pylori eradication: A randomized prospective study of triple therapy with or without ecabet sodium. *World J Gastroenterol* 2008; **14**: 908–912.

425 Armuzzi A, Cremonini F, Bartolozzi F *et al.* The effect of oral administration of Lactobacillus GG on antibiotic-associated gastrointestinal side-effects during *Helicobacter pylori* eradication therapy. *Aliment Pharmacol Ther* 2001; **15**: 163–169.

426 Cremonini F, Di Caro S, Covino M *et al.* Effect of different probiotic preparations on anti-*Helicobacter pylori* therapy-related side effects: a parallel group, triple blind, placebo-controlled study. *Am J Gastroenterol* 2002; **97**: 2744–2749.

427 Francavilla R, Lionetti E, Castellaneta SP *et al.* Inhibition of *Helicobacter pylori* infection in humans by Lactobacillus reuteri ATCC 55730 and effect on eradication therapy: A pilot study. *Helicobacter* 2008; **13**: 127–134.

428 Duman DG, Bor S, Ozutemiz O *et al.* Efficacy and safety of Saccharomyces boulardii in prevention of antibiotic-associated diarrhoea due to *Helicobacter pylori* eradication. *Eur J Gastroenterol Hepatol* 2005; **17**: 1357–1361.

429 Cindoruk M, Erkan G, Karakan T, Dursun A, Unal S. Efficacy and safety of Saccharomyces boulardii in the 14-day triple anti-*Helicobacter pylori* therapy: A prospective randomized placebo-controlled double-blind study. *Helicobacter* 2007; **12**: 309–316.

430 Sheu BS, Wu JJ, Lo CY *et al.* Impact of supplement with Lactobacillus- and Bifidobacterium-containing yogurt on triple therapy for *Helicobacter pylori* eradication. *Aliment Pharmacol Ther* 2002; **16**: 1669–1675.

431 Park SK, Park DI, Choi JS *et al.* The effect of probiotics on *Helicobacter pylori* eradication. *Hepatogastroenterology* 2007; **54**: 2032–2036.

432 Nista EC, Candelli M, Cremonini F *et al.* Bacillus clausii therapy to reduce side-effects of anti-*Helicobacter pylori* treatment: Randomized, double-blind, placebo controlled trial. *Aliment Pharmacol Ther* 2004; **20**: 1181–1188.

433 Myllyluoma E, Veijola L, Ahlroos T *et al.* Probiotic supplementation improves tolerance to *Helicobacter pylori* eradication therapy–a placebo-controlled, double-blind randomized pilot study. *Aliment Pharmacol Ther* 2005; **21**: 1263–1272.

434 Tursi A, Brandimarte G, Giorgetti GM, Modeo ME. Effect of *Lactobacillus casei* supplementation on the effectiveness and tolerability of a new second-line 10-day quadruple therapy after failure of a first attempt to cure *Helicobacter pylori* infection. *Med Sci Monit* 2004; **10**: CR662–CR666.

435 Ziemniak W. Efficacy of *Helicobacter pylori* eradication taking into account its resistance to antibiotics. *J Physiol Pharmacol* 2006; **57** Suppl 3: 123–141.

436 de Bortoli N, Leonardi G, Ciancia E *et al.* Helicobacter pylori eradication: A randomized prospective study of triple therapy versus triple therapy plus lactoferrin and probiotics. *Am J Gastroenterol* 2007; **102**: 951–956.

437 Sheu BS, Cheng HC, Kao AW *et al.* Pretreatment with Lactobacillus- and Bifidobacterium-containing yogurt can improve the efficacy of quadruple therapy in eradicating residual *Helicobacter pylori* infection after failed triple therapy. *Am J Clin Nutr* 2006; **83**: 864–869.

438 Tong JL, Ran ZH, Shen J, Zhang CX, Xiao SD. Meta-analysis: The effect of supplementation with probiotics on eradication rates and adverse events during *Helicobacter pylori* eradication therapy. *Aliment Pharmacol Ther* 2007; **25**: 155–168.

439 Meier R, Wettstein A, Drewe J, Geiser HR. Fish oil (Eicosapen) is less effective than metronidazole, in combination with pantoprazole and clarithromycin, for *Helicobacter pylori* eradication. *Aliment Pharmacol Ther* 2001; **15**: 851–855.

440 Gotoh A, Akamatsu T, Shimizu T *et al.* Additive effect of pronase on the efficacy of eradication therapy against *Helicobacter pylori*. *Helicobacter* 2002; **7**: 183–191.

441 Zullo A, de Francesco V, Scaccianoce G *et al.* Quadruple therapy with lactoferrin for *Helicobacter pylori* eradication: A randomised, multicentre study. *Dig Liver Dis* 2005; **37**: 496–500.

442 Tursi A, Elisei W, Brandimarte G, Giorgetti GM, Modeo ME, Aiello F. Effect of lactoferrin supplementation on the effectiveness and tolerability of a 7-day quadruple therapy after failure of a first attempt to cure *Helicobacter pylori* infection. *Med Sci Monit* 2007; **13**: CR187–CR190.

443 Zullo A, de Francesco V, Scaccianoce G *et al. Helicobacter pylori* eradication with either quadruple regimen with lactoferrin or levofloxacin-based triple therapy: a multicentre study. *Dig Liver Dis* 2007; **39**: 806–810.

7

Non-steroidal anti-inflammatory drug-induced gastro-duodenal toxicity

Alaa Rostom[1], Katherine Muir[2], Catherine Dubé[3], Emilie Jolicoeur[4], Michel Boucher[5], Peter Tugwell[6] and George Wells[7]

[1] Forzani & MacPhail Colon Cancer Screening Centre, University of Calgary, Calgary, Canada
[2] University of Toronto, Toronto, Canada
[3] Division of Gastroenterology, University of Calgary, Calgary, Canada
[4] Department of Gastroenterology, Montfort Hospital, Ottawa, Canada
[5] HTA Development, CADTH, Ottawa, Canada
[6] Department of Epidemiology and Community Medicine, University of Ottawa *and* Ottawa Hospital Research Institute, Ottawa, Canada
[7] Department of Epidemiology and Community Medicine and Cardiovascular Research Methods Centre, University of Ottawa, Ottawa, Canada

Introduction

This chapter was first written in 1999. At the time, evidence from non-clinical and early clinical trials suggested that the gastrointestinal (GI) safety of the newer cyclo-oxygenase-2 (COX-2) selective NSAIDs was such that a fundamental change in clinicians' choice from the use of standard NSAIDs with a gastroprotective agent to monotherapy with a COX-2 selective NSAID (COX-2 inhibitors) was on the horizon. However, much has changed since then in the field of non-steroidal anti-inflammatory drugs (NSAIDs). The release of the cyclo-oxygenase-2 selective inhibitors (COX-2s) brought about significant changes in the NSAID marketplace. Traditional non-selective NSAIDs (tNSAIDs) prescription numbers fell rapidly, to be replaced by COX-2 prescriptions. Additionally, overall NSAID prescriptions rose in number suggesting that clinicians were starting COX-2s on patients who where not considered candidates for tNSAIDs. The rise of COX-2s continued until 2004 when greater data regarding their cardiovascular and other toxicities became available, leading to the withdrawal of most of these agents from the market over the following years. Non-naproxen tNSAIDs were also suggested to have important cardiovascular toxicity leading to considerable uncertainty amongst clinicians treating patients with arthritis and other pain disorders as to the choice of agent to use.

Evidence-Based Gastroenterology and Hepatology, 3rd edition.
J. McDonald, A.K. Burroughs, B. Feagan, and M.B. Fennerty. © 2010
Blackwell Publishing Ltd

Background

Non-steroidal anti-inflammatory drugs (NSAIDs), including aspirin, are important agents in the management of patients with a variety of arthritic and inflammatory conditions [1]. Additionally, aspirin is important in the treatment and prevention of both myocardial infarction and stroke [2–5]. The efficacy of these agents is well described, making NSAIDs among the most frequently used medications, with an estimated world market in excess of $6 billion annually [6]. One cohort study found that short-term NSAIDs were prescribed for about 25% of Canadians, including about 4% for whom these agents were prescribed long term (defined in this study as ≥ 6 months) [7]; this equates to approximately 6.2 million short-term users, and 1.0 million long-term users of NSAID therapy. However, this substantially underestimates the true magnitude of NSAID uses since it does not include use of over the counter NSAIDs. A US cohort study, reported the point prevalence of NSAID use as 8.7% [8]. Low-dose ASA is extensively used for cardiovascular risk reduction. In addition, some evidence supports the use of these agents for the prevention of colorectal adenomas in at-risk individuals [9, 10].

NSAIDs including aspirin (ASA) cause a variety of gastrointestinal toxicities, which are associated with excess utilization of health care resources at a substantial cost [11]. Minor adverse effects such as nausea and dyspepsia are relatively common, but these clinical symptoms correlate poorly with serious adverse gastrointestinal events [12, 13]. Although, endoscopic ulcers, occurring with or without symptoms, can be documented in as many as 40% of chronic NSAID users [14], serious NSAID induced gastrointestinal toxicities are much less common [13]. Due to the vast numbers of individuals using these drugs, however, they have been linked directly to over 70,000 hospitalizations and over 7000 deaths annually in the USA alone [15]. NSAID use can also add significantly to the morbidity and mortality of chronic arthritic conditions. Among rheumatoid arthritis patients who are chronically using NSAIDs, the chance of hospitalization or death due to a gastrointestinal event is about 1.3 to 1.6% per year [15], accounting for about 2600 deaths and 20,000 hospitalizations each year [1]. These figures have led some to the suggestion that NSAID toxicity is among the "deadliest" of rheumatic disorders [15].

The serious gastrointestinal complications such as hemorrhage, perforation or death occur collectively with an incidence of about 2% per year in an average patient population on NSAIDs [13]. The relative risk of upper gastrointestinal hemorrhage or perforation with NSAID use varies in the literature from 4.7 in hospital based case control studies to 2.0 in cohort studies [16–18]. Gabriel *et al.* in a meta-analysis of 16 studies found that non-ASA NSAIDs were associated with a 2.7-fold increased risk of serious gastrointestinal events resulting in hospitalization [19]. Similarly, Langman *et al.* found that ASA and non-ASA NSAID use increased the risk of bleeding peptic ulcer 3.1-fold and 3.5-fold respectively [20]. In a recent large, prospective cohort study of 126,000 patients conducted over three years, MacDonald *et al.* found that NSAIDs increased the risk of any adverse gastrointestinal event 3.9-fold. However, NSAIDs appeared to raise the risk 8.0-fold, when only hemorrhage or perforation were considered [21], a level that is sufficiently high to imply causation. Armstrong *et al.* found that 60% of 235 consecutive patients presenting with a significant peptic ulcer complication were taking tNSAIDs, and nearly 80% of all ulcer related deaths occurred in NSAIDs users [22].

NSAIDs have also been linked to a variety of other gastrointestinal toxicities, including pyloric stenosis, small bowel ulcerations, strictures, lower gastrointestinal bleeds, and the exacerbation of colitis [6, 23–25]. Some experts suggest that the most effective means to prevent NSAID induced gastrointestinal toxicity is to discontinue the use of the NSAID, or to substitute an alternative non-NSAID analgesic [26]. However, this approach is clearly not always feasible, since a large proportion of NSAID users rely heavily on these medications, and a delicate balance exists between the therapeutic benefits and the risks of these drugs [27].

NSAIDs inhibit the enzyme cyclo-oxygenase (COX). This enzyme exists in two isoforms: COX-1 and COX-2. It is felt that NSAIDs exert their therapeutic anti-inflammatory and analgesic effects through the inhibition of inducible cyclo-oxygenase-2 (COX-2), whereas their gastric and renal toxicities arise from the inhibition of the constitutive COX-1

isoform [28, 29]. The anti-platelet effect of NSAIDs including ASA is mediated through inhibition of the COX-1 isoform. It has been recognized for some time that different NSAIDs have differing propensities toward gastroduodenal toxicity [21], and recently it has been proposed that those NSAIDs with the greatest affinity for COX-1 are associated with the highest risk of gastrointestinal toxicity. As a result of these observations, there has been a rapid development of new NSAIDs with increasing COX-2 selectivity, with claims of retained anti-inflammatory and analgesic activity, but with little gastrointestinal toxicity. However, increasing COX-2 selectivity may lead to increased prothrombotic effects and an increased risk of cardiovascular events. Extensive data now associate COX-2 inhibitors and non-naproxen tNSAIDs with an increased risk of cardiovascular events [30, 31], which has led regulatory authorities to introduce warning statements and advisories. Additionally, the COX-2 inhibitors, rofecoxib, valdecoxib and lumiracoxib have been withdrawn from the market because of cardiovascular, cutaneous, and hepatic adverse events respectively [7, 8, 32–34]. Health Canada and the Food and Drug Administration (FDA) require the product information for NSAIDs (tNSAIDs and COX-2 inhibitors) to include a warning of the increased incidence of cardiovascular (e.g. heart attack, stroke) and gastrointestinal (e.g. ulcer, bleeding) adverse events, as well as recommendations to limit use of the drug to the lowest effective dose for the shortest possible duration of treatment [8, 34].

A great deal of variability exists in the literature regarding the criteria by which an NSAID is classified as COX-2 selective and for the techniques used to make this determination. The most accepted technique involves determination of the COX-2 IC50 to COX-1 IC50 ratio (a ratio of the concentrations of the drug that results in 50% blockage of the COX-2 and COX-1 iso-enzymes) through a whole blood assay. A value below one indicates greater affinity for COX-2 inhibition than COX-1 inhibition. The lower the value, the greater the COX-2 selectivity. However, a ratio below 1 does not guarantee COX-2 selectivity in clinical practice, since other factors are at play, such as the COX-2 selectivity at target tissue such as the gastric mucosa, and the effect of clinically used dosages of the drug on its COX-2 selectivity (i.e. an agent may be COX-2 selective only at sub-therapeutic doses). Also, the reported COX-2 to COX-1 IC50 ratios for the available COX-2 selective NSAIDs differ from one report to another.

This chapter includes updates to two Cochrane collaboration systematic reviews on: the effects of pharmacologic interventions used to prevent the GI harms associated with the chronic use of non-selective tNSAIDs (diclofenac, ibuprofen, naproxen); the GI safety of COX-2s when used alone, as well as the influence of aspirin co-administration on GI harms, and the GI safety of a combined COX-2 proton pump inhibitor strategy.

Risk factors for NSAID related gastrointestinal toxicity

Several studies, meta-analyses and reviews have addressed the issue of risk factors for NSAID induced gastrointestinal toxicity. Increasing age (>65), previous peptic ulcer disease with or without previous hemorrhage and co-morbid medical illnesses, particularly heart disease, have been consistently shown to increase the risk of an adverse gastrointestinal event among patients on long-term NSAID therapy [13, 15, 17, 19, 35–39]. Using multiple logistic regression to adjust for risk factors simultaneously, Silverstein *et al.* found that among patients on chronic NSAIDs with none of these risk factors, only 0.4% developed a serious adverse gastrointestinal event at six months, whereas 9% of patients with all three risk factors experienced such an event [13]. Other risk factors have also been identified (Table 7.1). High doses of NSAIDs and the use of multiple NSAIDs increase the risk of adverse outcomes, as do the combined use of NSAIDs with corticosteroids, ASA, or warfarin [38, 40]. Specific NSAIDs (Table 7.2), and in some studies female gender is also associated with an increased risk of gastrointestinal toxicity [36–38, 41–44].

 The duration of NSAID use has been reported as a risk factor for gastrointestinal toxicity, with most studies suggesting that the risk is highest within the first month of use [16, 20, 42, 45, 46]. However there is increasing evidence to suggest that the risk of significant NSAID toxicity does not diminish with prolonged use beyond one month. Silverstein *et al.*, in their prospective study of misoprostol for the prevention of serious NSAID related gastrointestinal events, did not find a decreased risk with continued NSAID use [13]. Furthermore, in a large prospective cohort study of NSAID related gastrointestinal toxicity, MacDonald *et al.* found that there was a four-fold relative risk increase associated with the use of NSAIDs and that this risk was nearly constant over the three-year follow-up period [21]. Additionally these investigators found that a two-fold rela-

tive risk of gastrointestinal toxicity persisted for at least one year after the last exposure to NSAIDs.

 Compliance with NSAID use also appears to be a risk factor for gastrointestinal toxicity. Wynn *et al.* in a study of patient awareness of adverse effects and symptoms associated with NSAIDs, found that patients suffering an adverse gastrointestinal event had a higher rate of compliance (96%) with their NSAID use than those not suffering an event (70%) [47]. Similarly, Griffin *et al.* found that patients suffering a terminal NSAID related gastrointestinal event were more likely to have filled a prescription for an NSAID in the preceding month [16]. Symptoms, however, correlate quite poorly with the occurrence of endoscopic ulceration and adverse gastrointestinal events, and thus cannot be considered predictors of adverse gastrointestinal events [12, 13, 22, 40, 48].

 The role of *Helicobacter pylori* infection as a risk factor for NSAID related gastrointestinal toxicity is controversial and will be discussed in the following section.

Do endoscopic ulcers predict clinical events?

Gastrointestinal ulcers are established as the pathophysiologic correlate of clinical gastrointestinal events resulting from the chronic use of NSAIDs. For this reason endoscopically confirmed ulcers have been used as surrogate outcomes for clinical gastrointestinal events resulting from NSAID use. Endoscopic definitions of gastroduodenal ulcers are controversial [49], and do not equate with the pathological definition, which defines an ulcer as a loss of

Table 7.1 Risk factors for NSAID gastrointestinal toxicity.

Age >60
Previous peptic ulcer disease
Underlying medical conditions
Concomitant corticosteroid use
Concomitant anticoagulant therapy or ASA
High dose of NSAID or multiple NSAIDs
Type of NSAID
Duration of NSAID use/compliance
Helicobacter pylori – see text

Table 7.2 Individual NSAIDs and the risk of gastrointestinal events (relative to ibuprofen). Adapted from Henry *et al. BMJ* 1996 [43].

Drug	Relative risk
Azopropazone	9.2
Ketoprophen	4.2
Piroxicam	3.8
Tolmetin	3.0
Indomethacin	2.4
Naproxen	2.2
Diflunisal	2.2
Sulindac	2.1
Diclofenac	1.8
Aspirin	1.6
Fenoprofen	1.6
Ibuprofen	1.00
Dose: (Ibuprofen)	
Low	1.6
High	4.2

mucosal surface of sufficient depth to penetrate the muscularis mucosa [50]. In most clinical trials of NSAID prophylaxis, an endoscopic ulcer is defined as a break in the mucosal surface, usually greater than 3 mm in diameter with some appreciable depth. The strictness of these criteria has varied form study to study, with some authors requiring the use of an endoscopic measuring tool, or estimation based on the size of an open biopsy forceps to measure the ulcer diameter. Formal estimates of inter-observer variability among the endoscopists are often not presented, particularly in the larger multicentre trials. Some authors define an ulcer as the loss of mucosal surface of 5 mm or greater in diameter to better differentiate them from erosions and to achieve closer agreement with clinical events [49]. Varying definitions of endoscopic ulcers and the occasional use of composite endpoints all complicate comparison of results across studies.

Unfortunately, endoscopic ulcers are not ideal surrogate outcomes for clinical gastrointestinal events such as bleeding or perforation of an ulcer. In fact, the proportion of endoscopic ulcers that never become clinically symptomatic, is estimated to be as high as 85% [13, 51].

With the publication of several large randomized controlled trials (RCTs) that used actual clinical endpoints to measure the safety of COX-2 inhibitors and of misoprostol prophylaxis [13, 52, 53], it became possible to compare the reduction in clinical events with that of the reduction in endoscopic ulcers from the endoscopic studies [54–56]. Although these are indirect comparisons that have to be interpreted with caution, we have found in our systematic reviews that the standard NSAID arms of both the NSAID prophylaxis trials and the COX-2 trials were quite similar clinically, and demonstrated nearly identical NSAID ulcer and complication rates.

The relative risk reduction in endoscopic gastric ulcers with misoprostol prophylaxis and with COX-2 inhibitors is about 80%. In the clinical endpoint studies, the relative risk reductions in NSAID ulcer related perforations, obstructions and bleeding is about 50% with both these strategies. The consistency suggests that there is a relationship between the endoscopic and clinical endpoints. The relationship does not have to be 1:1. In fact based on our results, prophylactic agents and COX-2 inhibitors are 1.5–2.0 times more effective at reducing the risk of endoscopic ulcers than they are at reducing the risk of clinical endpoints. Unfortunately the studies using clinical gastrointestinal events as the primary outcome measure were not designed to look at the relationship of clinical events to endoscopic ulcers, and we used indirect comparisons to arrive at this result [13]. However, with the cautions described above, the reader can estimate what the expected reduction in clinical events would be based on the results of an endoscopic endpoint study, assuming the control groups are average risk arthritic patients requiring long-term NSAID use.

The role of *Helicobacter pylori* in NSAID associated ulcers

The causal role of *Helicobacter pylori* in the development of gastroduodenal ulcers has added a new perspective to the management of patients with gastrointestinal complaints [57–59]. NSAIDs are now thought to cause approximately 25% of gastroduodenal ulcers [60], and do so in the absence of *H. pylori* [61–64]. The study of the potential interaction between *H. pylori* and NSAIDs has been complicated by the following facts: (1) NSAID use is most frequent among elderly patients, the same group with the highest *H. pylori* prevalence in western populations [65, 66], (2) in the presence of both factors, it has been difficult to determine whether an ulcer is caused by NSAIDs with incidental *H. pylori*, or caused by *H. pylori* with incidental or exacerbating NSAIDs [67, 68], and (3) whereas one would expect, based on conventional thinking, an increased incidence of ulcers in the presence of these two well-established risk factors, some clinical and observational studies found that infection with *H. pylori* decreased the likelihood of ulcers or gastroduodenal injury in NSAID users [69–72]. Still other studies have found no effect of *H. pylori* infection on NSAID induced gastroduodenal injury [70, 73].

A systematic review published in 2002 has shed some light on our understanding of the clinical impact of the co-existence of *H. pylori* infection and NSAID use [74]. In this systematic review of observational studies of PUD in adult patients taking NSAIDs and of *H. pylori* infection and NSAID use in PUD bleeding, strict diagnostic criteria for the documentation of *H. pylori* infection and endoscopic ulcers were used. Twenty-five studies were included out of 61 potentially relevant publications. Sixteen studies with a total of 1625 patients assessed the effect of *H. pylori* infection on the risk of uncomplicated PUD in adult NSAID users. In these patients, *H. pylori* infection increased the risk of uncomplicated PUD 2.12-fold (95% CI: 1.68–2.67).

The interaction between *H. pylori* infection and NSAID exposure was derived from five age-matched controlled studies of chronic (>4 weeks) NSAID exposure. In the presence of *H. pylori* infection, the use of NSAIDs increased the risk of uncomplicated PUD 3.55-fold (95% CI: 1.26–9.96); while in the presence of NSAIDs, *H. pylori* infection increased the risk of PUD 3.53-fold (95% CI: 2.16–5.75). Compared to control patients without either NSAID or *H. pylori* exposure, the combined exposure to both factors increased the risk of uncomplicated PUD 6.36-fold (95% CI: 2.21–18.31) after correction for a zero event rate in *H. pylori* negative controls.

Nine case-control studies with 893 patients and 1002 controls assessed the effects of *H. pylori* infection and NSAID exposure on the risk of ulcer bleeding. *H. pylori* infection conferred a marginally increased risk, with an OR 1.67

(95% CI: 1.02–2.72), which was more pronounced when the analysis was limited to studies using serology for diagnosis of *H. pylori* infection (OR 2.16 (95% CI: 1.54–3.04)). Studies using patients with non-bleeding ulcers as controls (as opposed to either healthy or hospitalized non-ulcer controls) tended to be negative, but the results of a sensitivity analysis based on the type of controls were not presented. NSAID exposure, which was principally short term in these studies (<1 week and <1 month in six and two out of nine studies respectively), conferred an increased risk of ulcer bleeding (OR 4.79; 95% CI: 3.78–6.06), whereas the combined exposure to NSAIDs and *H. pylori* led to an increased risk of PUD bleed of 6.13 (95% CI: 3.93–9.56). These findings are in keeping with the hypothesis that short-term NSAID exposure renders "silent" *H. pylori*-related ulcers clinically manifest, a notion that has been suggested by others [75–77].

The authors of this systematic review support the conventional thinking that in peptic ulcer disease two sources of injuries are worse than one. However, the outcome of combined exposure to NSAIDs and *H. pylori* infection differs depending on the patient population (prior history of PUD or not), the type of NSAID exposure (first time or not, short term or long-term; ASA or non-ASA NSAID), the study outcome (ulcer healing, ulcer bleeding, ulcer prevention) and the co-administration of ulcer prophylaxis. Several recent randomized trials have addressed some of these issues.

Ulcer healing

Ulcer healing with omeprazole or ranitidine occurs more readily in the presence of *H. pylori* infection [78, 79]. As well, the presence of *H. pylori* enhances the ability of omeprazole to raise gastric pH among patients with duodenal ulcer [80]. However, Bianchi Porro *et al.* found that the presence of *H. pylori* did not statistically affect the healing rates at either four or eight weeks in a study of 100 chronic NSAID users with peptic ulcers [81].

In a group of 81 *H. pylori* positive ulcer patients with ongoing requirement for NSAIDs, Hawkey *et al.* observed that the addition of *H. pylori* eradication to a one-month course of omeprazole led to a significantly lower healing rate for gastric ulcers (50 vs 88% healing at four weeks and 72 vs 100% healing at eight weeks, for the *H. pylori* treated and omeprazole alone groups, respectively (p = 0.006)), while the rates of duodenal ulcer healing were similar in both groups [82].

Ulcer prevention in NSAID naive patients

Chan *et al.* randomized 100 *H. pylori* positive, NSAID naive, patients with no prior history of peptic ulcer, to receive either naproxen alone or *H. pylori* eradication (bismuth, tetracycline and metronidazole) followed by naproxen for eight weeks [83]. At eight weeks, the rate of ulcer recurrence was statistically lower in the triple therapy group (7% vs 26% in the naproxen alone group in the intention-to-treat analysis, p = 0.01), for a 74% relative risk reduction with *H. pylori* eradication. The importance of coexistent risk factors was highlighted by the fact that 73% of ulcer patients were older than 60 and that 73% of them also had co-morbidity.

In a more recent study, the same group enrolled 100 *H. pylori* positive, NSAID naive, patients with either a prior history of peptic ulcer (16% of the patients) or dyspepsia, to receive *H. pylori* eradication or omeprazole plus placebo for one week, followed by diclofenac 100 mg daily for six months [84]. Once again, in these NSAID naive patients, *H. pylori* eradication conferred a protective effect, leading to a significantly reduced incidence of both endoscopic ulcers (12.1% (95% CI: 3.1–21.1) vs 34.4% (21.1–47.7) in the eradication vs omeprazole alone groups respectively), and of clinical ulcers (4.2% (1.3–9.7) vs 27.1% (14.7–39.5) in the eradication vs omeprazole alone groups respectively) at six months. Of note, 17% of these patients had received low-dose ASA prior to enrolment.

Secondary ulcer prevention in patients on continuous NSAID

The role of *H. pylori* eradication for the prevention of recurrent upper gastrointestinal bleeding was studied by Chan *et al.* [85]. Four hundred *H. pylori* positive, chronic users of ASA or other NSAID, presenting with a bleeding peptic ulcer, were randomized to receive either *H. pylori* eradication or ulcer prophylaxis with omeprazole and followed up for six months for the recurrence of clinical events. In the group of patients on low-dose (80 mg daily) ASA, the probability of ulcer recurrence was similar among *H. pylori* treated patients and those on PPI prophylaxis. However, in patients on a non-ASA NSAID (naproxen 500 mg twice daily), *H. pylori* eradication did not confer the same magnitude of ulcer protection as omeprazole, so that the trial was terminated after the second interim analysis (probability of recurrence 18.8% vs 4.4% for the *H. pylori* eradication and omeprazole groups respectively (p = 0.005) at that point).

Hawkey *et al.* studied the role of *H. pylori* eradication in a group of 285 *H. pylori* positive patients with a history of ulcer or dyspepsia and ongoing requirement for NSAIDs [82], who were randomized to a one-week course of either *H. pylori* eradication or omeprazole plus placebo. All patients then received a three-week course of omeprazole for ulcer healing. During the follow-up period patients received continuous NSAIDs without ulcer prophylaxis. The probability of ulcer recurrence at six months was similar in both groups, and the study concluded that in chronic NSAID (non-ASA) users, *H. pylori* eradication did not confer a protective effect on ulcer recurrence.

In summary, we can conclude based on these recent RCTs, that *H. pylori* contributes to an excess ulcer risk in NSAID naive patients, whereas ulcers occurring in long-term NSAID users are probably largely caused by NSAIDs themselves, irrespective of *H. pylori* status. Therefore, the impact of *H. pylori* is likely to be manifest early in the course of NSAID exposure, either because these patients are prone to early ulcer complications with NSAIDs, or because the administration of NSAIDs has precipitated complications in pre-existing *H. pylori* ulcers. We can also conclude that the impact of *H. pylori* eradication is related to the amount of co-existing ulcerogenic factors; while its benefits are more obvious in conjunction with low-dose ASA administration, they are not significant in comparison to the ulcerogenic effects of "regular" NSAIDs and are less marked in the elderly or in the presence of co-morbidity.

Based on this evidence, it would seem appropriate to eradicate *H. pylori* in NSAID naive patients prior to starting chronic ASA or NSAID therapy. However, *H. pylori* eradication alone appears to be insufficient for ulcer prophylaxis in chronic non-ASA NSAID users.

Definition of terms

In the discussion that follows, we use the relative risk (RR) to indicate the likelihood of an outcome in subjects on treatment compared to those on placebo [86, 87]. For example a RR of 0.25, means that the treatment is associated with only 25% or 1/4 the probability of the outcome as compared to placebo. Expressed in another way, an RR of 0.25 means that the treatment reduces the "risk" of an event by 75% compared to placebo (1–0.25 = 0.75 or 75%). This relative risk reduction differs from the absolute risk reduction (ARR), the arithmetic difference in the proportion of patients with the outcome between the placebo and treatment groups. If the stated 95% confidence interval overlaps with 1, then the observed risk is not statistically significant. Several clinical endpoints are used in the chapter. The composite endpoint of perforation, obstruction or bleeding is referred to as POB; while a PUB refers to a POB or a symptomatic ulcer. Endoscopic ulcers refer to endoscopically detected ulcers as part of studies with predetermined endoscopy schedules. Non-selective traditional NSAIDs are referred to as tNSAIDs; and cyclo-oxygenase-2 inhibitors as COX-2s. The term NSAID is used when referring to the overall group including (tNSAIDs and COX-2s).

Misoprostol

Misoprostol is a synthetic prostaglandin E_1 analogue [88–91]. It reduces basal and stimulated gastric acid secretion through a direct effect on parietal cells [91], and reduces gastric damage caused by a variety of aggressive factors including bile salts and NSAIDs [92]. Misoprostol's protective effects are felt to be related to its ability to stimulate gastric bicarbonate and mucus secretion, and to maintain mucosal blood flow and the mucosal permeability barrier. Misoprostol also promotes epithelial proliferation in response to injury [88]. It appears that at doses of misoprostol sufficient to protect gastric mucosa, suppression of acid secretion also occurs [90]. However, since standard doses of H_2-receptor antagonists inhibit gastric acid secretion at least as effectively as misoprostol, and yet have not been shown to protect the gastric mucosa against NSAID induced ulceration (see next section), it is likely that mechanisms other than acid suppression are important for the prevention of gastric ulcers. Additionally, it has recently been suggested that misoprostol may be superior to PPIs for the prevention of NSAID induced gastric ulcers and gastroduodenal erosions [93, 94].

Misoprostol appears to be effective in preventing acute gastroduodenal injury induced by short courses of ASA and NSAIDs as measured by mucosal, or fecal blood loss, and by endoscopic injury scores [95–99]. However the clinical relevance of this effect is unclear, given the adaptation of gastroduodenal mucosa to acute injury with continued NSAID use [73, 100, 101].

Long-term efficacy of misoprostol

In our meta-analysis, we found 23 studies that assessed the long-term effect of misoprostol on the prevention of tNSAID ulcers [13, 33, 94, 102–121]. The dosage of misoprostol varied from 200 ug to 800 ug daily, and follow up ranged between 4 to 48 weeks.

Endoscopic ulcers

Eleven studies with 3641 patients compared the incidence of endoscopic ulcers, after at least three months, in misoprostol and placebo treated patients [94, 102, 103, 106, 110–113, 116, 118, 121]. The cumulative incidence of endoscopic gastric and duodenal ulcers with placebo was 15% and 6%, respectively. Misoprostol significantly reduced the relative risk of gastric ulcer and duodenal ulcers by 74% RR = 0.26; 95% CI: 0.17–0.39 random effects), and 58% (RR = 0.42; 95% CI: 0.22–0.81 random effects). These relative risks correspond to 12.0% and 3% absolute risk reductions for gastric and duodenal ulcers, respectively. The observed heterogeneity in these estimates was due to inclusion of all misoprostol doses in the analyses. Analysis of the misoprostol studies stratified by dose eliminated this heterogeneity.

Analysis by dose

All the studied doses of misoprostol significantly reduced the risk of endoscopic ulcers and a dose response relationship was demonstrated for endoscopic gastric ulcers (Figure 7.1). Six studies with 2461 patients used misoprostol 400 ug [103, 106, 111, 113, 116, 121], one study with 928 patients used 600 ug daily [116], and seven with 2423 patients used 800 ug daily [94, 102, 110–112, 116, 118]. Misoprostol 800 ug daily was associated with the lowest risk (RR = 0.17; 95% CI: 0.11–0.24) of endoscopic gastric ulcers when compared to placebo, whereas misoprostol 400 ug daily was associated with a relative risk of 0.42 (95% CI: 0.28–0.67 random effects model for heterogeneity). The

observed heterogeneity in the 400 ug dose group was the result of the addition of the Chan study (Chan 2001). This study compared the relatively more toxic naproxen with low dose misoprostol to nabumatone alone. In this study the risk of ulcers was inexplicably greater in the misoprostol group, but this result is probably based on the differences between the safety of the comparator tNSAIDS rather than on an effect of the prophylactic agent. In a sensitivity analysis, removal of the Chan study eliminates the observed heterogeneity without significantly altering the results, giving low dose misoprostol prophylaxis a RR of 0.39 (95% CI: 0.3–0.51). This difference between high and low-dose misoprostol was statistically significant (p = 0.0055). The observed risk for the intermediate misoprostol dose (600 ug

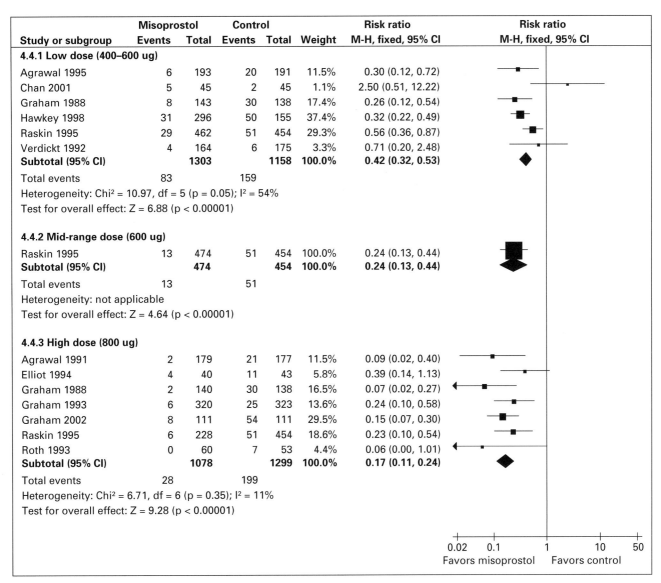

Figure 7.1 Misoprostol vs placebo for the prevention of gastric ulcers – efficacy by dose: Misoprosol 800 ug/day is superior to 400 or 600 ug/day for the prevention of endoscopically detected gastric ulcer.

daily) was not statistically significantly different from that observed for either the low or high dose. The pooled relative risk reduction of 78% (4.7% absolute risk difference, RR = 0.21; 95% CI: 0.09–0.49) for duodenal ulcers with misoprostol 800 ug daily was not statistically different from those observed with lower daily misoprostol dosages.

Studies including data with less than three months' tNSAID exposure

Eight studies, with 2206 patients, assessed the rates of endoscopic ulcers with misoprostol compared to placebo at 1–1.5 months [33, 104, 105, 107, 109, 110, 114, 119]. The pooling of these studies revealed an 81% relative risk reduction for gastric ulcers with misoprostol (RR = 0.17; 95% CI: 0.09–0.31) and a 72% relative risk reduction for duodenal ulcers (RR = 0.28; 95% CI: 0.14–0.56).

One study compared misoprostol to a newer cytoprotective agent, Dosmafate, for tNSAID prophylaxis and found no statistically significant difference in ulcer rates between the two agents [108].

Clinical ulcers

Only one RCT, the MUCOSA trial, evaluated the efficacy of misoprostol prophylaxis against clinically important tNSAID induced ulcer complications as the primary endpoint. In this study, of 8843 patients studied over six months, the overall GI event incidence was about 1.5% per year [13]. Misoprostol 800 ug/day was associated with a statistically significant 40% risk reduction (OR = 0.598; 95% CI: 0.364–0.982) in combined GI events (p = 0.049), representing a risk difference of 0.38% (from 0.95% to 0.57%).

Adverse effects

Misoprostol was associated with a small but statistically significant 1.6-fold excess risk of drop-out due to drug induced adverse effects, and an excess risk of drop-outs due to nausea (RR = 1.30; 95% CI: 1.08–1.55), diarrhea (RR = 2.36; 95% CI: 2.01–2.77), and abdominal pain (RR = 1.36; 95% CI: 1.20–1.55). In the MUCOSA trial, 732 out of 4404 patients on misoprostol experienced diarrhea or abdominal pain, compared to 399 out of 4439 on placebo for a relative risk of 1.82 associated with misoprostol (p <0.001). Overall, 27% of patients on misoprostol experienced one or more adverse effects [13].

When analyzed by dose, only misoprostol 800 ug daily showed a statistically significant excess risk of drop-outs due to diarrhea (RR = 2.45; 95% CI: 2.09–2.88) and abdominal pain (RR = 1.38; 95% CI: 1.17–1.63). Both misoprostol doses were associated with a statistically significant risk of diarrhea. However, the risk of diarrhea with 800 ug/day

(RR = 3.25; 95% CI: 2.60–4.06) was significantly higher than that seen with 400 ug/day (RR = 1.81 95% CI: 1.52–2.16) (p = 0.0012).

In conclusion, misoprostol prophylaxis significantly reduces the risk of ulcers as well as serious gastrointestinal events in patients on long-term NSAID therapy. **A1a** Misoprostol is more effective at reducing the risk of gastric than duodenal ulcers, and may be more effective than PPIs at reducing the risk of gastric ulcers. The use of misoprostol, particularly at higher doses, is associated with more frequent gastrointestinal adverse effects, often resulting in the patient discontinuing the medication, which is an important consideration, given the symptoms associated with NSAID use alone. The effectiveness outside of clinical trials of misoprostol for prevention of ulcer may be lower than figures which have been presented above. However, since misoprostol is the only prophylactic agent that has been directly shown to reduce serious NSAID related gastrointestinal complications, it should be considered as the first-line agent in the primary prophylaxis of NSAID complications, particularly in high risk groups. **A1a**

H₂-receptor antagonists

Treatment of NSAID induced ulcer

The efficacy of H₂-receptor antagonists in the treatment and prevention of NSAID related upper gastrointestinal toxicity has been exclusively evaluated in studies in which ulcers were defined endoscopically. In several early open label studies of cimetidine for healing of ulcers associated with the use of NSAIDs, it was shown that greater than 75% of gastric and duodenal ulcers could be healed with 12 weeks of therapy despite continued use of NSAIDs [122–126]. There was a trend toward improved efficacy with higher doses. However, in a randomized trial in which patients with NSAID – induced ulcers were randomized to receive standard dose ranitidine, or the more potent acid suppressor omeprazole, omeprazole was nearly twice as effective [127], although ranitidine was still somewhat effective [127, 128]. **A1a** O'Laughlin *et al.* found that ulcer size correlated inversely with healing rates. At eight weeks, ulcers with a diameter <5 mm were healed in greater than 90% of patients compared to 35% healing for ulcers >5 mm [129]. Hudson *et al.* reported similar observations [130]. The potency of acid suppression and initial ulcer size are important determinants of the rapidity of ulcer healing, and the continued use of NSAIDs in the presence of gastric acid may slow ulcer healing.

Prevention of NSAID- induced ulcers

Standard doses of H₂-receptor antagonists have been consistently shown to be effective for prevention of endoscopi-

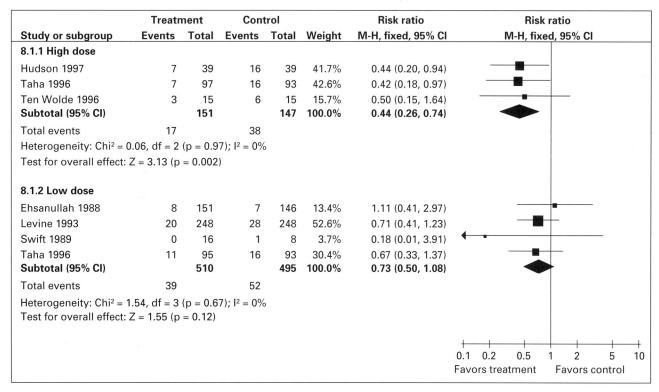

Study or subgroup	Treatment		Control		Weight	Risk ratio M-H, fixed, 95% CI	Risk ratio M-H, fixed, 95% CI
	Events	Total	Events	Total			
8.1.1 High dose							
Hudson 1997	7	39	16	39	41.7%	0.44 (0.20, 0.94)	
Taha 1996	7	97	16	93	42.6%	0.42 (0.18, 0.97)	
Ten Wolde 1996	3	15	6	15	15.7%	0.50 (0.15, 1.64)	
Subtotal (95% CI)		**151**		**147**	**100.0%**	**0.44 (0.26, 0.74)**	
Total events	17		38				
Heterogeneity: Chi² = 0.06, df = 2 (p = 0.97); I² = 0%							
Test for overall effect: Z = 3.13 (p = 0.002)							
8.1.2 Low dose							
Ehsanullah 1988	8	151	7	146	13.4%	1.11 (0.41, 2.97)	
Levine 1993	20	248	28	248	52.6%	0.71 (0.41, 1.23)	
Swift 1989	0	16	1	8	3.7%	0.18 (0.01, 3.91)	
Taha 1996	11	95	16	93	30.4%	0.67 (0.33, 1.37)	
Subtotal (95% CI)		**510**		**495**	**100.0%**	**0.73 (0.50, 1.08)**	
Total events	39		52				
Heterogeneity: Chi² = 1.54, df = 3 (p = 0.67); I² = 0%							
Test for overall effect: Z = 1.55 (p = 0.12)							

0.1 0.2 0.5 1 2 5 10
Favors treatment   Favors control

Figure 7.2 H_2-receptor antagonists compared to placebo for the prevention of gastric ulcers: While all doses of H_2-RAs are effective for reducing the incidence of endoscopically detected duodenal ulcers (figure not shown), only high doses of H_2-RAs (equivalent to ranitidine 300 mg bid) are effective for reducing the incidence of gastric ulcers.

cally defined duodenal ulcers, but not of gastric ulcers (Figure 7.2) [117, 131–140]. Koch *et al.* [141] in a meta-analysis of randomized trials that employed standard doses of H_2-receptor antagonists [131–133, 135, 137, 138] and Stalnikowicz *et al.* [14] were also unable to show a benefit for the prevention of gastric ulcers. Similarly, our meta-analysis of the standard dose H_2-receptor antagonist trials confirms that there is no statistically significant reduction in the relative risk of endoscopically defined gastric ulcers [54, 55].

Six trials that included 942 patients assessed the effect of standard dose H_2-RAs on the prevention of endoscopic tNSAID ulcers at one month [131–134, 138, 142], and five trials with 1005 patients assessed these outcomes at three months or longer [131, 134, 135, 140, 143]. Standard dose H_2-RAs are effective at reducing the risk of duodenal ulcers (RR = 0.24; 95% CI: 0.10–0.57, and RR = 0.36; 95% CI: 0.18–0.74 at one and three or more months respectively), but not of gastric ulcers (NS). One study did not have a placebo comparator and was not included in the pooled estimate [140].

Although achlorhydria has been reported not to prevent early NSAID induced gastric lesions [144], there is accumulating evidence that profound acid suppression can reduce acute NSAID and ASA induced gastric mucosal injury

[145–147]. Based on these observations, several investigators have tested the hypothesis that higher doses of H_2-receptor antagonists may achieve more consistent acid suppression and may therefore be effective for prevention of gastric ulcer among chronic NSAID users. We identified three RCTs that included 298 patients that assessed the efficacy of double dose H_2-RA for the prevention of tNSAID induced upper GI toxicity [130, 134, 148]. Double dose H_2-RAs when compared to placebo were associated with a statistically significant reduction in the risk of both duodenal (RR = 0.26; 95% CI: 0.11–0.65) and gastric ulcers (RR = 0.44; 95% CI: 026–0.74). This 56% relative risk reduction in gastric ulcer corresponds to a 12% absolute risk difference (from 23.1% to 11.3%). **A1c**

Analysis of the secondary prophylaxis studies alone yielded similar results.

Symptoms H_2-RAs, in standard or double doses, were not associated with an excess risk of total drop-outs, drop-outs due to adverse effects, or symptoms when compared to placebo. However, high dose H_2-RAs significantly reduced symptoms of abdominal pain when compared to placebo (RR = 0.57, 95% CI: 0.33–0.98).

H_2-RAs were generally quite well tolerated in the presented studies. Standard doses of these agents appear to be effective in preventing NSAID induced duodenal but not gastric ulcers. However, double dose H_2-receptor antagonists appear to be effective for healing and prevention of both gastric and duodenal ulcers in patients taking NSAIDs chronically. The clinical use of this class of drugs for the prevention of gastroduodenal ulceration may be questioned for several reasons. In terms of the trial results, the ulcer rates in the placebo groups of the famotidine studies are higher than are generally reported. Furthermore, since H_2-receptor antagonists are associated with tolerance to their acid suppressive effects [149–151], the long-term efficacy of these drugs must be questioned. Finally, even if effective for ulcer prevention, there is no economic or therapeutic advantage to using double doses of these drugs rather than standard doses of proton pump inhibitors that produce more potent and reliable acid suppression. **C5**

Proton pump inhibitors

Proton pump inhibitors (PPIs) block the final step of gastric acid secretion by inhibiting parietal cell H+-K+-ATPase. Direct evidence for the efficacy of PPIs in the primary or secondary prevention of clinically important NSAID induced upper gastrointestinal toxicity is lacking. Several factors have prompted interest in the use of PPIs for prophylaxis against NSAID induced ulcers: (1) dissatisfaction with the adverse effects of misoprostol; (2) the apparent efficacy of PPIs in healing NSAID ulcers; (3) the proven efficacy of PPIs in other acid-peptic disorders; (4) the attractive tolerability profile of PPIs.

PPIs appear to be effective for the prevention of early NSAID induced upper gastrointestinal injury assessed either endoscopically or through the detection of mucosal blood loss, in healthy volunteers given aspirin or naproxen

[145–147, 152]. However, as discussed previously the clinical relevance of these early lesions is in question.

Healing of ulcers with continued NSAID use

Omeprazole has been shown to heal both gastric and duodenal ulcers irrespective of continued NSAID use [79, 93, 127, 153–155]. Walan et al. in a double-blind trial, assessed the healing rates of benign gastric and prepyloric ulcers in 602 patients randomized to receive either omeprazole (40 mg or 20 mg) or ranitidine 150 mg bid [127]. In a subset of 58 patients with endoscopically documented ulcers who continued to take NSAIDs, the proportions of patients whose ulcers healed at eight weeks were: omeprazole 40 mg, 95% (similar to results for patients with non-NSAID ulcers), omeprazole 20 mg, 82% and ranitidine, 53%, (p < 0.05). These data suggest that selected patients with endoscopically documented NSAID ulcers can experience ulcer healing with omeprazole despite continued NSAID use. However, caution should be exercised in extrapolating these results to patients presenting with NSAID induced upper gastrointestinal hemorrhage. In these patients the decision to continue the NSAID must be individualized, since the safety and efficacy of omeprazole in this setting has not been assessed.

NSAID ulcer prevention

Six RCTs with 1259 patients assessed the effect of PPIs on the prevention of tNSAID induced upper GI toxicity [94, 113, 156–159].

PPIs significantly reduced the risk of both endoscopic duodenal (RR = 0.20; 95% CI: 0.10–0.39) and gastric ulcers (RR = 0.39; 95% CI: 0.31–0.50) compared to placebo (Figure 7.3) [94, 113, 156–159]. The results were similar for both primary and secondary prophylaxis trials. **A1a**

Study or subgroup	Treatment Events	Treatment Total	Control Events	Control Total	Weight	Risk ratio M-H, fxed, 95% CI	Risk ratio M-H, fixed, 95% CI
Bianchi Porro 2000	7	43	5	23	3.9%	0.75 (0.27, 2.10)	
Cullen 1998	3	83	9	85	5.4%	0.34 (0.10, 1.22)	
Ekstrom 1996	2	86	6	91	3.5%	0.35 (0.07, 1.70)	
Graham 2002	45	236	54	111	44.3%	0.39 (0.28, 0.54)	
Hawkey 1998	35	274	50	155	38.5%	0.40 (0.27, 0.58)	
Lai 2003	1	22	7	21	4.3%	0.14 (0.02, 1.02)	
Total (95% CI)		744		486	100.0%	0.39 (0.31, 0.50)	
Total events	93		131				
Heterogeneity: Chi² = 2.64, df = 5 (p = 0.75); I² = 0%							
Test for overall effect: Z = 7.79 (p < 0.00001)							

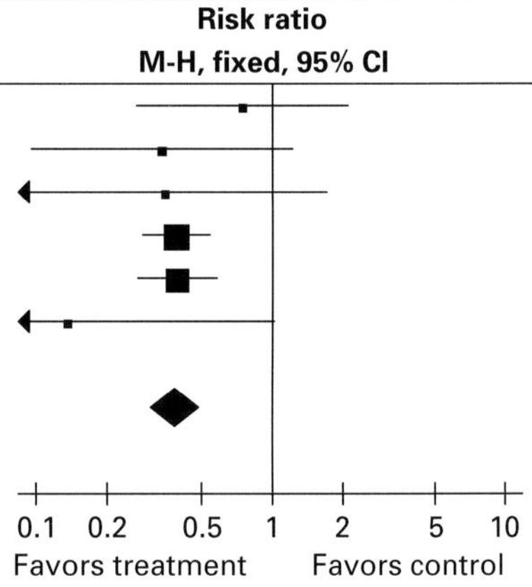

0.1   0.2   0.5   1   2   5   10
Favors treatment   Favors control

Figure 7.3 PPIs compared to placebo for the prevention of gastric ulcer in studies of eight weeks or longer duration. PPIs are effective for reducing the incidence of both gastric and duodenal ulcers. Data for gastric ulcers is shown.

Symptoms

Four omeprazole trials used the same composite endpoints to define treatment success [79, 113, 157, 158]. In these trials omeprazole significantly reduced "dyspeptic symptoms" as defined by the authors. In the combined analysis, drop-outs overall and drop-outs due to adverse effects were not different from placebo.

Head-to-head comparisons

Misoprostol vs H$_2$-RAs

Two trials with 600 patients compared misoprostol to ranitidine 150 mg twice daily [116, 120]. Misoprostol appears to be superior to standard dose ranitidine for the prevention of tNSAID induced gastric ulcers (RR = 0.12; 95% CI: 0.03–0.51) but not duodenal ulcers (RR = 1.00; 95% CI: 0.14–7.14). **A1a**

PPI vs H$_2$-RA

Yeomans *et al.* in a study of 425 patients, compared omeprazole 20 mg daily to ranitidine 150 mg twice daily for tNSAID prophylaxis [79]. In this study, omeprazole was superior to standard dose ranitidine for the prevention of both gastric (RR = 0.32; 95% CI: 0.17–0.62) and duodenal ulcers (RR = 0.11; 95% CI: 0.01–0.89). **A1a**

PPI vs misoprostol

Four trials with a total of 1478 patients [32, 94, 113, 115] compared a PPI to misoprostol. Two studies compared low dose misoprostol (400 ug) daily to a standard dose PPI [32, 113] or high dose misoprostol (800 ug) to lansoprazole 15 or 30 mg daily. PPIs are significantly more effective than misoprostol for the prevention of duodenal (RR = 0.25; 95% CI: 0.11–0.56), but not gastric (RR = 1.61; 95% CI: 0.88–3.06 random effects) or total gastroduodenal ulcers (RR = 0.90; 95% CI: 0.47–1.72 random effects). **A1a** The trial conducted by Hawkey *et al.* showed a non-significant trend towards greater benefit with misoprostol over omeprazole for the prevention of gastric ulcers, while the study reported by Graham *et al.* actually showed that misoprostol was superior to lansoprazole for the prevention of gastric ulcers. The pooled results mirrored these findings but did not demonstrate a statistically significant benefit of misopostol over PPIs (RR = 0.62; 95% CI: 0.33–1.18 random effects).

Symptoms

In the two head-to-head comparison of omeprazole and misoprostol [94, 113], PPIs were associated with signifi-

cantly fewer drop-outs overall (RR = 0.71; 95% CI: 0.52–0.97), as well as significantly fewer drop-outs due to adverse effects (RR = 0.48; 09% CI: 0.29–0.78). **A1a** When compared to H$_2$-RA used for less than two months, misoprostol caused significantly more drop-outs due to abdominal pain (RR = 3.00, 95% CI: 1.11, 8.14) and more symptoms of diarrhea (RR 2.03, 95% CI: 1.38, 2.99). **A1a** There were no significant differences in drop-outs due to adverse effects (RR 1.90, 95% CI: 0.77–4.67) or symptoms of abdominal pain or diarrhea between low dose H$_2$-RAs and PPIs. Misoprostol also appears to be associated with a lower quality of life amongst chronic tNSAID users compared to PPIs [79].

Summary

Collectively these studies demonstrate that PPIs are effective for healing both gastric and duodenal NSAID induced ulcers irrespective of continued NSAID use or *H. pylori* status. These agents also appear to be effective for the prevention of endoscopically diagnosed NSAID induced ulcers. In high risk GI patients (secondary prophylaxis), a study from Hong Kong suggested that strategies employing a COX-2 or an NSAID + PPI show similar efficacy at reducing re-bleeding events, though both strategies were associated with important re-bleeding rates [160, 161]. A second study performed in Hong Kong showed that for very high risk GI patients, a strategy of a COX-2+ a PPI was associated with very low re-bleeding rates [162]. **A1c**

The appropriate choice of therapy for secondary prophylaxis against NSAID ulcer recurrence among chronic NSAID users is unclear. Currently misoprostol is the only prophylactic agent of proven benefit for the prevention of NSAID induced clinical events. However, in reality most clinicians will prescribe a PPI to heal NSAID-induced ulcers, and will continue the same agent for secondary prophylaxis. Given the results of the OMNIUM and ASTRONAUT studies, this approach may be appropriate, but a degree of caution is indicated given the limitations of these studies, and the absence of direct evidence for effectiveness of PPIs for prevention of clinical gastrointestinal events. The cost-effectiveness of PPIs for the primary or secondary prophylaxis against NSAID induced upper gastrointestinal toxicity has not been established.

Cyclo-oxygenase-2 inhibitors

Since the publication of the last edition of this book, several endoscopic studies demonstrating the safety of COX-2 inhibitors, and several important clinical outcome studies similar to the misoprostol MUCOSA study have been published. In this section we will present the latest evidence for the GI safety of COX-2 inhibitors. We will concentrate on the following COX-2s: celecoxib, rofecoxib, etoricoxib, valdecoxib, and lumiracoxib.

NSAIDs are believed to exert their therapeutic anti-inflammatory and analgesic effects through the inhibition of inducible cyclo-oxygenase-2 (COX-2), whereas their gastric and renal toxicities, and antiplatelet effects appear to arise from the inhibition of the constitutive COX-1 isoform [28, 29]. This COX-2 hypothesis, along with the unfavorable safety profile of standard NSAIDs, has prompted the development of newer NSAIDs with selectivity for the COX-2 isoform.

Endoscopic ulcer trials

Cyclo-oxygenase-2s vs nonselective non-steroidal anti-inflammatory drugs

Seventeen studies with over 10,000 patients assessed the proportion of patients who developed endoscopic ulcers while taking a COX-2 compared to those taking a non-selective tNSAID [163–179]. There were seven studies that assessed celecoxib [163–165, 169, 175, 176, 178], three that assessed rofecoxib [166–168], two that assessed etoricoxib [173, 174], five that assessed valdecoxib [170–172, 177, 179], and two that assessed lumiracoxib [169, 175]. Some studies assessed more than one intervention [169, 175].

Endoscopically detected gastro-duodenal ulcers

Thirteen studies with a total of 7839 patients showed a 74% RRR (relative risk reduction) in combined gastro-duodenal ulcers with COX-2s versus tNSAIDs (RR = 0.26; 95% CI: 0.23–0.30) (Figure 7.4) [163–174, 180]. This represented a 16% absolute risk reduction (ARR) and NNT = 6. Addition of the FDA studies did not significantly alter the results (RR = 0.28; 95% CI: 0.24–0.32). **A1a**

Eleven studies with a total of 6726 patients compared the safety of a COX-2 to a comparator tNSAID for endoscopic gastric ulcers [163–172, 180]. The use of a COX-2 in this setting was associated with a 79% RRR in gastric ulcers (RR = 0.21; 95% CI: 0.18–0.25). This represented a 14% ARR in gastric ulcers with the use of COX-2s compared with tNSAIDs. (NNT = 7). Addition of the FDA studies did not significantly alter the results (RR = 0.26; 95% CI: 0.22–0.30). **A1a**

The same eleven studies also compared the proportions of duodenal ulcers that occurred while using a COX-2 versus a tNSAID [163–172, 180]. Compared to using a tNSAID, the use of a COX-2 was associated with a 66%

RRR in duodenal ulcers (RR = 0.34; 95% CI: 0.25–0.45) (Figure 7.4). This represented a 3% ARR (NNT = 33). **A1a** Addition of the FDA studies did not significantly alter the results (RR = 0.29; 95% CI: 0.23–0.38) Keeping in mind that tNSAID related gastric ulcers were more commonly observed than duodenal ulcers, a trend was observed for greater RRR and ARR for gastric ulcers than for duodenal ulcers with COX-2s, compared to tNSAIDs (RR = 0.21 vs 0.34, ARR of 14% vs 3%). This trend was consistent when celecoxib, rofecoxib and valdecoxib were analyzed separately.

Analysis by duration

The data presented above are for any dose and duration up to six months. Subgroup analysis of these studies on the basis of duration (1–3 months and 3–6 months) did not significantly alter the results.

Analysis by cyclo-oxygenase-2

Celecoxib

Five studies with a total of 2439 patients compared celecoxib to tNSAIDs, showing a 79% RRR in total gastro-duodenal ulcers (RR = 0.21; 95% CI: 0.16–0.28) with celecoxib [163–165, 169, 180]. Similar RRR were observed for gastric ulcers (RR = 0.20; 95% CI: 0.14–0.28) and duodenal ulcers alone (RR = 0.29; 95% CI: 0.18–0.47), as well as when the FDA studies were included (RR = 0.26; 95% CI: 0.21–0.32). **A1a**

Rofecoxib

Three studies with a total of 1526 patients compared rofecoxib to tNSAIDs [166–168]. In this case, a 74% RRR was seen with rofecoxib (RR = 0.26; 95% CI: 0.21–0.32). The results were similar when FDA studies were added to the analysis as well as when the analysis was done only for gastric ulcers (RR = 0.20; 95% CI: 0.15–0.26) or duodenal ulcers (RR = 0.36; 95% CI: 0.14–0.93 random effects). **A1a**

Etoricoxib

Two studies, with a total of 900 patients compared etoricoxib to tNSAIDs using the endpoint of endoscopic gastro-duodenal ulcers [173, 174]. These trials demonstrated a 64% RRR (RR = 0.37; 95% CI: 0.18–0.77 random effects) with etoricoxib. **A1a**

Valdecoxib

Three studies compared valdecoxib to tNSAIDs in 2045 patients and demonstrated a 70% RRR in gastro-duodenal ulcers (RR = 0.29; 95% CI: 0.21–0.39) with valdecoxib [170–172]. Similar RRR were observed when the analysis was done for gastric ulcers (RR = 0.24; 95% CI: 0.18–0.37) and duodenal ulcers alone (RR = 0.39; 95% CI: 0.21–0.70), and

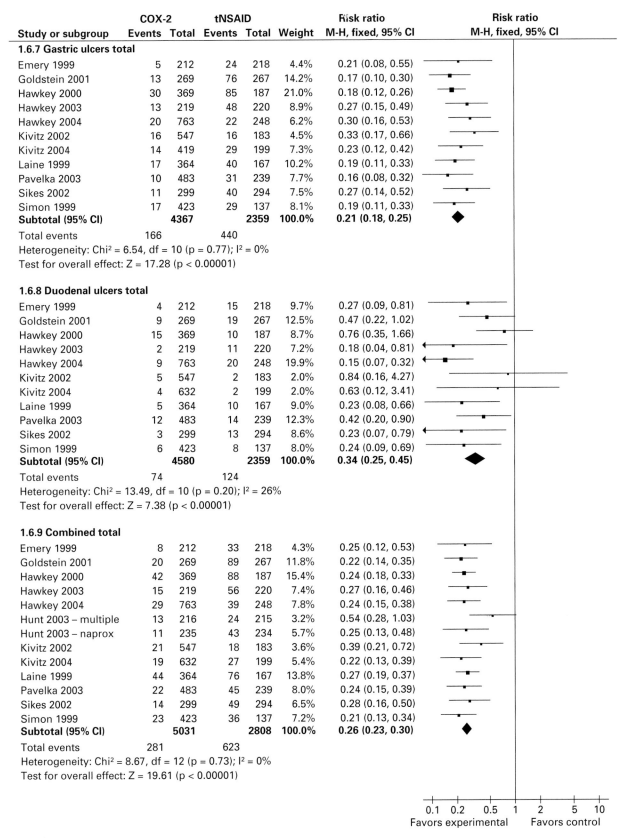

Figure 7.4 COX-2 inhibitors compared to tNSAIDs. Both low and high doses of COX-2s are associated with a significantly lower incidence of endoscopically detected gastric and duodenal ulcers compared to tNSAIDs. Data for "any" doses shown.

when the FDA studies were included in the gastro-duodenal ulcers analysis (RR = 0.30; 95% CI: 0.24–0.39). **A1a**

Lumiracoxib

Two studies with a total of 1376 patients compared lumiracoxib to tNSAIDs [180, 181]. Lumiracoxib was associated with a 74% RRR in gastro-duodenal ulcers (RR = 0.26; 95% CI: 0.18–0.39). Similar results were observed for gastric ulcers (RR = 0.25; 95% CI: 0.16–0.40) and duodenal ulcers (RR = 0.20; 95% CI: 0.09–0.43) when they were considered alone. **A1a**

Analysis by comparator non-steroidal anti-inflammatory drugs

Naproxen

Five studies compared either celecoxib or valdecoxib to naproxen in 2734 patients. These showed a 75% RRR in endoscopic gastro-duodenal ulcers in favour of the COX-2s (RR = 0.25; 95% CI: 0.20–0.32). Results were similar when the FDA studies were included in the analysis (RR = 0.27; 95% CI: 0.22–0.32) [163, 165, 168, 170, 174]. **A1a**

Ibuprofen

Six studies that included over 3800 patients (two rofecoxib [166, 167]; one etoricoxib [173]; two lumiracoxib [180, 181] and one valdecoxib [171]) showed a 73% RRR in gastro-duodenal ulcers with COX-2s compared with ibuprofen (RR = 0.27; 95% CI: 0.23–0.32). Results were similar when the FDA studies were included in the analysis (RR = 0.28; 95% CI: 0.23–0.32). **A1a**

Diclofenac

Three studies that included a total of 1596 patients demonstrated a 75% RRR in gastro-duodenal ulcers with COX-2s compared to diclofenac (RR = 0.25; 95% CI: 0.18–0.35). This effect was somewhat reduced when the FDA studies were included in the analysis (RR = 0.36; 95% CI: 0.27–0.47) [164, 171, 172]. **A1a**

Similar results were obtained when individual COX-2s were compared with the individual tNSAIDs.

Cyclo-oxygenase-2s vs placebo

Eight studies with a total of 4081 patients compared low and high-dose COX-2s to placebo [165–168, 170, 171, 173, 174]. Low dose COX-2s appeared to demonstrate no greater risk of gastric or gastro-duodenal ulcers than placebo. **A1a** However, there was a non-significant trend toward high dose COX-2s increasing the relative risk of gastric (RR = 1.22; 95% CI: 0.83–1.80) duodenal (RR = 1.29; 95% CI: 0.63–2.66), and combined gastro-duodenal ulcers (RR = 1.57; 95% CI: 0.96–2.56 random effects).

Clinical gastrointestinal events

Cyclo-oxygenase-2s vs non-selective non-steroidal anti-inflammatory drugs

Nine studies with a total of 94,294 patients assessed the safety of COX-2s by using the clinically important endpoint of ulcer complication, POB [52, 53, 182–188]. Three of these trials studied celecoxib [53, 182, 187], two studied rofecoxib [52, 183], two trials evaluated etoracoxib [186, 188], and one each evaluated valdecoxib [184] and lumiracoxib [185] separately. Overall, the use of these COX-2s was associated with a 57% RRR in POBs (RR, 0.43; 95% CI: 0.28–0.67 random effects), compared with using tNSAIDs (Figure 7.5). Removal of the combined analyses studies had no influence on the result (RR = 0.39; 0.29–0.53) and the inclusion of the FDA 12-month CLASS study data [53] did not alter the results (RR = 0.42; 95% CI: 0.33–0.54). The 60% RRR in these analyses represent an ARR of 0.4% (NNT = 250). **A1a**

Fourteen studies compared COX-2s with tNSAIDs by using PUB as the study endpoint [52, 53, 173, 182–192]. In this analysis, the use of a COX-2 was associated with a 57% RRR in PUBs (RR, 0.43; 95% CI, 0.34–0.55 random effects). Removal of the combined analyses studies eliminated the observed heterogeneity but had little effect on the point estimate (RR, 0.49; 95% CI, 0.41–0.58). Similarly, the use of the FDA CLASS data did not significantly alter the estimate (RR, 0.42; 95% CI: 0.33–0.53 random effects). **A1a**

Analyses stratified by cyclo-oxygenase-2s

Celecoxib

Four studies with 31,106 patients assessed the effect celecoxib versus tNSAIDs on clinical GI events (POBs or PUBs) [53, 182, 189]. Celecoxib use was associated with a 77% RRR in POBs (RR = 0.23; 95% CI: 0.07–0.76 random effects) and a 61% RRR in PUBs (RR = 0.39; 95% CI: 0.21–0.73 random effects). Removal of the combined analyses study [182] eliminated the heterogeneity observed in both the POB (RR = 0.42; 95% CI: 0.22–0.80) and PUBs (RR = 0.34; 95% CI: 0.22–0.80) analyses. The use of the FDA 12-month CLASS data did not alter the RR estimates for POBs or PUBs significantly. **A1a**

Rofecoxib

Four studies with 19,288 patients assessed the effect of rofecoxib versus tNSAIDs on clinical GI events (POBs or PUBs) [52, 183, 190, 192]. Rofecoxib use reduced the relative risk of POBs by 58% (RR = 0.42; 95% CI: 0.24–0.73) and the relative risk of PUBs by 56% (RR = 0.44; 95% CI: 0.34–0.58).

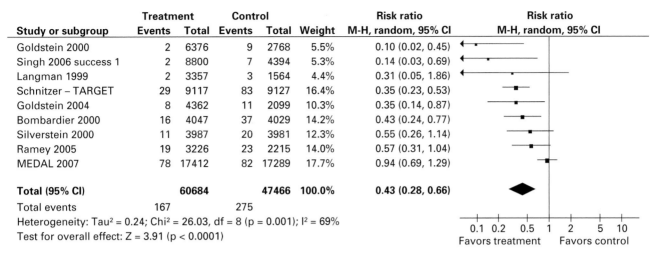

Study or subgroup	Treatment		Control		Weight	Risk ratio M-H, random, 95% CI	Risk ratio M-H, random, 95% CI
	Events	Total	Events	Total			
Goldstein 2000	2	6376	9	2768	5.5%	0.10 (0.02, 0.45)	
Singh 2006 success 1	2	8800	7	4394	5.3%	0.14 (0.03, 0.69)	
Langman 1999	2	3357	3	1564	4.4%	0.31 (0.05, 1.86)	
Schnitzer – TARGET	29	9117	83	9127	16.4%	0.35 (0.23, 0.53)	
Goldstein 2004	8	4362	11	2099	10.3%	0.35 (0.14, 0.87)	
Bombardier 2000	16	4047	37	4029	14.2%	0.43 (0.24, 0.77)	
Silverstein 2000	11	3987	20	3981	12.3%	0.55 (0.26, 1.14)	
Ramey 2005	19	3226	23	2215	14.0%	0.57 (0.31, 1.04)	
MEDAL 2007	78	17412	82	17289	17.7%	0.94 (0.69, 1.29)	
Total (95% CI)		**60684**		**47466**	**100.0%**	**0.43 (0.28, 0.66)**	
Total events	167		275				

Heterogeneity: Tau² = 0.24; Chi² = 26.03, df = 8 (p = 0.001); I² = 69%
Test for overall effect: Z = 3.91 (p < 0.0001)

Figure 7.5 COX-2 compared to tNSAIDs for clinically important ulcer complications. COX-2s are associated with significantly reduced incidence of POBs (perforation, obstructions or bleeding) than tNSAIDs. Removal of the MEDAL study eliminated the observed heterogeneity, likely stemming from the "real practice" design that allowed co-interventions such as PPIs. Data for PUBs (not shown) are similar.

Removal of the combined analysis study did not alter the point estimates. **A1a**

Valdecoxib

One combined analysis study with 6461 patients evaluated the effect of valdecoxib on POBs and PUBs [184]. Valdecoxib reduced the relative risk of POBs by 65% (RR = 0.35; 95% CI: 0.14–0.87) and the relative risk of PUBs by 77% (RR = 0.23; 95% CI: 0.15–0.36). **A1a**

Etoricoxib

Four studies with 10, 856 evaluated the effect of etoricoxib on POBs [186, 188] and PUBs [173, 191]. Etoricoxib demonstrated a non-significant trend in reducing the risk of POBs (RR = 0.82; 95% CI: 0.44–1.51 random effects), but it significantly reduced the RR of PUBs by 46% (RR = 0.64; 95% CI: 0.42–0.96). **A1a**

Lumiracoxib

One study with 18,244 patients demonstrated a significant 64% RRR in POBs (RR = 0.36; 95% CI: 0.24–0.55) and a 44% RRR in PUBs (RR = 0.56; 0.41–0.78) with the use of lumiracoxib, compared with using tNSAIDs [185]. **A1a**

Analysis by comparator non-steroidal anti-inflammatory drugs

In general, COX-2s appeared to maintain their safety advantage regardless of the comparator tNSAID. COX-2s were statistically superior to naproxen (RR = 0.34; 95% CI: 0.24–0.48), and ibuprofen (RR = 0.46; 95% CI: 0.30–0.71) for the POB endpoint. The data comparing COX-2s to diclofenac are predominately derived from two studies and heavily influenced by the CLASS trial data which showed no significant difference between celecoxib vs diclofenac [53, 182]. In the current analysis, celecoxib demonstrated a non-significant trend towards fewer POBs than diclofenac (RR = 0.31; 95% CI: 0.06–1.61) while a statistically significant 59% RRR in PUBs was observed (RR = 0.41; 95% 0.30–0.55). **A1a**

Cyclo-oxygenase-2s vs placebo

There are limited data, mostly derived from the combined analyses studies, comparing COX-2s with placebo for the clinical outcomes of POBs [182, 184] and PUBs [182–184, 189, 191]. In these analyses, the use of COX-2s was associated with non-significant trends toward an increased RR of POBs (RR = 2.66; 95% CI: 0.34–20.95) and PUBs (RR = 2.26; 95% CI: 0.96–5.33). These findings are supported by the APPROVe polyp prevention study, which demonstrated that over a three-year period, rofecoxib was associated with a statistically significant 4.9-fold increased risk of clinical ulcer complications compared to placebo [193].

Influence of acetylsalicylic acid co-administration on clinically important ulcer complications

Five trials allowed assessment of the effects of the co-administration of acetylsalicylic acid (ASA) with a COX-2 [53, 184, 185, 188, 194]. In a pooled subgroup analysis of over 18,000 patients taking ASA, there was no statistically significant difference in the RR of ulcer complications (POBs) between those in the COX-2 arms and those in the non-selective arms of these trials (RR =, 0.93; 95% CI: 0.68–1.27 for POBs). **A1a** A small advantage of COX-2s over tNSAIDs cannot be ruled out by these results because this subgroup analysis may lack adequate power. The PUB analysis showed a statistically significant benefit for COX-2+ASA vs tNSAID+ASA (RR = 0.72; 95% CI: 0.62–0.95), but data from one study could not be used in this analysis. In more than 40,000 patients in the COX-2 arms, patients taking ASA had a 3.46 (95% CI: 2.44–4.91) greater RR of POBs than COX-2 users not taking ASA. **A1a** Among 34,000 patients in the tNSAID arms of these studies, those taking ASA had a 1.65 greater RR of POBs than those not taking ASA, although this result was not statistically significant (95% CI: 0.76–3.57). These are *post hoc* subgroup analyses that may be subject to bias. Furthermore, the subgroup analysis within a tNSAID treatment group (e.g. COX-2 vs COX-2 + ASA) represents a non-randomized comparison in which differences could be influenced by factors other than ASA use.

Addition of a proton pump inhibitor to cyclo-oxygenase-2s

The comparative safety of a COX-2s compared to a tNSAID with a PPI has been addressed in high-risk patients with recent ulcer bleeding who were enrolled after ulcer healing and *H. pylori* eradication. Chan *et al.* [161] found recurrent ulcer bleeding at six months to occur in 4.9% of patients treated with celecoxib 200 mg twice daily and in 6.4% of those treated with diclofenac 75 mg twice daily plus omeprazole 20 mg daily. Lai *et al.* [195] found recurrent ulcer complications (bleeding and one case of severe pain) in 3.7% with celecoxib 200 mg daily and 6.3% with naproxen 750 mg daily plus lansoprazole 30 mg daily at a median follow-up of 24 weeks. These results suggest high risk patients have high rates of recurrent bleeding even with the protective strategy of a coxib or a tNSAID + PPI. **A1d**

The combination of a coxib and PPI was assessed in the same high-risk population in a subsequent one-year study by Chan *et al.* [162]. Recurrent ulcer bleeding occurred in 9% of patients who received celecoxib alone vs 0% in patients treated with celecoxib plus twice daily esomeprazole. The MEDAL Program also demonstrated that a coxib plus PPI resulted in significantly fewer upper GI clinical events (again, driven by a decrease in uncomplicated events) compared to a tNSAID plus PPI (RR = 0.62; 0.45–0.83) [188]. **A1d**

Symptoms and treatment withdrawals

Treatment withdrawals as a result of gastrointestinal side effects: cyclo-oxygenase-2s vs non-selective non-steroidal anti-inflammatory drugs

Twenty-one studies that included approximately 47,000 patients assessed the effect of COX-2s on patient withdraw-

als due to GI symptoms [52, 53, 163–165, 174, 179, 187, 189, 190–192, 196–204]. Overall, compared to tNSAIDs, COX-2s were associated with a significantly lower relative risk of withdrawals due to GI "side effects" (RR = 0.65; 95% CI: 0.57–0.73 random effects), withdrawals due to dyspepsia (RR = 0.37; 95% CI: 0.18–0.74), and due to abdominal pain (RR = 0.25; 95% CI: 0.13–0.49). **A1a** Compared to placebo, low dose COX-2s showed no statistically significant difference for these same endpoints, while high dose COX-2s were associated with a small but significantly increased relative risk of drop-outs due to GI "side effects" (RR = 1.74; 95% CI: 1.13–2.68) **A1a**

Adverse gastrointestinal symptoms with cyclo-oxygenase-2s compared with non-selective non-steroidal anti-inflammatory drugs

Twenty-eight studies that included approximately 60,000 patients assessed the effect of low or high dose COX-2s compared to tNSAIDs for treatment-related overall GI adverse effects, dyspepsia, nausea and abdominal pain [53, 163, 164, 169, 171, 172, 180, 185, 189–191, 197–199, 201, 203, 205–210]. Low dose COX-2s were associated with a lower relative risk of "GI symptoms" (RR = 0.78; 95% CI: 0.74–0.82); dyspepsia (RR = 0.83; 95% CI: 0.75–0.90); nausea (RR = 0.72; 95% CI: 0.64–0.82); and abdominal pain (RR = 0.64; 95% CI: 0.58–0.70). The results for high dose COX-2s were similar. **A1a**

Adverse gastrointestinal symptoms with cyclo-oxygenase-2s compared with placebo

Twenty studies with over 10,000 patients compared the occurrence of adverse GI symptoms between COX-2s and placebo. Low dose COX-2s were associated with a slight but statistically significant increased relative risk of overall "GI symptoms" (RR = 1.26; 95% CI: 1.13–1.42); dyspepsia (RR = 1.28; 95% CI: 1.08–1.51); nausea (RR = 1.24; 95% CI: 1.01–1.53); and abdominal pain (RR = 1.24; 95% CI: 1.02–1.52) [170, 171, 189–191, 201, 203–216]. The results for high dose COX-2s were similar. **A1a**

Summary

The results of these systematic reviews demonstrate that there are several therapeutic strategies available to reduce the incidence of tNSAID related upper GI harms. Large, well powered, studies have shown that strategies using either a tNSAID with misoprostol, or the use of a COX-2 inhibitor instead of a tNSAID reduce the incidence of endoscopically detected upper GI ulcerations, and clinically important UGI events such as bleeding. **A1a** Misoprostol in doses that prevent UGI ulcer complications is associated with important adverse effects that may limit its long-term use. Standard doses of H_2-RAs reduce the incidence of duodenal ulcers but not gastric ulcers. Double doses of H_2-RAs and standard dose PPIs reduce the incidence of duodenal as well as gastric ulcers, but because tachyphylaxis can occur with chronic H_2-RA use, a standard dose PPI strategy is preferred. **A1a C5** H_2-RAs and PPIs have not been directly assessed in large primary prevention clinical outcome studies powered to detect ulcer complications. However, in secondary prevention studies of high risk GI patients, tNSAIDs with a PPI, appear as effective as a COX-2s strategy at preventing clinical ulcer complications. In these high risk patients, these strategies were still associated with important ulcer relapse rates, suggesting that both strategies may provide incomplete protection for the secondary prevention of NSAID related ulcers. However, a recent study has shown that a strategy of combining a PPI with a COX-2s was superior to a COX-2s alone for the secondary prevention of ulcer complications, suggesting that a COX-2s+ PPI strategy is the preferred strategy in high risk GI patients. **A1d** Furthermore, the current meta-analysis, supported by the APPROVe polyp prevention study [193] has shown that while COX-2s offer greater GI safety than tNSAIDs as a group, COX-2s are associated with a statistically greater risk of clinical upper GI complications than is observed with placebo. **A1a**

The discovery that COX-2s are associated with important CVS harms has complicated the clinical use of NSAIDs significantly. Furthermore, in Canada all COX-2s except celecoxib, have been withdrawn from the market due to cardiovascular and other harms and it is unlikely that a new COX-2s will be released to market unless it is truly "cardiovascularly neutral" or it is combined with a "GI safe" antithrombotic agent. During this time of uncertainty, when physicians were actively switching patients back to tNSAIDs + a gastroprotective agent such as a PPI, it became increasingly clear that non-naproxen tNSAIDs were also associated with important CVS harms. A meta-analysis by Kearney *et al.* using an extensive set of RCT data derived from published and unpublished studies has suggested that, as a group, COX-2s are associated with an increased risk of CV outcomes when compared with placebo or naproxen, but not when compared with non-naproxen-non-ASA tNSAIDs [30], suggesting that non-naproxen-tNSAIDs share the cardiovascular harms of COX-2s. **A1a**

In light of the cardiovascular harm data relating to COX-2s, it is tempting to suggest combining these agents with ASA. However, the available data from this meta-analysis suggest that this strategy would likely undermine the GI safety advantage of COX-2s. In patients taking ASA, we found no statistically significant difference in POBs or PUBs in patients randomized to a COX-2 or a tNSAID. However, the analyses did not stratify the randomization for ASA use. Thus, it is possible that other patient-related

factors played a role in this result. Furthermore, although the analysis included about 7000 patients, it is still possible that a protective effect of COX-2s over tNSAIDs in this setting is present but not detected because of insufficient statistical power. We also found that the addition of ASA to a COX-2 significantly increased the risk of a POB 4.12 times over that observed with a COX-2 alone, and that the addition of ASA to a tNSAID demonstrated a non-significant 1.27 increased risk of POBs over the use of a tNSAID alone. These analyses represent non-randomized comparisons, and the group sizes were somewhat uneven (more patients in the COX-2 or tNSAID alone groups than in the groups with ASA). Nonetheless, the results are not entirely unexpected, because it has been known for some time that concomitant use of multiple tNSAIDs increases the risk of GI complications over a single tNSAID alone. These results are also in keeping with an RCT by Laine *et al.* [217], revealing that the incidence of endoscopically detected ulcers with rofecoxib and low-dose ASA was not lower than that seen with ibuprofen alone. However, it is clear that further study in this area is required to verify these findings, such as performance of a dedicated RCT or from analysis of individual patient data in systematic reviews. Further, adding ASA to a COX-2 implies that the COX-2s will not interfere with the effect of ASA. However, this hypothesis also requires further study, because there are suggestions that the use of a tNSAID might interfere with the action of ASA in this setting, although there appears to be less interference from selective COX-2s [218–222].

When COX-2s were released, they promised an era of improved GI safety, as well as an era of greater clinical simplicity, with the option of prescribing a single low risk agent when chronic NSAID use was required. However, with the greater understanding of the GI, cardiovascular, and other end organ safety profile of tNSAIDs and COX-2s, clinicians must now stratify their patients on the basis of GI, CVS, and other organ system risk factors and choose an NSAID strategy that minimizes a patient's overall risk. This has become especially difficult for patients who are known to be at high risk of GI and CVS harms.

Figure 7.6 presents an evidence-based algorithm for the use of long-term NSAID therapy according to individual gastrointestinal and cardiovascular risk. Since low-dose ASA is recommended for patients at increased cardiovascular risk [223, 224], the algorithm assumes the use of low-dose ASA in such patients. For patients with both low gastrointestinal and cardiovascular risk, a tNSAID alone may be acceptable. For patients with low gastrointestinal risk and high cardiovascular risk, naproxen may be preferred because of the potentially lower cardiovascular risk with this drug than with other tNSAIDs or COX-2 inhibitors. However, since these patients are assumed to be on low-dose ASA therapy, the combination of naproxen plus ASA would increase the gastrointestinal risk, and there-

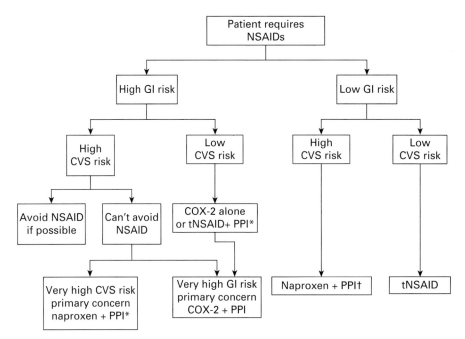

Figure 7.6 Algorithm for management of patients requiring long-term NSAID therapy (Canadian Association of Gastroenterology Consensus Conference).

*In high risk patients a COX-2 inhibitor and a tNSAID + PPI show similar reductions of rebleeding rates, but these reductions may be incomplete.

†In general, most patients on ASA + naproxen would need the addition of a PPI. However, for some patients at very low GI risk naproxen alone may be appropriate.

fore, the addition of a gastroprotective agent such as a PPI should be considered.

Long-term NSAID therapy is more complex in patients with high gastrointestinal risk. Testing for and eradicating *H. pylori* in patients at high risk of NSAID-related gastrointestinal bleeding should be considered, but this strategy will be insufficient without ongoing gastroprotection [159, 225–228]. In these patients, if cardiovascular risk is low, the use of a COX-2 inhibitor alone or a tNSAID with a PPI appear to offer similar protection from recurrent gastrointestinal bleeding, but this protection is incomplete. Therefore, for patients at very high risk of upper gastrointestinal events, the combination of a COX-2 inhibitor plus a PPI may offer the best gastrointestinal safety profile. When both gastrointestinal and cardiovascular risks are high, the optimal strategy is to avoid NSAID therapy if at all possible. If NSAID therapy is deemed to be necessary, then the clinician must prioritize the cardiovascular and gastrointestinal risks, recognizing that these patients are likely taking ASA for their cardiovascular risk. If gastrointestinal risk is the primary concern (i.e. a very high risk gastrointestinal patient), a COX-2 inhibitor plus a PPI is recommended. If the primary concern is cardiovascular risk, naproxen plus a PPI in patients on ASA would be preferred. However, gastrointestinal risk should be closely monitored as this strategy carries a higher gastrointestinal

risk than a COX-2 inhibitor plus a PPI in patients on ASA (Figure 7.6) [229].

References

1 Fries JF, Miller SR, Spitz PW, Williams CA, Hubert HB, Bloch DA. Identification of patients at risk for gastropathy associated with NSAID use. *Journal of Rheumatology* 1990; **20**(suppl): 12–19.

2 Patr o. Aspirin as an anti-platelet drug. *N Eng J Med* 1994; **330**: 1287–1294.

3 Stroke prevention in atrial fibrillation investigators. Stroke prevention in atrial fibrillation study: Final results. *Circulation* 1991; **84**: 527–539.

4 Steering Committee of the physicians' health study research group: Final report on the aspirin component of the ongoing physician's health study. *N Eng J Med* 1989; **321**: 129–135.

5 The SALT collaborative study group. Swedish aspirin low-dose trial of 75 mg aspirin as secondary prophylaxis after cerebrovascular ischemic events. *Lancet* 1991; **338**: 1345–49.

6 Wallace JL. Nonsteroidal anti-inflammatory drugs and gastroenteropathy: The second hundred years. *Gastroenterology* 1997; **112**(3): 1000–1016.

7 Barnard L, Lavoie D, Lajeunesse N. Increase in nonfatal digestive perforations and haemorrhages following introduction of selective NSAIDs: A public health concern. *Drug Saf* 2006; **29**(7): 613–620.

8 Roumie CL, Arbogast PG, Mitchel EF, Jr., Griffin MR. Prescriptions for chronic high-dose cyclooxygenase-2 inhibitors are often inappropriate and potentially dangerous. *J Gen Intern Med* 2005; **20**(10): 879–883.

9 Dube C, Rostom A, Lewin G *et al*. The use of aspirin for primary prevention of colorectal cancer: a systematic review prepared for the US Preventive Services Task Force. *Ann Intern Med* 2007; **146**(5): 365–375.

10 Rostom A, Dube C, Lewin G *et al*. Nonsteroidal anti-inflammatory drugs and cyclooxygenase-2 inhibitors for primary prevention of colorectal cancer: A systematic review prepared for the US Preventive Services Task Force. *Ann Intern Med* 2007; **146**(5):376–389.

11 Smalley WE, Griffin MR, Fought RL, Ray WA. Excess costs from gastrointestinal disease associated with nonsteroidal anti-inflammatory drugs. *J Gen Intern Med* 1996; **11**(8): 461–469.

12 Larkai E, Smith J, Lidsky M. Gastroduodenal mucosa and dyspeptic symptoms in arthritic patients during chronic non-steroidal anti-inflammatory drug use. *Am J Gastroenterol* 1987; **82**: 1153–1158.

13 Silverstein FE, Graham DY, Senior JR *et al*. Misoprostol reduces serious gastrointestinal complications in patients with rheumatoid arthritis receiving nonsteroidal anti-inflammatory drugs. A randomized, double-blind, placebo-controlled trial. *Ann Intern Med* 1995; **123**(4): 241–249.

14 Stalnikowicz R, Rachmilewitz D. NSAID-induced gastroduodenal damage: Is prevention needed? A review and metaanalysis. *J Clin Gastroenterol* 1993; **17**(3): 238–243.

15 Fries JF. NSAID gastropathy: The second most deadly rheumatic disease? Epidemiology and risk appraisal. *Journal of Rheumatology* 1991; **28**(Suppl): 6–10.

16 Griffin MR, Ray WA, Schaffner W. Nonsteroidal anti-inflammatory drug use and death from peptic ulcer in elderly persons. *Ann Intern Med* 1988; **109**(5): 359–363.

17 Bollini P, Rodriguez G, Gutthann S. The impact of research quality and study design on epidemiologic estimates of the effect of nonsteroidal anti-inflammatory drugs on upper gastrointestinal tract disease. *Arch Intern Med* 1992; **152**: 1289–1295.

18 McMahon AD, Evans JM, White G *et al*. A cohort study (with re-sampled comparator groups) to measure the association between new NSAID prescribing and upper gastrointestinal hemorrhage and perforation. *J Clin Epidemiol* 1997; **50**(3): 351–356.

19 Gabriel S, Jaakkimainen L, Bombardier C. Risk for serious gastrointestinal complications related to use of non-steroidal anti-inflammatory drugs: A meta-analysis. *Ann Intern Med* 1991; **115**: 787–796.

20 Langman MJ, Weil J, Wainwright P *et al*. Risks of bleeding peptic ulcer associated with individual non-steroidal anti-inflammatory drugs. *Lancet* 1994; **343**(8905): 1075–1078.

21 MacDonald T, Morant S, Robinson G. Association of upper Gastrointestinal toxicity of non-steroidal anti-inflammatory drugs with continued exposure: Cohort Study. *BMJ* 1997; **315**(22): 1333–1337.

22 Armstrong C, Blower A. Nonsteroidal antiinflammatory drugs and life threatening complications of peptic ulceration. *Gut* 1987; **28**(5): 527–532.

23 Kaufmann HJ, Taubin HL. Nonsteroidal anti-inflammatory drugs activate quiescent inflammatory bowel disease. *Ann Intern Med* 1987; **107**: 513–516.

24 Wallace JL. NSAID gastroenteropathy: Past, present and future. *Can J Gastroenterol* 1996; **10**(7): 451–459.

25 Matsuhashi N, Yamada A, Hiraishi M *et al*. Multiple strictures of the small intestine after long-term nonsteroidal anti-inflammatory drug therapy. *Am J Gastroenterol* 1992; **87**(9): 1183–1186.

26 Tannenbaum H, Davis P, Russell AS *et al*. An evidence-based approach to prescribing NSAIDs in musculoskeletal disease: a Canadian consensus. Canadian NSAID Consensus Participants. *CMAJ* 1996; **155**(1): 77–88.

27 Lichtenstein DR, Syngal S, Wolfe MM. Nonsteroidal antiinflammatory drugs and the gastrointestinal tract. The double-edged sword. *Arthritis & Rheumatism* 1995; **38**(1): 5–18.

28 Dvornik DM. Tissue selective inhibition of prostaglandin biosynthesis by etodolac. *Journal of Rheumatology* 1997; **47**(suppl): 40–47.

29 Robinson DR. Regulation of prostoglandin synthesis by anti-inflammatory drugs. *J Rheumatol* 1997; **24** (Suppl 47): 32–39.

30 Kearney PM, Baigent C, Godwin J, Halls H, Emberson J, Patrono C. Do selective cyclo-oxygenase-2 inhibitors and traditional non-steroidal anti-inflammatory drugs increase the risk of atherothrombosis? Meta-analysis of randomised trials. *Br Med J* 2006; **332**: 1302–1308.

31 McGettigan P, Henry D. Cardiovascular risk and inhibition of cyclooxygenase: a systematic review of the observational studies of selective and nonselective inhibitors of cyclooxygenase 2. *Journal of the American Medical Association* 2006; **296**(13): 1633–1644.

32 Stupnicki T, Dietrich K, Gonzalez-Carro P *et al*. Efficacy and tolerability of pantoprazole compared with misoprostol for the prevention of NSAID-related gastrointestinal lesions and symptoms in rheumatic patients. *Digestion* 2003; **68**(4): 198–208.

33 Melo GA, Roth SH, Zeeh J, Bruyn GA, Woods EM, Geis GS. Double-blind comparison of efficacy and gastroduodenal safety of diclofenac/misoprostol, piroxicam, and naproxen in the treatment of osteoarthritis. *Ann Rheum Dis* 1993; **52**(12): 881–885.

34 Watson DJ, Rahme E, Santanello NC. Increase in nonfatal digestive perforations and haemorrhages following introduction of selective NSAIDs: A public health concern. *Drug Saf* 2007; **30**(1): 89–90.

35 Hallas J, Lauritsen J, Villadsen HD, Gram LF. Nonsteroidal anti-inflammatory drugs and upper gastrointestinal bleeding, identifying high-risk groups by excess risk estimates. *Scand J Gastroenterol* 1995; **30**(5): 438–444.

36 Hansen JM, Hallas J, Lauritsen JM, Bytzer P. Non-steroidal anti-inflammatory drugs and ulcer complications: A risk factor analysis for clinical decision-making. *Scand J Gastroenterol* 1996; **31**(2): 126–130.

37 Laporte JR, Carne X, Vidal X, Moreno V. Upper gastrointestinal bleeding in relation to previous use of analgesics and non-steroidal anti-inflammatory drugs. *Lancet* 1991; **337**: 85–89.

38 Rodriguez LA. Nonsteroidal anti-inflammatory drugs, ulcers and risks: A collaborative meta-analysis. *Seminars in Arthritis & Rheumatism* 1997; **26**: 16–20.

39 Hochain P, Berkelmans I, Czernichow P et al. Which patients taking non-aspirin non-steroidal anti-inflammatory drugs bleed? A case-control study. *Eur J Gastroenterology & Hepatology* 1995; **7**(5): 419–426.

40 Scheiman JM. Nsaids, gastrointestinal injury, and cytoprotection. *Gastroenterol Clin North Am* 1998; **25**(2): 270–298.

41 Gutthann SP, Garcia RL, Raiford DS. Individual nonsteroidal antiinflammatory drugs and other risk factors for upper gastrointestinal bleeding and perforation. *Epidemiology* 1997; **8**(1): 18–24.

42 Henry D, Dobson A, Turner C. Variability in the risk of major gastrointestinal complications from nonaspirin nonsteroidal anti-inflammatory drugs. *Gastroenterology* 1993; **105**(4): 1078–1088.

43 Henry D, Lim LL, Garcia RL et al. Variability in risk of gastrointestinal complications with individual non-steroidal anti-inflammatory drugs: Results of a collaborative meta-analysis. *BMJ* 1996; **312**(7046): 1563–1566.

44 Smalley WE, Griffin MR. The risks and costs of upper gastrointestinal disease attributable to NSAIDs. *Gastroenterol Clin North Am* 1996; **25**(2): 373–396.

45 Carson JL, Strom BL, Morse ML, West SL. The relative gastrointestinal toxicity of the non-steroidal anti-inflammatory drugs. *Arch Intern Med* 1987; **147**: 1054–1059.

46 Griffin M, Piper J, Daughtery J, Snowden M. Non-steroidal anti-inflammatory drug use and increased risk for peptic ulcer disease in elderly persons. *Ann Intern Med* 1991; **114**: 257–263.

47 Wynne HA, Long A. Patient awareness of the adverse effects of non-steroidal anti-inflammatory drugs (NSAIDs). *Br J Clin Pharmacol* 1996; **42**(2): 253–256.

48 Jorde R, Burhol PG. Asymptomatic peptic ulcer disease. *Scand J Gastroenterol* 1987; **22**: 129–34.

49 Graham DY. High-dose famotidine for prevention of NSAID ulcers? *Gastroenterology* 1997; **112**(6): 2143–2145.

50 Robbins SL, Cotran RS, Kumar V. *Pathologic Basis of Disease*. 3rd ed. W.B. Saunders Company, Philadelphia, 1984.

51 Maetzel A, Ferraz MB, Bombardier C. The cost-effectiveness of misoprostol in preventing serious gastrointestinal events associated with the use of nonsteroidal antiinflammatory drugs. *Arthritis & Rheumatism* 1998; **41**(1): 16–25.

52 Bombardier C, Laine L, Reicin A et al. Comparison of upper gastrointestinal toxicity of rofecoxib and naproxen in patients with rheumatoid arthritis. VIGOR Study Group. *N Engl J Med* 2000; **343**(21): 1520–1528.

53 Silverstein FE, Faich G, Goldstein JL et al. Gastrointestinal toxicity with celecoxib vs nonsteroidal anti-inflammatory drugs for osteoarthritis and rheumatoid arthritis: The CLASS study: A randomized controlled trial. Celecoxib Long-term Arthritis Safety Study. *Journal of the American Medical Association* 2000; **284**(10): 1247–1255.

54 Rostom A, Wells G, Tugwell P, Welch V, Dube C, McGowan J. Prevention of NSAID-induced gastroduodenal ulcers. (update of Cochrane Database Syst Rev. 2000;(3):CD002296; 10908548). (Review). *Cochrane Database of Systematic Reviews* 2002 (4): CD002296.

55 Rostom A, Wells G, Tugwell P, Welch V, Dube C, McGowan J. The prevention of chronic NSAID induced upper gastrointestinal toxicity: a Cochrane collaboration metaanalysis of rand-omized controlled trials. *Journal of Rheumatology* 2000; **27**(9): 2203–2214.

56 Rostom A, Dube C, Jolicoeur E, Boucher M, Joyce J. *Evaluation Of Pharmacological Interventions For The Prevention Of Gastroduodenal Ulcers Associated With The Use Of Non Steroidal Antiinflammatory Drugs: A Systematic Review*. Canadian Coordinating Office for Health Technology Assessment (CCOHTA) 168. 2003. CCOHTA, Ottawa, Canada.

57 Van Der Hulst R, Rauws E, Koycu B. Recurrence after eradication of *Helicobacter pylori*: A prospective long-term follow-up study. *Gastroenterology* 1997; **113**: 1082–1086.

58 Rauws EJ, Tytgat GN. *Helicobacter pylori* in duodenal and gastric ulcer disease. *Baillieres Clinical Gastroenterology* 1995; **9**(3): 529–547.

59 Veldhuyzen van Zanten SJ, Sherman PM. *Helicobacter pylori* infection as a cause of gastritis, duodenal ulcer, gastric cancer and nonulcer dyspepsia: a systematic overview. *CMAJ* 1994; **150**(2): 177–185.

60 Kurata JH, Nogawa AN. Meta-analysis of risk factors for peptic ulcer. Nonsteroidal antiinflammatory drugs, *Helicobacter pylori*, and smoking. *J Clin Gastroenterol* 1997; **24**(1): 2–17.

61 Veldhuyzen Van Zanten S. Ulcers, *H. pylori*, NSAIDs, and dyspepsia. *Gastroenterology* 1997; **113**(Suppl 6): S90–S92.

62 Borody Tj, George LL, Brandl S. *Helicobacter pylori*-negative duodenal ulcer. *Am J Gastroenterol* 1991; **86**: 1154–1157.

63 Laine L, Martin-Sorensen M, Weinstein W. Nsaid-associated gastric ulcers do not require *H. pylori* for their development. *Am J Gastroenterol* 1992; **87**: 1398–1402.

64 McColl K, El-Nujumi A, Chittajullu R. A study of the pathogenesis of *Helicobacter pylori*-negative duodenal ulceration. *Gut* 1993; **34**: 762–768.

65 Dooley CP, Cohen H, Fitzgibbon Pl. Prevalence of *Helicobacter pylori* infection and histologic gastritis in asymptomatic persons. *N Engl J Med* 1989; **321**: 1562–1566.

66 Graham DY, Lidsky MD, Cox AM et al. Long-term nonsteroidal antiinflammatory drug use and *Helicobacter pylori* infection. *Gastroenterology* 1991; **100**(6): 1653–1657.

67 Sontag SJ. Guilty as charged: bugs and drugs in gastric ulcer. *Am J Gastroenterol* 1997; **92**(8): 1255–1261.

68 Graham DY. Nonsteroidal anti-inflammatory drugs, *Helicobacter pylori*, and ulcers: where we stand. *Am J Gastroenterol* 1996; **91**(10): 2080–2086.

69 Hudson N, Balsitis M, Filipowicz F. Effect of *Helicobacter pylori* colonization on gastric mucosal eicosanoid synthesis in patients taking Nsaids. *Gut* 1993; **34**: 748–751.

70 Laine L, Cominelli F, Sloane R, Casini-Raggi V, Marin-Sorensen M, Weinstein WM. Interaction of NSAIDs and *Helicobacter pylori* on gastrointestinal injury and prostaglandin production: A controlled double-blind trial. *Alimentary Pharmacology & Therapeutics* 1995; **9**(2): 127–135.

71 Konturek J, Dembinski A, Konturek SJ. Infection of *Helicobacter pylori* and gastric adaptation to continued administration of aspirin in humans. *Gastroenterology* 1998; **114**: 245–255.

72 Loeb DS, Talley NJ, Ahlquist DA, Carpenter HA, Zinsmeister AR. Long-term nonsteroidal anti-inflammatory drug use and gastroduodenal injury: The role of *Helicobacter pylori*. *Gastroenterology* 1992; **102**(6): 1899–1905.

73 Lipscomb GR, Wallis N, Armstrong G, Goodman MJ, Rees WD. Influence of *Helicobacter pylori* on gastric mucosal adaptation to

naproxen in man. *Digestive Diseases & Sciences* 1996; **41**(8): 1583–1588.

74 Huang JQ, Sridhar S, Hunt RH. Role of *Helicobacter pylori* infection and non-steroidal anti-inflammatory drugs in peptic-ulcer disease: A meta-analysis. *Lancet* 2002; **359**(9300): 14–22.

75 Soll AH. Pathogenesis of peptic ulcer and implications for therapy. *N Engl J Med* 1990; **322**: 909–916.

76 Soll AH. Consensus conference. Medical treatment of peptic ulcer disease. Practice guidelines. Practice Parameters Committee of the American College of Gastroenterology. *Journal of the American Medical Association* 1996; **275**(8): 622–629.

77 Somerville K, Faulkner G, Langman M. Non-steroidal anti-inflammatory drugs and bleeding peptic ulcer. *Lancet* 1986; **1**(8479): 462–464.

78 Hawkey CJ, Swannell AJ, Yeomans ND. Increased effectiveness of Omeprazole compared to ranitidine in non steroidal anti inflammatory drug (NSAID) users with reference to *H. pylori* status. *Gut* 1996; **39**(suppl 1): A33.

79 Yeomans ND, Tulassay Z, Juhasz L, Racz I, Howard J. A comparison of omeprazole with ranitidine for ulcers associated with nonsteroidal antiinflammatory drugs. *N Eng J Med* 1998; **338**(11): 719–726.

80 Labenz J, Tillenburg B, Peitz U, Idstrom JP. *Helicobacter pylori* augments the ph-increasing effect of omeprazole in patients with duodenal ulcer. *Gastroenterology* 1996; **110**: 725–732.

81 Porro GB, Parente F, Imbesi V. Role of *Helicobacter pylori* in ulcer healing and recurrence of gastric and duodenal ulcers in long term Nsaid users: Response to omeprazole dual therapy. *Gut* 1996; **39**: 22–26.

82 Hawkey CJ, Tulassay Z, Szczepanski L *et al.* Randomised controlled trial of *Helicobacter pylori* eradication in patients on non-steroidal anti-inflammatory drugs: HELP NSAIDs study. Helicobacter Eradication for Lesion Prevention. *Lancet* 1998; **352**(9133): 1016–1021.

83 Chan FK, Sung JJ, Chung SC *et al.* Randomised trial of eradication of *Helicobacter pylori* before non-steroidal anti-inflammatory drug therapy to prevent peptic ulcers. *Lancet* 1997; **350**(9083): 975–979.

84 Chan FKL, To KF, Wu JCY *et al.* Eradication of *Helicobacter pylori* and risk of peptic ulcers in patients starting long-term treatment with non-steroidal anti-inflammatory drugs: A randomised trial. *Lancet* 2002; **359**(9300): 9–13.

85 Chan FKL, Chung SC, Suen BY *et al.* Preventing recurrent upper gastrointestinal bleeding in patients with *Helicobacter pylori* infection who are taking low-dose aspirin or naproxen. *N Engl J Med* 2001; **344**(13): 967–973.

86 Fletcher RH, Fletcher SW, Wagner EH. *Clinical Epidemiology: The essentials.* 2nd ed. Williams & Wilkins, Baltimore, 1988.

87 Sackett DL, Haynes RB, Guyatt GH, Tugwell P. *Clinical Epidemiology: A basic sceince for clinical medicine.* 2nd ed. Little, Brown and Company, Toronto, 1998.

88 Levi S, Goodlad RA, Lee CY *et al.* Inhibitory effect of non-steroidal anti-inflammatory drugs on mucosal cell proliferation associated with gastric ulcer healing. *Lancet* 1990; **336**(8719): 840–843.

89 Smedfors B, Johansson C. Stimulation of dudenal bicarbonate secretion by misoprostol. *Digestive Diseases & Sciences* 1998; **31**(suppl): 96–100.

90 Walt RP. Misoprostol for the treatment of peptic ulcer and anti-inflammatory drug induced gastroduodenal ulceration. *N Eng J Med* 1992; **327**(22): 1575–1580.

91 Wilson DE, Quadros E, Rajapaksa T, Adams A. Effects of Misoprostol on gastric acid and mucus secretion in man. *Digestive Diseases & Sciences* 1986; **31**(suppl): 126–129.

92 Collins PW. Misoprostol: discovery, development, and clinical applications. *Med Res Rev* 1990; **10**: 149–172.

93 Hawkey CJ, Karrasch JA, Szczepanski L *et al.* Omeprazole compared to misoprostol for ulcers associated with nonsteroidal antiinflammatory drugs. *N Eng J Med* 1998; **338**(11): 727–734.

94 Graham DY, Agrawal NM, Campbell DR *et al.* Ulcer prevention in long-term users of nonsteroidal anti-inflammatory drugs: Results of a double-blind, randomized, multicenter, active- and placebo-controlled study of misoprostol vs lansoprazole. *Arch Intern Med* 2002; **162**(2): 169–175.

95 Cohen MM, Clark L, Armstrong L, D'Souza J. Reduction of aspirin-induced fecal blood loss with low-dose misoprostol tablets in man. *Digestive Diseases & Sciences* 1985; **30**(7): 605–611.

96 Lanza FL, Fakouhi D, Rubin A *et al.* A double-blind placebo-controlled comparison of the efficacy and safety of 50, 100, and 200 micrograms of misoprostol QID in the prevention of ibuprofen-induced gastric and duodenal mucosal lesions and symptoms. *Am J Gastroenterol* 1989; **84**(6): 633–636.

97 Ryan JR, Vargas R, Clay GA, McMahon FG. Role of misoprostol in reducing aspirin-induced gastrointestinal blood loss in arthritic patients. *Am J Med* 1987; **83**(1A): 41–46.

98 Silverstein FE, Kimmey MB, Saunders DR, Levine DS. Gastric protection by misoprostol against 1300 mg of aspirin. An endoscopic study. *Digestive Diseases & Sciences* 1986; **31**(Suppl 2): 137S–141S.

99 Hunt Jn, Smith Jl, Jiang CL, Kessler L. Effect of synthetic protoglandin E1 anologue on aspirin induced gastric bleeding and secretion. *Digestive Diseases & Sciences* 1983; **28**: 897–902.

100 Konturek JW, Dembinski A, Stoll R, Domschke W, Konturek SJ. Mucosal adaptation to aspirin induced gastric damage in humans. Studies on blood flow, gastric mucosal growth, and neutrophil activation. *Gut* 1994; **35**(9): 1197–1204.

101 Konturek JW, Dembinski A, Konturek SJ, Domschke W. *Helicobacter pylori* and gastric adaptation to repeated aspirin administration in humans. *Journal of Physiology & Pharmacology* 1997; **48**(3): 383–391.

102 Agrawal NM, Roth S, Graham DY *et al.* Misoprostol compared with sucralfate in the prevention of nonsteroidal anti-inflammatory drug-induced gastric ulcer. A randomized, controlled trial. *Ann Intern Med* 1991; **115**(3): 195–200.

103 Agrawal NM, Van KH, Erhardt LJ, Geis GS. Misoprostol coadministered with diclofenac for prevention of gastroduodenal ulcers. A one-year study. *Digestive Diseases & Sciences* 1995; **40**(5): 1125–1131.

104 Bocanegra TS, Weaver AL, Tindall EA *et al.* Diclofenac/misoprostol compared with diclofenac in the treatment of osteoarthritis of the knee or hip: A randomized, placebo controlled trial. Arthrotec Osteoarthritis Study Group. *Journal of Rheumatology* 1998; **25**(8): 1602–1611.

105 Bolten W, Gomes JA, Stead H, Geis GS. The gastroduodenal safety and efficacy of the fixed combination of diclofenac and

misoprostol in the treatment of osteoarthritis. *Br J Rheumatol* 1992; **31**(11): 753–758.

106 Chan FK, Sung JJ, Ching JY *et al.* Randomized trial of low-dose misoprostol and naproxen vs. nabumetone to prevent recurrent upper gastrointestinal haemorrhage in users of non-steroidal anti-inflammatory drugs. *Aliment Pharmacol Ther* 2001; **15**(1): 19–24.

107 Chandrasekaran AN, Sambandam PR, Lal HM *et al.* Double blind, placebo controlled trial on the cytoprotective effect of misoprostol in subjects with rheumatoid arthritis, osteoarthritis and seronegative spondarthropathy on NSAIDs. *J Assoc Physicians India* 1991; **39**(12): 919–921.

108 Cohen de Lara A, Gompel H, Baranes C *et al.* Two comparative studies of dosmalfate vs. misoprostol in the prevention of NSAID-induced gastric ulcers in rheumatic patients. *Drugs Today* 2000; **36** (Suppl A): 73–78.

109 Delmas PD, Lambert R, Capron MH. Misoprostol in the prevention of gastric erosions caused by nonsteroidal anti-inflammatory agents. *Revue du Rhumatisme* 1994; **2**: 126–131.

110 Elliott SL, Yeomans ND, Buchanan RR, Smallwood RA. Efficacy of 12 months' misoprostol as prophylaxis against NSAID-induced gastric ulcers. A placebo-controlled trial. *Scand J Rheumatol* 1994; **23**(4): 171–176.

111 Graham DY, Agrawal NM, Roth SH. Prevention of NSAID-induced gastric ulcer with misoprostol: multicentre, double-blind, placebo-controlled trial. *Lancet* 1988; **2**(8623): 1277–1280.

112 Graham DY, White RH, Moreland LW *et al.* Duodenal and gastric ulcer prevention with misoprostol in arthritis patients taking NSAIDs. Misoprostol Study Group. *Ann Intern Med* 1993; **119**(4): 257–262.

113 Hawkey CJ, Karrasch JA, Szczepanski L *et al.* Omeprazole compared with misoprostol for ulcers associated with nonsteroidal antiinflammatory drugs. Omeprazole versus Misoprostol for NSAID-induced Ulcer Management (OMNIUM) Study Group. *N Engl J Med* 1998; **338**(11): 727–734.

114 Henriksson K, Uribe A, Sandstedt B, Nord CE. *Helicobacter pylori* infection, ABO blood group, and effect of misoprostol on gastroduodenal mucosa in NSAID-treated patients with rheumatoid arthritis. *Digestive Diseases & Sciences* 1993; **38**(9): 1688–1696.

115 Jensen DM, Ho S, Hamamah S *et al.* A randomized study of omeprazole compared to misoprostol for prevention of recurrent ulcers and ulcer hemorrhage in high risk patients ingesting aspirin or NSAIDs (abstract). *Gastroenterology* 2000; **118**(4, Suppl 2, Pt 1): AGA A892.

116 Raskin JB, White RH, Jackson JE *et al.* Misoprostol dosage in the prevention of nonsteroidal anti-inflammatory drug-induced gastric and duodenal ulcers: a comparison of three regimens. *Ann Intern Med* 1995; **123**(5): 344–350.

117 Raskin JB, White RH, Jaszewski R, Korsten MA, Schubert TT, Fort JG. Misoprostol and ranitidine in the prevention of NSAID-induced ulcers: a prospective, double-blind, multicenter study. *Am J Gastroenterol* 1996; **91**(2): 223–227.

118 Roth SH, Tindall EA, Jain AK *et al.* A controlled study comparing the effects of nabumetone, ibuprofen, and ibuprofen plus misoprostol on the upper gastrointestinal tract mucosa. *Arch Intern Med* 1993; **153**(22): 2565–2571.

119 Saggioro A, Alvisi V, Blasi A, Dobrilla G, Fioravanti A, Marcolongo R. Misoprostol prevents NSAID-induced gastroduodenal lesions in patients with osteoarthritis and rheumatoid arthritis. *Ital J Gastroenterol* 1991; **23**(3): 119–123.

120 Valentini M, Cannizzaro R, Poletti M *et al.* Nonsteroidal antiinflammatory drugs for cancer pain: comparison between misoprostol and ranitidine in prevention of upper gastrointestinal damage. *J Clin Oncol* 1995; **13**(10): 2637–2642.

121 Verdickt W, Moran C, Hantzschel H, Fraga AM, Stead H, Geis GS. A double-blind comparison of the gastroduodenal safety and efficacy of diclofenac and a fixed dose combination of diclofenac and misoprostol in the treatment of rheumatoid arthritis. *Scand J Rheumatol* 1992; **21**(2): 85–91.

122 Bijlsma JW. Treatment of NSAID-induced gastrointestinal lesions with cimetidine: an international multicentre collaborative study. *Alimentary Pharmacology & Therapeutics* 1988; **2**(Suppl 1): 85–95.

123 Croker JR, Cotton PB, Boyle AC, Kinsella P. Cimetidine for peptic ulcer in patients with arthritis. *Ann Rheum Dis* 1980; **39**(3): 275–278.

124 Farah D, Sturrock RD, Russell RI. Peptic ulcer in rheumatoid arthritis. *Ann Rheum Dis* 1988; **47**(6): 478–480.

125 LoIudice TA, Saleem T, Lang JA. Cimetidine in the treatment of gastric ulcer induced by steroidal and nonsteroidal anti-inflammatory agents. *Am J Gastroenterol* 1981; **75**(2): 104–110.

126 O'Laughlin JC, Silvoso GR, Ivey KJ. Healing of aspirin-associated peptic ulcer disease despite continued salicylate ingestion. *Arch Intern Med* 1981; **141**(6): 781–783.

127 Walan A, Bader JP, Classen M, Lamers CB, Piper DW. Effect of omeprazole and ranitidine on ulcer healing and relapse rates in patients with benign gastric ulcers. *N Eng J Med* 1989; **320**(2): 69–75.

128 Mani V. Ranitidine in NSAID ulcers. *National Medical Journal of India* 1992; **5**(2): 69.

129 O'Laughlin JC, Silvoso GK, Ivey KJ. Resistance to medical therapy of gastric ulcers in rheumatic disease patients taking aspirin. A double-blind study with cimetidine and follow-up. *Digestive Diseases & Sciences* 1982; **27**(11): 976–980.

130 Hudson N, Taha AS, Russell RI *et al.* Famotidine for healing and maintenance in nonsteroidal anti-inflammatory drug-associated gastroduodenal ulceration. *Gastroenterology* 1997; **112**(6): 1817–1822.

131 Ehsanullah RS, Page MC, Tildesley G, Wood JR. Prevention of gastroduodenal damage induced by non-steroidal anti-inflammatory drugs: Controlled trial of ranitidine. *BMJ* 1988; **297**(6655): 1017–1021.

132 Robinson MG, Griffin JJ, Bowers J *et al.* Effect of ranitidine on gastroduodenal mucosal damage induced by nonsteroidal anti-inflammatory drugs. *Digestive Diseases & Sciences* 1989; **34**(3): 424–428.

133 Robinson M, Mills RJ, Euler AR. Ranitidine prevents duodenal ulcers associated with non-steroidal anti-inflammatory drug therapy. *Alimentary Pharmacology & Therapeutics* 1991; **5**(2): 143–150.

134 Taha AS, Hudson N, Hawkey CJ *et al.* Famotidine for the prevention of gastric and duodenal ulcers caused by nonsteroidal antiinflammatory drugs. *N Engl J Med* 1996; **334**(22): 1435–1439.

135 Levine LR, Cloud ML, Enas NH. Nizatidine prevents peptic ulceration in high-risk patients taking nonsteroidal anti-inflammatory drugs. *Arch Intern Med* 1993; **153**(21): 2449–2454.

136 Roth SH, Bennett RE, Mitchell CS, Hartman RJ. Cimetidine therapy in nonsteroidal anti-inflammatory drug gastropathy. Double-blind long-term evaluation. *Arch Intern Med* 1987; **147**(10): 1798–1801.

137 Bianchi Porro G., Pace F, Caruso I. Why are non-steroidal anti-inflammatory drugs important in peptic ulceration? *Alimentary Pharmacology & Therapeutics* 1987; **1**(suppl): 547S.

138 Berkowitz JM, Rogenes PR, Sharp JT, Warner CW. Ranitidine protects against gastroduodenal mucosal damage associated with chronic aspirin therapy. *Arch Intern Med* 1987; **147**(12): 2137–2139.

139 Simon B, Bergdolt H, Dammann H, Muller P. Ranitidine in the therapy and prevention of NSAR-induced (non-steroidal anti-rheumatic agents) gastroduodenal lesions in patients with rheumatism. *Zeitschrift fur Gastroenterologie* 1991; **29**(5): 217–221.

140 Simon B, Muller P. Nizatidine in therapy and prevention of non-steroidal anti-inflammatory drug-induced gastroduodenal ulcer in rheumatic patients. *Scandinavian Journal of Gastroenterology* 1994; **206**: 25–28.

141 Koch M, Dezi A, Ferrario F, Capurso I. Prevention of nonsteroidal anti-inflammatory drug-induced gastrointestinal mucosal injury. A meta-analysis of randomized controlled clinical trials. *Arch Intern Med* 1996; **156**(20): 2321–2332.

142 Van Groenendael JH, Markusse HM, Dijkmans BA, Breedveld FC. The effect of ranitidine on NSAID related dyspeptic symptoms with and without peptic ulcer disease of patients with rheumatoid arthritis and osteoarthritis. *Clin Rheumatol* 1996; **15**(5): 450–456.

143 Swift GL, Heneghan M, Williams GT, Williams BD, O'Sullivan MM, Rhodes J. Effect of ranitidine on gastroduodenal mucosal damage in patients on long-term non-steroidal anti-inflammatory drugs. *Digestion* 1989; **44**(2): 86–94.

144 Janssen M, Dijkmans BA, Vandenbroucke JP, Biemond I, Lamers CB. Achlorhydria does not protect against benign upper gastrointestinal ulcers during NSAID use. *Digestive Diseases & Sciences* 1994; **39**(2): 362–365.

145 Daneshmend TK, Stein AG, Bhaskar NK, Hawkey CJ. Abolition by omeprazole of aspirin induced gastric mucosal injury in man. *Gut* 1990; **31**(5): 514–517.

146 Scheiman JM, Behler EM, Loeffler KM, Elta GH. Omeprazole ameliorates aspirin-induced gastroduodenal injury. *Digestive Diseases & Sciences* 1994; **39**(1): 97–103.

147 Bergmann JF, Chassany O, Simoneau ML. Protection against aspirin induced gastric lesions by lansoprazole: Simultaneous evaluation of functional and morphologic responces. *Clinical Pharmacology & Therapeutics* 1992; **52**: 413–416.

148 Wolde S, Dijkmans BA, Janssen M, Hermans J, Lamers CB. High-dose ranitidine for the prevention of recurrent peptic ulcer disease in rheumatoid arthritis patients taking NSAIDs. *Alimentary Pharmacology & Therapeutics* 1996; **10**(3): 347–351.

149 Nwokolo CU, Prewett EJ, Sawyerr AM, Hudson M, Lim S, Pounder RE. Tolerance during 5 months of dosing with ranitidine, 150 mg nightly: A placebo-controlled, double-blind study. *Gastroenterology* 1991; **101**(4): 948–953.

150 Smith JT, Gavey C, Nwokolo CU, Pounder RE. Tolerance during 8 days of high-dose H2-blockade: placebo-controlled studies of 24-hour acidity and gastrin. *Alimentary Pharmacology & Therapeutics* 1990; **4**(suppl): 63.

151 Nwokolo CU, Smith JT, Gavey C, Sawyerr A, Pounder RE. Tolerance during 29 days of conventional dosing with cimetidine, nizatidine, famotidine or ranitidine. *Alimentary Pharmacology & Therapeutics* 1990; **4**(suppl): 45.

152 Oddsson E, Gudjonsson H, Thjodleifsson B. Comparison between ranitidine and omeprazole for protection against gastroduodenal damage caused by naproxen. *Scand J Gastroenterol* 1992; **27**(12): 1045–1048.

153 Lauritsen K, rutgersson K, Bolling E. Omeprazole 20 or 40 mg daily for healing of duodenal ulcer? A double blind comparative study. *European Journal of Gastroenterology & Hepatology* 1992; **4**: 995–1000.

154 Hawkey CJ, Swannell AJ, Eriksson S. Benefits of omeprazole over misoprostol in healing Nsaid associated ulcers. *Gastroenterology* 1996; **110**(4 suppl): A131.

155 Hawkey CJ, Foren I, Langstrom G. Omeprazole vs misoprostol: different effectiveness in healing gastric and duodenal ulcers vs erosions in Nsaid users: The Omnium study. *Gut* 1997; **40**(suppl): A1.

156 Bianchi Porro G, Lazzaroni M, Imbesi V, Montrone F, Santagada T. Efficacy of pantoprazole in the prevention of peptic ulcers, induced by non-steroidal anti-inflammatory drugs: A prospective, placebo-controlled, double-blind, parallel-group study. *Dig Liver Dis* 2000; **32**(3): 201–208.

157 Cullen D, Bardhan KD, Eisner M *et al.* Primary gastroduodenal prophylaxis with omeprazole for non-steroidal anti-inflammatory drug users. *Alimentary Pharmacology & Therapeutics* 1998; **12**(2): 135–140.

158 Ekstrom P, Carling L, Wetterhus S *et al.* Prevention of peptic ulcer and dyspeptic symptoms with omeprazole in patients receiving continuous non-steroidal anti-inflammatory drug therapy. A Nordic multicentre study. *Scand J Gastroenterol* 1996; **31**(8): 753–758.

159 Lai KC, Lam SK, Chu KM *et al.* Lansoprazole reduces ulcer relapse after eradication of *Helicobacter pylori* in nonsteroidal anti-inflammatory drug users–a randomized trial. *Aliment Pharmacol Ther* 2003; **18**(8): 829–836.

160 Chan FK, Hung LC, Suen BY *et al.* Celecoxib versus diclofenac plus omeprazole in high-risk arthritis patients: Results of a randomized double-blind trial. *Gastroenterology* 2004; **127**(4): 1038–1043.

161 Chan FK, Hung LC, Suen BY *et al.* Celecoxib versus diclofenac and omeprazole in reducing the risk of recurrent ulcer bleeding in patients with arthritis. *N Engl J Med* 2002; **347**(26): 2104–2110.

162 Chan FK, Wong VW, Suen BY *et al.* Combination of a cyclo-oxygenase-2 inhibitor and a proton-pump inhibitor for prevention of recurrent ulcer bleeding in patients at very high risk: a double-blind, randomised trial. *Lancet* 2007; **369**(9573): 1621–1626.

163 Goldstein JL, Correa P, Zhao WW *et al.* Reduced incidence of gastroduodenal ulcers with celecoxib, a novel cyclooxygenase-2 inhibitor, compared to naproxen in patients with arthritis. *Am J Gastroenterol* 2001; **96**(4): 1019–1027.

164 Emery P, Zeidler H, Kvien TK *et al.* Celecoxib versus diclofenac in long-term management of rheumatoid arthritis: Randomised double-blind comparison. *Lancet* 1999; **354**(9196): 2106–2111.

165 Simon LS, Weaver AL, Graham DY *et al.* Anti-inflammatory and upper gastrointestinal effects of celecoxib in rheumatoid arthri-

tis: A randomized controlled trial. *Journal of the American Medical Association* 1999; **282**(20): 1921–1928.

166 Laine L, Harper S, Simon T *et al.* A randomized trial comparing the effect of rofecoxib, a cyclooxygenase 2-specific inhibitor, with that of ibuprofen on the gastroduodenal mucosa of patients with osteoarthritis.Rofecoxib Osteoarthritis Endoscopy Study Group. *Gastroenterology* 1999; **117**(4): 776–783.

167 Hawkey C, Laine L, Simon T *et al.* Comparison of the effect of rofecoxib (a cyclooxygenase 2 inhibitor), ibuprofen, and placebo on the gastroduodenal mucosa of patients with osteoarthritis: A randomized, double-blind, placebo-controlled trial. The Rofecoxib Osteoarthritis Endoscopy Multinational Study Group. *Arthritis & Rheumatism* 2000; **43**(2): 370–377.

168 Hawkey CJ, Laine L, Simon T *et al.* Incidence of gastroduodenal ulcers in patients with rheumatoid arthritis after 12 weeks of rofecoxib, naproxen, or placebo: A multicentre, randomised, double blind study. *Gut* 2003; **52**(6): 820–826.

169 Hawkey CC, Svoboda P, Fiedorowicz-Fabrycy IF *et al.* Gastroduodenal safety and tolerability of lumiracoxib compared with Ibuprofen and celecoxib in patients with osteoarthritis. *J Rheumatol* 2004; **31**(9): 1804–1810.

170 Kivitz A, Eisen G, Zhao WW, Bevirt T, Recker DP. Randomized placebo-controlled trial comparing efficacy and safety of valdecoxib with naproxen in patients with osteoarthritis. *Journal of Family Practice* 2002; **51**(6): 530–537.

171 Sikes DH, Agrawal NM, Zhao WW, Kent JD, Recker DP, Verburg KM. Incidence of gastroduodenal ulcers associated with valdecoxib compared with that of ibuprofen and diclofenac in patients with osteoarthritis. *European Journal of Gastroenterology & Hepatology* 2002; **14**(10): 1101–1111.

172 Pavelka K, Recker DP, Verburg KM. Valdecoxib is as effective as diclofenac in the management of rheumatoid arthritis with a lower incidence of gastroduodenal ulcers: Results of a 26-week trial. *Rheumatology* 2003; **42**(10): 1207–1215.

173 Hunt RH, Harper S, Watson DJ *et al.* The gastrointestinal safety of the COX-2 selective inhibitor etoricoxib assessed by both endoscopy and analysis of upper gastrointestinal events. *Am J Gastroenterol* 2003; **98**(8): 1725–1733.

174 Hunt RH, Harper S, Callegari P *et al.* Complementary studies of the gastrointestinal safety of the cyclo-oxygenase-2-selective inhibitor etoricoxib. *Alimentary Pharmacology & Therapeutics* 2003; **17**(2): 201–210.

175 Kivitz AJ, Nayiager S, Schimansky T, Gimona A, Thurston HJ, Hawkey C. Reduced incidence of gastroduodenal ulcers associated with lumiracoxib compared with ibuprofen in patients with rheumatoid arthritis. *Alimentary Pharmacology & Therapeutics* 2004; **19**(11): 1189–1198.

176 FDA – Study 21 – Celebrex (http://www.fda.gov/cder/foi/adcomm/98/celebrex.htm) 1998.

177 FDA – Study 63 – FDA Drug Review (ND21-341) – Bextra (http://www.fda.gov/cder/foi/nda/2001/21-341_Bextra.htm) 2001.

178 FDA – Study 71 – Celebrex (http://www.fda.gov/cder/foi/adcomm/98/celebrex.htm) 1998.

179 FDA Study 47 – FDA Review (ND21-341) – Bextra (http://www.fda.gov/cder/foi/nda/2001/21-341_Bextra.htm) 2006.

180 Kivitz AJ, Nayiager S, Schimansky T, Gimona A, Thurston HJ, Hawkey C. Reduced incidence of gastroduodenal ulcers associated with lumiracoxib compared with ibuprofen in patients with rheumatoid arthritis. *Alimentary Pharmacology & Therapeutics* 2004; **19**(11): 1189–1198.

181 Hawkey CC, Svoboda P, Fiedorowicz-Fabrycy IF *et al.* Gastroduodenal safety and tolerability of lumiracoxib compared with Ibuprofen and celecoxib in patients with osteoarthritis. *J Rheumatol* 2004; **31**(9): 1804–1810.

182 Goldstein JL, Silverstein FE, Agrawal NM *et al.* Reduced risk of upper gastrointestinal ulcer complications with celecoxib, a novel COX-2 inhibitor. *Am J Gastroenterol* 2000; **95**(7): 1681–1690.

183 Langman MJ, Jensen DM, Watson DJ *et al.* Adverse upper gastrointestinal effects of rofecoxib compared with NSAIDs. *Journal of the American Medical Association* 1999; **282**(20): 1929–1933.

184 Goldstein JL, Eisen GM, Agrawal N, Stenson WF, Kent JD, Verburg KM. Reduced incidence of upper gastrointestinal ulcer complications with the COX-2 selective inhibitor, valdecoxib. *Alimentary Pharmacology & Therapeutics* 2004; **20**(5): 527–538.

185 Schnitzer TJ, Burmester GR, Mysler E *et al.* Comparison of lumiracoxib with naproxen and ibuprofen in the Therapeutic Arthritis Research and Gastrointestinal Event Trial (TARGET), reduction in ulcer complications: randomised controlled trial. *Lancet* 2004; **364**(9435): 665–674.

186 Ramey DR, Watson DJ, Yu C, Bolognese JA, Curtis SP, Reicin AS. The incidence of upper gastrointestinal adverse events in clinical trials of etoricoxib vs. non-selective NSAIDs: An updated combined analysis. *Current Medical Research & Opinion* 2005; **21**(5): 715–722.

187 Goldstein JL, Agrawal N, Eisen G *et al.* Significantly improved upper gastrointestinal (UGI) tolerability with celecoxib, a COX-2 specific inhibitor, compared with conventional NSAIDS. The Success-1 trial (abstract). *Gastroenterology* 2001; **120**: A105.

188 Laine L, Curtis SP, Cryer B, Kaur A, Cannon CP. Assessment of upper gastrointestinal safety of etoricoxib and diclofenac in patients with osteoarthritis and rheumatoid arthritis in the Multinational Etoricoxib and Diclofenac Arthritis Long-term (MEDAL) programme: a randomised comparison. *Lancet* 2007; **369**(9560): 465–473.

189 Zhao SZ, McMillen JI, Markenson JA *et al.* Evaluation of the functional status aspects of health-related quality of life of patients with osteoarthritis treated with celecoxib. *Pharmacotherapy* 1999; **19**(11): 1269–1278.

190 Geusens PP, Truitt K, Sfikakis P *et al.* A placebo and active comparator-controlled trial of rofecoxib for the treatment of rheumatoid arthritis. *Scand J Rheumatol* 2002; **31**(4): 230–238.

191 Leung AT, Malmstrom K, Gallacher AE *et al.* Efficacy and tolerability profile of etoricoxib in patients with osteoarthritis: A randomized, double-blind, placebo and active-comparator controlled 12-week efficacy trial. *Current Medical Research & Opinion* 2002; **18**(2): 49–58.

192 Lisse JR, Perlman M, Johansson G *et al.* Gastrointestinal tolerability and effectiveness of rofecoxib versus naproxen in the treatment of osteoarthritis: a randomized, controlled trial. *Ann Intern Med* 2003; **139**(7): 539–546.

193 Baron JA, Sandler RS, Bresalier RS *et al.* A randomized trial of rofecoxib for the chemoprevention of colorectal adenomas. *Gastroenterology* 2006; **131**(6): 1674–1682.

194 Singh G, Fort JG, Goldstein JL *et al.* Celecoxib versus naproxen and diclofenac in osteoarthritis patients: SUCCESS-I Study. *Am J Med* 2006; **119**(3): 255–266.

195 Lai KC, Chu KM, Hui WM *et al.* Celecoxib compared with lansoprazole and naproxen to prevent gastrointestinal ulcer complications. *Am J Med* 2005; **118**(11): 1271–1278.

196 Bensen WG, Fiechtner JJ, McMillen JI *et al.* Treatment of osteoarthritis with celecoxib, a cyclooxygenase-2 inhibitor: A randomized controlled trial. *Mayo Clin Proc* 1999; **74**(11): 1095–1105.

197 Matsumoto AK, Melian A, Mandel DR *et al.* A randomized, controlled, clinical trial of etoricoxib in the treatment of rheumatoid arthritis. *J Rheumatol* 2002; **29**(8): 1623–1630.

198 Cannon GW, Caldwell JR, Holt P *et al.* Rofecoxib, a specific inhibitor of cyclooxygenase 2, with clinical efficacy comparable with that of diclofenac sodium: Results of a one-year, randomized, clinical trial in patients with osteoarthritis of the knee and hip. Rofecoxib Phase III Protocol 035 Study Group. *Arthritis & Rheumatism* 2000; **43**(5): 978–987.

199 Saag K, van der HD, Fisher C *et al.* Rofecoxib, a new cyclooxygenase 2 inhibitor, shows sustained efficacy, comparable with other nonsteroidal anti-inflammatory drugs: A 6-week and a 1-year trial in patients with osteoarthritis. Osteoarthritis Studies Group. *Archives of Family Medicine* 2000; **9**(10): 1124–1134.

200 Collantes E, Curtis SP, Lee KW *et al.* A multinational randomized, controlled, clinical trial of etoricoxib in the treatment of rheumatoid arthritis (ISRCTN25142273). *BMC Family Practice* 2002; **3**(1): 10.

201 Makarowski W, Zhao WW, Bevirt T, Recker DP. Efficacy and safety of the COX-2 specific inhibitor valdecoxib in the management of osteoarthritis of the hip: A randomized, double-blind, placebo-controlled comparison with naproxen. *Osteoarthritis & Cartilage* 2002; **10**(4): 290–296.

202 Myllykangas-Luosujarvi R, Lu HS, Chen SL *et al.* Comparison of low-dose rofecoxib versus 1000 mg naproxen in patients with osteoarthritis. Results of two randomized treatment trals of six weeks duration. *Scand J Rheumatol* 2002; **31**(6): 337–344.

203 Kivitz AJ, Moskowitz RW, Woods E *et al.* Comparative efficacy and safety of celecoxib and naproxen in the treatment of osteoarthritis of the hip. *Journal of International Medical Research* 2001; **29**(6): 467–479.

204 Wiesenhutter CW, Boice JA, Ko A *et al.* Evaluation of the comparative efficacy of etoricoxib and ibuprofen for treatment of patients with osteoarthritis: A randomized, double-blind, placebo-controlled trial. *Mayo Clin Proc* 2005; **80**(4): 470–479.

205 Day R, Morrison B, Luza A *et al.* A randomized trial of the efficacy and tolerability of the COX-2 inhibitor rofecoxib vs ibuprofen in patients with osteoarthritis. Rofecoxib/Ibuprofen Comparator Study Group. *Arch Intern Med* 2000; **160**(12): 1781–1787.

206 McKenna F, Borenstein D, Wendt H, Wallemark C, Lefkowith JB, Geis GS. Celecoxib versus diclofenac in the management of osteoarthritis of the knee. *Scand J Rheumatol* 2001; **30**(1): 11–18.

207 Truitt KE, Sperling RS, Ettinger WH, Jr *et al.* A multicenter, randomized, controlled trial to evaluate the safety profile, tolerability, and efficacy of rofecoxib in advanced elderly patients with osteoarthritis. *Aging-Clinical & Experimental Research* 2001; **13**(2): 112–121.

208 Bensen W, Weaver A, Espinoza L *et al.* Efficacy and safety of valdecoxib in treating the signs and symptoms of rheumatoid arthritis: A randomized, controlled comparison with placebo and naproxen. *Rheumatology* 2002; **41**(9): 1008–1016.

209 Geusens P, Alten R, Rovensky J *et al.* Efficacy, safety and tolerability of lumiracoxib in patients with rheumatoid arthritis. *International Journal of Clinical Practice* 2004; **58**(11): 1033–1041.

210 Schnitzer TJ, Fricke J, Jr., Gitton X, Jayawardene S, Sloan VS. Lumiracoxib in the treatment of osteoarthritis, rheumatoid arthritis and acute postoperative dental pain: Results of three dose-response studies. *Current Medical Research & Opinion* 2005; **21**(1): 151–161.

211 Ehrich EW STM. Effect of specific COX-2 inhibition in osteoarthritis of the knee: A 6 week double blind, placebo controlled pilot study of rofecoxib. *Journal of Rheumatology* 1999; **26**(11): 2438–2447.

212 Schnitzer TJ TK. The safety profile, tolerability, and effective dose range of rofecoxib in the treatment of rheumatoid arthritis. *Clinical therapeutics* 1999; **21**(10): 1688–1702.

213 Williams GW. ERREHRLMYSZ. Treatment of osteoarthritis with a once-daily dosing regimen of celecoxib: A randomized, controlled trial. *JCR: Journal of Clinical Rheumatology* 2000; **6**(2): 65–74.

214 Gottesdiener K, Schnitzer T, Fisher C *et al.* Results of a randomized, dose-ranging trial of etoricoxib in patients with osteoarthritis. *Rheumatology* 2002; **41**(9): 1052–1061.

215 Grifka JK, Zacher J, Brown JP *et al.* Efficacy and tolerability of lumiracoxib versus placebo in patients with osteoarthritis of the hand. *Clinical & Experimental Rheumatology* 2004; **22**(5): 589–596.

216 Lehmann R, Brzosko M, Kopsa P *et al.* Efficacy and tolerability of lumiracoxib 100 mg once daily in knee osteoarthritis: A 13-week, randomized, double-blind study vs. placebo and celecoxib. *Current Medical Research & Opinion* 2005; **21**(4): 517–526.

217 Laine L, Maller ES, Yu C, Quan H, Simon T. Ulcer formation with low-dose enteric-coated aspirin and the effect of COX-2 selective inhibition: A double-blind trial. *Gastroenterology* 2004; **127**(2): 395–402.

218 Catella-Lawson F, Reilly MP, Kapoor SC *et al.* Cyclooxygenase inhibitors and the antiplatelet effects of aspirin. *N Engl J Med* 2001; **345**(25): 1809–1817.

219 Ouellet M, Riendeau D, Percival MD. A high level of cyclooxygenase-2 inhibitor selectivity is associated with a reduced interference of platelet cyclooxygenase-1 inactivation by aspirin. *Proc Natl Acad Sci USA* 2001; **98**(25): 14583–14588.

220 Baigent C, Patrono C. Selective cyclooxygenase 2 inhibitors, aspirin, and cardiovascular disease: A reappraisal. *Arthritis Rheum* 2003; **48**(1): 12–20.

221 Patrono C. Aspirin resistance: Definition, mechanisms and clinical read-outs. *J Thromb Haemost* 2003; **1**(8): 1710–1713.

222 Cipollone F, Rocca B, Patrono C. Cyclooxygenase-2 expression and inhibition in atherothrombosis. *Arterioscler Thromb Vasc Biol* 2004; **24**(2): 246–255.

223 Khan NA, McAlister FA, Rabkin SW *et al.* The 2006 Canadian Hypertension Education Program recommendations for the management of hypertension: Part II – Therapy. *Can J Cardiol* 2006; **22**(7): 583–593.

224 Pearson TA, Blair SN, Daniels SR *et al.* AHA Guidelines for Primary Prevention of Cardiovascular Disease and Stroke: 2002 Update: Consensus Panel Guide to Comprehensive Risk Reduction for Adult Patients Without Coronary or Other

Atherosclerotic Vascular Diseases. American Heart Association Science Advisory and Coordinating Committee. *Circulation* 2002; **106**(3): 388–391.

225 Chan FK, Chung SC, Suen BY *et al.* Preventing recurrent upper gastrointestinal bleeding in patients with *Helicobacter pylori* infection who are taking low-dose aspirin or naproxen. *N Engl J Med* 2001; **344**(13): 967–973.

226 Vergara M, Catalan M, Gisbert JP, Calvet X. Meta-analysis: Role of *Helicobacter pylori* eradication in the prevention of peptic ulcer in NSAID users. *Aliment Pharmacol Ther* 2005; **21**(12): 1411–1418.

227 Labenz J, Blum AL, Bolten WW *et al.* Primary prevention of diclofenac associated ulcers and dyspepsia by omeprazole or triple therapy in *Helicobacter pylori* positive patients: A randomised, double blind, placebo controlled, clinical trial. *Gut* 2002; **51**(3): 329–335.

228 Hunt R, Fallone C, Veldhuyzan van ZS *et al.* Canadian Helicobacter Study Group Consensus Conference: Update on the management of *Helicobacter pylori*–an evidence-based evaluation of six topics relevant to clinical outcomes in patients evaluated for *H. pylori* infection. *Can J Gastroenterol* 2004; **18**(9): 547–554.

229 Rostom A, Moayyedi P, Hunt R. Systematic Review: Canadian Consensus guidelines on long-term NSAID therapy and the need for gastroprotection. *Aliment Pharmacol Ther* 2009; **29**(5): 481–496. Epub 27 Nov 2008.

8

Acute non-variceal gastrointestinal hemorrhage: Treatment

Nicholas Church[1] and Kelvin Palmer[2]

[1] Centre for Liver and Digestive Disorders, Royal Infirmary of Edinburgh, Edinburgh, UK
[2] Gastrointestinal Unit, Western General Hospital, Edinburgh, UK

Introduction

Peptic ulcer is the commonest cause of acute non-variceal bleeding, accounting for approximately one-third of cases [1]. Other major causes such as gastroduodenal erosions, gastritis, esophagitis, Mallory–Weiss tears, and vascular malformations are not usually life-threatening and respond to conservative therapy.

Approximately 80% of cases pursue a benign course without re-bleeding in hospital and specific intervention is not required. The remaining 20% have severe bleeding due to erosion of a major artery. Most deaths from bleeding arise from this subgroup. Despite significant advances in resuscitation, diagnosis and therapy, the crude death rate from gastrointestinal bleeding has only marginally improved over five decades. Avery Jones in 1947 reported a hospital mortality rate of 16% [2], whilst a large audit of acute gastrointestinal bleeding performed in England in 1995 reported a very similar mortality rate of 14% [3]. The recent UK National audit of gastrointestinal bleeding included 6750 cases and reported an overall mortality of 10%, with a rate of 7% in those admitted to hospital because of bleeding, rising to 26% for inpatients [1]. This observation is disappointing but must, however, be tempered by the fact that the case mix of patients now admitted is very different to that of previous decades. For example, less than 2% of patients admitted with acute bleeding in 1947 were aged over 80 years, whilst approximately a quarter of patients currently admitted are octogenarians. There is a close relationship between increasing age and hospital mortality: increasing age is inevitably associated with a high prevalence of chronic disease, rendering patients susceptible to complications following major hemorrhage.

This chapter will review the evidence to support risk assessment and resuscitation, medical and endoscopic therapies for bleeding peptic ulcer, management when endoscopic therapy fails and treatment in the early post-endoscopy period.

Risk assessment and resuscitation

The risk of death following admission to hospital for gastrointestinal bleeding has been quantified by Rockall *et al.* [4]. Independent factors associated with a poor prognosis were identified from data derived from a large population of patients whose clinical course was observed following hospital admission and a scoring system was developed. This comprises three clinical variables, from which an initial clinical Rockall score is derived, and two endoscopic variables, for the complete score (Table 8.1). The Rockall score correlated well with observed mortality, but not re-bleeding, in a Dutch validation study [5].

As shown in Table 8.2, Rockall *et al.* showed a good correlation between the risk score, re-bleeding and hospital mortality. Deaths following admission to hospital because of acute gastrointestinal bleeding are rarely due to exsanguination. They are usually a consequence of postoperative complications when an urgent operation is undertaken, or of deterioration of co-morbid conditions.

In Rockall's study [4] 0.2% of 595 patients with a clinical score of zero died. This very low mortality has been observed in other studies in which the clinical Rockall score has been calculated both retrospectively [6], and prospectively [7]. This has led to the suggestion that patients with a clinical score of zero may be safely managed with early discharge and outpatient endoscopy. The safety or otherwise of this approach has not been tested in clinical trials.

In order to evaluate the use of the Rockall scoring system in patients at highest risk, Church *et al.* calculated scores for a series of 247 patients who had been entered into a randomized trial of endoscopic therapy for major peptic

Evidence-Based Gastroenterology and Hepatology, 3rd edition.
J. McDonald, A.K. Burroughs, B. Feagan, and M.B. Fennerty. © 2010
Blackwell Publishing Ltd

Table 8.1 The Rockall scoring system for risk of re-bleeding and death after admission to hospital for acute gastrointestinal bleeding.

Variable	Score			
	0	**1**	**2**	**3**
Age	<60 yr	60–79 yr	≥80 yr	
Shock	No shock Systolic BP > 100 Pulse <100	Tachycardia Systolic BP > 100 Pulse >100	Hypotension Systolic BP < 100	
Co-morbidity	Nil major		Cardiac failure, ischemic heart disease, any major co-morbidity	Renal failure, liver failure, disseminated malignancy
Diagnosis	Mallory–Weiss tear, no lesion and no SRH	All other diagnoses	Malignancy of upper GI tract	
Major SRH	None, or dark spot		Blood in upper GI tract, adherent clot, visible or spurting vessel	

SRH: Stigmata of recent hemorrhage.
Source: Rockall *et al.* [4].

Table 8.2 Correlation between Rockall score and re-bleeding and mortality.

Risk score	n	Re-bleed (%)	Mortality (%)
0	144	7 (5)	0 (0)
1	281	9 (3)	0 (0)
2	337	18 (5)	1 (0.2)
3	444	50 (11)	13 (3)
4	528	76 (14)	28 (5)
5	455	83 (24)	49 (11)
6	312	102 (33)	54 (17)
7	267	113 (44)	72 (27)
8+	190	101 (42)	78 (41)

ulcer bleeding in Scotland [8]. Following endoscopic therapy, the Rockall system did not adequately predict re-bleeding but accurately identified patients at high risk of death. The findings suggested that patients scoring 6 or above should be managed in a high dependency unit after endoscopic therapy.

A number of other risk scoring systems have been developed of which the best known is that developed by Blatchford *et al.* [9]. The Blatchford system differs from the other scores in two ways. First, the system was designed to predict a need for intervention to treat bleeding, rather than to quantify the risk of re-bleeding or death. Second, the score does not include endoscopic findings as a component and is therefore potentially useful in patient triage at the time of admission. Data were obtained from 1748 patients admitted following upper gastrointestinal bleed-ing in the west of Scotland. After logistic regression analysis a risk score was developed based on the admission hemoglobin, blood urea, pulse, systolic blood pressure, presentation with syncope, presentation with melena, evidence of hepatic disease and evidence of cardiac failure. Intervention was defined as the requirement for a blood transfusion, endoscopic therapy or surgery to control bleeding. Increasing scores correlated with the need for intervention. A receiver operator curve was plotted for a subsequent internal validation sample of 197 patients, and the score discriminated well with an area under the curve of 0.92 (95% CI: 0.88–0.95). The number of patients requiring each intervention was not reported and this limits an assessment of its utility and clinical relevance. External validation of this scoring system is required before it can be recommended for clinical use.

Optimum management of patients with major upper GI hemorrhage relies very much on a team approach, with appropriate use of drug therapy, endoscopic intervention, radiological intervention and surgery. Despite much evidence from randomized trials, the management of an individual patient still depends on clinical judgment. Endoscopy should only be undertaken once appropriate resuscitation has been achieved in order to minimize cardiorespiratory complications of the procedure [10]. For the majority of patients with peptic ulcer bleeding an endoscopy within 24 hours of presentation is appropriate, and there is no evidence to support emergency endoscopy for all comers. However, in the small proportion of cases with severe, life-threatening bleeding resulting in a failure to respond to resuscitation efforts, an immediate endoscopy may be required.

Management may be best undertaken in a specialized "bleeding unit" in which the patient is treated using agreed protocols and guidelines and with management decisions based upon endoscopic and surgical opinions. Relatively weak evidence derived from comparison of results in case series with historical controls suggests that this approach may achieve lower hospital mortality and more efficient use of resources than management by generalists working in conventional medical or surgical units [11, 12]. More recently a study by Sanders *et al.* described the outcomes of 900 patients with significant bleeding who were managed over a three-year period in a dedicated bleeding unit [13]. Rockall scores were calculated for all patients and outcomes were analyzed prospectively. Patients were stratified into groups at low, medium and high risk of death according to their Rockall score and outcomes were compared with those of the patients in Rockall's national audit [3] by calculation of standardized mortality ratios (SMR). Although there were more high-risk patients in the Sanders cohort, their overall mortality was significantly lower than that of the Rockall patients (SMR 0.63 (95% CI: 0.48–0.78)). The difference was most marked for patients at medium risk (Rockall score 4–6; SMR 0.56 (CI: 0.34–0.78)). However, it is worthy of note that if the SMRs had been calculated using the findings of the UK National Bleeding audit [1] the findings of this study may well have been negative. A trial in which patients with major bleeding have been randomized to management in either a specialized bleeding unit or a general medical or surgical ward has not been performed.

Specific therapy

For the 80% of patients who have relatively minor bleeding and who do not have major endoscopic stigmata of bleeding, supportive therapy including use of intravenous fluid and the management of co-morbidity (particularly cardiorespiratory disease) is sufficient.

Patients who present with clinical shock and who at endoscopy have an actively bleeding peptic ulcer have an 80% risk of continuing to bleed or re-bleed in hospital [14]. Those who have a non-bleeding visible vessel have a 50% risk of further hemorrhage [15]. The "visible vessel" represents a pseudoaneurysm of the involved artery, or adherent blood clot, plugging the arterial defect [16]. Patients who are found to have a tightly adherent blood clot over the ulcer usually have an underlying high-risk lesion and should also be regarded as being at considerable risk of further hemorrhage in hospital. Patients who at endoscopy have a clean ulcer base or who have black or red spots are at very little risk of re-bleeding.

It follows from these observations that patients with major endoscopic stigmata should be considered for spe-cific hemostatic treatment and only such patients should be included in clinical trials of therapy for gastrointestinal bleeding. This review will only consider those studies that exclusively include patients having a non-bleeding visible vessel, active hemorrhage, or tightly adherent blood clot as entry criteria.

The specific non-surgical approaches to hemostasis are drug therapy, endoscopic therapy and transcatheter arterial embolization.

Drug therapy

There are three principles underlying the use of drugs as agents which might stop active hemorrhage and prevent re-bleeding. The first of these is that the stability of a blood clot is poor in an acid environment [17]. Thus, agents that suppress acid secretion, including H_2-receptor antagonists (H_2-RA) and proton pump inhibitor (PPI) drugs might reduce re-bleeding. The second is that a blood clot may be stabilized by decreasing fibrinolytic mechanisms using agents such as tranexamic acid. The third approach is that, since major gastrointestinal bleeding is due to arterial erosion, reduction of arterial blood flow by agents such as somatostatin and octreotide could achieve hemostasis and prevent re-bleeding.

Acid suppressing drugs

The efficacy of H_2-RA in the management of acute upper gastrointestinal bleeding has been assessed in randomized trials [18, 19]. Unfortunately, no trial has shown benefit in terms of reduction of re-bleeding incidence or mortality. **A1c**

Experience involving the use of PPIs is inconsistent, but the evidence now supports their use in patients who have required endoscopic hemostasis. The largest trial involved 1147 patients who were randomized to receive omeprazole, (initially intravenously, then orally) or placebo [20]. No significant differences in hospital mortality, operation rate or re-bleeding were demonstrated. The study was not restricted to the high-risk patients who had endoscopic stigmata of recent hemorrhage. Accordingly, event rates were rather low in the placebo group, and this may have limited the power of the study to show a difference. **A1a**

Khuroo *et al.* randomized 220 bleeding ulcer patients who had major endoscopic stigmata to receive high dose oral omeprazole or placebo [21]. Although all patients had major stigmata of hemorrhage, an adherent clot in the ulcer base was reported in 57% of patients. Re-bleeding, the need for urgent surgery, blood transfusion, and mortality were all reduced in the actively treated group of patients (Table 8.3). The number of patients needed to treat with omeprazole to prevent one death was 25, and to prevent one opera-

Table 8.3 Omeprazole vs placebo for bleeding peptic ulcer.

Outcome	Omeprazole (n = 110)	Placebo (n = 110)	p value
Re-bleed (%)	12 (11)	40 (36)	<0.001
Surgery (%)	8 (8)	26 (23)	<0.001
Transfusion (mean units)	2.3	4.1	<0.001
Death	2	6	NS

Source: Khuroo *et al.* [21].

Table 8.4 Omeprazole vs placebo for bleeding peptic ulcer treated with endoscopic therapy.

Outcome	Omeprazole (n = 120)	Placebo (n = 120)	p value
Re-bleed (%)	8 (7)	27 (23)	<0.001
Surgery (%)	3 (3)	9 (8)	0.14
Transfusion (mean units +/– SD)	2.7 +/– 2.5	3.5 +/– 3.8	0.04
Length of stay <5 days (number of patients (%))	56 (47)	38 (32)	0.02
Death	5 (4)	12 (10)	0.13

Source: Lau *et al.* [26].

tion was seven. **A1c** This trial has been criticized because it included relatively young patients with relatively little co-morbidity and because endoscopic therapy was not administered to any patient. The observation that omeprazole reduced re-bleeding and surgery rates when no endoscopic therapy was performed suggested a beneficial effect of the PPI. This effect might, however, have been exaggerated by the fact that the majority of patients in the trial were bleeding from ulcers in which an adherent clot was found at endoscopy.

Two trials published back to back in the *Scandinavian Journal of Gastroenterology* [22, 23] examined the use of high dose intravenous omeprazole after endoscopic hemostasis. All patients had major peptic ulcer bleeding, but as in the trial by Khuroo *et al.* half the patients had adherent clot as the reported stigma of hemorrhage. The conclusions were that intravenous omeprazole infusion for three days following endoscopic therapy improved outcome. **A1d** Both trials used composite endpoints which were complex and ill-defined and both were discontinued early due to an unexplained imbalance in mortality in one of the trials [23], factors that weaken the impact of these results. Villanueva *et al.* randomized 86 patients following successful endoscopic hemostasis for peptic ulcer bleeding to either intravenous omeprazole or ranitidine. There were no differences between the groups for the endpoints of re-bleeding, surgery or death [24]. **A1d** In contrast, a similar small trial by Lin and colleagues [25] concluded that intravenous omeprazole was superior to cimetidine in terms of reduction of re-bleeding rates, but not those of surgery or death.

The most important recent trial was performed by Lau *et al.* [26]. Two hundred and forty patients in whom endoscopic therapy for major ulcer bleeding had been successful were randomized. All patients had high-risk ulcers with active bleeding or non-bleeding visible vessels, and were treated by adrenaline injection followed by heater probe thermocoagulation. Adherent clots were removed to allow therapy to the underlying vessel. The patients then received either an 80 mg bolus dose of intravenous omeprazole followed by an infusion of 8 mg per hour for 72 hours or

placebo. Re-bleeding rates, blood transfusion requirements and length of hospital stay were significantly reduced in the omeprazole group compared to placebo. **A1a** There was a trend toward fewer operations and deaths in the omeprazole group, but these differences were not statistically significant (Table 8.4). These results have been closely replicated in a similar sized trial by Zargar *et al.* in which an almost identical design to that of Lau *et al.* was used, except that pantoprazole was substituted for omeprazole [27]. This supports the likelihood that the observed outcomes of therapy with PPIs following endoscopic hemostasis are the result of a class effect of PPIs, rather than a specific response to omeprazole.

A subsequent trial by the Hong Kong group included 156 patients with peptic ulcers containing non-bleeding visible vessels or adherent clot in the ulcer base [28]. Patients were randomized to endoscopic therapy using adrenaline injection and heater probe thermocoagulation plus the previously published high dose intravenous PPI regimen, or to the PPI regimen alone. The probability of re-bleeding within 30 days of the index episode was significantly reduced in the combination therapy group, suggesting that PPI infusion in combination with endoscopic therapy is superior to PPI infusion alone. **A1c** Seventeen percent of patients with non-bleeding visible vessels re-bled in the PPI only group, and although a control group receiving no treatment was not included for ethical reasons, this represents a substantial improvement over the expected re-bleeding rate of 30–50% based on previous studies.

Following the publication of the trial by Lau *et al.* [26] the use of high dose intravenous PPI after successful endoscopic therapy for bleeding ulcer has become standard management in many centers in the UK and Europe. The 80 mg bolus and 8 mg per hour infusion regimen consistently raises intragastric pH above six for the majority of a 24-hour period [29]. It is not known, however, whether this optimum regimen is actually necessary following endoscopic therapy, and whether bolus intravenous or even oral PPI would suffice. A recent study has suggested that frequent oral PPI therapy with lansoprazole could raise intragastric pH to similar levels to those achieved by lansoprazole infusion. However, the confidence intervals were wide and the conclusion can be questioned [30]. Two small clinical studies have attempted to answer these questions.

Udd *et al.* [31] randomized 142 patients with ulcer bleeding to the high dose three-day intravenous omeprazole regimen or to a single daily bolus dose of 20 mg for three days. Rates of re-bleeding (8% for high dose vs 12% for standard dose), surgery (4% vs 7%) and death (6% vs 3%) were comparable between the groups. Only 102 patients had required endoscopic therapy, and approximately 30% of patients had an ulcer with a black base only. Thus, the number of high-risk ulcers in the trial was small, the event rates were low and the study may have lacked power to demonstrate a difference between the effects of the two treatments.

The effect of oral omeprazole following endoscopic therapy for bleeding peptic ulcer was studied by Javid *et al.* [32]. One hundred and sixty six patients with ulcers which were actively bleeding, and had non-bleeding visible vessels or adherent clots were treated with a combination of 1:10,000 adrenaline plus 1% polidocanol injection. They were then randomized to receive oral omeprazole 40 mg bd or placebo. Six (7%) of the 82 patients in the omeprazole group re-bled compared with 18 (21%) of the 84 patients in the placebo group (p = 0.02). **A1c** Surgery was required in two patients in the omeprazole group and seven patients in the placebo group (p = 0.17). One death occurred in the omeprazole group compared to two in the placebo group. The results are comparable to those achieved by Lau *et al.* with the high dose intravenous regimen [26]. It should be noted, however, that 40% of patients in this trial had ulcers with adherent clot, and the number of patients with high-risk lesions was therefore correspondingly lower than that in the Hong Kong study. A further high quality trial comparing the use of intravenous and oral omeprazole in high-risk ulcer bleeding patients is required.

The trials involving PPI therapy in ulcer bleeding are heterogeneous but have been subjected to several meta-analyses. The most comprehensive is the recently updated report from the Cochrane group [33]. This systematic review of 24 trials included 4373 patients with peptic ulcer bleeding who had been treated with PPIs compared with H_2-receptor antagonists or placebo. Seven trials included high-risk patients following endoscopic therapy, and four of these used high dose PPI infusion in the active therapy arm. Overall results demonstrated a reduction in re-bleeding (OR 0.49; 95% CI: 0.37–0.65, NNT 13), surgery (OR 0.61; 95% CI: 0.48–0.78, NNT 34) and requirement for further endoscopic hemostatic therapy (OR 0.32; 95% CI: 0.20–0.51,

NNT 10). Mortality was not reduced (OR 1.01; 95% CI: 0.74–1.40). However, in a subgroup analysis, mortality in PPI groups was significantly reduced in Asian patients (OR 0.35; 95% CI: 0.16–0.74, NNT 34) and in the high-risk patients entered into the endoscopic therapy trials (OR 0.53; 95% CI: 0.31–0.91, NNT 50).

The more pronounced PPI treatment effect observed in Asian patients is likely to be the result of a combination of lower mean age, reduced parietal cell mass and a greater proportion of slow metabolisers of PPIs. There is a need to further evaluate the use of PPI therapy in non-Asian populations, but in our view the available evidence supports the routine use high dose intravenous PPI therapy for 72 hours following endoscopy in those patients who have required hemostatic therapy. **A1a**

As PPI therapy has become more widely used in acute peptic ulcer bleeding it has become common practice to institute intravenous PPI therapy before endoscopy is undertaken. This approach is not evidence based and to try to determine whether PPI prior to endoscopy was beneficial, Lau *et al.* randomized 638 patients with overt clinical signs of upper GI bleeding to high dose IV PPI or to placebo infusion before endoscopy was performed [34]. Patients who were taking aspirin were excluded as they were randomized into a concurrent study. One hundred and eighty seven patients in the omeprazole arm and 190 patients in the placebo arm were found to be bleeding from peptic ulcers. Fewer patients pre-treated with omeprazole were actively bleeding at endoscopy, resulting in a reduced need for endoscopic therapy (22.5% vs 36.8%, RR 0.61; 95% CI: 0.44–0.84) and a shorter hospital stay (median 3 days (range 1–43) vs 3 days (1–54), p = 0.003). Despite these findings, the important outcomes of re-bleeding, surgery and mortality were unchanged. The conclusion was that PPI therapy prior to endoscopy reduced the proportion of patients found to have stigmata of hemorrhage, with consequent resource savings. These results are encouraging, but do not show a benefit in terms of clinical outcomes and may not be applicable generally. The principal criticism of this trial is the exclusion of patients requiring long-term aspirin therapy. In addition, 60% of patients presenting with upper GI bleeding in Hong Kong are found to have peptic ulcer compared to 50% or lower in Western populations, in whom the effect of general prescription of PPIs before endoscopy is likely to be significantly less apparent. Further studies in non-Asian populations are required.

Tranexamic acid

Two meta-analyses have been published examining the role of tranexamic acid for gastrointestinal bleeding [35, 36]. The most recent by Gluud *et al.* [36] included 1754 patients from seven placebo controlled trials. Pooled analysis demonstrated a reduction in all cause mortality for patients treated with tranexamic acid (5% vs 8%, RR 0.61; 95% CI: 0.42–0.89). Rates of further bleeding, surgery and blood transfusion were unaffected.

The largest study included in the meta-analysis was undertaken by the Nottingham group [37]. Seven hundred and seventy-five patients presenting to hospital because of acute gastrointestinal bleeding were randomized to receive oral cimetidine, tranexamic acid or placebo. No significant difference in bleeding or operation rates was demonstrated, but there was a rather surprising large difference in mortality. Mortality was 7.7% in cimetidine treated patients, 6.3% in tranexamic acid treated patients and 13.5% in those treated with placebo. The mortality rate of 13.5% in the placebo treated group is greater than that expected for conservatively treated patients based on the results of other studies. Furthermore, other studies do not demonstrate benefit from the use of cimetidine. It is possible that more high-risk patients were inadvertently randomized to the placebo group in this study.

The meta-analyses included trials in which many patients did not have major endoscopic stigmata of bleeding. In addition, there were significant differences in methodology, doses and routes of administration of tranexamic acid and adjunctive therapy, and few patients received endoscopic therapy and PPI administration. Therefore, it is unlikely that the patients studied can be seen as representative of the current population, and further randomized trials in high-risk patients are required before tranexamic acid can be recommended as a standard therapy for peptic ulcer bleeding.

Somatostatin and octreotide

Somatostatin and its analogs have two actions which are theoretically valuable in the management of ulcer bleeding, namely inhibition of acid secretion and reduction of splanchnic blood flow. Mesenteric blood flow falls dramatically during infusions of somatostatin but it is not clear whether this is principally due to vasoconstriction of major blood vessels or peripheral arterioles.

There have been 14 controlled trials of somatostatin versus other therapy in the management of patients presenting with acute gastrointestinal bleeding [38–51]. Two meta-analyses suggest that somatostatin but not octreotide has a primary hemostatic role and reduces the need for surgical intervention [52, 53]. However, scrutiny of the relevant trials reveals many problems. Many of the studies were small and inclusion criteria varied widely from gastritis to major active bleeding. In common with the studies of tranexamic acid, the somatostatin trials were conducted before the widespread use of endoscopic therapy and PPI administration.

Currently, the evidence for routine use of somatostatin is weak and further studies are needed before this agent can be advocated as therapy for acute non-variceal gastrointestinal bleeding.

Endoscopic therapy

Many therapeutic endoscopic treatments have been used to try to stop active ulcer bleeding and prevent re-bleeding. These can be classified into three basic endoscopic approaches (Table 8.5).

Thermal approaches involving laser, the heater probe and electrocoagulation by monopolar or bipolar probes attempt to induce thermocoagulation with thrombosis of the bleeding point. In experimental bleeding ulcers these approaches are more effective than injection treatments [54]. However, there is currently no good model of acute peptic ulcer bleeding. Experiments in animals were historically based upon observation or intervention following superficial mucosal injury, which is different from erosion of arteries by chronic or acute peptic ulceration. A novel pig model has recently been developed, which appears to resemble the real life situation of an actively bleeding peptic ulcer more closely, although the element of chronic inflammation cannot be reproduced [55]. This model could facilitate the development of new endoscopic therapeutic methods. Injection therapy may produce tamponade by the injection of a relatively large volume of fluid into a rigid compartment, compressing the bleeding artery. Vasoconstriction induced by dilute adrenaline, endarteritis induced by sclerosants, dehydration following absolute alcohol injection or a direct effect upon blood clot formation following injection of thrombin or fibrin glue are other putative mechanisms. Mechanical clips, staples and sewing

Table 8.5 Endoscopic therapy.

Modality	Type
Thermal	Argon laser
	Nd-YAG laser
	Heater probe
	Electrocoagulation
	Argon plasma coagulation
Injection	Adrenaline
	Sclerosants
	Alcohol
	Thrombin
	Fibrin glue
Mechanical	Hemoclips
	Staples
	Sutures

attempt to produce hemostasis by clamping the bleeding arterial lesion. Many clinical trials of endoscopic therapy for non-variceal bleeding have been published. The quality of these trials varies greatly. In general, the number of patients randomized in any one study is small and clinicians managing the patients have not been blinded to the type of endoscopic therapy. Only one trial has included a placebo control intervention for endoscopic therapy [56].

Thermal methods

Laser photocoagulation

Lasers were the first endoscopic therapeutic modality shown to be effective in managing acute non-variceal gastrointestinal bleeding. Initial experience involved the use of argon lasers but it subsequently became clear that the tissue characteristics of thermal injury achieved by Nd-YAG were more appropriate. There have been a number of trials involving lasers for peptic ulcer bleeding [57–68]. Most of these studies show that laser treatment significantly reduced the rates of re-bleeding, transfusion requirement and operation rate. One trial showed significant improvement in hospital mortality [60].

Endoscopic laser therapy was found to be relatively safe with few complications; in particular, gastrointestinal perforation was rare. However, since the technique is difficult, relatively expensive and because other approaches are at least as effective, laser therapy for peptic ulcer bleeding is no longer used.

Heater probe

The heater probe transmits preset amounts of energy to the bleeding point via a Teflon tipped catheter. A powerful water jet is used to clean the ulcer base, help visualize the bleeding point and also to prevent the probe sticking to the bleeding point. Hemostasis is achieved by coaptive coagulation, using both tamponade and the application of heat. Best results are achieved using large sized probes. There have been two trials in which the heater probe has been compared to conservative therapy [69, 70]. Both showed benefit in terms of further bleeding, and surgery, and one published only in abstract form [71] demonstrated a trend towards reduction in mortality (Table 8.6). **A1d**

The heater probe is "user friendly". Its capacity to apply thermal energy by tangential application and its powerful water jet are particular advantages. Perforations have occurred following treatment, although these are unusual, and are of the order of 1% [71]. In general, medium power settings (20–30 joules) are used, but it is not possible to be prescriptive concerning the total amount of energy that should be applied. Most authorities consider that treatment should be continued until active hemorrhage is stopped and until the treated area is blackened and cavitated.

Table 8.6 Heater probe for gastrointestinal bleeding.

Study	Group	Re-bleed	Surgery	Mortality
Fullarton 1989 [69]	HP (n = 20)	0	0	0
	Sham (n = 23)	22[a]	13[b]	0
Jensen 1988 [70]	BICAP	44	33	3
	HP	22[c]	3[c]	3
	Nil	72	41	9
	n (total) = 94			

[a] p = 0.05.
[b] p = 0.23.
[c] p < 0.05.
HP: heater probe; BICAP: bipolar electrocoagulation.

Electrocoagulation

Monopolar electrocoagulation uses a metal ball-tipped probe. An electrical circuit is completed by a plate attached to the patient. Application of energy is rather haphazard and perforations and a death were reported in early series. Consequently this device is no longer used. Multipolar electrocoagulation is based upon transmission of electrical energy between adjacent electrodes. The BICAP has eight separate electrodes over its surface. Early studies from the UK involving small numbers of patients showed no benefit for active treatment compared to conservative therapy. Subsequently, however, trials from the UK and the USA showed improved outcomes including primary hemostasis, re-bleeding, the need for surgery and transfusion requirements with bipolar electrocoagulation compared to conventionally treated patients (Table 8.7) [72–75]. The efficacy of the heater probe and BICAP appear to be comparable with similar low complication rates [71, 76]. **A1d**

Argon plasma coagulation

This procedure is based upon coagulation through a jet of argon gas. Relatively superficial thermal damage is achieved. The method is particularly applicable to mucosal and superficial bleeding lesions and its final role may be in dealing with vascular malformations such as gastric antral vascular ectasia. One small trial has shown that argon plasma coagulation is comparable in efficacy to heater probe therapy for ulcer hemostasis [77]. A second trial compared the argon plasma coagulator with combination injection of adrenaline and polidocanol [78]. Again the two approaches were equally effective. Nevertheless the tissue damage characteristics of argon plasma coagulation are less than ideal for managing arterial bleeding, and it will probably prove to be less appropriate for managing peptic ulcer bleeding than contact methods.

Table 8.7 Electrocoagulation for gastrointestinal bleeding.

Study	Group	n	Re-bleed (%)	Surgery (%)	Mean units transfused
O'Brien 1987 [72]	Bipolar probe	101	17 (17)[c]	7 (7)	4.6[d]
	Nil	103	34 (33)	10 (10)	7.3
[a]Laine 1987 [73]	MPEC	21	—	3 (14)[e]	2.4[f]
	Sham	23	—	10 (43)	5.4
Brearley 1987 [74]	Bipolar probe	20	6 (30)	—	—
	Nil	21	8 (38)	—	—
[b]Laine 1988 [75]	MPEC	37	7 (19)[g]	3 (8)	1.6[g]
	Sham	37	15 (41)	11 (30)	3.0

[a] Study included ulcers, Mallory–Weiss tears and vascular malformations.
[b] Study was restricted to ulcers with non-bleeding visible vessels. See also Jensen [70], Table 8.6.
[c] $p = 0.01$.
[d] $p = 0.13$.
[e] $p = 0.049$.
[f] $p = 0.002$.
[g] $p < 0.05$.
MPEC: multipolar electrocoagulation.

Conclusions

Thermal methods of hemostasis were shown to be superior to conservative management in two meta-analyses. In the study of Cook *et al.* [79] the odds ratio for prevention of re-bleeding was 0.48 (95% CI: 0.32–0.76); and for avoidance of surgery was 0.47 (95% CI: 0.27–0.80). Similarly, in the study of Henry and White [80], the odds ratio for prevention of bleeding was 0.32 (95% CI: 0.22–0.41) and for the avoidance of surgery was 0.31 (95% CI: 0.19–0.43). **A1d** Thermal contact methods (heater probe and bipolar coagulation) are technically easier to undertake than laser techniques. There are insufficient data to determine whether the heater probe is better than the BICAP.

The safety profile of thermal modalities is generally very good. Perforations are unusual and treatment induced exacerbation of bleeding is not usually clinically important.

Injection therapy

Injection treatment is simple to perform and is the cheapest available hemostatic modality. A large range of injection materials have been studied and it is difficult to prove that any one of these is superior to the others.

Dilute adrenaline

In 1988 Chung *et al.* reported a controlled trial in which patients with active ulcer bleeding were randomized to

Table 8.8 Adrenaline for gastrointestinal bleeding.

Outcome	Adrenaline n = 34	Conservative n = 34
Primary hemostasis (%)	34 (100)	—[a]
Surgery (%)	5 (15)	14 (41)
Mortality (%)	3 (9)	2 (6)

[a] Twenty patients stopped bleeding spontaneously.
Source: Chung et al. [81].

receive endoscopic injection with 1:10,000 adrenaline or were treated conservatively [81]. Primary hemostasis was achieved in all injected patients and the need for subsequent urgent surgery was significantly reduced (Table 8.8). **A1d** Re-bleeding occurred in 24% of injected patients, suggesting that although dilute adrenaline did stop active bleeding, its effects were temporary.

It seemed logical to combine an injection of adrenaline with that of an agent which might cause permanent sealing of the bleeding arterial defect. For this reason a series of trials were undertaken in which adrenaline injection was combined with a range of sclerosants.

The results of trials in which a combination of adrenaline plus sclerosants were compared to conservative therapy are summarized in Table 8.9 [82–85]. All showed that active bleeding stopped more rapidly in treated patients, that re-

Table 8.9 Adrenaline plus sclerosants for gastrointestinal bleeding.

Study	Group	n	Rebleed (%)	Surgery (%)	Mortality (%)
Panès 1987 [82]	Adr + Pol + Cim	55	3 (5)	3 (5)	2 (4)
	Cim	58	25 (43)	20 (34)	4 (7)
Rajgopal 1991 [83]	Adr + Eth	56	7 (13)	6 (11)	2 (4)
	Nil	53	25 (47)	13 (25)	3 (6)
Balanzo 1988 [84]	Adr + Pol	36	7 (19)	7 (19)	—
	Nil	36	15 (42)	15 (42)	—
Oxner 1992 [85]	Adr + Eth	48	8 (17)	4 (8)	4 (8)
	Nil	45	21 (47)	8 (18)	9 (20)

Adr: adrenaline; Pol: polidocanol; Eth: ethanolamine; Cim: cimetidine.

bleeding rates were less, and that the need for surgery was reduced. No single trial, however, was powerful enough to determine whether mortality was affected. A subsequent meta-analysis, involving thermal contact devices, laser and injection therapy performed by Cook *et al.* [79] did show a modest reduction in mortality, although this was statistically significant only for laser therapy. **A1a**

Sclerosants

The sclerosants that have been studied are polidocanol, 5% ethanolamine oleate and 3% sodium tetradecyl sulphate. There are no controlled trials in which outcome has been assessed in patients randomized to sclerosants versus conservative (no injection) therapy. Several trials compared the efficacy of sclerosants with other endoscopic therapies. Benedetti *et al.* [86] showed similar efficacy for polidocanol and thrombin injection in patients presenting with a range of bleeding lesions. Strohm *et al.* [87] randomized patients to one of four treatment arms (fibrin glue, 1% polidocanol, dilute adrenaline or adrenaline plus polidocanol) and showed no advantage for any one approach. Rutgeerts *et al.* showed no difference in outcome for patients treated by polidocanol or Nd-YAG laser therapy [88]. In general these studies suffer from the problem of small sample size and they probably lacked statistical power.

A series of case reports documented complications of injection by sclerosant [89, 90], particularly perforation and necrosis of the upper gastrointestinal tract. These complications did not occur following adrenaline injection and indeed the latter seems remarkably safe. Fears concerning the possible systemic affects of circulating adrenaline have not translated into cardiovascular mishaps [91]. Since complications are mainly due to sclerosant injection, it was important to confirm the importance of combining the sclerosant with the adrenaline injection. Whilst the logic of attempting to induce endarteritis using sclerosants was reasonable, experiments in animals did not demonstrate that this could be achieved by injection using ethanolamine or absolute alcohol [92]. **C** Three trials have compared the efficacy of injection by adrenaline alone versus a combination of adrenaline plus a sclerosant [93–95], and a further two have compared adrenaline to adrenaline plus alcohol [96, 97]. As shown in Table 8.10, these five studies did not show that combination treatment was superior to injection by adrenaline alone. **A1c** No study has directly compared outcome in patients randomized to dilute adrenaline or to a sclerosant.

Since the addition of sclerosants to an injection of adrenaline offers no proven advantage over injecting adrenaline alone, and because sclerosants have the potential to cause significant local complications following injection, they should no longer be employed as part of the injection treatment regimen.

Alcohol

The efficacy of injecting absolute alcohol into bleeding ulcers has been examined in several clinical trials. Two of these (Table 8.11) [98, 99] randomized patients to alcohol injection or to conservative therapy and showed benefit in terms of reduction in re-bleeding rates and need for surgical intervention. **A1d**

In a randomized controlled trial, Lin *et al.* [100] reported that alcohol injection stopped active bleeding and prevented re-bleeding in 86% of patients whose ulcers were injected, and this result was similar to the proportion of bleeding ulcers responding to injection with 3% sodium

Table 8.10 Adrenaline vs adrenaline plus sclerosant in gastrointestinal bleeding.

Study	Group	n	Primary hemostasis	Re-bleed (%)	Surgery (%)	Transfusion (units +/− range)	Mortality (%)
Chung 1993 [93]	Adr + STD	101	98	14 (14)		—	—
	Adr	99	93	16 (16)		—	—
Villanueva 1993 [94]	Adr + Pol	33	32	7 (21)	5 (15)	2	1 (3)
	Adr	30	29	3 (10)	4 (13)	2	2 (7)
Choudari 1994 [95]	Adr + Eth	52	—	7 (14)	4 (8)	8	0 (0)
	Adr	55	—	8 (15)	4 (7)	9	1 (2)
Lin 1993 [96]	Adr + Alc	32	32	5 (16)	2 (6)	—	2 (6)
	Adr	32	31	11 (36)	1 (3)	—	0 (0)
Chung 1996 [97]	Adr + Alc	79	75	6 (8)	9 (11)	2 (0–23)	7 (9)
	Adr	81	79	9 (11)	12 (15)	3 (0–20)	4 (5)

Adr: adrenaline; STD: sodium tetradecyl sulphate; Alc: alcohol; Eth: ethanolamine; Pol: polidocanol.

Table 8.11 Alcohol vs conservative therapy for gastrointestinal bleeding.

Study	Group	n	Re-bleeding (%)	Surgery (%)	Mortality (%)
Pascu 1989 [98]	Alcohol	65	1 (2)[a]	1 (2)[a]	2 (3)
	Conservative	78	17 (22)	17 (22)	10 (13)
Lazo 1992 [99]	Alcohol	25	2 (8)[b]	1 (4)[c]	—
	Conservative	14	8 (57)	7 (50)	—

[a] p = 0.0007.
[b] p < 0.001.
[c] p < 0.05.

chloride, 50% dextrose, or normal saline. Only one small study [101] has attempted to compare the efficacy of alcohol with dilute adrenaline injection, but this study lacked statistical power to demonstrate differences in the effects of these interventions, should any exist.

The evidence that alcohol stops active bleeding and prevents re-bleeding is stronger than that for the sclerosants. Unfortunately, the potential for adverse effects is higher for alcohol than for adrenaline. Deep ulcers commonly follow alcohol injection and perforations have occurred [102]. Two trials have examined the need to combine alcohol injection with adrenaline and found no beneficial effect over the injection of adrenaline alone (Table 8.10) [96, 97].

Whilst alcohol injection is an effective hemostatic therapy, current evidence suggests that the magnitude of its effect is probably similar to that achieved by injection with adrenaline alone. Because of its propensity for causing adverse effects, alcohol injection is not recommended as treatment for ulcer bleeding.

Thrombin and fibrin glue

The most attractive endoscopic approach is to directly cause blood clot formation by injecting thrombogenic substances. In the 1980s small trials examined the efficacy of bovine thrombin and showed little benefit compared to other modalities.

In 1996 Kubba et al. [103] reported a comparison of endoscopic injection therapy using a combination of adrenaline plus human thrombin with dilute adrenaline injection alone (Table 8.12). A proportion of randomized patients had active bleeding at the time of randomization, while the remainder had non-bleeding visible vessels. Re-bleeding and mortality were significantly reduced in the group receiving combination therapy compared to patients receiving adrenaline alone. The number of patients needed to be treated with combination therapy rather than adrenaline alone to prevent one death is approximately 14. Paradoxically, no statistically significant differences in the

Table 8.12 Adrenaline plus thrombin vs adrenaline alone for gastrointestinal bleeding 1.

Outcome	Adrenaline + thrombin	Adrenaline alone
n	70	70
Re-bleed (%)	3 (4)	14 (20)[a]
Transfusion (units)	7	5
Surgery (%)	3 (4)	5 (7)
Mortality (%)	0 (0)	7 (10)[b]

[a] p < 0.005.
[b] p < 0.013.
Source: Kubba *et al.* [103].

Table 8.13 Adrenaline plus thrombin vs adrenaline alone for gastrointestinal bleeding 2.

Outcome	Adrenaline + thrombin	Adrenaline alone
n	32	32
Re-bleed (%)	2 (6)	4 (13)
Transfusion (units)	3.14	3.94
Surgery (%)	5 (16)	4 (13)
Mortality (%)	0 (0)	0 (0)

Source: Balanzo *et al.* [104].

Table 8.14 Heater probe plus thrombin vs heater probe plus placebo for gastrointestinal bleeding.

Outcome	Heater probe plus thrombin	Heater probe plus placebo
n	127	120
Rebleed (%)	19 (15)	17 (15)
Surgery (%)	16 (13)	13 (11)
Mortality (%)	8 (6)	14 (12)

Source: Church *et al.* [56].

Table 8.15 Fibrin glue vs adrenaline injection for gastrointestinal bleeding.

Outcome	Fibrin glue	Hypertonic saline/adrenaline
n	64	63
Rebleed (%)	7 (11)	14 (22)
Surgery (%)	4 (6)	7 (11)
Mortality (%)	1 (2)	4 (6)

Source: Song *et al.* [105].

need for surgical operation and the overall rate of hemostasis were demonstrated. Indeed, deaths in this study all occurred, as is usually the case, in patients who had significant co-morbidity. Complications in this study were minimal. Although this was not a direct comparison of adrenaline versus thrombin, it did strongly suggest that human thrombin is an effective modality.

Balanzo *et al.* [104] randomized 64 ulcer bleeding patients to adrenaline injection or adrenaline plus thrombin in a similar, but smaller trial. There were no differences in the rates of primary hemostasis, re-bleeding, surgery or death (Table 8.13).

To further investigate the use of thrombin as a potential adjunct to standard endoscopic therapy Church *et al.* randomized 247 patients to treatment with heater probe plus thrombin injection or to heater probe plus placebo injection [56]. This trial included only patients with bleeding peptic ulcers who were at high-risk for re-bleeding and death, and was the first trial to include placebo endoscopic therapy. Initial hemostasis was achieved in 97% of patients in both groups, and the rates of re-bleeding, surgery and mortality were similar (Table 8.14). The results of this trial do not suggest that thrombin is any more effective than placebo

when combined with the heater probe for endoscopic hemostasis. **A1a**

Fibrin glue is a mixture of fibrinogen and thrombin which is injected through a double-channeled endoscopy needle. Its effect was studied by Song *et al.* in a trial of 127 patients with bleeding ulcers and major stigmata of hemorrhage [105]. Patients were randomized to injection of fibrin glue or hypertonic saline-adrenaline. There were no significant differences between rates of re-bleeding, surgery and death (Table 8.15). **A1c** This trial is the only one which has compared the efficacy of fibrin glue directly with that of another endoscopic therapeutic modality.

In a large multicenter European study (Table 8.16) [106] 850 patients were randomized to endoscopic injection with dilute adrenaline plus a single injection of fibrin glue, to adrenaline and repeated injection of fibrin glue given at daily intervals according to the discretion of the endoscopists, or to adrenaline plus 1% polidocanol. Re-bleeding rates were lowest in patients treated by repeated injection. The rate of serious re-bleeding requiring major blood transfusion or surgical operation was significantly reduced in patients receiving repeated injections of glue compared to the polidocanol treated group. **A1a** A total of seven perforations occurred in this study and these were distributed equally amongst the treatment modalities.

The most recent trial involving fibrin glue randomized 135 patients to injection of adrenaline plus fibrin glue or to

Table 8.16 Adrenaline plus fibrin glue vs adrenaline plus polidocanol for gastrointestinal bleeding.

Outcome	Adr + rep FG	Adr + single FG	Adr + Pol
n	284	285	281
Re-bleed (%)	41 (16)	51 (19)	58 (21)[a]
Transfusion (units)	3.7	3.2	3.3
Surgery (%)	9 (3)	13 (5)	13 (5)
Perforation (%)	2 (1)	2 (1)	3 (1)
Mortality (30 day) (%)	12 (4)	15 (5)	13 (5)

[a] $p < 0.036$.

Adr: adrenaline; FG: fibrin glue; Pol: polidocanol.
Source: Rutgeerts *et al.* [106].

adrenaline alone [107]. Endoscopy was repeated daily with retreatment of stigmata until the ulcer base contained flat pigmented spots or was clean. The rate of re-bleeding in the combination group was not significantly different from that in the single agent group (24% vs 22%). Rates for surgery were also similar (10% vs 6%), and mortality was 3% in both groups. **A1c**

The evidence regarding the use of thrombogenic substances is conflicting. There is evidence of benefit in some studies, but not in others, and currently there is not enough evidence to recommend thrombin or fibrin glue over other injection agents. Thrombin is derived from pooled plasma, and although viral (or other infective agent) transmission has not been reported, this is a possibility. Acute complications are infrequent and no adverse effects have been apparent in terms of systemic coagulation.

Human thrombin is not currently commercially available. It is relatively inexpensive, although more costly than adrenaline.

Mechanism of action and volume of injection

The mechanism of injection therapy is not completely understood. It is thought to work at least in part by exerting a tamponade effect resulting from the injection of a volume of fluid into the rigid ulcer base. This possibility is supported by the study reported by *Lin et al.* [100] who compared injection of normal saline, 3% NaCl solution, 50% glucose/water solution and pure alcohol in 200 patients with actively bleeding ulcers or non-bleeding visible vessels. There were no statistical differences between rates of initial hemostasis, re-bleeding, and surgery for any group. Larger injected volumes were required to achieve initial hemostasis in the saline and glucose/water groups, suggesting that tamponade was an important factor. These

results are challenged by those of Laine and Estrada [108]. In this study patients with high-risk ulcers were randomized to injection of normal saline (n = 48), or to bipolar electrocoagulation (n = 52). Twenty nine percent of patients in the saline group had recurrent bleeding compared with 12% of those treated with the BICAP. The saline-treated patients required significantly more blood, but there were no differences in length of hospital stay or mortality. It is likely that tamponade does not completely explain the mechanism of injection therapy, and active agents should continue to be used.

The optimum volume of injection is not known. Small volumes of alcohol and sclerosants are required in order to reduce the risk of perforation. Much larger volumes of saline and adrenaline can be used without major complications. In the trial by Lin *et al.* [100] discussed above, the mean injection volume in the saline group was 15 ml. Laine and Estrada injected a mean volume of 30 ml [108]. A further trial by Lin *et al.* compared large with relatively small volume injection [109]. One hundred and fifty six ulcer bleeding patients were randomized to injection of 5–10 ml of adrenaline (the small volume group) or injection of 13–20 ml (the large volume group). Re-bleeding occurred in 31% of the small volume patients compared with 15% in the large volume group. The other usual endpoints were similar. The conclusion of this trial is that larger volume injection of adrenaline is safe and more likely to prevent re-bleeding than injection of a smaller volume. These results are supported by those of two other groups. Park *et al.* [110] randomized 72 patients with high-risk stigmata of bleeding to either 15–25 ml adrenaline injection (mean volume 19.4 ml) or to 35–45 ml injection (mean volume 41.1 ml). The overall rates of re-bleeding were significantly lower in the large volume group (0% vs 17.1%, $p < 0.05$), this effect being entirely due to a reduction in re-bleeding from ulcers in the gastric body. There was one perforation in the large volume group, but no other complications. The largest trial was performed by Liou *et al.* [111]. Two hundred and twenty eight patients with actively bleeding ulcers were randomized to receive either a 20 ml, 30 ml or 40 ml total volume adrenaline injection. Initial hemostasis was achieved in almost all patients. Recurrent bleeding occurred in a significantly greater proportion of patients in the 20 ml injection group. Those patients treated with the 40 ml injection had increased rates of perforation and injection related abdominal pain (Table 8.17). The conclusion was that 30 ml was the optimal volume of adrenaline injection for treatment of actively bleeding ulcers.

Conclusion

Injection therapy is effective and safe. The optimum injection regimen should include 1:10,000 adrenaline, which

Table 8.17 Optimal volume of adrenaline for peptic ulcer bleeding.

Outcome	Adrenaline 20 ml (%)	Adrenaline 30 ml (%)	Adrenaline 40 ml (%)
n	76	76	76
Initial hemostasis	74 (97.4)	75 (98.7)	76 (100)
Recurrent bleeding	15/74 (20.3)[a]	4/75 (5.3)	2/72 (2.8)
Perforated ulcer	0 (0)	0 (0)	4 (5.3)[b]
Surgical intervention	4 (5.3)	2 (2.6)	5 (6.6)
Transfusion requirement (units)	4.7 +/− 3.4	4.5 +/− 3.2	4.2 +/− 3.6
Total hospital stay (days)	10.8 +/− 3.3	9.7 +/− 3.5	10.2 +/− 3.1
Deaths from bleeding	0 (0)	0 (0)	0 (0)
Thirty-day mortality	3 (3.9)	2 (2.6)	4 (5.3)
Injection related abdominal pain	2 (2.6)	5 (6.6)	51 (67.1)[c]

[a] $p < 0.01$ vs 30 ml and 40 ml groups.
[b] $p < 0.05$ vs the 20 ml and 30 ml groups.
[c] $p < 0.001$ vs the 20 ml and 30 ml groups.
Source: Liou *et al.* [111].

stops active hemorrhage. Studies suggest that a volume of at least 13 ml should be injected. Re-bleeding rates are not convincingly reduced by the addition of agents such as thrombin or a thrombin–fibrinogen mixture. Sclerosants and alcohol should not be used, since there is no evidence that they are beneficial and they increase the risk of serious complications.

Comparison of injection and thermal treatments

A number of small trials have compared injection with thermal therapies. In general, the two modalities appear to have similar efficacy.

Six trials have compared heater probe with injection (Table 8.18) [112–117]. The two trials reported by Lin *et al.* [112, 113] showed that heater probe treatment was more effective in achieving primary hemostasis. These authors noted the heater probe to be better when ulcers were difficult to approach, since it can be applied tangentially. They also found the water jet to be useful in the presence of spurting bleeding. It may be argued that alcohol is a less appropriate injection therapy than adrenaline, which may account for the apparent superiority of the heater probe in these studies. This view was supported by the findings of Chung *et al.* [114]. They concluded that heater probe and adrenaline were equally effective, but that initial hemostasis was more easily achieved with adrenaline. Choudari *et al.* [115] compared the heater probe with adrenaline plus ethanolamine and found no differences between the modalities. The remaining two trials by Saeed *et al.* [116] and Llach *et al.* [117] support this conclusion. Laine [118] showed that electrocoagulation and injection with ethanol

were equivalent, although the size of this trial was suboptimal. **A1c**

Two trials involved the Nd-YAG laser. Carter *et al.* [119] compared laser with adrenaline and Pulanic *et al.* [120], in a much larger trial, compared laser with polidocanol. Neither showed a difference in outcome.

Current evidence does not allow a conclusion to be drawn on whether injection or thermal treatment is superior as a single modality. We advocate the heater probe as the thermal method of choice. Some situations, particularly those involving awkwardly placed posterior duodenal ulcers, lend themselves better to use of the heater probe than to injection therapy.

Mechanical clips

The hemoclip was first used for non-variceal bleeding by Japanese investigators in the early 1970s [121]. Early clips were difficult to apply, but since modifications were introduced in the late 1980s the device has gained favor as the endoscopic method most analogous to under-running an ulcer at operative surgery. Various types of clips have been evaluated but of the most frequently used devices only the Olympus Hemoclip and the Cook TriClip have been investigated in human studies [122].

Hemoclip

The Olympus Hemoclip is the most widely used clipping device, and has the largest evidence base. Three large case series [123–125] support hemoclips as a safe and effective method for the treatment of bleeding peptic ulcer, and

Table 8.18 Comparison of heater probe with injection therapy.

Study	Group	n	Primary hemostasis (%)	Re-bleed (%)	Surgery (%)	Mortality (%)
Lin 1988 [112]	HP	42	42 (100)	5 (12)	—	—
	PA	36	29 (81)	6 (22)	—	—
Lin 1990 [113]	HP	45	44 (98)[a]	8 (18)	3 (7)[b]	1 (2)[c]
	PA	46	31 (67)	2 (7)	2 (4)	0
	Control	46	—	—	12 (26)	7 (15)
Chung 1991 [114]	HP	64	53 (83)[d]	6/53 (11)	14 (22)	4 (6)
	Adr	68	65 (96)	11 (17)	14 (21)	2 (3)
Choudari 1992 [115]	HP	60	—	9 (15)	7 (12)	3 (5)
	Adr + Eth	60	—	8 (13)	7 (12)	2 (3)
Saeed 1993 [116]	HP	39	35 (90)	4 (10)	—	—
	Ethanol	41	33 (81)	5 (12)	—	—
Llach 1996 [117]	HP	53	—	3 (6)	2 (4)	1 (2)
	Adr + Pol	51	—	2 (4)	2 (4)	1 (2)

[a] $p = 0.0004$.
[b] $p = 0.0024$ ($p = 0.027$ between control and HP; $p = 0.012$ between PA and HP).
[c] $p = 0.002$ ($p = 0.031$ between control and HP; $p = 0.018$ between control and PA).
[d] $p < 0.05$.
HP: heater probe; PA: pure alcohol; Adr: adrenaline; Eth: ethanolamine; Pol: polidocanol.

there are eight randomized trials of reasonable size comparing clips to other hemostatic therapies (Table 8.19) [126–133]. Other trials combining hemoclips with injection therapy are discussed in a later section.

The first randomized trial was published by Chung et al. in 1999 [126]. Primary hemostasis was achieved in over 95% of patients. Re-bleeding and surgery rates were lower in the hemoclip groups but these were not statistically significant. Three patients had complications, all in the adrenaline only group. In one patient severe bleeding requiring surgical operation was precipitated; two patients developed submucosal hematoma. Cipoletta et al. [127] randomized 113 patients with endoscopic stigmata of hemorrhage to heater probe thermocoagulation or to application of hemoclips. A mean of three clips per patient were used with up to six being required in some cases. Re-bleeding was dramatically reduced in the hemoclip group. Surgery and mortality rates were similar in the two groups and there were no complications.

The two previous trials suggested clips to be effective, with re-bleed rates below 3% in the clip only groups. However, subsequent studies have been less encouraging. Lin et al. [128] achieved primary hemostasis in only 85% of patients in a group of patients treated with clips versus 100% of those treated with the heater probe ($p = 0.01$). The following year the same group compared ulcer bleeding patients treated by hemoclip placement with patients in

whom heater probe thermocoagulation and adrenaline injection were used. The rate of primary hemostasis was lower in the hemoclip group (95.1% vs 100%) but this difference was not statistically significant [129]. Gevers et al. [130] performed a similar trial to Chung et al. [126] in which patients were randomized to injection with adrenaline and polidocanol, hemoclip application or a combination of the two. Patients treated with clips had lower primary haemostasis rates but this did not reach statistical significance. A composite endpoint defined as the overall failure rate was significantly higher in the hemoclip alone group than in the injection and combination groups (34%, 6% and 25% respectively, $p = 0.01$). Patients in the other three trials [131–133] fared better, although clips were only demonstrated to be superior to injection in terms of a reduction in rebleeding in the trial by Chou et al. [131]. There were no other differences in any category.

Hemoclips have been the subject of two recently published meta-analyses [134, 135]. The first of these [134] was restricted to trials comparing the hemoclip alone with other hemostatic techniques. Twelve randomized trials were identified, including all those mentioned above, in addition to four other small trials which studied patients who were not bleeding from high-risk peptic ulcers. In a pooled analysis considering only those patients with bleeding peptic ulcer, 351 patients were treated with hemoclips and 348 patients received another form of therapy. Initial hemosta-

Table 8.19 Hemoclip for peptic ulcer bleeding.

Study	Group	n	Primary hemostasis (%)	Re-bleeding (%)	Surgery (%)	Death (%)
Chung 1999 [126]	HC	41	40 (97.5)	1 (2.5)	2 (4.9)	1 (2.4)
	Adr injection	41	39 (95.1)	6 (15.4)	6 (14.6)	1 (2.4)
	HC + Adr	42	41 (97.6)	4 (9.8)	1 (2.4)	1 (2.4)
Cipolletta 2001 [127]	HC	56	50 (89.3)	1 (2.0)[a]	2 (3.6)	2 (3.6)
	HP	57	49 (86.0)	12 (24.5)	4 (7.0)	2 (3.5)
Lin 2002 [128]	HC	40	34 (85.0)[b]	3 (8.8)	2 (5.0)	2 (5.0)
	HP	40	40 (100.0)	2 (5.0)	1 (2.5)	1 (2.5)
Gevers 2002 [130]	HC	35	29 (82.9)	7 (24.1)	0 (0)	0 (0)
	Adr + Pol	34	33 (97.1)	5 (15.2)	0 (0)	0 (0)
	HC + Adr + Pol	32	29 (90.6)	5 (17.2)	0 (0)	3 (9.4)
Lin 2003 [129]	HC	46	39 (95.1)	4 (10.3)	0 (0)	2 (4.3)
	HP + Adr	47	47 (100.0)	3 (6.4)	2 (4.3)	1 (2.1)
Chou 2003 [131]	HC	39	39 (100.0)	4 (10.3)[c]	2 (5.1)	1 (2.6)
	Distilled water	40	39 (97.5)	11 (28.2)	5 (12.5)	2 (5.0)
Shimoda 2003 [132]	HC	42	42 (100.0)	4 (9.5)	0 (0)	3 (7.1)
	Alc	42	42 (100.0)	6 (14.3)	0 (0)	1 (2.4)
	HC + Alc	42	42 (100.0)	3 (7.1)	0 (0)	1 (2.4)
Ljubicic 2004 [133]	HC	31	30 (96.8)	2 (6.7)	1 (3.2)	1 (3.2)
	Pol	30	29 (96.7)	4 (13.8)	1 (3.3)	0 (0)

[a] $p < 0.05$.

[b] $p = 0.01$.

[c] $p = 0.04$.

HC: hemoclip; Adr: adrenaline; Pol: polidocanol; Alc: pure alcohol.

sis was lower in the clips group when compared to controls, but this was not significant (92% vs 96%, OR 0.58; 95% CI: 0.19–1.75). There was a non-significant trend towards a reduction in rebleeding in the clip group (8.5% vs 15.5%, OR 0.56; 95% CI 0.30–1.05), and no other differences were identified. **A1a**

Sung *et al*. [135] reported a more wide ranging study in which the main difference to the Yuan study was the inclusion of a number of trials comparing hemoclips in combination with injection to injection therapy alone. There was total of 1156 patients in 15 trials and several subgroup analyses were performed. Comparing hemoclips alone to injection therapy alone, re-bleeding rates were lower in patients treated with clips (9.5% vs 19.6%, RR 0.49; 95% CI: 0.30–0.79). There was also a significant reduction in the need for emergency surgery (2.3% vs 7.4%, RR 0.37; 95% CI: 0.15–0.90). A similar effect was not surprisingly demonstrated when clips combined with injection were compared to injection therapy alone (8.3% vs 18.0%, RR 0.47; 95% CI: 0.28–0.76 for re-bleeding; 1.3% vs 6.3%, RR 0.23: 95% CI: 0.08–0.70 for surgery). Despite these results, an

effect on mortality was not demonstrated. In another analysis, clips were found to have equivalent efficacy to thermal therapies for all the usual endpoints (definitive hemostasis 81.5% vs 81.2%, RR 1.00; 95% CI: 0.77–1.31). The conclusion that can be drawn from both meta-analyses is that hemoclips are probably equivalent to other forms of endoscopic therapy, and may be superior to injection therapy alone when the clips are optimally applied. **A1a**

The major difficulty with hemoclip placement occurs when ulcers are difficult to reach and tangential application is required. In the Sung meta-analysis, the ulcer locations most associated with failure of clip application were the posterior duodenal bulb, the posterior wall of the stomach and the high lesser curve of the stomach – precisely the areas where the highest risk lesions are found. Initial clip applicators resulted in problems with clip alignment, but a rotating applicator is now in general use. Further problems arise when clips are applied to the fibrous base of a chronic ulcer, as in this situation it may not be possible to adequately compress the bleeding vessel. In the trial by Lin *et al*. [128] a surveillance endoscopy was performed 72 hours after therapy. Hemoclips had been successfully placed in 31 patients, but at 72 hours the clip was still attached to the ulcer base in only 10 patients. This could have accounted for the disappointing performance of the clip group, and perhaps clips with a more powerful clamping mechanism would improve the efficacy of the device. Further trials with improved clips are required.

Triclip

The Cook triclip was developed to try to overcome the difficulties encountered with tangential application reported with the hemoclip. As its name suggests the clip comprises three prongs instead of two. The triclip can be rotated in a similar way to the hemoclip. Trials involving the triclip are few in number.

Following experimental studies suggesting the device to be effective [136], a pilot study in human subjects was carried out by Chan *et al.* in 2004 [137]. Twenty seven high-risk ulcer bleeding patients were treated with triclips. Initial hemostasis was achieved in 22 (81.5%) but at repeat endoscopy 24 hours later four (14.8%) were oozing from the treated site, giving an overall definitive hemostasis rate of only 66.7%. At the second endoscopy clips were found to be dislodged in 11 patients (40.7%). It was noted that if more than one clip was required, the three prong design could make the application of a second clip difficult. Further disappointing results were reported following a randomized trial by Lin *et al.* comparing the triclip with the hemoclip in 100 ulcer patients with active bleeding or non-bleeding visible vessels [138]. Primary hemostasis rates were significantly lower in the triclip group (76% vs 94%, p = 0.011). This difference was principally due to failure of triclip application in ulcers which were difficult to reach on the lesser curve and posterior wall of the stomach and in the posterior duodenum. Outcomes for the other endpoints were similar. The conclusion was that the hemoclip is superior to the triclip for high-risk ulcers in difficult to reach sites. **A1c**

Conclusion

Mechanical clips appear to be similar in efficacy to other endoscopic hemostatic modalities and there are few reports of adverse events following their use. Several devices are in clinical use, but the evidence in human subjects to date supports the use of the hemoclip. The major limitation of clipping devices relates to suboptimal deployment of clips in the posterior duodenum and high lesser curve of the stomach. With future development and modifications to clip applicators these difficulties may be overcome.

Combination of injection, thermal and mechanical treatments

The mechanisms leading to hemostasis associated with thermal treatment and injection therapy may differ, providing a rationale for combining a thermal modality with injection treatment. **C** Currently, only two small studies have shown a benefit from use of such a combination. The first trial by Lin *et al.* [139] used the gold probe, a bipolar coagulation probe containing an injection needle in the center. Using this device heat and injection therapy may be applied without removing the probe from the ulcer. Ninety six patients were randomized to receive injection alone, coagulation alone or combination therapy. Re-bleeding rates were lower in the combination group compared to the injection alone and coagulation alone groups (7% vs 36%, p = 0.01 and 7% vs 30%, p = 0.04 respectively). **A1c** The volume of blood transfused in the combination group was also significantly lower. Although this small trial demonstrated a beneficial outcome following combination endoscopic therapy, the results were not confirmed by the subsequent trial of Bianco *et al.* reported in 2004 [140]. This group randomized 114 patients with high-risk bleeding to initial injection of adrenaline followed by coagulation, again using the gold probe, or to gold probe therapy alone. In the event of failure of primary hemostasis in either group, repeat therapy using both injection and coagulation was applied. There were trends towards a reduction in re-bleeding, surgery and mortality in the combination group. The study probably lacked power to demonstrate statistically significant differences between the groups, should they exist, but the numbers were too small for these to reach statistical significance. There were 19 patients with active bleeding in each arm. Initial hemostasis was possible in only 68.4% of these patients treated with gold probe alone, compared to 100% in the combination group (p = 0.02), suggesting that combination therapy was advantageous when active bleeding was present.

A similar trend relates to a finding within a study reported by Chung *et al.* [141]. This study involved randomization of appropriate ulcer bleeding patients to injection therapy using 1 : 10,000 adrenaline or to a combination of adrenaline plus the heater probe (Table 8.20). Although there was no overall difference in outcome between patients randomized to either arm, a post hoc subgroup analysis did reveal positive findings. Sixty patients had active spurting hemorrhage from large ulcers, and within this group the primary hemostatic effect of both treatments was similar. However, the need for operation was significantly reduced in the group treated by heater probe and injection. The number of surgical endpoints was very small, and this observation from subgroup analysis requires confirmation in further trials.

Five trials have examined the combination of mechanical clips with injection compared to injection therapy alone [126, 130, 132, 142, 143]. The combined results of these trials are included in the meta-analysis by Sung *et al.* [135] and the results of the first three trials are shown in Table 8.19. Park *et al.* [142] randomized 90 patients to either a combination of adrenaline injection plus one of hemoclip or band ligation or to adrenaline injection as monotherapy. Re-bleeding rates were significantly lower in the combination group (4.5% vs 20.5%, p = 0.024). **A1c** A separate analysis of the individual effects of clips or bands was not included in the published data. The most recent trial was of the same design, but restricted the mechanical component of the combination therapy group to the hemoclip [143]. One hundred and eight patients were randomized and both the

re-bleeding and surgery rates were significantly reduced in the combination therapy group (3.8% vs 21%, p = 0.008 for re-bleeding; 0% vs 9%, p = 0.02 for surgery). **A1c** The authors reported technical difficulty in the application of clips to ulcers in the posterior duodenum and high lesser curve of the stomach. However, with good technique it was possible to place clips in all patients.

Two meta-analyses have been performed to try to confirm the suspicion that combination therapy was superior to single modality treatment [144, 145]. The results are shown in Table 8.21. Calvet *et al.* [144] showed that rates of re-bleeding, surgery and mortality were significantly reduced when an additional therapy (either injection, thermal or mechanical) was added to adrenaline injection. Of the 16 trials included (1673 patients), 11 studied additional injection therapy, a sclerosant being used in eight of these. Perforations were seen in six of 558 patients in the combination group, but these were not all related to sclerosant injection. Patients with active bleeding were most likely to benefit from combination therapy. The more extensive study by Marmo *et al.* [145] included 2472 patients in 20 trials. Again, rebleeding and surgery rates were significantly lower in patients treated with combination endoscopic therapy. There was a trend towards mortality reduction but this did not achieve statistical significance. This study attempted to explore the differences between the outcomes of combination therapy and injection, thermal and mechanical monotherapy by dividing the trials into subgroups. The resulting analysis suggested that combination therapy was superior to injection monotherapy, but not to either thermal or mechanical monotherapy. However, the numbers of patients in the thermal and mechanical subgroups were small, and the study is not sufficiently powered to make this conclusion definitive.

The current evidence suggests that adrenaline injection for peptic ulcer bleeding should be combined with a second therapeutic modality. **A1d** Further trials are needed before it is possible to recommend any particular additional therapy over the others.

Table 8.20 Adrenaline plus heater probe vs adrenaline alone for gastrointestinal bleeding.

Outcome	Adrenaline + heater probe	Adrenaline alone
Overall	n = 136	n = 134
Primary hemostasis (%)	135 (99)	131 (98)
Re-bleed (%)	5 (4)	12 (9)
Transfusion (units)	3	2
Surgery (%)	8 (6)	14 (11)
Mortality (%)	8 (6)	7 (5)
Subgroup with spurting hemorrhage	n = 32	n = 28
Primary hemostasis (%)	31 (97)	25 (89)
Re-bleed (%)	2 (6)	6 (21)
Transfusion (units)	4	5
Surgery (%)	2 (6)	8 (29)[a]
Mortality (%)	Not stated	Not stated

[a]p = 0.03.
Source: Chung *et al.* [141].

Table 8.21 Meta-analyses of combination endoscopic therapy.

Study	Category	Single therapy	Combination therapy	OR	95% CI
Calvet 2004 [144]	Re-bleeding	18.4%	10.6%	0.53	0.40–0.69
	Surgery	11.3%	7.6%	0.64	0.46–0.90
	Death	5.1%	2.6%	0.51	0.31–0.84
Marmo 2007 [145]	Re-bleeding	15.6%	9.7%	0.59	0.44–0.80
	Surgery	9.1%	6.8%	0.66	0.49–0.89
	Death	5.0%	3.8%	0.68	0.46–1.02

Endoscopic therapy for ulcers with adherent blood clot

There is debate concerning the appropriate intervention when blood clot is tightly adherent to an ulcer base. To remove a clot seems counterintuitive in the situation of acute bleeding, but to leave it *in situ* prevents accurate categorisation of stigmata of hemorrhage, and may prevent correct application of endoscopic therapy.

Lin *et al.* [146] showed that when clot is tightly adherent after washing for 10 seconds with Water Pik irrigation, the re-bleed rate is 25%. Factors independently associated with re-bleeding in this situation are the presence of shock, co-morbid disease and hemoglobin at presentation of <10 g/dl. In the trial by Sung *et al.* [28] clot was defined as adherent only after five minutes irrigation with the 3.2 mm heater probe. Patients received high dose PPI infusion plus or minus endoscopic therapy. Of 39 patients with adherent clot only one (in the combination group) re-bled, suggesting that when clot is truly adherent to an ulcer base a PPI infusion may be all that is required. Bleau *et al.* published a small trial in which patients with adherent clot were randomized to pre-injection with adrenaline followed by clot removal and thermocoagulation of a visible vessel, or to medical therapy with PPI [147]. The patients in the endoscopic therapy group had a significantly lower re-bleeding rate, although the numbers were small (56 patients). A similar but very small trial (32 patients) has been reported by Jensen *et al.* [148]. The results again indicate that clot removal and therapy to the underlying stigmata is a safe and effective strategy. However, it should be noted that both the Bleau and the Jensen trials were terminated prematurely. The Jensen trial was also a subgroup analysis of a larger trial which was, therefore, not designed primarily to study outcomes in relation to adherent clot. Despite these limitations, Jensen's group included both trials in a meta-analysis of six studies including 240 patients which was published in 2005 [149]. Of the other four trials included, only two had been published in peer-reviewed journals. There was significant heterogeneity with regard to methodology and in particular the type, dose and delivery of medical therapy. The conclusion was that there was a significant reduction in re-bleeding rate for the endoscopic therapy group compared to those treated with medical therapy alone (5 of 61 (8.2%) vs 21 of 85 (24.7%); RR 0.35; 95% CI: 0.14–0.83). **A1c** Other outcomes were unaffected. Further trials specifically designed to address the question of whether or not to remove adherent clot are required before this approach can be advocated.

Elective repeat endoscopic therapy

It is not yet clear whether electively repeating endoscopy and hemostatic therapy in the absence of clinical or endo-scopic signs of re-bleeding is a useful strategy. There are six trials which include patients receiving repeated endoscopic therapy [106, 107, 150–153] and four of these have specifically addressed the question of the efficacy of endoscopic retreatment [150–153]. The trial by Pescatore *et al.* [107] reported no clear benefit from the use of an elective repeat endoscopy approach. A similar conclusion was reached by Messmann *et al.* in a study of 105 patients who had required endoscopic therapy for bleeding ulcers. Patients were randomized to daily repeat endoscopy with re-treatment of persistent stigmata, or to close observation. There was no difference between the groups for any of the usual endpoints [150]. In contrast to these results, Rutgeerts *et al.* reported a clear positive trend towards reduction in re-bleeding in patients treated with programmed repeat endoscopic therapy [106]. Villanueva *et al.* randomized 104 patients in whom endoscopic hemostasis had been achieved following injection of adrenaline, to repeat endoscopy or to observation [151]. There were trends towards a better outcome in the repeat endoscopy group, but statistically significant reductions in re-bleeding, surgery and mortality were not demonstrated.

Two trials suggested that repeat endoscopic therapy significantly reduces re-bleeding rates. The very small trial by Saeed *et al.* included only 40 patients [152], but Chiu *et al.* randomized 194 patients following endoscopic hemostasis using adrenaline injection and heater probe thermocoagulation [153]. One hundred patients underwent a scheduled repeat endoscopy and 35 of these required further endoscopic therapy. The remaining 94 patients were observed closely. All patients received intravenous omeprazole 40 mg twice daily for 72 hours following endoscopy. The mean total volume of adrenaline injected in the repeat endoscopy group was 11.1 ml compared with 9.1 ml in the control group (p = 0.008). The mean total joules of heater probe therapy in the two groups were 95.3 and 110.2 respectively. Re-bleeding rates were significantly lower in the repeat endoscopy group compared to the control group (5% vs 14%, p = 0.034). There was also a trend towards reduction in the requirement for surgery (1% vs 6%, p = 0.05). Mortality rates were similar in the two groups.

Two meta-analyses examining the above trials have been published [154, 155]. Both suggest that elective repeat endoscopy significantly reduces re-bleeding (12% vs 18.2%; OR 0.64; 95% CI: 0.44–0.95) [155], but has no beneficial effect on the rates of surgery or mortality. **A1c**

Complications of repeat endoscopic therapy including sedation related cardiorespiratory adverse events, and heater probe related perforation have not been reported. However, in the trials by the Hong Kong group, perforation of the duodenum following repeat thermal therapy with the heater probe occurred in 3% [114] and 4.5% [156] of cases. This is considerably higher than the overall heater probe related perforation rate and suggests that aggressive repeat thermal therapy in the duodenum should be avoided. In many cases repeat endoscopic therapy is not required at the time of second look endoscopy, and a cost-benefit analysis of a policy of elective repeat endoscopic therapy is required. Currently, the total number of patients studied is small, but the available evidence indicates that elective repeat endoscopic therapy may be beneficial in patients at high-risk of re-bleeding or surgery. Repeat endoscopy should also be considered in cases where the endoscopist is not convinced that adequate hemostasis has been achieved at the time of the initial endoscopy.

Failure of endoscopic therapy

It may be argued that endoscopists can adversely affect outcome in patients who fail endoscopic therapy. Repeated unsuccessful therapeutic endoscopy, large blood transfusion and delayed surgical operation in those who ultimately fail attempted endoscopic hemostasis may all increase the risk of death. A number of studies have reported factors associated with failure of endoscopic therapy. These have been summarized in a paper by Elmunzer et al. [157]. Independent pre-endoscopic predictors of failure were hemodynamic instability and the presence of co-morbid disease. Endoscopic factors associated with a poor outcome were active bleeding, large ulcer size, posterior duodenal ulcer and high lesser curve gastric ulcer. Although none of these predictors is particularly surprising, it is interesting to note that patient age appears to have no independent effect on outcome. It should be noted that none of the patients in the studies reviewed were treated with high dose PPI infusions, and combination endoscopic therapy was not universal. Thus, the results may not be generalisable to current practice, but could be used to aid decisions regarding elective repeat endoscopy and to focus future trials to ensure that only high-risk patients are included.

Unfortunately, we cannot reliably predict who will fail and who will respond to endoscopic therapy, and even in the highest risk group of patients, who present with active spurting hemorrhage from large posterior duodenal ulcers, endoscopic hemostasis can be achieved in approximately 70% of patients [158]. Currently, it is not possible to accurately define a subgroup of patients in whom endoscopic therapy should not be attempted. What is clear, however, is that patients who have actively bleeding, large posterior duodenal ulcers should be considered to be at very high-risk of requiring urgent operation.

The management of re-bleeding after failed endoscopic therapy has been examined by Lau et al. [156]. Of 3473 patients admitted with bleeding peptic ulcers, 1169 underwent endoscopic therapy in an attempt to achieve hemostasis. Primary hemostasis was achieved in a remarkable 98.5% of patients. One hundred of these re-bled after endo-

Table 8.22 Repeat endoscopic therapy vs surgery for patients who re-bleed.

Outcome	Endoscopic therapy	Surgery
n	48	44
Transfusion (units)	8	7
Complications (no. of pts) (%)	7 (15)	16 (36)[a]
Mortality (30-day) (%)	5 (10)	8 (18)

[a]p = 0.03.
Source: Lau et al. [156].

scopic therapy and 92 were randomized to receive endoscopic retreatment or to emergency surgery. The characteristics of the two groups of patients were similar, including the median transfusion requirements before randomization. Endoscopic retreatment consisted of a combination of adrenaline injection plus the heater probe. Overall, more complications occurred in the group randomized to surgery and there was no significant difference in 30-day mortality between the two groups (Table 8.22). This paper suggests that endoscopic retreatment rather than immediate, urgent surgery may be undertaken in patients who re-bleed after endoscopic hemostatic therapy. **A1c**

In cases when endoscopic therapy fails, transcatheter arterial embolization (TAE) may offer an alternative to immediate surgery in selected patients. Two retrospective case series in patients who had failed endoscopic therapy or were re-bleeding after surgery for peptic ulcer disease have reported high levels of technical success, definitive haemostasis rates of 65–72% and no significant complications [159, 160]. **B** Occasionally it is not possible to advance a microcatheter to the bleeding site. In this situation embolization with N-butyl-2-cyanoacrylate has been shown to be effective and safe [161, 162]. There are no randomized, controlled trials comparing embolization to emergency surgery, but two retrospective analyses have been published. Ripoll et al. [163] reviewed 70 patients with refractory ulcer bleeding, 31 of whom were managed by embolization. The patients in this group were elderly (75.2 vs 63.3 years), had a high incidence of heart disease (67.7% vs 20.5%) and many were coagulopathic (25.8 vs 5.1%). These considerations probably accounted for the decision to perform TAE rather than operative surgery. The rates of both re-bleeding and mortality following salvage therapy were similar (29.0% vs 23.1% for re-bleeding and 25.8% vs 20.5% for death), suggesting that TAE could be an acceptable alternative to urgent surgery. There were no complications relating to TAE. The second review analyzed 91 patients who had failed endoscopic therapy [164]. Forty patients were treated with TAE and the remainder underwent surgery. Again the patients in the TAE group were older with more co-morbid conditions. Mortality at 30 days was 3% in the TAE group compared with 14% in the surgery arm. **B** This difference did not reach statistical significance but was seen as an encouraging trend. These results are promising and a randomized trial of TAE versus surgery following failed endoscopic hemostasis for bleeding peptic ulcer is warranted.

Endoscopic therapy: summary

Endoscopic therapy for non-variceal hemorrhage is safe and effective, and should be used in the 20% of patients who have major endoscopic stigmata of recent hemorrhage. Thermal hemostasis is effective using either the heat probe or multipolar electrocoagulation. No injection agent has been convincingly shown to be superior to dilute adrenaline solution. Injection of larger volumes may improve outcome. The hemoclip is an effective and safe mechanical device which would benefit from technical development. The addition of a second therapeutic modality to adrenaline injection improves outcome, and it is likely that combination therapy is the best approach for patients with active, spurting hemorrhage. Re-bleeding should be treated first by further endoscopic intervention, although clinical judgment should dictate when urgent surgery is required for specific high-risk cases. Transcatheter arterial embolization may be considered as an alternative to urgent surgery but this requires further study.

Intravenous infusion of proton pump inhibitor drugs is recommended following successful endoscopic hemostasis. There is little evidence currently that other drug therapies are effective.

References

1 UK Comparative audit of upper gastrointestinal bleeding and the use of blood. London: British Society of Gastroenterology; 2007. Available from http://www.bsg.org.uk/pdf_word_docs/blood_audit_report_07.pdf.

2 Avery Jones F. Haematemesis and melaena with special reference to bleeding peptic ulcer. *Br Med J* 1947; **ii**: 441–446.

3 Rockall TA, Logan RFA, Devlin HB *et al*. Incidence of and mortality from acute upper gastrointestinal hemorrhage in the United Kingdom. *Br Med J* 1995; **311**: 222–226.

4 Rockall TA, Logan RFA, Devlin HB *et al*. Risk assessment after acute upper gastrointestinal hemorrhage. *Gut* 1996; **38**: 316–321.

5 Vreeburg EM, Terwee CB, Snel P *et al*. Validation of the Rockall risk scoring system in upper gastrointestinal bleeding. *Gut* 1999; **44**: 331–335.

6 Phang TS, Vornik V, Stubbs R. Risk assessment in upper gastrointestinal haemorrhage: implications for resource utilization. *NZ Med J* 2000; **113**: 331–333.

7 Sanders DS, Carter MJ, Goodchap RJ *et al*. Prospective validation of the Rockall risk scoring system for upper GI hemorrhage in subgroups of patients with varices and peptic ulcers. *Am J Gastroenterol* 2002; **97**(3): 630–635.

8 Church NI, Dallal HJ, Masson J *et al*. Validity of the Rockall scoring system after endoscopic therapy for bleeding peptic ulcer: A prospective cohort study. *Gastrointest Endosc* 2006; **63**: 606–612.

9 Blatchford O, Murray WR, Blatchford M. A risk score to predict need for treatment for upper-gastrointestinal haemorrhage. *Lancet* 2000; **356**: 1318–1321.

10 Barkun A, Bardou M, Marshall JK. Consensus recommendations for managing patients with nonvariceal upper gastrointestinal bleeding. *Ann Intern Med* 2003; **139**(10): 843–857.

11 Holman RAE, Davis M, Gough KR *et al*. Value of centralised approach in the management of haematemesis and melaena: Experience in a district general hospital. *Gut* 1990; **31**: 504–508.

12 Sanderson JD, Taylor RFH, Pugh S *et al*. Specialised gastrointestinal units for the management of upper gastrointestinal bleeding. *Postgrad Med J* 1990; **66**: 654–656.

13 Sanders DS, Perry MJ, Jones SGW *et al*. Effectiveness of an upper-gastrointestinal haemorrhage unit: a prospective analysis of 900 consecutive cases using the Rockall score as a method of risk standardisation. *Eur J Gastroenterol Hepatol* 2004; **16**: 487–494.

14 Bornman PC, Theodorou N, Shuttleworth RD *et al*. Importance of hypovolaemic shock and endoscopic signs in predicting recurrent hemorrhage from peptic ulceration: A prospective evaluation. *Br Med J* 1985; **291**: 245–247.

15 Griffiths WJ, Neumann DA, Welsh DA. The visible vessels as an indicator of uncontrolled or recurrent gastrointestinal hemorrhage. *N Engl J Med* 1979; **300**: 1411–1413.

16 Swain CP, Storey DW, Bown SG. Nature of the bleeding vessel in recurrently bleeding gastric ulcers. *Gastroenterology* 1986; **90**: 595–606.

17 Patchett SE, Enright l, Afdhal N *et al*. Clot lysis by gastric juice; an *in vitro* study. *Gut* 1989; **30**: 1704–1707.

18 Walt RP, Cottrell J, Mann SG *et al*. Continuous intravenous famotidine for hemorrhage from peptic ulcer. *Lancet* 1992; **340**: 1058–1062.

19 Collins R, Langman M. Treatment with histamine H_2 antagonists in acute upper gastrointestinal hemorrhage: Implications of randomized trials. *N Engl J Med* 1985; **313**: 660–666.

20 Daneshmend TK, Hawkey CJ, Langman MJS *et al*. Omeprazole versus placebo for acute upper gastrointestinal bleeding: randomized double blind controlled trial. *Br Med J* 1992; **304**: 143–147.

21 Khuroo MS, Yattoo GN, Javid G *et al*. A comparison of omeprazole and placebo for bleeding peptic ulcer. *N Engl J Med* 1997; **336**: 1054–1058.

22 Schaffalitzky de Muckadell OB, Havelund T, Harling H *et al*. Effect of omeprazole on the outcome of endoscopically treated bleeding peptic ulcers: Randomized double blind placebo controlled multicenter study. *Scand J Gastroenterol* 1997; **32**(4): 320–327.

23 Hasslegren G, Lind T, Lundell L *et al*. Continuous intravenous infusion of omeprazole in elderly patients with peptic ulcer

bleeding: Results of a placebo controlled multicentre study. *Scand J Gastroenterol* 1997; **32**(4): 328–333.

24 Villanueva C, Balanzo J, Torras X *et al.* Omeprazole versus rani-tidine as adjunct therapy to endoscopic injection in actively bleeding ulcers: A prospective randomized study. *Endoscopy* 1995; **27**: 308–312.

25 Lin HJ, Lo WC, Lee FY *et al.* A prospective randomized com-parative trial showing that omeprazole prevents re-bleeding in patients with bleeding peptic ulcer after successful endoscopic therapy. *Arch Intern Med* 1998; **158**: 54–58.

26 Lau JYW, Sung JY, Lee KKC *et al.* Effect of intravenous omepra-zole on recurrent bleeding after endoscopic treatment of bleed-ing peptic ulcers. *N Engl J Med* 2000; **343**: 310–316.

27 Zargar SA, Javid G, Khan BA *et al.* Pantoprazole infusion as adjuvant therapy to endoscopic treatment in patients with peptic ulcer bleeding: Prospective randomized controlled trial. *J Gastroenterol Hepatol* 2006; **21**: 716–721.

28 Sung JJY, Chan FKL, Lau JYW *et al.* The effect of endoscopic therapy in patients receiving omeprazole for bleeding ulcers with nonbleeding visible vessels or adherent clots. *Ann Intern Med* 2003; **139**: 237–243.

29 Hasselgren G, Keelan M, Kirdeikis P *et al.* Optimization of acid suppression for patients with peptic ulcer bleeding: An intra-gastric pH-metry study with omeprazole. *Eur J Gastroenterol Hepatol* 1998; **10**: 601–606.

30 Laine L, Shah A, Bemanian S. Intragastric pH with oral vs intravenous bolus infusion proton-pump inhibitor therapy in patients with bleeding ulcers. *Gastroenterology* 2008; **134**(7): 1836–1841.

31 Udd M, Mietinnen P, Palmu A *et al.* Regular-dose versus high-dose omeprazole in peptic ulcer bleeding: A prospective rand-omized double-blind study. *Scand J Gastroenterol* 2001; **36**(12): 1332–1338.

32 Javid G, Masoodi I, Zargar SA *et al.* Omeprazole as adjuvant therapy to endoscopic combination injection sclerotherapy for treating bleeding peptic ulcer. *American Journal of Medicine* 2001; **111**(4): 280–284.

33 Leontiadis GI, Sharma VK, Howden CW. Proton pump inhibi-tor therapy for peptic ulcer bleeding: Cochrane Collaboration meta-analysis of randomized controlled trials. *Mayo Clin Proc* 2007; **82**(3): 286–296.

34 Lau JY, Leung WK, Wu JC *et al.* Omeprazole before endoscopy in patients with gastrointestinal bleeding. *N Engl J Med* 2007; **356**(16): 1631–1640.

35 Henry DA, O'Connell DL. Effect of fibrinolytic inhibitors on mortality from upper gastrointestinal hemorrhage. *Br Med J* 1989; **298**: 1142–1146.

36 Gluud LL, Kilngenberg SL, Langholz SE. Systematic review: Tranexamic acid for upper gastrointestinal bleeding. *Aliment Pharmacol Ther* 2008; **27**(9): 752–758.

37 Barer D, Ogilvie A, Henry D *et al.* Cimetidine and tranexamic acid in the treatment of acute upper-gastrointestinal-tract bleed-ing. *N Engl J Med* 1983; **308**(26): 1571–1575.

38 Sommerville KW, Henry DA, Davies JG *et al.* Somatostatin in treatment of haematemesis and melaena. *Lancet* 1985; **i**: 130–132.

39 Magnusson I, Ihre T, Johansson C *et al.* Randomized double blind trial of somatostatin in the treatment of massive upper gastrointestinal hemorrhage. *Gut* 1985; **26**: 221–226.

40 Basso N, Bagarani M, Bracci F *et al.* Ranitidine and somatostatin. Their effects on bleeding from the upper gastrointestinal tract. *Arch Surg* 1986; **121**: 833–835.

41 Coraggio F, Scarpato P, Spina M *et al.* Somatostatin and raniti-dine in the control of iatrogenic hemorrhage of the upper gas-trointestinal tract. *Br Med J* 1984; **289**: 224.

42 Coraggio F, Bertini G, Catalona A *et al.* Clinical controlled trial of somatostatin with ranitidine and placebo in the control of peptic hemorrhage of the upper gastrointestinal tract. *Digestion* 1989; **43**: 190–195.

43 Galmiche JP, Cassigneul J, Faivre J *et al.* Somatostatin in peptic ulcer bleeding. Results of a double blind controlled trial. *Int J Clin Pharmacol Res* 1983; **III**: 379–387.

44 Saperas E, Pique JM, Perez-Ayuso R *et al.* Somatostatin com-pared with cimetidine in the treatment of bleeding peptic ulcer without visible vessel. *Aliment Pharmacol Ther* 1988; **2**: 153–159.

45 Kayasseh L, Gyr K, Keller U *et al.* Somatostatin and cimetidine in peptic ulcer hemorrhage. A randomized controlled trial. *Lancet* 1980; **i**: 844–846.

46 Antonioli A, Gandolfo M, Rigo GP *et al.* Somatostatin and cime-tidine in the control of acute upper gastrointestinal bleeding. A controlled multicentre study. *Hepato-gastroenterol* 1986; **33**: 71–74.

47 Tulassay Z, Gupta R, Papp J *et al.* Somatostatin versus cimeti-dine in the treatment of actively bleeding duodenal ulcer: A prospective, randomized, controlled trial. *Am J Gastroenterol* 1989; **84**: 6–9.

48 Torres AJ, Landa I, Hernandez F *et al.* Somatostatin in the treat-ment of severe upper gastrointestinal bleeding: A multicentre controlled trial. *Br J Surg* 1986; **73**: 786–789.

49 Wagner PK, Rothmund M, Gronniger J. Secretin and somato-statin in treatment of acute upper gastrointestinal hemorrhage: A randomized trial. *Klin Wochenschr* 1983; **61**: 285–289.

50 Goletti O, Sidoti F, Lippolis PV *et al.* Omeprazole versus raniti-dine and somatostatin in the treatment of acute severe gas-troduodenal hemorrhage. *Br J Surg* 1992; **79**(Suppl): S123.

51 Christiansen J, Ottenjann R, Von Arx F. Placebo-controlled trial with the somatostatin analogue sms 201-995 in peptic ulcer bleeding. *Gastroenterology* 1989; **97**: 568–574.

52 Jenkins SA, Poulianos G, Coraggio F *et al.* Somatostatin in the treatment of non-variceal upper gastrointestinal bleeding. *Dig Dis Sci* 1998; **16**: 214–224.

53 Imperiale TF, Birgisson S. Somatostatin or octreotide compared with H$_2$ antagonists and placebo in the management of acute non-variceal upper gastrointestinal hemorrhage: A meta-analy-sis. *Ann Intern Med* 1997; **127**: 1062–1071.

54 Rutgeerts P, Geboes K, Vantrappen G. Experimental studies of injection therapy for severe nonvariceal bleeding in dogs. *Gastroenterology* 1989; **97**: 601–621.

55 Hu B, Chung SC, Sun LC *et al.* Developing an animal model of massive ulcer bleeding for assessing endoscopic hemostatic devices. *Endoscopy* 2005; **37**(9): 847–851.

56 Church NI, Dallal HJ, Masson J *et al.* A randomized trial com-paring heater probe plus thrombin with heater probe plus placebo for bleeding peptic ulcer. *Gastroenterology* 2003; **125**(2): 396–404.

57 Vallon AG, Cotton PB, Laurence BH *et al.* Randomized trial of endoscopic argon laser photocoagulation in bleeding peptic ulcers. *Gut* 1981; **22**: 228–233.

58 Swain CP, Bown SG, Storey DW *et al.* Controlled trial of argon laser photocoagulation in bleeding peptic ulcer. *Lancet* 1981; **ii**: 1313–1316.

59 Jensen DM, Machicado GA, Tapia JL *et al.* Controlled trial of endoscopic argon laser for severe ulcer hemorrhage. *Gastroenterology* 1984; **86**: 1125.

60 Swain CP, Salmon PR, Kirkham JS. Controlled trial of Nd-YAG laser photocoagulation in bleeding peptic ulcers. *Lancet* 1986; **i**: 1113–1117.

61 Krejs GJ, Little KH, Westergaard H. Laser photocoagulation for the treatment of acute peptic ulcer bleeding. *N Engl J Med* 1987; **316**: 1618–1621.

62 Rhode H, Thon K, Fischer M. Results of a defined concept of endoscopic Nd-YAG laser therapy in patients with upper gastrointestinal bleeding. *Br J Surg* 1980; **67**: 360.

63 Rutgeerts P, Vantrappen G, Broeckhaert L. Controlled trial of YAG laser treatment of upper digestive hemorrhage. *Gastroenterology* 1982; **83**: 410–416.

64 Macleod I, Mills PR, Mackenzie JF. Neodymium yttrium aluminium garnet laser photocoagulation for major hemorrhage from peptic ulcers and single vessels. *Br Med J* 1983; **286**: 345–358.

65 Homer AC, Powell S, Vacary FR. Is Nd-YAG laser treatment for upper gastrointestinal bleeds of benefit in a district general hospital? *Postgrad Med J* 1985; **61**: 19–22.

66 Trudeau W, Siepler JK, Ross K *et al.* Endoscopic Nd-YAG laser photocoagulation of bleeding ulcers with visible vessels. *Gastrointest Endosc* 1985; **31**: 138.

67 Buset M, Des Marez B, Vandermeeran A. Laser therapy for non bleeding visible vessel in peptic ulcer hemorrhage: A prospective randomized study. *Gastrointest Endosc* 1988; **34**: 173.

68 Matthewson K, Swain CP, Bland M *et al.* Randomized comparison of Nd-YAG laser, heater probe and no endoscopic therapy for bleeding peptic ulcers. *Gastroenterology* 1990; **98**: 1234–1244.

69 Fullarton GM, Birnie GG, MacDonald A *et al.* Controlled trial of heater probe treatment in bleeding peptic ulcers. *Br J Surg* 1989; **76**: 541–544.

70 Jensen DM, Machicado GA, Kovacs TOG. Controlled randomized study of heater probe and BICAP for hemostasis of severe ulcer bleeding. *Gastroenterology* 1988; **94**: A208.

71 Wong SKH, YU L-M, Lau JYW *et al.* Prediction of therapeutic failure after adrenaline injection plus heater probe treatment in patients with bleeding peptic ulcer. *Gut* 2002; **50**: 322–325.

72 O'Brien JD, Day SJ, Burnham WR. Controlled trial of small bipolar probes in bleeding peptic ulcers. *Lancet* 1986; **i**: 464–468.

73 Laine L. Multipolar electrocoagulation in the treatment of active upper gastrointestinal tract hemorrhage. A prospective controlled trial. *N Engl J Med* 1987; **316**: 1613–1617.

74 Brearley S, Hawker PC, Dykes PW *et al.* Peri-endoscopic bipolar diathermy coagulation of visible vessels using a 3.2mm probe – a randomized clinical trial. *Endoscopy* 1987; **19**: 160–163.

75 Laine L. Multipolar electrocoagulation for the treatment of ulcers with non bleeding visible vessels: a prospective, controlled trial. *Gastroenterology* 1988; **94**: A246.

76 Papp JP. Heat probe versus BICAP in the treatment of upper gastrointestinal bleeding. *Am J Gastroenterol* 1987; **82**: 619–621.

77 Cipolletta L, Bianco MA, Rotondano G *et al.* Prospective comparison of argon plasma coagulator and heater probe in the endoscopic treatment of major peptic ulcer bleeding. *Gastrointest Endosc* 1998; **48**(2): 191–195.

78 Skok P, Krizman I, Skok M. Argon plasma coagulation versus injection sclerotherapy in peptic ulcer hemorrhage-a prospective, controlled study. *Hepatogastroenterology* 2004; **51**(55): 165–170.

79 Cook DJ, Guyatt GH, Salena BJ *et al.* Endoscopic therapy for acute non-variceal hemorrhage: A meta-analysis. *Gastroenterology* 1992; **102**: 139–148.

80 Henry DA, White I. Endoscopic coagulation for gastrointestinal bleeding. *N Engl J Med* 1988; **318**: 186–187.

81 Chung SCS, Leung JWC, Steele RJC. Endoscopic injection of adrenaline for actively bleeding ulcers: A randomized trial. *Br Med J* 1988; **296**: 1631–1633.

82 Panes J, Viver J, Forne M *et al.* Controlled trial of endoscopic sclerosis in bleeding peptic ulcers. *Lancet* 1987; 1292–1294.

83 Rajgopal C, Palmer KR. Endoscopic injection sclerosis: Effective treatment for bleeding peptic ulcer. *Gut* 1991; **32**: 727–729.

84 Balanzo J, Sainz S, Such J. Endoscopic hemostasis by local injection of epinephrine in bleeding ulcers. A prospective randomized trial. *Endoscopy* 1988; **20**: 289–291.

85 Oxner RBG, Simmonds NJ, Gertner DJ *et al.* Controlled trial of endoscopic injection treatment for bleeding peptic ulcers with visible vessels. *Lancet* 1992; **339**: 966–968.

86 Beneditti G, Sablich R, Lacchin T. Endoscopic injection sclerotherapy in non-variceal upper gastrointestinal bleeding. A comparative study of epinephrine and thrombin. *Endoscopy* 1990; **22**: 157–159.

87 Strohm WD, Rommele UE, Barton E *et al.* Injection therapy of bleeding ulcers with fibrin or polidocanol. *Dtsch Med Wochenschr* 1994; **119**: 249–256.

88 Rutgeerts P, Vantrappen G, Brockaert L *et al.* Comparison of endoscopic polidocanol injection and YAG laser for bleeding peptic ulcers. *Lancet* 1989; **i**: 1164–1167.

89 Levy J, Khakoo S, Barton R *et al.* Fatal injection sclerotherapy of a bleeding peptic ulcer. *Lancet* 1991; **337**: 504 (letter).

90 Loperfido S, Patelli G, La Torre L. Extensive necrosis of gastric mucosa following injection therapy of a bleeding peptic ulcer. *Endoscopy* 1990; **22**: 785–786 (letter).

91 Sung JY, Chung SC, Low JM *et al.* Systemic absorption of epinephrine after endoscopic submucosal injection in patients with bleeding peptic ulcers. *Gastrointest Endosc* 1993; **39**(1): 20–22.

92 Rajgopal C, Lessells AM, Palmer KR. Mechanisms of action of injection therapy for bleeding peptic ulcer. *Br J Surg* 1992; **79**: 782–784.

93 Chung SCS, Leung JWC, Leoug HT *et al.* Adding a sclerosant to endoscopic epinephrine injection in actively bleeding ulcers: Randomized trial. *Gastrointest Endosc* 1993; **39**: 611–615.

94 Villanueva C, Balanzo C, Espinos JC. Endoscopic injection therapy of bleeding ulcer: A prospective and randomized comparison of adrenaline alone or with polidocanol. *J Clin Gastroenterol* 1993; **17**: 195–200.

95 Choudari CP, Palmer KR. Endoscopic injection therapy for bleeding peptic ulcer: A comparison of adrenaline alone with adrenaline plus ethanolamine oleate. *Gut* 1994; **35**: 608–610.

96 Lin HJ, Perng CL, Lee SD. Is sclerosant injection mandatory after an epinephrine injection for arrest of peptic ulcer haemor-

rhage? A prospective, randomised, comparative study. *Gut* 1993; **34**(9): 1182–1185.

97 Chung SC, Leong HT, Chan AC *et al*. Epinephrine or epinephrine plus alcohol for injection of bleeding ulcers: a prospective randomized trial. *Gastrointest Endosc* 1996; **43**(6): 591–595.

98 Pascu O, Draghici A, Acalovschi I. The effect of endoscopic hemostasis with alcohol on the mortality rate of non-variceal upper gastrointestinal hemorrhage: A randomized prospective study. *Endoscopy* 1989; **21**: 53–55.

99 Lazo MD, Andrade R, Medina MC *et al*. Effect of injection sclerosis with alcohol on the re-bleeding rate of gastroduodenal peptic ulcers with nonbleeding visible vessels: A prospective, controlled trial. *Am J Gastroenterol* 1992; **87**(7): 843–846.

100 Lin HJ, Perng CL, Lee FY. Endoscopic injection for the arrest of peptic ulcer hemorrhage: Final results of a prospective, randomized, comparative trial. *Gastrointest Endosc* 1993; **39**: 15–19.

101 Chiozzini G, Bortoluzzi F, Pallini P *et al*. Controlled trial of absolute ethanol vs epinephrine as injection agent in gastroduodenal bleeding. *Gastroenterology* 1989; **96**: A86.

102 Nakagawa K, Asaki S, Sato T. Endoscopic treatment of bleeding peptic ulcers. *World Journal of Surgery* 1989; **13**(2): 154–157.

103 Kubba AK, Murphy W, Palmer KR. Endoscopic injection for bleeding peptic ulcer: A comparison of adrenaline with adrenaline plus human thrombin. *Gastroenterology* 1996; **111**: 623–628.

104 Balanzo J, Villanueva C, Sainz S *et al*. Injection therapy of bleeding peptic ulcer. A prospective, randomized trial using epinephrine and thrombin. *Endoscopy* 1990; **22**: 157–159.

105 Song SY, Chung JB, Moon YM *et al*. Comparison of the hemostatic effect of endoscopic injection with fibrin glue and hypertonic saline-epinephrine for peptic ulcer bleeding: A prospective randomized trial. *Endoscopy* 1997; **29**: 827–833.

106 Rutgeerts P, Rauws E, Wara P *et al*. Randomized trial of single and repeated fibrin glue compared with injection of polidocanol in treatment of bleeding peptic ulcer. *Lancet* 1997; **350**: 692–696.

107 Pescatore P, Jornod P, Borovicka J *et al*. Epinephrine versus epinephrine plus fibrin glue injection in peptic ulcer bleeding: A prospective randomized trial. *Gastrointest Endosc* 2002; **55**: 348–353.

108 Laine L, Estrada R. Randomized trial of normal saline solution injection versus bipolar electrocoagulation for treatment of patients with high-risk bleeding ulcers: Is local tamponade enough? *Gastrointest Endosc* 2002; **55**(1): 6–10.

109 Lin HJ, Hsieh YH, Tseng GY *et al*. A prospective, randomized trial of large- versus small-volume endoscopic injection of epinephrine for peptic ulcer bleeding. *Gastrointest Endosc* 2002; **55**(6): 615–619.

110 Park CH, Lee SJ, Park JH *et al*. Optimal injection volume of epinephrine for endoscopic prevention of recurrent peptic ulcer bleeding. *Gastrointest Endosc* 2004; **60**: 875–880.

111 Liou TC, Lin SC, Wang HY, Chang WH. Optimal injection volume of epinephrine for endoscopic treatment of peptic ulcer bleeding. *World J Gastroenterol* 2006; **12**(19): 3108–3113.

112 Lin HJ, Tsai YT, Lee SD *et al*. A prospectively randomized trial of heat probe thermocoagulation versus pure alcohol injection in nonvariceal peptic ulcer hemorrhage. *Am J Gastroenterol* 1988; **83**(3): 283–286.

113 Lin HJ, Lee FY, Kang WM *et al*. Heat probe thermocoagulation and pure alcohol injection in massive peptic ulcer hemorrhage: A prospective, randomized controlled trial. *Gut* 1990; **31**: 753–757.

114 Chung SCS, Leung JWC, Sung JY *et al*. Injection or heat probe for bleeding ulcer? *Gastroenterology* 1991; **100**: 33–37.

115 Choudari CP, Rajgopal C, Palmer KR. Comparison of endoscopic injection therapy versus the heater probe in major peptic ulcer hemorrhage. *Gut* 1992; **33**(9): 1159–1161.

116 Saeed ZA, Winchester CB, Michaletz PA *et al*. A scoring system to predict re-bleeding after endoscopic therapy of nonvariceal upper gastrointestinal hemorrhage, with a comparison of heat probe and ethanol injection. *Am J Gastroenterol* 1993; **88**(11): 1842–1849.

117 Llach J, Bordas JM, Salmeron JM *et al*. A prospective randomized trial of heater probe thermocoagulation versus injection therapy in peptic ulcer hemorrhage. *Gastrointest Endosc* 1996; **43**(2 Pt 1): 117–120.

118 Laine L. Multipolar electrocoagulation versus injection therapy in the treatment of bleeding peptic ulcers. *Gastroenterology* 1990; **99**: 1303–1306.

119 Carter R, Anderson JR. Randomized trial of adrenaline injection and laser photocoagulation in the control of hemorrhage from peptic ulcer. *Br J Surg* 1994; **81**: 869–871.

120 Pulanic R, Vucelic B, Rosandic M *et al*. Comparison of injection sclerotherapy and laser photocoagulation for bleeding peptic ulcers. *Endoscopy* 1995; **27**(4): 291–297.

121 Hayashi T, Yonezawa M, Kawabara T. The study on staunch clip for the treatment by endoscopy. *Gastroenterol Endosc* 1975; **17**; 92–101.

122 Maiss J, Hochberger J, Schwab D. Hemoclips: Which is the pick of the bunch? *Gastrointest Endosc* 2008; **67**(1): 40–42.

123 Binmoeller KF, Thonke F, Soehendra N. Endoscopic hemoclip treatment for gastrointestinal bleeding. *Endoscopy* 1993; **25**(2): 167–170.

124 Yokohata T, Takeshima H, Fukushima R *et al*. Limitations of Endoscopy Injection Therapy and efficacy of Endoscopic Hemoclipping in the Treatment of Bleeding Gastric Ulcer. *Japanese Abdominal Emergency Medical Society Magazine* 1996; **16**: 1113–1119.

125 Nagayama K, Tazawa J, Sakai Y *et al*. Efficacy of Endoscopic Clipping for Bleeding Gastroduodenal Ulcer: Comparison with Topical Ethanol Injection. *Am J Gastroenterol* 1999; **94**: 2897–2901.

126 Chung IK, Ham JS, Kim HS *et al*. Comparison of the hemostatic efficacy of the endoscopic hemoclip method with hypertonic saline-epinephrine injection and a combination of the two for the management of bleeding peptic ulcers. *Gastrointest Endosc* 1999; **49**(1): 13–18.

127 Cipoletta L, Bianco MA, Marmo R *et al*. Endoclips versus heater probe in preventing early recurrent bleeding from peptic ulcer: A prospective and randomized trial. *Gastrointest Endosc* 2001; **53**: 147–151.

128 Lin HJ, Hsieh YH, Tseng GY *et al*. A prospective, randomized trial of endoscopic hemoclip versus heater probe thermocoagulation for peptic ulcer bleeding. *Am J Gastroenterol* 2002; **97**: 2250–2254.

129 Lin HJ, Perng CL, Sun IC, Tseng GY. Endoscopic hemoclip versus heater probe thermocoagulation plus hypertonic saline-epinephrine injection for peptic ulcer bleeding. *Dig Liver Dis* 2003; **35**(12): 898–902.

130 Gevers AM, De Goede E, Simoens M *et al*. A randomized trial comparing injection therapy with hemoclip and with injection combined with hemoclip for bleeding ulcers. *Gastrointest Endosc* 2002; **55**(4): 466–469.

131 Chou YC, Hsu PL, Lai KH *et al*. A prospective, randomized trial of endoscopic hemoclip placement and distilled water injection for treatment of high-risk bleeding ulcers. *Gastrointest Endosc* 2003; **57**: 324–328.

132 Shimoda R, Iwakiri R, Sakata H *et al*. Evaluation of endoscopic hemostasis with metallic hemoclips for bleeding gastric ulcer: comparison with endoscopic injection of absolute ethanol in a prospective, randomized study. *Am J Gastroenterol* 2003; **98**: 2198–2202.

133 Ljubicic N, Supanc V, Vrsalovic M. Efficacy of endoscopic clipping for actively bleeding peptic ulcer: Comparison with polidocanol injection therapy. *Hepatogastroenterology* 2004; **51**: 408–412.

134 Yuan H, Wang C, Hunt RH. Endoscopic clipping for acute nonvariceal upper-GI bleeding: a meta-analysis and critical appraisal of controlled trials. *Gastrointest Endosc* 2008; **68**: 339–51.

135 Sung JJ, Tsoi KK, Lai LH *et al*. Endoscopic clipping versus injection and thermo-coagulation in the treatment of non-variceal upper gastrointestinal bleeding: A meta-analysis. *Gut* 2007; **56**: 1364–1373.

136 Jensen DM, Machicado GA, Hirabayashi K. Randomized controlled study of 3 different types of hemoclips for hemostasis of bleeding canine acute gastric ulcers. *Gastrointest Endosc* 2006; **64**: 768–773.

137 Chan CY, Yau KK, Siu WT *et al*. Endoscopic hemostasis by using the TriClip for peptic ulcer hemorrhage: A pilot study. *Gastrointest Endosc* 2008; **67**: 35–39.

138 Lin HJ, Lo WC, Cheng YC, Perng CL. Endoscopic hemoclip versus triclip placement in patients with high-risk peptic ulcer bleeding. *Am J Gastroenterol* 2007; **102**: 539–543.

139 Lin HJ, Tseng GY, Perng CL *et al*. Comparison of adrenaline injection and bipolar electrocoagulation for the arrest of peptic ulcer bleeding. *Gut* 1999; **44**: 715–719.

140 Bianco MA, Rotondano G, Marmo R *et al*. Combined epinephrine and bipolar probe coagulation vs. bipolar probe coagulation alone for bleeding peptic ulcer: a randomized, controlled trial. *Gastrointest Endosc* 2004; **60**: 910–915.

141 Chung SCS, Lau JY, Sung JJ. Randomized comparison between adrenaline injection alone and adrenaline injection plus heat probe treatment for actively bleeding peptic ulcers. *Br Med J* 1997; **314**: 1307–1311.

142 Park CH, Joo JE, Kim HS *et al*. A prospective, randomized trial comparing mechanical methods of hemostasis plus epinephrine injection to epinephrine injection alone for bleeding peptic ulcer. *Gastrointest Endosc* 2004; **60**: 173–179.

143 Lo CC, Hsu PI, Lo GH *et al*. Comparison of hemostatic efficacy for epinephrine injection alone and injection combined with hemoclip therapy in treating high-risk bleeding ulcers. *Gastrointest Endosc* 2006; **63**: 767–773.

144 Calvet X, Vergara M, Brullet E *et al*. Addition of a second endoscopic treatment following epinephrine injection improves outcome in high-risk bleeding ulcers. *Gastroenterology* 2004; **126**: 441–450.

145 Marmo R, Rotondano G, Piscopo R *et al*. Dual therapy versus monotherapy in the endoscopic treatment of high-risk bleeding ulcers: A meta-analysis of controlled trials. *Am J Gastroenterol* 2007; **102**: 279–289.

146 Lin HJ, Wang K, Perng CL *et al*. Natural history of bleeding peptic ulcers with a tightly adherent blood clot: A prospective observation. *Gastrointest Endosc* 1996; **43**: 470–473.

147 Bleau BL, Gostout CJ, Sherman KE *et al*. Recurrent bleeding from peptic ulcer associated with adherent clot: A randomized study comparing endoscopic treatment with medical therapy. *Gastrointest Endosc* 2002; **56**(1): 1–6.

148 Jensen DM, Kovacs TOG, Jutabha R *et al*. Randomized trial of medical or endoscopic therapy to prevent recurrent ulcer hemorrhage in patients with adherent clots. *Gastroenterology* 2002; **123**: 407–413.

149 Kahi CJ, Jensen DM, Sung JJ *et al*. Endoscopic therapy versus medical therapy for bleeding peptic ulcer with adherent clot: A meta-analysis. *Gastroenterology* 2005; **129**: 855–862.

150 Messmann H, Schaller P, Andus T *et al*. Effect of programmed endoscopic follow-up examinations on the re-bleeding rate of gastric or duodenal peptic ulcers treated by injection therapy: A prospective, randomized controlled trial. *Endoscopy* 1998; **30**(7): 583–589.

151 Villanueva C, Balanzo J, Torras X *et al*. Value of second-look endoscopy after injection therapy for bleeding peptic ulcer: A prospective and randomized trial. *Gastrointest Endosc* 1994; **40**(1): 34–39.

152 Saeed ZA, Cole RA, Ramirez FC *et al*. Endoscopic retreatment after successful initial hemostasis prevents ulcer re-bleeding: A prospective randomized trial. *Endoscopy* 1996; **28**(3): 288–294.

153 Chiu PWY, Lam CYW, Lee SW *et al*. Effect of scheduled second therapeutic endoscopy on peptic ulcer re-bleeding: A prospective randomized trial. *Gut* 2003; **52**: 1403–1407.

154 Marmo R, Rotondano G, Bianco MA *et al*. Outcome of endoscopic treatment for peptic ulcer bleeding: Is a second look necessary? A meta-analysis. *Gastrointest Endosc* 2003; **57**: 62–67.

155 Chiu PWY, Lau TS, Kwong KH *et al*. Impact of programmed second endoscopy with appropriate re-treatment on peptic ulcer re-bleeding: A systematic review. *Ann Coll Surg* 2003; **7**: 106–115.

156 Lau JYW, Sung JJY, Lam Y *et al*. Endoscopic retreatment compared with surgery in patients with recurrent bleeding after initial endoscopic control of bleeding ulcers. *N Engl J Med* 1999; **340**: 751–756.

157 Elmunzer BJ, Young SD, Inadomi JM *et al*. Systematic review of the predictors of recurrent hemorrhage after endoscopic hemostatic therapy for bleeding peptic ulcers. *Am J Gastroenterol* 2008; **103**: 2625–2632.

158 Choudari CP, Rajgopal C, Elton RA *et al*. Failures of endoscopic therapy for bleeding peptic ulcers; an analysis of risk factors. *Am J Gastroenterol* 1994; **89**: 1968–1972.

159 Holme JB, Nielson DT, Funch-Jensen P, Mortensen FV. Transcatheter arterial embolization in patients with bleeding duodenal ulcer: An alternative to surgery. *Acta Radiol* 2006; **47**(3): 244–247.

160 Larssen L, Moger T, Bjornbeth BA *et al*. Transcatheter arterial embolization in the management of bleeding duodenal ulcers:

A 5.5-year retrospective study of treatment and outcome. *Scand J Gastroenterol* 2008; **43**(2): 217–222.

161 Lee CW, Liu KL, Wang HP *et al*. Transcatheter arterial embolization of acute upper gastrointestinal tract bleeding with N-butyl-2-cyanoacrylate. *J Vasc Interv Radiol* 2007; **18**(2): 209–216.

162 Jae HJ, Chung JW, Jung AY *et al*. Transcatheter arterial embolization of nonvariceal upper gastrointestinal bleeding with N-butyl-2-cyanoacrylate. *Korean J Radiol* 2007; **8**(1): 48–56.

163 Ripoll C, Banares R, Beceiro I *et al*. Comparison of transcatheter arterial embolization and surgery for treatment of bleeding peptic ulcer after endoscopic treatment failure. *J Vasc Interv Radiol* 2004; **15**: 447–450.

164 Eriksson LG, Ljungdahl M, Sundbom M, Nyman R. Transcatheter arterial embolization versus surgery in the treatment of upper gastrointestinal bleeding after therapeutic endoscopy failure. *J Vasc Interv Radiol* 2008; **19**(10): 1413–1418.

9   Functional dyspepsia

Sander Veldhuyzen van Zanten

Division of Gastroenterology, Department of Medicine, University of Alberta, Edmonton, Canada

Introduction

In this chapter the diagnosis of functional dyspepsia and efficacy of therapeutic interventions will be evaluated. Functional dyspepsia, often referred to as non-ulcer dyspepsia, is an important health problem with a very high prevalence in the general population. Data from Sweden and Canada show that 5–7% of all consultations in primary care are for the symptom of dyspepsia [1, 2]. In Sweden, up to 98% of patients receive a prescription if they consult a physician for dyspepsia [1]. Consequently, for the health care system the cost of medications, which are often prescribed for long periods of time, adds significantly to the already substantial expenditures for consultations and diagnostic investigations. The following topics will be reviewed: definition of functional dyspepsia, evaluation and diagnostic tests, methodology of trials, and pharmacological treatments including antacids, H2-receptor antagonists, proton pump inhibitors (PPIs), prokinetic agents, anti-*Helicobacter* therapy and antidepressant therapy.

Definition of functional dyspepsia

There is agreement that the cardinal feature of functional dyspepsia is unexplained pain or discomfort centered in the upper part of the abdomen. Epigastric pain or discomfort may be accompanied by other symptoms such as excessive burping or belching, nausea, bloating, postprandial fullness, early satiety, or burning sensations. Increasingly, investigators have accepted the definition of the Rome Working Party which has now been revised three times [3, 4, 5].

Evidence-Based Gastroenterology and Hepatology, 3rd edition.
J. McDonald, A.K. Burroughs, B. Feagan, and M.B. Fennerty. © 2010
Blackwell Publishing Ltd

The general definitions of dyspepsia and functional dyspepsia have remained unchanged, but in Rome III major changes have been introduced. For a diagnosis of functional dyspepsia to be made, it is required that investigations, usually upper gastrointestinal endoscopy, have not revealed abnormalities such as ulcers that could explain the symptoms of the dyspepsia. The Rome criteria continue to exclude the symptoms of heartburn and acid regurgitation as these are considered to be diagnostic of gastro-esophageal reflux disease (GERD). Although there is consensus that "dominant" symptoms of heartburn and acid regurgitation make a diagnosis of GERD likely, it is less clear how heartburn should be handled if it is of severity equal to or less than epigastric pain. Furthermore, heartburn and acid regurgitation are often present as associated symptoms in patients who otherwise fit the dyspepsia diagnostic criteria. In the context of functional dyspepsia the recent publication on the definition of gastro-esophageal reflux Disease (the "Montreal definition") is very relevant [6].

The criteria proposed by the Rome III working group included very significant changes [5]. It was proposed that for research studies the term functional dyspepsia should be replaced by more distinctively defined disorders, for which there was felt to be increasing evidence in the literature. The two new proposed diagnostic categories are: (1) meal-induced dyspeptic symptoms (PDS, postprandial dyspepsia symptoms); and (2) epigastric pain (EPS, epigastric pain syndrome). This new subclassification is supported by some studies in which factor analysis supported a division into four symptom subgroups: epigastric pain, epigastric burning, postprandial fullness and early satiation [7]. Furthermore, some studies from a tertiary referral center also reported significant weight loss (10%) as a feature of functional dyspepsia, especially in patients complaining of early satiety [7, 8], but at this time these findings are not considered to be generalizable. Given that the overall empiric evidence surrounding the definitions of most functional GI disorders including functional dyspepsia is weak, it remains to be seen whether any new classification will indeed help research in this area to move forward. To date the utilization of the Rome III functional dyspepsia definitions appears to be low.

There is evidence, especially in primary care, that excluding heartburn from the dyspepsia syndrome does not fit with the conceptual framework for dyspepsia used by primary care physicians [9]. This is especially true for uninvestigated dyspepsia patients who are commonly seen in primary care. The Canadian Dyspepsia Working Group has developed a definition for dyspepsia that includes heartburn and acid regurgitation [9]. There is some empiric support for the latter definition, as a few studies in *Helicobacter pylori* infected patients have demonstrated that cure of the infection not only led to a decrease in epigastric pain but also in symptoms of heartburn in a small but definite proportion of patients [10, 11, 12]. Other studies in primary care have included similar broad definitions of dyspepsia [13].

Diagnosis of functional dyspepsia

There is consensus that there is so much overlap in symptoms among patients with duodenal and gastric ulcers, GERD and functional dyspepsia that it is impossible to make a definitive diagnosis based on symptoms alone. This is supported by the results from the Canadian Prompt Endoscopy (CADET-PE) Study [14]. In this study, 1014 patients underwent endoscopy within ten days without having received acid suppressive therapy. There was a marked overlap in symptoms and it was impossible to distinguish between individuals with ulcers, esophagitis, or functional dyspepsia based on symptoms. In both the Enter and STARS studies reflux esophagitis was the most frequent reason for exclusion, despite the fact that the study entry criteria for heartburn were strict [15, 16]. In essence, functional dyspepsia is a diagnosis of exclusion, and in the setting of clinical trials generally requires an upper gastrointestinal endoscopy to exclude other diseases. In practice, physicians often decide on a trial of empiric therapy for patients presenting with dyspepsia, without worrying about a definitive diagnosis of a particular disease. This strategy is often attractive, given that the treatments for duodenal and gastric ulcers, GERD and functional dyspepsia are similar. The current standard of practice is a trial of acid suppressive therapy. Therefore, subclassification into separate diseases is not always necessary and in primary care may not be feasible. The decision whether or not to refer a patient for further investigation, usually either an upper gastrointestinal endoscopy or a barium study, is based on the severity of the presenting symptoms, age of the patient and on the presence or absence of "alarm symptoms" such as weight loss, evidence of bleeding or anemia, dysphagia and vomiting.

Subgroups of dyspepsia and overlap with GERD

The description of subgroups of dyspepsia has become popular despite evidence of the existence of considerable overlap among them. The Rome II classification recognized four subgroups: ulcer-like dyspepsia, reflux-like dyspepsia, dysmotility-like dyspepsia, and unclassified dyspepsia [17, 18]. An attractive, although not empirically proven feature of the Rome II classification was that the terms non-ulcer, reflux-like and dysmotility like dyspepsia conform with clinical beliefs about the pathophysiology of functional dyspepsia [4]. However, a study by Talley *et al.* demonstrated considerable overlap among the different subgroups [18], as did the CADET-PE Study [14]. Over the last few years functional dyspepsia trials have become increasingly strict in excluding patients with heartburn symptoms, and there is evidence that the treatment response rate using a proton pump inhibitor is lower when heartburn exclusion criteria become stricter [15, 16]. For example, in the STARS I study patients were excluded if they had >2 days with any heartburn symptom [16]. However, in contrast in the itopride Phase II trial it was unclear how heartburn symptoms were handled [19]. This is especially relevant since there was a suggestion that patients with heartburn showed a better response.

Increasingly, endoscopy negative GERD is now recognized as a distinct entity. This is a difficult issue for the methodology of trials of functional dyspepsia. In practice the preferred operational definition excludes patients with heartburn and/or regurgitation, based on severity and frequency criteria for these symptoms. An example of how this approach can be operationalized is the inclusion of patients who have heartburn no more than one day a week that is, at most, mild in severity.

What constitutes a normal endoscopy has been poorly defined in the literature. It is especially important to determine whether or not patients are, or were recently taking, acid suppressive therapy, as the use of these agents can mask the presence of esophagitis or ulcers. It would be ideal for trials of functional dyspepsia treatment to require that patients are not allowed to have consumed acid suppressive therapy for at least four weeks before the endoscopy. After withdrawal from acid suppressive therapy, it may take longer than four weeks for endoscopic abnormalities to become visible; however, a four-week period of avoidance of acid suppressive therapy seems a reasonable compromise as was recommended in the Montreal GERD definition publication [6].

Diagnostic investigation: endoscopy or radiographs?

Referral for endoscopy is indicated for older patients presenting with new-onset dyspepsia. Formerly, the recommendation was to use age >45 years as an indication for investigations, but it seems likely that this can be increased to 50 years or perhaps even higher [20, 21, 22]. This cutoff age is largely driven by the incidence of gastric cancer in the population where one practices. Interestingly, the Scottish guidelines have removed all age criteria, as there are insufficient data to support them [23]. In primary care, upper gastrointestinal barium studies are still commonly used to rule out peptic ulcer disease and esophageal or gastric cancer in patients with dyspepsia. The technical review of the American Gastroenterology Association (AGA) on dyspepsia summarizes the consistent evidence of the superiority of upper gastrointestinal endoscopy for detection of structural abnormalities [20]. Radiographs are still frequently used because of their lower cost, wider availability in the community and the speed with which the procedure can be arranged. Often there is a significant waiting time before patients can be seen after they are referred to a gastroenterologist. "Open access endoscopy" is one method by which delay in diagnostic endoscopy can be reduced. The AGA technical review assessed whether patients with new onset of symptoms should be investigated or treated empirically and came to the conclusion that the evidence is equivocal [20]. For example, in the study by Bytzer *et al.*, empiric treatment was compared with direct endoscopy in patients presenting with dyspepsia [24]. Patients in the endoscopy arm were more satisfied, and subsequent health care costs were significantly lower in this group. There is further evidence that a patient's quality of life is improved following a normal endoscopy [24]. This is largely due to alleviation of fear of a serious underlying disease when the dyspepsia symptoms persisted. However, a recommendation that endoscopy should be done in all or most patients presenting with dyspepsia would probably be too costly for most health care systems. A more rational approach therefore seems to be to stratify patients according to their risk of having serious underlying disease. Factors that can be considered are age of the patient, background prevalence of serious disease, especially of esophageal and gastric cancer, and the presence or absence of alarm symptoms. The recent significant increase in the incidence of esophageal adenocarcinoma in the West will likely drive the demand for gastroscopy, which although resource intensive is relatively easy to perform [25].

Methodological problems in trials of functional dyspepsia

In order to determine whether a treatment does more good than harm, valid and reliable outcome measures must be used in clinical trials. In the case of functional dyspepsia the lack of definite structural or pathophysiological abnormalities which explain the origin of the symptoms of functional dyspepsia has hampered the development of such measures. Clinical trials must use outcome measures that rely on the recording of symptoms and their severity, as is the case in other functional gastrointestinal disorders. A systematic review of drug treatment of functional dyspepsia evaluated the quality of clinical trials in this field [26]. Few studies used validated outcome measures, and methodological weaknesses were apparent in several trials. Problems included a lack of definition of functional dyspepsia, unclear inclusion and exclusion criteria, suboptimal study design and short duration of treatment. The most important problem in randomized controlled trials of interventions for functional dyspepsia is the lack of consensus on outcome measures. Only a small number of outcome measures have been validated. In the systematic review of studies on functional dyspepsia, only 5 of 52 studies used a validated outcome measure [26]. In a recent systematic review on outcome measures in functional dyspepsia and GERD 26 ways of measuring outcomes were identified [27]. Of these 12 only assessed symptoms (unidimensional) and 14 assessed both symptoms and quality of life (multidimensional). Eleven questionnaires assessed both frequency and severity of dyspepsia, and ten were felt to be sufficiently validated [27].

Subjective endpoints, such as recording of symptoms and their severity, used to measure a clinical outcome in a trial should fulfill four requirements [28]: (1) the range of symptoms included should be important to, and representative of, the disease process; (2) the measurements should be reproducible (producing consistent results when repeated in subjects who have not changed); (3) the measurements should be responsive (able to detect change); (4) changes in the measurement should reflect a real change in general health status.

Ideally, a separate study is required to demonstrate that an instrument meets these requirements, prior to its use in a randomized controlled trial. However, when dealing with symptoms, their severity and frequency, the face validity of their use is generally high. What is less clear is how one determines what amount of improvement is clinically important. The latter point is important because it drives the definition of what constitutes a patient responder. Both the Rome II and III working parties on design of clinical trials recommended the use of a primary outcome measure that integrates the global overall severity of symptoms, although it did not specify how this should be done [4, 5]. A common method to measure overall severity of symptoms is by using four, five or seven-point Likert scales. The Rome II report on study design provides a detailed discussion of the different scales that can be used [4, 29]. The Rome III working party went further in supporting the use of adequate or satisfactory relief as a suitable primary outcome measure [5]. These outcome measures have been used in large clinical trials evaluating the use of alosetron and tegaserod in irritable bowel syndrome [5]. These outcome measures have methodological shortcomings. They do not allow a comparison of post-treatment scores to baseline severity, making it impossible to determine the true effect size [30]. Furthermore, patients who reported severe or mild symptoms at baseline are considered the same if they report adequate or satisfactory relief during the study [30].

Another important weakness of many trials has been the relatively short duration of treatment. The duration of treatment was four weeks or less in 44 trials evaluated in the

systematic review of 52 studies [26]. It was eight weeks or longer in only four studies. Only seven studies had a follow-up period (varying from 3 to 52 weeks) after treatment was discontinued.

The short duration of treatment is surprising given the known chronicity of the symptoms of functional dyspepsia. The placebo response rate is high in clinical trials in patients with functional dyspepsia and other functional gastrointestinal disorders, such as irritable bowel syndrome. In the systematic review of trials of functional dyspepsia it varied from 13–73% [26]. Studies should also report the proportion of patients who become asymptomatic, since the placebo response is lowest for this outcome [30]. This approach permits a good estimate of true effect size. An explanation for the high placebo response rate may be the reassurance effect of a "normal" endoscopy. Fear of cancer is a frequent reason for concern among patients with functional dyspepsia undergoing gastroscopy [20, 22]. Wiklund *et al.* measured quality of life and gastrointestinal symptoms just prior to endoscopy and seven days later [31]. In patients in whom no significant endoscopic abnormalities were found overall quality of life improved, although there was little change in the severity of individual gastrointestinal symptoms. This observation supports the concept that endoscopy has a powerful placebo effect through reassurance of patients. However, a Dutch study did not confirm these findings [32]. The higher satisfaction with care in the study by Bytzer *et al.* may also be explained by a reassurance effect [24].

Functional versus uninvestigated dyspepsia

It is important to distinguish between uninvestigated dyspepsia and functional dyspepsia. The diagnosis of functional dyspepsia is generally considered to require an endoscopy. Most studies to date have dealt with investigated dyspepsia. Studies of uninvestigated dyspepsia will include a proportion of patients with duodenal or gastric ulcer, esophagitis and, rarely, gastric cancer. The frequency with which structural abnormalities are found has changed over the past decade [20]. With the declining prevalence of duodenal and gastric ulcers, reflux esophagitis is now by far the most common abnormality. Its prevalence ranges from 20% to 40% among patients and is far more common than duodenal and gastric ulcers which were present in 3% and 4% of patients in the CADET-PE Study [14]. However, these rates clearly depend on the prevalence of these disorders in the population being studied. Gastric cancer is rare below the age of 50 years [20, 33]. In most endoscopic dyspepsia studies the rate of functional dyspepsia is high and varies between 30% and 60% [20]. In this chapter we will focus on patients with investigated dyspepsia, that is functional dyspepsia. Given the problems in study design, especially the large variation in the way outcome measures have been used, it is difficult to do quantitative meta-analysis. Over the past few years, several meta-analyses have been reported including Cochrane reviews. Although several of these systematic reviews have statistically combined results of individual trials, it is important to stress that this is usually done by transforming the various outcome measures. For example, in one of the Cochrane meta-analyses, all outcomes of included studies were dichotomized into improved versus not improved [34]. No evidence has been provided that such an approach is valid, although some kind of transformation is required if one wants to combine studies which have used substantially different outcome measures. This author also believes that it is important that studies report the proportion of patients who become asymptomatic in the active and placebo treated patient groups [30]. This is the hardest outcome measure for which the placebo response is also the lowest. This does help to allow estimation of true effect size.

Drug treatment

Antacids

Over-the-counter medications, especially antacids, are commonly prescribed as first-line treatment. Many patients will probably have tried these medications before consulting a physician. As several reviews have been written on the use of antacids, the details of individual studies will not be discussed here. Clinical trials have generally not shown significant benefit from antacids [20, 35, 36]. The frequently cited and methodologically strong randomized controlled trial reported by Nyren et al. did not show benefit of antacids over placebo over a three-week treatment period [36].

H2-receptor antagonists

Over the past few years, four systematic reviews have evaluated the use of H2-blockers in functional dyspepsia [3, 37–39]. The number of studies that met the inclusion criteria varied in these reviews. All four came to the same conclusion: that there is some evidence that these agents provide benefit in functional dyspepsia patients (see Box 9.1). However, it is important to point out several methodological issues. The reason why the results for H2-blockers have varied is that several of the included studies which showed benefit probably included GERD patients. This factor may explain why the meta-analysis by Dobrilla et al. showed a therapeutic gain of 18% of active treatment over placebo [37]. Two methodologically strong studies did not show a benefit of either cimetidine or nizatidine over placebo [36, 40]. It is also worth pointing out that most studies have used low doses of H2-receptor antagonists (H2-RA), for example ranitidine 150 mg twice a day. It is possible that higher doses of H2-RA might yield larger and more consistent treatment effects, but this needs to be assessed in future studies. Finally there is also evidence that the reported benefit of H2-blockers is larger in methodologically weaker studies [41]. One of the likely explanations for this is contamination with patients who have GERD. Many of the included studies were vague concerning this particular inclusion criterion [41].

BOX 9.1 Results of meta-analyses of clinical trials of treatment of functional dyspepsia with H2-blockers

(1) Dobrilla et al.: Therapeutic gain H2-blockers compared with placebo 18% [34].
(2) Bytzer: Therapeutic gain H2-blockers compared with placebo 22% [36].
(3) Soo et al.: Relative risk reduction of ongoing dyspepsia of H2-blockers compared with placebo 22% [30].
(4) Redstone et al.: Odds ratio studies of H2-blockers compared with placebo reporting complete relief from epigastric pain 1·8 (95% CI: 1.2–2.8) [35]. Odds ratio studies of H2-blockers compared with placebo reporting global improvement dyspepsia symptoms 1·48 (95% CI: 0.9–2.3)

Proton pump inhibitors

PPIs have largely overtaken the use of H2-RAs in the treatment of acid related-disorders. The first large studies were the BOND-OPERA studies which evaluated the role of PPI therapy in functional dyspepsia [42]. Over a four-week period, 1262 functional dyspepsia patients received either omeprazole (20 mg or 10 mg) or placebo. Complete relief of symptoms was achieved in 38% of patients on omeprazole 20 mg, 36% on omeprazole 10 mg, and 28% on placebo (p < 0.001). The absolute risk reduction (ARR) of 10% and 8% correspond to an NNT (the number of patients needed to treat with omeprazole to yield one additional patient with a complete response) of 10 for 20 mg omeprazole and 12 for 10 mg omeprazole. Subgroup analysis suggested that patients with ulcer-like and reflux-like dyspepsia benefited from omeprazole therapy, while patients fulfilling the criteria for dysmotility-like dyspepsia did not. Although it is generally not felt useful to make a diagnosis of specific dyspepsia subgroups, the results of this study suggest that use of the two subgroups – ulcer-like and reflux-like dyspepsia – may help predict a response to PPI therapy. Interestingly, although overt reflux patients were supposed to have been excluded, a proportion of patients reported heartburn as their most bothersome symptom. This is one of the reasons why in recent years the study entry criteria have become much more stringent for reflux symptoms. Moayyedi et al. conducted a systematic review on the effectiveness of PPIs in treatment of functional dyspepsia [43]. Eight trials were identified that compared PPI therapy with placebo in a total of 3293 patients. Response is expressed as the Relative Risk (RR) of having ongoing symptoms, which clinically is not the most user friendly way of expressing efficacy, although it is sound methodologically. For clinicians it is easier to understand that patients treated with a specific intervention are more likely to have improved or become asymptomatic relative to those who received a placebo, rather than considering a decreased risk of ongoing symptoms. The relative risk of remaining dyspeptic with PPI therapy versus placebo was 0.86 (95% CI: 0.78–0.95; p = .003, random-effects model) with a number needed to treat of 9 (95% CI: 5–25). The response rate in PPI treated patients was 33% compared to 23% for placebo. The placebo response rate was lowest in studies that used absence of symptoms as the primary outcome measure. There was statistically significant heterogeneity between trials. As expected, the presence of heartburn was a predictor of response. No benefit was seen in the subgroup that met the dysmotility criteria.

In another recent meta-analysis performed by Wong et al. seven studies with a total of 3725 patients met inclusion criteria [44]. Use of PPIs was more effective than placebo for reducing symptoms in patients, expressed as a relative risk reduction RRR of 10.3%; (95% CI: 2.7–17.3%). The number needed to treat is 15 (95% CI: 9–57). In subgroup analysis a significant difference in the benefit was observed for patients with ulcer-like (RRR, 13%; 95% CI: 7–18%) and reflux-like dyspepsia (RRR, 20%; 95% CI: 2–34%), but not in those with dysmotility-like dyspepsia (RRR, 5.%; 95% CI: –11–19%) and unspecified dyspepsia (RRR, –8.0%; 95% CI: –24–6%).

The practical bottom line for use of PPIs in functional dyspepsia is that it is reasonable to give patients a trial of 4–8 weeks of therapy, with the understanding that heartburn is a predictor of response and that the majority of patients will not respond.

Use of prokinetic agents

The following prokinetic agents will be discussed: domperidone, cisapride, itopride and tegaserod.

Domperidone

Prokinetics have been evaluated in functional dyspepsia because of the hypothesis that disturbed gastrointestinal motility may in part be responsible for the symptoms of dyspepsia. Domperidone is a dopamine receptor antagonist, which has shown a benefit in several randomized placebo controlled trials in patients with functional dyspepsia. However, as a systematic review pointed out, many of these trials enrolled only small numbers of patients and had other important methodological weaknesses [45]. These data can certainly not be considered as being conclusive.

Cisapride

This a prokinetic agent with 5-HT4 -agonist activity specifically targeted patients with dysmotility-like dyspepsia. The drug had also been proved to be effective in patients with mild GERD and in patients with delayed gastric emptying. Due to rare but serious cardiac side effects this drug has now been removed from most markets. The four systematic reviews that have looked at the efficacy of cisapride in functional dyspepsia all came to the same conclusion: that there was some evidence that the drug did improve dyspepsia symptoms [34, 39, 41, 45]. However, several of the cisapride studies suffered from serious methodological weaknesses, which made the conclusions about efficacy tentative. Furthermore, on funnel plots there was also evidence of a publication bias, almost certainly due to the fact that there was an overrepresentation of small studies with positive results [34].

Itopride

Recently a comprehensive clinical trial program evaluated the use of itopride in the treatment of functional dyspepsia [9, 46]. Itopride, similarly to cisapride, is a benzamide

derivative. It exerts its activity by inhibition of the dopamine D2 receptor and acetylcholinesterase.

The phase-II trial published in the *New England Journal of Medicine* received a lot of attention as it reported positive results in favor of itopride [19]. However, the results of two simultaneously conducted phase-III clinical trials involving 1170 patients unfortunately did not show a difference between itopride and placebo groups [46]. In the two phase-III studies the two primary outcome measures were global patient assessment measured on a five-point scale and two questions of the Leeds Dyspepsia Questionnaire (LDQ) [47]: the severity of pain in the upper abdomen and feeling of upper abdominal fullness. On the global scale, to be considered as a responder the patient had to become symptom free or to have reported a marked improvement. Either a one or two-point improvement on each of the two LDQ questions was used as a primary endpoint. Itopride was not more effective than placebo for any of these outcome measures. The only difference for the LDQ questions that did show a significant change was a two-point improvement in one of the two phase II studies (the International Study, 62% vs 53%, p = 0.04), but this was not seen in the North American trial (47% vs 45%). No significant difference was found in the proportion of patients who reported complete absence of symptoms after eight weeks of itopride treatment (16.1% vs 13.7% in the international trial and 8.9% vs 6.6% in the North American trial). Further development of itopride for use in functional dyspepsia has been halted.

Tegaserod

Tegaserod is a selective serotonin type 4 receptor agonist that has been comprehensively studied in irritable bowel syndrome, especially in the subgroup of patients with constipation dominant symptoms, where it has shown efficacy using the endpoint of satisfactory relief. Its use has also been studied in two trials of patients with dysmotility-like functional dyspepsia [48]. For this diagnosis patients needed to have postprandial fullness, early satiety and/or bloating. As in the tegaserod IBS trial program satisfactory relief (>50% of the time) was used as a primary outcome measure. In addition, a composite score of average daily severity (measured on a seven-point scale, which had to show >1 point improvement) of the three inclusion criteria symptoms was used. The program only included women and the combined studies included 2667 patients. In one study, improvement in tegaserod treated patients of borderline statistical significance was observed, but this improvement was not observed in the second study. When the results of the two studies were combined there was a 4.6% increase in days with satisfactory relief. This difference, in the author's opinion, is not clinically meaningful, especially in view of the fact that diarrhea as an adverse effect requiring study discontinuation was experienced more commonly with tegaserod than with placebo (4.1% vs 0.3%) [48]. Unfortunately, tegaserod was withdrawn from the market in 2007 because of a small increase in cardiovascular events in post-marketing surveillance.

In summary currently there is no convincing evidence for use of prokinetic agents in treatment of functional dyspepsia.

Anti-*Helicobacter* therapy

The prevalence of *H. pylori* in functional dyspepsia varies from 30% to 70%, but this is in large part dependent on known risk factors for *H. pylori* infection: age, socioeconomic status and race [49, 50]. Due to differences in study design and problems with selection bias, it is still unclear whether the prevalence of *H. pylori* infection is increased in patients with functional dyspepsia compared with normal controls, although a meta-analysis suggested that it is [51]. A hotly debated issue over the past 15 years has been the question of whether cure of *H. pylori* infection leads to a sustained improvement in symptoms of functional dyspepsia.

Related to this is the question of whether testing and treating for *H. pylori* infection is a worthwhile strategy in patients presenting with uninvestigated dyspepsia. Such testing can be done without the need for endoscopy by using a urea breath test or *Helicobacter* serology. A detailed discussion about this approach is beyond the scope of this chapter, which deals with functional dyspepsia, but there is evidence that it may lead to long term symptom improvement in a proportion of patients [10, 11, 12, 20].

Although there have been differences in the methodological quality of anti-*Helicobacter* therapy functional dyspepsia studies several high quality studies with large sample sizes have also been conducted [41]. A Cochrane meta-analysis on this topic was updated in 2006 [52]. Importantly, in this systematic review dyspepsia outcome measures were dichotomized into minimal remaining or resolved symptoms versus same or worse symptoms. Twenty-one trials met inclusion criteria, of which eighteen trials compared antisecretory dual or triple therapy with placebo antibiotics +/− antisecretory therapy. The study duration varied from 3 to 12 months. For the combined sample of 3566 patients there was a 10% relative risk reduction in the *H. pylori* eradication group (95% CI: 6–14%) compared to placebo. This translates to a number needed to treat to cure one case of dyspepsia of 14 (95% CI: 10–25). Based on these data it appears that there is a small but statistically significant benefit in curing *H. pylori* infection in infected non-ulcer dyspepsia patients. It is important to keep in mind that the overall contribution of *H. pylori* infection to functional dyspepsia is small and that despite cure of the infection many patients will have ongoing dyspepsia symptoms. It is possible that the benefit is mainly limited to patients who have an underlying ulcer diathesis, but at the moment there is no reliable method to identify this subgroup of patients. Given that *H. pylori* is a true pathogen that leads to peptic ulcer disease in 5–15% of infected individuals and is associated with gastric cancer in up to 1% of patients, it seems reasonable that patients with chronic dyspepsia symptoms who come to endoscopy are tested for the infection and treated if positive.

Use of antidepressants

Functional dyspepsia patients who do not respond to H2-RAs, PPIs, prokinetic agents and anti-*Helicobacter* therapy (if positive) are a difficult group to treat. As with IBS patients antidepressant therapy has been tested in this patient group. However, the overall evidence in favor of their use, when obvious psychopathology is absent, is weak. A Cochrane review identified only four trials, each of which used different psychological interventions so that no formal pooling of results was possible [53]. All trials reported that psychological interventions provided benefit in improving dyspepsia symptoms. An identified weakness in all trials was the use of statistical techniques that adjusted for baseline differences between groups. This was likely necessary to compensate for small sample sizes [53]. Unadjusted data was not statistically significant. The other problems in the included studies were low recruitment and high drop-out rates. The authors concluded that there were insufficient data to determine whether psychological interventions were effective in functional dyspepsia.

Recently, a study was reported in 166 functional dyspepsia patients who were randomized to treatment for eight weeks with either placebo or the serotonin and norepinephrine reuptake inhibitor venlafaxine (two weeks, 75 mg once daily, four weeks, 150 mg once daily, and two weeks, 75 mg once daily) [54]. There was no difference in the proportion of venlafaxine treated patients who were symptom-free after eight weeks of treatment or at 20 weeks after inclusion, when compared to placebo (37% versus 39%).

Given the limited amount of available data the use of antidepressant therapy can not be recommended for functional dyspepsia patients.

Conclusion

There are methodological shortcomings in many functional dyspepsia treatment trials, but their quality has improved over the last five years, in large part due to contributions of the pharmaceutical industry who have conducted many large-scale studies. There are no large sample size trials which compare the main treatment options for which there is supporting evidence: H2-receptor antagonists, PPIs and anti-*Helicobacter* therapy for patients who are *H. pylori* posi-

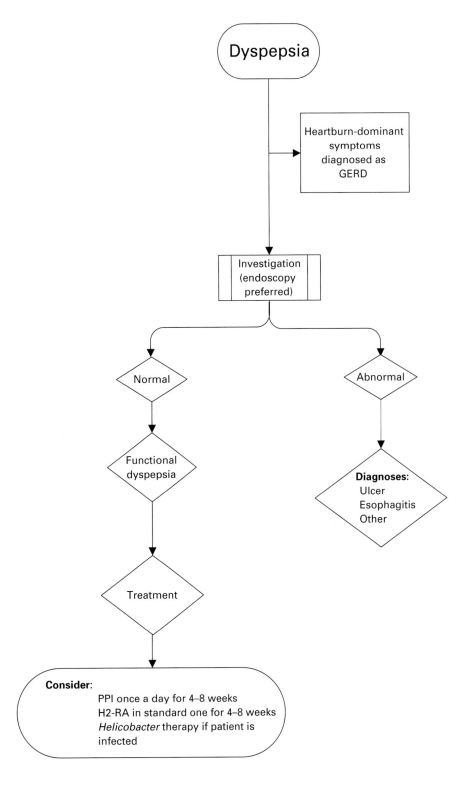

Figure 9.1 Algorithm for dyspepsia.

tive. An algorithm that may serve as a useful guide is presented in Figure 9.1. It is reasonable to give functional dyspepsia patients a trial of acid suppression with either an H2-RA or a PPI. Evidence for effectiveness of PPIs is stronger. For all these treatments it is possible that patients with unrecognized GERD represent the main group who respond to acid suppression, or that associated heartburn is a driver of response. There is evidence that cure of *H. pylori* infection will lead to a sustained improvement of functional dyspepsia symptoms in a small proportion of patients. Given that *H. pylori* is a true pathogen, capable of producing peptic ulcers and sometimes gastric cancer it is advisable that patients coming for endoscopy are tested for *H. pylori* and treated if positive. There is no evidence that supports the use of currently available prokinetic agents and similarly the evidence for use of antidepressants is also weak.

References

1 Nyrén O, Lindberg G, Lindstrom E *et al. Economic Costs of Functional Dyspepsia. Pharmacoconomics* 1992; **1**(5): 312–324.

2 Chiba N, Bernard L, O'Brien BJ *et al.* A Canadian physician survey of dyspepsia management. *Can J Gastroenterol* 1998; **12**: 183–190.

3 Talley NJ, Colin-Jones D, Koch KL *et al.* Functional dyspepsia: a classification with guidelines for diagnosis and management. *Gastroenterol Int* 1991; **4**: 145–160.

4 Talley NJ, Stanghellinin V, Heading RC, Koch KL, Malageleda JR, Tytgat GNJ. Functional gastroduodenal disorders. *Gut* 1999; **45**(suppl. II): 37–42.

5 Irvine EJ, Whitehead WE, Chey WD *et al.* Design of treatment trials for functional gastrointestinal disorders. *Gastroenterology* 2006; **130**(5): 1538–1551.

6 Vakil N, Veldhuyzen van Zanten S, Kahrilas P, Dent J, Jones R, the Global Consensus Group. The Montreal definition and classification of gastroesophageal reflux disease: a global evidence-based consensus. *Am J Gastroenterol* 2006; **101**(8): 1900–1920.

7 Fischler B, Tack J, De Gucht V *et al.* Heterogeneity of symptom pattern, psychosocial factors, and pathophysiological mechanisms in severe functional dyspepsia. *Gastroenterology* 2003; **124**(4): 903–910.

8 Tack J, Jones MP, Karamanolis G, Coulie B, Dubois D. Symptom pattern and pathophysiological correlates of weight loss in tertiary-referred functional dyspepsia. *Neurogastroenterol Motil.* 2009 30. (Epub ahead of print).

9 Veldhuyzen van Zanten SJ, Flook N, Chiba N *et al.* An evidence-based approach to the management of uninvestigated dyspepsia in the era of *Helicobacter pylori.* Canadian Dyspepsia Working Group. *Can Med Assoc J* 2000; **162**(12 suppl.): S3–23.

10 Chiba N, Van Zanten SJ, Sinclair P, Ferguson RA, Escobedo S, Grace E. Treating *Helicobacter pylori* infection in primary care patients with uninvestigated dyspepsia: the Canadian adult dyspepsia empiric treatment – *Helicobacter pylori* positive (CADET-Hp) randomised controlled trial. *BMJ* 2002; **324**: 1012–1016.

11 Moayyedi P, Feltbower R, Brown J *et al.* Effect of population screening and treatment for *Helicobacter pylori* on dyspepsia and quality of life in the community: a randomised controlled trial. Leeds HELP Study Group. *Lancet* 2000; **355**: 1665–1669.

12 Wildner-Christensen M, Moller Hansen J, Schaffalitzky De Muckadell OB. Rates of dyspepsia one year after *Helicobacter pylori* screening and eradication in a Danish population. *Gastroenterology* 2003; **125**: 372–379.

13 van Marrewijk CJ, Mujakovic S, Fransen GA *et al.* Effect and cost-effectiveness of step-up versus step-down treatment with antacids, H2-receptor antagonists, and proton pump inhibitors in patients with new onset dyspepsia (DIAMOND study):

a primary-care-based randomised controlled trial. *Lancet* 2009; **373**(9659): 215–225.

14 Thomson AB, Barkun AN, Armstrong D *et al.* The prevalence of clinically significant endoscopic findings in primary care patients with uninvestigated dyspepsia: the Canadian Adult Dyspepsia Empiric Treatment – Prompt Endoscopy (CADET-PE) study. *Aliment Pharmacol Ther* 2003; **17**: 1481–1491.

15 Veldhuyzen van Zanten S, Armstrong D, Chiba N *et al.* Esomeprazole 40 mg once a day in patients with functional dyspepsia: the randomized, placebo-controlled "ENTER" trial. *Am J GE* 2006; **101**: 2096–2106.

16 Talley NJ, Vakil N, Lauritsen K *et al.* and STARS I Study Group. Randomized-controlled trial of esomeprazole in functional dyspepsia patients with epigastric pain or burning: does a 1-week trial of acid suppression predict symptom response? *Aliment Pharmacol Ther* 2007; **26**(5): 673–682.

17 Talley NJ, Zinsmeister AR, Schleck CD *et al.* Dyspepsia and dyspepsia subgroups: a population-based study. *Gastroenterology* 1992; **102**: 1259–1268.

18 Talley NJ, Weaver AL, Tesmer DL *et al.* Lack of discriminant value of dyspepsia subgroups in patients referred for upper endoscopy. *Gastroenterology* 1993; **105**: 1378–1386.

19 Holtmann G, Talley N, Liebregts T, Adam B and Parow C. A placebo-controlled trial of itopride in functional dyspepsia. *N Engl J Med* 2006; **354**: 832–840.

20 Talley NJ, Silverstein MC, Agreus L *et al.* AGA Technical review: evaluation of dyspepsia. *Gastroenterology* 1998; **114**: 582–595.

21 Veldhuyzen van Zanten SJO. Can the age limit for endoscopy be increased in dyspepsia patients who do not have alarm symptoms? *Am J Gastroenterol* 1999; **94**: 9–11.

22 Axon ATR. Chronic dyspepsia: who needs endoscopy? *Gastroenterology* 1997; **112**: 1376–1380.

23 Scottish Intercollegiate Guideline Network (SIGN) *Clinical Guidelines No. 68, Dyspepsia.* A national clinical guideline. March 2003. www.sign.ac.uk (accessed September 2003).

24 Bytzer P, Hansen JM, Schaffalitzky de Muckadell OB. Empirical H2-blocker therapy or prompt endoscopy in management of dyspepsia. *Lancet* 1994; **343**; 811–816.

25 Brown LM, Devesa SS. Epidemiologic trends in esophageal and gastric cancer in the United States. *Surg Oncol Clin N Am* 2002; **11**: 235–256.

26 Veldhuyzen van Zanten SJO, Cleary C, Talley NJ *et al.* Drug treatment of functional dyspepsia: a systematic analysis of trial methodology with recommendations for design of future trials. *Am J Gastroenterol* 1996; **91**: 660–671.

27 Fraser A, Delaney B, Moayyedi P. Symptom-based outcome measures for dyspepsia and GERD trials: a systematic review. *Am J Gastroenterol* 2005; **100**(2): 442–452.

28 Guyatt GH, Veldhuyzen van Zanten SJO, Feeney DH *et al.* Measuring quality of life in clinical trials. A taxonomy and review. *Can Med J Assoc* 1989; **140**: 1441–1448.

29 Veldhuyzen van Zanten S, Talley N, Bytzer P, Klein K, Whorwell P, Zinsmeister A. *Design of treatment trials for the functional gastrointestinal disorders.* Rome II The Functional Gastrointestinal Disorders. Printed Allen Press, Inc, Lawrence, KS, 1999; Chapter 11: 577–622.

30 Veldhuyzen van Zanten S. Pitfalls in designing trials of functional dyspepsia: the ascent and demise of itopride. *Gut* 2008; **57**(6): 723–724.

31 Wiklund I, Glise H, Jerndal PI *et al.* Does endoscopy have a positive impact on quality of life in dyspepsia? *Gastrointest Endosc* 1998; **47**: 449–454.

32 van Kerkhoven LA, van Rossum LG, van Oijen MG, Tan AC, Laheij RJ, Jansen JB. Upper gastrointestinal endoscopy does not reassure patients with functional dyspepsia. *Endoscopy* 2006; **38**(9): 879–885.

33 Christie J, Shepherd NA, Codling BW *et al.* Gastric cancer below the age of 55: implications for screening patients with uncomplicated dyspepsia. *Gut* 1997; **41**: 513–517.

34 Soo S, Moayyedi P, Deeks J, Delaney B, Innes M, Forman D. Pharmacological interventions for non-ulcer dyspepsia. *Cochrane Database Syst Rev* 2000; **2**: CD01960.

35 Talley NJ. Drug treatment of functional dyspepsia. *Scand J Gastroenterol* 1991; **26**(S182): 47–60.

36 Nyren O, Adami HO, Bates S *et al.* Absence of therapeutic benefit from antacids or cimetidine in non-ulcer dyspepsia. *N Engl J Med* 1986; **314**: 339–343.

37 Dobrilla G, Comberlato L, Steele A *et al.* Drug treatment of functional dyspepsia. A meta-analysis of randomized controlled clinical trials. *J Clin Gastroenterol* 1989; **11**: 169–177.

38 Redstone HA, Barrowman N, Veldhuyzen van Zanten SJO. H2-receptor antagonists in the treatment of functional (nonulcer) dyspepsia: a meta-analysis of randomized controlled clinical trials. *Aliment Pharmacol Ther* 2001; **15**: 1291–1299.

39 Bytzer P. H2-receptor antagonists and prokinetics in dyspepsia: a critical review. *Gut* 2002; **50**(suppl. 4): iv: 58–62.

40 Hansen JM, Bytzer P, Schaffalitzky de Muckadell OB. Placebo-controlled trial of cisapride and nizatidine in unselected patients with functional dyspepsia. *Am J Gastroenterol* 1998; **93**: 368–374.

41 Abraham NS, Moayyedi P, Daniels B, Veldhuyzen van Zanten SJO. Systematic review: the methodological quality of trials affects estimates of treatment efficacy in functional (non-ulcer) dyspepsia. *Aliment Pharmacol Ther* 2004; **19**(6): 631–641.

42 Talley NJ, Meineche-Schmidt V, Pare P *et al.* Efficacy of omeprazole in functional dyspepsia: double-blind, randomized placebo-controlled trials (the Bond and Opera studies). *Aliment Pharmacol Ther* 1998; **12**: 1055–1065.

43 Moayyedi P, Delaney BC, Vakil N, Forman D, Talley NJ. The efficacy of proton pump inhibitors in nonulcer dyspepsia: a systematic review and economic analysis. *Gastroenterology* 2004; **127**(5): 1329–1337.

44 Wang WH, Huang JQ, Zheng GF *et al.* Effects of proton-pump inhibitors on functional dyspepsia: a meta-analysis of randomized placebo-controlled trials. *Clin Gastroenterol Hepatol* 2007; **5**(2): 178–185.

45 Veldhuyzen van Zanten SJ, Jones MJ, Verlinden M, Talley NJ. Efficacy of cisapride and domperidone in functional (nonulcer) dyspepsia: a meta-analysis. *Am J Gastroenterol* 2001; **96**: 689–696.

46 Talley NJ, Tack J, Ptak Th, Gupta R, Giguère M. Itopride in functional dyspepsia: results of two phase-III multicenter randomized, double-blind, placebo-controlled trials. *Gut* 2008; **57**(6): 740–746.

47 Fraser A, Delaney BC, Ford AC, Qume M, Moayyedi P. The Short-Form Leeds Dyspepsia Questionnaire validation study. *Aliment Pharmacol Ther* 2007; **25**: 477–486.

48 Vakil N, Laine L, Talley NJ *et al.* Tegaserod treatment for dysmotility-like functional dyspepsia: results of two randomized, controlled trials. *Am J Gastroenterol* 2008; **103**(8): 1906–1919. Epub 4 July 2008.

49 Graham DY, Malaty HM, Evans DG *et al.* Epidemiology of *H. pylori* in an asymptomatic population in the United States: effect of age, race and socioeconomic status. *Gastroenterology* 1991; **100**: 1495–1501.

50 Veldhuyzen van Zanten SJO. *H. pylori*, socioeconomic status, marital status and occupation. *Aliment Pharmacol Ther* 1995; **9**(S2): 41–44.

51 Armstrong D. *H. pylori* and dyspepsia. *Scand J Gastroenterol* 1996; **31**(suppl. 215): 38–47.

52 Moayyedi P, Soo S, Deeks J *et al.* Eradication of *Helicobacter pylori* for non-ulcer dyspepsia. *Cochrane Database Syst Rev*. 19 April 2006 (2): CD002096.

53 Soo S, Moayyedi P, Deeks J, Delaney B, Lewis M, Forman D. Psychological interventions for non-ulcer dyspepsia. *Cochrane Database Syst Rev*. 18 April 2005 (2): CD002301.

54 van Kerkhoven LA, Laheij RJ, Aparicio N *et al.* Effect of the antidepressant venlafaxine in functional dyspepsia: a randomized, double-blind, placebo-controlled trial. *Clin Gastroenterol Hepatol* 2008; **6**(7): 746–752.

10 Celiac disease: Diagnosis, treatment and prognosis

James Gregor and Michael Sai Lai Sey
Department of Medicine, University of Western Ontario, London, Ontario, Canada

Since its first description in children by Gee [1] over a century ago, the term celiac disease has been used interchangeably with such designations as primary malabsorption, gluten-sensitive enteropathy, and non-tropical or celiac sprue. Due to the protean nature of its clinical manifestations and their consistent improvement with appropriate therapy, few medical conditions can rival celiac disease for both the frustration and gratification experienced by clinicians and patients.

The first clinical description of celiac disease in adults was provided by Thaysen [2] in 1932. In the early 1950s, Dicke first reported a putative link between the disease and the ingestion of certain grains [3]. Over the next decade the characteristic intestinal lesion was described in both surgical specimens [4] and those obtained using the newly developed peroral suction biopsy technique [5].

Epidemiology

Celiac disease is most common in western Europeans and in immigrants from this area to North America and Australia; it is less common in non-Caucasoids, and although reported in Indians, Arabs, Hispanics, Israeli Jews, Sudanese and people of Cantonese extraction, it is very rare in those of Afro-Caribbean extraction. The true prevalence of celiac disease remains difficult to ascertain, and the prevalence varies with the intensity of screening [6].

Until the advent of new, accurate serologic tests, celiac disease was presumed to be a rare entity, with a prevalence of 1:1500 in Europe and 1:3000 in the USA [7]. The recognition of atypical presentations of disease has led to intensified serologic screening followed by intestinal biopsy, and

this protocol has revealed a true prevalence ranging from 1:300 in the UK [8] to 1:150 in Ireland [9, 10] In the USA, screening of blood from 2000 blood donors has found a prevalence of raised anti-endomysial antibodies of 1:250 [11], while a retrospective cohort of 3654 school-aged subjects in Finland estimated a prevalence approaching 1 in 99 [12]. The suggestion has been made that celiac disease detected by screening is not silent, but rather undetected, given the range of pathology and symptomatology that correlate with this disease [13, 14].

Clinical manifestations

The clinical manifestations of celiac disease are largely due to nutrient malabsorption, with iron-deficiency anemia being the most common presenting finding in an adult celiac patient [15]. Other symptoms, such as severe abdominal pain, nausea and vomiting are much less common. Although some patients may even complain of constipation, most describe increased stool volume. The diarrhea of celiac disease is classically described as high volume, pale, loose to semi-formed and foul-smelling. However, in many cases it is watery, probably due to the effects of malabsorbed fat and its bacterial degradation products on the secretory mechanisms of intestinal mucosal cells. A high fat content may produce an oily or frothy appearance and a high gas content can make the stools difficult to flush from the toilet bowl.

Constitutional symptoms of fatigue, weakness and weight loss, often despite a history of hyperphagia, are common. Many of these symptoms can be attributed to the presence of nutritional deficiencies. In some patients, insufficient calories and protein are absorbed to meet nutritional requirements and weight loss and muscle wasting ensue. Specific deficiencies resulting in anemia, bleeding diathesis, tetany, neuropathy and dermatitis can also occur.

Given the genetic and immunological factors felt to be important in the pathogenesis of the disease, it is not sur-

Evidence-Based Gastroenterology and Hepatology, 3rd edition.
J. McDonald, A.K. Burroughs, B. Feagan, and M.B. Fennerty. © 2010
Blackwell Publishing Ltd

prising that investigators have sought and reported an association between celiac disease and over 100 medical conditions [16]. By far the most common of these is dermatitis herpetiformis. This pruritic rash is typically papulovesicular and characterized by IgA deposits at the dermal-epidermal junction. If adequate biopsies are performed, villous atrophy has been identified in up to 95% of these patients. In support of the validity of this association is the observation that the characteristic blistering skin lesions tend to improve in response to a gluten-free diet, although at a slower rate (up to two years) than the intestinal lesions [17].

Lymphocytic infiltration of the epithelium of the colon and even stomach has been widely reported in celiac disease. Recent data suggest, however, that the majority of patients with microscopic or collagenous colitis do not have serological evidence of disease [18].

Type I diabetes mellitus has been described in up to 5% of patients with celiac disease [16] and a similar proportion of insulin dependent diabetics has been reported to have occult villous atrophy [19, 20]. Autoimmune thyroid disease and selective IgA deficiency [21] also appear to be more prevalent in patients with celiac disease. Studies linking celiac disease to other autoimmune diseases such as ulcerative colitis [22], primary biliary cirrhosis [23] and sclerosing cholangitis [24] are primarily family studies or small case series.

Screening studies suggest an increased prevalence (up to 7%) of celiac disease in patients with Down's syndrome [25, 26]. In one study this generated an odds ratio as high as 100, compared to the general population [27]. However, due to the small number of celiac patients diagnosed in the groups with Down's syndrome, a statistically significantly increased prevalence has not been demonstrated uniformly.

Pathology

Celiac disease primarily affects the mucosal layer of the small intestine, often involving only duodenum and jejunum, with damage decreasing in severity more distally. In severe disease, the entire length of the small bowel may be involved, and there have even been occasional reports of abnormalities of the gastric and rectal mucosa [14]. The characteristic lesion includes lymphocytic infiltration of the lamina propria and, in particular, the surface epithelium, resulting in villous atrophy and crypt hyperplasia. The degree of villous damage ranges from mere blunting to total atrophy. The degree and extent of disease involvement grossly correlates with the severity of gastrointestinal symptoms [28]. In some studies the prevalence of asymptomatic celiac disease is four-fold greater than the prevalence of symptomatic disease [29].

Historically, the gold standard for the diagnosis of celiac disease has required not only the identification of the typical histological lesion, but also clinical and histological improvement with appropriate dietary therapy. It has been clearly demonstrated in human subjects that the instillation into the small bowel of wheat, rye, or barley flour or their alcohol-soluble protein components, "prolamins", produces both clinical symptoms and histological lesions [30].

Wheat gluten must be processed into alcohol soluble prolamins in order to develop antigenicity. Although the exact epitope(s) within gluten remain unknown, the generation of this epitope from the antigenic wheat protein is accomplished by a brush border enzyme known as tissue transglutaminase (tTG). Once the epitope has been generated by the tTG enzyme, the enzyme itself becomes one of the targets of the autoimmune response [14].

Although the environmental trigger of wheat gluten is implicated in the development of this disease, it is apparent that genetic factors also play a prominent role. Concordance between identical twins approaches 100%, and first-degree relatives of celiac disease have a 10% prevalence of CD, which is higher than that cited in the general population [15]. Current theories of disease pathogenesis therefore focus on the interaction between the antigen (wheat gluten) and the HLA predisposition of affected individuals. Over 95% of patients with CD express the HLA DQ (a1*501, β1*02) heterodimer (HLA-DQ2). This class II MHC molecule exists on antigen-presenting cells, including the gluten-sensitive T helper cells, which preferentially present gluten-derived gliadin peptide epitopes to intestinal mucosal T cells. A Th1/Th0 type inflammatory response is mounted, thus producing the observed mucosal damage. One of the targets of this autoimmune response is the tTG brush border enzyme which generates the gluten-derived epitope. An anti-tTG assay may therefore be used to screen populations for celiac disease [14, 15].

Much of the fundamental research relating to celiac disease in recent years has focused on the immunologic and genetic factors associated with sensitivity to gliadin and the other prolamins. In clinical practice the diagnosis and treatment of the disease are well-defined. Thus most of the recently published clinical research has addressed a few specific questions, namely:

(1) Diagnosis: the role of the anti-endomysial antibody and the anti-tissue transglutaminase antibody for screening populations at risk, diagnosing symptomatic individuals and following the response to a gluten-free diet.

(2) Treatment: whether oats (or specifically the oat prolamin avenin) can safely be consumed by patients with celiac disease or dermatitis herpetiformis.

(3) Prognosis: whether patients are at an increased risk of malignancy and other autoimmune diseases, and whether adherence to a gluten-free diet reduces that risk.

Serological testing

In patients with typical signs, symptoms and laboratory parameters the diagnosis of celiac disease is usually made by performing a mucosal biopsy of the small bowel. Though the differential diagnosis of villous injury is long (including tropical sprue, lymphoma, cows' milk induced enteritis, Zollinger–Ellison syndrome, Whipple's disease, eosinophilic gastroenteritis, bacterial overgrowth, and even viral gastroenteritis), in most patients the diagnosis is not in doubt. From the 1950s until the introduction of flexible endoscopic equipment, specimens were usually obtained using peroral suction instruments, a cumbersome procedure which was uncomfortable for the patient. With the recognition of the immunological nature of the disease it was predictable that serological testing would be developed and evaluated to simplify diagnosis and to facilitate the institution of screening programs in areas of high prevalence.

A number of serological tests have been developed employing antireticulin antibodies (ARA), antigliadin antibodies (AGA), anti-smooth muscle endomysium antibodies (EMA) and, more recently, anti-tissue transglutaminase antibodies (tTG). Given that the pathogenesis of celiac disease appears to involve the interaction between cereal grain gluten, or more specifically the alcohol-soluble gliadins, it is not surprising that many of the early reports have focused on AGA as the primary serological test. As is often the case following the introduction of a new diagnostic test, the initial promise has to some degree yielded to acknowledgement of the test's limitations. Most studies have examined both the IgG and IgA subsets of AGA [31, 32]. The data demonstrate reasonable sensitivity (69–91%) but poor specificity (2–79%) for the IgG antibody, suggesting that it may be a general marker for increased gut permeability of any cause rather than an important factor in disease pathogenesis. The IgA AGA has improved specificity (90–94%) at the expense of sensitivity (66–87%).

The development of the anti-endomysial antibody test has produced a renewed interest in serological diagnosis. Initial reports suggested almost perfect test accuracy in subjects not restricted to a gluten-free diet. Because it employs an IgA antibody, it is acknowledged that the test may be falsely negative in a celiac patient with associated IgA deficiency. The test is generally performed on serum diluted at 1:10 and 1:20 concentrations, using an immunofluorescence technique. The substrate used is derived from monkey esophagus, which has the disadvantages of being expensive (US$20–40) and morally controversial. Recently, studies have shown that using human umbilical cord as a substrate (UCA) produces similar test results [33–36].

One of the largest studies evaluating the EMA assay involved 22 pediatric gastroenterology centers throughout Italy [37]. Almost 4000 children underwent testing with both AGA (IgA and IgG) and IgA EMA. "Gold standard" biopsies had been obtained from all patients with a diagnosis of celiac disease who had not yet been placed on dietary therapy (n = 688) and from those with compatible gastrointestinal symptoms who subsequently were given a different diagnosis (n = 797). Limiting the analysis to these two groups, the EMA assay was more sensitive than the IgG AGA assay (94% vs 90%) and more specific than the IgA AGA assay (97 vs 90%), both differences being statistically significant. Healthy first-degree relatives (n = 599) were also studied. Of the 46 positive EMA results (7.6%), 32 underwent biopsy. Ninety percent of these patients were found to have pathological changes consistent with a diagnosis of celiac disease. In patients on a strict gluten-free diet (n = 96) it was found that 81% were negative for EMA, suggesting that the test may have a role in monitoring intestinal response after diagnosis.

One useful way of summarizing the utility of a test is to consider both its positive and negative likelihood ratios (LR). In Bayesian analysis the appropriate LR (depending on the positivity or negativity of the test) is multiplied by the estimated pretest odds to determine the likelihood that a particular condition is present or absent. Positive LRs greater than 10 and negative LRs less than 0.1 are generally agreed to be quite useful. Consider an example of a patient with non-specific symptoms and a family history of celiac disease in whom the pretest likelihood of celiac disease was estimated to be 8% (odds of 2:23). Using the LRs from the large Italian study [37] of 31 and 0.06 respectively, the post-test likelihood of celiac disease after a positive test would be 65% and after a negative test 0.5%. In a patient with more specific symptoms and therefore a higher pretest probability estimated at 50%, a positive test would produce a post-test likelihood of 97% while a negative test would reduce this likelihood to 6%. Similarly, if one screened the general population (with a prevalence of 0.25%) the post-test probabilities would be much different at 8% and 0.02% respectively, significantly lower than a high risk or symptomatic population.

There have been many studies from several countries [29, 33–49] that have evaluated the diagnostic accuracy of EMA. Though varied in sample size, ranging from 35 to 1485 children and adults, the majority have consistently found a positive LR greater than 10 and negative LR less than 0.1.

The discovery of tissue transglutaminase (tTG) as the antigen recognized by EMA has led to the development of assays to directly detect the tTG antibody. Since tTG assays utilize ELISA, they offer several advantages over conventional immunofluorscence based EMA, which is more labour intensive, subjective in nature and require a limited substrate (monkey esophagus or umbilical cord).

In a 2005 systematic review of the diagnostic performance of serologic tests for celiac disease, the sensitivity and specificity of tTG was found to be comparable to EMA [50]. Rigorous studies utilizing duodenal biopsies as the gold standard were included in the review and weighted sensitivities and specificities were calculated separately for EMA (EMA-monkey esophagus, EMA-umbilical cord) and tTG (tTG-human recombinant (tTG-HR), tTG-guinea pig (rTG-GP)) in children and adults. The sensitivity and specificity for EMA was found to be approximately 96% and 100% respectively, with the exception of EMA-umbilical cord which had a sensitivity of only 90% in adults. In comparison, tTG-HR had a sensitivity and specificity of approximately 96% and 99% respectively. The performance of tTG-GP was inferior to tTG-HR, with a sensitivity and specificity of approximately 90% and 95% respectively.

Subsequent to this systematic review, numerous articles have been published regarding the test performance of tTG (Table 10.1) [51–60]. As in the systematic review, sensitivities and specificities in these studies generally exceed 90%. In the largest study, Hopper *et al.* prospectively biopsied 2000 adult patients referred for gastroscopy and determined the sensitivity and specificity of tTG to be 91% [53]. These results represent the lower end of the spectrum for tTG sensitivity and specificity, which is likely a function of

the study design. Unlike other studies, Hopper *et al.* selected a group of general gastroenterology patients who had a low risk for celiac disease, thus minimizing their ascertainment bias. In addition, the prospective nature of their study is consistent with the general observation that prospective studies often yield results of lesser magnitudes than retrospective ones. Lastly, unlike studies that biopsy only those in the control group who have positive serology, Hopper *et al.* biopsied all patients, resulting in the diagnosis of six cases of seronegative celiac disease. Studies that do not biopsy all patients fail to detect false negatives, resulting in a falsely elevated sensitivity.

Although non-invasive and relatively inexpensive, tTG is unlikely to replace endoscopy for the diagnosis of celiac disease. The primary limitation of this marker is its imperfect sensitivity. Several studies have documented a significant reduction in the sensitivity of tTG in patients with low grade lesions [50, 53]. In one report, the sensitivity of tTG decreased from 100% for patients with Marsh 3c lesions to 86% for patients with Marsh 3a [53]. In addition, since the most commonly utilized tTG assays detect the IgA immunoglobulin, patients with selective IgA deficiency may receive false negative results. Since selective IgA deficiency is associated with a 10–20-fold increased risk for celiac disease, this population represents a significant cohort of patients who are at risk [61]. Preliminary trials of IgG-tTG are limited in size and have reported mixed results, with

Table 10.1 Sensitivity and specificity of tTG in recent studies utilizing small bowel biopsy as gold standard for celiac disease.

Study	Subjects	% Celiac	Sn (%)	Sp (%)	+LR[a]	−LR[b]
Leach *et al.* 2008 [51]	115 children with GI symptoms	28	93	90	9	0.08
Fabbro *et al.* 2008 [52]	102 pediatric and adult untreated celiac patients and 155 controls	40	100	100	100	.01
Hopper *et al.* 2008 [53]	2000 adult patients referred for gastroscopy	4	91	91	10	0.10
Poddar *et al.* 2008 [54]	333 children referred for possible celiac disease	59	94	97	31	0.06
Niveloni *et al.* 2007 [55]	141 adults referred for possible small bowel disease	43	95	98	38	0.05
Basso *et al.* 2006 [56]	204 children referred for possible malabsorption	50	94–98[c]	96–98[c]	24–48[c]	0.02–0.06[c]
Yachha *et al.* 2006 [57]	23 children with celiac and 41 controls	36	74	100	74	0.26
Reeves *et al.* 2006 [58]	254 children and adults referred for GI symptoms	10	88	84	6	0.14
Collin *et al.* 2005 [59]	126 pediatric and adult patients with celiac disease and 106 controls	54	94	99	94	0.06
Van Meensel *et al.* 2004 [60]	75 pediatric and adult patients with celiac disease and 70 controls	52	91–97[c]	96–100[c]	13–97[c]	0.03–0.09[c]

[a] Calculated using sensitivity/1-specificity and assuming specificity = 99% when reported as 100%.
[b] Calculated using 1-sensitivity/specificity and assuming sensitivity = 99% when reported as 100%.
[c] >1 tTG assays utilized.

sensitivities and specificities ranging from 23 to 100 and 89 to 100, respectively [50, 58, 61]. Even in the absence of IgA deficiency, a small population of seronegative celiac patients exists, which would not be detectable with tTG assays. As a result of these limitations, tTG will likely remain as an adjunct to endoscopy for the diagnosis of celiac disease rather than a replacement.

Therapy

The mainstay of therapy for celiac disease is a lifelong gluten-free diet. Because biopsy findings suggesting celiac disease may also be compatible with other conditions, some clinicians advocate a follow-up biopsy to confirm remission after implementation of a gluten-free diet. However, most are satisfied with a symptomatic response. In addition to a gluten-free diet, supplemental vitamins such as iron, folic acid, or vitamin K should be given where deficiencies are documented. Calcium and vitamin D may be deficient, and consideration may be given to measuring bone mineral density, particularly in women. Although it is suggested that the institution of a gluten-free diet protects against increasing bone loss, some patients may be candidates for hormone replacement or bisphosphonate therapy [62].

Poor dietary compliance is the most common reason for failure of a gluten-free diet. However, the complications of intestinal lymphoma and adenocarcinoma must be considered. Patients with persistent symptoms in whom other diagnoses are excluded are described as having refractory sprue [63]. There are considerable uncontrolled data to support the use of corticosteroids for this indication. Anecdotal evidence suggests that azathioprine [64] and cyclosporine [65] may also be effective in patients who do not respond to corticosteroids. In one known case of steroid-refractory celiac disease, infliximab followed by azathioprine was successfully used to induce and maintain remission [66]. In a subset of patients with refractory celiac disease, there is an increase in aberrant intraepithelial lymphocytes. Denoted refractory celiac disease type II, these patients have a significantly increased lifetime risk for enteropathy associated T cell lymphoma. Due to its resistance to conventional treatment regimens the prognosis is poor, with a five-year survival of less than 50% [67]. Emerging research into novel treatment strategies have been disappointing. In an open label phase II pilot study, Al-Toma et al. [68] evaluated the use of cladribine, a cytotoxic purine nucleoside, to treat type II refractory celiac disease. Of the 17 patients enrolled in the study, six demonstrated a clinical improvement (weight, diarrhea, hypoalbuminemia), 10 developed a histological improvement, and six had a decrease in aberrant T cells. Although one patient developed complete clinical and histological

recovery, seven patients still developed fatal enteropathy associated T cell lymphoma and one died secondary to complications of emaciation. The authors concluded that cladribine may induce clinical and histological improvement in a minority of patients but does not prevent T cell lymphoma and may in fact precipitate it.

Currently, the greatest controversy pertaining to therapy is the safety of including modest amounts of oats in the diet. Historically, wheat and rye were the first grains with demonstrated toxicity in celiac patients, followed subsequently by reports of toxicity with oats and barley. Similar injurious effects were not found with corn, rice and potatoes [69]. Biologic plausibility exists for the safety of oats, which stems from three primary difference between the gluten found in oat (avenin) and wheat (gliadin), barley (hordein) and rye (secalin) [70]. First, oat avenin is unique because it does not share substantial sequence homology with wheat gliadin, barley hordein, or rye secalin. Second, barley hordeins and rye secalins are antigenically related to wheat gliadin, whereas oat avenin is not. Third, oat avenin accounts for a smaller fraction of total protein as compared to wheat gliadin, barley hordein, or rye secalin. Thus, even if oat avenin were toxic in celiac disease, it would take a larger quantity to bring about the same effect as for wheat, barley, or rye. In vitro studies, however, have produced mixed results, with some studies demonstrating an immune response to avenin whereas others do not [71–73].

Despite this, clinical evidence is now accumulating to demonstrate a lack of toxicity of oats in newly diagnosed patients with celiac disease and in celiac disease patients in remission. In the largest study to date, Janathuinen et al. randomized 52 celiac patients on stable gluten free diets and 40 newly diagnosed celiac patients to a conventional gluten free diet (GFD) versus a GFD that included oats [74]. Patients in the established celiac disease group were followed for six months, while the newly diagnosed celiac group were followed for one year in terms of symptoms, BMI, laboratory parameters (hemoglobin, iron studies, albumin) and duodenal histology. Mean oat consumption was approximately 50 g per day. Upon completion of the study, there was no significant difference in symptoms, BMI, laboratory parameters, or histology. All previously established celiac patients remained in remission and all newly diagnosed celiac patients were in remission at one year except for one in the control group. Six patients in the oats group withdrew from the study citing pruritis, abdominal complaints, or unspecified reason for withdrawing, although this was similar to the control group.

To provide long-term evidence for the safety of oats, a five-year follow-up study of the same patients was conducted [75]. Of the original 81 patients (39 oats, 42 controls) who had completed the initial study, 63 were recruited into the follow-up study (4 and 14 drop-outs in oat and control arm, respectively). Among the remaining 35 patients in the oat group, 12 patients had stopped consuming oats, citing the following reasons: uncertainty regarding the long-term safety of oats (nine patients), flatulence (one patient) and rash (two patients). The remaining 23 patients in the oat group and 28 in the control group were subsequently enrolled in the study. During the five-year interval, mean oat consumption was 34 g/day, with approximately two-thirds of patients consuming oats at least once a week. Similar to the original study, there was no significant difference in duodenal histology scores between those who consumed oats versus a conventional gluten-free diet. Although this study provides the first evidence of long-term safety of oats, it can be criticized for its high attrition rate. This is concerning as it may represent a substantial portion of symptomatic patients who were not accounted for.

To assess the safety of high doses of oats, Storsrud et al. challenged 20 celiac patients to a high dose oat diet [76]. During the two-year study period, patients were periodically assessed for symptoms, biochemical nutritional markers, EMA and duodenal histology. Fifteen patients completed the study, consuming on average 93 g of oat/day. Similar to previous studies, there was no significant change in symptoms, biochemistry, EMA, or duodenal histology after exposure to oats. Three patients withdrew from the study for non-medical reasons and two withdrew due to abdominal distension and flatulence. Follow-up histology for both patients did not reveal any evidence of relapse and their symptoms were attributed to the increase in dietary fiber from the oats.

Despite the encouraging data supporting the safety of oats, significant concern remains due to the possibility of contamination with wheat, rye and barley. From the planting to the harvesting and manufacturing stage, multiple opportunities for contamination exist. In a 2008 study of 134 oat products from Canada, USA and Europe, 109 were found to be contaminated with wheat, barley, or rye [77]. The study utilized the new R5-ELISA assay, which replaced the conventional barley insensitive ω–ELISA. Similarly, another study utilizing the R5-ELISA assay to examine four lots of oats from three brands found that only three lots were gluten free [78]. To address the issue of contamination, government and advisory bodies are beginning to implement purity standards for the production of pure oats. Recently, the Canadian Celiac Association, in conjunction with Health Canada and Agriculture Canada, established strict planting, harvesting, processing and testing criteria to facilitate the production of pure oats. Safety data for pure oats manufactured under these guidelines are lacking and future studies are needed to ensure the safety of these products.

For the time being, the ultimate decision regarding whether to incorporate oats into the gluten free diet will have to be made on a case by case basis. Although numerous studies support the safety of oats, the strength of the evidence is generally limited by the small sample size. In addition, rare case reports have emerged describing cases of oat intolerance. In a 2003 case report, Lundin et al. [79] described a patient who developed diarrhea and villous atrophy during an oat challenge. During her oat challenge, her histology progressed from Marsh 1 to Marsh 3A. Elimination of oats from her diet resulted in resolution of her histology to Marsh 1. During a second oat challenge, her symptoms returned and she subsequently developed Marsh 3b lesions. Since the purity of the oats was confirmed by the barley insensitive w–ELISA assay in this case, it is plausible that her relapse was secondary to barley contamination although this cannot be confirmed. A minority of oat samples were further analyzed by western blot and mass spectrometry. Of six samples subject to additional testing, one was found to be contaminated. Thus, in deciding whether to include oats in the gluten-free diet, one must weigh the nutritional benefit of oats against the risk of contamination and the rare possibility of true oat intolerance.

Prognosis

Celiac disease, if left unrecognized and untreated, has the potential to result in severe complications which are for the most part secondary to malnutrition. When appropriate dietary therapy is instituted, the prognosis for celiac disease is usually good; however, untreated, the morbidity and mortality, and the risk of certain malignancies has been postulated to be increased in a celiac population. Past studies have suggested an increase in age-adjusted mortality attributable to the disease itself [28]. However, these studies may have been biased because of the inclusion of substantial numbers of untreated patients. More recent studies have suggested that at least short-term survival is not different from that of the general population [16]. Despite this finding there is evidence, both from retrospective and cohort studies, which suggests an increased risk of certain malignancies [80]. A recent retrospective Italian study identified seven malignancies in a cohort of 549 celiac patients followed for a mean of seven years [81].

Immunological stimulation and increased permeability are among the characteristics of the gut in celiac disease which lend biological credence to the possibility that celiac patients are at increased risk for malignancies such as lymphoma and adenocarcinoma of the small bowel. Although the epidemiological studies are heterogeneous in their design and findings, most of the epidemiological evidence to date confirms a general increase in morbidity. The left-hand column of Table 10.2 summarizes some of the data from these studies.

Most of the reports are based on case-control studies. This design is particularly subject to problems with *bias* and *confounding*. A *selection bias* toward the inclusion of

Table 10.2 A subjective assessment of current evidence attempting to establish a causal or non-causal relationship (see text).

	Hypothesis	
	Untreated celiac causes gastro-intestinal malignancy/lymphoma	Oats may be consumed as part of a gluten-free diet
Criteria		
Biological plausibility	Yes	Yes
Study designs	Case-control/cohort	Randomized controlled
Study consistency	**Moderate**	Good
Control groups used	Yes	Yes
Group similarity	**Questionable**	Yes
Adequate follow-up	Yes	**Questionable**
Temporal relationship	Probable	Yes
Exposure gradient	**Not shown**	**Questionable**
Strength of association	Strong	Strong
Precision of estimate	**Poor**	Good

particularly ill or refractory patients is one of the most frequently cited criticisms of the studies, which show a mortality rate that is increased as much as 3.4-fold over that of the general population [82–85] and complicating malignancy rates as high as 14% [83]. *Measurement bias* is another potential problem. Patients presenting with abdominal symptoms secondary to a malignancy may be more likely to undergo investigations like small bowel biopsy, which could lead to a diagnosis of celiac disease. Finally, some of the risk factors for celiac disease such as ethnic/geographic origin or immune markers (e.g. the class II HLA antigens HLA-DR3 and HLA-DQw2) could potentially be independent risk factors for certain diseases.

Despite these concerns, it is unlikely that the excess risk of small bowel lymphoma and adenocarcinoma seen in most studies can be explained by methodological flaws. In the early 1980s, a British registry collected data on approximately 400 cases of celiac disease and various cancers. The data were analyzed and compared to individual cancer rates in the local population [86]. Of the 259 histologically-confirmed tumors, slightly more than half of these were lymphomas, the majority of which had arisen in the small bowel. Two-thirds were discovered after the diagnosis of celiac disease was established at a mean interval of 7.3 years. A number of other studies have shown similarly high rates of lymphoma with death rates due to this complication varying from 2.6% to 8.9%, translating into relative risks of 25–122 with respect to the general population [87].

Of non-lymphomatous malignancies only those of the gastrointestinal tract were seen in excess, compared to the general population. A statistically significant increased risk of adenocarcinomas of the pharynx, esophagus and small bowel was observed. The relative risk of pharyngeal or esophageal cancer was relatively small (five to six) and could possibly be explained by confounding risk factors. However, the relative risk of small bowel carcinoma, a rare malignancy in the general population, was markedly increased at 83 (95% confidence limits 46–117).

Another British series of 210 patients reported in 1976 [88] produced similar results. It was followed by a prospective cohort study published in 1989 [89] which also demonstrated increased cancer risk. The patients were a priori divided into three groups: patients following a strict gluten-free diet (n = 108), patients intermittently adherent or adherent less than five years (n = 56) and patients not adhering to any dietary restrictions (n = 46). Increased risk was seen overall for cancers of the mouth, pharynx and esophagus (ratio of observed to expected (O/E) approached 10). The increase in risk was particularly strong for non-Hodgkin's lymphoma (n = 9; O/E = 42.7). For these cancers there was a statistically significant reduced risk for the strict gluten-free diet group. In a follow-up article by the same author [90] on the same cohort of patients, *excess morbidity* for those not observing a gluten-free diet was confirmed.

Retrospective cohort and genetic studies on celiac patients who develop malignancy has yielded information on possible prognostic indicators of malignant disease. Refractory sprue, or celiac disease which does not respond to dietary treatment, is a negative prognostic indicator, possibly because of the ongoing immune stimulation which may predispose to malignant transformation. Non-response to therapy may be present from diagnosis or after a period of response to dietary therapy, but is always a negative prognostic indicator [90]. A confounding factor may exist in that other disease types that produce villous atrophy and inflammatory infiltrates may be present, such as ulcerative jejunitis or jejunoileitis or mesenteric lymph node cavitation syndrome, and thus the diagnosis of underlying celiac disease may be questionable. Genetic prognostic indicators are less well studied still. A small case study of six refractory sprue patients demonstrated the replacement of the normal IEL population with morphologically normal and phenotypically abnormal cells with intracytoplasmic CD3, no surface CD3, CD4, CD8 or TCR, and restricted TCR γ gene rearrangements. On this basis, the authors posited a spectrum of disease ranging from celiac disease to refractory sprue to enteropathy-associated T cell lymphoma (EATL), with refractory sprue being the transitional disease state between celiac disease and malignancy [91]. The same study showed a poorer prognosis for the three patients with the aberrant phenotype TCR γ gene rearrangement, intracytoplasmic CD3+, surface CD8−, and a better prognosis (in terms of treatment response to diet and steroid therapy) for the three patients without this phenotype. This finding could be of practical importance, as non-response to treatment, coupled with the above phenotype implying a poor prognosis, would warrant closer follow-up for the implicated patient. Non-response to treatment in the absence of this phenotype would suggest non-compliance with dietary therapy.

The risk of malignancy in patients with dermatitis herpetiformis has also been studied. One study used a retrospective cohort design [92] to evaluate 109 patients who were followed for 13 years at one clinic, with almost complete follow-up. Seven patients (6.4%) developed a malignancy, three of which were lymphomas, one without small intestinal involvement. This translated into a relative risk of lymphoma of 100. The overall relative risk of malignancy was 2.38 (95% confidence intervals 1.22–3.56). However, in those patients adhering to a gluten-free diet, no increased risk was seen. A subsequent Finnish study [93] of 305 patients in whom 81% were compliant with a gluten-free diet also showed no excess risk of malignancy, with the exception of non-Hodgkin's lymphoma (n = 4) (RR = 10, 95% confidence intervals 2.8–26.3). A cohort study of 487 patients with dermatitis herpetiformis reported a 2% incidence of lymphoma while on a normal diet or a gluten-free diet for less than five years [94].

In contrast to these results, another retrospective cohort study originating in Finland [16] compared 335 celiac patients to age and sex-matched controls with other gastrointestinal disease and normal villous architecture. A statistically significant increased incidence of endocrine disease (12%) and connective tissue disease (7%) was observed, but no increased incidence of malignancy was detected. Notably, no cases of small bowel adenocarcinoma or non-Hodgkin's lymphoma were identified. This negative finding may be accounted for by either the relatively short mean follow-up (3.1 years) or the high rate of dietary compliance with a strict gluten-free diet (83%).

Though debate persists on the magnitude and type of cancer for which untreated celiac patients are at risk, there is general acceptance among clinicians that the risk is significant enough to warrant lifelong strict dietary compliance even in asymptomatic patients. This concern is foremost among those advocating that oats should not be included in a gluten-free diet [95]. Table 10.2 suggests that the evidence supporting the view that the inclusion of modest amounts of oats in a celiac diet is safe may actually be stronger than the data demonstrating an increased cancer risk in celiac patients.

Strict dietary therapy is warranted in adolescent and pediatric populations alone on the sole basis of prevention of morbidity, even if the questions of malignancy and mortality are set aside. A large retrospective cohort analysis of 909 pediatric and adolescent celiac patients, 1268 control subjects and 163 patients with Crohn's disease was under-

taken to determine the effect of duration of gluten exposure on the development of autoimmune disease in patients with celiac disease [96]. The prevalence of autoimmune disorders was noted to be significantly increased in the celiac population (14%) with respect to the control population (2.8%) but not with respect to the Crohn's disease population (12.9%). When the celiac population was subdivided into groups according to age at diagnosis, a surrogate for duration of gluten exposure, it was noted that the first group (<2 years at diagnosis; 5.1% prevalence) did not have a significantly different prevalence of autoimmune disease compared to the control group, but that the second group (2–10 years; 17.0% prevalence) and the third group (>10 years; 23.8% prevalence) did have a significantly increased comparative prevalence of autoimmune disease. Furthermore, a logistic regression model predicted increased odds of developing autoimmunity of 1.1% per year of diagnosis delay, with the expected numbers derived from this model correlating well with the observed study numbers. A second analysis of a subset of the 374 celiac disease patients who were diagnosed before the age of two years was subdivided on the basis of exposure to a gluten challenge following diagnosis, and those exposed to gluten for an additional "challenge" period following diagnosis were susceptible to an increased prevalence of autoimmune disorders. The implications of this study support early clinical diagnosis with serologic and histologic confirmation, and avoidance of prolonged exposure to gluten, even in the form of a gluten challenge.

This study has been challenged by a subsequent, similar study in an adult population [95]. This retrospective cohort analysis analyzed 605 controls and 422 celiac disease patients. Although the prevalence of autoimmunity was three-fold higher in the celiac population than in controls, the duration of gluten exposure did not correlate with the development of autoimmunity in an adult population. The two studies may be reconciled by the pathogenesis of the disease; it is possible that immune modulation and gluten exposure play a role in the development of disease early in life, and that once exposure has occurred in youth, circulating autoantibodies to various organs arise and the risk of later development of autoimmune disorders is subsequently increased in the adult celiac population [97].

Other complications of celiac disease exist in addition to those listed above, but are more rarely seen than autoimmune disease and malignancy. These include refractory sprue, which often requires immunosuppressive therapy. Ulcerative jejunoileitis manifesting as chronic ulcers of the small and occasionally large bowel can rarely occur and can lead to the diagnosis of celiac disease [80]. This condition can be difficult to distinguish from intestinal lymphoma and may actually progress to this disease. Collagenous sprue, an even more rare complication of celiac disease, is histologically distinguished by a thick subepithelial band of collagen. No effective therapy has been described and patients generally go on to parenteral alimentation [6, 98].

Conclusion

The gold standard for the diagnosis of celiac disease remains the small bowel biopsy. Serological testing, particularly the anti-endomysial antibody and tissue transglutaminase, can be very useful in the appropriate clinical situation to diagnose the disease and to monitor the response to a gluten-free diet. The threshold for initial and follow-up biopsy, if necessary, should be low given the limitations of the test and the general ease of upper gastrointestinal endoscopy and biopsy. A gluten-free diet remains the cornerstone of management. The available evidence suggests that a substantial proportion of patients will tolerate a moderate amount of oats in their diet with the appropriate clinical follow-up. To prevent symptomatic recurrences, nutritional deficiencies (particularly bone disease), and malignant and autoimmune complications, a strict gluten-free diet should be encouraged in all patients.

References

1 Gee S. On the coeliac affection. *St Barth Hosp Rep* 1888; **24**: 17–20.

2 Thaysen TEH. *Non-Tropical Sprue*. Levin & Munksgaard, Copenhagen, 1932.

3 Dicke WK, Weijers HA, van de Kamer JH. Coeliac disease. II: The presence in wheat of a factor having a deleterious effect in cases of coeliac disease. *Acta Paediatr Scand* 1953; **42**: 34–42.

4 Paulley LW. Observations on the aetiology of idiopathic steatorrhea. *Br Med J* 1954; **2**: 1318–1321.

5 Rubin CE, Brandborg LL, Phelps PC *et al.* Studies of coeliac disease I. The apparent identical and specific nature of the duodenal and proximal jejunal lesion in coeliac disease and idiopathic sprue. *Gastroenterology* 1960; **38**: 28–49.

6 Trier JS. Coeliac sprue. *N Engl J Med* 1991; **325**: 1709–1719.

7 Fasano, A. Where have all the American celiacs gone? *Acta Paediatrica* Suppl 1996; **412**: 20–24.

8 Hin H, Bird G, Fisher P, Mahy N, Jewell D. Coeliac disease in primary care: A case finding study. *BMJ* 1999; **318**: 164–167.

9 Mylotte M, Egan-Mitchell B, McCarthy CE, McNicholl B. Coeliac disease in the west of Ireland. *BMJ* 1973; **3**: 498–499.

10 Catassi C, Fabiani E, Ratsch IM *et al.* The coeliac iceberg in Italy: A multicentre antigliadin antibodies screening for coeliac disease in school-age subjects. *Acta Paediatr Suppl* 1996; **412**: 29–35.

11 Not T, Horvath K, Hill ID *et al.* Celiac disease risk in the USA: High prevalence of anti-endomysium antibodies in healthy blood donors. *Scand J Gastroenterol* 1998; **33**: 494–498.

12 Maki M, Mustalahti K *et al.* Prevalence of Celiac Disease among Children in *Finland. NEJM* 2003; **348**: 2517–2524.

13 Johnston SD, Watson RG, McMillan SA, Slaon J, Love AH. Coeliac disease detected by screening is not silent – simply unrecognized. *QJM* 1998; **91**: 853–860.

14 Ciclitira, PJ. AGA Technical Review on Celiac Sprue. AGA Practice Guidelines. *Gastroenterology* 2001; **120**(6): 1–26.

15 Farrell RJ, Kelly, CP. Celiac Sprue. *NEJM* 2002; **346**(3): 180–188.

16 Collin R, Reunala T, Pukkala E *et al.* Coeliac disease – associated disorders and survival. *Gut* 1994; **35**: 1215–1218.

17 Hardman C, Garioch JJ, Leonard JN *et al.* Absence of toxicity of oats in patients with dermatitis herpetiformis. *N Engl J Med* 1997; **337**: 1884–1887.

18 Bohr J, Tysk C, Yang P *et al.* Autoantibodies and immunoglobulins in collagenous colitis. *Gut* 1996; **39**: 73–76.

19 Mäki M, Huupponen T, Holm K *et al.* Seroconversion of reticulin autoantibodies predicts coeliac disease in insulin dependent diabetes mellitus. *Gut* 1995; **36**: 239–242.

20 Rensch MJ, Merenich JA, Lieberman M *et al.* Gluten-sensitive enteropathy in patients with insulin-dependent diabetes mellitus. *Ann Intern Med* 1996; **124**: 564–567.

21 Rittmeyer C, Rhoads JM. IgA deficiency causes false-negative endomysial antibody results in coeliac disease. *J Pediatr Gastroenterol Nutr* 1996; **23**: 504–506.

22 Shah A, Mayberry JF, Williams G *et al.* Epidemiological survey of coeliac disease and inflammatory bowel disease in first-degree relatives of coeliac patients. *Q J Med* 1990; **74**: 283–288.

23 Logan RF, Finlayson NDC, Weir DG. Primary biliary cirrhosis and coeliac disease: An association? *Lancet* 1978; **i**: 230–233.

24 Hay JE, Wiesner RH, Shorter R *et al.* Primary sclerosing cholangitis and coeliac disease. *Ann Intern Med* 1988; **109**: 713–717.

25 George EK, Mearin ML, Bouquet J *et al.* High frequency of coeliac disease in Down's syndrome. *J Pediatr* 1996; **128**: 555–557.

26 Bonamico M, Rasore-Quartino A, Mariani P *et al.* Down syndrome and coeliac disease: Usefulness of antigliadin and anti-endomysium antibodies. *Acta Paediatr* 1996; **85**: 1503–1505.

27 Gale L, Wimalaratna H, Brotodihargo A *et al.* Down's syndrome is strongly associated with coeliac disease. *Gut* 1997; **40**: 492–496.

28 Trier JS. *Coeliac Sprue and Refractory Sprue*. WB Saunders, Toronto 1998.

29 Grodzinsky E. Screening for coeliac disease in apparently healthy blood donors. *Acta Paediatr* 1996; **412**(Suppl): 36–38.

30 van de Kamer JH, Weijers HA, Dicke WK. Coeliac disease. IV. An investigation into the injurious constituents of wheat in connection with their action on patients with coeliac disease. *Acta Paediatr Scand* 1953; **42**: 223–231.

31 Berger R, Schmidt G. Evaluation of six anti-gliadin antibody assays. *J Immunol Methods* 1996; **91**: 77–86.

32 Chartrand LJ, Agulnik J, Vanounou T *et al.* Effectiveness of antigliadin antibodies as a screening test for coeliac disease in children. *Can Med Assoc J* 1997; **157**: 527–533.

33 Volta U, Molinaro N, De Franceshi L *et al.* IgA anti-endomysial antibodies on human umbilical cord tissue for coeliac disease screening save both money and monkeys. *Dig Dis Sci* 1995; **40**: 1902–1905.

34 Kolho KL, Savilahti E. IgA endomysium antibodies on human umbilical cord: an excellent diagnostic tool for coeliac disease in childhood. *J Pediatr Gastroenterol Nutr* 1997; **24**: 563–567.

35 Carroccio A, Cavataio F, Iacono G et al. IgA anti-endomysial antibodies on the umbilical cord in diagnosing coeliac disease. Sensitivity, specificity, and comparative evaluation with the traditional kit. Scand J Gastroenterol 1996; 31: 759–763.

36 Yiannakou JY, Dell'Olio D, Saaka M, et al. Detection and characterization of anti-endomysial antibody in celiac disease using human umbilical cord. Int Arch Allergy Immunol 1997 (Feb); 112(2): 140–144.

37 Cataldo F, Ventura A, Lazzari R et al. Anti-endomysium antibodies and coeliac disease: Solved and unsolved questions. An Italian multicentre study. Acta Paediatr 1995; 84: 1125–1131.

38 Sulkanen S, Halttunen T, Laurila K et al. Tissue transglutaminase autoantibody enzyme-linked immunosorbent assay in detecting celiac disease. Gastroenterology 1998; 115: 1322–13228.

39 Grodzinsky E, Jansson G, Skogh T et al. Anti-endomysium and anti-gliadin antibodies as serological markers for coeliac disease in childhood: A clinical study to develop a practical routine. Acta Paediatr 1995; 84: 294–298.

40 Vogelsang H, Genser D, Wyatt J et al. Screening for coeliac disease: A prospective study on the value of noninvasive tests. Am J Gastroenterol 1995; 90: 394–398.

41 Pacht A, Sinai N, Hornstein L. The diagnostic reliability of anti-endomysial antibody in coeliac disease: The north Israel experience. Isr J Med Sci 1995; 31: 218–220.

42 Stern M, Teuscher M, Wechmann T. Serological screening for coeliac disease: Methodological standards and quality control. Acta Paediatr Suppl 1996; 412: 49–51.

43 Valdimarsson T, Franzen L, Grodzinsky E. Is small bowel biopsy necessary in adults with suspected coeliac disease and IgA anti-endomysium antibodies? 100% positive predictive value for coeliac disease in adults. Dig Dis Sci 1996; 41: 83–87.

44 Ascher H, Hahn-Zoric M, Hanson LÅ et al. Value of serologic markers for clinical diagnosis and population studies of coeliac disease. Scand J Gastroenterol 1996; 31: 61–67.

45 Sacchetti L, Ferrajolo A, Salerno G et al. Diagnostic value of various serum antibodies detected by diverse methods in childhood coeliac disease. Clin Chem 1996; 42: 1838–1842.

46 de Lecea A, Ribes-Koninckx C, Polanco I, Calvete JF. Serological screening (antigliadin and anti-endomysium antibodies) for non-overt coeliac disease in children of short stature. Acta Paediatr 1996; 412(Suppl): 54–55.

47 Bottaro G, Volta U, Spina M et al. Antibody pattern in childhood coeliac disease. J Pediatr Gastroenterol Nutr 1997; 24: 559–562.

48 Atkinson K, Tokmakajian S, Watson W. Evaluation of the endomysial antibody for coeliac disease: Operating properties and associated cost implications in clinical practice. Can J Gastroenterol 1997; 11: 673–677.

49 Corazza GR, Biagi F, Andreani ML et al. Screening test for coeliac disease. Lancet 1997; 349: 325–326.

50 Rostom A, Dube C, Cranney A, Saloojee N, SY R, Garrity C et al. The diagnostic accuracy of serologic tests for celiac disease: A systematic review. Gastroenterology 2005; 128: S38–S46.

51 Leach ST, Brekhna A, Day AS. Coeliac disease screening in children: assessment of a novel anti-gliadin antibody assay. J Clin Lab Anal 2008; 22: 327–333.

52 Fabbro E, Rubert L, Quaglia S, Ferrara F, Kiren V, Ventura A et al. Uselessness of anti-actin antibody in celiac disease screening. Clinica Chimica Acta 2008; 390: 134–137.

53 Hopper AD, Hadjivassiliou M, Hurlstone DP, Lobo AJ, McAlindon ME, Egner W et al. What is the role of serologic testing in celiac disease? A prospective, biopsy-confirmed study with economic analysis. Clin Gastroenterol Hepatol 2008; 6: 314–320.

54 Poddar U, Thapa BR, Nain CK, Singh K. Is tissue transglutaminase autoantibody the best for diagnosing celiac disease in children of developing countries? J Clin Gastroenterol 2008; 42: 147–151.

55 Niveloni S, Sugai E, Cabanne A, Vazquez H, Argonz J, Smecuol E et al. Antibodies against synthetic deamidated gliadin peptides as predictors of celiac disease: prospective assessment in an adult population with a high pretest probability of disease. Clin Chem 2007; 53: 2186–2192.

56 Basso D, Guariso G, Fasolo M, Pittoni M, Schiavon S, Fogar P. A new indirect chemiluminescent immunoassay to measure anti–tissue transglutaminase antibodies. J Pediatr Gastroenterol Nutr 2006; 43: 613–618.

57 Yachha SK, Aggarwal R, Srinivas RA, Srivastava A, Somani SK, Itha S. Antibody testing in Indian children with celiac disease. Indian J Gastroenterol 2006; 25: 132–135.

58 Reeves GEM, Squance ML, Duggan AE, Murugasu RR, Wilson RJ, Wong RC et al. Diagnostic accuracy of coeliac serological tests: A prospective study. Gastroenterol Hepatol 2006; 18: 493–501.

59 Collin P, Kaukinen K, Vogelsang H, Korponay-Szabo I, Sommer R, Schreier E. Anti-endomysial and antihuman recombinant tissue transglutaminase antibodies in the diagnosis of celiac disease: A biopsy-proven European multicentre study. Eur J Gastroenterol Hepatol 2005; 17: 85–91.

60 Van Meensel B, Hiele M, Hoffman I, Vermeire S, Rutgeerts P, Geboes K et al. Diagnostic accuracy of ten second-generation (human) tissue transglutaminase antibody assays in celiac disease. Clin Chem. 2004; 50: 2125–2135.

61 Villalta D, Alessio MG, Tampoia M, Tonutti E, Brusca I, Bagnasco M. Testing for IgG class antibodies in celiac disease patients with selective IgA deficiency. A comparison of the diagnostic accuracy of 9 IgG anti-tissue transglutaminase, 1 IgG anti-gliadin and 1 IgG anti-deamidated gliadin peptide antibody assays. Clinica Chimica Acta 2007; 382: 95–99.

62 Valdimarsson T, Löfman O, Toss G et al. Reversal of osteopenia with diet in adult coeliac disease. Gut 1996; 38: 322–327.

63 Trier JS. Coeliac sprue and refractory sprue. Gastroenterology 1978; 75: 307–308.

64 Sinclair TS, Kumar PJ, Dawson AM. Azathioprine responsive villous atrophy. Gut 1983; 24: A494 (abstract).

65 Longstreth GF. Successful treatment of refractory sprue with cyclosporine. Ann Intern Med 1993; 119: 1014–1016.

66 Gillett HR, Arnott IDR et al. Successful infliximab treatment for Steroid-Refractory Celiac Disease: A Case Report. Gastroenterology 2002; 122: 800–805.

67 Rubio-Tapia A, Kelly DG, Lahr BD, Dogan A, Wu TT, Murray JA. Clinical Staging and Survival in Refractory Celiac Disease: A Single Center Experience. Gastroenterology 2009; 136: 99–107.

68 Al-Toma A, Goerres MS, Meijer JWR et al. Cladribine therapy in refractory celiac disease with aberrant T cells. Clin Gastroenterol Hepatol 2006; 4: 1322–1327.

69 Schmitz J. Lack of oats toxicity in celiac disease (editorial). BMJ 1997; 314: 159–160.

70 Thompson T. Do oats belong in a gluten-free diet? *J Am Diet Assoc* 1997; **97**: 1413–1416.

71 Arentz-Hansen H, Fleckenstein B, Molberg O, Scott H, Koning F, Jung G *et al*. The molecular basis for oat intolerance in patients with celiac disease. *PLOS Med* 2004; **1**: 84–92.

72 Kilmartin C, Lynch S, Abuzakouk M, Wieser H, Feighery C. Avenin fails to induce a Th1 response to celiac tissue following in vitro culture. *Gut* 2003; **52**: 47–52.

73 Picarelli A, Di Tola M, Sabbatella L *et al*. Immunologic evidence of no harmful effect of oats in celiac disease. *Am J Clin Nutr* 2001; **74**: 137–140.

74 Janatuinen EK, Pikkaraines PH, Kemppainen TA, Kosma VM, Jarvinen RMK, Uusitupa IJ *et al*. A comparison of diets with and without oats in adults with celiac disease. *N Engl J Med*; **333**: 1033–1037.

75 Janatuinen EK, Kemppainen TA, Julkunen RJK, Kosma VM, Maki M, Heikkinen M *et al*. No harm from five year ingestion of oats in coelic disease. *Gut* 2002; **50**: 332–335.

76 Storsrud S, Olsson M, Lenner RA, Nilsson LA, Nilsson O, Kilander A. Adults celiac patients do tolerate large amounts of oats. *Eur J Clin Nutr* 2003; **57**: 163–169.

77 Hernando A, Mujico JR, Mena MC, Lombadia M, Mendez E. Measurement of wheat gluten and barley hordeins in contaminated oats from Europe, the United States, and Canada by sandwich R5 ELISA. *Eur J Gastroenterol Hepatol* 2008; **20**: 545–554.

78 Thompson, T. Gluten contamination of commercial oat products in the United States. *N Engl J Med* 2004; **351**: 2021–2022.

79 Lundin KEA, Nilsen EM, Scott HG, Loberg EM, Gjoen A, Bratlie J *et al*. Oats induced villous atrophy in coelic disease. *Gut* 2003; **52**: 1649–1652.

80 Holmes GKT. Coeliac disease and malignancy. *J Pediatr Gastroenterol Nutr* 1997; **24**: S20–S24.

81 Tursi A, Elisei W, Giorgetti GM, Brandimarte G, Aiello F. Complications in Celiac Disease Under Gluten-Free Diet. *Blood* 2008; **112**(13): 5103–5110.

82 Nielsen OH, Jacobsen O, Pedersen EF *et al*. Non-tropical sprue: malignant diseases and mortality rate. *Scand J Gastroenterol* 1985; **20**: 13–18.

83 Logan RF, Rifkind EA, Turner ID *et al*. Mortality in coeliac disease. *Gastroenterology* 1989; **97**: 265–271.

84 Ferguson A, Kingstone K. Coeliac disease and malignancies. *Acta Paediatr* 1996; **412**(Suppl): 78–81.

85 Harris OD, Cooke WT, Thompson H *et al*. Malignancy in adult coeliac disease and idiopathic steatorrhoea. *Am J Med* 1967; **42**: 899–912.

86 Swinson CM, Coles EC, Slavin G *et al*. Coeliac disease and malignancy. *Lancet* 1983; **i**: 111–115.

87 Mathus-Vliegen EMH. Coeliac disease and lymphoma: Current status. *Neth J Med* 1996; **49**: 212–220.

88 Holmes GKT, Stokes PL, Sorahan TM *et al*. Coeliac disease, gluten-free diet, and malignancy. *Gut* 1976; **17**: 612–619.

89 Holmes GKT, Prior P, Lane MR *et al*. Malignancy in coeliac disease – effect of a gluten free diet. *Gut* 1989; **30**: 333–338.

90 Holmes GKT. Coeliac disease and malignancy. *Digest Liver Dis* 2002; **34**: 229–237.

91 Cellier C, Delabesse E, Helmer C, Patey N, Matuchansky C, Jabri B *et al*. Refractory sprue, coeliac disease and enteropathy-associated T-cell lymphoma. *Lancet* 2000; **356**: 202–208.

92 Leonard JN, Tucker WFG, Fry JS *et al*. Increased incidence of malignancy in dermatitis herpetiformis. *Br Med J* 1983; **286**: 16–18.

93 Collin P, Pukkala E, Reunala T. Malignancy and survival in dermatitis herpetiformis: A comparison with coeliac disease. *Gut* 1996; **38**: 528–530.

94 Lewis HM, Renaula RL, Garioch JN, Leonard JN, Fry JS, Collin P *et al*. Protective effect of gluten-free diet against development of lymphoma in dermatitis herpetiformis. *Br J Dermatol* 1996; **135**: 363–367.

95 Branski D, Shine M. Oats in coeliac disease (Letter). *N Engl J Med* 1996; **334**: 865–866.

96 Ventura A, Magazzu G, Greco L. Duration of exposure to gluten and risk for autoimmune disorders in patients with celiac disease. *Gastroenterology* 1999; **117**: 297–303.

97 Ventura A, Maguzu G, Gerarduzzi T, Greco L. Coeliac disease and the risk of autoimmune disorders. Author reply. *Gut* 2002; **51**(6): 897–898.

98 Trier JS. Complications of coeliac sprue and potentially related diseases with similar intestinal histopathology. *Gastroenterology* 1978; **75**: 314–315.

11 Crohn's disease

Brian G Feagan and John WD McDonald

Robarts Clinical Trials, Robarts Research Unit, University of Western Ontario, London, Ontario, Canada

Introduction

The use of non-specific, anti-inflammatory drugs, such as the 5-aminosalicylates, glucocorticoids and antimetabolites was the foundation of the current management of Crohn's disease (CD). However, recent advances in molecular biology have yielded novel approaches which may be more relevant to the pathophysiology of the disease. This review offers an evidence-based approach to the management of active CD and of interventions that have been evaluated for maintenance therapy.

Induction of remission

An ideal treatment for active CD should rapidly and reliably induce remission of symptoms. In clinical trials the most frequently used metric is a decrease in the Crohn's Disease Activity Index (CDAI) of from 50 to 100 points with a final score below 150 [1, 2]. A substantial placebo response (20–30%) is observed in short-term (8–16 week) studies. Four classes of drugs have been most frequently evaluated for treatment of active disease: 5-aminosalicylates (5-ASA), glucocorticoids, antibiotics and monoclonal antibodies.

5-aminosalicylates

The prototypic 5-ASA compound sulfasalazine has been used to treat CD for more than 40 years [3]. Although highly effective for ulcerative colitis, randomized trials showed that sulfasalazine was only marginally superior to a placebo for the induction of remission in active CD (see

Evidence-Based Gastroenterology and Hepatology, 3rd edition.
J. McDonald, A.K. Burroughs, B. Feagan, and M.B. Fennerty. © 2010
Blackwell Publishing Ltd

Figure 11.1) [4, 5]. **Alc** Since the sulfa-related adverse effects of sulfasalazine often limit the maximum drug dose that can be administered, the development of 5-ASA formulations which lack a sulfa moiety and which target specific regions of the gastrointestinal tract raised the possibility that greater efficacy was possible. Multiple randomized controlled trials (RCTs) have compared the newer 5-ASA compounds with either a placebo (see Table 11.1) or an active treatment (sulfasalazine, glucocorticoids). Although many of these trials were at a high risk of a type II statistical error due to a small sample size, some definite conclusions can be derived.

Initial experience with 5-ASA doses of 1–5 g/day showed no clear benefit over a placebo [6, 7]. These negative studies led to the evaluation of higher dose regimens. Singleton and colleagues allocated over 300 patients with moderate disease activity to receive either 1 g, 2 g or 4 g of Pentasa daily or a placebo for a period of 16 weeks [8]. Although 5-ASA was well tolerated, only a modest benefit of treatment was observed; 43% of the patients who received 4 g/day of Pentasa entered remission as compared with 18% of those who were assigned to the placebo (absolute risk reduction (ARR) 25%, number needed to treat (NNT) 4; $p = 0.017$). **Alc** No improvement over placebo was observed for those individuals who received the lower doses of 5-ASA. Subgroup analyses failed to identify any specific predictors of response. Pentasa was well tolerated; more patients who received the placebo were withdrawn from treatment due to adverse events than those who received the highest dose of the active drug.

Although this trial suggested a benefit of high dose 5-ASA therapy, a cautionary note was raised subsequently by the principal investigator, who described a second evaluation of Pentasa in 232 patients [15]. Data from this trial and a third unpublished study performed by Hanauer and associates have been combined in a meta-analysis, which suggested that patients assigned to 4 g/day Pentasa (n = 304) improved on average only 18 points more on the CDAI score than those who received a placebo (n = 311)

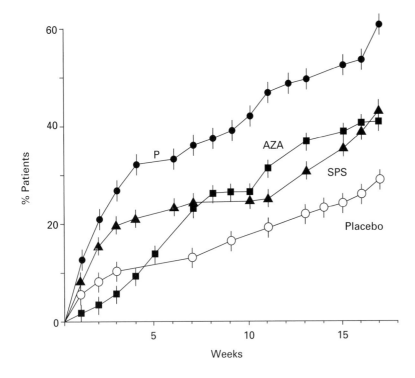

No. significant

Prednisone (P)		85	74	57	52		58	57	54	55	52	50	45	44		43	41	40
Sulfasalazine (SPS)	74	65	62	50			58				56		55		51	48	25
Azathioprine (AZA)		39	38	37	34	43		51	45		44	43		40		37	35
Placebo			77		72			69		67		64		62	60	59	58	57

Figure 11.1 Cumulative percentage of patients in remission week by week: comparison of prednisone, sulfasalazine, azathioprine and placebo. Remission is defined as Crohn's Disease Activity Index (CDAI) less than 150 and continuing below 150 through week 17 (life-table using Kaplan-Meier method). Adapted with permission from Summers RW *et al. Gastroenterology* 1979; **77**: 847–694.

[16]. **Ala** No difference in remission rates was observed. Readers should be aware that a minimum clinically important difference in CDAI score is approximately 50 points.

No trials of adequate power have compared the efficacy of the newer 5-ASA drugs and sulfasalazine. However, several studies have compared 5-ASA to glucocorticoid therapy for induction of remission (see Table 11.1). Schölmerich randomized 62 patients to receive either 5-ASA at a dose of 2 g/day or a standard tapering regimen of methyl prednisolone [9]. In this 24-week trial 73% of the 5-ASA-treated patients failed therapy compared with 34% of those who received methyl prednisolone (ARR 39%, NNT = 3; p = 0.0019). **Alc** The authors concluded that treatment with 5-ASA, although well tolerated, was inferior to steroid therapy. Martin *et al.* compared a 3 g/day dose of Salofalk to a standard oral prednisone regimen [10]. Although a similar proportion of individuals in the two treatment groups entered remission (47% 5-ASA vs 46% prednisone; p = 0.59), an analysis of the change in mean CDAI and quality of life scores demonstrated a more rapid improvement in patients treated with prednisone. A study by Thomsen and colleagues provides important information on the relative efficacy of glucocorticoids and 5-ASA

[12]. In this methodologically rigorous trial 182 patients with active disease were assigned to receive either 9 mg/day of a controlled ileal release preparation of budesonide (a locally active steroid) or 4 g/day of Pentasa. Following 16 weeks of treatment, 62% of budesonide treated patients were in remission compared with only 36% of the patients who received 5-ASA (ARR 26%, NNT = 4, p < 0.01). **Ald**

What conclusions can be drawn from these trials? The existing data show that the newer 5-ASA compounds are not more effective than sulfasalazine and are, at best, only marginally superior to a placebo for the induction of remission. A single clinical trial has demonstrated the superiority of budesonide over high dose 5-ASA, with no increased frequency of adverse events. Although many clinicians prescribe 5-ASA compounds as first-line therapy for mild disease activity and treat those patients who fail to achieve a remission with glucocorticoids, the wisdom of this approach is questionable. Although the reluctance of physicians to expose individuals to glucocorticoid therapy is understandable, the likelihood of a response to the newer 5-ASA formulations is so low that the strategy is inefficient. Most patients will ultimately require the more potent agents discussed below to induce remission. In any event,

Table 11.1 Response rates of remission in studies comparing 5-ASA to placebo or glucocorticoid therapy.

Study	Drug dose	No. of patients	Duration (weeks)	Placebo	% remission 5-ASA	GL
NCCDS (1979) [4]	SPS 4–6 g/day	236	17	30	43	—
ECCDS (1984) [5]	SPS 3 g/day	159	18	38	50	82
Rasmussen et al. (1987) [6]	Pentasa 1.5 g/day	67	16	30	40	—
Mahida et al. (1990) [7]	Pentasa 1.5 g/day	40	6	—	—	—
Singleton et al. (1993) [8]	Pentasa 1, 2, 4 g	310	16	18 placebo vs 4g 18	43	—
Schölmerich et al. (1990) [9]	Pentasa 2 g	62	24	—	27	66
Martin et al. (1990) [10]	Salofalk 3 g/day	55	12	—	47	46
Maier et al. (1990) [11]	Salofalk 3 g/day	52	12	—	83	88
Thomsen et al. (1996) [12]	Pentasa 4 g	182	16	—	36	62
Prantera et al. (1992) [13]	Asacol 4 g, 5-ASA microgranules	94	12	—	60	61
Gross (1995) [14]	Salofalk 4.5 g	34	8	—	40	56.3

Source: Feagan B. *Eur J Surg* 1998; **164**: 903–909.

SFS: sulfasalazine; GL: glucocorticoids; 5-ASA: 5-aminosalicylate; NCCDS: National Cooperative Crohn's Disease Study; ECCDS: European Cooperative Crohn's Disease Study.

if a 5-ASA drug is used for induction of remission in patients with mild disease the best evidence supports the use of sulfasalazine. **Alc**

Glucocorticoids

Conventional steroids

The conventional glucocorticoid compounds, prednisone and 6-methyl prednisolone, are highly effective drugs for the treatment of active CD. The National Cooperative Crohn's Disease Study (NCCDS) and the European Cooperative Crohn's Disease Study (ECCDS) both showed that approximately 70% of patients who are treated with 40–60 mg/day of prednisone for 3–4 months enter remission, compared with 30% of patients treated with placebo (see Figure 11.1) [4, 5]. **Ala**

Budesonide

Glucocorticoids have pluripotent actions on the immune system, including effects on the synthesis of inflammatory mediators, cellular immunity and neutrophil function [17]. Since the glucocorticoid receptor is widely expressed in tissues, the biological actions of these drugs are not restricted to the immune system. Unpleasant cosmetic effects (acne, moon faces and bruising) and more serious effects, such as metabolic disturbances (hypertension, metabolic bone disease and diabetes) are common and limit the usefulness of these agents [18]. An ideal glucocorticoid should retain the efficacy of conventional glucocorticoid drugs, while minimizing systemic effects. One possible means of achieving this objective is to specifically target the

bowel wall as the therapeutic compartment of interest [19]. The development of budesonide as a treatment for active CD is an example of this approach.

Budesonide is a novel glucocorticoid with a potency approximately five times that of prednisone. The systemic effects of budesonide are reduced in comparison to conventional steroid drugs as a result of extensive first pass metabolism to inactive compounds. Thus, a high local anti-inflammatory effect on mucosal surfaces is possible with low systemic activity [20]. Proof of this concept was first demonstrated in asthma therapy, where topical budesonide was shown to be highly effective, with few or no systemic adverse effects [21]. An oral controlled ileal release formulation of budesonide was developed for the treatment of active CD of the ileum and right colon. A Canadian multicenter dose finding study found that, first, 9 mg/day of budesonide was more effective than a placebo for the induction of remission in patients with moderately active CD (51% vs 20%, p < 0.001 ~ and, second, the proportion of patients experiencing glucocorticoid-related adverse effects with this drug was not greater than with placebo treatment (26% 9 mg budesonide vs 26% placebo, p > 0.05) [22]. **Alc** In a second study, Rutgeerts and colleagues compared 9 mg/day of budesonide with a standard prednisolone regimen [23]. Although a favorable trend in response rate was observed in favor of prednisolone therapy, the difference in efficacy between the treatment groups was not large (65% vs 52%, p = 0.12). There were fewer glucocorticoid-related adverse events in patients who received budesonide (budesonide 29%, prednisolone 55%, ARR 26%, NNT = 4, p = 0.003). **Alc** Finally, as described earlier, Thomsen and colleagues have shown that 9 mg/day of budesonide is more effective than 4 g/day of 5-ASA and is equally well tolerated [12]. Data from the studies have been summarized in a Cochrane review by Seow and colleagues, who estimated that budesonide was approximately 15% less effective than conventional glucocorticoid therapy, but was much less likely to cause glucocorticoid-related adverse events [24]. **A1a** Thus, budesonide is an attractive alternative to 5-ASA or prednisone for induction of remission in patients whose disease is restricted to the appropriate anatomical sites.

Antibiotics

A substantial body of experimental evidence supports the notion that bacteria play an important role in initiating and/or sustaining the pathological inflammatory reaction in the bowel wall [25, 26]. Antibiotics have been used empirically for the treatment of active CD for many years, and review articles and textbooks of medicine commonly advocate their use. However, few good data exist to support this endorsement. The Cooperative Crohn's Disease Study in Sweden compared 800 mg/day of metronidazole to 1.5 g/day of sulfasalazine in 78 patients with active disease [27]. A 25% response rate for both treatments was shown. Accordingly, it is debatable whether these results are more consistent with an equivalent benefit of metronidazole or the lack of any therapeutic effect for either treatment. The largest trial of metronidazole, carried out by Sutherland and colleagues, randomized patients to receive metronidazole (10 or 20 mg/kg per day) or a placebo for 16 weeks (n = 105) [28]. Metronidazole therapy produced a dose-dependent decrease of disease activity (decrease in CDAI: metronidazole 20 mg/kg 97, 10 mg/kg 60, placebo 1; p = 0.001). However, no difference in remission rate was observed (proportion in remission: placebo 25%, metronidazole 10 mg/kg 36%, 20 mg/kg 27%). Thus, the controlled data that support the efficacy of metronidazole are not impressive. **A1d**

More recently the quinolone antibiotic ciprofloxacin has been used in combination with metronidazole. Prantera and colleagues randomized 41 patients to receive combined antibiotics (ciprofloxacin 500 mg twice daily and 250 mg of metronidazole four times daily) or methyl prednisolone 0.7–1.0 mg/kg for 12 weeks [29]. A statistically significant difference in patients entering remission was not demonstrated (combined antibiotic therapy 10/22 (46%), steroid therapy 12/19 (63%), p > 0.05). The small number of patients in this trial does not permit any definitive conclusion regarding the value of combined antibiotic therapy; however, the 17% difference in remission rates in favor of methyl prednisolone is most consistent with a clinically meaningful treatment advantage in favor of glucocorticoid therapy. **A1d**

Steinhart *et al.* conducted a double-blind study of oral ciprofloxacin and metronidazole (both 500 mg twice daily), or placebo for eight weeks in 134 patients with active CD of the ileum, right colon or both [30]. All patients received oral budesonide 9 mg once daily. At week 8, 21 patients (33%) assigned to antibiotics were in remission, compared with 25 patients (38%) in the placebo group (p = 0.55; absolute difference –5%, 95% CI –21 to 11%). **A1a** An interaction (p = 0025) between treatment allocation and disease location on treatment response was identified. Among patients with disease of the colon, 9 of 17 (53%) were in remission after treatment with antibiotics, compared with 4 of 16 (25%) of those who received placebo (p = 0.10). Discontinuation of therapy because of adverse events occurred in 13 of 66 (20%) patients treated with antibiotics, compared with 0 of 68 in the group who received placebo (p < 0.001). In patients with active CD of the ileum, the addition of ciprofloxacin and metronidazole to budesonide was an ineffective intervention.

Although this antibiotic combination may improve outcome when there is involvement of the colon, the evidence supporting this possibility comes only from a *post hoc* analysis of a small number of patients and was not statistically significant. The section on antituberculous therapy for maintenance describes a trial conducted by Selby and colleagues that may also lend some credibility to the concept that alteration of bacterial flora may yet prove to be helpful for induction of remission [31].

In summary, of the traditional and most widely used interventions glucocorticoids are the most effective treatment for inducing clinical remission of active CD. For those patients whose disease is confined to the terminal ileum and/or right colon, budesonide is an attractive alternative to the conventional glucocorticoids because of the lower incidence of adverse events. Sulfasalazine is modestly effective in patients with mild disease activity. Although the newer 5-ASA compounds and antibiotics are used by many clinicians to treat patients with milder forms of the disease, current data do not provide good evidence for the efficacy of these drugs.

Treatment of therapy-resistant or steroid-dependent patients

Munkholm and colleagues have documented the natural history of an acute exacerbation of CD in a cohort of patients from Copenhagen county [32]. One year after an initial course of treatment a high proportion (56%) of their patients were either therapy resistant (20%) or steroid dependent (36%). This observation has led many clinicians to conclude that earlier and more aggressive treatment with immunosuppressives may be warranted in selected patients.

Conventional immunosuppressive drugs

Three drugs or classes of drugs have been most frequently used: the purine antimetabolites (azathioprine (AZA)/6-mercaptopurine), cyclosporin and methotrexate.

Purine antimetabolites

Until recently the use of the purine antimetabolites for the treatment of refractory patients was not widely accepted, perhaps because of the inconsistent results obtained from the early randomized trials of these drugs. However, more recent studies have for the most part confirmed their efficacy. One of the more important trials was conducted by Candy *et al.*, who randomized 63 patients with active CD to receive a standard tapering induction regimen of prednisone over three months and either AZA 2.5 mg/kg daily or a placebo for 15 months [33]. Although no early (three months) benefit of AZA was identified with respect to remission rates (CDAI < 150 and no prednisone), the proportion of patients who remained in remission over the entire follow-up time was greater in the AZA group (42% vs 7%, ARR 35%, NNT = 3; p = 0.001). **A1c** This result is consistent with observational data that suggest that the purine anti-metabolites require a minimum of three months to show a treatment effect. In an attempt to overcome this theoretical limitation Sandborn *et al.* did a small, uncontrolled study in which patients with active CD received an intravenous 1800 mg loading dose of AZA [34]. This strategy rapidly achieved stable erythrocyte concentrations of the thiol metabolites, which are believed to be responsible for the immunosuppressive effects of AZA. Despite this promising finding, a subsequent RCT which evaluated 96 patients showed equally low (eight week) remission rates in patients who received either loading or conventional AZA regimens (25% vs 24%), in spite of achieving steady state nucleotide levels by week 2 [35]. **A1d** Furthermore, the proportion of patients entering remission did not increase after eight weeks of treatment. It should be noted that all patients in this study received oral AZA in a dose of 2 mg/kg and that the proportion of these patients who entered remission and withdrew completely from steroids was only 24%, a figure roughly comparable with the expected response to a placebo in many induction of remission studies. The data are consistent with a slow onset of effect for the purine antimetabolites.

The data from the RCTs which have evaluated the purine antimetabolites for the treatment of active CD in adults have been summarized in a meta-analysis in which the pooled ARR for AZA treatment for induction of remission is approximately 20% (NNT = 5) (see Figure 11.2) [36]. **A1d** In the majority of these studies patients were receiving concomitant corticosteroid therapy. A steroid-sparing

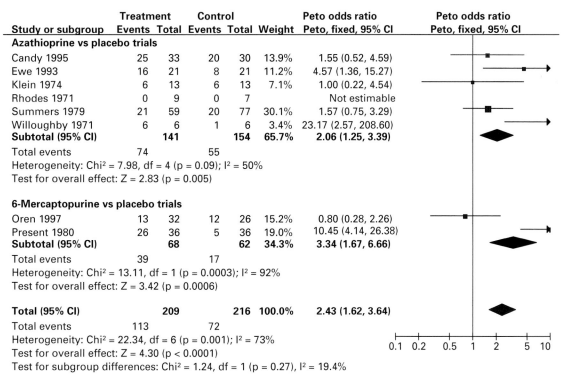

Figure 11.2 Azathioprine or 6-mercaptopurine for inducing remission in Crohn's disease. Source: *Cochrane Database Syst Rev* 2009; **4**: CD000545. Azathioprine or 6-mercaptopurine for induction of remission in Crohn's disease. Prefontaine E, Macdonald JK, Sutherland LR. Department of Community Health Sciences, University of Calgary, Health Sciences Centre, Calgary, Canada. Update of: *Cochrane Database Syst Rev* 2000; **2**: CD000545.

effect was also demonstrated in this analysis: the NNT for steroid sparing (the NNT for AZA to permit one additional patient to reduce steroids to < 10 mg/day) was estimated to be 3. These results should be interpreted with a degree of caution, since important clinical heterogeneity exists among the studies in their definitions of treatment response, duration and the use of cointerventions. No single, large, well-designed trial that resulted in a clinically and statistically significant benefit compared with placebo exists. Nevertheless, the meta-analysis suggests that some beneficial effect is present on disease activity, and the use of these drugs can be recommended for treatment of patients who fail to respond to steroid therapy or develop steroid dependence.

Cyclosporine

The emergence of this drug as a standard therapy for organ transplantation led to large-scale evaluations for the treatment of chronically active CD. The results of four RCTs (see Figure 11.3 [37]) have shown that the therapeutic index for cyclosporin is low, if there is any efficacy [38–41]. **A1c** The study of Brynskov *et al.* [39], which demonstrated only a modest benefit, used a high cyclosporin dose (7.6 mg/kg per day), which cannot be recommended for chronic treatment, since the risk of nephrotoxicity is unacceptably high [42]. The three trials that assessed a dose of cyclosporin that is tolerable for long-term treatment (5 mg/kg per day) showed no benefit with this drug [38–40]. Thus, cyclosporin is not a practical therapy for long-term management. Although uncontrolled studies have suggested that short-duration, high-dose intravenous therapy may be beneficial in patients with refractory CD, data from controlled trials would be required to support a recommendation for widespread use [43, 44]. These trials are unlikely to be performed given the demonstrated efficacy and safety of other agents.

Methotrexate

The success of low dose (5–25 mg/weekly) methotrexate as a treatment for rheumatoid arthritis led to its evaluation in patients with chronically active CD. In 1989, Kozarek *et al.* reported the results of an open study in which two-thirds of patients with steroid refractory disease showed an improvement in symptoms and a concomitant reduction in prednisone requirements [45]. **B4** Some patients demonstrated an endoscopic remission. A controlled trial was subsequently conducted in which 141 patients who had failed previous attempts to discontinue prednisone were randomized to receive either methotrexate 25 mg/weekly intramuscularly or a placebo for 16 weeks [46]. All of the patients received 20 mg of prednisone per day at the initiation of the trial; a standardized prednisone withdrawal regimen was then used. Patients who responded to therapy discontinued prednisone entirely 12 weeks following randomization. A significant benefit of methotrexate therapy was observed for the primary outcome measure, the proportion of patients who were completely withdrawn from prednisone and in clinical remission as defined by a CDAI score of < 150 points (methotrexate 39%, placebo 19%, ARR 20%, NNT = 5; p = 0.025) (see Figure 11.4). **A1a** Improvements in the median prednisone dose, Health Related Quality of Life and mean CDAI scores, and concentration of serum acute phase reactants were also associated with methotrexate therapy. In this short-term trial, no serious toxicity was observed, although withdrawals from treatment due to nausea were more common with methotrexate.

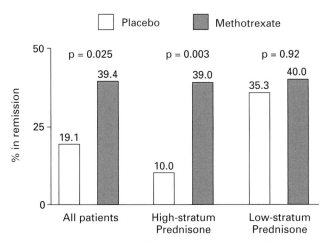

Figure 11.4 Percentages of patients in remission at week 16 according to study group and stratum of daily prednisone dose before entry into the study. The high prednisone stratum was receiving a daily dose of more than 20 mg prednisone, and the low prednisone stratum a daily dose of 20 mg or less more than two weeks before randomization. The actual percentages are shown above the bars. P values were derived by the Mantel-Haenszel chi-square test, with adjustment for study center. Reproduced with permission from Feagan BG *et al. N Engl J Med* 1995; **332**: 292–297.

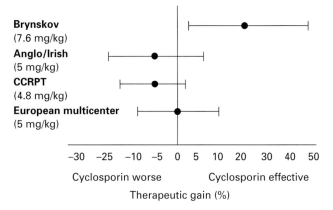

Figure 11.3 Point estimates (•) and 95% confidence limits (I–I) of the therapeutic gain (% response cyclosporin–% response placebo) for four RCTs of cyclosporin for Crohn's disease. Reproduced with permission from Feagan B. *Inflamm Bowel Dis* 1995; **1**: 335–339.

Novel immunosuppressive drugs

New knowledge of the human immune system and the growth of the biotechnology industry have combined to yield an abundance of new treatments for chronic inflammatory diseases. The development of anti-TNF alpha (infliximab, adalimumab, certolizumab) and anti-integrin antibodies (natalizumab) as therapies for CD are examples of the development of this new technology.

Anti TNF alpha antibodies

Tumor necrosis factorα (TNF) is a proinflammatory cytokine which plays an important part in the pathophysiology of CD [47]. Following the successful treatment of a young woman with a chimeric anti-TNF-α antibody by investigators in Amsterdam, a series of controlled studies were initiated with several different chimeric or humanized monoclonal antibodies [48].

Infliximab Targan and colleagues carried out a multicenter dose finding study that evaluated 108 patients whose disease was refractory to other forms of treatment [49]. Patients with moderately severe disease received one of three doses of infliximab (5, 10, 20 mg/kg) or a placebo administered as a single intravenous infusion. Patients continued to receive other treatments at a fixed dose. The primary endpoint of the study was the occurrence of a clinical response as defined by a decrement of 70 points in the CDAI score from the baseline value. No dose-response relationship was identified; 81.5% of infliximab-treated patients responded compared with 16.7% of those who received the placebo (ARR 65%, NNT = 2; p < 0.001). **A1a** Minor allergic reactions to the antibody occurred infrequently, but clinically significant adverse effects were not encountered in this short-term study.

In a second pivotal trial Present and colleagues evaluated the efficacy of infliximab for the treatment of patients with fistulizing CD (no previous controlled trials had evaluated this population of patients) [50]. The patients studied had active, fistulizing disease for a minimum of three months prior to randomization. Concomitant treatment with steroids, 6-mercaptopurine or AZA, and antibiotics was permitted although the dose of these cointerventions was maintained at a stable level throughout the trial. The primary measure of response was a 50% reduction in the number of open fistulae. Ninety-four patients received three intravenous infusions of either a placebo or one of two dose regimens of antibody (5 or 10 mg/kg) during a total of 18 weeks of follow-up. Patients treated with infliximab were significantly more likely to respond (61.9% vs 25.8%, ARR 36.1%, NNT = 3; p = 0.002). **A1a** The response to treatment was rapid and in many cases dramatic. Again, no dose-response relationship was identifiable.

Adalimumab Adalimumab was developed as a human recombinant immunoglobulin G1 anti-TNF monoclonal antibody for subcutaneous administration. In the CLASSIC-1 trial 299 patients with moderate to severe CD naive to anti-TNF therapy were randomized to receive subcutaneous injections at weeks 0 and 2 of adalimumab 40 mg/20 mg, 80 mg/40 mg, or 160 mg/80 mg, or placebo [51]. The optimal induction dosing regimen for adalimumab in this study was 160 mg at week 0 followed by 80 mg at week 2, which produced clinical remission in 36% of patients compared to the rate of 12% observed in the placebo group. (NNT = 4, p = 0.001). Adalimumab was well tolerated.

Certolizumab Certolizumab pegol is a pegylated humanized Fab' fragment that binds tumor necrosis factor alpha. In the PRECISE-1 study 662 adults with moderate to severe Crohn's disease were randomly assigned to receive either 400 mg of certolizumab pegol or placebo subcutaneously at weeks 0, 2 and 4 and then every four weeks [52]. Response rates at week 6 were 35% in the certolizumab group and 27% in the placebo group (p = 0.02), although remission rates were not significantly different in the two groups. **A1a** Serious adverse events were reported in 10% of patients in the certolizumab group and 7% of those in the placebo group. *Post hoc* analysis of the health-related, quality of life data (self-administered IBDQ questionnaire) from 290 patients showed improvement in emotional well-being and systematic symptoms in certolizumab treated patients at all intervals up to 12 weeks.

Natalizumab

Natalizumab is a recombinant, humanized, monoclonal antibody against the alpha4 integrin. A systematic Cochrane review has summarized the results of pooled data from four randomized trials that investigated the ability of natalizumab, in a variety of dose regimens to induce remission in a total of 1641 patients with moderately to severely active disease [53–57]. Natalizumab (300 mg or 3 to 4 mg/kg) is effective for induction of clinical response and remission in patients with moderately to severely active disease. This benefit was statistically significant for one, two and three infusion treatments, although there was a trend toward increased benefit with additional infusions of natalizumab. The NNT for induction of remission or clinical response varied according to the infusion regimen and outcome and ranged from approximately 4 to 10. For example, pooled data from three studies that included 2456 patients showed that the number of patients required to be treated with a single infusion of natalizumab to produce clinical response at four weeks was eight. Subgroup analysis demonstrated significantly greater clinical response and remission rates for natalizumab compared with placebo in patients in whom active disease was characterized by elevated C-reactive protein levels and active disease despite the use of immunosuppressants or prior anti-tumor necrosis factor therapy.

There were no statistically significant differences between natalizumab and placebo treated patients in the proportions of patients who withdrew due to adverse events or those who experienced serious adverse events. However, the included trials lacked adequate power to detect serious adverse effects that occur infrequently. When two patients with multiple sclerosis treated with natalizumab in combination with interferon beta-1a, and one patient with Crohn's disease treated with natalizumab in combination with azathioprine developed progressive multifocal leukoencephalopathy (PML) resulting in two patient deaths, a considerable degree of alarm arose about the safety of this preparation [58–60]. A retrospective investigation was conducted to assess the risk of PML in natalizumab treated patients and no new cases were identified. The incidence of PML has been estimated to be 1 case per 1000 patients (95% CI: 0.2–2.8 per 1000) in this population who received a mean of 17.9 monthly doses of natalizumab [61]. Subsequently, the FDA (US) has approved the use of this antibody for induction of remission in Crohn's disease.

Combination therapy with anti-TNF alpha antibodies and methotrexate or azathioprine for induction and maintenance of remission

Two important randomized trials have been performed to compare the effectiveness of infliximab alone or in combination with immunomodulator therapy (azathioprine or methotrexate) for induction and maintenance of remission.

In the SONIC trial 508 patients who were immunosuppressant and anti-TNF naive, and whose mean disease duration was approximately two years, were randomized to receive infliximab plus a placebo (IFX + Pl), azathioprine plus a placebo (AZA + Pl), or infliximab plus azathioprine (IFX + AZA) [62]. The primary endpoint of steroid-free clinical remission at 26 weeks was achieved as follows: IFX + Pl 44.4, AZA + Pl 30.6, and IFX + AZA 56.8 (p < 0.05 for all comparisons). The predefined secondary endpoint of complete mucosal healing was also observed significantly more frequently in infliximab than in azathioprine treated patients. The SONIC trial clearly showed benefit from combined anti-TNF alpha and antimetabolite therapy over monotherapies with these agents.

In the COMMIT study 126 patients with active disease (mean CDAI 208) requiring steroid therapy were randomized to receive standard infliximab induction and maintenance therapy (IFX 5 mg/kg weeks 1, 3 and 7 and q 8 weeks) with either a placebo (IFX + Pl) or methotrexate 25 mg subcutaneously weekly (IFX + MTX) [63]. Prednisone therapy was tapered after the first week to be discontinued by week 14. The combination of IFX and MTX, although safe, was no more effective than IFX alone. Treatment

failure rates (percent) at 50 weeks were virtually identical: IFX + Pl 29.8, IFX + MTX 30.6, p = 0.63). This study showed that infliximab combined with initial prednisone therapy can result in very high steroid-free clinical remission rates at one year that are not improved with the addition of methotrexate therapy.

The results of these two trials should not be interpreted as showing that infliximab combined with azathioprine is an effective approach, while the combination with methotrexate is not. No "head-to-head" comparison has been made. The selection of patients and the use of concomitant therapy, particularly prednisone, were quite different in the SONIC and COMMIT trials. All patients in the COMMIT trial received corticosteroids as part of the induction regimen, and remission was achieved in a very high proportion of patients, compared to the rate observed in the SONIC study. It may not be possible to significantly increase the remission rate associated with anti-TNF alpha therapy in combination with steroids by the addition of methotrexate therapy under these circumstances. It is possible that combined therapy with infliximab and methotrexate is more effective than therapy with infliximab alone in other circumstances, for example in the absence of concomitant steroid therapy.

Conventional 'step-up' versus 'top-down' approach to use of immunosuppressive agents for induction and maintenance of remission

It is clear that anti-TNF alpha antibodies are effective for induction of remission of CD in a patient population refractory to other treatments and that serious short-term toxicity is uncommon. However, potential safety concerns include the formation of autoantibodies, the risk of infusion reactions with re-treatment, and a possible increased risk of lymphoproliferative disease. Therefore, the conventional approach to induction of remission in patients with active Crohn's disease has been to employ initial therapy with corticosteroids, adding immunosuppressive medications when patients become resistant to or dependent on steroid therapy. D'Haens *et al.* compared this approach with the use of early combined immunosuppression in an open label, randomized trial in 133 patients who were randomized to receive three infusions of infliximab (5 mg/kg at weeks 0, 2 and 6) combined with azathioprine (with additional treatments with infliximab and if necessary steroids) or conventional management with corticosteroids, followed in sequence by azathioprine and infliximab [64]. At 26 weeks 60% of patients who received early combined immunosuppression were in remission without corticosteroids and without surgical resection, compared to 35.9% for patients receiving conventional management (ARR = 24%, 95% CI: 7.3–40.8, p = 0.0062, NNT = 4). **Ala** These differences were maintained at 52 weeks. Furthermore, mucosal healing at two years was twice as likely to occur in patients assigned to combined immuno-suppressive therapy. Serious adverse events were not significantly more frequent in the early combined immunosuppression group. These results suggest that early combined immunosuppression may yield significantly better outcomes than the conventional approach of adding the more potent immunosuppressive agents in a stepwise approach when induction of remission is not achieved, or when patients become steroid dependent. However, many clinicians and patients are reluctant to adopt this type of aggressive strategy until more long-term efficacy and safety data are available. It may be that outcomes can be improved following an approach that recognizes in a timely fashion when particular therapies have not achieved specific, clinically relevant outcomes and advances to the next therapeutic "step" when this occurs. A cluster randomized trial has been organized to test this hypothesis [65]. Forty centers in Belgium and Canada will be randomized to utilize either a conventional or accelerated step-up approach to management of active Crohn's disease.

Probiotics

A single small randomized trial that included only 11 patients failed to show any benefit of probiotics for induction of remission [66]. There are no methodologically randomized trials of adequate size to permit any conclusions about the efficacy of this approach.

Maintenance of remission

The objectives of maintenance therapy are to prevent the recurrence of symptoms, to reduce the risk of complications, and to avoid the need for surgery and hospitalization. One year after a medically induced remission of CD approximately 30–40% of patients will experience a relapse of disease; and following surgery symptoms recur at a rate of approximately 15% per year [67]. The failure of the maintenance therapy components of the NCCD [4] and ECCDS [5] trials to demonstrate a long-term benefit of sulfasalazine or conventional, low dose glucocorticoid therapy led to the extensive evaluation of the newer 5-ASA and budesonide for this indication. **A1c**

5-aminosalicylates

The second edition of this textbook summarized data from over twenty randomized trials of 5-ASA compounds for maintenance of remission of medically or surgically induced remission of Crohn's disease. Although some randomized trials and early meta-analyses had suggested modest benefit, subsequent larger trials did not. Our overall review of the trials and meta-analysis led us to conclude

that it was increasingly difficult to recommend chronic use of 5-ASA therapy for Crohn's disease. More recently Akobeng and Gardener performed a Cochrane review on the use of 5-ASA for maintenance of medically induced remission [68]. The reviewers concluded on the basis of data from seven trials that included 1500 patients that there is no evidence to suggest that 5-ASA preparations are superior to placebo for the maintenance of medically-induced remission in patients with Crohn's disease, and that additional randomized trials of this agent are not justified (see Figure 11.5). **A1a** We concur with this conclusion, given that there are several other agents that are proven to be effective for this purpose.

On the other hand, Doherty *et al.* performed a Cochrane review of the use of 5-ASA for the prevention of relapse after surgically induced remission and concluded on the basis of five trials that included 652 patients that 5-ASA is modestly effective for this purpose with an RR of 0.76 (95% CI: 0.62–0.94) (see Figure 11.6) [69]. **A1a** The NNT to prevent a single clinical recurrence within 12 months was 12. However, it should be noted that the largest and methodologically rigorous trial performed by Lochs and colleagues did not demonstrate efficacy for this intervention [70].

Budesonide

The efficacy of budesonide for induction of remission in CD suggested that chronic therapy might be an effective and safe maintenance strategy. Four randomized placebo controlled trials have evaluated the use of either 6 mg/day or 3 mg/day of budesonide for one year of treatment [71–73]. The first three studies were of similar design, following treatment of active CD with either budesonide, prednisolone or a placebo. Patients who responded to treatment were randomized to receive either one of the two doses of budesonide or a placebo. Patients who responded to treatment were randomized to receive either one of the two doses of budesonide or placebo. No other treatments for CD were permitted. The primary outcome measure of these studies was the proportion of symptomatic relapses of CD as defined by a 60 point increase in the CDAI and a minimum CDAI score of 200 at the time of the disease exacerbation.

Greenberg *et al.* (n = 105) found that the median time to relapse or withdrawal from treatment differed significantly between the three treatment groups: budesonide-treated patients remained in remission longer than those who received the placebo (178 days 6 mg vs 124 days 3 mg vs 39 days placebo; p = 0.027) [71]. However, the treatment effect was not durable. The greatest difference in remission rates was observed three months after randomization, whereas at one year no significant differences were present (39% 6 mg vs 30% 3 mg vs 33% placebo). **A1a** Budesonide therapy

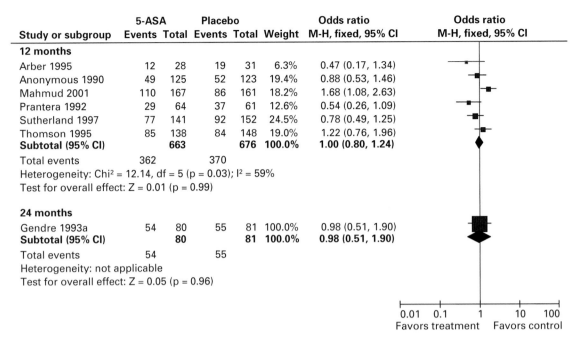

Study or subgroup	5-ASA Events	Total	Placebo Events	Total	Weight	Odds ratio M-H, fixed, 95% CI
12 months						
Arber 1995	12	28	19	31	6.3%	0.47 (0.17, 1.34)
Anonymous 1990	49	125	52	123	19.4%	0.88 (0.53, 1.46)
Mahmud 2001	110	167	86	161	18.2%	1.68 (1.08, 2.63)
Prantera 1992	29	64	37	61	12.6%	0.54 (0.26, 1.09)
Sutherland 1997	77	141	92	152	24.5%	0.78 (0.49, 1.25)
Thomson 1995	85	138	84	148	19.0%	1.22 (0.76, 1.96)
Subtotal (95% CI)		**663**		**676**	**100.0%**	**1.00 (0.80, 1.24)**
Total events	362		370			

Heterogeneity: Chi² = 12.14, df = 5 (p = 0.03); I² = 59%
Test for overall effect: Z = 0.01 (p = 0.99)

	5-ASA Events	Total	Placebo Events	Total	Weight	Odds ratio M-H, fixed, 95% CI
24 months						
Gendre 1993a	54	80	55	81	100.0%	0.98 (0.51, 1.90)
Subtotal (95% CI)		**80**		**81**	**100.0%**	**0.98 (0.51, 1.90)**
Total events	54		55			

Heterogeneity: not applicable
Test for overall effect: Z = 0.05 (p = 0.96)

Figure 11.5 Oral 5-aminosalicylic acid for maintenance of medically-induced remission in Crohn's disease. Source: Akobeng AK, Gardener E. Oral 5-aminosalicylic acid for maintenance of medically-induced remission in Crohn's disease. *Cochrane Database of Systematic Reviews* 2005; Issue 1. Art. No.: CD003715. DOI: 10.1002/14651858.CD003715.pub2.

Review: interventions for prevention of post-operative recurrence of Crohn's disease
Outcome: clinical recurrence (at study completion)
Comparison: 5-ASA versus placebo

Study or Subgroup	5-ASA Events	Total	Placebo Events	Total	Weight	Risk ratio M-H, fixed, 95% CI
Brignola 1995	7	44	10	43	7.7%	0.68 (0.29, 1.63)
Hanauer 2004	26	44	31	40	24.8%	0.76 (0.57, 1.03)
Lochs 2000	36	152	50	166	36.5%	0.79 (0.54, 1.14)
McLeod 1995	27	87	31	76	25.3%	0.76 (0.50, 1.15)
Sutherland 1997	3	31	8	35	5.7%	0.42 (0.12, 1.46)
Total (95% CI)		**358**		**360**	**100.0%**	**0.75 (0.61, 0.92)**
Total events	99		130			

Heterogeneity: Chi² = 0.96, df = 4 (p = 0.92); I² = 0%
Test for overall effect: Z = 2.79 (p = 0.005)

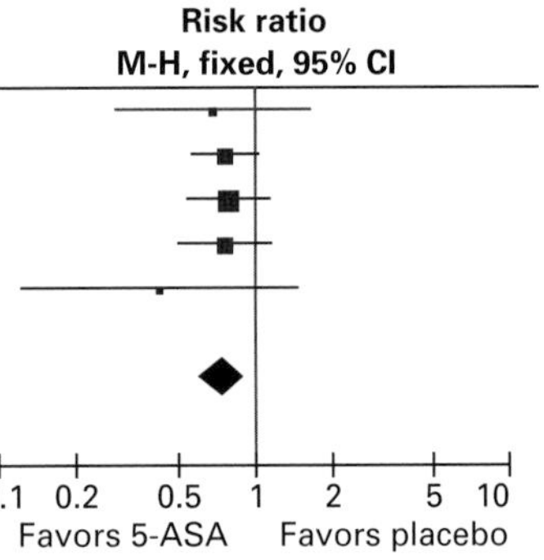

Figure 11.6 Interventions for prevention of post-operative recurrence of Crohn's disease. Source: Doherty G *et al.* Interventions for prevention of post-operative recurrence of Crohn's disease. *Cochrane Database of Systematic Reviews* 2009; Issue 4. Art. No.: CD006873. DOI: 10.1002/14651858. CD006873.pub2.

was well tolerated. No differences were observed among the treatment groups in the proportion of patients who experienced adverse events (78% 6 mg vs 70% 3 mg vs 89% placebo). Although glucocorticoid-related adverse events occurred more frequently in patients who were treated with budesonide, the proportion of patients who reported these events decreased throughout the follow-up period and the most common steroid-related adverse event identified was easy bruising. A dose-dependent depression of the plasma cortisol concentration was noted in the budesonide-treated groups.

Similar results were obtained by Lofberg and colleagues (n = 90) who observed that the median time to relapse or discontinuation of therapy was 258 days for the 6 mg/day group, 139 days for the 3 mg/day group, and 92 days for the patients who received a placebo (p = 0.021) [72]. Again, the time in remission was significantly prolonged for those patients who received budesonide, but the therapeutic effect was not sustained. At 12 months following randomization, 41%, 26% and 37% of the 6 mg/day, 3 mg/ day, and placebo group respectively remained in remission (p = 0.44). **Ala** Thirty-eight percent of those patients who had received 6 mg/day reported glucocorticoid-related adverse events compared with 20% of those who received 3 mg/day and 12% of those who received the placebo.

The third trial, by Ferguson *et al.*, which evaluated the smallest number of patients (n = 75), failed to demonstrate any benefit of budesonide treatment [73]. The median time to relapse or discontinuation of therapy was 272 days in the 6 mg/day group, 321 days in the 3 mg/day group, and 290 days in the placebo group (p = 0.80). **Alc** A similar proportion of patients in the three treatment groups experienced glucocorticoid-related adverse events (18% 6 mg/day vs 36% 3 mg/day and 15% placebo; p = 0.79).

An analysis of the pooled data from these studies and additional studies in a Cochrane review showed that budesonide 6 mg daily was no more effective than placebo for maintenance of remission at three months (RR 1.25; 95% CI: 1.00–1.58; p = 0.05), six months (RR 1.15; 95% CI: 0.95–1.39; p = 0.14), or 12 months (RR 1.13; 95% CI: 0.94–1.35; p = 0.19) [74]. **Ala** Adverse events were more frequent in patients treated with 6 mg of budesonide compared with placebo (RR 1.49; 95% CI: 1.01–2.19; p = 0.05), but not in patients using lower doses of budesonide. These events were relatively minor and did not result in increased rates of study withdrawal. Abnormal adrenocorticoid stimulation tests were seen more frequently in patients receiving both 6 mg daily (RR 2.88; 95% CI: 1.72–4.82; p < 0.0001) and 3 mg daily (RR 2.73; 95% CI: 1.34–5.57; p = 0.006) compared with placebo.

Two additional randomized trials that used endoscopic relapse following surgery as endpoints have not demonstrated significant prolongation of remission with this therapy. Hellers *et al.* randomized 129 patients following ileal or ileocecal resection to receive budesonide 6 mg daily or a placebo [5, 75]. Ileocolonoscopy, including biopsy, was carried out 3 and 12 months after surgery. The frequency of endoscopic recurrence did not differ between the groups. **Ala** The investigators reported a subgroup analysis which suggested that recurrence at 12 months was lower in patients who had undergone surgery for control of disease activity rather than for stricture (budesonide 32%, placebo 65%; p = 0.047). However, this *post hoc* analysis should be viewed with caution.

Ewe *et al.* randomized 88 patients to receive budesonide 3 mg (pH-modified release formulation) or a placebo for one year [76]. Endoscopic recurrence at 3 and 12 months was the primary measure of efficacy. The recurrence rate was not reduced by active treatment (budesonide 57%, placebo 70%; p = 0.2). Survival analysis also failed to show prolongation of remission with active therapy. **Alc**

Given the lack of sustained benefit observed in any of these trials we do not recommend continued budesonide therapy for patients who have entered remission during treatment with this intervention.

Antituberculous therapy

A systematic review of antituberculous therapy for maintenance of remission in CD demonstrated a possible small benefit in patients in whom remission was induced by steroid [77].

However, this observation was derived from a meta-analysis of subgroups from only two trials involving 90 patients, and the authors of the review do not recommend this form of therapy in the absence of further trials. More recently Selby reported the results from a trial in which 213 patients were randomized to receive, in addition to a 16-week tapering course of prednisolone, either a placebo or a combination of clarithromycin, rifabutin and clofazimine [31]. Relapse rates were not significantly different over the next two years. The remission rate at 16 weeks, however, was significantly higher in the antibiotic group than in the placebo group (antibiotic 0.66, placebo 0.5, p = 0.02). This outcome was not the predetermined outcome for this study, but it does lend some continuing interest in the concept that altering bacterial flora may eventually prove to be beneficial in Crohn's disease.

Nitroimadazole antibiotics

Rutgeerts and colleagues have performed three randomized trials that evaluated metronidazole for postoperative maintenance therapy [78]. In the first study, 66 patients were randomized to two weeks of therapy with 20 mg/kg per day of metronidazole or placebo within one week of surgical resection of all visible disease. Following 12 weeks of therapy endoscopic recurrence occurred in 52% of patients assigned to metronidazole compared with 75% of those who received placebo (p = 0.09). **Alc** Furthermore, a significant effect was shown for clinical recurrence at one year (4% for metronidazole vs 25% for placebo (p = 0.046). However, peripheral neuropathy was common, making continuous therapy impracticable. A second trial of a potentially less neurotoxic nitroimadazole, ornidazole, also suggested a maintenance benefit of antibiotic therapy; unfortunately clinically relevant neuropathy was also observed [79]. More recently, a third trial evaluated the combination of azathioprine and metronidazole versus metronidazole monotherapy and observed a lower endoscopic recurrence rate at 12 months in the combined therapy group (combined therapy 43.7%, metronidazole monotherapy 69%, p = 0.048) [80]. These trials indicate that manipulation of the endogenous bacterial flora with antibiotics may ultimately prove to be an effective strategy for the prevention of postoperative recurrence. Unfortunately, the problems of antibiotic resistance and neuropathy mitigate against the use of nitroimadazole antibiotics as long-term treatments.

Probiotics

A Cochrane review has concluded that there is no evidence to suggest that probiotics are beneficial for the maintenance of remission in CD [81]. However, the reported studies enrolled small numbers of patients and may have lacked statistical power to show differences should they exist. Larger trials are required to determine if probiotics are of benefit in Crohn's disease.

Azathioprine

A systematic review published by Prefontaine *et al.* included seven trials of azathioprine therapy and one of 6-mercaptopureine therapy [82].

Seven trials of azathioprine therapy and one of 6-mercaptopurine were included in the review. Azathioprine and 6-mercaptopurine had a positive effect on maintaining remission (see Figure 11.7). The Peto odds ratio (OR) for maintenance of remission with azathioprine was 2.32 (95% CI: 1.55–3.49) with a NNT of 6. The Peto OR for maintenance of remission with 6-mercaptopurine was 3.32 (95% CI: 1.40–7.87) with NNT of 4. Higher doses of azathioprine improved response. A steroid sparing effect with azathioprine was noted, with a Peto OR of 5.22 (95% CI: 1.06–25.68) and NNT of 3 for quiescent disease. Withdrawals due to adverse events were more common in patients treated with azathioprine (Peto OR 3.74; 95% CI: 1.48–9.45, NNT = 20) than with placebo. Common events for withdrawal included pancreatitis, leukopenia, nausea, "allergy" and infection.

Study or subgroup	Treatment Events	Total	Control Events	Total	Weight	Peto odds ratio Peto, fixed, 95% CI	Peto odds ratio Peto, fixed, 95% CI
Azathioprine dose 2.5 mg/kg/day							
Candy 1995	14	25	2	20	11.3%	7.12 (2.11, 23.99)	
Summers 1979	16	19	15	20	7.1%	1.73 (0.37, 8.05)	
Subtotal (95% CI)		**44**		**40**	**18.3%**	**4.13 (1.59, 10.71)**	
Total events	30		17				
Heterogeneity: Chi² = 2.00, df = 1 (p = 0.16); I² = 50%							
Test for overall effect: Z = 2.92 (p = 0.004)							
Azathioprine dose 2.0 mg/kg/day							
D'Haens 2007	18	32	9	29	16.5%	2.73 (1.00, 7.45)	
Lemann 2005	38	40	36	43	8.8%	3.17 (0.80, 12.54)	
O'Donoghue 1978	13	23	8	27	13.4%	2.95 (0.97, 9.00)	
Rosenberg 1975	7	10	4	10	5.6%	3.16 (0.57, 17.62)	
Willoughby 1971	4	5	2	5	2.9%	4.48 (0.41, 49.42)	
Subtotal (95% CI)		**110**		**114**	**47.2%**	**3.01 (1.66, 5.45)**	
Total events	80		59				
Heterogeneity: Chi² = 0.15, df = 4 (p = 1.00); I² = 0%							
Test for overall effect: Z = 3.64 (p = 0.0003)							
Azathioprine dose 1.0 mg/kg/day							
Summers 1979	37	54	65	101	34.5%	1.20 (0.60, 2.41)	
Subtotal (95% CI)		**54**		**101**	**34.5%**	**1.20 (0.60, 2.41)**	
Total events	37		65				
Heterogeneity: not applicable							
Test for overall effect: Z = 0.52 (p = 0.60)							
Total (95% CI)		**208**		**255**	**100.0%**	**2.32 (1.55, 3.49)**	
Total events	147		141				
Heterogeneity: Chi² = 7.75, df = 7 (p = 0.36); I² = 10%							
Test for overall effect: Z = 4.05 (p < 0.0001)							
Test for subgroup differences: Chi² = 5.60, df = 2 (p = 0.06), I² = 64.3%							

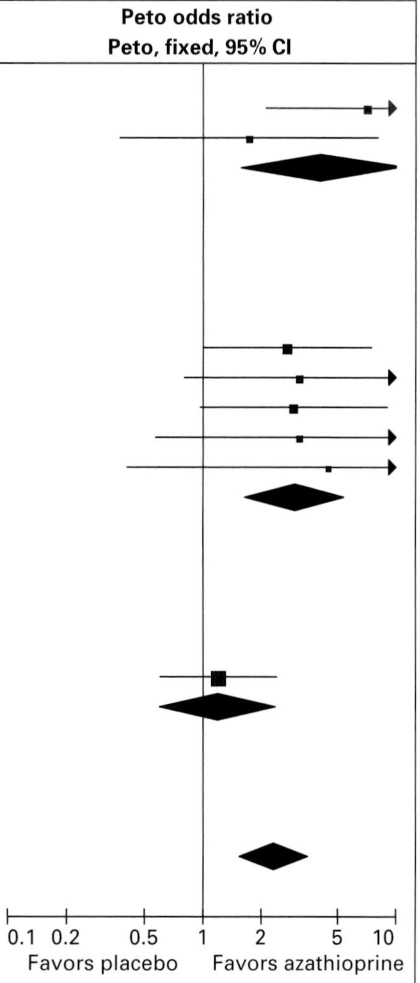

0.1 0.2   0.5   1   2   5   10
Favors placebo   Favors azathioprine

Figure 11.7 Azathioprine or 6-mercaptopurine for maintenance of remission in Crohn's disease. Source: Prefontaine E *et al.* Azathioprine or 6-mercaptopurine for maintenance of remission in Crohn's disease. *Cochrane Database of Systematic Reviews* 2009; Issue 1. Art. No.: CD000067. DOI: 10.1002/14651858.CD000067.pub2.
Review: azathioprine or 6-mercaptopurine for maintenance of remission in Crohn's disease.
Comparison: 5-ASA versus placebo.
Outcome: maintenance of remission.

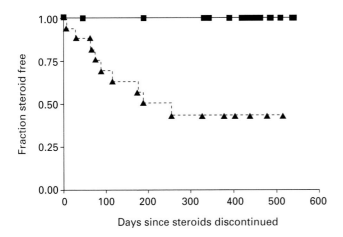

Figure 11.8 Time (days) off of corticosteroid treatment after initial discontinuation, depicted as a Kaplan-Meier survival curve. ■ 6-mercaptopurine; ▲ controls; p < 0.0001 Adapted from Markowitz et al. [83].

Markowitz *et al.* conducted a study that included 55 children (age 13 +/− 2 years) who were randomized within eight weeks of initial diagnosis to receive treatment with 6-mercaptopurine (1.5 mg/kg per day) or a placebo for 18 months in addition to prednisone (40 mg/day), with prednisone dosage withdrawal based on a defined schedule [83]. Although remission was induced in 89% of both groups, only 9% of the remitters in the 6-mercaptopurine group relapsed compared with 47% of controls (p = 0.007) (see Figure 11.8). **A1c** In the 6-mercaptopurine group, the duration of steroid use was shorter (p < 0.001) and the cumulative steroid dose was lower at 6, 12 and 18 months (p < 0.01).

Growth was comparable in both groups. No clinically significant adverse events occurred, although mild leukopenia and increases in aminotransferase activity were noted in the 6-mercaptopurine group; 6-mercaptopurine decreased the need for corticosteroids and decreased the frequency of relapses.

Minor toxicity, such as nausea, fatigue, skin rash, fever and arthralgias, is relatively common with the purine antimetabolites. Asymptomatic elevation of liver and pancreatic enzymes also occur frequently. Clinically important pancreatitis occurs in 3% of patients. Although leukopenia, defined by a white blood cell count of < 3.8, develops in approximately 20% of patients per year, infection associated with severe neutropenia is uncommon [84]. Whether therapeutic drug monitoring can improve efficacy and/or reduce toxicity remains controversial and is being investigated by a National Institute for Health sponsored RCT [85, 86]. In the USA, the Food and Drug Administration has recommended genotype testing prior to the initiation of treatment so that patients with low thiopurine methyltransferase activity can be identified. These individuals develop profound leukopenia following treatment with

either agent. No studies have compared this strategy to the usual clinical practice of initiating treatment with a relatively low drug dose and following the white blood cell count each week.

Recent research has identified an association between purine antimetabolites and the occurrence of lymphoma. The meta-analysis performed by Kandiel *et al.* suggests a four-fold increased risk [87]. The prospective observational cohort study of the CESAME study group enrolled 29,486 patients with IBD (60% Crohn's disease) from the practices of 680 gastroenterologists. The multivariate-adjusted hazard ratio of lymphoproliferative disorder between patients receiving thiopurines and those who had never received the drug was 5.28 (2.01–13.9, p = 0.0007) [88].

In summary, AZA or 6-mercaptopurine are moderately effective for maintenance of remission in adults and children and are relatively well tolerated. However, concerns about a significantly increased risk of lymphoma in patients receiving these agents appear to be increasing.

Methotrexate

The efficacy of methotrexate in a dose of 15 mg per week for maintaining remission was evaluated in 76 patients with quiescent CD. Patients who entered remission and were totally withdrawn from steroids during the induction phase of the trial of methotrexate for induction of remission described above and additional patients who entered remission on a similar regimen outside the trial were randomized to receive methotrexate 15 mg weekly (40 patients) or a placebo (36 patients) for 40 weeks [89]. Methotrexate was effective for maintaining remission (proportion in remission at 40 weeks: methotrexate 65%, placebo 38.9%, ARR 0–26, NNT 4; p = 0.01) [89]. **A1c** The survival data for maintenance of remission are shown in Figure 11.9. Methotrexate also reduced the requirement for prednisone use (methotrexate 27.5%, placebo 58.3%, p = 0.01) and mean disease activity (CDAI) score at week 40 (methotrexate 135 ± 16, placebo 196 ± 18; p = 0.005). Only one methotrexate-treated patient withdrew because of nausea and no serious adverse events occurred. A low dose of methotrexate is safe and effective for maintaining remission in patients who have responded to methotrexate for inducing remission of active disease. The available data regarding the short-term efficacy of methotrexate have been summarized in a recently published systematic review [90].

The adverse event profile of low dose methotrexate is well established [91]. The most common minor adverse effect is nausea, which tends to develop for a period of 24–48 hours after the weekly injection. This problem, which occurs in at most 15% of patients, can usually be managed by coadministration of oral folate (1 mg every day), use of antinauseants around the time of dosing (metoclopramide, odansetron), or, uncommonly, dose reduction. As with the

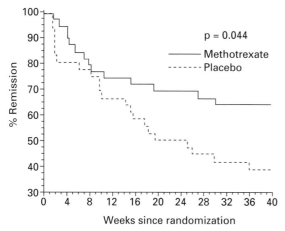

Figure 11.9 Methotrexate for maintenance of remission Crohn's disease. With permission from Feagan BG *et al.* A comparison of methotrexate with placebo for the maintenance of remission in Crohn's disease. North American Crohn's Study Group Investigators. *N Engl J Med* 2000; **342**(22): 1627–1632.

purine antimetabolites, leukopenia and associated opportunistic infections occur uncommonly. Methotrexate is teratogenic and must not be given to women of childbearing potential who are not using effective contraceptive measures. This issue is the most important limitation to the use of the drug. Hepatotoxicity was first documented in psoriatic patients. Subsequent understanding of pharmacokinetics and the conversion to weekly, from daily, dosing has virtually eliminated this problem. Patients should be monitored according to the American Rheumatological Association guidelines, paraphrased as follows: (1) avoid treating patients with risk factors for hepatotoxicity (obesity, diabetes, excessive alcohol use); and (2) measure transaminases every 4–6 weeks [92]. If, over the course of one year, more than half of the transaminase values are abnormal, take a liver biopsy before continuing treatment. Finally, no good data indicate that methotrexate is associated with malignancy.

Monoclonal antibodies

Behm and Bickston performed a Cochrane review of randomized trials of four different anti-TNF-a agents [94]: infliximab in three trials [95–97], CDP571 in three trials [98–100], adalimumab in two trials [101, 102], and certolizumab in one trial [103]. The authors decided not to statistically combine the data from trials involving different anti-TNF-a agents because of differences in drug administration, patient demographics, definitions of disease activity, and differences in clinical endpoints and study durations. These authors demonstrated that infliximab

maintains clinical remission (RR 2.50; 95% CI: 1.64–3.80), maintains clinical response (RR 1.66; 95% CI: 1.00–2.76), has corticosteroid-sparing effects (RR 3.13; 95% CI: 1.25–7.81) and maintains fistula healing (RR 1.87; 95% CI: 1.15–3.04) in patients with Crohn's disease with a response to infliximab induction therapy. There were no significant differences in remission rates between infliximab doses of 5 mg/kg or 10 mg/kg. Similarly, the results from a single randomized trial show that adalimumab maintains clinical remission (RR 3.28; 95% CI: 2.13–5.06), clinical response (RR 2.69; 95% CI: 1.88–3.86), and has corticosteroid-sparing effects (4.25; 95% CI: 1.57–11.47) in patients with Crohn's disease who have responded to or entered remission with adalimumab induction therapy. There were no significant differences in remission rates between adalimumab 40 mg weekly or every other week. Certolizumab pegol maintains clinical remission (RR 1.68; 95% CI: 1.30–2.16) and maintains clinical response (RR 1.74; 95% CI: 1.41–2.13) in patients who have responded to certolizumab induction therapy. The authors of the Cochrane review concluded that the evidence does not support the use of CDP571 for the maintenance of remission in Crohn's disease.

It can be calculated that the NNT, the number of patients needed to be treated with an anti-TNF alpha agent rather than placebo for approximately one year to maintain remission and achieve steroid sparing is in the range of 4 to 5. For maintenance of healing of fistulae it appears to be approximately 10. It has also been demonstrated that this form of maintenance therapy maintains health-related quality of life and reduces the need for hospitalization and surgery [104, 105]. It appears that scheduled maintenance therapy with infliximab is more effective that episodic treatment for maintaining clinical response or remission, and reducing the need for hospitalization and surgery. It also reduces the proportion of patients who form antibodies against anti-TNF alpha from 28% observed with episodic treatment to 6–9% observed with infliximab in 10 mg/kg and 5 mg/kg doses.

These benefits of maintenance therapy need to be considered in the light of knowledge about risk of infection and malignancy. The overall serious infection rates in the treatment groups summarized in the Cochrane review were in the range of 2.8–4% and did not differ significantly from the rates observed in placebo-treated patients. Recent data from the TREAT™ Registry revealed no increased risk of serious infections with infliximab after adjusting for disease severity and corticosteroid use (RR 0.99; 95% CI: 0.64–1.54) [106]. Tuberculosis and opportunistic infections have been associated with the use of these agents and are usually the result of disease reactivation [107, 108]. Since the introduction of appropriate screening methods (identification of high-risk patients, tuberculin testing, chest radiography) the incidence of tuberculosis has declined [109]. With respect to opportunistic infection, aspergillosis, listeriosis and Pneumonocystis carinii infections have been reported [110–112]. The estimated rate of opportunistic infection is estimated at 0.43 cases per 1000 patient exposures. Data from the TREAT™ Registry have not shown a significant increase of malignancy in patients with inflammatory bowel disease treated with anti-TNF alpha therapy [113]. A link between anti-TNF-a therapy and malignancy in patients with Crohn's disease remains unproven, unlike the evidence described above that azathioprine or 6-mercaptopurine therapy increase the risk for development of lymphoma. The apparent relative safety of the TNF alpha agents with respect to serious infections is in contrast with observed data in the TREAT™ Registry for a significant association of serious infections with the use of steroids and narcotics.

Combined immunosuppression therapy versus anti-TNF alpha alone for induction and maintenance

The evidence is presented above in the section on induction of remission that the combination of infliximab and azathioprine is more effective than infliximab alone for maintenance of steroid free clinical and endoscopic remission at one year [62]. There is no evidence that the combination of infliximab and methotrexate is more effective than infliximab alone in patients with active disease who are treated initially with conventional doses of corticosteroids in a tapering regimen [63].

Omega-3 fatty acids

Omega-3 fatty acids are polyunsaturated long-chain fatty acids derived from fish. Diets high in marine fish oils increase the concentrations of the omega-3 fatty acids, eicosapentaenoic acid and docosahexaenoic acid, in cell membranes. As a consequence, the concentration of the pro-inflammatory eicosanoid precursor, arachidonic acid is reduced, which theoretically should attenuate inflammatory responses [114–115].

A preliminary randomized controlled trial by Belluzzi and colleagues evaluated the efficacy of an omega-3 fatty acid formulation in 78 patients with CD who were at a high risk for the development of a relapse [116]. Patients were randomly assigned to receive either 4–5 g/day of omega-3 fatty acids or placebo for one year. At the end of treatment, 59% of the patients assigned to active treatment remained in remission as compared with 26% of those who received placebo (p < 0.001). **A1c** The only adverse event attributed to treatment was diarrhea, which occurred in 10% of patients. No serious adverse events were observed.

Please review

A second study published in the same year did not show benefit of omega-3 fatty acids [117]. Subsequently two large-scale trials that included 761 patients have evaluated this approach [118]. In EPIC-1 383 patients who had been in remission for 3 to 12 months, and in EPIC-2, 379 patients who entered remission during a standardized 16-week tapering course of prednisone or budesonide, were randomized to receive 4 mg/d of the encapsulated fatty acids or a triglyceride oil placebo for one year. Although the treatment was well tolerated, the proportions of patients who experienced relapse did not differ between the treatment groups in either trial (EPIC-1: omega-3 fatty acids 31.6%, placebo 35.7%, p = 0.30; EPIC-2: omega-3 fatty acids 47.8%, placebo 48.8%, p = 0.48).

A Cochrane review of six studies has concluded that omega-3 fatty acids are safe but probably ineffective for maintenance of remission of CD [119]. Although the use of this approach is often attractive to patients, the evidence indicates that it is not effective for maintaining remission in Crohn's disease, and patients should be advised on the benefits of other proven interventions.

Summary

An algorithm for the treatment of Crohn's disease is given in Figure 11.10 and Figure 11.11. Figure 11.10 summarizes the conventional stepwise approach, and Figure 11.11 provides detail on a more aggressive accelerated stepwise approach that is currently under evaluation with respect to the possibility that careful monitoring of response at specified intervals and the earlier addition of azathioprine or methotrexate and anti-TNF blockers results in better and earlier outcomes. The evidence is not yet available to support one approach as being superior to the other. We no longer recommend the use of 5-aminosalicylates for induction of remission. Patients with moderately severe disease and involvement of the terminal ileum and or right colon may be treated with budesonide at a dose of 9 mg/day. Patients with more extensive colonic involvement, those who fail to respond to budesonide or those with severe disease activity should receive either prednisone or parenteral steroids. Failure to achieve control of disease activity with these drugs (therapy-resistant disease) is an indication for addition of azathioprine (or 6-mercaptopurine), methotrexate, infliximab or surgery. Individuals who respond to glucocorticoid therapy should be withdrawn from steroid therapy over a 12–16 week period. In those patients who fail to successfully discontinue prednisone without a reactivation of disease activity (steroid-dependent disease), the introduction of either azathioprine, (or 6-mercaptopurine) or methotrexate treatment is warranted. The use of an anti-TNF alpha agent is indicated for patients who do not respond to one of these drugs. Furthermore, individuals who experience early or frequent relapses of the disease are candidates for long-term therapy with one

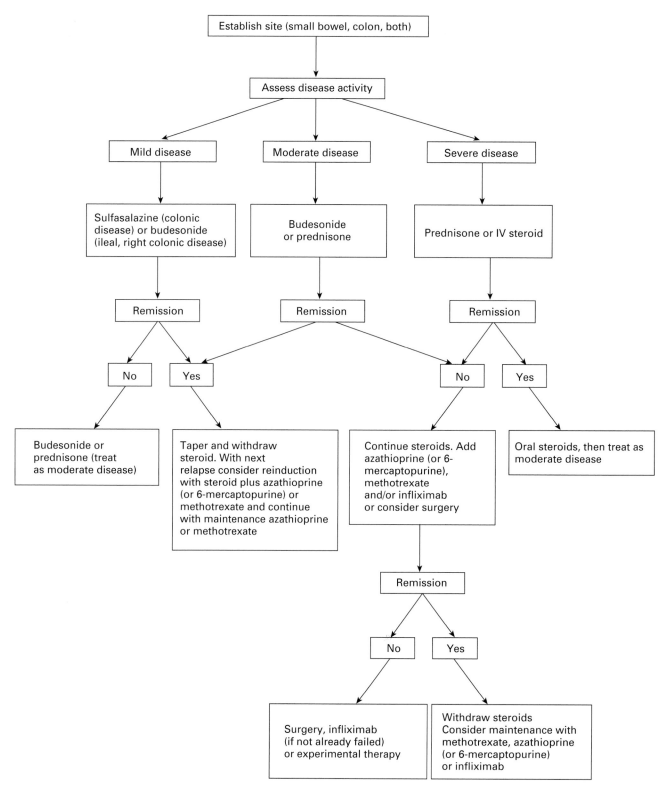

Figure 11.10 Therapeutic algorithm for 'accelerated step-wise' approach to treatment of active luminal Crohn's disease.

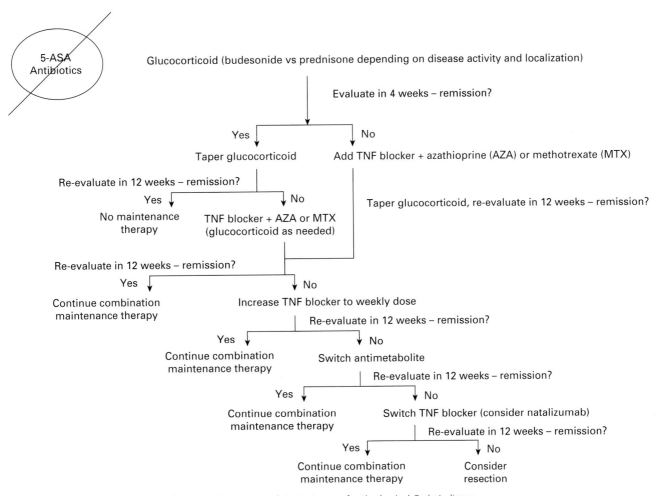

Figure 11.11 Therapeutic algorithm for conventional approach to treatment of active luminal Crohn's disease.

of the purine antimetabolites, methotrexate or an anti-TFN agent. Natalizumab therapy may be considered for patients who fail to respond to these agents, in jurisdictions where it is approved. Surgery remains a highly effective therapy for patients with limited disease who are experiencing adverse effects of medical therapy.

Although our existing medical management is relatively effective for induction of remission of CD, and improves the quality of life of the majority of patients, current therapy for maintenance of remission is less effective. A substantial proportion of patients still experience morbidity from chronically active disease, complications, or adverse effects of drug therapy. Many patients require surgery and a majority undergo more than one resection. At the present time there is insufficient evidence to support the use of any available drug for maintenance of remission following surgery. 5-ASA products may have a small benefit but are probably not cost-effective for this purpose. Metronidazole may also have some benefit, but its use is limited by toxic-

ity. In the future it is highly likely that drugs will become available which are able to favorably modify the natural history of the disease.

References

1 Feagan BG, McDonald JW, Koval JJ. Therapeutics and inflammatory bowel disease: a guide to the interpretation of randomized controlled trials. *Gastroenterology*; **110**(1): 275–283.

2 Sandborn WJ, Feagan BG, Hanauer SB *et al.* A review of activity indices and efficacy endpoints for clinical trials of medical therapy in adults with Crohn's disease. *Gastroenterology* 2002; **122**(2): 512–530.

3 Azad Khan AK, Piris J, Truelove SC. An experiment to determine the active therapeutic moiety of sulphasalazine. *Lancet* 1977; **2**(8044): 892–895.

4 Summers RW, Switz DM, Sessions JT Jr *et al.* National Cooperative Crohn's Disease Study: results of drug treatment. *Gastroenterology* 1979; **77**(4 Pt 2): 847–869.

5 Malchow H, Ewe K, Brandes JW *et al*. European Cooperative Crohn's Disease Study (ECCDS): results of drug treatment. *Gastroenterology* 1984; **86**(2): 249–266.

6 Rasmussen SN, Lauritsen K, Tage-Jensen U *et al*. 5-Aminosalicylic acid in the treatment of Crohn's disease. A 16-week double-blind, placebo-controlled, multicentre study with Pentasa. *Scand J Gastroenterol* 1987; **22**(7): 877–883.

7 Mahida YR, Jewell DP. Slow-release 5-amino-salicylic acid (Pentasa) for the treatment of active Crohn's disease. *Digestion* 1990; **45**(2): 88–92.

8 Singleton JW, Hanauer SB, Gitnick GL *et al*. Mesalamine capsules for the treatment of active Crohn's disease: results of a 16-week trial. Pentasa Crohn's Disease Study Group. *Gastroenterology* 1993; **104**(5): 1293–1301.

9 Scholmerich J, Jenss H, Hartmann F, The German 5-ASA Study Group. Oral 5-aminosalicyclic acid versus 6-methylprednisolone in active Crohn's disease. *Can J Gastroenterol* 1990; **4**: 446–451.

10 Martin F, Sutherland L, Beck I *et al*. Oral 5-ASA versus prednisone in short term treatment of Crohn's disease: a multicentre controlled trial. *Can J Gastroenterol* 1990; **4**: 452–457.

11 Maier K, Frick H-J, von Gaisberg U, Teufel T, *et al*. Clinical efficacy of oral mesalazine in Crohn's disease. *Can J Gastroenterol* 1990; **4**(1): 13–18.

12 Thomsen OO, Cortot A, Jewell D *et al*. Budesonide CIR is more effective than mesalazine in active Crohn's disease. A 16-week, international randomized, double-blind multicentre trial. *ACA Abstracts* 1996; **112**: A1104.

13 Prantera C, Pallone F, Brunetti G, Cottone M, Miglioli M. Oral 5-aminosalicylic acid (Asacol) in the maintenance treatment of Crohn's disease. The Italian IBD Study Group. *Gastroenterology* 1992; **103**(2): 363–368.

14 Gross V, Andus T, Fischbach W *et al*. Comparison between high dose 5-aminosalicylic acid and 6-methylprednisolone in active Crohn's ileocolitis. A multicenter randomized double-blind study. German 5-ASA Study Group. *Z Gastroenterol* 1995; **33**(10): 581–584.

15 Singleton J. Second trial of mesalamine therapy in the treatment of active Crohn's disease. *Gastroenterology* 1994; **107**(2): 632–633.

16 Hanauer SB, Stromberg U. Oral Pentasa in the treatment of active Crohn's disease: A meta-analysis of double-blind, placebo-controlled trials. *Clin Gastroenterol Hepatol* 2004; **2**(5): 379–388.

17 Fahey JV, Guyer PM, Munck A. Mechanisms of anti-inflammatory actions of glucocorticoids. In: Weissman G, ed. *Advances in Inflammation Research*. Raven Press, New York, 1981.

18 Singleton JW, Law DH, Kelley ML Jr, Mekhjian HS, Sturdevant RA. National Cooperative Crohn's Disease Study: adverse reactions to study drugs. *Gastroenterology* 1979; **77**(4 Pt 2): 870–882.

19 Hamedani R, Feldman RD, Feagan BG. Review article: drug development in inflammatory bowel disease: budesonide – a model of targeted therapy. *Aliment Pharmacol Ther* 1997; **11**(Suppl. 3): 98–107; discussion 107–108.

20 Brattsand R. Overview of newer glucocorticosterod preparations for inflammatory bowel disease. *Can J Gastroenterol* 1990; **4**: 407–414.

21 Pauwels RA, Lofdahl CG, Postma DS *et al*. Effect of inhaled formoterol and budesonide on exacerbations of asthma.

Formoterol and Corticosteroids Establishing Therapy (FACET) International Study Group. *N Engl J Med* 1997; **337**(20): 1405–1411.

22 Greenberg GR, Feagan BG, Martin F *et al*. Oral budesonide for active Crohn's disease. Canadian Inflammatory Bowel Disease Study Group. *N Engl J Med* 1994; **331**(13): 836–841.

23 Rutgeerts P, Lofberg R, Malchow H *et al*. A comparison of budesonide with prednisolone for active Crohn's disease. *N Engl J Med* 1994; **331**(13): 842–845.

24 Seow CH, Benchimol EI, Griffiths AM, Otley AR, Steinhart AH. Budesonide for induction of remission in Crohn's disease. *Cochrane Database Syst Rev* 2008; **3**(3): CD000296.

25 Herfarth HH, Mohanty SP, Rath HC, Tonkonogy S, Sartor RB. Interleukin 10 suppresses experimental chronic, granulomatous inflammation induced by bacterial cell wall polymers. *Gut* 1996; **39**(6): 836–845.

26 Duchmann R, Schmitt E, Knolle P, Meyer zum Buschenfelde KH, Neurath M. Tolerance towards resident intestinal flora in mice is abrogated in experimental colitis and restored by treatment with interleukin-10 or antibodies to interleukin-12. *Eur J Immunol* 1996; **26**(4): 934–938.

27 Ursing B, Alm T, Barany F *et al*. A comparative study of metronidazole and sulfasalazine for active Crohn's disease: the cooperative Crohn's disease study in Sweden. II. Result. *Gastroenterology* 1982; **83**(3): 550–562.

28 Sutherland L, Singleton J, Sessions J *et al*. Double blind, placebo controlled trial of metronidazole in Crohn's disease. *Gut* 1991; **32**(9): 1071–1075.

29 Prantera C, Zannoni F, Scribano ML *et al*. An antibiotic regimen for the treatment of active Crohn's disease: a randomized, controlled clinical trial of metronidazole plus ciprofloxacin. *Am J Gastroenterol* 1996; **91**(2): 328–332.

30 Steinhart AH, Feagan BG, Wong CJ *et al*. Combined budesonide and antibiotic therapy for active Crohn's disease: a randomized controlled trial. *Gastroenterology* 2002; **123**(1): 33–40.

31 Selby W, Pavli P, Crotty B *et al*. Two-year combination antibiotic therapy with clarithromycin, rifabutin, and clofazimine for Crohn's disease. *Gastroenterology* 2007; **132**(7): 2313–2319.

32 Munkholm P, Langholz E, Davidsen M, Binder V. Disease activity courses in a regional cohort of Crohn's disease patients. *Scand J Gastroenterol* 1995; **30**(7): 699–706.

33 Candy S, Wright J, Gerber M, Adams G, Gerig M, Goodman R. A controlled double blind study of azathioprine in the management of Crohn's disease. *Gut* 1995; **37**(5): 674–678.

34 Sandborn WJ, Van OEC, Zins BJ, Tremaine WJ, Mays DC, Lipsky JJ. An intravenous loading dose of azathioprine decreases the time to response in patients with Crohn's disease. *Gastroenterology* 1995; **109**(6): 1808–1817.

35 Sandborn WJ, Tremaine WJ, Wolf DC *et al*. Lack of effect of intravenous administration on time to respond to azathioprine for steroid-treated Crohn's disease. North American Azathioprine Study Group. *Gastroenterology* 1999; **117**(3): 527–535.

36 Prefontaine E, Macdonald JK, Sutherland LR. Azathioprine or 6-mercaptopurine for induction of remission in Crohn's disease. *Cochrane Database Syst Rev* 2009; **4**(4): CD000545.

37 Feagan B. Cyclosporin has no proven role as a therapy for Crohn's disease. *Inflamm Bowel Dis* 1995; **1**: 335–339.

38 Feagan BG, McDonald JW, Rochon J *et al*. Low-dose cyclosporine for the treatment of Crohn's disease. The Canadian Crohn's

Relapse Prevention Trial Investigators. *N Engl J Med* 1994; **330**(26): 1846–1851.

39 Brynskov J, Freund L, Rasmussen SN *et al.* A placebo-controlled, double-blind, randomized trial of cyclosporine therapy in active chronic Crohn's disease. *N Engl J Med* 1989; **321**(13): 845–850.

40 Jewell DP, Lennard-Jones JE, Cyclosporin Study Group of Great Britain and Ireland. Oral cyclosporin for chronic active Crohn's disease: a multicentre controlled trial. *Eur J Gastroenterol Hepatol* 1994; **6**: 499–505.

41 Stange EF, Modigliani R, Pena AS, Wood AJ, Feutren G, Smith PR. European trial of cyclosporine in chronic active Crohn's disease: a 12-month study. The European Study Group. *Gastroenterology* 1995; **109**(3): 774–782.

42 Feutren G, Mihatsch MJ. Risk factors for cyclosporine-induced nephropathy in patients with autoimmune diseases. International Kidney Biopsy Registry of Cyclosporine in Autoimmune Diseases. *N Engl J Med* 1992; **326**(25): 1654–1660.

43 Hanauer SB, Smith MB. Rapid closure of Crohn's disease fistulas with continuous intravenous cyclosporin A. *Am J Gastroenterol* 1993; **88**(5): 646–649.

44 Present DH, Lichtiger S. Efficacy of cyclosporine in treatment of fistula of Crohn's disease. *Dig Dis Sci* 1994; **39**(2): 374–380.

45 Kozarek RA, Patterson DJ, Gelfand MD, Botoman VA, Ball TJ, Wilske KR. Methotrexate induces clinical and histologic remission in patients with refractory inflammatory bowel disease. *Ann Intern Med* 1989; **110**(5): 353–356.

46 Feagan BG, Rochon J, Fedorak RN *et al.* Methotrexate for the treatment of Crohn's disease. The North American Crohn's Study Group Investigators. *N Engl J Med* 1995; **332**(5): 292–297.

47 Van Deventer SJ. Tumour necrosis factor and Crohn's disease. *Gut* 1997; **40**(4): 443–448.

48 Derkx B, Taminiau J, Radema S *et al.* Tumour-necrosis-factor antibody treatment in Crohn's disease. *Lancet* 1993; **342**(8864): 173–174.

49 Targan SR, Hanauer SB, van Deventer SJ et al. A short-term study of chimeric monoclonal antibody cA2 to tumor necrosis factor alpha for Crohn's disease. Crohn's Disease cA2 Study Group. *N Engl J Med* 1997; **337**(15): 1029–1035.

50 Present DH, Rutgeerts P, Targan S *et al.* Infliximab for the treatment of fistulas in patients with Crohn's disease. *N Engl J Med* 1999; **340**(18): 1398–1405.

51 Hanauer SB, Sandborn WJ, Rutgeerts P *et al.* Human anti-tumor necrosis factor monoclonal antibody (adalimumab) in Crohn's disease: the CLASSIC-I trial. *Gastroenterology* 2006; **130**(2): 323–333; quiz 591.

52 Sandborn WJ, Feagan BG, Stoinov S *et al.* Certolizumab pegol for the treatment of Crohn's disease. *N Engl J Med* 2007; **357**(3): 228–238.

53 MacDonald JK, McDonald JW. Natalizumab for induction of remission in Crohn's disease. *Cochrane Database Syst Rev* 2007; **1**(1): CD006097.

54 Ghosh S, Goldin E, Gordon FH *et al.* Natalizumab for active Crohn's disease. *N Engl J Med* 2003; **348**(1): 24–32.

55 Targan SR, Feagan BG, Fedorak RN *et al.* Natalizumab for the treatment of active Crohn's disease: results of the ENCORE Trial. *Gastroenterology* 2007; **132**(5): 1672–1683.

56 Gordon FH, Lai CW, Hamilton MI *et al.* A randomized placebo-controlled trial of a humanized monoclonal antibody to alpha4 integrin in active Crohn's disease. *Gastroenterology* 2001; **121**(2): 268–274.

57 Sandborn WJ, Colombel JF, Enns R *et al.* Natalizumab induction and maintenance therapy for Crohn's disease. *N Engl J Med* 2005; **353**(18): 1912–1925.

58 Kleinschmidt-DeMasters BK, Tyler KL. Progressive multifocal leukoencephalopathy complicating treatment with natalizumab and interferon beta-1a for multiple sclerosis. *N Engl J Med* 2005; **353**(4): 369–374.

59 Langer-Gould A, Atlas SW, Green AJ, Bollen AW, Pelletier D. Progressive multifocal leukoencephalopathy in a patient treated with natalizumab. *N Engl J Med* 2005; **353**(4): 375–381.

60 Van Assche G, Van Ranst M, Sciot R *et al.* Progressive multifocal leukoencephalopathy after natalizumab therapy for Crohn's disease. *N Engl J Med* 2005; **353**(4): 362–368.

61 Yousry TA, Major EO, Ryschkewitsch C *et al.* Evaluation of patients treated with natalizumab for progressive multifocal leukoencephalopathy. *N Engl J Med* 2006; **354**(9): 924–933.

62 Sandborn WJ, Rutgeerts PJ, Reinisch W *et al.* One year data from the Sonic study: a randomized, double-blind trial comparing infliximab and infliximab plus azathioprine to azathioprine in patients with Crohn's disease naive to immunomodulators and biologic therapy. *Gastroenterology* 2009; **136**(5 Suppl. 1): 751f.

63 Feagan BG, McDonald JWD, Panaccione R *et al.* A randomized trial of methotrexate (MTX) in combination with infliximab (IFX) for the treatment of Crohn's disease (CD). *Gastroenterology* 2008; **135**: 294.

64 D'Haens G, Baert F, van Assche G *et al.* Early combined immunosuppression or conventional management in patients with newly diagnosed Crohn's disease: an open randomised trial. *Lancet* 2008; **371**(9613): 660–667.

65 Trial of a Treatment Algorithm for the Management of Crohn's Disease (REACT). Available at: http://www.clinicaltrials.gov/ct2/show/NCT01030809?term=react&rank=7. Accessed 26 January 2010.

66 Schultz M, Timmer A, Herfarth HH, Sartor RB, Vanderhoof JA, Rath HC. Lactobacillus GG in inducing and maintaining remission of Crohn's disease. *BMC Gastroenterology* 2004; **4**: 5.

67 Lapidus A, Bernell O, Hellers G, Lofberg R. Clinical course of colorectal Crohn's disease: a 35-year follow-up study of 507 patients. *Gastroenterology* 1998; **114**(6): 1151–1160.

68 Akobeng AK, Gardener E. Oral 5-aminosalicylic acid for maintenance of medically-induced remission in Crohn's disease. *Cochrane Database Syst Rev* 2005; **1**(1): CD003715.

69 Doherty G, Bennett G, Patil S, Cheifetz A, Moss AC. Interventions for prevention of post-operative recurrence of Crohn's disease. *Cochrane Database Syst Rev* 2009; **4**(4): CD006873.

70 Lochs H, Mayer M, Fleig WE *et al.* Prophylaxis of postoperative relapse in Crohn's disease with mesalamine: European Cooperative Crohn's Disease Study VI. *Gastroenterology* 2000; **118**(2): 264–273.

71 Greenberg GR, Feagan BG, Martin F *et al.* Oral budesonide as maintenance treatment for Crohn's disease: a placebo-controlled, dose-ranging study. Canadian Inflammatory Bowel Disease Study Group. *Gastroenterology* 1996; **110**(1): 45–51.

72 Lofberg R, Danielsson A, Suhr O *et al*. Oral budesonide versus prednisolone in patients with active extensive and left-sided ulcerative colitis. *Gastroenterology* 1996; **110**(6): 1713–1718.

73 Ferguson A, Campieri M, Doe W, Persson T, Nygard G. Oral budesonide as maintenance therapy in Crohn's disease – results of a 12-month study. Global Budesonide Study Group. *Aliment Pharmacol Ther* 1998; **12**(2): 175–183.

74 Benchimol EI, Seow CH, Otley AR, Steinhart AH. Budesonide for maintenance of remission in Crohn's disease. *Cochrane Database Syst Rev* 2009; **1**(1): CD002913.

75 Hellers G, Cortot A, Jewell D *et al*. Oral budesonide for prevention of postsurgical recurrence in Crohn's disease. The IOIBD Budesonide Study Group. *Gastroenterology* 1999; **116**(2): 294–300.

76 Ewe K, Bottger T, Buhr HJ, Ecker KW, Otto HF. Low-dose budesonide treatment for prevention of postoperative recurrence of Crohn's disease: a multicentre randomized placebo-controlled trial. German Budesonide Study Group. *Eur J Gastroenterol Hepatol* 1999; **11**(3): 277–282.

77 Borgaonkar M, MacIntosh D, Fardy J, Simms L. Anti-tuberculous therapy for maintaining remission of Crohn's disease. *Cochrane Database Syst Rev* 2000; **2**(2): CD000299.

78 Rutgeerts P, Hiele M, Geboes K *et al*. Controlled trial of metronidazole treatment for prevention of Crohn's recurrence after ileal resection. *Gastroenterology* 1995; **108**(6): 1617–1621.

79 Rutgeerts P. Strategies in the prevention of post-operative recurrence in Crohn's disease. *Best Pract Res Clin Gastroenterol* 2003; **17**(1): 63–73.

80 D'Haens GR, Vermeire S, Van Assche G *et al*. Therapy of metronidazole with azathioprine to prevent postoperative recurrence of Crohn's disease: a controlled randomized trial. *Gastroenterology* 2008; **135**(4): 1123–1129.

81 Rolfe VE, Fortun PJ, Hawkey CJ, Bath-Hextall F. Probiotics for maintenance of remission in Crohn's disease. *Cochrane Database Syst Rev* 2006; **4**(4): CD004826.

82 Prefontaine E, Sutherland LR, Macdonald JK, Cepoiu M. Azathioprine or 6-mercaptopurine for maintenance of remission in Crohn's disease. *Cochrane Database Syst Rev* 2009; **1**(1): CD000067.

83 Markowitz J, Grancher K, Kohn N, Lesser M, Daum F. A multicenter trial of 6-mercaptopurine and prednisone in children with newly diagnosed Crohn's disease. *Gastroenterology* 2000; **119**(4): 895–902.

84 Present DH, Meltzer SJ, Krumholz MP, Wolke A, Korelitz BI. 6-Mercaptopurine in the management of inflammatory bowel disease: short- and long-term toxicity. *Ann Intern Med* 1989; **111**(8): 641–649.

85 Reuther LO, Sonne J, Larsen NE *et al*. Pharmacological monitoring of azathioprine therapy. *Scand J Gastroenterol* 2003; **38**(9): 972–977.

86 NCT00521950. Cost-Effectiveness of TPMT Pharmacogenetics (TOPIC). 2007; Available at: http://www.clinicaltrials.gov/ct2/show/NCT00521950?term=TPMT&rank=1. Accessed 27 January 2010.

87 Kandiel A, Fraser AG, Korelitz BI, Brensinger C, Lewis JD. Increased risk of lymphoma among inflammatory bowel disease patients treated with azathioprine and 6-mercaptopurine. *Gut* 2005; **54**(8): 1121–1125.

88 Beaugerie L, Brousse N, Bouvier AM *et al*. Lymphoproliferative disorders in patients receiving thiopurines for inflammatory bowel disease: a prospective observational cohort study. *Lancet* 2009; **374**(9701): 1617–1625.

89 Feagan BG, Fedorak RN, Irvine EJ *et al*. A comparison of methotrexate with placebo for the maintenance of remission in Crohn's disease. North American Crohn's Study Group Investigators. *N Engl J Med* 2000; **342**(22): 1627–1632.

90 Alfadhli AA, McDonald JW, Feagan BG. Methotrexate for induction of remission in refractory Crohn's disease. *Cochrane Database Syst Rev* 2005; **1**(1): CD003459.

91 McKendry RJ. The remarkable spectrum of methotrexate toxicities. *Rheum Dis Clin North Am* 1997; **23**(4): 939–954.

92 Kremer JM, Alarcon GS, Lightfoot RW Jr *et al*. Methotrexate for rheumatoid arthritis. Suggested guidelines for monitoring liver toxicity. American College of Rheumatology. *Arthritis Rheum* 1994; **37**(3): 316–328.

93 Bernatsky S, Clarke AE, Suissa S. Hematologic malignant neoplasms after drug exposure in rheumatoid arthritis. *Arch Intern Med* 2008; **168**(4): 378–381.

94 Behm BW, Bickston SJ. Tumor necrosis factor-alpha antibody for maintenance of remission in Crohn's disease. *Cochrane Database Syst Rev* 2008; **1**(1): CD006893.

95 Hanauer SB, Feagan BG, Lichtenstein GR *et al*. Maintenance infliximab for Crohn's disease: the ACCENT I randomised trial. *Lancet* 2002; **359**(9317): 1541–1549.

96 Sands BE, Anderson FH, Bernstein CN *et al*. Infliximab maintenance therapy for fistulizing Crohn's disease. *N Engl J Med* 2004; **350**(9): 876–885.

97 Sandborn WJ, Feagan BG, Hanauer SB *et al*. An engineered human antibody to TNF (CDP571) for active Crohn's disease: a randomized double-blind placebo-controlled trial. *Gastroenterology* 2001; **120**(6): 1330–1338.

98 Rutgeerts P, D'Haens G, Targan S *et al*. Efficacy and safety of retreatment with anti-tumor necrosis factor antibody (infliximab) to maintain remission in Crohn's disease. *Gastroenterology* 1999; **117**(4): 761–769.

99 Feagan BG, Sandborn WJ, Lichtenstein G, Radford-Smith G, Patel J, Innes A. CDP571, a humanized monoclonal antibody to tumour necrosis factor-alpha, for steroid-dependent Crohn's disease: a randomized, double-blind, placebo-controlled trial. *Aliment Pharmacol Ther* 2006; **23**(5): 617–628.

100 Sandborn WJ, Feagan BG, Radford-Smith G *et al*. CDP571, a humanised monoclonal antibody to tumour necrosis factor alpha, for moderate to severe Crohn's disease: a randomised, double blind, placebo controlled trial. *Gut* 2004; **53**(10): 1485–1493.

101 Sandborn WJ, Hanauer SB, Rutgeerts P *et al*. Adalimumab for maintenance treatment of Crohn's disease: results of the CLASSIC II trial. *Gut* 2007; **56**(9): 1232–1239.

102 Colombel JF, Sandborn WJ, Rutgeerts P *et al*. Adalimumab for maintenance of clinical response and remission in patients with Crohn's disease: the CHARM trial. *Gastroenterology* 2007; **132**(1): 52–65.

103 Schreiber S, Khaliq-Kareemi M, Lawrance IC *et al*. Maintenance therapy with certolizumab pegol for Crohn's disease. *N Engl J Med* 2007; **357**(3): 239–250.

104 Loftus EV, Feagan BG, Colombel JF *et al*. Effects of adalimumab maintenance therapy on health-related quality of life of patients

with Crohn's disease: patient-reported outcomes of the CHARM trial. *Am J Gastroenterol* 2008; **103**(12): 3132–3141.

105 Feagan BG, Panaccione R, Sandborn WJ *et al*. Effects of adalimumab therapy on incidence of hospitalization and surgery in Crohn's disease: results from the CHARM study. *Gastroenterology* 2008; **135**(5): 1493–1499.

106 Lichtenstein GR, Feagan BG, Cohen RD *et al*. Serious infections and mortality in association with therapies for Crohn's disease: TREAT registry. *Clin Gastroenterol Hepatol* 2006; **4**(5): 621–630.

107 Long R, Gardam M. Tumour necrosis factor-alpha inhibitors and the reactivation of latent tuberculosis infection. *CMAJ* 2003; **168**(9): 1153–1156.

108 Keane J, Gershon S, Wise RP *et al*. Tuberculosis associated with infliximab, a tumor necrosis factor alpha-neutralizing agent. *N Engl J Med* 2001; **345**(15): 1098–1104.

109 Gardam MA, Keystone EC, Menzies R *et al*. Anti-tumour necrosis factor agents and tuberculosis risk: mechanisms of action and clinical management. *Lancet Infect Dis* 2003; **3**(3): 148–155.

110 Warris A, Bjorneklett A, Gaustad P. Invasive pulmonary aspergillosis associated with infliximab therapy. *N Engl J Med* 2001; **344**(14): 1099–1100.

111 Gluck T, Linde HJ, Scholmerich J, Muller-Ladner U, Fiehn C, Bohland P. Anti-tumor necrosis factor therapy and Listeria monocytogenes infection: report of two cases. *Arthritis Rheum* 2002; **46**(8): 2255–2257; author reply 2257.

112 Tai TL, O'Rourke KP, McWeeney M, Burke CM, Sheehan K, Barry M. Pneumocystis carinii pneumonia following a second infusion of infliximab. *Rheumatology* (Oxford) 2002; **41**(8): 951–952.

113 Lichtenstein GR, Cohen RD, Feagan BG *et al*. Safety of infliximab and other Crohn's disease therapies – Treat™ Registry data with nearly 20,000 patient-years of follow-up. *Gastroenterology* 2007; **132**(4 Suppl. 2): A178.

114 Endres S, Ghorbani R, Kelley VE *et al*. The effect of dietary supplementation with n-3 polyunsaturated fatty acids on the synthesis of interleukin-1 and tumor necrosis factor by mononuclear cells. *N Engl J Med* 1989; **320**(5): 265–271.

115 Teitelbaum JE, Allan Walker W. Review: the role of omega-3 fatty acids in intestinal inflammation. *J Nutr Biochem* 2001; **12**(1): 21–32.

116 Belluzzi A, Brignola C, Campieri M, Pera A, Boschi S, Miglioli M. Effect of an enteric-coated fish-oil preparation on relapses in Crohn's disease. *N Engl J Med* 1996; **334**(24): 1557–1560.

117 Lorenz-Meyer H, Bauer P, Nicolay C *et al*. Omega-3 fatty acids and low carbohydrate diet for maintenance of remission in Crohn's disease. A randomized controlled multicenter trial. Study Group Members (German Crohn's Disease Study Group). *Scand J Gastroenterol* 1996; **31**(8): 778–785.

118 Feagan BG, Sandborn WJ, Mittmann U *et al*. Omega-3 free fatty acids for the maintenance of remission in Crohn disease: the EPIC Randomized Controlled Trials. *JAMA* 2008; **299**(14): 1690–1697.

119 Turner D, Zlotkin SH, Shah PS, Griffiths AM. Omega-3 fatty acids (fish oil) for maintenance of remission in Crohn's disease. *Cochrane Database Syst Rev* 2009; **1**(1):CD006320.

12 Ulcerative colitis

Derek P Jewell[1], Lloyd R Sutherland[2], John WD McDonald[3] and Brian G Feagan[3]

[1] Experimental Medicine Division, John Radcliffe Hospital, Oxford, UK
[2] Department of Community Health Sciences, University of Calgary Health Sciences Centre, Calgary, Canada
[3] Robarts Clinical Trials, Robarts Research Unit, University of Western Ontario, London, Ontario, Canada

Introduction

Patients with ulcerative colitis have a variety of questions for those practitioners who treat their disease. This chapter focuses on the evidence on which decisions relating to patient advice (prognosis for the first attack, extension of disease, risk of cancer) and treatment options should be made. Our recommendations are based wherever possible on evidence from published population-based studies and randomized controlled clinical trials. Where several clinical trials have addressed the same question we have frequently used meta-analyses to summarize the results.

Histological diagnosis

The diagnosis of ulcerative colitis and Crohn's disease, together with accurate differentiation between them and other inflammatory diseases of the colon relies on a combination of clinical, radiological, endoscopic and histological features. Accurate histological interpretation is crucial but is confounded by at least four major problems:

• Variability in assessing normal colorectal histology and assessing minimal degrees of inflammation.
• Considerable overlap in the histological changes of most colonic inflammatory conditions.
• Accuracy and reproducibility of many of the histological features commonly used for diagnosis have not been determined.
• Absence of standard nomenclature.

Recently, a working party of the British Society of Gastroenterology has published guidelines for the biopsy diagnosis of suspected chronic inflammatory bowel disease

[1]. Databases were searched for papers relating to reproducibility, sensitivity and specificity of histological features used for the differential diagnosis of inflammatory bowel disease (IBD). Only those achieving moderate reproducibility (a minimum κ statistic of 0.4 or a percentage agreement of 80% or more) were included. Precise definitions of mucosal architectural changes, lamina propria cellularity, neutrophil infiltration and epithelial cell abnormalities were derived from the systematic review of the literature. Then the quality of the evidence for these features with respect to differential diagnosis was rated according to the criteria recommended by the evidence-based working party. Features for which the literature review provided high quality evidence for their use in differential diagnosis are shown in Figure 12.1. These histopathological criteria formed the basis of guidelines for clinical practice, thereby helping to ensure uniformity and consistency of reporting. Subsequently, a workshop was set up to examine the value of these guidelines [2]. A group of histopathologists was asked to report on a series of colonoscopic biopsies from 60 patients. The group consisted of 13 pathologists with a special interest in IBD and 12 general pathologists. Following this, there was a discussion with regard to the evidence-based guidelines, and the biopsy specimens were then renumbered and re-reported. For ulcerative colitis, the accuracy of reporting was similar in both the first and second rounds, and there was little difference between the expert pathologists and the generalists. However, there was improved accuracy in reporting Crohn's disease following discussion of the guidelines: for the experts accuracy improved from 56% to 64% and for the general pathologists from 50% to 60%. The same workshop was also able to show that multiple, as opposed to single, biopsies led to better and more reproducible diagnoses, especially for Crohn's disease. Thus, the introduction of evidence-based guidelines and training in their use are helpful, predominantly for Crohn's disease, but result in a more accurate histopathological diagnosis only in one in ten colonoscopic series reported.

Evidence-Based Gastroenterology and Hepatology, 3rd edition.
J. McDonald, A.K. Burroughs, B. Feagan, and M.B. Fennerty. © 2010
Blackwell Publishing Ltd

Review: Ulc. Colitis: induction of remission, 5-ASA
Comparison: 5-ASA vs placebo
Outcome: Failure to induce global/clinical remission

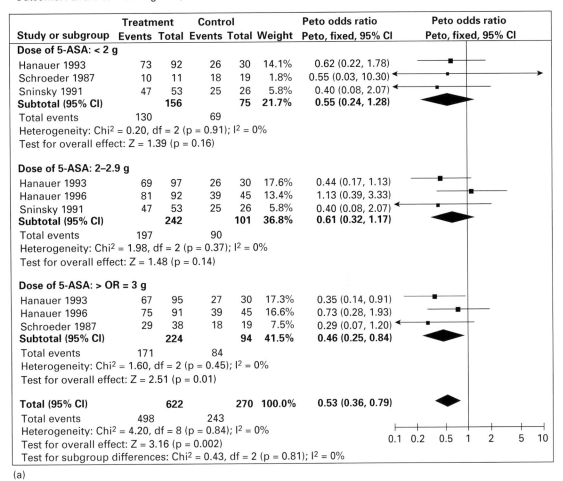

Study or subgroup	Treatment Events	Total	Control Events	Total	Weight	Peto odds ratio Peto, fixed, 95% CI
Dose of 5-ASA: < 2 g						
Hanauer 1993	73	92	26	30	14.1%	0.62 (0.22, 1.78)
Schroeder 1987	10	11	18	19	1.8%	0.55 (0.03, 10.30)
Sninsky 1991	47	53	25	26	5.8%	0.40 (0.08, 2.07)
Subtotal (95% CI)		**156**		**75**	**21.7%**	**0.55 (0.24, 1.28)**
Total events	130		69			
Heterogeneity: Chi² = 0.20, df = 2 (p = 0.91); I² = 0%						
Test for overall effect: Z = 1.39 (p = 0.16)						
Dose of 5-ASA: 2–2.9 g						
Hanauer 1993	69	97	26	30	17.6%	0.44 (0.17, 1.13)
Hanauer 1996	81	92	39	45	13.4%	1.13 (0.39, 3.33)
Sninsky 1991	47	53	25	26	5.8%	0.40 (0.08, 2.07)
Subtotal (95% CI)		**242**		**101**	**36.8%**	**0.61 (0.32, 1.17)**
Total events	197		90			
Heterogeneity: Chi² = 1.98, df = 2 (p = 0.37); I² = 0%						
Test for overall effect: Z = 1.48 (p = 0.14)						
Dose of 5-ASA: > OR = 3 g						
Hanauer 1993	67	95	27	30	17.3%	0.35 (0.14, 0.91)
Hanauer 1996	75	91	39	45	16.6%	0.73 (0.28, 1.93)
Schroeder 1987	29	38	18	19	7.5%	0.29 (0.07, 1.20)
Subtotal (95% CI)		**224**		**94**	**41.5%**	**0.46 (0.25, 0.84)**
Total events	171		84			
Heterogeneity: Chi² = 1.60, df = 2 (p = 0.45); I² = 0%						
Test for overall effect: Z = 2.51 (p = 0.01)						
Total (95% CI)		**622**		**270**	**100.0%**	**0.53 (0.36, 0.79)**
Total events	498		243			
Heterogeneity: Chi² = 4.20, df = 8 (p = 0.84); I² = 0%						
Test for overall effect: Z = 3.16 (p = 0.002)						
Test for subgroup differences: Chi² = 0.43, df = 2 (p = 0.81); I² = 0%						

(a)

Figure 12.1 Evidence-based features for histological diagnosis of colonic biopsy specimens. Note: all features have the highest quality of evidence except for: (a) evidence of diagnostic value from single studies only and (b) no published evidence of accuracy or reproducibility. IBD: inflammatory bowel disease; UC: ulcerative colitis; CD: Crohn's disease.

Prognosis

Population-based studies

The importance of recognizing that the prognosis for referred patients differs from that of a regional population was recognized by Truelove and Pena over three decades ago [3]. They found that the survival of patients who were referred to Oxford (UK) from other regions was significantly reduced compared with that of patients who actually resided in the Oxford catchment area.

There are several population-based studies on the prognosis for patients with ulcerative colitis. Sinclair and associates described the prognosis of 537 patients with ulcerative colitis, seen between 1967 and 1976 in northeastern Scotland [4]. They found a high proportion of cases with distal

disease (70%). The overall mortality and surgical resection rates in the first attack were both 3%. During this period of time, the mortality for severe, first-time attacks was 23%. However, there were only modest differences in the observed and expected mortality for the ulcerative colitis population. The colectomy rate after five years was 8%.

The prognosis and mortality associated with ulcerative colitis in Stockholm county were reported by Persson *et al.* [5]. In their review of 1547 patients followed from 1955 to 1984, they found that the mortality in the patient population was higher than that expected in the general population. After 15 years of follow-up, the survival rate was 94% of that expected based on the age and sex of the study population. The relative survival rates differed more for patients with pancolitis than for patients with proctitis, but the confidence intervals overlapped. While ulcerative colitis was the most important influence on the increased

Review: Ulc. Colitis: maintenance of remission, 5-ASA
Comparison: 5-ASA vs placebo
Outcome: Failure to maintain clinical or endoscopic remission

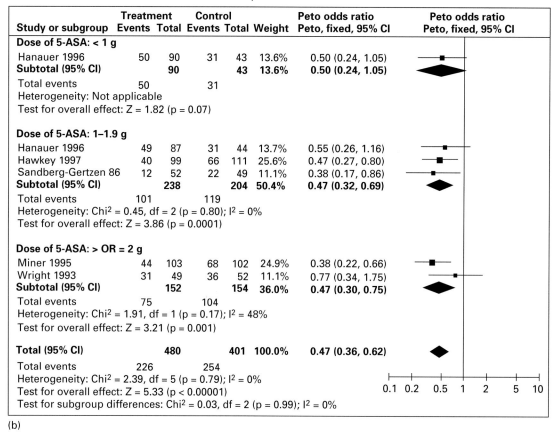

(b)

Figure 12.1 *Continued*

mortality, deaths from colorectal cancer, asthma and non-alcoholic liver disease were also increased.

Danish investigators have also reported the results of their population-based assessment of the prognosis of ulcerative colitis. Their population included 1161 patients with ulcerative colitis followed for up to 25 years (median 11 years) [6]. Of the 1161 patients, 235 underwent colectomy. Interestingly, 60 of these patients presented with proctosigmoiditis initially. The cumulative colectomy rate was 9%, 24%, 30% and 32% at 1, 10, 15 and 25 years respectively, after diagnosis. At any one time, nearly half of the clinic population was in remission. Prognostic factors associated with frequent relapses included: the number of relapses in the first three years after diagnosis and the year of diagnosis (1960s vs 1970s vs 1980s). Surprisingly, signs and symptoms of weight loss or fever were associated with fewer relapses on follow-up. A recent report on the same inception cohort of patients, published nearly ten years after these initial observations, has shown that overall life expectancy is normal for patients with ulcerative colitis, but patients over 50 years of age with extensive colitis at diagnosis have an increased mortality within the first two years, due to colitis-associated postoperative complications and co-morbidity [7].

Another report by the same investigators focused on the prognosis in children with ulcerative colitis [8]. Eighty of the 1161 patients in the cohort were children who presented with more extensive disease compared with adults. The cumulative colectomy rate did not differ from that of adults (29% at 20 years). At any interval from diagnosis, the majority of children were thought to be in remission.

Two prospective population studies are in progress in Europe (the European Collaborative Study on Inflammatory Bowel Diseases and the Inflammatory Bowel South Eastern Norway (IBSEN) cohort) but only one-year, follow-up data have so far been reported [9, 10].

Extension of disease

Ayres and associates reported their experience with extension of disease in 145 patients presenting with proctitis or proctosigmoiditis, followed prospectively for a median of 11 years. By life-table analysis, extension occurred in 16%

and 31% of patients at five and ten years' follow-up respectively. Extension was associated with a clinical exacerbation of disease in most cases, but no specific clinical factors were associated with disease extension [11].

Much higher rates of progression have been reported, largely in retrospective non-population-based series. However, in the IBSEN cohort, 22% of 130 patients with a new diagnosis of ulcerative colitis had progressed to more extensive disease during the first year of follow-up [12]. The most recent study from Italy included 273 patients with proctitis [13]. It is retrospective and not population-based (patients were identified in 13 hospitals) but it is the largest cohort yet reported. Overall, proximal extension occurred in 27.1% during clinical and endoscopic follow-up: 20% at five years and 54% at ten years. However, the disease only extended into the sigmoid in the majority and into the splenic flexure in only 10% of the patients. An interesting observation was that smoking protected against disease progression on univariate analysis.

While research for the most part has focused on extension of disease, Langholz and colleagues report a much more dynamic pattern. After 25 years of follow-up, 53% of patients with limited disease had extension of disease, but in 75% of patients with extensive disease, the disease boundary had regressed [14]. This dynamic process, if confirmed by others, could have implications in terms of cancer surveillance programs. One potential explanation for these findings is that in the early years of the study, disease extent was assessed by radiological techniques.

Cancer surveillance (see also Chapter 17)

Although ulcerative colitis is a premalignant condition, the proportion of patients who develop cancer is small. In a population study using a retrospectively assembled cohort of patients the cumulative risk at 20 years of disease was about 7% and rose to 12% at 30 years [15]. This study is likely to have included all or nearly all patients with ulcerative colitis in two regions of England and one of Sweden and referral bias is probably minimal. Follow-up was both of long duration (17–38 years) and thorough (97%). On the other hand, in centers with an aggressive policy of colectomy, no increased cancer risk has been seen [16]. In all studies, length of history and extent of disease are important factors. Thus, left-sided colitis carries only a slightly increased risk while extensive colitis increases the risk about 20 times over that of an age and sex-matched population. Whether early age of onset of ulcerative colitis is an independent risk factor is controversial. Children tend to have extensive disease and have greater life expectancy than adults; they are, therefore, more likely to be at risk.

There is some controversy concerning the role of colonoscopic surveillance in detection of cancer. Most centers carry out colonoscopy in patients with extensive disease 8–10 years after diagnosis. Even at that stage, a few patients with dysplasia or a frank carcinoma will be identified. However, the subsequent pick-up rate during the surveillance program is small (about 11%) and in one center only two cancers were detected in 200 patients over a 20-year period [17]. Furthermore, cancers can develop outside the screening program. Thus, the need for colonoscopic surveillance has been questioned and no controlled study has shown that surveillance reduces mortality. However, in the published studies, the five-year survival rates for cancers detected in asymptomatic patients have been considerably higher than was observed in those presenting with symptoms. **B4 C5**

A second controversial area is the management of patients with endoscopically visible lesions. Where such lesions are associated with dysplasia in the adjacent mucosa (dysplasia-associated lesions or masses (DALMs)) the incidence of cancer appears to be very high and prophylactic colectomy is recommended [18, 19]. However, polyps for which there is no associated dysplasia in adjacent mucosa do not appear to carry this high risk of cancer, and in such cases conservative management rather than colectomy is recommended [20, 21]. **B4 C5**

Reviewing the evidence for dysplasia surveillance, Riddell recommended obtaining three to four biopsies every 10 cm [22]. Annual colonoscopy is probably ideal, but two-yearly colonoscopy with intervening flexible sigmoidoscopy in alternate years is a compromise. Dysplasia detected at the initial screening colonoscopy should lead to colectomy, as there is a high chance of concomitant cancer. Indeed, most clinicians advocate colectomy whenever dysplasia is found, even when it is low grade. There is no doubt that such a policy abolishes the cancer risk but justification for it for patients with low grade dysplasia remains controversial [23, 24]. The development of molecular markers may help to resolve the issue.

Treatment

The treatment of ulcerative colitis can be conveniently discussed for each category or class of medications, and in terms of either induction or maintenance of remission.

Aminosalicylates

With the discovery of sulfasalazine by Svartz [25], the first effective agent for the treatment of ulcerative colitis became available. The first trial that established the efficacy of sulfasalazine for the induction of remission was reported in 1962 [26]. **A1c** Misiewicz and colleagues were the first to study its efficacy as maintenance therapy [27]. An early

Review: Ulc. Colitis: induction of remission, 5-ASA
Comparison: 5-ASA vs sulfasalazine
Outcome: Failure to induce global/clinical remission

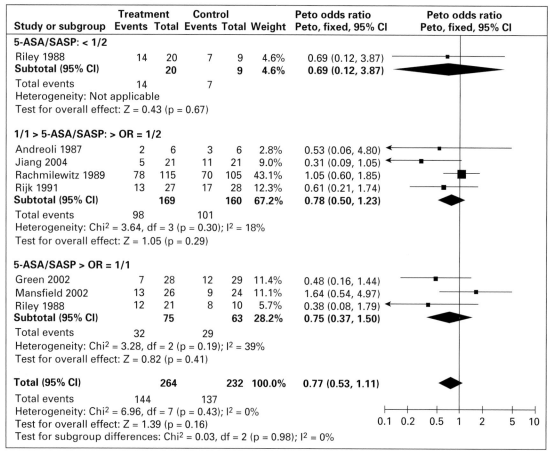

Study or subgroup	Treatment Events	Total	Control Events	Total	Weight	Peto odds ratio Peto, fixed, 95% CI	Peto odds ratio Peto, fixed, 95% CI
5-ASA/SASP: < 1/2							
Riley 1988	14	20	7	9	4.6%	0.69 (0.12, 3.87)	
Subtotal (95% CI)		**20**		**9**	**4.6%**	**0.69 (0.12, 3.87)**	
Total events	14		7				
Heterogeneity: Not applicable							
Test for overall effect: Z = 0.43 (p = 0.67)							
1/1 > 5-ASA/SASP: > OR = 1/2							
Andreoli 1987	2	6	3	6	2.8%	0.53 (0.06, 4.80)	
Jiang 2004	5	21	11	21	9.0%	0.31 (0.09, 1.05)	
Rachmilewitz 1989	78	115	70	105	43.1%	1.05 (0.60, 1.85)	
Rijk 1991	13	27	17	28	12.3%	0.61 (0.21, 1.74)	
Subtotal (95% CI)		**169**		**160**	**67.2%**	**0.78 (0.50, 1.23)**	
Total events	98		101				
Heterogeneity: Chi² = 3.64, df = 3 (p = 0.30); I² = 18%							
Test for overall effect: Z = 1.05 (p = 0.29)							
5-ASA/SASP > OR = 1/1							
Green 2002	7	28	12	29	11.4%	0.48 (0.16, 1.44)	
Mansfield 2002	13	26	9	24	11.1%	1.64 (0.54, 4.97)	
Riley 1988	12	21	8	10	5.7%	0.38 (0.08, 1.79)	
Subtotal (95% CI)		**75**		**63**	**28.2%**	**0.75 (0.37, 1.50)**	
Total events	32		29				
Heterogeneity: Chi² = 3.28, df = 2 (p = 0.19); I² = 39%							
Test for overall effect: Z = 0.82 (p = 0.41)							
Total (95% CI)		**264**		**232**	**100.0%**	**0.77 (0.53, 1.11)**	
Total events	144		137				
Heterogeneity: Chi² = 6.96, df = 7 (p = 0.43); I² = 0%							
Test for overall effect: Z = 1.39 (p = 0.16)							
Test for subgroup differences: Chi² = 0.03, df = 2 (p = 0.98); I² = 0%							

Figure 12.2 Failure to induce clinical or endoscopic remission in ulcerative colitis. Randomized controlled clinical trials of mesalamine (5-ASA) and sulfasalazine (SASP): (a) mesalamine (Expt) versus placebo (Ctrl), (b) mesalamine (Expt) versus sulfasalazine (Ctrl). (Source: Sutherland LR *et al. Cochrane Database Syst Rev* 2006; 2: CD000543 [34]).

randomized trial in the UK established the importance of continuous therapy [28]. **Alc** Azad Khan and the Oxford group established that 2 g/day of sulfasalazine provided the optimal trade-off between efficacy and adverse effects [29].

The finding that mesalamine (5-ASA) is the active moiety of sulfasalazine stimulated a decade of trials of induction and maintenance of remission [30, 31]. Numerous aminosalicylate delivery systems have been developed. These include drugs that release 5-ASA upon bacterial splitting of the azo bond (for example sulfasalazine, olsalazine and balsalazide), pH dependent release formulations (for example Asacol (pH 7) and Claversal/Mesasal/Salofalk (pH 6)), and a microsphere preparation (Pentasa) [32].

The efficacy of oral mesalamine has been evaluated by meta-analyses of randomized controlled trials [33–35]. As shown in Figure 12.2a, mesalamine is more effective than placebo for the induction of remission (pooled odds ratio 0.51; CI: 0.35–0.76) [34]. **Ala** The newer 5-ASA preparations

were not significantly more effective than sulfasalazine, however, for active disease (pooled odds ratio 0.75; CI: 0.50–1.13) (see Figure 12.2b). On the other hand, adverse events were less frequently noted with mesalamine than with sulfasalazine: the number of patients needed to treat (NNT) with mesalamine rather than sulfasalazine to avoid an adverse event in one patient is approximately 7. **Ala**

Figure 12.3a illustrates the results of a meta-analysis that demonstrates the superiority of aminosalicylates over placebo for maintenance of remission (pooled odds ratio 0.47; CI: 0.36–0.62) [35]. **Ala** Conflicting results were obtained in studies comparing sulfasalazine with mesalamine for maintenance therapy. The overall results are shown in Figure 12.3b; sulfasalazine appeared to be more effective than mesalamine (pooled odds ratio 1.29; CI: 1.05–1.57). **Ala** When only studies with a minimum of 12 months' follow-up were included in the analysis, however, there was no statistically significant advantage for sulfasalazine (pooled odds ratio 1.15; CI: 0.89–1.50). There are a number

Review: Ulc. Colitis: maintenance of remission, 5-ASA
Comparison: 5-ASA vs sulfasalazine
Outcome: Failure to maintain clinical or endoscopic remission

Study or subgroup	Treatment Events	Total	Control Events	Total	Weight	Peto odds ratio Peto, fixed, 95% CI
Andreoli 1987	3	7	1	6	0.8%	3.11 (0.32, 30.11)
Ardizzone 1995	20	44	27	44	5.7%	0.53 (0.23, 1.22)
Ireland 1988	35	82	21	82	9.6%	2.13 (1.12, 4.05)
Kiilerich 1992	61	114	55	112	14.7%	1.19 (0.71, 2.01)
Kruis 1995	39	108	13	40	6.9%	1.17 (0.55, 2.50)
McIntyre 1988	20	41	14	38	5.1%	1.62 (0.67, 3.92)
Mulder 1988	19	42	20	36	5.1%	0.67 (0.27, 1.61)
Nilsson 1995	88	161	76	161	20.9%	1.35 (0.87, 2.08)
Rijk 1992	14	23	11	23	3.0%	1.67 (0.53, 5.27)
Riley 1988	20	50	23	50	6.4%	0.78 (0.36, 1.73)
Rutgeerts 1989	90	167	70	167	21.7%	1.61 (1.05, 2.48)
Total (95% CI)		839		759	100.0%	1.29 (1.05, 1.57)

Total events 409 331
Heterogeneity: $Chi^2 = 12.61$, df = 10 (p = 0.25); $I^2 = 21\%$
Test for overall effect: Z = 2.47 (p = 0.01)

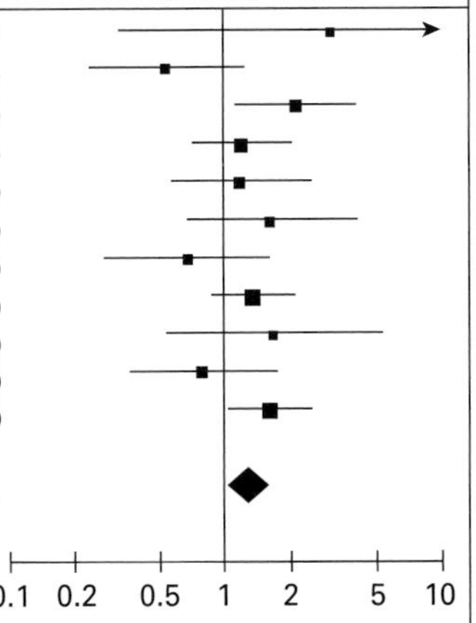

Figure 12.3 Failure to maintain clinical or endoscopic remission in ulcerative colitis. Randomized controlled clinical trials of mesalamine (5-ASA) and sulfasalazine (SASP): (a) mesalamine (Expt) versus placebo (Ctrl), (b) mesalamine (Expt) versus sulfasalazine (Ctrl). (Source: Sutherland LR et al. *Cochrane Database Syst Rev* 2006; 4: CD000544 [35]).

of possible explanations for this discrepancy. First, the observation in the overall analysis may be correct: sulfasalazine may be a more effective delivery system than mesalamine. Second, the analysis that was restricted to studies with 12 months' follow-up might have lacked sufficient statistical power to detect a small difference in efficacy. Third, the high drop-out rate with olsalazine therapy might have biased the overall results against mesalamine. Finally, it is possible that the comparison studies suffered from selection bias. With the exception of one trial, the inclusion criteria included tolerance to sulfasalazine [36]. This factor would tend to minimize the occurrence of adverse events with sulfasalazine therapy.

Several oral 5-ASA preparations are available, but two warrant special mention. Olsalazine and balsalazide appear to be approximately as effective as sulfasalazine and mesalamine in the treatment of active ulcerative colitis and in the maintenance of remission. There have been concerns about the development of secretory diarrhea with olsalazine [37, 38], due to interference with Na^+/K^+-ATPase, but the frequency of this adverse effect can be minimized by taking the medication in divided doses with meals [39, 40]. Moreover, systemic absorption of 5-ASA and its metabolites is less with olsalazine than with mesalamine, which might translate into a smaller risk of nephropathy [41, 42]. Several randomized controlled trials have demonstrated a slight (and statistically insignificant) advantage of balsalazide (in a dosage of 6.75 g/day) to sulfasalazine 3 g/day or mesalamine 2.4 g/day in the treatment of active ulcerative colitis. **Ald** The newer agent may provide relief of symptoms and sigmoidoscopic healing more quickly than mesalamine [43–45], and may be better tolerated [46]. Balsalazide 3 g/day appears to be as effective as mesalamine 1.2 g/day at maintaining remission, and may provide better relief of nocturnal symptoms in the first three months of maintenance therapy [47]. It should be noted that these observations suggesting small advantages of balsalazide over mesalamine depend on *post hoc* subgroup analyses of relatively small groups of patients and should be interpreted with some caution.

Topical therapy is a logical option for patients with disease limited to the distal colon. In theory, it presents a high concentration of mesalamine to the affected area, while minimizing systemic absorption. Marshall and Irvine have published two meta-analyses of topical therapy [48, 49]. The first analysis established that topical mesalamine was effective for both induction and maintenance therapy in patients with distal disease [48]. **Alc** The second analysis found that mesalamine was more effective than topical corticosteroids for the induction of remission [49]. **Alc** Foam enemas can reliably deliver mesalamine to the rectum and sigmoid colon, and sometimes even to the descending colon, in healthy individuals and patients with ulcerative colitis [50–53]. Foam enemas are superior to placebo, and are at least as easily tolerated and effective as liquid enemas [54–56]. Gel enemas may be better tolerated than foam preparations [57]. Mesalamine suppositories have been shown to be effective for the maintenance of remission of ulcerative proctitis [58]. **Ald**

Some patients may benefit from a combination of oral and topical 5-ASA preparations. A small randomized trial performed by Safdi et al. suggested that combined topical and oral 5-aminosalicylate therapy may be more effective than oral therapy alone [59]. This result was confirmed by Marteau *et al.* in a large randomized, double-blind, placebo-controlled trial in which 127 patients with mild to moderately active colitis were randomized to receive either a 5-aminosalicylate enema or a placebo enema for the first four weeks of treatment with oral 5-ASA 4 g/day [60]. At eight weeks the observed remission rates were: 5-ASA enema 64%, placebo enema 43%, p = 0.03.

Corticosteroids

Corticosteroids remain the standard therapy for moderate to severe ulcerative colitis. Truelove and Witts were the first to undertake a randomized, controlled trial of cortisone in patients with active colitis, and showed that 100 mg/day, followed by tapering over six weeks, was an effective treatment [61]. **Alc** Lennard-Jones and associates reported similar efficacy for prednisone [62]. It appears that once daily dosage yields similar effectiveness as divided doses of the medication [63].

The assumption that there is no additional benefit from the use of more than 40 mg/day of prednisone is based on a small randomized trial conducted by Baron and colleagues [64]. This trial compared the outcomes of 58 outpatients who were randomized to 20, 40, or 60 mg of prednisone per day. Although either 40 or 60 mg/day yielded better results than 20 mg/day, no difference in results was observed in patients given 40 versus 60 mg/day. The study included too few patients, however, to have sufficient statistical power to rule out a relative benefit from the 60 mg dose. **Ald**

Budesonide is a potent second-generation corticosteroid with 90% first pass metabolism, resulting in decreased systemic toxicity [65]. A randomized, controlled trial demonstrated that a targeted colonic release formulation of budesonide appeared to be as effective as prednisolone

and exhibited a more favorable adverse event profile [66]. **Ald**

Budesonide enemas have also been used for active distal disease. A meta-analysis published by Marshall and Irvine documented that they are as effective as conventional steroid enemas [67]. **Alc** The only published trial comparing budesonide enemas with 5-ASA enemas revealed no differences in endoscopic or histopathologic scores between the treatment groups, but the clinical remission rate was greater with 5-ASA (60% vs 38%, p = 0.03) [67].

Most reported trials have demonstrated no benefit for corticosteroids in the maintenance of remission of ulcerative colitis [68–70].

Azathioprine and 6-mercaptopurine

Most trials of anti-metabolite drugs in ulcerative colitis have been small. There is no evidence that azathioprine (2–5 mg/kg/day) combined with prednisolone induces remission more effectively than steroids alone [71]. **Alc**

Nevertheless, azathioprine has been shown to have a steroid-sparing effect at doses between 1.5 and 2.5 mg/kg/day, and the major indication for this drug in ulcerative colitis is for patients who require continuing steroid therapy [72, 73].

In the double-blind, randomized, controlled trial conducted by Jewell and Truelove, patients who had gone into remission during the acute stage were weaned off steroids and given either placebo or maintenance therapy with azathioprine for one year [71]. Overall, azathioprine offered no statistically significant advantage over placebo for reducing the relapse rate. There may have been some benefit to azathioprine, however, in the subgroup of patients who were treated for relapsing disease, as opposed to those who presented with their first episode of colitis, as illustrated in Table 12.1. Specifically, 9 of 24 azathioprine-treated patients in the former group had no relapse during

Table 12.1 Clinical course during trial in two treatment groups of patients according to whether patients entered trial in first attack of ulcerative colitis or in relapse.

No. of relapses	Admitted in first attack		Admitted in relapses	
	Azathioprine group	Control group	Azathioprine group	Control group
0	7	6	9	3
1–2	5	6	8	7
3 or failed	4	3	7	15
Total	16	15	24	25
Significance of differences[a]		NS	p = 0.055	

[a] Fisher's exact test.
Reproduced from Jewell DP *et al. BMJ* 1974; iv: 627–630 [71].

follow-up, compared with 3 of 25 patients given placebo. More detailed *post hoc* analysis revealed that only seven patients in the azathioprine group experienced at least three relapses or failed therapy, compared with 15 patients in the placebo group (p = 0.055). These analyses should be interpreted with caution because they represent *post hoc* subgroup analyses of small numbers of patients.

Hawthorne and colleagues conducted an azathioprine withdrawal trial that suggested a benefit for this drug in the maintenance of remission [74]. In this study, patients who were in long-term remission while taking azathioprine were randomized to continue with the medication or take placebo. During the subsequent year of follow-up, patients receiving placebo relapsed significantly more often than did those who remained on azathioprine. **A1d** It should be pointed out, however, that this type of trial design cannot be used to estimate the size of the treatment effect from an intervention. It is possible that only a small proportion of patients can be maintained in remission with azathioprine, and that most of these patients would relapse if the drug were withdrawn. More recently, Sood *et al.* randomized 35 patients with newly diagnosed ulcerative colitis, all of whom received corticosteroids to induce remission, to receive either sulfasalazine and azathioprine, or sulfasalazine and a placebo for one year [75]. Four patients (23.5%) who received azathioprine suffered relapse of disease, compared to 10 (55.6%) who received sulfasalazine alone (p < 0.05). **A1d** This is somewhat stronger evidence that azathioprine is beneficial for maintenance of remission in ulcerative colitis, but the results should be confirmed with a larger study.

A single small randomized trial reported by Maté-Jimenez *et al.* using 6-mercaptopurine rather than azathioprine showed 6-mercaptopurine to be more effective than methotrexate or 5-ASA for induction and maintenance of remission in ulcerative colitis (see below) [76]. **A1d**

Methotrexate

There have been anecdotal reports of the steroid-sparing effects of methotrexate in patients with chronic active ulcerative colitis. In a double-blind, randomized, controlled trial 67 patients with steroid-dependent disease were randomized to either oral methotrexate 12.5 mg per week (30 patients) or placebo (37 patients) for nine months [77]. No benefit was demonstrated for methotrexate in terms of disease activity, remission rate or steroid dosage. **A1c** The dosage of methotrexate employed in this study, however, was smaller than those used in case reports (up to 25 mg intramuscularly per week). A subsequent small study using oral methotrexate at a dose of 15 mg/week in steroid-dependent ulcerative colitis found that the dosage of corticosteroids could be reduced acutely but that the benefit was not maintained over the subsequent 76 weeks [76]. In

this study Maté-Jimenez *et al.* compared 6-mercaptopurine (1.5 mg/kg), methotrexate (15 mg orally weekly), and 5-ASA (3 g daily) for induction and maintenance of remission in 34 steroid-dependent patients with ulcerative colitis [76]. They reported that 6-mercaptopurine was more effective than either methotrexate or 5-ASA for both induction and maintenance of remission in these patients. **A1d** Larger studies using higher doses of methotrexate would be of interest.

Cyclosporin

There have been no randomized controlled trials of oral cyclosporin in patients with ulcerative colitis, and case reports have not suggested impressive efficacy. Anecdotal reports of benefit from intravenous cyclosporin led to a randomized controlled trial by Lichtiger and associates, involving 20 patients with severe ulcerative colitis unresponsive to 7–10 days of intravenous hydrocortisone therapy [78]. Patients received either cyclosporin (4 mg/kg) or placebo by continuous intravenous infusion. Nine of the eleven cyclosporin-treated patients went into remission without surgery, compared with none of the patients in the placebo group. Moreover, five of the placebo-treated patients achieved remission after receiving intravenous cyclosporin. **A1d**

Since publication of Lichtiger's trial, intravenous cyclosporin has been extensively used for severe disease. Response rates between 60% and 85% have been reported outside of controlled trials, but many patients subsequently relapse and require colectomy [79, 80]. **B4** Nevertheless, intravenous cyclosporin may be useful especially for patients experiencing their first episode of severe colitis and for those who need time before deciding to undergo surgery. Although most clinical investigators have continued to use 4 mg/kg intravenously, 2 mg/kg was as effective as the higher dose in a randomized trial of 73 patients with severe colitis [81]. **A1c** Further trials are necessary to determine the optimal length of treatment and especially to decide what to do with the responders. Many clinicians discontinue cyclosporin and add azathioprine on the basis that this approach may provide sufficient time for azathioprine to become effective while the corticosteroids are being tapered. For patients who either refuse intravenous corticosteroids or who have previously had major adverse effects (for example psychoses), no difference in effectiveness was demonstrated in a small randomized trial between intravenous cyclosporin as monotherapy and intravenous hydrocortisone [82]. **A1d**

Several clinical trials have shown that oral cyclosporin is not an effective maintenance therapy in patients with steroid-resistant ulcerative colitis who achieved remission with either intravenous or oral cyclosporine [83–85]. Most patients either relapsed (and underwent colectomy) or required corticosteroid therapy. Uncontrolled trials suggest that azathioprine may be effective in maintaining remission in patients whose disease remitted with intravenous cyclosporine [86–88]. **B4**

Topical cyclosporine has been used for patients with resistant proctitis or distal colitis. Enemas containing 250 mg of the drug have yielded minimal plasma concentrations and no systemic adverse effects. Small clinical series have been reported from Copenhagen, the Mayo Clinic and Oxford. These patients had failed to respond to oral or topical mesalamine, corticosteroids or antimetabolites. Approximately 70% of the patients seemed to improve with topical cyclosporin, although many relapsed when treatment was discontinued. **B4** No formal clinical trial has been conducted in patients with resistant proctitis, largely because of the negative results found by Sandborn and colleagues in a small randomized controlled trial [89]. **A1d** Because this study enrolled only 40 patients, it may not have had sufficient power to exclude a small therapeutic benefit. Furthermore, Sandborn's trial differed from the open series in that it involved patients with active distal colitis instead of resistant proctitis.

Nicotine

Cigarette smoking seems to protect against the development of ulcerative colitis; ex-smokers and non-smokers are at increased risk [90]. Three randomized controlled trials have examined the efficacy of transdermal nicotine, given concurrently with mesalamine and/or corticosteroids, in the treatment of ulcerative colitis [91–93]. Pullan and associates found that the nicotine patch was more effective than placebo (49% vs 24%) for the induction of remission [91]. Sandborn and colleagues showed that nicotine was superior to placebo (39% vs 9%) at producing clinical improvement [92]. The NNT to induce remission or result in clinical improvement in these two trials was 4 and 3 respectively. **A1c**

A six-week trial failed to demonstrate any benefit of transdermal nicotine over prednisolone 15 mg/day [93]. A more recent randomized controlled trial involving patients with left-sided ulcerative colitis that relapsed despite taking mesalamine 1 g twice daily, compared nicotine patches with prednisone, each given for five weeks [94]. The study found that the rate of relapse after nicotine was less than with prednisone (20% vs 60%), and that patients in the latter group relapsed earlier. **A1d**

Two pilot studies found that nicotine enemas were effective for distal colitis, and randomized controlled trials are warranted [95, 96].

Thomas and associates reported the only randomized controlled trial of transdermal nicotine as maintenance therapy for ulcerative colitis [97]. The study demonstrated no benefit of nicotine 15 mg/day over placebo over a six-

month period, but this may be explained by poor compliance with the patch. **A1d**

New agents

Many new approaches are being developed for the treatment of moderate to severe ulcerative colitis. Several have now been evaluated in randomized trials.

Apheretic techniques

Apheretic techniques, in which leukocytes are removed by passing venous blood through absorption columns, have been widely reported to be effective, but virtually all the data are anecdotal, mainly from Japan. A single, small, randomized, controlled trial has been carried out in which 19 ulcerative colitis patients were randomized to receive apheresis or a sham procedure in addition to continuing their conventional therapy [98]. Apheresis appeared to be significantly more "effective" than the sham procedure (remission rates: apheresis 8/10, sham procedure 3/9, p < 0.05) and was well tolerated.

However, in a randomized trial in which 168 patients were randomized in a 2:1 ratio to receive apheresis with the Adacolumn Apheresis System or sham apheresis for nine weeks of treatment, clinical remission rates (Mayo score 0–2, with scores of 0 on rectal bleeding and 0 or 1 on endoscopic examination) were: apheresis 17%, sham-treated 11%, p = 0.36. Clinical response was also observed to be similar in the two groups: apheresis 44%, sham-treated 39%, p = 0.62 [99]. Similar results were obtained in a smaller trial conducted in Europe and Japan. This form of therapy is not effective for patients with moderate to severe ulcerative colitis. **A1c**

Anti-integrin monoclonal antibodies

Monoclonal antibodies to adhesion molecules, (a4ß7 integrin) have also been investigated in clinical trials, based on the hypothesis that inhibiting the recruitment of lymphocytes into the lamina propria might lead to a downregulation of the inflammation. Feagan et al. carried out a randomized placebo controlled trial of two doses (0.5 and 2.0 mg/kg) of the humanized $\alpha_4\beta_7$ anti-body MLN02 in 181 patients with mildly to moderately active ulcerative colitis (median Ulcerative Colitis Clinical Score 7, median Modified Baron Score 3, minimum disease extent 25 cm) [100]. Remission rates two weeks after the two infusions were significantly greater in the MLN02-treated patients (MLN02 0.5 mg/kg 33%, 2.0 mg/kg 34%, placebo 15%; p = 0.03). **A1a** A single patient experienced mild angioedema following MLN02 infusion. Further studies of this agent are required.

Anti-interleukin-2 receptor antibodies

Based on the favorable experience with intravenous cyclosporine, it is plausible that inhibition of interleukin-2 by other, better tolerated, agents might be an effective therapeutic strategy. Preliminary studies that evaluated two different humanized monoclonal anti-bodies to the interleukin-2 receptor yielded promising results [101, 102]. However, this approach was not effective in a randomized, placebo-controlled dose ranging trial of daclizumab, a humanized antibody to the interleukin-2 receptor (CD25) in 159 patients with moderately severe colitis. The remission rates at week 8 were: daclizumab 1 mg/kg 2%, daclizumab 2 mg/kg 7% and placebo 10% (p = 0.11, 0.73 respectively, for comparisons of daclizumab doses with placebo). **Alc**

Anti-tumor necrosis factor (TNF) monoclonal antibodies

The anti-tumor necrosis factor (TNF) strategies have primarily been directed towards Crohn's disease. Following many anecdotal reports of the use of infliximab for severe ulcerative colitis not responding to intravenous corticosteroids [103], and the reporting of two small randomized trials [104, 105], more definitive studies have been reported, and the results have been summarized in a Cochrane Review [106].

This systematic review included a meta-analysis of data from the two trials performed by Rutgeerts et al. that included 728 patients with moderate to severe ulcerative colitis refractory to conventional treatment using corticosteroids and/or immunosuppressive agents [107]. Infliximab (three intravenous infusions at 0, 2 and 6 weeks) was more effective than placebo in inducing clinical remission (Relative Risk (RR) 3.22; 95% CI: 2.18–4.76); inducing endoscopic remission (RR 1.88; 95% CI: 1.54–2.28); and in inducing clinical response (RR 1.99; 95% CI: 1.65–2.41) at eight weeks. A single infusion of infliximab was also more effective than placebo in reducing the need for colectomy within 90 days after infusion (RR 0.44; 95% CI: 0.22–0.87). **A1a** Severe adverse effects appear to be rare if patients are screened for latent tuberculosis.

Alpha interferon

Pegylated interferon alpha in one of two doses (0.5 micrograms/kg or 1.0 micrograms/kg) infused weekly for 12 weeks was compared with placebo in a randomized trial in 60 patients who continued to receive conventional therapies (5-ASA, steroids, azathioprine) in stable doses [108]. A trend toward benefit with the lower dose of interferon was reported, but further studies are required. **Ald**

Epidermal and fibroblast growth factors

Sinha et al. randomized 12 patients with active left-sided colitis or proctitis to receive daily enemas of the potent mitogenic epidermal growth factor (EGF), and 12 to receive placebo enemas for 14 days [109]. All patients received oral mesalamine. At two weeks 10 of the 12 patients given EGF enemas were in clinical remission, as compared with 1 of 12 in the control group p < 0.001). **Ald** At the two-week assessment, disease-activity scores, sigmoidoscopic scores and histologic scores were all significantly better in the EGF group than in the placebo group (p < 0.01 for all comparisons), and this benefit was maintained at 4 weeks and at 12 weeks. Sandborn et al. conducted a randomized, placebo-controlled trial of the fibroblast growth factor repifermin at doses of 1–50 micrograms/kg infused daily for five days in patients with active ulcerative colitis who were receiving 5-ASA, steroids or azathioprine [110]. They found this agent to be safe but not effective at these doses. **Ald**

Probiotics

A popular theory regarding the pathogenesis of IBD contends that chronic inflammation is the result of an abnormal host response to the endogenous microflora. Thus, a sound rationale exists for attempts to modify host bacteria in the hope that this will down-regulate the pathological immune response [111]. Experiments in rodents have demonstrated the potential of this approach and preliminary studies in humans have been reported [112, 113]. Earlier studies evaluated single strains of non-pathogenic E. coli for maintenance of remission [114].

Kruis [109] randomly assigned 120 patients with ulcerative colitis in remission to receive either 1.5 g/day of 5-ASA or identically appearing tablets that contained *Escherichia coli* strain Nissle 1917 [115]. At the end of this one-year study 11.3% of patients who received 5-ASA relapsed as compared with 16.0% of those who received the probiotic (p > 0.05). **Alc** No serious adverse events were associated with active treatment. This study can be criticized because of the very low relapse rate observed in the control group, despite the rather modest dose of 5-ASA that was used. Moreover, the trial was not designed as a formal non-superiority study and therefore lacked sufficient statistical power to assess whether the treatments were clinically equivalent.

Rembacken et al. randomized 116 patients with active disease to receive 5-ASA or the E. coli strain [114]. Treatment was continued for one year. At the end of the trial 73% of the patients who had entered remission with conventional therapy relapsed as compared with 67% of those assigned to the probiotic (p > 0.05). The authors concluded that the two strategies were of equivalent efficacy. **Alc** In a randomized trial that was designed as a formal non-superiority study, 109 randomized 327 patients with quiescent disease to 200 mg once daily of the probiotic or 500 mg three times daily of 5-ASA for 12 months of treatment. The rate of relapse was 45% in patients who received E. coli Nissle 1917 compared with 36% (absolute difference 9%) in favor of 5-ASA and met the investigators' prespecified criterion for therapeutic equivalence [116]. **Ala**

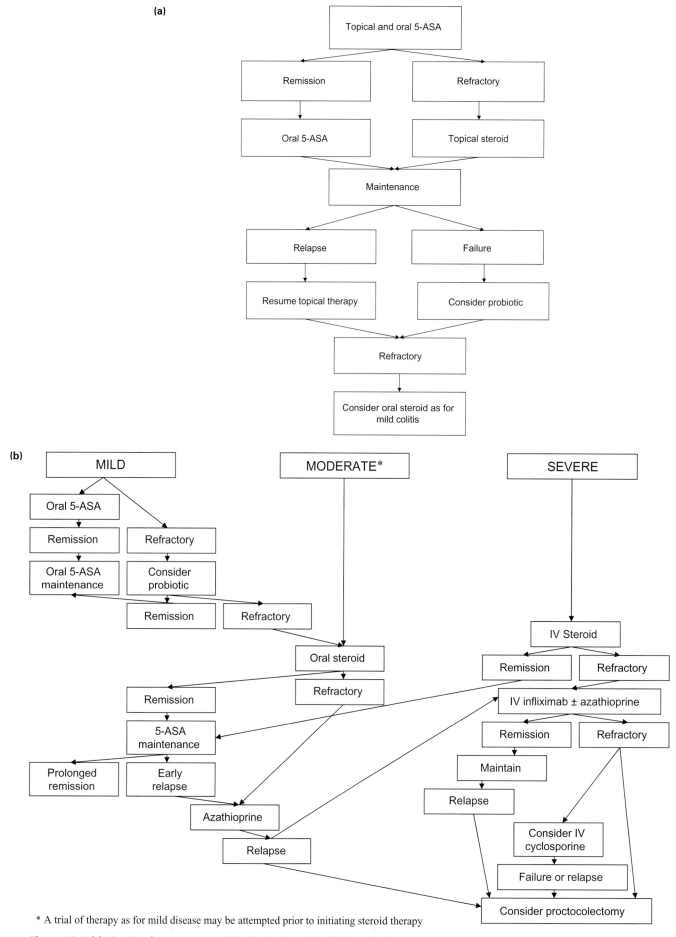

Figure 12.4 **(a)** Algorithm for management of distal ulcerative colitis. **(b)** Algorithm for management of more extensive ulcerative colitis.

In summary, these results from relatively large randomized trials provide evidence that probiotics are useful for maintenance of remission in ulcerative colitis. **A1c**

More recently the probiotic preparation VSL #3 that contains a high concentration of eight lyophilized bacterial strains was compared to a placebo containing lyophilized maize powder for induction of remission in 47 patients with mild or moderately active ulcerative colitis [117]. A majority of patients continued with mesalamine therapy alone (VSL #3 89.6%, placebo 67.1%), or in combination with immunosuppressants (VSL #3 6.4%, placebo 21.4%). Clinical remission was observed significantly more frequently in the VSL #3 treated groups (VSL #3 42.9%, placebo 15.7%, p < 0.001). No major adverse events were encountered. This study provides evidence that probiotics may be useful as an adjunct to conventional therapy for induction of remission of mild to moderately active ulcerative colitis. **A1d**

Surgery

Colectomy with construction of an ileal pouch-anal anastomosis has become the operation of choice for ulcerative colitis in major centers. Precise details of pouch construction may affect the eventual functional outcome, although a "J" pouch with 20 cm limbs and a stapled anastomosis 1.0–1.5 cm above the dentate line is the best for most patients [118–120]. Pouch dysfunction remains a frequent problem, and is often due to "pouchitis". The management of this disorder is addressed in Chapter 13.

Algorithm for management of ulcerative colitis

When endoscopic evaluation leads to the diagnosis of distal ulcerative colitis, the evidence for efficacy of interventions to induce and maintain remission supports the management algorithm shown in Figure 12.4a.

Therapy should be initiated with topic and oral 5-ASA preparations. If the disease enters remission, maintenance therapy with an oral 5-ASA preparation should be continued. If the disease relapses, topical therapy may be resumed and may be continued for maintenance of remission. Distal disease that is refractory to a topical 5-ASA preparation may be treated with a topical steroid preparation. Although there is evidence that the 5-ASA preparations are more effective, and there is no good evidence that switching to topical steroids is effective, the latter approach is a logical one that may be successful in some patients. Failure to respond to oral and topical 5-ASA should also lead to consideration of adding a probiotic preparation (*E. coli* Nissile 1917 or VSL #3). Patients in whom distal disease is refractory to these interventions should be considered for interventions proven to be effective for mild but more extensive disease, as outlined in Figure 12.4b.

The choice of interventions for treatment of more extensive colitis should be made after classifying the clinical disease severity as mild, moderate or severe. Mild disease should be treated with an oral 5-ASA. If the disease is refractory to this approach the addition of the probiotic preparation VSL #3 may be considered. If remission is achieved with these interventions the 5-ASA preparation, and possibly the probiotic, should be continued for maintenance therapy.

Moderately severe disease, and mild disease that is refractory to 5-ASA and probiotic therapy, should be treated with oral steroid. It is appropriate to treat some patients with moderately severe disease initially as outlined for mild disease, rather than initiating corticosteroid therapy, but the patients should be closely monitored for an increase in severity that would be a strong indication for steroid therapy. If remission is achieved maintenance therapy with oral 5-ASA is continued. Refractory colitis and early or frequently relapsing disease should lead to a consideration of introducing azathioprine therapy.

Severe colitis should be treated with IV steroids for a minimum of five days. Severe colitis that is refractory to IV steroids, and moderately severe disease that is refractory to or relapses on the regimen outline above, may be treated with IV Remicade as the next line of induction therapy. If remission is achieved maintenance therapy with Remicade and/or azathioprine should be considered.

Patients with severe or moderately severe disease that is either refractory to IV Remicade or relapses in spite of maintenance therapy, should be advised to consider proctocolectomy. This option, rather than immunosuppressive therapy with Remicade or azathioprine, may also be selected by some patients with less severe refractory or frequently relapsing disease. IV cyclosporine is another alternative therapy that may be considered for some patients with severe refractory disease who are reluctant to proceed to surgery, but the risk of severe adverse effects is relatively high, and a majority of such patients will eventually undergo proctocolectomy.

References

1 Jenkins D, Balsitis M, Gallivan S *et al.* Guidelines for the initial biopsy diagnosis of suspected chronic idiopathic inflammatory bowel disease. The British Society of Gastroenterology Initiative. *J Clin Pathol* 1997; **50**(2): 93–105.

2 Bentley E, Jenkins D, Campbell F, Warren B. How could pathologists improve the initial diagnosis of colitis? Evidence from an international workshop. *J Clin Pathol* 2002; **55**(12): 955–960.

3 Truelove SC, Pena AS. Course and prognosis of Crohn's disease. *Gut* 1976; **17**(3): 192–201.

4 Sinclair TS, Brunt PW, Mowat NA. Nonspecific proctocolitis in northeastern Scotland: a community study. *Gastroenterology* 1983; **85**(1): 1–11.

5 Persson PG, Bernell O, Leijonmarck CE, Farahmand BY, Hellers G, Ahlbom A. Survival and cause-specific mortality in inflammatory bowel disease: a population-based cohort study. *Gastroenterology* 1996; **110**(5): 1339–1345.

6 Langholz E, Munkholm P, Davidsen M, Binder V. Course of ulcerative colitis: analysis of changes in disease activity over years. *Gastroenterology* 1994; **107**(1): 3–11.

7 Winther KV, Jess T, Langholz E, Munkholm P, Binder V. Survival and cause-specific mortality in ulcerative colitis: follow-up of a population-based cohort in Copenhagen County. *Gastroenterology* 2003; **125**(6): 1576–1582.

8 Langholz E, Munkholm P, Krasilnikoff PA, Binder V. Inflammatory bowel diseases with onset in childhood. Clinical features, morbidity, and mortality in a regional cohort. *Scand J Gastroenterol* 1997; **32**(2): 139–147.

9 Moum B, Ekbom A, Vatn MH *et al.* Clinical course during the 1st year after diagnosis in ulcerative colitis and Crohn's disease. Results of a large, prospective population-based study in southeastern Norway, 1990–93. *Scand J Gastroenterol* 1997; **32**(10): 1005–1012.

10 Witte J, Shivananda S, Lennard-Jones JE *et al.* Disease outcome in inflammatory bowel disease: mortality, morbidity and therapeutic management of a 796-person inception cohort in the European Collaborative Study on Inflammatory Bowel Disease (EC-IBD). *Scand J Gastroenterol* 2000; **35**(12): 1272–1277.

11 Ayres RC, Gillen CD, Walmsley RS, Allan RN. Progression of ulcerative proctosigmoiditis: incidence and factors influencing progression. *Eur J Gastroenterol Hepatol* 1996; **8**(6): 555–558.

12 Moum B, Ekbom A, Vatn MH, Elgjo K. Change in the extent of colonoscopic and histological involvement in ulcerative colitis over time. *Am J Gastroenterol* 1999; **94**(6): 1564–1569.

13 Meucci G, Vecchi M, Astegiano M *et al.* The natural history of ulcerative proctitis: a multicenter, retrospective study. Gruppo di Studio per le Malattie Infiammatorie Intestinali (GSMII). *Am J Gastroenterol* 2000; **95**(2): 469–473.

14 Langholz E, Munkholm P, Davidsen M, Nielsen OH, Binder V. Changes in extent of ulcerative colitis: a study on the course and prognostic factors. *Scand J Gastroenterol* 1996; **31**(3): 260–266.

15 Gyde SN, Prior P, Allan RN *et al.* Colorectal cancer in ulcerative colitis: a cohort study of primary referrals from three centres. *Gut* 1988; **29**(2): 206–217.

16 Langholz E, Munkholm P, Davidsen M, Binder V. Colorectal cancer risk and mortality in patients with ulcerative colitis. *Gastroenterology* 1992; **103**(5): 1444–1451.

17 Lynch DA, Lobo AJ, Sobala GM, Dixon MF, Axon AT. Failure of colonoscopic surveillance in ulcerative colitis. *Gut* 1993; **34**(8): 1075–1080.

18 Blackstone MO, Riddell RH, Rogers BH, Levin B. Dysplasia-associated lesion or mass (DALM) detected by colonoscopy in long-standing ulcerative colitis: an indication for colectomy. *Gastroenterology* 1981; **80**(2): 366–374.

19 Butt JH, Konishi F, Morson BC, Lennard-Jones JE, Ritchie JK. Macroscopic lesions in dysplasia and carcinoma complicating ulcerative colitis. *Dig Dis Sci* 1983; **28**(1): 18–26.

20 Engelsgjerd M, Farraye FA, Odze RD. Polypectomy may be adequate treatment for adenoma-like dysplastic lesions in chronic ulcerative colitis. *Gastroenterology* 1999; **117**(6): 1288–1294; discussion 1488–1491.

21 Rubin PH, Friedman S, Harpaz N *et al.* Colonoscopic polypectomy in chronic colitis: conservative management after endoscopic resection of dysplastic polyps. *Gastroenterology* 1999; **117**(6): 1295–1300.

22 Riddell RH. Cancer surveillance in IBD does not work: the argument against. In: Tytgat GNJ, Bartelsman JFWM, Deventer SJH, eds. *Inflammatory Bowel Diseases Great Britain.* Kluwer Academic, London, 1995: 690–700.

23 Lim CH, Axon AT. Low-grade dysplasia: nonsurgical treatment. *Inflamm Bowel Dis* 2003; **9**(4): 270–272; discussion 273–275.

24 Ullman TA. Patients with low-grade dysplasia should be advised to undergo colectomy. *Inflamm Bowel Dis* 2003; **9**(4): 267–269; discussion 273–275.

25 Svartz N. Salazopyrin, a new sulfanilaminde preparation. A. Therapeutic results in rheumatic polyarthritis. B. Therapeutic results in ulcerative colitis. C. Toxic manifestations in treatment with sulfanilamide preparations. *Acta Med Scand* 1942; **110**: 557–590.

26 Baron JH, Connell AM, Lennard-Jones JE, Jones FA. Sulphasalazine and salicylazosulphadimidine in ulcerative colitis. *Lancet* 1962; **1**(7239): 1094–1096.

27 Misiewicz JJ, Lennard-Jones JE, Connell AM, Baron JH, Avery Jones F. Controlled trial of sulphasalazine in maintenance therapy for ulcerative colitis. *Lancet* 1965; **285**(7378): 185–188.

28 Dissanayake AS, Truelove SC. A controlled therapeutic trial of long-term maintenance treatment of ulcerative colitis with sulphazalazine (Salazopyrin). *Gut* 1973; **14**(12): 923–926.

29 Azad Khan AK, Piris J, Truelove SC. An experiment to determine the active therapeutic moiety of sulphasalazine. *Lancet* 1977; **2**(8044): 892–895.

30 Azad Khan AK, Howes DT, Piris J, Truelove SC. Optimum dose of sulphasalazine for maintenance treatment in ulcerative colitis. *Gut* 1980; **21**(3): 232–240.

31 van Hees PA, Bakker JH, van Tongeren JH. Effect of sulphapyridine, 5-aminosalicylic acid, and placebo in patients with idiopathic proctitis: a study to determine the active therapeutic moiety of sulphasalazine. *Gut* 1980; **21**(7): 632–635.

32 Williams CN. Overview of 5-ASA in the therapy of IBD. In: Sutherland LR, Collins SM, Martin F, eds. *Bowel Disease: Basic Research, Clinical Implications and Trends in Therapy.* Kluwer Academic, Dordecht, 1994.

33 Sutherland LR, Roth DE, Beck PL. Alternatives to sulfasalazine: a meta-analysis of 5-ASA in the treatment of ulcerative colitis. *Inflamm Bowel Dis* 1997; **3**: 65–78.

34 Sutherland L, Roth D, Beck P, May G, Makiyama K. Oral 5-aminosalicylic acid for inducing remission in ulcerative colitis. *Cochrane Database Syst Rev* 2000; **2**(2): CD000543.

35 Sutherland L, Roth D, Beck P, May G, Makiyama K. Oral 5-aminosalicylic acid for maintenance of remission in ulcerative colitis. *Cochrane Database Syst Rev* 2002; **4**(4): CD000544.

36 Rao SS, Dundas SA, Holdsworth CD, Cann PA, Palmer KR, Corbett CL. Olsalazine or sulphasalazine in first attacks of ulcerative colitis? A double blind study. *Gut* 1989; **30**(5): 675–679.

37 Nilsson A, Danielsson A, Lofberg R *et al.* Olsalazine versus sulphasalazine for relapse prevention in ulcerative

colitis: a multicenter study. *Am J Gastroenterol* 1995; **90**(3): 381–387.

38 Travis SP, Tysk C, de Silva HJ, Sandberg-Gertzen H, Jewell DP, Jarnerot G. Optimum dose of olsalazine for maintaining remission in ulcerative colitis. *Gut* 1994; **35**(9): 1282–1286.

39 Wadworth AN, Fitton A. Olsalazine. A review of its pharmacodynamic and pharmacokinetic properties, and therapeutic potential in inflammatory bowel disease. *Drugs* 1991; **41**(4): 647–664.

40 Jarnerot G. Withdrawal rates because of diarrhoea in Dipentum-treated patients with ulcerative colitis are low when Dipentium is taken with food and dose titrated. *Gastroenterology* 1996; **110**: A932.

41 Gionchetti P, Campieri M, Venturi A et al. Systemic availability of 5-aminosalicylic acid: comparison of delayed release and an azo-bond preparation. *Aliment Pharmacol Ther* 1996; **10**(4): 601–605.

42 Stoa-Birketvedt G, Florholmen J. The systemic load and efficient delivery of active 5-aminosalicylic acid in patients with ulcerative colitis on treatment with olsalazine or mesalazine. *Aliment Pharmacol Ther* 1999; **13**(3): 357–361.

43 Green JR, Lobo AJ, Holdsworth CD et al. Balsalazide is more effective and better tolerated than mesalamine in the treatment of acute ulcerative colitis. The Abacus Investigator Group. *Gastroenterology* 1998; **114**(1): 15–22.

44 Levine DS, Riff DS, Pruitt R et al. A randomized, double blind, dose-response comparison of balsalazide (6.75 g), balsalazide (2.25 g), and mesalamine (2.4 g) in the treatment of active, mild-to-moderate ulcerative colitis. *Am J Gastroenterol* 2002; **97**(6): 1398–1407.

45 Pruitt R, Hanson J, Safdi M et al. Balsalazide is superior to mesalamine in the time to improvement of signs and symptoms of acute mild-to-moderate ulcerative colitis. *Am J Gastroenterol* 2002; **97**(12): 3078–3086.

46 Green JR, Mansfield JC, Gibson JA, Kerr GD, Thornton PC. A double-blind comparison of balsalazide, 6.75 g daily, and sulfasalazine, 3 g daily, in patients with newly diagnosed or relapsed active ulcerative colitis. *Aliment Pharmacol Ther* 2002; **16**(1): 61–68.

47 Green JR, Gibson JA, Kerr GD et al. Maintenance of remission of ulcerative colitis: a comparison between balsalazide 3 g daily and mesalazine 1.2 g daily over 12 months. ABACUS Investigator group. *Aliment Pharmacol Ther* 1998; **12**(12): 1207–1216.

48 Marshall JK, Irvine EJ. Rectal aminosalicylate therapy for distal ulcerative colitis: a meta-analysis. *Aliment Pharmacol Ther* 1995; **9**(3): 293–300.

49 Marshall JK, Irvine EJ. Rectal corticosteroids versus alternative treatments in ulcerative colitis: a meta-analysis. *Gut* 1997; **40**(6): 775–781.

50 Brown J, Haines S, Wilding IR. Colonic spread of three rectally administered mesalazine (Pentasa) dosage forms in healthy volunteers as assessed by gamma scintigraphy. *Aliment Pharmacol Ther* 1997; **11**(4): 685–691.

51 Wilding IR, Kenyon CJ, Chauhan S et al. Colonic spreading of a non-chlorofluorocarbon mesalazine rectal foam enema in patients with quiescent ulcerative colitis. *Aliment Pharmacol Ther* 1995; **9**(2): 161–166.

52 Campieri M, Corbelli C, Gionchetti P et al. Spread and distribu-

tion of 5-ASA colonic foam and 5-ASA enema in patients with ulcerative colitis. *Dig Dis Sci* 1992; **37**(12): 1890–1897.

53 Pokrotnieks J, Marlicz K, Paradowski L, Margus B, Zaborowski P, Greinwald R. Efficacy and tolerability of mesalazine foam enema (Salofalk foam) for distal ulcerative colitis: a double-blind, randomized, placebo-controlled study. *Aliment Pharmacol Ther* 2000; **14**(9): 1191–1198.

54 Campieri M, Paoluzi P, D'Albasio G, Brunetti G, Pera A, Barbara L. Better quality of therapy with 5-ASA colonic foam in active ulcerative colitis. A multicenter comparative trial with 5-ASA enema. *Dig Dis Sci* 1993; **38**(10): 1843–1850.

55 Ardizzone S, Doldo P, Ranzi T et al. Mesalazine foam (Salofalk foam) in the treatment of active distal ulcerative colitis. A comparative trial vs Salofalk enema. The SAF-3 study group. *Ital J Gastroenterol Hepatol* 1999; **31**(8): 677–684.

56 Malchow H, Gertz B, CLAFOAM Study group. A new mesalazine foam enema (Claversal Foam) compared with a standard liquid enema in patients with active distal ulcerative colitis. *Aliment Pharmacol Ther* 2002; **16**(3): 415–423.

57 Gionchetti P, Ardizzone S, Benvenuti ME et al. A new mesalazine gel enema in the treatment of left-sided ulcerative colitis: a randomized controlled multicentre trial. *Aliment Pharmacol Ther* 1999; **13**(3): 381–388.

58 d'Albasio G, Paoluzi P, Campieri M et al. Maintenance treatment of ulcerative proctitis with mesalazine suppositories: a double-blind placebo-controlled trial. The Italian IBD Study Group. *Am J Gastroenterol* 1998; **93**(5): 799–803.

59 Safdi M, DeMicco M, Sninsky C et al. A double-blind comparison of oral versus rectal mesalamine versus combination therapy in the treatment of distal ulcerative colitis. *Am J Gastroenterol* 1997; **92**(10): 1867–1871.

60 Marteau P, Probert CS, Lindgren S et al. Combined oral and enema treatment with Pentasa (mesalazine) is superior to oral therapy alone in patients with extensive mild/moderate active ulcerative colitis: a randomised, double blind, placebo controlled study. *Gut* 2005; **54**(7): 960–965.

61 Truelove SC, Witts LJ. Cortisone in ulcerative colitis; final report on a therapeutic trial. *BMJ* 1955; **2**(4947): 1041–1048.

62 Lennard-Jones JE, Longmore AJ, Newell AC, Wilson CW, Jones FA. An assessment of prednisone, salazopyrin, and topical hydrocortisone hemisuccinate used as out-patient treatment for ulcerative colitis. *Gut* 1960; **1**: 217–222.

63 Powell-Tuck J, Bown RL, Lennard-Jones JE. A comparison of oral prednisolone given as single or multiple daily doses for active proctocolitis. *Scand J Gastroenterol* 1978; **13**(7): 833–837.

64 Baron JH, Connell AM, Kanaghinis TG, Lennard-Jones JE, Jones AF. Out-patient treatment of ulcerative colitis. Comparison between three doses of oral prednisone. *BMJ* 1962; **2**(5302): 441–443.

65 Brattsand R. Overview of newer glucocorticosterod preparations for inflammatory bowel disease. *Can J Gastroenterol* 1990; **4**: 407–414.

66 Lofberg R, Danielsson A, Suhr O et al. Oral budesonide versus prednisolone in patients with active extensive and left-sided ulcerative colitis. *Gastroenterology* 1996; **110**(6): 1713–1718.

67 Lemann M, Galian A, Rutgeerts P, Van Heuverzwijn R, Cortot A, Viteau JM et al. Comparison of budesonide and 5-aminosalicylic acid enemas in active distal ulcerative colitis. *Aliment Pharmacol Ther* 1995; **9**(5): 557–562.

68 Truelove SC, Witts LJ. Cortisone and corticotrophin in ulcerative colitis. *BMJ* 1959; **1**(5119): 387–394.

69 Truelove SC, Hambling MH. Treatment of ulcerative colitis with local hydrocortisone hemisuccinate sodium; a report on a controlled therapeutic trial. *BMJ* 1958; **2**(5103): 1072–1077.

70 Lennard-Jones JE, Misiewicz JJ, Connell AM, Baron JH, Jones FA. Prednisone as maintenance treatment for ulcerative colitis in remission. *Lancet* 1965; **1**(7378): 188–189.

71 Jewell DP, Truelove SC. Azathioprine in ulcerative colitis: final report on controlled therapeutic trial. *BMJ* 1974; **4**(5945): 627–630.

72 Rosenberg JL, Wall AJ, Levin B, Binder HJ, Kirsner JB. A controlled trial of azathioprine in the management of chronic ulcerative colitis. *Gastroenterology* 1975; **69**(1): 96–99.

73 Kirk AP, Lennard-Jones JE. Controlled trial of azathioprine in chronic ulcerative colitis. *BMJ* (Clin Res Ed) 1982; **284**(6325): 1291–1292.

74 Hawthorne AB, Logan RF, Hawkey CJ et al. Randomised controlled trial of azathioprine withdrawal in ulcerative colitis. *BMJ* 1992; **305**(6844): 20–22.

75 Sood A, Kaushal V, Midha V, Bhatia KL, Sood N, Malhotra V. The beneficial effect of azathioprine on maintenance of remission in severe ulcerative colitis. *J Gastroenterol* 2002; **37**(4): 270–274.

76 Mate-Jimenez J, Hermida C, Cantero-Perona J, Moreno-Otero R. 6-mercaptopurine or methotrexate added to prednisone induces and maintains remission in steroid-dependent inflammatory bowel disease. *Eur J Gastroenterol Hepatol* 2000; **12**(11): 1227–1233.

77 Oren R, Arber N, Odes S et al. Methotrexate in chronic active ulcerative colitis: a double-blind, randomized, Israeli multicenter trial. *Gastroenterology* 1996; **110**(5): 1416–1421.

78 Lichtiger S, Present DH, Kornbluth A et al. Cyclosporine in severe ulcerative colitis refractory to steroid therapy. *N Engl J Med* 1994; **330**(26): 1841–1845.

79 Hyde GM, Thillainayagam AV, Jewell DP. Intravenous cyclosporin as rescue therapy in severe ulcerative colitis: time for a reappraisal? *Eur J Gastroenterol Hepatol* 1998; **10**(5): 411–413.

80 Jewell DP, Hyde GM. Severe ulcerative colitis: cyclosporin or colectomy? A European view. In: Modigliani R, ed. *IBD and Salicylates-3*. Wells Medical, Tunbridge Wells, UK, 1998.

81 Van Assche G, D'Haens G, Noman M et al. Randomized, double-blind comparison of 4 mg/kg versus 2 mg/kg intravenous cyclosporine in severe ulcerative colitis. *Gastroenterology* 2003; **125**(4): 1025–1031.

82 D'Haens G, Lemmens L, Geboes K et al. Intravenous cyclosporine versus intravenous corticosteroids as single therapy for severe attacks of ulcerative colitis. *Gastroenterology* 2001; **120**(6): 1323–1329.

83 Treem WR, Cohen J, Davis PM, Justinich CJ, Hyams JS. Cyclosporine for the treatment of fulminant ulcerative colitis in children. Immediate response, long-term results, and impact on surgery. *Dis Colon Rectum* 1995; **38**(5): 474–479.

84 Gurudu SR, Griffel LH, Gialanella RJ, Das KM. Cyclosporine therapy in inflammatory bowel disease: short-term and long-term results. *J Clin Gastroenterol* 1999; **29**(2): 151–154.

85 Rowe FA, Walker JH, Karp LC, Vasiliauskas EA, Plevy SE, Targan SR. Factors predictive of response to cyclosporin treatment for severe, steroid-resistant ulcerative colitis. *Am J Gastroenterol* 2000; **95**(8): 2000–2008.

86 Fernandez-Banares F, Bertran X, Esteve-Comas M et al. Azathioprine is useful in maintaining long-term remission induced by intravenous cyclosporine in steroid-refractory severe ulcerative colitis. *Am J Gastroenterol* 1996; **91**(12): 2498–2499.

87 Actis GC, Bresso F, Astegiano M et al. Safety and efficacy of azathioprine in the maintenance of ciclosporin-induced remission of ulcerative colitis. *Aliment Pharmacol Ther* 2001; **15**(9): 1307–1311.

88 Domenech E, Garcia-Planella E, Bernal I et al. Azathioprine without oral ciclosporin in the long-term maintenance of remission induced by intravenous ciclosporin in severe, steroid-refractory ulcerative colitis. *Aliment Pharmacol Ther* 2002; **16**(12): 2061–2065.

89 Sandborn WJ, Tremaine WJ, Schroeder KW et al. A placebo-controlled trial of cyclosporine enemas for mildly to moderately active left-sided ulcerative colitis. *Gastroenterology* 1994; **106**(6): 1429–1435.

90 Calkins BM. A meta-analysis of the role of smoking in inflammatory bowel disease. *Dig Dis Sci* 1989; **34**(12): 1841–1854.

91 Pullan RD, Rhodes J, Ganesh S et al. Transdermal nicotine for active ulcerative colitis. *N Engl J Med* 1994; **330**(12): 811–815.

92 Sandborn WJ, Tremaine WJ, Offord KP et al. Transdermal nicotine for mildly to moderately active ulcerative colitis. A randomized, double-blind, placebo-controlled trial. *Ann Intern Med* 1997; **126**(5): 364–371.

93 Thomas GA, Rhodes J, Ragunath K et al. Transdermal nicotine compared with oral prednisolone therapy for active ulcerative colitis. *Eur J Gastroenterol.Hepatol* 1996; **8**(8): 769–776.

94 Guslandi M, Tittobello A. Outcome of ulcerative colitis after treatment with transdermal nicotine. *Eur J Gastroenterol Hepatol* 1998; **10**(6): 513–515.

95 Sandborn WJ, Tremaine WJ, Leighton JA et al. Nicotine tartrate liquid enemas for mildly to moderately active left-sided ulcerative colitis unresponsive to first-line therapy: a pilot study. *Aliment Pharmacol Ther* 1997; **11**(4): 663–671.

96 Green JT, Thomas GA, Rhodes J et al. Nicotine enemas for active ulcerative colitis – a pilot study. *Aliment Pharmacol Ther* 1997; **11**(5): 859–863.

97 Thomas GA, Rhodes J, Mani V et al. Transdermal nicotine as maintenance therapy for ulcerative colitis. *N Engl J Med* 1995; **332**(15): 988–992.

98 Sawada K, Kusugam K, Suzuki Y et al. Multicenter randomized double blind controlled trial for ulcerative colitis therapy with leukocytapheresis. *Gastroenterology* 2003; **124**(4 Suppl. 1): A67–68.

99 Sands BE, Sandborn WJ, Feagan B et al. A randomized, double-blind, sham-controlled study of granulocyte/monocyte apheresis for active ulcerative colitis. *Gastroenterology* 2008; **135**(2): 400–409.

100 Feagan BG, Greenberg GR, Wild G et al. Treatment of ulcerative colitis with a humanized antibody to the alpha4beta7 integrin. *N Engl J Med* 2005; **352**(24): 2499–2507.

101 Van Assche G, Dalle I, Noman M et al. A pilot study on the use of the humanized anti-interleukin-2 receptor antibody daclizumab in active ulcerative colitis. *Am J Gastroenterol* 2003; **98**(2): 369–376.

102 Creed TJ, Norman MR, Probert CS *et al.* Basiliximab (anti-CD25) in combination with steroids may be an effective new treatment for steroid-resistant ulcerative colitis. *Aliment Pharmacol Ther* 2003; **18**(1): 65–75.

103 Gornet JM, Couve S, Hassani Z *et al.* Infliximab for refractory ulcerative colitis or indeterminate colitis: an open-label multicentre study. *Aliment Pharmacol Ther* 2003; **18**(2): 175–181.

104 Probert CS, Hearing SD, Schreiber S *et al.* Infliximab in moderately severe glucocorticoid resistant ulcerative colitis: a randomised controlled trial. *Gut* 2003; **52**(7): 998–1002.

105 Ochsenkuhn T, Sackmann M, Goke B. Infliximab for acute, not steroid-refractory ulcerative colitis: a randomized pilot study. *Eur J Gastroenterol Hepatol* 2004; **16**(11): 1167–1171.

106 Lawson MM, Thomas AG, Akobeng AK. Tumour necrosis factor alpha blocking agents for induction of remission in ulcerative colitis. *Cochrane Database Syst Rev* 2006; **3**: CD005112.

107 Rutgeerts P, Sandborn WJ, Feagan BG *et al.* Infliximab for induction and maintenance therapy for ulcerative colitis. *N Engl J Med* 2005; **353**(23): 2462–2476.

108 Tilg H, Vogelsang H, Ludwiczek O *et al.* A randomised placebo controlled trial of pegylated interferon alpha in active ulcerative colitis. *Gut* 2003; **52**(12): 1728–1733.

109 Sinha A, Nightingale J, West KP, Berlanga-Acosta J, Playford RJ. Epidermal growth factor enemas with oral mesalamine for mild-to-moderate left-sided ulcerative colitis or proctitis. *N Engl J Med* 2003; **349**(4): 350–357.

110 Sandborn WJ, Sands BE, Wolf DC *et al.* Repifermin (keratinocyte growth factor-2) for the treatment of active ulcerative colitis: a randomized, double-blind, placebo-controlled, dose-escalation trial. *Aliment Pharmacol Ther* 2003; **17**(11): 1355–1364.

111 Shanahan F. Probiotics and inflammatory bowel disease: from fads and fantasy to facts and future. *Br J Nutr* 2002; **88**(Suppl. 1): S5–9.

112 McCarthy J, O'Mahony L, O'Callaghan L *et al.* Double blind, placebo controlled trial of two probiotic strains in interleukin 10 knockout mice and mechanistic link with cytokine balance. *Gut* 2003; **52**(7): 975–980.

113 Madsen KL. Inflammatory bowel disease: lessons from the IL-10 gene-deficient mouse. *Clin Invest Med* 2001; **24**(5): 250–257.

114 Rembacken BJ, Snelling AM, Hawkey PM, Chalmers DM, Axon AT. Non-pathogenic *Escherichia coli* versus mesalazine for the treatment of ulcerative colitis: a randomised trial. *Lancet* 1999; **354**(9179): 635–639.

115 Kruis W, Schutz E, Fric P, Fixa B, Judmaier G, Stolte M. Double-blind comparison of an oral *Escherichia coli* preparation and mesalazine in maintaining remission of ulcerative colitis. *Aliment Pharmacol Ther* 1997; **11**(5): 853–858.

116 Kruis W, Fric P, Pokrotnieks J *et al.* Maintaining remission of ulcerative colitis with the probiotic *Escherichia coli* Nissle 1917 is as effective as with standard mesalazine. *Gut* 2004; **53**(11): 1617–1623.

117 Sood A, Midha V, Makharia GK *et al.* The probiotic preparation, VSL#3 induces remission in patients with mild-to-moderately active ulcerative colitis. *Clin Gastroenterol Hepatol* 2009; **7**(11): 1202–1209, 1209.e1.

118 Romanos J, Samarasekera DN, Stebbing JF, Jewell DP, Kettlewell MG, Mortensen NJ. Outcome of 200 restorative proctocolectomy operations: the John Radcliffe Hospital experience. *Br J Surg* 1997; **84**(6): 814–818.

119 Setti-Carraro P, Ritchie JK, Wilkinson KH, Nicholls RJ, Hawley PR. The first 10 years' experience of restorative proctocolectomy for ulcerative colitis. *Gut* 1994; **35**(8): 1070–1075.

120 McIntyre PB, Pemberton JH, Wolff BG, Beart RW, Dozois RR. Comparing functional results one year and ten years after ileal pouch–anal anastomosis for chronic ulcerative colitis. *Dis Colon Rectum* 1994; **37**(4): 303–307.

13 Pouchitis after restorative proctocolectomy

Darrell S Pardi and William J Sandborn

Inflammatory Bowel Disease Clinic, Division of Gastroenterology and Hepatology, Mayo Clinic, Rochester, USA

Introduction

Approximately 30% of patients with ulcerative colitis will require colectomy for fulminant or medically refractory disease, or because of dysplasia or another complication [1, 2]. The preferred operation for most patients is a restorative proctocolectomy, also known as a total proctocolectomy with ileal pouch anal anastomosis (IPAA). Although many studies have shown excellent quality of life in patients who have undergone IPAA, complications are common after this operation [3, 4]. Pouchitis, an idiopathic inflammatory condition in the pouch, is the most common, occurring in up to 60% of patients after IPAA for ulcerative colitis [1–7]. It has been estimated that the number of patients with pouchitis in the USA will reach 30,000–45,000 persons, or a prevalence of 12–18/100,000 [8]. Thus, pouchitis has emerged as an important third form of inflammatory bowel disease (IBD).

Despite these facts, criteria for diagnosis, classification and measurement of disease activity in pouchitis are still evolving. The previous lack of consensus on these issues hampered the design and conduct of randomized trials of proposed interventions, and medical therapy for pouchitis was largely empirical. This lack of consensus also makes it difficult to analyse the existing literature due to differing definitions or categories of disease and differing criteria for response or remission. In 1994, the Pouchitis Disease Activity Index (PDAI), an instrument to measure disease activity and efficacy of therapy, was developed [9]. This index facilitated clinical research in pouchitis, and there are now 13 controlled trials, and many more uncontrolled

studies, of various agents for induction and maintenance therapy in pouchitis. The medical therapies reported to be of benefit for pouchitis are shown in Table 13.1. This chapter will assist physicians and surgeons in becoming familiar with the diagnosis and classification of pouchitis, and will review the results from reports of empirical medical therapies and controlled trials, and the rationale for using various treatments.

Diagnosis and classification

Pouchitis is suggested by variable clinical symptoms, including increased stool frequency, decreased stool consistency, abdominal cramping, fecal urgency, tenesmus, incontinence, and occasionally rectal bleeding, fever or extra-intestinal manifestations such as arthralgias. Since these symptoms are non-specific, a clinical suspicion of pouchitis should be confirmed by endoscopy and biopsy of the pouch [1]. Endoscopic examination shows inflammatory changes, which may include mucosal edema, granularity, contact bleeding, loss of vascular pattern, hemorrhage and ulceration [10]. Histologic examination shows acute inflammation with neutrophil infiltration and occasionally mucosal ulceration, superimposed on a background of chronic changes including villous atrophy, crypt hyperplasia and chronic inflammatory cell infiltration [11, 12]. Endoscopic examination of the neo-terminal ileum above the ileal pouch should be normal. Significant inflammation in this location is suggestive of Crohn's disease [10]. In addition, the anal transition zone, or rectal cuff, should also be inspected endoscopically [10]. Inflammation here is termed cuffitis, and can exist with or without pouchitis.

The PDAI is a quantitative 19-point index of pouchitis activity based on clinical symptoms and findings on endoscopy and histology (Table 13.2). Active pouchitis is defined as a PDAI score ≥ 7 points and remission is defined as a

Evidence-Based Gastroenterology and Hepatology, 3rd edition.
J. McDonald, A.K. Burroughs, B. Feagan, and M.B. Fennerty. © 2010
Blackwell Publishing Ltd

Table 13.1 Treatments reported to be beneficial for pouchitis.

Antibiotics
- Single antibiotics
  Ciprofloxacin, metronidazole, amoxicillin/clavulanate, erythromycin, tetracycline, rifaximin
- Combination antibiotics
  Ciprofloxacin + metronidazole, ciprofloxacin + rifaximin, ciprofloxacin + tinidazole

Probiotic bacteria
- Lactobacilli, Bifidobacteria, Streptococci (VSL#3)
- *Escherichia coli* strain Nissle 1917

5-Aminosalicylates
- Mesalamine enemas
- Oral mesalamine
- Sulfasalazine

Corticosteroids
- Conventional corticosteroid enemas
- Budesonide suppositories
- Budesonide enemas
- Oral corticosteroids

Immune modifier agents
- Cyclosporin enema
- Azathioprine, 6-mercaptopurine
- Infliximab

Nutritional agents
- Short chain fatty acids enemas or suppositories
- Glutamine suppositories
- Dietary fiber (pectin, methylcellulose, inulin)

Oxygen radical inhibitors
- Allopurinol

Antidiarrheal/antimicrobial
- Bismuth carbomer enemas
- Bismuth subsalicylate

Modified with permission from Mahadevan and Sandborn. *Gastroenterology* 2003; **124**: 1636–1650.

Table 13.2 Pouchitis disease activity index (PDAI).

Clinical criteria	Score
Stool frequency	
Usual postop stool frequency	0
1–2 stools/day > postop usual	1
3 or more stools/day > postop usual	2
Rectal bleeding	
None or rare	0
Present daily	1
Fecal urgency/abdominal cramps	
None	0
Occasional	1
Usual	2
Fever (temperature > 100.5° F)	
Absent	0
Present	1
Endoscopic criteria	
Edema	1
Granularity	1
Friability	1
Loss of vascular pattern	1
Mucus exudate	1
Ulceration	1
Histological criteria	
Polymorph infiltration	
Mild	1
Moderate + crypt abscess	2
Severe + crypt abscess	3
Ulceration per low power field (average)	
<25%	1
≥25% < 50%	2
≥50%	3

Pouchitis is defined as a total PDAI score > 7 points.
Adapted with permission from Sandborn WJ *et al. Mayo Clin Proc* 1994; **69**: 409–415.

PDAI score < 7 points, assuming other causes of pouch inflammation have been excluded.

Patients with pouchitis can be classified according to disease activity (mild, moderate, or severe), symptom duration, disease pattern or response to antibiotics [1]. Duration can be classified as acute (<4 weeks) or chronic (≥4 weeks). Disease pattern can be classified as infrequent (1–2 episodes per year), relapsing (≥3 episodes per year), or continuous. Relapsing pouchitis is also considered a form of chronic pouchitis, even if the symptoms during a single episode do not last for four weeks on therapy. Finally, pouchitis can be classified as antibiotic-responsive, dependent or refractory.

Treatment with antibiotics

Rationale

The fact that pouchitis typically does not occur until the diverting ileostomy is closed and luminal contents flow through the pouch suggests that bacterial antigens are important in driving the inflammatory process. However, it is not clear whether pouchitis occurs due to overgrowth of commensal bacteria or the presence of abnormal bacteria [13–17]. After IPAA, the primary function of the terminal ileum changes from absorption to storage, and bacterial overgrowth occurs by design, with bacterial concentrations increasing to levels that are intermediate between those seen with an end ileostomy and in the colon [18, 19]. There is no correlation between fecal bacterial concentrations and histologic changes of acute inflammation [18, 19], suggesting that pouchitis and bacterial overgrowth are not directly related. However, anaerobic bacterial overgrowth of the pouch is associated with transformation of the ileal mucosa to a "colon-like" morphology (with villous atrophy, and chronic inflammatory cell infiltration) [18, 20]. Furthermore, the flora in pouch effluent has a higher ratio of anaerobes to aerobes and more Bacteroides and Bifidobacteria than effluent from subjects with an end ileostomy [19, 21]. However, in other studies, total aerobes and some pathogenic bacteria (*Clostridium perfringens* and hemolytic strains of *Escherichia coli*) may be increased, while total anaerobes are decreased [22]. Thus, pouch anaerobic bacterial overgrowth may indirectly set the stage for pouchitis to the extent that "colon-like" ileal mucosa may be more susceptible to a recurrence of UC. Strategies directed towards reducing fecal concentrations of anaerobic bacteria through the use of antibiotics may be useful in treating pouchitis.

Clinical results

Antibiotics are the standard medical therapy for pouchitis, based on a small number of controlled trials as well as overwhelming clinical evidence that antibiotics are effective. Previously, the most commonly used antibiotic for pouchitis was metronidazole [19, 23–26], with most patients responding to doses of 750–1500 mg/day within 1–2 days. The first controlled trial of metronidazole was a small, placebo-controlled crossover trial [27]. Each patient had a seven-day washout period before crossing over to the second therapy. Metronidazole was better than placebo at improving the daily stool frequency, although the overall change was small, and there was no significant difference in endoscopic or histologic improvement. A second small controlled trial compared two weeks of treatment with metronidazole 20 mg/kg/day with ciprofloxacin 1000 mg/day in patients with acute pouchitis [28]. Both drugs significantly reduced the PDAI score, but ciprofloxacin had a greater reduction with fewer side effects. Based on this study, other reports of the effectiveness of ciprofloxacin [25], and the high risk of adverse effects seen during metronidazole treatment (33–55%, including nausea, vomiting, abdominal discomfort, headache and skin rash [27–29]), ciprofloxacin has become the antibiotic of choice for most patients with active pouchitis. **A1d** Amoxicillin/clavulanic acid, erythromycin, tetracycline and topical metronidazole have also been reported to be of benefit [1]. Rifaximin, a non-absorbed oral antibiotic, was not superior to placebo in a small randomized clinical trial [30]. **A1d**

In patients who do not respond to a single antibiotic, treatment with combination antibiotics, such as ciprofloxacin and rifaximin [31], ciprofloxacin and metronidazole [32], or ciprofloxacin and tinidazole [33] have been reported beneficial in open-label studies.

Patients with relapsing pouchitis may require chronic maintenance antibiotic therapy. Given the risk of adverse effects with prolonged metronidazole therapy, these patients are usually treated with ciprofloxacin at doses ranging from 250 mg every third day up to 1000 mg/day, although many can be controlled with 250 mg every 1–2 days.

Treatment with probiotics

Rationale

As mentioned above, there is extensive evidence implicating changes in the pouch bacterial milieu in the pathogenesis of pouchitis. Thus, strategies directed at altering the relative balance of bacteria using probiotic therapy may be useful in treating or preventing pouchitis.

Clinical results

Three controlled trials have been performed [34–36]. The first two studies randomized patients with chronic pouchitis in remission after induction therapy with antibiotics to treatment with either an oral probiotic preparation (VSL-3, which contains strains of lactobacilli, bifidobacteria and streptococci) or placebo for 9–12 months [34, 35]. The relapse rates in the VSL-3 groups were 10–15% compared with 94–100% with placebo. In a third study, patients undergoing colectomy and IPAA were randomized to prophylactic therapy with VSL-3 or placebo for one year [36]. The rate of developing pouchitis during the first year was 10% in the VSL-3 group and 40% in the placebo group. **A1d** In this study, VSL-3 also reduced the stool frequency of patients without clinical pouchitis. Finally, an open-label study of VSL-3 suggested efficacy for the treatment of mildly active acute pouchitis [37], and a case report of two patients suggested that another probiotic, *E. coli* Nissle 1917, may be of benefit for the treatment of active pouchitis and for maintenance therapy [38].

In contrast, an open-label study of VSL-3 in clinical practice was less encouraging [39]. In this uncontrolled report of 31 patients with antibiotic-dependent chronic pouchitis treated at a referral center, <20% were able to maintain remission on VSL-3 during eight months of follow-up.

Treatment with anti-inflammatory and immune modifier agents

Rationale

Pouchitis may represent a recurrence of IBD in the ileal pouch. Data to support this view include: an increased frequency of pouchitis in patients with UC compared to those with familial polyposis; an increased frequency of pouchitis in patients who have extra-intestinal manifestations of UC, primary sclerosing cholangitis (PSC) or antineutrophil cytoplasmic antibodies (pANCA); and a decreased frequency of pouchitis in current smokers. Strategies directed towards empirical medical therapy with agents known to be efficacious in IBD may be useful in treating pouchitis. Unfortunately, few controlled trials have been reported to provide evidence for the efficacy of these approaches.

Clinical results

Uncontrolled studies suggest that topical mesalamine (enemas or suppositories), sulfasalazine and oral mesalamine may be beneficial for active pouchitis [19, 26, 40–42]. Uncontrolled reports also have suggested that oral and topical corticosteroids may be of benefit in pouchitis [19, 26, 42, 43]. Budesonide suppositories resulted in clinical and endoscopic improvement, and decreased pouch concentrations of inflammatory mediators, in a small study in acute pouchitis [44]. A randomized controlled trial of budesonide enemas versus oral metronidazole showed equivalent efficacy, but fewer side effects from budesonide [29]. **A1d** Oral controlled release budesonide has also been reported to be effective for the treatment of pouchitis in uncontrolled reports. In one study, budesonide (9 mg/day for eight weeks) induced remission in 72% of patients not responding to one month of ciprofloxacin or metronidazole [45]. In another small open-label series [46], budesonide therapy induced a 60% response rate in patients refractory to antibiotics. **B4**

Cyclosporin enemas were reported to be beneficial in one patient with active chronic pouchitis [47]. Two studies involving 11 patients with IPAA who underwent liver transplantation for PSC have reported on the clinical course of pouchitis [48, 49]. Five of 11 patients had chronic pouchitis following transplantation, despite immunosuppression with cyclosporin or tacrolimus, prednisone, and azathioprine, suggesting that immunosuppression may not be efficacious for pouchitis, at least in this population. **B4** Two small reports have suggested a beneficial effect of azathioprine in patients with Crohn's disease and an IPAA [50, 51]. Recently, infliximab has been reported to be of benefit in patients with pouchitis [51, 52]

and patients with Crohn's disease of the ileoanal pouch [53, 54, 55].

Treatment with nutritional agents

Rationale

In a well-functioning ileal pouch, the bacterial flora produce short chain fatty acids (SCFA), including acetate, propionate and butyrate at concentrations similar to those in the colon of healthy controls, and increased compared with stomal SCFA concentrations in ileostomy patients [18, 56]. Some [57, 58], but not all [18], studies have reported that patients with pouchitis have significantly lower concentrations of SCFAs than healthy patients with IPAAs, perhaps from dilution [57]. Strategies directed at administering SCFA enemas or suppositories, or dietary fiber that is fermented to SCFA, may theoretically be useful in treating pouchitis. Another nutritional approach to improving pouch function is through use of non-fermentable dietary fiber, with the goal of improving stool consistency.

Clinical results

A case report using SCFA enemas containing sodium acetate, propionate and butyrate reported success in active chronic pouchitis [59]. However, SFCA enemas were of little or no benefit in two other reports of patients with active pouchitis [60, 61]. A fourth study, in patients with active chronic pouchitis, reported improvement in 3/9 patients treated with sodium butyrate suppositories compared with 6/10 patients treated with glutamine suppositories [58]. **B4** Inulin, a dietary fiber that is fermented to SCFAs, increases fecal butyrate concentrations and lowers fecal pH, concentrations of *Bacteroides fragilis*, and concentrations of some secondary bile acids in patients with IPAA compared to those treated with placebo [62]. However, the effectiveness of inulin for the treatment of active pouchitis is unclear. A crossover trial with pectin (a soluble fermentable fiber) and Citrucel (a methyl cellulose-based non-fermentable fiber) found that neither improved stool frequency, pouch function, bloating or stool consistency after IPAA [63]. Thus, these small studies suggest that neither SCFA enemas or suppositories, nor fiber, are highly effective therapies for active pouchitis.

Treatment with allopurinol

Rationale

During construction of the ileal pouch, the mesenteric vessels may be divided to avoid tension on the pouch-anal anastomosis [64]. This ligation of the blood supply has the potential to cause ischemic injury to the pouch, and oxygen free radical formation is known to be one of the mechanisms by which ischemic injury occurs [26]. However, there are little or no objective data demonstrating that pouch ischemia occurs in many patients with pouch dysfunction. If ischemia did contribute to the pathogenesis of pouchitis, then medical therapy directed toward reducing oxygen free radical formation, such as the xanthine oxidase inhibitor allopurinol, might be a useful strategy for the treatment of pouchitis.

Clinical results

An uncontrolled study reported that oral allopurinol induced clinical improvement in 4/8 patients with active acute pouchitis and maintained remission despite the withdrawal of suppressive antibiotic therapy in 7/14 patients with chronic pouchitis [65]. However, a randomized, double blind, placebo-controlled trial of allopurinol for the prophylaxis of pouchitis in 184 patients undergoing IPAA was negative [66]. **A1a** Additionally, there was no difference in overall pouch function between these two groups. These findings do not support the idea that ischemic damage and free radical injury contribute to the pathogenesis of pouchitis.

Treatment with bismuth

Rationale

Bismuth has both antimicrobial and antidiarrheal properties, and has been useful in the treatment of traveler's diarrhea. A controlled trial suggested that bismuth citrate may be comparable with mesalamine for the treatment of left-sided UC [67]. Given the benefit of bismuth for traveler's diarrhea, and its potential benefit in UC, therapeutic trials of bismuth in pouchitis seemed reasonable.

Clinical results

An uncontrolled study of bismuth carbomer enemas suggested beneficial effects in chronic pouchitis [68]. However, a small randomized controlled trial in active chronic pouchitis showed no benefit compared with placebo [69]. **A1d** In this study, the placebo response rate was high, and thus it is possible that bismuth carbomer and the xanthan gum used for the placebo were both effective therapies. Furthermore the study may have lacked power to demonstrate a significant difference, should one exist. An uncontrolled maintenance study of bismuth carbomer foam enemas in patients with pouchitis demonstrated minimal systemic absorption of bismuth, no toxicity and possible

continued clinical benefit in patients with chronic pouchitis after treatment for 9–128 weeks [70]. Further support for a potential therapeutic effect of bismuth in pouchitis comes from an uncontrolled study of oral bismuth subsalicylate tablets, which suggested a beneficial effect in 11/13 patients with active chronic pouchitis [71]. **B4** Adequately powered controlled trials, using an inactive placebo, are needed to determine whether bismuth has a role in the treatment of pouchitis.

Treatment algorithm for pouchitis

An algorithmic approach to treatment of pouchitis is shown in Figure 13.1. A presumptive diagnosis of pouchitis in patients with compatible symptoms should be confirmed by pouch endoscopy and biopsy. After the diagnosis is confirmed, treatment with ciprofloxacin or metronidazole is initiated. Responding patients who experience recurrent episodes and are able to tolerate the medication should be re-treated with the same regimen. Some patients with recurrent pouchitis (e.g. ≥3 episodes per year or recurrence within one or two months of stopping antibiotic therapy) will benefit from long-term suppressive or maintenance antibiotic therapy. If patients who require suppressive antibiotic therapy develop bacterial resistance after prolonged treatment, cycling of three or four antibiotics may be beneficial. Probiotic therapy can also be considered in patients with chronic pouchitis as an alternative to maintenance antibiotic therapy. Those patients who do not respond to a single antibiotic are usually tried on another antibiotic or combination antibiotics. If this strategy is ineffective, therapy with oral budesonide or aminosalicylate products, or topical pouch therapy with mesalamine or steroids, can be considered. In more refractory cases, azathioprine, 6-mercaptopurine or even infliximab may be useful. Some patients may require combination therapy with multiple agents, as for some patients with IBD, although there are no data to support this approach. There are few data and there is limited rationale to support empirical therapy with SCFA enemas, glutamine suppositories, inulin or allopurinol. A small number of patients will be refractory to all forms of medical therapy, and these patients should be referred to a surgeon for consideration of permanent ileostomy with pouch exclusion or excision.

Response to treatment of pouchitis (natural history)

In patients with IPAA for UC, the cumulative risk of developing at least one episode of pouchitis is approximately 30–60% [1]. Of those patients who develop pouchitis, approximately 35% have one or two episodes per year

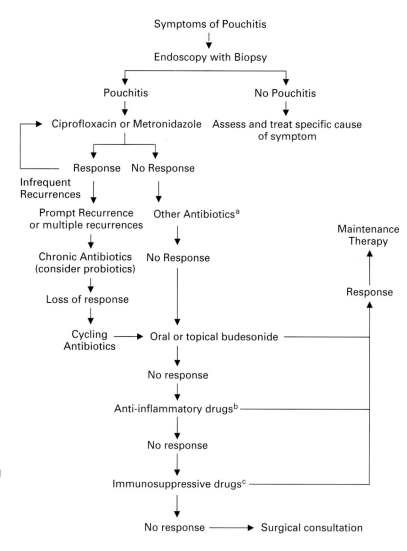

Figure 13.1 Treatment algorithm for pouchitis. Rifaximin[a]; amoxicillin/clavulanate; erythromycin; tetracycline; and cycling of multiple antibiotics. Bismuth subsalicylate[b], mesalamine enemas; sulfasalazine; and oral mesalamine. Budesonide[c], steroid enemas; oral steroids; azathioprine. (Reproduced with permission from Mahadevan U and Sandborn WJ. *Gastroenterology* 2003; **124**: 1636–1650).

which respond to treatment with antibiotics, 50% relapse more frequently (≥3 episodes per year) but still respond to antibiotics, and 15% require maintenance therapy and have been classified as having chronic pouchitis [8]. Of patients with chronic pouchitis, some require surgical exclusion or excision of the pouch. An algorithm showing the clinical course of pouchitis in IPAA patients is shown in Figure 13.2.

Conclusion

Small controlled trials have demonstrated the efficacy of ciprofloxacin and metronidazole for acute pouchitis and budesonide enemas for active chronic pouchitis. Three trials suggested that probiotic bacteria may be useful in maintaining remission of chronic pouchitis and as prophylaxis against developing pouchitis. Controlled trials of rifaximin, bismuth carbomer and allopurinol did not demonstrate

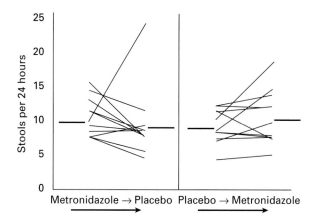

Figure 13.2 Clinical outcome with regard to pouchitis in 100 patients with ulcerative colitis (UC) undergoing proctocolectomy with ileal pouch-anal anastomosis (IPAA). (Reproduced with permission from Sandborn WJ. In: *Trends in Inflammatory Bowel Disease*. Kluwer Academic, Lancaster, UK, 1997).

efficacy. Uncontrolled studies suggest possible benefit from other antibiotics, sulfasalazine, mesalamine, corticosteroids and bismuth. There are few data suggesting that immune modifiers, SCFA enemas or inulin are of benefit.

Natural history studies suggest that most patients with pouchitis respond to a short course of antibiotic therapy. Some patients with chronic pouchitis require suppressive medical therapy with antibiotics or probiotics, and some will require permanent ileostomy with pouch exclusion or excision. Additional randomized, double blind placebo-controlled trials are needed to determine the efficacy of empirical medical therapies currently being used in patients with pouchitis.

References

1 Sandborn WJ, Pardi DS. Clinical management of pouchitis. *Gastroenterology* 2004; **127**: 1809–1814.

2 Fazio VW, Ziv Y, Church JM *et al.* Ileal pouch-anal anastomosis: Complications and function in 1005 patients. *Ann Surg* 1995; **222**: 120–127.

3 Marcello PW, Roberts PL, Schoetz DJ Jr *et al.* Long-term results of the ileoanal pouch procedure. *Arch Surg* 1993; **128**: 500–504.

4 Hueting WE, Buskens E, van der Tweel I *et al.* Results and complications after ileall pouch anal anastomosis: A meta-analysis of 43 observational studies comprising 9317 patients. *Dig Surg* 2005; **22**: 69–79.

5 Simchuk EJ, Thirlby RC. Risk factors and true incidence of pouchitis in patients after ileal pouch-anal anastomoses. *World J Surg* 2000; **24**: 851–856.

6 Salemans JM, Nagengast FM, Lubbers EJ *et al.* Postoperative and long-term results of ileal pouch-anal anastomosis for ulcerative colitis and familial polyposis coli. *Dig Dis Sci* 1992; **37**: 1882–1889.

7 Meagher AP, Farouk R, Dozois RR *et al.* J ileal pouch-anal anastomosis for chronic ulcerative colitis: Complications and long-term outcome in 1310 patients. *Br J Surg* 1998; **85**: 800–803.

8 Sandborn WJ. (1997) Pouchitis: Definition, risk factors, frequency, natural history, classification, and public health perspective. In: McLeod RS (ed.) *Trends in inflammatory bowel disease.* Kluwer Academic, Lancaster, UK, 1997.

9 Sandborn WJ, Tremaine WJ, Batts KP *et al.* Pouchitis after ileal pouch-anal anastomosis: a Pouchitis Disease Activity Index. *Mayo Clin Proc* 1994; **69**: 409–415.

10 Pardi DS, Shen B. Endoscopy in the management of patients after ileal pouch surgery for ulcerative colitis. *Endoscopy* 2008; **40**: 529–533.

11 Moskowitz RL, Shepherd NA, Nicholls RJ. An assessment of inflammation in the reservoir after restorative proctocolectomy with ileoanal ileal reservoir. *Int J Colorectal Dis* 1986; **1**: 167–174.

12 Shepherd NA, Jass JR, Duval I *et al.* Restorative proctocolectomy with ileal reservoir: Pathological and histochemical study of mucosal biopsy specimens. *J Clin Pathol* 1987; **40**: 601–607.

13 Sandborn WJ. Pouchitis following ileal pouch-anal anastomosis: Definition, pathogenesis and treatment. *Gastroenterology* 1994; **107**: 1856–60.

14 Duffy M, O'Mahony L, Coffey JC *et al.* Sulfate-reducing bacteria colonize pouches formed for ulcerative colitis but not for familial adenomatous polyposis. *Dis Colon Rectum* 2002; **45**: 384–388.

15 Gosselink MP, Schouten WR, van Lieshout LM *et al.* Eradication of pathogenic bacteria and restoration of normal pouch flora: Comparison of metronidazole and ciprofloxacin in the treatment of pouchitis. *Dis Colon Rectum* 2004; **47**: 1519–1525.

16 Gionchetti P, Rizzello F, Venturi A *et al.* Antibiotic combination therapy in patients with chronic, treatment-resistant pouchitis. *Aliment Pharmacol Ther* 1999; **13**: 713–718.

17 Kmiot WA, Youngs D, Tudor R *et al.* Mucosal morphology, cell proliferation and faecal bacteriology in acute pouchitis. *Br J Surg* 1993; **80**: 1445–1449.

18 Sandborn WJ, Tremaine WJ, Batts KP *et al.* Fecal bile acids, short-chain fatty acids, and bacteria after ileal pouch-anal anastomosis do not differ in patients with pouchitis. *Dig Dis Sci* 1995; **40**: 1474–1483.

19 Shepherd NA, Hulten L, Tytgat GN *et al.* Pouchitis. *Int J Colorectal Dis* 1989; **4**: 205–229.

20 Natori H, Utsunomiya J, Yamamura T *et al.* Fecal and stomal bile acid composition after ileostomy or ileoanal anastomosis in patients with chronic ulcerative colitis and adenomatosis coli. *Gastroenterology* 1992; **102**: 1278–1288.

21 Nasmyth DG, Godwin PG, Dixon MF *et al.* Ileal ecology after pouch-anal anastomosis or ileostomy. A study of mucosal morphology, fecal bacteriology, fecal volatile fatty acids, and their interrelationship. *Gastroenterology* 1989; **96**: 817–824.

22 Gosselink MP, Schouten WR, van Lieshout LM *et al.* Eradication of pathogenic bacteria and restoration of normal pouch flora: Comparison of metronidazole and ciprofloxacin in the treatment of pouchitis. *Dis Colon Rectum* 2004; **47**: 1519–1525.

23 McLeod RS, Taylor DW, Cohen Z, Cullen JB. Single-patient randomised clinical trial. Use in determining optimum treatment for patient with inflammation of Kock continent ileostomy reservoir. *Lancet* 1986; **1**: 726–728.

24 Zuccaro G Jr, Fazio VW, Church JM et al. Pouch ileitis. *Dig Dis Sci* 1989; **34**: 1505–1510.

25 Hurst RD, Molinari M, Chung TP et al. Prospective study of the incidence, timing and treatment of pouchitis in 104 consecutive patients after restorative proctocolectomy. *Arch Surg* 1996; **131**: 497–500; discussion 501–2.

26 Tytgat GN, van Deventer SJ. Pouchitis. *Int J Colorectal Dis* 1988; **3**: 226–228.

27 Madden MV, McIntyre AS, Nicholls RJ. Double-blind crossover trial of metronidazole versus placebo in chronic unremitting pouchitis. *Dig Dis Sci* 1994; **39**: 1193–1196.

28 Shen B, Achkar JP, Lashner BA et al. A randomized clinical trial of ciprofloxacin and metronidazole to treat acute pouchitis. *Inflamm Bowel Dis* 2001; **7**: 301–305.

29 Sambuelli A, Boerr L, Negreira S et al. Budesonide enema in pouchitis – a double-blind, double-dummy, controlled trial. *Aliment Pharmacol Ther* 2002; **16**: 27–34.

30 Isaacs KL, Sandler RS, Abreu M et al. Rifaximin for the treatment of active pouchitis: A randomized, double-blind, placebo-controlled pilot study. *Inflamm Bow Dis* 2007; **13**: 1250–1255.

31 Gionchetti P, Rizzello F, Venturi A et al. Antibiotic combination therapy in patients with chronic, treatmentresistant pouchitis. *Aliment Pharmacol Ther* 1999; **13**: 713–718.

32 Mimura T, Rizzello F, Helwig U et al. Four week open-label trial of metronidazole and ciprofloxacin for the treatment of recurrent or refractory pouchitis. *Aliment Pharmacol Ther* 2002; **16**: 909–917.

33 Shen B, Fazio VW, Remzi FH et al. Combined ciprofloxacin and tinidazole therapy in the treatment of chronic refractory pouchitis. *Dis Colon Rectum* 2007; **50**: 498–508.

34 Gionchetti P, Rizzello F, Venturi A et al. Oral bacteriotherapy as maintenance treatment in patients with chronic pouchitis: A double-blind, placebo-controlled trial. *Gastroenterology* 2000; **119**: 305–309.

35 Mimura T, Rizzello F, Helwig U et al. Once daily high dose probiotic therapy (VSL#3) for maintaining remission in recurrent or refreactory pouchitis. *Gut* 2004; **53**: 108–114.

36 Gionchetti P, Rizzello F, Helwig U et al. Prophylaxis of pouchitis onset with probiotic therapy: A double-blind, placebo-controlled trial. *Gastroenterology* 2003; **124**: 1202–1209.

37 Gionchetti P, Rizzello F, Morselli C et al. High-dose probiotics for the treatment of active pouchitis. *Dis Colon Rectum* 2007; **50**: 2075–2084.

38 Kuzela L, Kascak M, Vavrecka A. Induction and maintenance of remission with nonpathogenic Escherichia coli in patients with pouchitis. *Am J Gastroenterol* 2001; **96**: 3218–3219.

39 Shen B, Brzezinski A, Fazio VW et al. Maintenance therapy with a probiotic in antibiotic-dependent pouchitis: Experience in clinical practice. *Aliment Pharmacol Ther* 2005; **22**: 721–728.

40 Miglioli M, Barbara L, Di Febo G et al. Topical administration of 5-aminosalicylic acid: A therapeutic proposal for the treatment of pouchitis. *N Engl J Med* 1989; **320**: 257.

41 Belluzzi A, Campieri M, Gionchetti P et al. Acute pouchitis: 5-aminosalicylic acid and budesonide suppositories effectiveness on inflammatory mediator production. *Gastroenterology* 1993; **104**: A665.

42 Keighley MRB. Review article: the management of pouchitis. *Aliment Pharmacol Ther* 1996; **10**: 449–457.

43 Sagar PM, Pemberton JH. Ileo-anal pouch function and dysfunction. *Dig Dis* 1997; **15**: 172–188.

44 Belluzzi A, Campieri M, Miglioli M et al. Evaluation of flogistic pattern in "pouchitis" before and after the treatment with budesonide. *Gastroenterology* 1992; **102**: A593.

45 Gionnchetti P, Rizello F, Poggioli G et al. Oral budesonide in the treatment of chronic refractory pouchitis. *Aliment Pharmacol Ther* 2007; **25**: 1231–1236.

46 Chopra A, Pardi DS, Loftus EV et al. Budesonide in the treatment of inflammatory bowel disease: The first year of experience in clinical practice. *Inflamm Bow Dis* 2006; **12**: 29–32.

47 Winter TA, Dalton HR, Merrett MN et al. Cyclosporin A retention enemas in refractory distal ulcerative colitis and "pouchitis". *Scand J Gastroenterol* 1993; **28**: 701–704.

48 Zins BJ, Sandborn WJ, Penna CR et al. Pouchitis disease course after orthotopic liver transplantation in patients with primary sclerosing cholangitis and an ileal pouch-anal anastomosis. *Am J Gastroenterol* 1995; **90**: 2177–2181.

49 Rowley S, Candinas D, Mayer AD et al. Restorative proctocolectomy and pouch anal anastomosis for ulcerative colitis following orthotopic liver transplantation. *Gut* 1995; **37**: 845–847.

50 Berrebi W, Chaussade S, Bruhl AL et al. Treatment of Crohn's disease recurrence after ileoanal anastomosis by azathioprine. *Dig Dis Sci* 1993; **38**: 1558–1560.

51 MacMillan F, Warner A. Efficacy of immunosuppressive therapy for the treatment of chronic pouchitis following ileal pouch-anal anastomosis. *Am J Gastroenterol* 1999; **94**: 2677.

52 Calabrese C, Gionchetti P, Rizello F et al. Short-term treatment with infliximab in chronic refractory pouchitis and ileitis. *Aliment Pharmacol Ther* 2008; **27**: 759–764.

53 Viscido A, Habib Fl, Kohn A et al. Infliximab in refractory pouchitis complicated by fistulae following ileo-anal pouch for ulcerative colitis. *Aliment Pharmacol Ther* 2003; **17**: 1263–1271.

54 Ricart E, Panaccione R, Loftus EV et al. Successful management of Crohn's disease of the ileoanal pouch with infliximab. *Gastroenterology* 1999; **117**: 429–432.

55 Colombel JF, Ricart E, Loftus EV et al. Management of Crohn's disease of the ileoanal pouch with infliximab. *Am J Gastroenterol* 2003; **98**: 2239–2244.

56 Nasmyth DG, Godwin PG, Dixon MF et al. Real ecology after pouch-anal anastomosis or ileostomy. A study of mucosal morphology, fecal bacteriology, fecal volatile fatty acids, and their interrelationship. *Gastroenterology* 1989; **96**: 817–824.

57 Clausen MR, Tvede M, Mortensen PB. Short-chain fatty acids in pouch contents from patients with and without pouchitis after ileal pouch-anal anastomosis. *Gastroenterology* 1992; **103**: 1144–1153.

58 Wischmeyer P, Pemberton JH, Phillips SE. Chronic pouchitis after ileal pouch-anal anastomosis: Responses to butyrate and glutamine suppositories in a pilot study. *Mayo Clin Proc* 1993; **68**: 978–981.

59 den Hoed PT, van Goch JJ, Veen HF, Ouwendijk RJ. Severe pouchitis successfully treated with short-chain fatty acids. *Can J Surg* 1996; **39**: 168–169.

60 de Silva HJ, Ireland A, Kettlewell M et al. Short-chain fatty acid irrigation in severe pouchitis. *N Engl J Med* 1989; **321**: 1416–1417.

61 Tremaine WJ, Sandborn WJ, Phillips SF et al. Short chain fatty acid enema therapy for treatment-resistant pouchitis following ileal pouch anal anastomosis for ulcerative colitis. *Gastroenterology* 1994; **106**: 784.

62 Welters CF, Heineman E, Thunnissen FB et al. Effect of dietary inulin supplementation on inflammation of pouch mucosa in patients with an ileal pouch-anal anastomosis. *Dis Colon Rectum* 2002; **45**: 621–627.

63 Thirlby RC, Kelly R. Pectin and methyl cellulose do not affect intestinal function in patients after ileal pouch-anal anastomosis. *Am J Gastroenterol* 1997; **92**: 99–102.

64 Smith L, Friend WG, Medwell SJ. The superior mesenteric artery. The critical factor in the pouch pull-through procedure. *Dis Colon Rectum* 1984; **27**: 741–744.

65 Levin KE, Pemberton JH, Phillips SF et al. Role of oxygen free radicals in the etiology of pouchitis. *Dis Colon Rectum* 1992; **35**: 452–456.

66 Joelsson M, Andersson M, Bark T et al. Allopurinol as prophylaxis against pouchitis following ileal pouch-anal anastomosis

for ulcerative colitis. A randomized placebo controlled double-blind study. *Scand J Gastroenterol* 2001; **36**: 1179–1184.

67 Pullan RD, Ganesh S, Mani V et al. Comparison of bismuth citrate and 5aminosalicylic acid enemas in distal ulcerative colitis: A controlled trial. *Gut* 1993; **34**: 676–679.

68 Gionchetti P, Rizzello F, Venturi A et al. Long-term efficacy of bismuth carbomer enemas in patients with treatment resistant chronic pouchitis. *Aliment Pharmacol Ther* 1997; **11**: 673–678.

69 Tremaine WJ, Sandborn WJ, Wolff BG et al. Bismuth carbomer foam enemas for active chronic pouchitis: a randomized, double blind, placebo-controlled trial. *Aliment Pharmacol Ther* 1997; **11**: 1041–1046.

70 Tremaine WJ, Sandborn WJ. Safety of long term open treatment with bismuth carbomer foam enemas for chronic pouchitis. *Gastroenterology* 1997; **112**: A1105.

71 Tremaine WJ, Sandborn WJ, Kenan ML. Bismuth subsalicylate tablets for chronic antibiotic-resistant pouchitis. *Gastroenterology* 1998; **114**: A1101.

14 Microscopic colitis: Collagenous and lymphocytic colitis

Johan Bohr[1], Robert Löfberg[2] and Curt Tysk[1]
[1]Department of Gastroenterology, Örebro University Hospital, Örebro, Sweden
[2]IBD Unit, HMQ Sophia Hospital, Karolinska Institute, Stockholm, Sweden

Microscopic colitis is characterised clinically by chronic, non-bloody diarrhea, a macroscopically normal or near-normal colonic mucosa and specific histopathologic features. Collagenous colitis and lymphocytic colitis constitute the two main forms of microscopic colitis. Collagenous colitis was first described by Lindström in 1976. The name emphasized the subepithelial collagenous band which characterises this disease [1]. The term lymphocytic colitis was introduced by Lazenby *et al.* in 1989, to reflect the fact that the major feature of lymphocytic colitis was an increased number of intraepithelial lymphocytes [2].

Epidemiology

Collagenous colitis was initially regarded as being rare, until the first epidemiologic studies showed incidence rates of 1.8/100,000 and 2.3/100,000 inhabitants and a prevalence of 15.7/100,000 inhabitants [3, 4]. Recent epidemiologic studies, however, show that collagenous colitis is more common, and incidence figures of 4.6/100,000 to 6.2/100,000 inhabitants have been reported (Table 14.1) [5–9]. Patients with collagenous colitis are typically middle-aged women, the average age at diagnosis being around 65 years, and the female: male ratio is approximately 7:1 (Figure 14.1) [3–5]. However, 25% of 163 patients were diagnosed before the age of 45 years so the diagnosis must be considered even in younger patients with chronic watery diarrhoea [10]. A few children below the age of 12 have been reported [11].

Epidemiologic data for lymphocytic colitis have now been reported from five different regions in Europe and North America (Table 14.1) [5–9]. The data have been fairly

consistent in the more recent studies, in which an annual incidence of 4 to 5.5 per 100,000 inhabitants has been reported. The incidence of collagenous and lymphocytic colitis is close to the incidence of Crohn's disease and combined rates for collagenous colitis and lymphocytic colitis approach the incidence of ulcerative colitis. The data illustrate that these conditions are more common than was considered earlier. Microscopic colitis may be diagnosed in 10% of patients investigated for chronic non-bloody diarrhea, and in 20% of such patients older than 70 years [12]. The average age at onset of symptoms in lymphocytic colitis is approximately 60 to 65 years, but the female predominance is less pronounced than is reported for collagenous colitis (Figure 14.2).

Histopathology

Collagenous colitis

The following histopathologic features are the hallmarks of collagenous colitis:
• Diffuse non-continuous thickening of a subepithelial collagen layer beneath the basement membrane (See colour plate 14.1) with the thickness of the subepithelial layer measuring at least 10 µm on a well-orientated section of the mucosa (in comparison to 0–3 µm in normal tissue)
• Chronic inflammation in the lamina propria dominated by lymphocytes and plasma cells
• Flattening and vacuolisation of the epithelial cells and detachment of the surface epithelium
• Intraepithelial lymphocyte infiltration may be present, although this feature is not as prominent as in lymphocytic colitis [2, 13].

Cryptitis does not exclude the diagnosis of collagenous colitis [14]. In the matrix containing the thickened collagen layer collagen type I, III and VI and fibronectine have been identified [15, 16]. The histopathologic findings are mainly

Evidence-Based Gastroenterology and Hepatology, 3rd edition.
J. McDonald, A.K. Burroughs, B. Feagan, and M.B. Fennerty. © 2010
Blackwell Publishing Ltd

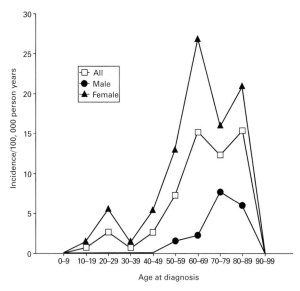

Figure 14.1 Age and sex-specific incidence of collagenous colitis. Reprinted with permission from Olesen *et al. Gut* 2004; **53**: 346–350 [6].

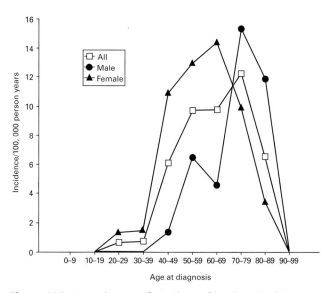

Figure 14.2 Age and sex-specific incidence of lymphocytic colitis. Reprinted with permission from Olesen *et al. Gut* 2004; **53**: 346–350 [6].

Table 14.1 Annual incidence per 100,000 inhabitants of collagenous and lymphocytic colitis in population based epidemiological studies.

Region and study period	Collagenous colitis	Lymphocytic colitis
Örebro, Sweden, 1984–88 [3]	0.8	
Örebro, Sweden, 1989–93 [3]	2.7	
Örebro, Sweden, 1993–95 [6]	3.7	3.1
Örebro, Sweden, 1996–98 [6]	6.1	5.7
Örebro, Sweden 1999–2004 [8]	5.2	5.5
Terrassa, Spain, 1993–97 [4]	2.3	3.7
Iceland, 1995–99 [5]	5.2	4.0
Olmsted, USA 1985–89 [7]	0.3	0.5
Olmsted, USA 1990–93 [7]	1.6	1.0
Olmsted, USA 1994–97 [7]	3.9	6.4
Olmsted, USA 1997–2001 [7]	6.2	12.9
Calgary, Canada 2002–2004 [9]	4.6	5.4

located in the colon and the rectum. The collagen layer is most prominent in the proximal colon, and may be absent in the rectal mucosa in between 18–73% of biopsy specimens [4, 5, 17, 18]. However, an increased subepithelial collagen layer in the stomach and duodenum as well as in the terminal ileum, so called collagenous gastritis and collagenous enterocolitis, has been reported occasionally [19–28].

Lymphocytic colitis

The histopathologic diagnostic criteria of lymphocytic colitis are:
- Epithelial lesions
- An increase in intraepithelial lymphocytes (>20 lymphocytes per 100 epithelial cells)
- Infiltration of the lamina propria with lymphocytes and plasma cells, in the absence of an increase of the collagen layer (See colour plate 14.2) [2, 29]

An increased number of intraepithelial T-lymphocytes may also be seen in the terminal ileum [28].

A recent blinded and independent study of the observer variability in diagnosing microscopic colitis histopathologically, showed that the interobserver agreement with final diagnostic categories was 91% [30], indicating that the histopathologic criteria are consistent and reproducible.

Etiology and pathophysiology

The etiology of microscopic colitis is largely unknown. At present, both collagenous and lymphocytic colitis are considered to be caused by an abnormal immunologic reaction to various mucosal insults in predisposed individuals.

Genetics

Data on genetics are sparse. A small number of familial cases with collagenous and lymphocytic colitis, and with mixed collagenous and lymphocytic colitis has been reported [31–35]. Twelve percent of patients with lymphocytic colitis reported a family history of other bowel disorders such us inflammatory bowel disease, celiac disease or collagenous colitis [12]. A recent study showed a significant association between both collagenous colitis and lymphocytic colitis and HLA-DR3-DQ2 [36]. Another study showed that HLA-DQ2 or DQ1,3 were seen more frequently in microscopic colitis than in controls, which indicate that there may be a partly genetic background for the diseases [37]. However, other studies have shown less strong associations [38], and there is no association found between NOD2/CARD15 gene polymorphisms and collagenous colitis [39].

Reaction to a luminal agent

The increased number of T-lymphocytes in the epithelium has supported the theory that collagenous colitis may be caused by an abnormal immunologic reaction to a luminal agent [40–42]. The observation, that diversion of the fecal stream by an ileostomy normalises or reduces the characteristic histopathologic changes in collagenous colitis, further supports this theory [43]. Recurrence of symptoms and histopathologic changes were seen after closure of ileostomy. Furthermore, abnormalities of colonic histology resembling lymphocytic colitis have been reported in untreated celiac disease [44].

A recent cytokine study in both collagenous and lymphocytic colitis demonstrated a T_H1-cytokine profile, with increased IFN-γ and TNFα, and normal levels of IL-2, IL-4 and IL-10 [45]. A down-regulation of E-cadherin and ZO-1 was observed, and another study demonstrated a decrease in occludin and claudin-4 expression [46]; both events might result in an impaired function of tight junctions. Taha *et al.* found a significant correlation between the increased concentrations of eosinophil cationic protein and albumin in rectal perfusate, indicating a disturbed mucosal permeability [47].

Infectious agent

The sudden onset of the disease in some patients, and the effects of various antibiotics support a possible infectious cause [10]. An association with microscopic colitis and infections with *Campylobacter jejuni* [48] and *Clostridium difficile* [49–51] has been reported. In another study, *Yersinia enterocolitica* was detected in three of six patients prior to the collagenous colitis diagnosis, and a serologic study showed that antibodies to *Yersinia species* were more common in collagenous colitis patients than in healthy controls [52, 53]. "Brainerd diarrhea" is the term applied to an outbreak of chronic watery diarrhea characterised by acute onset and prolonged duration [54]. An infectious cause has been suspected but the responsible agent has not been identified. Colonic biopsies in these patients show epithe-

Table 14.2 Drugs reported in association with microscopic colitis.

Lymphocytic colitis	Collagenous colitis
Ticlopidine [57–59]	Lanzoprazole [60, 61]
Cyclo 3 Fort [62–64]	NSAID [55]
Ranitidine [65]	Cimetidine [66]
Vinburnine [67]	
Tardyferon [68]	
Flutamide [59]	
Acarbose [69]	
Piroxicam [70]	
Levodopa-benserazide [71]	
Carbamazepine [12, 72, 73]	
Sertraline [12]	
Paroxetine [12]	
Oxetorone [74]	
Lanzoprazole [61, 75]	

lial lymphocytosis similar to lymphocytic colitis but the surface epithelial lesions are absent.

Drugs

There are several reports of drug-induced microscopic colitis, especially lymphocytic colitis (Table 14.2). Most reports concern ticlopidine and Cyclo 3 Fort. In a case-control study the use of NSAIDs was significantly more common in collagenous colitis patients than in controls, and discontinuation of NSAIDs was followed by improvement of the diarrhea in some patients [55]. Others found that use of NSAIDs at presentation was associated with a greater need for 5-ASA and steroid therapy, possibly reflecting a more resistant form of disease, but withdrawal of NSAIDs did not improve clinical symptoms in that study [56]. The increased use of NSAIDs in collagenous colitis observed in collagenous colitis patients compared to controls is possibly due to the occurrence of concomitant arthritis. The number of reported cases of drug-induced microscopic colitis is small and chance associations are possible. It is, however, important to assess concomitant drug use in patients and consider withdrawal of drugs that may worsen the condition.

Autoimmunity

Both collagenous and lymphocytic colitis are associated with autoimmune diseases. An autoimmune pathogenesis has therefore been proposed, possibly initiated by a foreign luminal agent that causes an immunologic cross-reaction with an endogenous antigen. A study of autoantibodies and immunoglobulins in collagenous colitis showed that the mean level of IgM in collagenous colitis patients was significantly increased [76], similar to observations in primary biliary cirrhosis. A specific autoantibody in collagenous colitis has not been reported.

Bile acids

Data on bile acid malabsorption in microscopic colitis are conflicting. In one study no association was found [77], whereas others found bile acid malabsorption in 27–44% of patients with collagenous colitis and in 9–60% of patients with lymphocytic colitis [78–80]. The coexistence of bile acid malabsorption seems to worsen the diarrhea in patients with collagenous colitis [78]. These observations are the rationale for recommendations of bile acid binding treatment, which was reported effective in a majority of patients with microscopic colitis and concomitant bile acid malabsorption [78, 80]. Even patients without bile acid malabsorption may respond to this treatment. This emphasises the possibility of a causative agent in the fecal stream, and the therapeutic effect may possibly be related to binding of luminal toxins [81].

Nitric oxide

Colonic nitric oxide (NO) production is greatly increased in active microscopic colitis caused by an up-regulation of inducible nitric oxide synthase (iNOS) in the colonic epithelium [82–84]. The levels of NO correlated with clinical activity and histopathologic status of the colonic mucosa; i.e. patients in histopathologic remission had normal levels of colonic NO in contrast to increased levels in patients with histologic active disease [84, 85]. The role of NO in microscopic colitis is uncertain. NO is an inflammatory mediator but whether its role is proinflammatory or protective remains unclear. Nitric oxide may furthermore be involved in the diarrheal pathophysiology as infusion in the colon of N^G-monomethyl-L-arginine, an inhibitor of NOS, reduced colonic net secretion by 70% and the addition of L-arginine increased colonic net secretion by 50% [86].

Secretory or osmotic diarrhea

Diarrheal pathophysiology in collagenous colitis has been regarded as secretory, caused by the epithelial lesions, the inflammatory infiltrate in the lamina propria and the collagenous band that may be a barrier for reabsorption of electrolytes and water [46, 87]. Furthermore, an impaired epithelial barrier function due to down-regulation of tight junction molecules was found to contribute to diarrheal pathophysiology [46]. Studies on the influence of fasting on diarrhea in collagenous colitis indicated, however, that osmotic diarrhea was predominant [88]. Many patients

report that fasting reduces their diarrhea in accordance with this observation.

Clinical features and diagnosis

The main symptom in collagenous colitis is non-bloody diarrhea that may be accompanied by nocturnal diarrhea, fecal incontinence, crampy abdominal pain and distension [10]. Weight loss of up to 5 kg is common initially and occasionally is even more pronounced. Serious dehydration is rare, although 25% of patients report 10 or more daily stools, and stool volumes up to 5 litres have been reported. Mucus or blood in the stools is unusual. In some patients the onset of the disease may be as sudden as that of infectious diarrhea [10].

In most cases the clinical course is chronic, relapsing and benign [89, 90]. Serious complications are uncommon, although a number of patients with colonic perforation have been reported [91–94], and perforation seems to be related to "mucosal tears" that can be seen at colonoscopy [95–98]. The risk of developing colorectal cancer in collagenous colitis is not increased [89, 99]. In a follow-up study, 63% of patients had lasting remission after 3.5 years [100]. Another cohort study showed that all patients were improved 47 months after the diagnosis and only 29% of these required medications [101]. In a number of collagenous colitis patients, however, remission is difficult to achieve, and such patients have usually tried different medications unsuccessfully [10, 43].

Patients with collagenous colitis often have concomitant diseases. Up to 40% have one or more associated autoimmune diseases. The most common are rheumatoid arthritis, thyroid disorders, celiac disease, asthma/allergy and diabetes mellitus. Crohn's disease or ulcerative colitis concomitant with collagenous colitis have occasionally been reported [10, 102]. Lymphocytic colitis is clinically indistinguishable from collagenous colitis and the predominant symptom is chronic watery diarrhea. In a recent report, however, it was found that symptoms in lymphocytic colitis were milder and more likely to disappear than in collagenous colitis [59]. Similar to collagenous colitis, lymphocytic colitis has also been reported in association with autoimmune diseases [59]. The prognosis of lymphocytic colitis is good [103]. There is no increased mortality and no increased risk of subsequent bowel malignancy reported. A benign course was reported in 27 cases with resolution of diarrhea and normalization of histology in over 80% of the patients within 38 months [104]. Others reported that the clinical course was a single attack in 63% of the patients with a median duration of six months from onset of symptoms to remission [12].

Only microscopic assessment of colonic mucosal biopsies can verify the diagnosis of collagenous or lymphocytic colitis. Merely non-specific, minor laboratory abnormalities are found, and there are at present no blood tests available for screening purposes. Analyses of P-ANCA [76] or serum procollagen III propeptide are of no diagnostic value in collagenous colitis [105]. Stool examinations reveal no pathologic organisms though increased excretion of fecal leukocytes in more than half of the collagenous colitis patients has been reported [26]. Barium enema and endoscopy are usually normal, though subtle endoscopic changes such as mucosal edema, granularity or erythema may be seen in up to 30% of cases [10, 12]. Pancolonoscopy must be preferred to sigmoidoscopy as the thickened collagenous layer in collagenous colitis may be absent in a considerable percentage of rectal biopsy specimens [18]. The use of confocal laser endomicroscopy may aid in diagnosing collagenous colitis [106, 107].

One or two diseases?

It has been questioned whether lymphocytic colitis and collagenous colitis are the same disease in different stages of development or two different but related conditions, as they have a similar clinical expression and similar histopathologic features, except for the subepithelial collagenous layer in collagenous colitis. Conversion of lymphocytic colitis to collagenous colitis or the opposite has been reported [7, 108], but the fact that conversion happens fairly seldom, and differences in sex ratio and HLA pattern [38] makes it more likely that collagenous colitis and lymphocytic colitis are two separate but related entities.

Treatment of microscopic colitis

The enigmatic etiology of microscopic colitis has led to a wide range of anti-diarrheal and anti-inflammatory drugs being evaluated for medical treatment. A relatively small number of controlled trials has been conducted, and recommendations on therapy have mainly been based on retrospective reports and uncontrolled data [10, 109]. The benign course of microscopic colitis in general has led to suggestions of an algorithm with a "step-up" type of approach to medical treatment, depending on clinical response and outcome in the individual patient. Milder symptoms may be well controlled using drugs such as loperamide or cholestyramine [78, 110]. However, in patients with moderate to intense symptoms potent anti-inflammatory treatment is required. In a retrospective study, the degree of lamina propria inflammation in colonic biopsies was found to predict the response to therapy, and greater inflammation may indicate the need for corticosteroid therapy [56]. A finding of a substantial degree of

inflammation at the time of diagnosis may thus aid in clinical decision-making.

Randomised controlled trials

Treatment of collagenous colitis and lymphocytic colitis has been evaluated in randomised, controlled trials (RCTs). Cochrane reviews performed in 2008 identified all published reports on the treatment of microscopic colitis between 1970 and 2007 [111, 112]. For collagenous colitis there are ten randomised trials, seven of which were placebo controlled, of which five studied budesonide [113–117], one prednisolone [118], and one bismuth subsalicylate [119]. One trial compared mesalazine to mesalazine + cholestyramine [120], and there was one trial of probiotics [121] and one of Boswellia serrata [122]. There are three completed randomised controlled studies in lymphocytic colitis: of budesonide [123], bismuth subsalicylate (includes also collagenous colitis) [119], and mesalazine compared to mesalazine + cholestyramine (includes also collagenous colitis) [120]. A number of these trials are described in some details below.

Budesonide
The use of oral preparations of budesonide has been well proven for induction of remission in active ileocolonic Crohn's disease. This glucocorticosteroid has a high potency and a rapid first pass metabolism, rendering it active topically with less systemic effects than are observed with conventional steroids. A total of 94 patients with collagenous colitis were enrolled in three placebo-controlled trials of budesonide 9 mg daily for six to eight weeks (Table 14.3). Fifty patients received active budesonide therapy. The pooled odds ratio for clinical response with budesonide was 12.32 (95% CI: 5.53–27.46), with a number needed to treat of two patients. Most responders experienced a decrease in the number of loose stools after two to four weeks of therapy. After cessation of active therapy most patients were reported to experience a flare-up of symptoms. Histological improvement was significant in all three trials. A decrease in the grade of infiltration of lamina propria mononuclear cells was observed in most patients, whereas a reduction in the thickness of the collagen layer was found less consistently. One of the trials demonstrated a significant decrease of the collagen band in the sigmoid colon, with almost a normalisation of the mean thickness to 10.2 μm [115]. In a placebo-controlled trial of budesonide in lymphocytic colitis (9 mg daily for six weeks) [123] 21 of 41 enrolled patients received active treatment, which was more effective than placebo with respect to clinical (p = 0.004; NNT = 3) and histopathological (p = 0.04; NNT = 3) response [112].

In two trials studying maintenance treatment with budesonide in collagenous colitis, 80 patients who had

Table 14.3 Data from four randomized, placebo-controlled trials of oral budesonide in collagenous colitis and lymphocytic colitis.

Author Year	Number	Dosage	Clinical response budesonide vs placebo	Histologic response budesonide vs placebo	Adverse effects
Collagenous colitis					
Baert et al. 2002 [113]	28	9 mg/day Budenofalk 8 weeks	Improvement: 8/14 vs 3/14 (p = 0.05)	Reduction of lamina propria inflammation in 9/13 vs 4/12 (p < 0.001)	Mild
Miehlke et al. 2002 [114]	45	9 mg/day Entocort 6 weeks	Remission: 15/23 vs 0/22 (p < 0.0001)	Improvement in 17/23 vs 5/22 (p < 0.01).	Mild
Bonderup et al. 2003 [115]	20	9 mg/day Entocort 8 weeks	Respons: 10/10 vs 2/10 (p < 0.001)	Reduction of overall inflammation (p < 0.01)	None
Lymphocytic colitis					
Miehlke et al. 2007 [123]	41	9 mg/day Budenofalk 6 weeks	Remission: 18/21 vs 8/20 p = 0.004	Response in 11/15 vs 4/12 p = 0.04	Mild

responded to open-label treatment with budesonide, were randomised to active treatment or placebo. Clinical response was maintained in 83% of patients receiving active treatment, compared to 28% receiving placebo [111]. There was, however, no difference in the median time to relapse (39 days versus 38 days) in the two groups after stopping treatment [117].

Bismuth subsalicylate

In a small pilot trial with oral bismuth subsalicylate 2.4 g daily vs placebo for eight weeks, patients with collagenous colitis given active treatment were more likely to improve clinically (p = 0.003) as well as histologically (p = 0.003). Patients with lymphocytic colitis given bismuth subsalicylate had no clinical or histological improvement, compared to placebo.

Other anti-inflammatory compounds

Sulphasalazine and mesalazine have been extensively used in microscopic colitis, and in a recent trial, 64 patients with collagenous or lymphocytic colitis were randomised to mesalazine 2.4 g/day or mezalazine 2.4 g/day + cholestyramine 4 g/day for six months. A high remission rate was seen in both treatment arms, with 85% of patients with lymphocytic colitis and 91% of patients with collagenous colitis in remission at the end of the study. Combined therapy was superior in collagenous colitis and induced an earlier clinical response in both diseases [120]. Retrospective assessments of sulphasalazine and mesalazine have reported benefit in 34–50% of the patients [10, 109]. Antibiotics such as metronidazole and erythromycin have been used, but have not been studied in controlled trials.

Two studies showed no statistical evidence for the effectiveness of Boswellia serrata extract, or probiotics, although these small studies probably lacked power [121, 122].

Retrospective evaluations have shown that oral prednisolone may be effective with a reported response rate in open studies of 70 to 80%. The effect, however, is generally not sustained after withdrawal, and the dose required to maintain remission is often unacceptably high(>20 mg per day) [10]. A small RCT on prednisolone, showed no statistically significant effect but the duration of the trial (two weeks) was probably too short.

Recommended therapy

Based on a meta-analysis and RCTs, short or medium time therapy with oral budesonide is the drug of choice for the treatment of collagenous and lymphocytic colitis in patients with significant symptoms that cannot be controlled with loperamide, cholestyramine or aminosalicylates. **A1c** Oral budesonide may even be more efficacious than conventional systemic corticosteroids (e.g. prednisolone) [124]. Local effects of budesonide on the terminal ileum may be of importance in explaining this apparent advantage. Budesonide has a benign safety profile, as proven in other IBD-conditions, but it would be prudent to taper the dose to the minimum necessary for controlling symptoms in patients with microscopic colitis if more than eight weeks of therapy is required. **C5** As mentioned above, there was no difference in the median time to relapse between budesonide and placebo after stopping treatment [117]. Most candidates for longer term budesonide treatment are females aged 50–70 years, a group with an increased risk for osteoporosis. In this respect, budesonide has been demonstrated to have less impact than prednisolone on bone mineral density in patients with Crohn's disease during treatment for up to two years [125]. Budesonide therapy given on demand may be an attractive option for long-term control of symptoms. **C5** Although we have positive experience from this approach in our own clinical practice, controlled data are lacking. Bismuth subsalicylate therapy may be an alternative to budesonide, but it is not available in all countries due to toxicity concerns. **A1d**

Severe attacks of microscopic colitis are rare, but a small number of patients may require hospitalisation, intravenous steroid therapy, bowel rest and total parenteral nutrition. For steroid-refractory or steroid dependent patients immunomodulators may be of value. In an uncontrolled trial azathioprine therapy resulted in partial or complete remission in eight of nine patients with microscopic colitis [126]. **B4** In another uncontrolled trial low dose methotrexate (median dose 7.5 mg/week) showed benefit in 16 of 19 patients with prednisolone-refractory collagenous colitis [127]. **B4**

Surgical treatment

If medical therapy fails and alternative diagnoses are ruled out surgery may be considered in a patient with intractable microscopic colitis. Split ileostomy was conducted successfully in nine women with collagenous colitis [43] and successful outcomes both in collagenous colitis and lymphocytic colitis have been reported after total or subtotal colectomy [128–132]. **B4**

References

1 Lindström CG. "Collagenous colitis" with watery diarrhoea – a new entity? *Pathol Eur* 1976; **11**(1): 87–89.
2 Lazenby AJ, Yardley JH, Giardiello FM, Jessurun J, Bayless TM. Lymphocytic ("microscopic") colitis: A comparative histopathologic study with particular reference to collagenous colitis. *Hum Pathol* 1989; **20**(1): 18–28.
3 Bohr J, Tysk C, Eriksson S, Järnerot G. Collagenous colitis in Orebro, Sweden, an epidemiological study 1984–1993. *Gut* 1995; **37**(3): 394–397.
4 Fernandez-Banares F, Salas A, Forne M, Esteve M, Espinos J, Viver JM. Incidence of collagenous and lymphocytic colitis: A 5-year population- based study. *Am J Gastroenterol.* 1999; **94**(2): 418–423.
5 Agnarsdottir M, Gunnlaugsson O, Orvar KB *et al.* Collagenous and lymphocytic colitis in Iceland. *Dig Dis Sci* 2002; **47**(5): 1122–1128.
6 Olesen M, Eriksson S, Bohr J, Jarnerot G, Tysk C. Microscopic colitis: A common diarrhoeal disease. An epidemiological study in Orebro, Sweden, 1993-1998. *Gut* 2004 Mar; **53**(3): 346–350.
7 Pardi DS, Loftus EV, Jr., Smyrk TC *et al.* The epidemiology of microscopic colitis: A population based study in Olmsted County, Minnesota. *Gut* 2007 (Apr); **56**(4): 504–508.
8 Wickbom A, Nyhlin N, Eriksson S, Bohr J, Tysk C. Collagenous colitis and lymphocytic colitis in Örebro, Sweden 1999-2004; A continuous epidemiological study. *Gut* 2006; **55**(suppl V): A111.

9 Williams JJ, Kaplan GG, Makhija S *et al.* Microscopic colitis-defining incidence rates and risk factors: A population-based study. *Clin Gastroenterol Hepatol* 2008 (Jan); **6**(1): 35–40.
10 Bohr J, Tysk C, Eriksson S, Abrahamsson H, Järnerot G. Collagenous colitis: a retrospective study of clinical presentation and treatment in 163 patients. *Gut* 1996; **39**(96): 846–851.
11 Gremse DA, Boudreaux CW, Manci EA. Collagenous colitis in children. *Gastroenterology* 1993; **104**(3): 906–909.
12 Olesen M, Eriksson S, Bohr J, Jarnerot G, Tysk C. Lymphocytic colitis: A retrospective clinical study of 199 Swedish patients. *Gut* 2004 (Apr); **53**(4): 536–41.
13 Levy AM, Yamazaki K, Van Keulen VP *et al.* Increased eosinophil infiltration and degranulation in colonic tissue from patients with collagenous colitis. *Am J Gastroenterol* 2001; **96**(5): 1522–1528.
14 Jessurun J, Yardley JH, Giardiello FM, Hamilton SR, Bayless TM. Chronic colitis with thickening of the subepithelial collagen layer (collagenous colitis): histopathologic findings in 15 patients. *Hum Pathol* 1987; **18**(8): 839–848.
15 Flejou JF, Grimaud JA, Molas G, Baviera E, Potet F. Collagenous colitis. Ultrastructural study and collagen immunotyping of four cases. *Arch Pathol Lab Med* 1984; **108**(12): 977–982.
16 Aigner T, Neureiter D, Muller S, Kuspert G, Belke J, Kirchner T. Extracellular matrix composition and gene expression in collagenous colitis. *Gastroenterology* 1997; **113**(1): 136–143.
17 Tanaka M, Mazzoleni G, Riddell RH. Distribution of collagenous colitis: Utility of flexible sigmoidoscopy. *Gut* 1992; **33**(1): 65–70.
18 Offner FA, Jao RV, Lewin KJ, Havelec L, Weinstein WM. Collagenous colitis: A study of the distribution of morphological abnormalities and their histological detection. *Hum Pathol* 1999; **30**(4): 451–457.
19 Eckstein RP, Dowsett JF, Riley JW. Collagenous enterocolitis: A case of collagenous colitis with involvement of the small intestine. *Am J Gastroenterol* 1988; **83**(7): 767–771.
20 Stolte M, Ritter M, Borchard F, Koch-Scherrer G. Collagenous gastroduodenitis on collagenous colitis. *Endoscopy* 1990; **22**(4): 186–187.
21 Lewis FW, Warren GH, Goff JS. Collagenous colitis with involvement of terminal ileum. *Dig Dis Sci* 1991; **36**(8): 1161–1163.
22 Meier PN, Otto P, Ritter M, Stolte M. Collagenous duodenitis and ileitis in a patient with collagenous colitis. *Leber Magen Darm.* 1991; **21**(5): 231–232.
23 McCashland TM, Donovan JP, Strobach RS, Linder J, Quigley EM. Collagenous enterocolitis: A manifestation of gluten-sensitive enteropathy. *J Clin Gastroenterol* 1992; **15**(1): 45–51.
24 Chatti S, Haouet S, Ourghi H *et al.* Collagenous enterocolitis. Apropos of a case and review of the literature. *Arch Anat Cytol Pathol* 1994; **42**(3-4): 149–153.
25 Veress B, Lofberg R, Bergman L. Microscopic colitis syndrome. *Gut* 1995 Jun; **36**(6): 880–886.
26 Zins BJ, Tremaine WJ, Carpenter HA. Collagenous colitis: Mucosal biopsies and association with fecal leukocytes. *Mayo Clin Proc* 1995; **70**(5): 430–433.
27 Pulimood AB, Ramakrishna BS, Mathan MM. Collagenous gastritis and collagenous colitis: A report with sequential histological and ultrastructural findings. *Gut* 1999; **44**(6): 881–885.

28 Padmanabhan V, Callas PW, Li SC, Trainer TD. Histopathological features of the terminal ileum in lymphocytic and collagenous colitis: A study of 32 cases and review of literature. *Mod Pathol* 2003; **16**(2): 115–119.

29 Bogomoletz WV. Collagenous, microscopic and lymphocytic colitis. An evolving concept. *Virchows Arch* 1994; **424**(6): 573–579.

30 Limsui D, Pardi DS, Smyrk TC *et al.* Observer variability in the histologic diagnosis of microscopic colitis. *Inflamm Bowel Dis* 2009; **15**: 35–38.

31 van Tilburg AJ, Lam HG, Seldenrijk CA *et al.* Familial occurrence of collagenous colitis. A report of two families. *J Clin Gastroenterol* 1990; **12**(3): 279–285.

32 Abdo AA, Zetler PJ, Halparin LS. Familial microscopic colitis. *Can J Gastroenterol* 2001; **15**(5): 341–343.

33 Freeman HJ. Familial occurrence of lymphocytic colitis. *Can J Gastroenterol* 2001; **15**(11): 757–760.

34 Jarnerot G, Hertervig E, Granno C *et al.* Familial occurrence of microscopic colitis: a report on five families. *Scand J Gastroenterol* 2001 (Sep); **36**(9): 959–62.

35 Thomson A, Kaye G. Further report of familial occurrence of collagenous colitis. *Scand J Gastroenterol* 2002; **37**(9): 1116.

36 Koskela RM, Karttunen TJ, Niemela SE, Lehtola JK, Ilonen J, Karttunen RA. Human leucocyte antigen and TNFalpha polymorphism association in microscopic colitis. *Eur J Gastroenterol Hepatol* 2008 (Apr); **20**(4): 276–282.

37 Fine KD, Do K, Schulte K *et al.* High prevalence of celiac sprue-like HLA-DQ genes and enteropathy in patients with the microscopic colitis syndrome. *Am J Gastroenterol* 2000; **95**(8): 1974–1982.

38 Giardiello FM, Lazenby AJ, Yardley JH *et al.* Increased HLA A1 and diminished HLA A3 in lymphocytic colitis compared to controls and patients with collagenous colitis. *Dig Dis Sci* 1992; **37**(4): 496–499.

39 Madisch A, Hellmig S, Schreiber S, Bethke B, Stolte M, Miehlke S. NOD2/CARD15 gene polymorphisms are not associated with collagenous colitis. *Int J Colorectal Dis* 2007 (Apr); **22**(4): 425–428.

40 Giardiello FM, Lazenby AJ. The atypical colitides. *Gastroenterol Clin North Am* 1999; **28**(2): 479–490.

41 Stampfl DA, Friedman LS. Collagenous colitis: Pathophysiologic considerations. *Dig Dis Sci* 1991; **36**(6): 705–711.

42 Armes J, Gee DC, Macrae FA, Schroeder W, Bhathal PS. Collagenous colitis: jejunal and colorectal pathology. *J Clin Pathol* 1992; **45**(9): 784–787.

43 Järnerot G, Tysk C, Bohr J, Eriksson S. Collagenous colitis and fecal stream diversion. *Gastroenterology* 1995; **109**(2): 449–455.

44 Fine KD, Lee EL, Meyer RL. Colonic histopathology in untreated celiac sprue or refractory sprue: Is it lymphocytic colitis or colonic lymphocytosis? *Hum Pathol* 1998; **29**(12): 1433–1440.

45 Tagkalidis PP, Gibson P, Bhathal PS. Microscopic colitis demonstrates a TH1 mucosal cytokine profile. *J Clin Pathol* 2007; **60**: 382–387.

46 Burgel N, Bojarski C, Mankertz J, Zeitz M, Fromm M, Schulzke JD. Mechanisms of diarrhea in collagenous colitis. *Gastroenterology* 2002; **123**(2): 433–443.

47 Taha Y, Carlson M, Thorn M, Loof L, Raab Y. Evidence of local eosinophil activation and altered mucosal permeability in collagenous colitis. *Dig Dis Sci* 2001; **46**(4): 888–897.

48 Perk G, Ackerman Z, Cohen P, Eliakim R. Lymphocytic colitis: A clue to an infectious trigger. *Scand J Gastroenterol* 1999; **34**(1): 110–112.

49 Vesoulis Z, Lozanski G, Loiudice T. Synchronous occurrence of collagenous colitis and pseudomembranous colitis. *Can J Gastroenterol* 2000; **14**(4): 353–358.

50 Khan MA, Brunt EM, Longo WE, Presti ME. Persistent Clostridium difficile colitis: A possible etiology for the development of collagenous colitis. *Dig Dis Sci* 2000; **45**(5): 998–1001.

51 Byrne MF, McVey G, Royston D, Patchett SE. Association of Clostridium difficile Infection With Collagenous Colitis. *J Clin Gastroenterol* 2003; **36**(3): 285.

52 Makinen M, Niemela S, Lehtola J, Karttunen TJ. Collagenous colitis and Yersinia enterocolitica infection. *Dig Dis Sci* 1998; **43**(6): 1341–1346.

53 Bohr J, Nordfelth R, Järnerot G, Tysk C. Yersinia species in collagenous colitis: A serologic study. *Scand J Gastroenterol* 2002; **37**(6): 711–714.

54 Bryant DA, Mintz ED, Puhr ND, Griffin PM, Petras RE. Colonic epithelial lymphocytosis associated with an epidemic of chronic diarrhea. *Am J Surg Pathol* 1996; **20**(9): 1102–1109.

55 Riddell RH, Tanaka M, Mazzoleni G. Non-steroidal anti-inflammatory drugs as a possible cause of collagenous colitis: A case-control study. *Gut* 1992; **33**(5): 683–686.

56 Abdo A, Raboud J, Freeman HJ *et al.* Clinical and histological predictors of response to medical therapy in collagenous colitis. *Am J Gastroenterol* 2002; **97**(5): 1164–1168.

57 Brigot C, Courillon-Mallet A, Roucayrol AM, Cattan D. Lymphocytic colitis and ticlopidine. *Gastroenterol Clin Biol* 1998; **22**(3): 361–362.

58 Berrebi D, Sautet A, Flejou JF, Dauge MC, Peuchmaur M, Potet F. Ticlopidine induced colitis: a histopathological study including apoptosis. *J Clin Pathol* 1998; **51**(4): 280–283.

59 Baert F, Wouters K, D'Haens G *et al.* Lymphocytic colitis: A distinct clinical entity? A clinicopathological confrontation of lymphocytic and collagenous colitis. *Gut* 1999; **45**(3): 375–381.

60 Wilcox GM, Mattia A. Collagenous colitis associated with lansoprazole. *J Clin Gastroenterol* 2002; **34**(2): 164–166.

61 Thomson RD, Lestina LS, Bensen SP, Toor A, Maheshwari Y, Ratcliffe NR. Lansoprazole-associated microscopic colitis: A case series. *Am J Gastroenterol* 2002; **97**(11): 2908–2913.

62 Pierrugues R, Saingra B. Lymphocytic colitis and Cyclo 3 fort: 4 new cases. *Gastroenterol Clin Biol* 1996; **20**(10): 916–917.

63 Beaugerie L, Luboinski J, Brousse N *et al.* Drug induced lymphocytic colitis. *Gut* 1994; **35**(3): 426–428.

64 Bouaniche M, Chassagne P, Landrin I, Kadri N, Doucet J, Bercoff E. Lymphocytic colitis caused by Cyclo 3 Fort. *Rev Med Interne* 1996; **17**(9): 776–778.

65 Beaugerie L, Patey N, Brousse N. Ranitidine, diarrhoea, and lymphocytic colitis. *Gut* 1995; **37**(5): 708–711.

66 Duncan HD, Talbot IC, Silk DB. Collagenous colitis and cimetidine. *Eur J Gastroenterol Hepatol* 1997; **9**(8): 819–820.

67 Chauveau E, Prignet JM, Carloz E, Duval JL, Gilles B. Lymphocytic colitis likely attributable to use of vinburnine (Cervoxan). *Gastroenterol Clin Biol* 1998; **22**(3): 362.

68 Bouchet-Laneuw F, Deplaix P, Dumollard JM *et al.* Chronic diarrhea following ingestion of Tardyferon associated with lymphocytic colitis. *Gastroenterol Clin Biol*. 1997; **21**(1): 83–84.

69 Piche T, Raimondi V, Schneider S, Hebuterne X, Rampal P. Acarbose and lymphocytic colitis. *Lancet* 2000; **356**(9237): 1246.

70 Mennecier D, Gros P, Bronstein JA, Thiolet C, Farret O. Chronic diarrhea due to lymphocytic colitis treated with piroxicam beta cyclodextrin. *Presse Med* 1999; **28**(14): 735–737.

71 Rassiat E, Michiels C, Sgro C, Yaziji N, Piard F, Faivre J. Lymphocytic colitis due to Modopar. *Gastroenterol Clin Biol* 2000; **24**(8–9): 852–853.

72 Mahajan L, Wyllie R, Goldblum J. Lymphocytic colitis in a pediatric patient: a possible adverse reaction to carbamazepine. *Am J Gastroenterol* 1997; **92**(11): 2126–2127.

73 Linares Torres P, Fidalgo Lopez I, Castanon Lopez A, Martinez Pinto Y. Lymphocytic colitis as a cause of chronic diarrhea: Possible association with carbamazepine. *Aten Primaria* 2000; **25**(5): 366–367.

74 Macaigne G, Boivin JF, Chayette C, Cheaib S, Deplus R. Oxetorone-associated lymphocytic colitis. *Gastroenterol Clin Biol* 2002; **26**(5): 537.

75 Ghilain JM, Schapira M, Maisin JM *et al.* Lymphocytic colitis associated with lansoprazole treatment. *Gastroenterol Clin Biol* 2000; **24**(10): 960–962.

76 Bohr J, Tysk C, Yang P, Danielsson D, Järnerot G. Autoantibodies and immunoglobulins in collagenous colitis. *Gut* 1996; **39**(1): 73–76.

77 Eusufzai S, Löfberg R, Veress B, Einarsson K, Angelin B. Studies on bile acid metabolism in collagenous colitis: No evidence of bile acid malabsorption as determined by the SeHCAT test. *Eur J Gastroenterol Hepatol* 1992; **4**(4): 317–321.

78 Ung KA, Gillberg R, Kilander A, Abrahamsson H. Role of bile acids and bile acid binding agents in patients with collagenous colitis. *Gut* 2000; **46**(2): 170–175.

79 Ung KA, Kilander A, Willen R, Abrahamsson H. Role of bile acids in lymphocytic colitis. *Hepatogastroenterology* 2002; **49**(44): 432–437.

80 Fernandez-Banares F, Esteve M, Salas A, Forne TM *et al.* Bile acid malabsorption in microscopic colitis and in previously unexplained functional chronic diarrhea. *Dig Dis Sci* 2001; **46**(10): 2231–2238.

81 Andersen T, Andersen JR, Tvede M, Franzmann MB. Collagenous colitis: are bacterial cytotoxins responsible? *Am J Gastroenterol* 1993; **88**(3): 375–377.

82 Lundberg JON, Herulf M, Olesen M *et al.* Increased nitric oxide production in collagenous and lymphocytic colitis. *Eur J Clin Invest* 1997; **27**(10): 869–871.

83 Perner A, Andresen L, Normark M, Rask-Madsen J. Constitutive expression of inducible nitric oxide synthase in the normal human colonic epithelium. *Scand J Gastroenterol* 2002; **37**(8): 944–948.

84 Olesen M, Middelveld R, Bohr J *et al.* Luminal nitric oxide and epithelial expression of inducible and endothelial nitric oxide synthase in collagenous and lymphocytic colitis. *Scand J Gastroenterol* 2003 Jan; **38**(1): 66–72.

85 Bonderup OK, Hansen JB, Madsen P, Vestergaard V, Fallingborg J, Teglbjaerg PS. Budesonide treatment and expression of inducible nitric oxide synthase mRNA in colonic mucosa in collagenous colitis. *Eur J Gastroenterol Hepatol* 2006 (Oct); **18**(10): 1095–1099.

86 Perner A, Andresen L, Normark M *et al.* Expression of nitric oxide synthases and effects of L-arginine and L-NMMA on

87 nitric oxide production and fluid transport in collagenous colitis. *Gut* 2001; **49**(3): 387–394.

87 Rask-Madsen J, Grove O, Hansen MG, Bukhave K, Scient C, Henrik-Nielsen R. Colonic transport of water and electrolytes in a patient with secretory diarrhea due to collagenous colitis. *Dig Dis Sci* 1983; **28**(12): 1141–1146.

88 Bohr J, Järnerot G, Tysk C, Jones I, Eriksson S. Effect of fasting on diarrhoea in collagenous colitis. *Digestion* 2002; **65**(1): 30–34.

89 Bonderup OK, Folkersen BH, Gjersoe P, Teglbjaerg PS. Collagenous colitis: A long-term follow-up study. *Eur J Gastroenterol Hepatol.* 1999; **11**(5): 493–495.

90 Madisch A, Miehlke S, Lindner M, Bethke B, Stolte M. Clinical course of collagenous colitis over a period of 10 years. *Z Gastroenterol* 2006 (Sep); **44**(9): 971–974.

91 Taylor S, Haggitt R, Bronner M. Colonic perforation complicating colonoscopy in collagenous colitis. *Gastroenterology* 1999; **116**: A938.

92 Freeman HJ, James D, Mahoney CJ. Spontaneous peritonitis from perforation of the colon in collagenous colitis. *Can J Gastroenterol* 2001; **15**(4): 265–267.

93 Bohr J, Larsson LG, Eriksson S, Jarnerot G, Tysk C. Colonic perforation in collagenous colitis: An unusual complication. *Eur J Gastroenterol Hepatol* 2005 (Jan); **17**(1): 121–124.

94 Allende DS, Taylor SL, Bronner MP. Colonic Perforation as a Complication of Collagenous Colitis in a Series of 12 Patients. *Am J Gastroenterol* 2008; **103**: 2598–2604.

95 Cruz-Correa M, Milligan F, Giardiello FM *et al.* Collagenous colitis with mucosal tears on endoscopic insufflation: A unique presentation. *Gut* 2002; **51**(4): 600.

96 Yarze JC. Finding mucosal tears in collagenous colitis during colonoscopic insufflation. *Gut* 2003 (Apr); **52**(4): 613–614.

97 Sherman A, Ackert JJ, Rajapaksa R, West AB, Oweity T. Fractured colon: an endoscopically distinctive lesion associated with colonic perforation following colonoscopy in patients with collagenous colitis. *J Clin Gastroenterol* 2004 (Apr); **38**(4): 341–345.

98 Wickbom A, Lindqvist M, Bohr J *et al.* Colonic mucosal tears in collagenous colitis. *Scand J Gastroenterol* 2006 (Jun); **41**(6): 726–729.

99 Chan JL, Tersmette AC, Offerhaus GJ, Gruber SB, Bayless TM, Giardiello FM. Cancer risk in collagenous colitis. *Inflamm Bowel Dis* 1999; **5**(1): 40–43.

100 Goff JS, Barnett JL, Pelke T, Appelman HD. Collagenous colitis: Histopathology and clinical course. *Am J Gastroenterol* 1997; **92**(1): 57–60.

101 Bonner GF, Petras RE, Cheong DM, Grewal ID, Breno S, Ruderman WB. Short- and long-term follow-up of treatment for lymphocytic and collagenous colitis. *Inflamm Bowel Dis* 2000; **6**(2): 85–91.

102 Pokorny CS, Kneale KL, Henderson CJ. Progression of collagenous colitis to ulcerative colitis. *J Clin Gastroenterol* 2001; **32**(5): 435–438.

103 Sveinsson OA, Orvar KB, Birgisson S, Agnarsdottir M, Jonasson JG. Clinical features of microscopic colitis in a nation-wide follow-up study in Iceland. *Scand J Gastroenterol* 2008 (Mar); **4**: 1–6.

104 Mullhaupt B, Guller U, Anabitarte M, Guller R, Fried M. Lymphocytic colitis: clinical presentation and long term course. *Gut* 1998; **43**(5): 629–633.

105 Bohr J, Jones I, Tysk C, Järnerot G. Serum procollagen III propeptide is not of diagnostic predictive value in collagenous colitis. *Inflamm Bowel Dis* 1995; **1**: 276–279.

106 Kiesslich R, Hoffman A, Goetz M *et al. In vivo* diagnosis of collagenous colitis by confocal endomicroscopy. *Gut* 2006 (Apr); **55**(4): 591–592.

107 Zambelli A, Villanacci V, Buscarini E, Bassotti G, Albarello L. Collagenous colitis: a case series with confocal laser microscopy and histology correlation. *Endoscopy* 2008 (Jul); **40**(7): 606–608.

108 Bowling TE, Price AB, al-Adnani M, Fairclough PD, Menzies-Gow N, Silk DB. Interchange between collagenous and lymphocytic colitis in severe disease with autoimmune associations requiring colectomy: A case report. *Gut* 1996; **38**(5): 788–791.

109 Pardi DS, Ramnath VR, Loftus EV, Jr., Tremaine WJ, Sandborn WJ. Lymphocytic colitis: clinical features, treatment, and outcomes. *Am J Gastroenterol* 2002; **97**(11): 2829–2833.

110 Pardi DS, Smyrk TC, Tremaine WJ, Sandborn WJ. Microscopic colitis: A review. *Am J Gastroenterol* 2002; **97**(4): 794–802.

111 Chande N, McDonald JWD, MacDonald JK. Interventions for treating collagenous colitis. *Cochrane Database of Systematic Reviews* 2008, Issue 2. Art. No.: CD003575. DOI: 10.1002/14651858.CD003575.pub5.

112 Chande N, McDonald JWD, MacDonald JK. Interventions for treating lymphocytic colitis. *Cochrane Database of Systematic Reviews* 2008, Issue 2. Art. No.: CD006096. DOI: 10.1002/14651858. CD006096.pub3.

113 Baert F, Schmit A, D'Haens G *et al.* Budesonide in collagenous colitis: a double-blind placebo-controlled trial with histologic follow-up. *Gastroenterology* 2002; **122**(1): 20–25.

114 Miehlke S, Heymer P, Bethke B *et al.* Budesonide treatment for collagenous colitis: A randomized, double-blind, placebo-controlled, multicenter trial. *Gastroenterology* 2002; **123**(4): 978–984.

115 Bonderup OK, Hansen JB, Birket-Smith L, Vestergaard V, Teglbjaerg PS, Fallingborg J. Budesonide treatment of collagenous colitis: A randomised, double blind, placebo controlled trial with morphometric analysis. *Gut* 2003; **52**(2): 248–251.

116 Miehlke S, Madisch A, Bethke B *et al.* Budesonide for maintenance treatment of collagenous colitis – a randomized, double-blind, placebo-controlled trial. *United European Gastroenterology Week 2007.* 2007: No. PS-M-13.

117 Bonderup OK, Hansen JB, Teglbjoerg PS, Christensen LA, Fallingborg JF. Long-term budesonide treatment of collagenous colitis: a randomised, double-blind, placebo-controlled trial. *Gut* 2009 (Jan); **58**(1): 68–72.

118 Munck LK, Kjeldsen J, Philipsen E, Fischer Hansen B. Incomplete remission with short-term prednisolone treatment in collagenous colitis: A randomised study. *Scand J Gastroenterol* 2003; **38**(6): 606–610.

119 Fine KD, Ogunji F, Lee E, Lafon G, Tanzi M. Randomized, double blind, placebo-controlled trial of bismuth subsalicylate for microscopic colitis. *Gastroenterology* 1999; **116**(4): A880.

120 Calabrese C, Fabbri A, Areni A, Zahlane D, Scialpi C, Di Febo G. Mesalazine with or without cholestyramine in the treatment of microscopic colitis: randomized controlled trial. *J Gastroenterol Hepatol* 2007 (Jun); **22**(6): 809–814.

121 Wildt S, Munck LK, Vinter-Jensen L *et al.* Probiotic treatment of collagenous colitis: A randomized, double-blind, placebo-controlled trial with Lactobacillus acidophilus and Bifidobacterium animalis subsp. Lactis. *Inflamm Bowel Dis* 2006 May; **12**(5): 395–401.

122 Madisch A, Miehlke S, Eichele O *et al.* Boswellia serrata extract for the treatment of collagenous colitis. A double-blind, randomized, placebo-controlled, multicenter trial. *Int J Colorectal Dis* 2007 (Dec); **22**(12): 1445–14451.

123 Miehlke S, Madisch A, Bethke B *et al.* Budesonide in lymphocytic colitis – a randomized, double-blind, placebo-controlled trial. *Gastroenterology* 2007; **132**(4, Suppl 2): A131–A132.

124 Lanyi B, Dries V, Dienes HP, Kruis W. Therapy of prednisone-refractory collagenous colitis with budesonide. *Int J Colorectal Dis* 1999; **14**(1): 58–61.

125 Schoon EJ, Bollani S, Mills PR *et al.* Bone mineral density in relation to efficacy and side effects of budesonide and prednisolone in Crohn's disease. *Clin Gastroenterol Hepatol* 2005 (Feb); **3**(2): 113–121.

126 Pardi DS, Loftus EV, Jr., Tremaine WJ, Sandborn WJ. Treatment of refractory microscopic colitis with azathioprine and 6-mercaptopurine. *Gastroenterology* 2001; **120**(6): 1483–1484.

127 Riddell J, Hillman L, Chiragakis L, Clarke A. Collagenous colitis: Oral low-dose methotrexate for patients with difficult symptoms: Long-term outcomes. *J Gastroenterol Hepatol.* 2007 (Oct); **22**(10): 1589–1593.

128 Alikhan M, Cummings OW, Rex D. Subtotal colectomy in a patient with collagenous colitis associated with colonic carcinoma and systemic lupus erythematosus. *Am J Gastroenterol* 1997; **92**(7): 1213–1215.

129 Yusuf TE, Soemijarsih M, Arpaia A, Goldberg SL, Sottile VM. Chronic microscopic enterocolitis with severe hypokalemia responding to subtotal colectomy. *J Clin Gastroenterol* 1999; **29**(3): 284–288.

130 Williams RA, Gelfand DV. Total proctocolectomy and ileal pouch anal anastomosis to successfully treat a patient with collagenous colitis. *Am J Gastroenterol.* 2000; **95**(8): 2147.

131 Varghese L, Galandiuk S, Tremaine WJ, Burgart LJ. Lymphocytic colitis treated with proctocolectomy and ileal J-pouch-anal anastomosis: report of a case. *Dis Colon Rectum* 2002; **45**(1): 123–126.

132 Riaz AA, Pitt J, Stirling RW, Madaan S, Dawson PM. Restorative proctocolectomy for collagenous colitis. *J R Soc Med* 2000; **93**(5): 261.

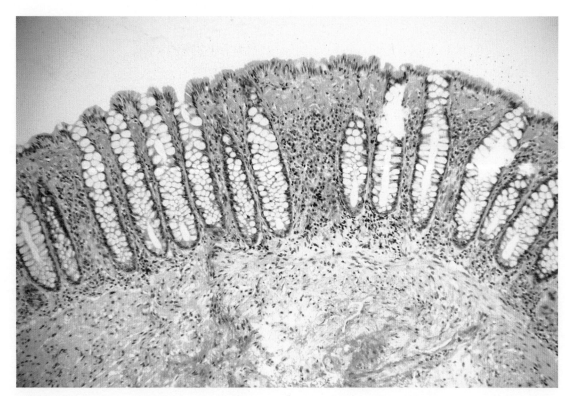

Plate 14.1 Biopsy from colon showing typical features of collagenous colitis-increased subepithelial collagen layer, inflammation of lamina propria and epithelial lesions with intraepithelial lymphocytes.

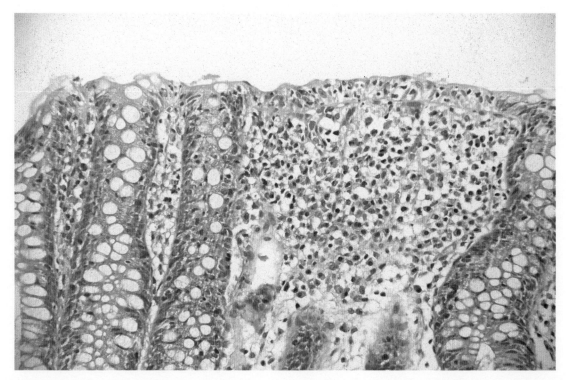

Plate 14.2 Biopsy from colon showing typical features of lymphocytic colitis-epithelial lesions with intraepithelial lymphocytes and inflammation in the lamina propria.

15 Drug-induced diarrhea

Bincy P Abraham and Joseph H Sellin
Section of Gastroenterology and Hepatology, Baylor College of Medicine, Houston, USA

Drug induced diarrhea

More than 700 drugs have been implicated as causing diarrhea, accounting for approximately 7% of all drug adverse effects [1]. However, the mechanism of action by which certain drugs contribute to this adverse effect is not well known. Drug-induced diarrhea is frequently suspected in patients who develop it soon after starting a new medication. However, there is usually only circumstantial evidence to support the link. The medication is usually stopped, and when the diarrhea resolves, the side effect will be attributed to that medication. The basic mechanisms are rarely investigated in these cases. Therefore, our understanding of specific drug-induced diarrheas may vary from solid understanding, to reasonable hypothesis, to considerable conjecture.

Although it is clear that drug-induced diarrhea is common, employing an evidence-based approach to this topic quickly creates considerable conundrums. Evidence-based medicine focuses on both the accuracy of diagnosis and the efficacy of treatment. Both are problematic for drug-induced diarrhea.

For well-established (i.e. "old") drugs, there rarely are controlled trials to quantify and characterize the association between a specific agent and diarrhea. The information for these drugs is derived from cohort or case-control studies. Although these studies may provide weaker evidence than controlled trials due to potential for biases in statistical analysis, they do provide better evidence than case-reports or case-series that lack control groups. For newer drugs that have gone through clinical trials, the assessment of adverse events permits a reasonable opportunity to characterize the frequency of drug-associated

Evidence-Based Gastroenterology and Hepatology, 3rd edition.
J. McDonald, A.K. Burroughs, B. Feagan, and M.B. Fennerty. © 2010
Blackwell Publishing Ltd

diarrhea. However, even with clinical trials, there may be a considerable variability in the incidence of an adverse event such as diarrhea. This variability may depend on the underlying disease, the definition of the adverse event, and the type of clinical trial. For example, most randomized controlled trials (RCTs) are short in duration, thus magnifying or minimizing an adverse effect in reference to the time a patient is exposed to the drug, compared to long-term follow-up observational studies. Also, diarrhea as an adverse event is rarely defined clearly. Thus, a minimal change in consistency and a significant increase in stool volume would both be labeled "diarrhea".

Evidence of the mechanisms underlying the diarrhea elicited by a specific drug may be elusive and serendipitous. For example, theophylline has been a standard for eliciting intestinal secretion in basic physiology. Thus, the effects of xanthine oxidase inhibitors are well understood. Similarly, as molecular-designed agents move from the bench to the bedside, there may be considerable understanding of the underlying mechanism. However, for many drugs, the purported mechanisms are based on small fragmentary studies or simple speculation. Table 15.1 lists drugs that cause diarrhea, according to the frequency with which they produce this adverse effect.

In order to have a basic understanding on what mechanisms played a role in contributing to diarrhea, the patient's stool characteristics can provide some clues. Diarrhea can be broadly categorized based on the following stool characteristics: (1) watery, a category that includes changes in ion transport, shortened transit time, or increased motility (2) inflammatory, and (3) fatty. This review will examine the mechanism of drug-induced diarrhea within these broad classifications. However, as with other diarrheas, the process is frequently multifactorial. The gastrointestinal tract is regulated through the integration of paracrine, immune, neural, and endocrine systems that coordinate changes in mucosal and muscular function and adapt to changing conditions (see Figure 15.1) [2]. These systems involve mechanisms that regulate mucosal permeability,

Table 15.1 Drugs that cause diarrhea.

Drugs that cause diarrhea in ≥ 20% of patients
Alpha-glucosidase inhibitors
Biguanides
Auronafin (gold salt)
Colchicine
Diacerein
Highly active antiretroviral therapy
Prostaglandins
Tyrosine kinase inhibitors

Drugs that cause diarrhea in ≥ 10 % of patients
Antibiotics
Chemotherapeutic agents
Cholinergic drugs
Cisapride (off the market)
Digoxin
Immunosuppressives agents
Metoclopramide
Orlistat (lipase inhibitor)
Osmotic laxatives
Poorly or non-absorbable carbohydrates
Selective serotonin reuptake inhibitors
Ticlopidine

Drugs that occasionally cause diarrhea
5-aminosalicylates (especially olsalazine)
Acetylcholinesterase inhibitors
Anticholinergics
Caffeine
Calcitonin
Carbamazepine
Chenodeoxycholic acid
Cholestyramine
Cholinesterase inhibitors
Cimetidine
Ferrous sulfate preparations (rare)
Flavanoid related veinotonic agents
HMG-CoA reductase inhibitors
Irinotecan
Isotretinoin
Levodopa-benserazide
Magnesium antacids
Methyldopa
Motilin agonists
Non-steroidal anti-inflammatory drugs
Octreotide
Penicillamine
Prebiotics
Proton pump inhibitors
Tacrine
Tegaserod (off the market)
Theophylline
Thyroid hormones

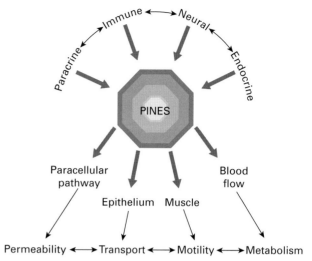

Figure 15.1 "PINES" regulatory system in the intestine. The regulatory system of the intestine integrates *paracrine*, *immune*, *neural*, and endocrine systems and produces coordinated changes in mucosal and muscular function that permit adaptive responses to changing conditions. The regulatory system can widen or narrow the paracellular pathway that governs passive transmucosal permeation of electrolytes, accelerate or retard the transepithelial movement of nutrients and electrolytes by affecting membrane channels and pumps, relax or contract the various muscle layers in the intestine, and increase or decrease mucosal blood flow. Acting simultaneously, these mechanisms regulate mucosal permeability, intestinal transport, and the motility and metabolism of the gut. (From Sellin JH (1997) Small intestine: Functional anatomy, fluid and electrolyte absorption. In: Feldman M and Schiller LR (eds) *Gastroenterology and Hepatology. The Comprehensive Visual Reference*, vol. 7. Current Medicine, Philadelphia, 1997. p. 1.11.)

intestinal transport, and the motility and metabolism of the gut [2]. Medications may influence this regulatory system through these different pathways and contribute to diarrhea. This influence may be part of the pharmacologic effect of the drug. In other cases there may be an allergic reaction, or possibly a pharmacogenomic component. Diarrhea may be an appropriate physiologic response to the drug. On occasion, the drug may cause direct tissue injury.

Clinically, if drug-induced diarrhea is suspected, the simplest approach is to switch to an alternative medication or treat with an antidiarrheal agent. Novel approaches for certain drug-associated diarrheas have been shown to be effective in treatment. In some cases, diarrhea may resolve with continued use.

Thus, for most examples of drug-induced diarrhea, therapeutic trials are not relevant. Only where there are no satisfactory alternatives, as is the case for some anti-cancer therapies, is there sufficient impetus to understand the mechanisms of drug-induced diarrhea. Thus, there probably has been more significant and novel evidence in drug-induced diarrhea obtained in the field of oncology.

Watery diarrhea

Watery diarrheas have been classified as either secretory or osmotic to explain underlying pathophysiology. However, the clinical utility of this classification has not been rigorously tested.

Osmotic diarrhea

Osmotic diarrheas can occur from intentional use of a drug as part of its mechanism of action, or unintentionally. Poorly absorbed solute traps fluid in the lumen, and these unabsorbable solutes account for osmotic activity of stool water [2].

The most common medications associated with osmotic diarrhea are magnesium containing salts and laxatives such as sodium phosphates and long-chain polyethylene glycols, e.g. Miralax (Schering-Plough, Kenilworth, NJ) used for treatment of constipation, and for pre-colonoscopy colon purging [3, 4]. Their cathartic action results from poor absorption in the gastrointestinal tract, leading to osmotically mediated water retention, stimulating peristalsis [4]. The usual dose of magnesium salts produces 300 to 600 ml of stool within six hours [4]. Sodium phosphates cause osmotic diarrhea, but without producing an osmotic gap [5].

Used for constipation and for the treatment of hepatic encephalopathy, lactulose is a synthetic non-absorbable disaccharide that is known to cause diarrhea through this mechanism. Poorly-absorbed fructose, found in fruit juices and carbonated beverages, and non-absorbable sorbitol and mannitol, found in sugar-free candies and gums, may not cause diarrhea until 24 to 48 hours after ingestion. Acarbose and miglitol, used for the treatment of diabetes, prevent the breakdown of carbohydrates to monosaccharides by inhibition of intestinal alpha-glucosidase, causing diarrhea. In a multicenter RCT of 286 patients comparing acarbose to placebo, tolbutamide and tolbutamide-plus-acarbose in NIDDM, 27% of patients taking acarbose and 35% taking acarbose + tolbutamide complained of diarrhea in comparison to 6% of patients taking placebo or tolbutamide (p < 0.05) [6]. Diarrhea is minimized by starting therapy at low doses (50 mg three times daily), and tends to decrease with time [7]. In the large-scale, multinational study investigating different doses of acarbose (from 25 mg tid to 200 mg tid) good patient tolerability and compliance was observed, even at the highest dose [8]. The study also confirmed the marked tendency for adverse effects to decline after 4–6 weeks.

Interestingly, in a post-market surveillance study of almost 20,000 patients (both NIDDM and IDDM, only 3.2% of those taking acarbose complained of diarrhea [9]. What can explain this difference between the surveillance study and the RCT? During RCT, there may be more attention directed toward minimal changes in signs and symptoms. Acarbose-associated diarrhea is most common in the early phase of treatment. Finally, surveillance generally separates out those subjects who had already discontinued acarbose because of diarrhea.

The prebiotics fructo-oligosaccharides and inulins, available in nutritional supplements and in functional foods, have been used for treatment of antibiotic-induced diarrhea at dose ranges of 4–10 g per day [10]. When given to healthy volunteers, doses higher than 30 g daily of these prebiotics caused significant gastrointestinal discomfort (flatulence, cramping, diarrhea) through fermentation in the colon and production of an osmotic effect in the intestinal lumen [11, 12]. If the dosage is split this usually alleviates the symptoms. Diagnosis can usually be made by checking fecal pH; a pH less than 6 is highly suggestive of carbohydrate malabsorption.

Some formulas for enteral nutrition are hypertonic and may induce osmotic diarrhea by a mechanism similar to dumping syndrome. Changing to an isotonic formula or slowing the infusion rate usually resolves the diarrhea [4].

Once recognized, the treatment of osmotic diarrhea is simple. Removal of the osmotic agent usually resolves this adverse effect. Loperamide or tincture of opium can be added, especially in the case of enteral nutrition. Dose reduction or dose splitting can also help. In some cases, such as acarbose, the diarrhea usually resolves over time with continued use.

Secretory diarrhea

Secretory diarrhea, on the other hand, produces voluminous stools that persist despite fasting. Drug-induced secretory diarrhea results from a medication either increasing the active secretion of ions and thus pulling fluid into the lumen, or from decreasing the absorption of large amounts of water and electrolytes in the gut lumen. In secretory diarrhea, a minimal osmotic gap is found. Specifically, drugs induce a secretory diarrhea by two main mechanisms: the inhibition of Na^+ absorption and the stimulation of $Cl^-/HCO3^-$ secretion. These changes may occur through either a direct effect on the transporter or changes in intracellular second messengers that alter the function of the transporter.

The Na^+ pump (Na^+, K^+-ATPase) is the final common pathway for Na^+ absorption; inhibition of the Na^+ pump blocks Na^+ (and fluid) absorption and this may cause diarrhea. Digoxin's therapeutic target is the cardiac Na^+, K^+-ATPase. However, inhibition of intestinal or colonic Na^+ pumps may cause diarrhea, most frequently at supratherapeutic drug levels, especially in elderly patients [3]. In fact, digoxin was the second commonest cause of diarrhea in a study of 100 elderly patients [13]. Similarly, auranofin, used previously for rheumatoid arthritis, caused diarrhea in up to 74% of patients, requiring discontinuation in 14% of them [3]. By reducing K⁺ conductance and inhibiting calcium channels, the class I antiarrhythmic drugs quinidine and propafenone impede transepithelial Na⁺ and water absorption causing diarrhea in 8–30% of patients [14]. Lubiprostone was initially developed as a treatment for constipation, specifically because of its properties as a ClC2 channel opener; however, it is still unclear what specific role the ClC2 channel has in intestinal secretion.

Olsalazine, used in the treatment of ulcerative colitis, causes diarrhea in 12–25% of patients through the stimulation of bicarbonate and sodium chloride secretion in the ileum [1, 15]. Similar azo compounds sulfasalazine and mesalazine may also cause diarrhea, but less frequently. The mechanism is unclear, but may involve a direct effect on anion transporters, rather than an anti-inflammatory action [16].

Some drugs cause a secretory diarrhea by altering intracellular signaling cascades, increasing cyclic AMP, cyclic GMP or calcium. The phosphodiesterase inhibitor, theophylline, causes diarrhea by increasing cyclic AMP, opening chloride channels and increasing secretion [17]. In our hypercaffeinated society, coffee is used as a "drug" by many, causing "Starbucks® diarrhea" through this similar mechanism. Caffeine administration in amounts ordinarily contained in many beverages and medications (75 to 300 mg) resulted in striking net secretion in the jejunum and in the ileum [18]. Prostaglandin analogs can cause diarrhea through many pathways, including altered permeability, motility, electrolyte transport and by affecting peptides that stimulate secretion [17]. Misoprostol specifically stimulates epithelial Cl⁻ secretion through cyclic AMP, resulting in intraluminal fluid accumulation and diarrhea, which usually occurs within the first two weeks of treatment [3].

A secretory type of diarrhea limited the clinical use of chenodeoxycholic acid, a bile acid initially used to dissolve cholesterol gallstones. Early studies showed that the mechanism of secretory diarrhea in chenodeoxycholic acid therapy was due to a rise in intracellular cyclic AMP levels. However, recent *in vitro* studies using much lower doses of bile acids suggest a mechanism involving activation of luminal K⁺ channels and Cl⁻ secretion mediated through increased intracellular Ca⁺⁺ levels [19, 20]. Another dihydroxy bile acid, ursodiol causes diarrhea much less frequently. Presumably this difference is due to the alternative configuration of the hydroxyl groups compared to chenodeoxycholic acid. However, there are some reports of ursodiol causing diarrhea. A meta-analysis of ursodiol and its adverse effects revealed that diarrhea was the single most frequent adverse drug event in patients treated for gallstone disease, with an incidence of 2–9% [21]. If and when ursodiol is associated with diarrhea, there are two possible

mechanisms: an increase in the secretion of all bile salts including chenodeoxycholic acid and/or luminal conversion of ursodiol to chenodeoxycholic acid by intestinal bacteria (Alan Hoffman, personal communication). In primary biliary cirrhosis patients, on the other hand , diarrhea was rarely reported, in five large-scale randomized trials. No report of ursodiol-induced diarrhea was found in the largest placebo-controlled randomized study of its use in primary sclerosing cholangitis [21].

These conflicting data highlight some of the challenges of evaluating adverse events of RCTs.

First of all, is this a real difference in that the incidence of diarrhea is truly higher in gallstone disease than in PBC/PSC. Perhaps bile salt metabolism is different in gallstone disease, where there is an increased conversion of ursodiol to chenodeoxycholic acid which is a potent secretagogue. The gallbladder in patients with gallstones is likely to be hypo-functional and may be altered in its contractility in response to a meal or in its concentrating capacity, thus allowing more bile acid to enter the duodenum per ursodiol dose. In addition, ursodiol may be stimulatory to the inflamed bowel, while neutral or inhibitory to the bowel of patients with gallstones (Roger Soloway, personal communication). Alternatively, the design of RCTs may account for the difference. The definition of diarrhea as an adverse event, the focus on a more serious disease, or an already increased baseline bowel movement frequency in patients with PSC are possible examples of this factor.

Used as an old home remedy, castor oil is hydrolyzed in the small bowel by the action of lipases into glycerol and the active agent, ricinoleic acid, which acts primarily in the colon to stimulate secretion of fluid and electrolytes by increasing cyclic AMP and speeding intestinal transit [22, 23].

Stimulant laxatives such as diphenylmethane derivatives and anthraquinones induce their effect by inducing a limited low-grade inflammation in the small and large bowel to promote accumulation of water and electrolytes and stimulate intestinal motility. This occurs through activation of prostaglandin-cyclic AMP and NO-cyclic GMP pathways, platelet-activating factor production and, perhaps, inhibition of Na⁺,K⁺-ATPase [4]. Anthraquinone laxatives are poorly absorbed in the small bowel, are activated in the colon, and produce giant migrating colonic contractions as well as water and electrolyte secretion. Other laxatives or stool softeners such as docusate (dioctyl sodium sulfosuccinate), can cause diarrhea when taken in large quantities, by stimulating fluid secretion by the small and large intestine [24]. Clinicians should thus be aware that surreptitious use of laxative may be the cause of diarrhea in patients who present with this complaint. Table 15.2 lists a number of commonly used laxatives.

Diarrhea associated with medullary carcinoma of the thyroid suggested that calcitonin may cause a secretory

Table 15.2 Stimulant laxatives.

Anthraquinones
Diphenylmethane derivatives (bisacodyl)
Oxyphenisatin – withdrawn for hepatotoxicity
Phenolphthalein – withdrawn for carcinogenicity
Ricinoleic acid (castor oil)
Sodium picosulfate – available outside US
Sodium dioctyl sulfosuccinate (docusate)

type of diarrhea. Calcitonin in high doses can induce a secretory diarrhea in 1–3% of patients. Studies involving intravenous infusions showed prompt and marked increase in jejunal secretion of water, sodium, chloride and potassium, and reduced absorption of bicarbonate, which was reversed immediately with discontinuation of the infusion [25, 26]. However, in clinical practice, the use of salmon calcitonin for treatment of osteoporosis rarely causes diarrhea (Vassilopoulou-Sellin, R. personal communication) [27]. This paradox highlights the variable and sometimes unpredictable pattern of drug-induced diarrhea.

Colchicine, besides causing secretory diarrhea through the inhibition of Na^+,K^+-ATPase activity, is a microtubule inhibitor and may induce diarrhea by interfering with the migration of epithelial cells from the crypt to the villus and/or interfere with intracellular trafficking of specific transport proteins [17].

The biguanide metformin, used in the treatment of type II diabetes, has an effect on the brush border, reducing disaccharidase activity and leading to malabsorptive diarrhea in 10–53% of patients [28, 29].

Animal studies have found that metformin or the older biguanide phenformin inhibits intestinal glucose absorption in a dose-dependent manner through effects on mucosal and serosal glucose transfer mechanisms [30–33]. Based on a systematic review evaluating common adverse events of metformin monotherapy in type II diabetes mellitus, patients receiving metformin are 3.4 times more likely to develop diarrhea compared to those taking placebo (p = 0.002) [34]. Most cases are transient and mild, but even in severe cases, lowering the dose usually resolves the diarrhea [35]. In clinical trials, only 5% of study participants discontinued metformin because of gastrointestinal side effects [34]. There have also been cases of metformin causing late-onset chronic diarrhea in whom discontinuation of the drug resolved the diarrhea [36]. Larger studies of 405 type II diabetics show that metformin was independently associated with chronic diarrhea with an odds ratio of 3.08 (CI: 1.29–7.36, p < 0.02) [37]. In a diabetic clinic, metformin was found to be the most common cause of diarrhea based on a questionnaire based survey of 285 randomly selected diabetic patients [38]. Diarrhea in a diabetic patient may be related to the disease process itself. However, diabetic diarrhea usually occurs in type I diabetes for which metformin is not a treatment.

Some have speculated that anticholinergic drugs, which most often cause constipation by reducing intestinal motility, as well as the proton pump inhibitor omeprazole, can cause a secretory diarrhea. Although the proposed mechanism for diarrhea is thought to be bacterial overgrowth leading to bacterial deconjugation of primary bile salts to dihydroxy bile acids causing net fluid and electrolyte secretion in the colon, there is no substantial evidence to confirm this explanation [3]. In fact, a Cochrane systemic review showed no statistically significant difference in diarrhea occurrence in patients treated with PPI for reflux disease either at maintenance dose (PPI 1.1%, vs placebo 3.3% , RR 0.34; 95% CI:0.04 to 3.18) or at healing dose for esophagitis (PPI 5.2% vs placebo 2%, p = 0.11) [39]. A recent article suggesting a link between PPI use and small bowel bacterial overgrowth contributing to diarrhea predominant IBS shows that there is a common assumption among gastroenterologists that PPI can cause diarrhea, that is not necessarily supported by evidence [40].

Diarrhea is a common adverse effect with molecularly targeted agents. Epidermal growth factor receptor tyrosine kinase inhibitor, erlotinib, and other tyrosine kinase inhibitors such as sorafenib, imatinib and bortezomib cause diarrhea in up to 60% of patients [41]. Erbitux® (cetuximab), used for the treatment of EGFR-expressing, metastatic colorectal carcinoma and squamous cell carcinoma of the head and neck and Iressa® (geftinib), used for non-small cell lung cancer, can cause diarrhea in 48–67% of patients, depending on dose [42, 43]. EGF can activate PI 3-kinase and the lipid products of this enzyme inhibit calcium-dependent Cl-transport in T84 human colonic epithelial cells [44, 45]. EGF-receptor inhibitors may cause diarrhea by blocking this inhibitory loop and causing secretion. Diarrhea can easily be managed by loperamide, dose reduction or treatment interruptions [41].

Flavopiridol, a cyclin-dependent kinase inhibitor, has undergone several clinical trials as an anti-tumor agent, with secretory diarrhea as a dose-limiting factor. Adding cholestyramine and loperamide as a prophylactic antidiarrheal treatment allowed for use of higher doses [46]. Diarrhea may be related to flavopiridol binding to the gut mucosa acting as a modest secretagogoue. Cholestyramine, by binding flavopiridol, eases the adverse effect [47]. Pharmacogenomics may play a role in drug-induced diarrhea. For example, those with extensive hepatic glucorinidation metabolism experienced less diarrhea than others [48]. The hepatic metabolism of the drug decreases the toxic metabolites that causes intestinal secretion. In this clinical study, mild cases of diarrhea were controlled by loperamide, whereas more severe diarrhea was controlled by octreotide infusion and reduction of flavopiridol dosages in subsequent cycles [48].

Disordered or deregulation motility

Although not as elegantly delineated as epithelial transport changes, disordered or deregulated motility can also cause diarrhea. Prokinetic agents reduce intestinal contact time between luminal fluid and the epithelium. The decreased amount of time chyme is exposed to intestinal epithelium can limit absorption, and ultimately lead to diarrhea [2]. Cisapride and tegaserod are 5-HT$_4$-receptor agonists that stimulate motility and accelerate gastrointestinal transit. However, both of these drugs have been removed from the market due to potential cardiotoxicity.

Cholinergic drugs such as bethanecol, used for urinary retention and neurogenic bladder, have broad muscarinic effects via cholinergic receptors in the smooth muscle of the urinary bladder and the gastrointestinal tract [4, 49]. The effect of acetylcholine on smooth muscle of the gastrointestinal tract is mediated by two types of G protein-coupled muscarinic receptors, M$_2$ and M$_3$ in [4]. The activation of the M$_3$ receptor increases intracellular Ca^{2+} mediated by the G$_q$-PLC-IP$_3$ pathway [4, 28]. This results in increased gastrointestinal and pancreatic secretions, as well as increased peristalsis.

Acetylcholinesterase inhibitors, such as those used for Alzheimer's disease, allow acetylcholine to accumulate in the synaptic and neuromuscular junctions. These drugs enhance contractile effects producing diarrhea in up to 14% of patients [1, 3]. RCTs comparing donepezil to placebo for the treatment of Alzheimer's disease revealed diarrhea incidence of 15% with donepazil compared to 10% in placebo [50]. The Cochrane Review of the use of donepazil with over 1000 patients revealed that diarrhea occurred more frequently in donepazil treated patients (OR 2.78; 95% CI: 2.10, 3.69) [51]. In another Cochrane Review of the three anticholinesterases (donepezil, galantamine and rivastigmine) used for Alzheimer's dementia, the odds ratio for diarrhea with the use of anticholinesterases in comparison to placebo was 1.91 (95% CI: 1.59, 2.3) [52].

Neostigmine, used off-label for acute colonic pseudo-obstruction (Ogilvie's syndrome) and paralytic ileus, also can cause diarrhea [4]. Irinotecan, a chemotherapeutic agent, can cause severe diarrhea from cholinergic-like syndrome through the inhibition of acetylcholinesterase [3].

Motilin, a peptide hormone found in the gastrointestinal M cells, and in some enterochromaffin cells of the upper small bowel, is a potent contractile agent of the upper GI tract. The effects of motilin can be mimicked by macrolide antibiotics, especially erythromycin, and can cause diarrhea. In addition to its motilin agonistic effect, erythromycin at lower doses (40–80 mg) may also entail cholin-

ergic involvement, although the mechanisms are not well understood [4].

Just as in thyrotoxicosis, excess levothyroxine therapy can accelerate small and large intestinal transit, causing diarrhea [53–55]. Ticlopidine, an inhibitor of platelet aggregation, can cause diarrhea through many processes, including reported cases of lymphocytic colitis. However, increased motility is thought to be the principal mechanism based on manometric readings of jejunal motility revealing abnormal motility patterns [56].

The treatment of watery diarrhea includes discontinuation of the offending medication. Maintaining hydration is important to prevent dehydration from the amount of fluid loss. Loperamide, lomotil and bismuth subsalicylate can help relieve the symptom.

Inflammatory diarrhea

Drug induced inflammatory diarrheas fall into several broad categories. Perhaps the most important is the disruption of colonic flora and precipitation of *Clostridum difficile* colitis. Other mechanisms include the direct damage to the integrity of the mucosa that occurs with NSAIDs and polyene antibiotics, stimulation of low grade inflammation causing microscopic colitis, disruption of the balance between proliferation and apoptosis with a resulting compromise of epithelial integrity seen with immunosuppressives and chemotherapeutic agents, and vascular compromise as occurs with ergotamine and cocaine.

Antibiotics account for 25% of drug-induced diarrhea [1]. The most well-known complication is pseudomembranous colitis due to *Clostridium difficile*, especially seen with the antibiotics clindamycin, amoxicillin, ampicillin, and cephalosporins [3]. *Clostridium difficile* causes diarrhea by secreting enterotoxin A, which adheres to the brush-border membrane of enterocytes inducing an inflammatory response, and cytotoxin B that induces direct mucosal damage [2, 57]. Diarrhea may occur a few days after antibiotic therapy is initiated and up to eight weeks after discontinuation. In the appropriate clinical setting, diagnosis is based on detection of toxin in the stool. Endoscopy reveals raised white to yellow plaques covering a normal or moderately erythematous colonic mucosa [57]. Recently, non-antibiotic associated community acquired *C. difficile* has become more frequent with the use of acid reducing agents and immunosuppressives. Lansoprazole, and in the elderly, histamine antagonist use, are reported to be significant risk factors for carriage of *C. difficile*, increasing the risk of developing pseudomembranous colitis [3, 58]. In fact, a meta-analysis to assess risk factors for recurrent *C. difficile* infection revealed that use of concomitant antacid medications increased the risk by two fold (OR: 2.15; 95% CI: 1.13–4.08; p = 0.019) [59].

There has been a rise in the incidence of *C. difficile* colitis in hospitalized patients with inflammatory bowel disease [60]. This may be attributable to the use of immunosuppressives and biologic agents [61]. Treatment is discussed in detail in Chapter 20 of this book.

Through multifactorial mechanisms, diarrhea occurs in 3 – 9% of patients treated with the non-steroidal anti-inflammatory drugs (NSAIDs), especially the older drugs mefenamic acid and flufenamic acid [1, 62–64]. Thirty nine percent (34 of 87) of patients in a six-week study given meclofenamate at doses of 200 to 400 mg per day experienced diarrhea [65].

Since NSAIDs stimulate *in vitro* absorption (increased Na^+ absorption and decreased Cl^- secretion), other mechanisms must be involved in diarrhea [66]. NSAIDS most likely cause diarrhea through increased permeability and direct mucosal damage [67]. Histologic findings include prominent apoptosis and increased intraepithelial lymphocyte counts [68]. NSAIDs have been associated with both microscopic and pseudomembranous colitis. Ileal disease mimicking Crohn's disease has also been described.

Maiden and others have quantitatively analyzed by capsule endoscopy NSAID-induced pathology in 40 subjects taking diclofenac. Images revealed new pathology in 27 subjects (68%), with common lesions of mucosal breaks, bleeding, erythema and denuded mucosa, and the majority have concurrent lesions. These patients also had elevated fecal calprotectin (a marker for inflammation) levels from baseline. This study provides both biochemical and direct evidence of macroscopic injury to the small intestine from NSAID use [69]. In a case-control study of 105 cases of newly-diagnosed colitis based on endoscopic and histologic findings, 78 patients (74%) were taking NSAIDs or salicylates prior to or during the development of their disease [70]. These studies support NSAIDs as an important class of drugs in causing colitis.

Acute proctocolitis has been documented in four separate cases of NSAID etiology, with the use of flufenamic acid, mefenamic acid, naproxen and ibuprofen. Symptoms and signs resolved in all cases with removal of the drug, but a rapid relapse occurred in three of the five patients who were subsequently rechallenged with the NSAID [71].

NSAIDs have also been implicated in causing collagenous colitis. Based on a case-control study of 31 patients with collagenous colitis and 31 controls, the use of NSAIDs was significantly more common in the study group (19/31) vs (4/31) in the control group (p < 0.02) [72].

Auranofin causes secretory diarrhea, but enterocolitis can also occur with relatively low dosages [62]. Over 30 cases have been reported of gold therapy causing severe enterocolitis. This adverse effect was unrelated to dosage, occurred within three months of beginning treatment and persisted despite withdrawal of the drug [3, 73].

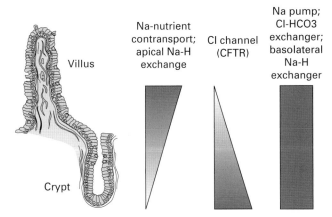

Figure 15.2 Gradients from crypt to villus. There is a significant spatial geometry of transport proteins along the crypt-villus (crypt-surface) axis. Some transport molecules are found at relatively constant concentrations along the axis, some exhibit a greater density in the base of the crypt, and others exhibit a greater density toward the villus or surface. (Adapted from Sellin JH (2002) Chapter 87: Intestinal electrolyte absorption and excretion. In: Feldman M, Friedman LS and Sleisenger MH (eds) *Gastrointestinal and Liver Disease: Pathophysiology/Diagnosis/Management*, 7th edn. Saunders, Philadelphia, 2002. Figure 87.3, p. 1695.)

Penicillamine has been shown in a few cases to cause acute proctosigmoiditis [62].

Inflammatory diarrhea can also be caused by immunosuppressive and chemotherapeutic agents. The balance between absorption and secretion may be disrupted by a change in the balance between mature villus and immature crypt cells (see Figure 15.2). This loss of intestinal epithelial homeostasis with some superficial necrosis causes an imbalance between absorptive, secretory, and motility functions of the gut contributing to diarrhea [17, 24, 57]. Epithelial apoptosis of more than five apoptotic bodies (per 100 crypts) is considered an increase above normal. NSAIDS and sodium phosphate bowel preparations cause 12 to 24 apoptotic bodies [58]. Chemotherapeutic agents, especially fluorouracil can cause greater than 100 apoptotic bodies [58]. These agents usually cause diarrhea in a dose-related fashion. It is most commonly seen with fluoropyrimidines (fluorouracil, irinotecan, methotrexate and cisplatin), the fluorouracil prodrug capecitabine and the combination treatment uracil-tegafur [1]. The patient's symptoms can range in severity from mild diarrhea to severe necrotizing enterocolitis [24].

Transplant immunosuppressives frequently cause diarrhea. This may be due to a similar apoptotic enteropathy. Mycophenolic acid may shift the balance between the pro and antiapoptotic factors Bcl-2 and Bax, leading to changes in mucosal homeostasis, and may also alter chloride secretion (Sellin, J unpublished observations).

Irinotecan can cause acute or delayed diarrhea in 50–88% of patients. Immediate-onset diarrhea is caused by acute cholinergic effects and usually responds rapidly to atropine. The delayed onset diarrhea usually occurs 24 hours to several days after administration, can be unpredictable, occurs at all dose levels and is worse with combination regimens with intravenous fluorouracil and leucovorin [41]. Several hypotheses have been proposed to explain the underlying mechanism. Evidence of a direct toxic effect on intestinal epithelium was provided by animal studies. Mice treated with irinotecan had intestinal wall thinning with epithelial vacuolation, vascular dilatation, an inflammatory cell infiltrate and evidence of apoptosis in the ileum [74, 75]. These studies led to the discovery of bacterial β-glucoronidase which deconjugates the irinotecan metabolite SN38 glucuronide causing its direct effect on the intestinal epithelium [24, 76].

Multiple agents have been studied in an attempt to reverse irinotecan-induced diarrhea. In humans, the use of the oral antibiotic, neomycin, which decreases β-glucuronidase activity in the intestinal lumen, resulted in good control of irinotecan-induced diarrhea in seven colorectal cancer patients [77]. The Chinese herb Hange-Shashito (TJ-14), a natural inhibitor of the β-glucuronidase activity of bacterial microflora, has also been shown to prevent the delayed diarrhea from irinotecan [78]. Probenecid, a biliary inhibitor of irinotecan and SN-38 secretion, has been shown to reduce irinotecan intestinal toxicity in mice, but no evidence has confirmed this observation in humans [79]. Oral cyclosporin (to reduce SN38 and SN38G clearance into the small bowel lumen) used with irinotecan in a phase I clinical trial, prevented severe diarrhea. Only one patient out of 37 experienced grade 3 diarrhea, and grade 4 diarrhea did not occur [80]. At increased pH, equilibrium favors the less toxic carboxylate form of the irinotecan metabolite SN-38. Reduced cellular damage and diarrhea was noted with bicarbonate administration in hamsters given irinotecan [81]. Phase II clinical trials also suggested benefit from sodium bicarbonate supplementation for irinotecan-induced severe delayed diarrhea [82].

Oxaliplatin combined with fluorouracil and irinotecan makes diarrhea even more common than the incidence observed with either agent alone [41]. Diarrhea can also result from an increase in opportunistic infections: invasive bacterial infections such as tuberculosis and yersinosis; ulcerating viral infections such as cytomegalovirus and herpes simplex; and invasive parasitic infections such as amebiasis and strongyloides. Neutropenic enterocolitis may also complicate chemotherapy in neutropenic patients with leukemia. This is especially associated with cytosine arabinoside, cisplatin, vincristine, adriamycin, fluorouracil and mercaptopurine [58].

Isotretinoid used for acne has been associated with inflammatory diarrheas [1]. Histology from these patients often shows acute focal superficial inflammatory infiltrate of the mucosa. HMG-CoA reductase inhibitors such as sim-

vastatin, lovastatin and pravastatin cause an inflammatory diarrhea in less than 5% of patients [1].

Several drugs have also been linked to microscopic colitis. These include NSAIDS, carbamazepine, ticlopidine, flutamide, and the selective serotonin receptor inhibitors, especially paroxetine and sertraline [1, 58].

Management of inflammatory diarrhea includes treatment of intercurrent infections such as CMV, antibiotic associated colitis, dose reduction of the etiologic agent, or cautious use of empiric therapy. Loperamide, diphenoxylate, deodorized tincture of opium and octreotide are effective for diarrhea from fluoropyridimoles [3]. Acetorphan, an enkephalinase inhibitor that blocks epithelial cyclic AMP mediated secretion, has shown moderate activity in clinical trials in patients with irinotecan-induced diarrhea [83]. Budesonide and octreotide have been used to slow intestinal motility and decrease water and electrolyte movement through the bowel [84–86].

Fatty diarrhea

Fatty diarrhea occurs in the clinical setting of weight loss and steatorrhea. This is caused by either maldigestion or malabsorption. Table 15.3 lists several medications that can cause this adverse effect. Highly active antiretroviral therapy has been known to cause steatorrhea, although the mechanisms have not been elucidated [87].

Interestingly, in a study of 33 HIV patients who underwent evaluation for diarrhea, over 90% had steatorrhea, irrespective of HAART therapy (20/21 patients not on HAART vs 10/12 patients on HAART) [87]. Thus, the specificity of steatorrhea secondary to HAART may be called into question.

Of the nucleoside analog reverse transcriptase inhibitors, didanosine causes diarrhea in 17–28% of patients, espe-

Table 15.3 Drugs inducing steatorrhea.

Aminoglycosides
Auranofin
Biguanides[a]
Cholestyramine
Colchicine
Highly active antiretroviral therapy[a]
Laxatives
Methyldopa
Octreotide
Orlistat (lipase inhibitor)[b]
Polymixin, bacitracin
Tetracyclines

[a] ≥20% incidence of diarrhea.
[b] >10% incidence of diarrhea.

cially in the buffered formulations [57]. Enteric-coated tablets decrease this incidence. Abacavir can produce diarrhea, especially in association with a hypersensitivity reaction that occurs in 3–5% of treated individuals [88, 89]. Diarrhea, among other symptoms, appears one to four weeks after initiation of therapy, and usually resolves within one to two days after discontinuation. Re-challenge with the drug, even at a decreased dose, may cause the return of symptoms within hours with increased severity [88].

Virtually all protease inhibitors cause diarrhea. Ritonavir causes diarrhea in up to 52% of patients [90, 91]. Adverse effects appear to be more common in patients with more advanced HIV/AIDS, and in patients with higher plasma drug levels. Effects are greatest at the beginning of therapy, before ritonavir induces an increase in its own metabolism [88]. Combination therapy, especially lopinavir with ritonavir increases the risk of diarrhea [88]. *In vitro* studies showed that several protease inhibitors inhibited lipase significantly at or below physiological concentrations [92]. Thus, besides the use of antidiarrheal medications such as loperamide that have been shown to control diarrhea, the use of pancrealipase with protease inhibitors may in theory reduce or eliminate steatorrhea in these patients [88, 92].

Orlistat, used as a prescription gastrointestinal lipase inhibitor for weight loss, is now available over the counter as "alli" (2007, GlaxoSmithKline, Pennsylvania) which contains half the prescription dose. Those using this drug can have malabsorptive diarrhea if fat intake is high. Of those taking orlistat, 60–80% experience steatorrhea in a dose-related mechanism [93]. This resolves when fat intake is reduced to 45g per day [93].

Olestra is a lipid that possesses properties of conventional fats and oils, but is neither digested nor absorbed. Olestra was approved by the FDA in January 1996 for use in snacks such as potato chips and crackers [94]. Although consumers complained of "diarrhea", a randomized control trial using higher than consumption doses showed no effect on stool frequency, but a modest stool softening effect measured by stool viscosity in subjects consuming olestra compared to controls [94].

Long-term use of oral antibacterials such as neomycin, polymixin and bacitracin can also cause malabsorptive diarrhea. These antibiotics damage the small intestinal mucosa, leading to a reduction of the enzyme activity of enterocytes [3, 49, 68]. They may also bind bile acids in the intestinal lumen and reduce the absorption of fat [1]. In *in vitro* transport studies, both neomycin and amphotericin act as membrane detergents, functionally "dissolving" the apical memberane of enterocytes or colonocytes. Administering 1g of neomycin with a test meal to five healthy subjects caused a marked increase in fatty acid and bile acid in their aspirated intestinal contents [95]. However, a subsequent study of 2g per day dose of neomycin given

to four patients revealed no evidence of steatorrhea, although daily stool weight increased in three or four patients [96].

Cholestyramine usually causes constipation, but in doses of 24–30g per day may cause steatorrhea [1]. Animal studies show that increasing the dietary amount of cholestyramine markedly increased the excretion of both free and esterified fat in the stool [97].

Octreotide, used as an antidiarrheal, has a paradoxical effect at higher doses, causing steatorrhea in 5–13% of patients by a possible synergistic inhibition of biliary and pancreatic function through decreased bicarbonate and lipase secretion [1, 98]. L-dopa, allopurinol, tetracycline and NSAIDs, especially mefanamic acid, can cause steatorrhea through changes in jejunal mucosa [28, 66].

Several medications have been implicated for inducing steatorrhea in addition to other types of diarrhea. For example, in addition to its effects on intestinal transit, levothyroxine has been implicated in bile acid malabsorption because of abnormal selenohomocholyltaurine (SeHCAT) testing. This test can be used to diagnose bile acid malabsorption as a cause of chronic diarrhea, but it best predicts the benefit of cholestyramine in these patients [99]. However, this adverse effect of levothyroxine may be a secondary effect of increased motility. Colchicine can cause secretory and inflammatory diarrhea, but can also cause malabsorption in large doses by causing villous atrophy [3]. Three out of twelve patients evaluated for gastrointestinal effects of the long-term use of colchicine prophylaxis for recurrent polyserositis developed mild steatorrhea [100].

Chemotherapeutic agents, besides causing inflammatory diarrhea, can damage immature epithelial cells in the crypts causing functionally compromised mature enterocytes. This effect leads to decreased nutrient absorptive capacity and potentially a malabsorptive diarrhea [3]. Rapamycin administration in rabbits showed significantly decreased jejunal and ileal villous surface areas and decreased fat and cholesterol uptake, possibly contributing to malabsorption [101].

Treatment of drug induced steatorrhea may require dose reduction or withdrawal of the drug. In some cases such as diarrhea due to metformin, continued symptoms may resolve with time even if the drug is continued, as the gastrointestinal system adjusts to the drug. Antidiarrheals such as loperamide and probiotics may help. In the case of antiretroviral drugs, soluble fiber and L-glutamine have been found to be helpful [102]. If prolonged, replacement of fat soluble vitamins maybe needed.

Conclusion

Ideally, decisions about diagnosis or therapy should be evidence-based; however, as emphasized above, there is frequently a dearth of high quality evidence to guide the clinician in the area of drug-induced diarrhea. Determining the etiology of drug induced diarrhea depends on a careful history to identify the offending agent. Any history of drug allergies or intolerances, and any new prescription medications taken within the six to eight weeks prior to symptom onset may reveal the etiology. One should always consider prescription as well as non-prescription drugs, nutritional supplements, excessive caffeine consumption and artificial sweeteners found in diet foods as potential causes. Most cases of drug-induced diarrhea resolve spontaneously within a few days after withdrawal of the drug, or with dose reduction. If diarrhea is severe or persistent, patient management should include replenishment of any fluid and electrolyte deficits with oral hydration or, if warranted, with intravenous fluids. Non-specific antidiarrheal agents can reduce stool frequency and stool weight as well as decrease abdominal cramps. Opiates (loperamide, diphenoxylate with atropine), intraluminal agents (bismuth subsalicylate) and adsorbents (kaolin) also can help reduce the fluidity of bowel movements [2, 58]. A low residue diet, specific treatment as described in above sections such as antibiotics for *C. difficile* colitis, and reduction of fat intake for patients taking orlistat, can also help. Probiotics as possible treatment or prevention have not been well studied, but future studies may prove to be useful.

References

1 Chassany O, Michaux A, Bergmann JF. Drug-Induced Diarrhoea. *Drug Safety* 2000; **22**: 53–72.

2 Schiller LR, Sellin JH. (2006) Diarrhea. In Feldman M, Friedman LS, Brandt LJ et al., eds. *Gastrointestinal and Liver Disease*. Saunders, Philadelphia, 2006: 159–181.

3 Ratnaike RN, Jones TE. Mechanisms of drug-induced diarrhoea in the elderly. *Drugs & Aging* 1998; **13**: 245–253.

4 Pasricha PJ. (2006) Treatment of disorders of bowel motility and water flux; antiemetics: Agents used in biliary and pancreatic disease. In Brunton LL, Lazo JS, Parker KL, eds. *Goodman & Gilman's The Pharmacological Basis of Therapeutics*. McGraw-Hill, New York, 2006.

5 Binder HJ. The gastroenterologist's osmotic gap: Fact or fiction? *Gastroenterology* 1992; **103**, 702–704.

6 Coniff RF, Shapiro JA, Seaton TB et al. Multicenter, placebo-controlled trial comparing acarbose (BAY g 5421) with placebo, tolbutamide, and tolbutamide-plus-acarbose in non-insulin-dependent diabetes mellitus. *Am J Med* 1995; **98**: 443–451.

7 Santeusanio F, Compagnucci P. A risk-benefit appraisal of acarbose in the management of non-insulin-dependent diabetes mellitus. *Drug Saf* 1994; **11**: 432–444.

8 Fischer S, Hanefeld M, Spengler M et al. European study on dose-response relationship of acarbose as a first-line drug in non-insulin-dependent diabetes mellitus: Efficacy and safety of low and high doses. *Acta Diabetol* 1998; **35**: 34–40.

9 Spengler M, Cagatay M. The use of acarbose in the primary-care setting: Evaluation of efficacy and tolerability of acarbose by postmarketing surveillance study. *Clin Invest Med* 1995; **18**: 325–331.

10 PDR Health: Prebiotics. http://www.pdrhealth.com/drug_info/nmdrugprofiles/nutsupdrugs/pre_0326.shtml. Accessed 11 June 2008.

11 Marteau, P, Seksik P. Tolerance of probiotics and prebiotics. *J Clin Gastroenterology* 2004; **38**: S67–S69.

12 Briet F, Achour L, Flourié B et al. Symptomatic response to varying levels of fructo-oligosaccharides consumed occasionally or regularly. *Eur J Clin Nutr* 1995; **49**(7): 501–507.

13 Pentland B, Pennington CR. Acute diarrhoea in the elderly. *Age and Ageing* 1980; **9**: 90–92.

14 Plass H, Charisius M,, Wyskovsky W et al. Class I antiarrhythmics inhibit Na+ absorption and Cl- secretion in rabbit descending colon epithelium. *Arch Pharmacol* 2005; **371**: 492–499.

15 Kles KA, Vavricka SR, Turner JR et al. Comparative analysis of the in vitro prosecretory effects of balsalazide, sulfasalazine, olsalazine, and mesalamine in rabbit distal ileum. *Inflammatory Bowel Diseases* 2005; **11**: 253–257.

16 Pamukcu R, Hanauer SB, Change EB. Effect of disodium azodisalicylate on electrolyte transport in rabbit ileum and colon *in vitro*. Comparison with sulfasalazine and 5-aminosalicylic acid. *Gastroenterology* 1988; **95**: 975–981.

17 Sellin JH. The pathophysiology of diarrhea. *Clin Transplantation* 2001; **15**: 2–10.

18 Wald A, Back C, Bayless TM. Effect of caffeine on the human small intestine. *Gastroenterology* 1976; **71**: 738–742.

19 Mauricio AC, Slawik M, Heitzmann D et al. Deoxycholic acid (DOC) affects the transport properties of distal colon. *Pflugers Arch* 2000; **439**: 532–540.

20 Venkatasubramanian J, Selvaraj N, Carlos M et al. Differences in Ca2+ signaling underlie age-specific effects of secretagogues on colonic Cl- transport. *Am J Physiol Cell Physiol* 2001; **280**: C646–C658.

21 Hempfling W, Dilger K, Beuers, U. Ursodeoxycholic acid – adverse effects and drug interactions *Alimentary Pharmacology & Therapeutics* 2003; **18**: 963–972.

22 Racusen LC, Binder HJ. Ricinoleic acid stimulation of active anion secretion in colonic mucosa of the rat. *J Clin Invest* 1979; **63**: 743–749.

23 Ramakrishna BS, Mathan M, Mathan VI. Alteration of colonic absorption by long-chain unsaturated fatty acids. Influence of hydroxylation and degree of unsaturation. *Scand J Gastroenterol* 1994; **29**: 54–58.

24 Solomon R, Cherny NI. Constipation and diarrhea in patients with cancer. *The Cancer Journal* 2006; **12**: 355–364.

25 Gray TK, Bieberdorf FA, Fordtran JS. Thyrocalcitonin and the jejunal absorption of calcium, water, and electrolytes in normal subjects. *Journal of Clinical Investigation* 1973; **52**: 3084–3088.

26 Kisloff B, Moore EW. Effects of intravenous calcitonin on water, electrolyte, and calcium movement across *in vivo* rabbit jejunum and ileum. *Gastroenterology* 1977; **72b**: 462–468.

27 Miacalcin® calcitonin-salmon (2007) In: *Physician Desk Reference*. Thomson PDR; 2253–2254.

28 Bateman DN. (1991) Gastrointestinal disorders. In: Davies DM, eds. *Textbook of adverse drug reactions*. Oxford University Press, New York, 1991: 230–244.

29 Berchtold P, Dahlqvist A, Gustafson A, *et al.* Effects of a biguanide (metformin) on vitamin B12 and folic acid absorption and intestinal enzyme activities. *Scand. J. Gastroenterol* 1971; **6**: 751.

30 Czyzyk A, Tawecki J, Sadowski J *et al.* Effect of biguanides on intestinal absorption of glucose. *Diabetes* 1968; **17**: 492–498.

31 Kruger FA, Altschuld RA, Hollobaugh SL *et al.* Studies on the site and mechanism of action of phenformin. II. Phenformin inhibition of glucose transport by rat intestine. *Diabetes* 1970; **19**: 50–52.

32 Ikeda T, Iwata K, Murakami H. Inhibitory effect of metformin on intestinal glucose absorption in the perfused rat intestine. *Biochem Pharmacol* 2000; **59**: 887–890.

33 Wilcock C, Bailey CJ. Reconsideration of inhibitory effect of metformin on intestinal glucose absorption. *J Pharm Pharmacol* 1991; **43**: 120–121.

34 Saenz A, Fernandez-Esteban I, Mataix A *et al.* (2005) Metformin monotherapy for type 2 diabetes mellitus. *Cochrane Database of Systematic Reviews*, Issue 3. Art. No.: CD002966. DOI: 10.1002/14651858.CD002966.pub3.

35 DeFronzo RA, Goodman AM. Efficacy of metformin in patients with non-insulin-dependent diabetes mellitus. *N Engl J Med* 1995; **333**: 541–549.

36 Foss MT, Clement KD. Metformin as a cause of late-onset chronic diarrhea. *Pharmacotherapy* 2001; **21**: 1422–1424.

37 Bytzer P, Talley NJ, Jones MP *et al.* Oral hypoglycaemic drugs and gastrointestinal symptoms in diabetes mellitus. *Aliment Pharmacol Ther* 2001; **15**: 137–142.

38 Dandona P, Fonseca V, Mier A *et al.* Diarrhea and metformin in a diabetic clinic. *Diabetes Care* 1983; **6**: 472–474.

39 Donnellan C, Sharma N, Preston C, Moayyedi P. (2004) Medical treatments for the maintenance therapy of reflux oesophagitis and endoscopic negative reflux disease. *Cochrane Database of Systematic Reviews*. Issue 4. Art. No.: CD003245. DOI: 10.1002/14651858.CD003245.pub2.

40 Brennan M, Spiegel R, Chey WD *et al.* Bacterial overgrowth and irritable bowel syndrome: Unifying hypothesis or a spurious consequence of proton pump inhibitors? *Am J Gastro* 2008; **103**: 2972–2976.

41 Benson AB 3rd, Ajani JA, Catalano RB *et al.* Recommended guidelines for the treatment of cancer treatment-induced diarrhea. *J Clin Oncol* 2004; **22**: 2918.

42 Erbitux® (Cetuximab) Package Insert. (2007) ImClone Systems Incorporated, New York, and Bristol-Myers Squibb Company, Princeton.

43 Iressa® (geftinib) Package Insert. (2004) AstraZeneca, Wilmington.

44 Uribe JM, Keely SJ, Traynor-Kaplan AE *et al.* Phosphatidylinositol 3-Kinase mediates the inhibitory effect of epidermal growth factor on calcium-dependent chloride secretion. *Journal of Biological Chemistr* 1996; **271**: 26588–26595.

45 Uribe JM, Gelbmann CM, Traynor-Kaplan AE *et al.* Epidermal growth factor inhibits Ca2+ -dependent Cl- transport in T84 human colonic epithelial cells. *Am J Physiol* 1996; **271**: C914–C922.

46 Zhai S, Senderowicz AM, Sausville EA *et al.* Flavopiridol, a Novel Cyclin-Dependent Kinase Inhibitor, in Clinical Development. *Ann Pharmacother* 2002; **36**: 905–911.

47 Kahn ME, Senderowicz A, Sausville EA *et al.* Possible mechanisms of diarrheal side effects associated with the use of a novel chemotherapeutic agent, flavopiridol. *Clin Cancer Res* 2001; **7**: 343–349.

48 Innocenti F, Stadler WM, Iyer L *et al.* Flavopiridol Metabolism in Cancer Patients Is Associated with the Occurrence of Diarrhea. *Clinical Cancer Research* 2000; **6**: 3400–3405.

49 Andersson KE. Current Concepts in the Treatment of Disorders of Micturition. *Drugs* 1988; **35**: 477.

50 Pierre N, Tariot PN, Cummings JL *et al.* A randomized, double-blind, placebo-controlled study of the efficacy and safety of donepezil in patients with Alzheimer's disease in the nursing home setting. *J Am Geriatr Soc* 2005; **49**: 1590–1599.

51 Birks J, Harvey RJ. (2006) Donepezil for dementia due to Alzheimer's disease. *Cochrane Database of Systematic Reviews*. Issue 1. Art. No.: CD001190. DOI: 10.1002/14651858.CD001190.pub2.

52 Birks J. (2006) Cholinesterase inhibitors for Alzheimer's disease. *Cochrane Database of Systematic Reviews*. Issue 1. Art. No.: CD005593. DOI: 10.1002/14651858.CD005593.

53 Nayak B, Burman K. Thyrotoxicosis and Thyroid Storm. *Endocrinol Metab Clin N Am* 2006; **35**: 663–686.

54 Wasan SM, Sellin JH, Vassilopoulou-Sellin R. (2005) The Gastrointestinal Tract and Liver in Thyrotoxicosis. In Braverman LE, Utiger RD, eds. *Werner & Ingbar's The Thyroid: A Fundamental and Clinical Text.* Lippincott Williams & Wilkins, Philadelphia, 2005. 589–594.

55 Wegener M, Wedmann B, Langhoff T *et al.* Effect of hyperthyroidism on the transit of a caloric solid-liquid meal through the stomach, the small intestine, and the colon in man. *J Clin Endocrinol Metab* 1992; **75**: 745–749.

56 Guédon C, Bruna T, Ducrotté P *et al.* Severe diarrhea caused by Ticlid associated with disorders of small intestine motility. *Gastroenterol Clin Biol* 1989; **13**: 934–937.

57 Gervasio JM. (2005) Diarrhea and Constipation. In Tisdale JE & Miller DA, eds. *Drug-Induced Diseases: Prevention, Detection, and Management.* American Society of Health Systems Pharmacists, Bethesda, 2005 501–514.

58 Parfitt JR, Driman DK. Pathological effects of drugs on the gastrointestinal tract: A review. *Human Pathology* 2007; **38**: 527–536.

59 Garey KW, Sethi S, Yadav Y, Dupont HL. Meta-analysis to assess risk factors for recurrent Clostridium difficile infection. *J Hosp Infect* 2008; **70**: 298–304.

60 Rodemann JF, Dubberke ER, Reske KA *et al.* Incidence of Clostridium difficile infection in inflammatory bowel disease. *Clinical Gastroenterology & Hepatology* 2007; **5**: 339–344.

61 Issa M, Vijayapal A, Graham MB *et al.* Impact of Clostridium difficile on inflammatory bowel disease. *Clinical Gastroenterology and Hepatology* 2007; **5**: 345–351.

62 D'Arcy PF, Griffin JP. *Iatrogenic Diseases.* Oxford University Press, New York, 1986: 573.

63 Hill, AG. (1966) Clinical trials of the fenamates: Review of flufenamic acid in rheumatoid arthritis. In Kendall PH, ed. *Annuals of Physical Medicine* (suppl.) Bailliere, Tindall and Cassell, London: 87–92.

64 Holmes EL. (1966) Pharmacology of the fenamates: Experimental observations on flufenamic, mefenamic and meclofenamic acids. IV.Toleration by normal human subjects. In Kendall PH, ed. *Annuals of Physical Medicine* (suppl). Bailliere, Tindall and Cassell, London: 36–49.

65 Ward JR, Bolzan JA, Brame CL *et al.* Sodium meclofenamate dose determining studies. *Curr Therap* 1978; *Res* **23**(suppl): S60–S65.

66 Langridge-Smith JE, Rao MC, Field M. Chloride and sodium transport across bovine tracheal epithelium: Effects of secretagogues and indomethacin. *Pflugers Arch* 1984; **402**: 42–47.

67 Gullikson GW, Sender M, Bass P. Laxative-like effects of nonsteroidal anti-inflammatory drugs on intestinal fluid movement and membrane integrity. *J Pharmacol Exp Ther* 1982; **220**: 236–242.

68 Price AB. Pathology of drug-associated gastrointestinal disease. *J Clin Pharmacol* 2003; **56**: 477–482.

69 Maiden L, Thjodleifsson B, Theodors A *et al.* A quantitative analysis of NSAID-induced small bowel pathology by capsule enteroscopy. *Gastroenterology* 2005; **128**: 1172–1178.

70 Gleeson MH, Davis AJM. Non-steroidal anti-inflammatory drugs, aspirin and newly diagnosed colitis: A case-control study. *Alimentary Pharmacology & Therapeutics* 2003; **17**: 817–825.

71 Ravi S, Keat AC, Keat EC. Colitis caused by non-steroidal anti-inflammatory drugs. *Postgrad Med J* 1986; **62**: 773–776.

72 Riddell RH, Tanaka M, Mazzoleni G. Non-steroidal anti-inflammatory drugs as a possible cause of collagenous colitis: A case-control study. *Gut* 1992; **33**: 683–686.

73 Jackson CW, Haboubi NY, Whorwell PJ *et al.* Gold induced enterocolitis *Gut* 1986; **27**: 452–456.

74 Ikuno N, Soda H, Watanabe M *et al.* Irinotecan (CPT-11) and characteristic mucosal changes in the mouse ileum and cecum. *J. Natl. Cancer Inst* 1995; **87**: 1876–1883.

75 Guffroy M, Hodge T. Re: Irinotecan (CPT-11) and characteristic mucosal changes in the mouse ileum and cecum (letter, comment). *J Natl Cancer Inst* 1996; **88**: 1240–1241.

76 Goumas P, Naxakis S, Christopoulou A *et al.* Octreotide acetate in the treatment of fluorouracil-induced diarrhea. *Oncologist* 1998; **8**: 50.

77 Diederik FS, Kehrer A, Sparreboom J, Verweij P *et al.* Modulation of irinotecan-induced diahrrea by cotreatment with Neomycin in cancer patients. *Clinical Cancer Research* 2001; **7**: 1136–1141.

78 Sakata Y, Suzuki H, Kamataki T. Preventive effect of TJ-14, a kampo (Chinese herb) medicine, on diarrhoea induced by irinotecan hydrochloride (CPT-11). *Gan. To Kagaku Ryoho* 1994; **21**: 1241–1244.

79 Horikawa M, Kato Y, Sugiyama Y. Reduced gastrointestinal toxicity following inhibition of the biliary excretion of irinotecan and its metabolites by probenecid in rats. *Pharm Res* 2002; **19**: 1345–1353.

80 Chester JD, Joel SP, Cheeseman SL *et al.* Phase I and pharmacokinetic study of intravenous irinotecan plus oral ciclosporin in patients with fluorouracil-refractory metastatic colon cancer. *Journal of Clinical Oncology* 2003; **21**: 1125–1132.

81 Ikegami T, Ha L, Arimori K. Intestinal alkalization as a possible preventive mechanism in irinotecan (CPT-11)-induced diarrhoea. *Cancer Res* 2002; **62**: 179–187.

82 Takeda Y, Kobayashi K, Akiyama Y *et al.* Prevention of irinotecan (CPT-11)-induced diarrhoea by oral alkalization combined with control of defecation in cancer patients. *Int J Cancer* 2001; **92**: 269–275.

83 Saliba F, Hagipantelli R, Misset JL *et al.* Pathophysiology and therapy of irinotecan-induced delayed-onset diarrhea in patients with advanced colorectal cancer: A prospective assessment. *J Clin Oncol* 1998; **16**: 2745.

84 Lenfers BH, Loeffler TM, Droege CM *et al.* Substantial activity of budesonide in patients with irinotecan (CPT-11) and 5-fluorouracil induced diarrhoea and failure of loperamide treatment. *Ann Oncol* 1999; **10**: 1251–1253.

85 Barbounis V, Koumakis G, Vassilomanolakis M *et al.* Control of irinotecan-induced diarrhoea by octreotide after loperamide failure. *Support Care Cancer* 2001; **9**: 258–260.

86 Pro B, Lozano R, Ajani JA. Therapeutic response to octreotide in patients with refractory CPT-11 induced diarrhoea. *Invest New Drugs* 2001; **19**: 341–343.

87 Poles M, Fuerst M, McGowan I *et al.* HIV-related diarrhea is multifactorial and fat malabsorption is commonly present, independent of HAART. *Am J Gastroenterology* 2001; **96**: 1831–1837.

88 Vella S, Floridia M. (2004) Antiviral Therapy. In: Cohen J, Powderly WG, Berkley SF *et al.* eds. *Infectious Diseases*. Mosby, New York, 2004: 1387–1394.

89 Kessler HA, Johnson J, Follansbee S *et al.* Abacavir expanded access program for adult patients infected with human immunodeficiency virus type 1. *Clin Infect Dis* 2004; **34**: 535–542.

90 Danner SA, Carr A, Leonard JM *et al.* A short-term study of the safety, pharmacokinetics, and efficacy of ritonavir, an inhibitor of HIV-1 protease. European-Australian Collaborative Ritonavir Study Group. *N Engl J Med* 1995; **333**: 1528–1533.

91 Cameron DW, Heath-Chiozzi M, Danner S *et al.* Randomised placebo-controlled trial of ritonavir in advanced HIV-1 disease. The Advanced HIV Disease Ritonavir Study Group. *Lancet* 1998; **351**: 543–549.

92 Terese M, Wignot RP, Stewart KJ *et al.* *In Vitro* Studies of the Effects of HAART Drugs and Excipients on Activity of Digestive Enzymes. *Pharm Res* 2004; **21**: 420–427.

93 Sjostrom L, Rissanen A, Andersen T *et al.* Randomised placebo-controlled trial of orlistat for weight loss and prevention of weight regain in obese patients. *Lancet* 1998; **352**: 167–173.

94 McRorie J, Zorich N, Riccardi K *et al.* Effects of olestra and sorbitol consumption on objective measures of diarrhea: Impact of stool viscosity on common gastrointestinal symptoms. *Regulatory Toxicology and Pharmacology* 2000; **31**: 59–67.

95 Thompson GR, Barrowman J, Gutierrez L *et al.* Action of neomycin on the intraluminal phase of lipid absorption. *J Clin Invest* 1971; **50**: 319–323.

96 Sedaghat A, Samuel P, Crouse JR *et al.* Effects of neomycin on absorption, synthesis, and/or flux of cholesterol in man. *J Clin Invest* 1975; **55**: 12–21.

97 Harkins RW, Hagerman LM, Sarett HP. Absorption of dietary fats by the rat in cholestyramine-induced steatorrhea. *J Nutr* 1965; **87**: 85–92.

98 Nakamura T, Kudoh K, Takebe K *et al.* Octreotide decreases biliary and pancreatic exocrine function, and induces steatorrhea in healthy subjects. *Internal Medicine* 1994; **33**: 593–596.

99 Raju GS, Dawson B, Bardhan KD. Bile acid malabsorption associated with Graves' disease. *J Clin Gastroenterol* 1994; **19**: 54–56.

100 Ehrenfeld M, Levy M, Sharon P *et al.* Gastrointestinal effects of long-term colchicine therapy in patients with recurrent polyse-

rositis (familial Mediterranean fever). *Dig Dis Sci* 1982; **27**: 723–727.

101 Dias VC, Madsen KL, Mulder KE *et al.* Oral administration of rapamycin and cyclosporine differentially alter intestinal function in rabbits. *Dig Dis Sci* 1998; **43**: 2227–2236.

102 Heiser CR, Ernst JA, Barret JT *et al.* Probiotics, soluble fiber and L-Glutamine (GLN) reduce nelfinavir (NFV)- or lopinavir/ritonavir (LPV/r)-related diarrhea. *J Int Assoc Physicians AIDS Care (Chic Ill)* 2004; **3**: 121–130.

16 Metabolic bone disease in gastrointestinal disorders

Ann Cranney[1], Alaa Rostom[2], Catherine Dubé[3], Rachid Mohamed[3], Peter Tugwell[4], George Wells[5] and John WD McDonald[6]

[1]Canadian Protective Medical Association *and* Clinical Epidemiology, Ottawa Hospital Research Institute *and* Faculty of Medicine, University of Ottawa, Ottawa, Canada
[2]Forzani and MacPhail Colon Cancer Screening Centre, University of Calgary, Calgary, Canada
[3]Division of Gastroenterology, University of Calgary, Calgary, Canada
[4]Department of Medicine and Epidemiology, University of Ottawa, Ottawa, Canada
[5]Department of Epidemiology and Community Medicine and Cardiovascular Research Methods Centre , University of Ottawa, Ottawa, Canada
[6]Robarts Clinical Trials, Robarts Research Unit, University of Western Ontario, London, Ontario, Canada

Introduction

Metabolic bone disease is seen in patients suffering from a variety of gastrointestinal disorders, including chronic liver disease, inflammatory bowel disease (IBD), and malabsorption syndromes such as celiac disease. In the setting of gastrointestinal disorders, bone disease can be broadly divided into osteoporosis and osteomalacia. Osteoporosis is a systemic skeletal disorder of reduced bone mass per unit volume (i.e. bone density) and disrupted micro-architecture, resulting in decreased bone strength and an increased risk of fragility fractures mainly of the hip, wrist and vertebrae [1]. Bone mass is a major determinant of bone strength. Osteomalacia, however, is characterized by defective mineralization of bone matrix, usually due to a disturbance of vitamin D and calcium homeostasis. It is clinically associated with pain, bone fractures, muscle weakness, difficulty walking and, radiologically, with pseudofractures (radiolucent bands perpendicular to surface of cortical bone) and loss of trabeculae.

There are two types of bone: cortical, which primarily makes up the long bones, and trabecular bone, which makes up most of the axial skeleton. Bone formation and resorption is a continuous process in which osteoblasts are responsible for the formation of new bone including the mineralization of bone, and osteoclasts are responsible for bone resorption. Metabolic bone disease results from abnormalities in the normal remodeling cycle. Osteoporosis is associated with disability, impaired quality of life and osteoporotic fractures can be associated with increased mortality [2].

Evidence-Based Gastroenterology and Hepatology, 3rd edition.
J. McDonald, A.K. Burroughs, B. Feagan, and M.B. Fennerty. © 2010
Blackwell Publishing Ltd

This chapter will focus on metabolic bone disease associated with chronic liver disease, IBD, celiac disease and will review corticosteroid-induced osteoporosis and the potential link between proton pump inhibitors and osteoporotic fractures.

Assessment of bone mass

Age-related bone loss begins during the fourth decade, and in women there is an accelerated bone loss at the time of menopause (5–15% in the initial five years after menopause), due to declines in estrogen. Perimenopausal bone loss is characterized by increased bone resorption and bone loss is greater at trabecular bone sites compared to cortical sites. Women experience greater rates of bone loss than men and their lifetime risk of an osteoporotic fracture is about 15% compared with 5% in men [3]. Osteoporosis can be detected by measurement of bone mineral density. Bone density is the most accurate predictor of fracture risk and it is a useful guide for monitoring therapy [4]. Prospective trials have established the ability of bone density to predict site-specific fractures [5]. For each reduction in bone density of the hip by 1 standard deviation (SD) from the mean for young normal individuals, the risk of hip fracture increases by a factor of 1.5–2.6 [6]. In men, low bone mineral density (BMD) has been demonstrated to be predictive of vertebral fractures [7]. In a prospective study which included 1690 men, it was estimated that a 1 SD decrease in femoral neck bone density was associated with a two-fold increase in risk of a traumatic fracture [8]. Increasing age and a history of a previous vertebral fracture are very important predictors of fracture.

Bone mass can be evaluated at a number of sites, such as the proximal femur, spine and distal radius. The most commonly used technique to evaluate BMD is dual energy X-ray absorptiometry (DXA). The reproducibility, accuracy and precision of DXA are excellent, with a coefficient of variation of 2%. Another technique, quantitative computed tomography (QCT), provides a three-dimensional image which makes it possible to separate trabecular and cortical bone. The accuracy of QCT is not as good (5–15%) as DXA, and is associated with a higher radiation dose.

Bone mineral content (BMC) is the total amount of mineralized tissue (g) in the bone scan, usually normalized to the length of the scan path (grams per mineral per centimeter of bone or g/cm). BMD, on the other hand, is the amount of mineralized tissue in the scanned area (g/cm^2). BMD can be expressed as a T-score (comparison of the patient's bone density with the peak bone mass in young normal individuals) or Z-score (comparison of patient's BMD to other age-matched controls). Individuals with a T-score or BMD less than 1 SD below the mean in young adults are considered to be osteopenic, while those with a BMD less than 2.5 SD below the young normal value are osteoporotic [1]. A study group on densitometry hosted by the World Health Organization (WHO) in 1993 defined these four diagnostic thresholds based on reference populations of healthy young women. Since these thresholds are based on young women, this definition does not account for biological variation and age-related bone loss and many have argued against the use of T-scores.

In addition to BMD, bone strength and fracture risk depend on other skeletal and non-skeletal factors such as trabecular micro-architecture and muscle strength. As a result, there has been a shift to the development of fracture risk prediction models which incorporate BMD, age and other clinical factors.

The increased use of DXA has resulted in more gastroenterology patients being diagnosed with osteoporosis. However, it is not clear what a diagnosis of osteopenia in gastrointestinal patients means in terms of increased fracture risk. On the basis of BMD, osteomalacia cannot be distinguished from osteoporosis.

Hepatic osteodystrophy

Hepatic osteodystrophy, or chronic liver disease-associated metabolic bone disease, was previously thought to arise mainly in cholestatic liver diseases, as a result of calcium and vitamin D malabsorption. However, hepatic osteodystrophy has now been described in association with most types of chronic liver diseases, whether cholestatic or non-cholestatic [9]. Increased bone loss and/or increased incidence of fractures have been described in primary biliary cirrhosis (PBC) [10], primary sclerosing cholangitis (PSC) [11], alcoholic liver disease (ALD) [12, 13], autoimmune hepatitis (AIH) [14], hemochromatosis [15, 16], as well as viral cirrhosis [17–20]. Additionally, hepatic osteodystrophy has important clinical repercussions in the early period after liver transplant, where immobilization, co-morbidity, corticosteroids and immunosuppressive drugs further reduce an already compromised bone mass [10], resulting in spontaneous vertebral fractures [21, 22].

Prevalence

The prevalence of hepatic osteodystrophy varies from 13–56% [11, 17, 23, 24], while the incidence of fractures in ambulatory and non-alcoholic patients with chronic liver disease ranges from 6–18%. The prevalence of vertebral fractures ranges from 7–44% and is approximately twice that of age and sex-matched controls, with the highest rates in those individuals with AIH [17, 23–25]. The degree of bone loss correlates with the severity of the cirrhosis and increasing age, making patients with endstage liver disease the group most at risk of fractures [5, 23, 26]. The situation in PBC is becoming less clear as some studies show an association with osteoporosis and fractures [24, 25, 27], while some recent studies including a prospective cohort study showed an association with age, postmenopausal status and BMI, but not with cirrhosis or serum bilirubin [28]. While another showed no increased risk of fractures in PBC [29]. Similarly, a study in PSC showed that bone mineral density did not correlate with the severity of the disease [30].

The fracture risk in chronic liver disease was best studied by Diamond *et al.*, in a case-control study of 115 patients with chronic liver disease (72 men and 43 women), who were matched for age, sex and menopausal status with healthy controls [23]. The etiology of the chronic liver disease was ALD (n = 40), chronic active hepatitis (n = 27), hemochromatosis (n = 25), PBC (n = 10), and PSC (n = 13). Fifty-two percent of the patients were cirrhotic, while 30% had clinical and biochemical evidence of hypogonadism. It is important to note that, in men, hypogonadism correlates with the degree of liver dysfunction. All patients were ambulatory and none were on cholestyramine, vitamin D, estrogen, or calcium. From the data in this study, the relative risk (RR) of either spinal or peripheral fractures can be calculated, based on the absolute number of fractures (as opposed to the number of patients with fractures). In men this RR is 3.03 (95% CI: 1.35–11.09), while in women the RR is 2.13 (95% CI: 1.38–7.46). These authors did a stepwise regression analysis to define the main predictors of fracture and osteoporosis. Variables used were: age, sex, gonadal status, presence of cirrhosis, type of liver disease, liver function, 25(OH) D$_3$ level and parathyroid hormone (PTH) level. Lumbar spine bone density, liver dysfunction and hypogonadism were the main predictors of spinal fracture, while hypogonadism and the presence of cirrhosis were the main predictors of peripheral fractures. There was no association with serum PTH or 25-hydroxy-vitamin D$_3$.

Because of the potential for impaired absorption of calcium and vitamin D [31, 32], as well as impaired hepatic uptake and metabolism of vitamin D [33], osteomalacia was initially thought to be the major cause of hepatic osteodystrophy in cholestatic liver diseases [33, 34]. However, it then became evident that bone disease was still prevalent despite treatment with calcium and vitamin D, and that most patients with cholestatic liver disease and osteopenia did not have low 25-hydroxyvitamin D_3 levels [11] or histomorphometric characteristics of osteomalacia [26, 35, 36]. Osteoporosis appears to be the major metabolic bone disease found with chronic liver disease.

The mechanisms responsible for the osteoporosis in this setting are uncertain, and evidence exists for both decreased bone formation [26, 37–39] and increased bone resorption [11, 35, 40]. The presence of cirrhosis seems to play an important role through several mechanisms. Testosterone, 25-hydroxy-vitamin D, and insulin-like growth factor 1 (IGF-1) levels are all reduced in advanced liver disease and correlate inversely with the degree of osteopenia [17, 23]. As well, bone mass starts to increase within six months to a year after liver transplantation [10]. Other factors may also affect bone metabolism independently of cirrhosis: bone formation is directly suppressed by alcohol [13, 41], and possibly by iron in hemochromatosis. The majority of patients with advanced PBC are also postmenopausal females, which adds to the list of pathogenic factors of hepatic osteodystrophy [23]. Malnutrition, treatment with corticosteroids [14, 42] or immunosuppressive agents plays a role in some cases.

Treatment

Osteomalacia

Osteomalacia secondary to vitamin D deficiency is characterized by low serum 25-hydroxy-vitamin D (25(OH) D < 25 nmol/L), low or normal calcium, low phosphate and elevated alkaline phosphatase and usually increased serum parathyroid hormone levels. Based on measurement of 25(OH) D level and bone histomorphometry, osteomalacia can be successfully treated and prevented with combined calcium and vitamin D supplementation (oral or parenteral) [43, 44]. **B4** Vitamin D does not need to be given as its 25-hydroxy metabolite, since the capacity of the liver to hydroxylate vitamin D is maintained, even in advanced liver disease. However, since its absorption and/or hepatic uptake may be decreased, sufficient doses should be administered [32]. Successful treatment of osteomalacia has been achieved with calcium and either oral vitamin D_2 2000–4000 IU daily, intramuscular vitamin D_2 150,000 IU weekly [43], or oral 25-hydroxy-D_3 1000–4000 IU daily [44], for a duration of 3–6 months. **B4**

Osteoporosis

The evidence for interventions for the treatment of osteoporosis in chronic liver disease is summarized in Tables 16.1 and 16.2. There are a number of observational trials and randomized controlled trials (RCTs), most of which have relatively small numbers of patients.

Vitamin D and calcium Therapy with vitamin D has been studied in osteoporotic patients with either cholestatic [40, 51] or non-cholestatic liver disease [12] and low 25(OH) D levels. Uncontrolled studies in PBC (Table 16.1) suggest that normalization of 25(OH) D levels failed to arrest bone loss [40] or to prevent spontaneous fractures. **B4** In one of these two reports, improvements in bone mass occurred only in patients whose calcium absorption increased as a result of therapy [51]. However, in an RCT of 18 abstinent patients with alcoholic liver disease, Mobarhan *et al.* showed that normalization of 25(OH) D levels was associated with a significant increase in BMD after a mean duration of 10 months (Table 16.2) [12]. **A1d** Unfortunately, a bone biopsy to rule out osteomalacia was done in only 9 of 18 patients.

Shiomi *et al.* studied the efficacy of 1,25-dihydroxy-vitamin D_3 (0.5 micrograms) on lumbar spine BMD in 76 individuals with cirrhosis secondary to hepatitis B or C infection. The results suggested that calcitriol may be effective for increasing bone mass at the lumbar spine over a 12-month period [52]. **B4**

Calcium supplementation appeared to prevent or diminish bone loss compared with untreated controls [53].

Antiresorptive and anabolic agents A retrospective study of 107 females with PBC suggested that hormone replacement therapy (HRT) is associated with a significant reduction of annual bone loss (Table 16.1) [50]. **B4** A small RCT of HRT compared to vitamin D supplements showed statistically significant improvement in BMD of LS and FN with HRT [55], and a small prospective non-randomized study showed a significant 2.25% improvement in LS BMD with one year of HRT compare with vitamin D alone (0.87%) [46]. Another small prospective study showed a non-significant trend towards less FN bone loss and fewer fractures with HRT [54].

In another non-randomized study, four years of clodronate and calcium/vitamin D3 supplements did not significantly improve osteoporosis or osteopenia in menopausal PBC patients but reduced "natural bone loss" [45].

Table 16.2 summarizes the results of randomized trials of a variety of other interventions. Guanabens *et al.*, in a two-year RCT of 32 women with PBC, compared cyclical etidronate at a dose of 400 mg for two weeks every 78 days, to sodium fluoride (NaF) 50 mg per day [59]. In the fluoride-treated group, the bone density of the lumbar spine decreased by 1.94% and the femoral neck decreased by 1.4%. By contrast, etidronate increased bone mass in the lumbar spine by 0.53% and femoral neck BMD was stable and was better tolerated. **A1d**

Table 16.1 Case series of interventions for hepatic osteodystrophy.

Study	Disease (no. of patients)	Therapy (duration)	Measurement (site)	Comments
Floreani et al. (2007) [45]	PBC (100)	oral calcium carbonate (1000 mg/day) + vit D3 (880 IU/day) + i.m. disodium clodronate 100 mg every 10 days) (four years)	DXA LS (L2-L4).	Clodronate + calcium/vitamin D3 supplements did not significantly improve osteoporosis or osteopenia, but reduced "natural bone loss"
Pereira et al. (2004) [46]	PBC (42)	Transdermal HRT vs oral vitamin D supplement (one year)	DXA LS	2.25% increase in BMD with HRT vs 0.87% with vitamin D
Floreani et al. (1997) [47]	PBC (34)	1,25(OH)2-D$_3$ 1 micrograms/day × 5d, calcitonin 40 U IM 3/week x four weeks every three months CaCO$_3$ 1–5 g/day × four weeks (three years)	DPA (LS)	Reduced bone loss in treated (uncontrolled)
Riemens et al. (1996) [48]	OLT (53)	1-OHD 1 microgram/day; Ca 1 g/day; etidronate 400 mg/day 2/15 week (one year)	DPA (LS)	No reduction in bone loss compared with historical controls
Neuhaus et al. (1995) [49]	OLT (150)	25-OH-D$_3$ 0.25–0.5 micrograms/day ± Ca 1 g/day ± NaF 25 mg/day (two years)	DXA (LS/FN)	Reduced bone loss in any of the treatment groups compared with untreated controls
Crippin et al. (1994) [50]	PBC (107)	Estrogen (low dose oral or patch) (one year)	DPA (LS)	Reduction in bone loss in estrogen group
Matloff et al. (1982) [51]	PBC (10)	25-OH-D$_3$ 40–120 micrograms/day (one year)	PBA (radius)	Normalization of 25-OH-D levels but ongoing bone loss and fractures
Herlong et al. (1982) [40]	PBC (15)	25-OH-D$_3$ 50–100 micrograms/day (one year)	PBA (radius)	Normalization of 25-OH-D levels but ongoing bone loss
Wagonfeld et al. (1976) [33]	PBC (8)	PO or SC D vs 25-OH-D$_3$ 100–200 micrograms/day (three months)	X-ray and PBA (hand)	Failure of oral or parenteral vitamin D to normalize 25-OH-D or to prevent accelerated bone loss

PBC: primary biliary cirrhosis; OLT: orthotopic liver transplantation; CAH: chronic active hepatitis; ALD: alcoholic liver disease; HA: hydroxyapatite; NaF: sodium fluoride; UDCA: ursodeoxycholic acid; DPA: dual photon absorptiometry; DXA: dual X-ray absorptiometry; PBA: photon beam absorptiometry; SPA: single photon absorptiometry; LS: lumbar spine; FN: femoral neck; 25-OH-D$_3$: 25-hydroxy-vitamin D$_3$; PO: per os; SC: subcutaneous; IM: intramuscular.

Wolfhagen et al. compared etidronate plus calcium with calcium alone in a randomized trial in 12 women with PBC on corticosteroids [61]. There was a statistically significant difference in the percentage change in mean lumbar BMD between the etidronate and calcium-treated groups (etidronate + 0.4%, calcium –3.0%, p = 0.01) [61]. **Ald** In a randomized trial that was not blinded, Shiomi et al. evaluated etidronate in 45 women with cirrhosis due to underlying viral hepatitis and also found a statistically significant difference in the percentage change in lumbar spine BMD [57]. Guanabens et al. compared alendronate with etidronate in an RCT of 36 women with PBC [56]. After two years, both treatments increased bone density but the increase was significantly greater in women on alendronate. **Ald**

Camisasca et al. [60] evaluated the effect of a six-month course of calcitonin 40 IU every other day, given subcutaneously in a trial with a crossover design. The control group received 1 IU of porcine calcitonin (no metabolic effect).

Both groups received calcium and 100,000 IU of parenteral vitamin D$_2$ (n = 25). Treatments were administered for six months with a three-month washout. There was no difference in bone density between the two treatment groups in either of the crossover periods. It is possible that this study was inadequately powered to detect a statistically significant difference. **Ald**

In another trial of 22 women with PBC followed for two years, Guanabens et al. [62] compared NaF to calcium in a two-year RCT. In the NaF group, the bone density of the lumbar spine increased by 2.9% compared with the control group in which it decreased by 6.6%. However, there was a high frequency of adverse effects, mainly gastrointestinal. Since NaF therapy was also less effective than etidronate in another study, this intervention is not recommended.

In summary, both cholestatic and non-cholestatic types of liver disease may be complicated by metabolic bone

Table 16.2 Randomized trials of interventions for hepatic osteodystrophy.

Study	Disease (no. of patients)	Intervention (duration)	Measurement (site)	Comments
Boone *et al.* (2006) [54]	PBC (31)	Two years' estrogen/progestin	DXA, FN	High treatment drop-out rate Less bone loss with treatment, and no fractures vs two with placebo (NS)
Ormarsdottir *et al.* (2004) [55]	PBC (18)	Two years' transdermal oestradiol + medroxyprogesterone vs vitimin D	DXA, LS, FN	BMD increased with HRT at LS, and FN (p < 0.05)
Guanabens *et al.* (2003) [56]	PBC (36)	Two-year cyclical etidronate vs alendronate	DXA, LS, FN	Both treatments increased BMD, but increases with alendronate were significantly larger
Shiomi *et al.* (2002) [57]	Viral hepatitis (50)	Two years' cyclical etidronate	DXA LS	Significant reduction in bone loss in etidronate treated group
Lindor *et al.* (2000) [58]	PBC (67)	One year cyclical etidronate	DXA LS, FN	No significant difference from placebo
Shiomi *et al.* (1999) [52]	Cirrhosis, PBC and secondary to hepatitis B and C (76)	0.5 micrograms calcitriol twice daily 15 months	DXA (LS)	Significant reduction in bone loss in calcitriol group
Guanabens *et al.* (1997) [59]	PBC (32)	Etidronate 400 mg/day 2/15 week vs NaF 50 mg/day (two years)	DPA (LS)	Significant reduction in bone loss in etidronate group
Camisasca *et al.* (1994) [60]	PBC (25)	Carbicalcitonin 40 U SC every day vs porcine calcitonin IU SC 2/week (15 months)	DPA (LS)	No difference between groups
Wolfhagen *et al.* (1997) [61]	PBC (12)	Etidronate 400 mg/day × two weeks + Ca 500 mg/day, 11/13 week vs Ca 500 mg/day (one year)	DXA (LS/FN)	Significant reduction in LS bone loss in etidronate group
Guanabens *et al.* (1992) [62]	PBC (22)	NaF 50 mg/day vs placebo (two years)	DPA (LS)	Significant reduction in bone loss in NaF group
Lindor *et al.* (1995) [63]	PBC (88)	UDCA 13–15 mg/kg/day (three years)	DPA (LS)	No difference between groups
Stellon *et al.* (1985) [64]	CAH (36)	HA 8 g/day (two years) X-ray/SPA	Reduced bone loss in HA group	
Mobarhan *et al.* (1984) [12]	ALD (18)	D2 50 000 U 2–3×/wk *v* 25-OHD 20–50 micrograms/day vs control (one year)	DPA (LS)	Significant increase in BMD compared to baseline in all groups a crossover design

PBC: primary biliary cirrhosis; OLT: orthotopic liver transplantation; CAH: chronic active hepatitis; ALD: alcoholic liver disease; HA: hydroxyapatite; NaF: sodium fluoride; UDCA: ursodeoxycholic acid; DPA: dual photon absorptiometry; DXA: dual X-ray absorptiometry; PBA: photon beam absorptiometry; SPA: single photon absorptiometry; LS: lumbar spine; FN: femoral neck; 25-OH-D_3: 25-hydroxy-vitamin D_3; PO: per os; SC: subcutaneous; IM: intramuscular.

disease, predominately osteoporosis. The prevalence of bone disease increases with the degree of cirrhosis. Accelerated bone loss is most severe after liver transplantation. Patients with advanced liver disease, awaiting transplantation, on prolonged corticosteroid therapy or with a history of fragility fractures, should be investigated with BMD testing. **C5** Low 25-(OH) D_3 levels should be cor-rected and calcium supplementation given. Bisphosphonates should be considered in patients with known osteoporosis or vertebral fractures, based on the evidence from a number of small randomized trials. **A1a** Testosterone therapy should be considered in males with hypogonadism. **C5**

There is a need for population-based studies of fracture risk in patients with chronic liver disease.

Inflammatory bowel disease

Prevalence

The importance of metabolic bone disease in patients with IBD has been recognized for some time. However, the point prevalence of bone disease in this population varies greatly from one study to another, with estimates as low as 5% to as high as 78%. This variation reflects a number of factors, including the definition of osteoporosis used, the site of bone density measurement and the heterogeneous nature of the IBD population. Furthermore, morphometric vertebral deformities also appear to be relatively common and are seen in 25% of both Crohn's disease, and ulcerative colitis patients [65]. A list of potential factors that need to be considered when evaluating studies in this area is provided in Table 16.3.

In a well-conducted study, Abitbol et al. [66] evaluated the BMD of 84 consecutive patients with IBD (34 Crohn's disease, 50 ulcerative colitis, excluding proctitis). Overall, 43% had osteopenia in the lumbar spine. Steroid users were at significantly greater risk of osteopenia (58% vs 28% in non-users, p = 0.03). Six patients with a mean age of 50 had vertebral crush fractures (mean Z-score was −1.63). Five patients were found to have low 25(OH) D_3 levels; however, the cause of this deficiency was felt to be extra-intestinal in all but one case. Multiple regression analysis of the lumbar spine Z-score revealed a significant correlation between osteopenia and age, cumulative corticosteroid dose, inflammatory status as assessed by the erythrocyte sedimentation rate (ESR), and low osteocalcin levels (r^2 = 0.76, p < 0.05).

The rate of bone loss in IBD has been studied in several longitudinal studies [67–73]. In the majority of the studies the annual rate of bone loss appears to be greater in the spine than at the radius, and varies from 2% to 6%. Schulte et al. studied the rate of BMD change in 80 IBD patients and found that the annual rate of bone loss was small (0.8%/year for spine) [71]. Corticosteroid use [67] and low body mass index [68] were found, in some studies, to affect bone mass negatively. Overall, metabolic bone disease is an important problem among patients with IBD, with an estimated prevalence in the range of 45%.

Malabsorption of calcium and vitamin D because of small bowel disease appears to play a minor role in the pathogenesis of metabolic bone disease in IBD. Both low and normal 25(OH) D levels have been documented in patients with Crohn's disease and there is no clear correlation between vitamin D levels and bone mass [74, 75]. Osteomalacia appears to be much less common than osteoporosis in IBD. Hessov et al. did a bone biopsy and serum 25(OH) D determinations on 36 randomly selected Crohn's disease patients with previous surgical resections (mean length 105 cm). Only two patients were found to have below normal 25-hydroxy-vitamin D_3 levels and/or histomorphometric evidence of osteomalacia. However, the mean trabecular bone volume was reduced in this group compared with controls, suggestive of osteoporosis. This finding did not correlate with any of the measured clinical characteristics, including length of resection and serum 25(OH) D level [76]. Another bone histomorphometry study in IBD revealed decreased bone formation without evidence of osteomalacia [77].

Comparisons between Crohn's disease and ulcerative colitis patients suggest that osteoporosis may be more prevalent in the former [78–80]. However, careful review of these publications suggests that the analysis may not have been fully controlled for the effects of disease activity and/or steroid use. Jahnsen et al. in an age and sex-matched cross-sectional study of 60 Crohn's disease patients, 60 ulcerative colitis patients and 60 controls, found no differences in BMD between the patients with ulcerative colitis and the controls [79]. However, Crohn's disease patients had significantly lower BMD. Overall 16% of ulcerative colitis patients and controls had Z-scores <−1 compared with 23% of Crohn's disease patients [79]. However, significantly more Crohn's disease than ulcerative colitis patients used corticosteroids (72% vs 47%), and smoked (57% vs 28%). Although disease activity was not specifically addressed in this study, 53% of the ulcerative colitis group had left-sided disease, with 40% having proctosigmoiditis or less. As well, the BMD of Crohn's disease patients who were not using steroids was not significantly different from that of the other two groups. Ghosh et al. [78] evaluated 30 IBD patients at the time of diagnosis and found that those with Crohn's disease had significantly lower bone density than those with ulcerative colitis. The mean lumbar spine Z-score for Crohn's disease patients

Table 16.3 Factors influencing interpretation of studies of bone disease in gastrointestinal patients.

Definition of osteopenia	Z-scores of ≤ 1 (? T-scores of −1 to −2.5)
Diagnostic method	X-ray, SPA, DPA, QCT, DXA, US
Results expressed (outcome)	BMD, BMC, radiological or clinical fracture (vertebral or non-vertebral)
Bone site studied	Spine, forearm, femoral neck or total hip
High risk patients	Included or excluded
Control of confounders	Smoking, steroid use, BMI

SPA: single photon absorptiometry; QCT: quantitative computed tomography; DPA: dual photon absorptiometry; DXA: dual energy X- ray absorptiometry; BMD: bone mineral density; BMC: bone mineral content.

was −1.06 versus −0.03 for those with ulcerative colitis. However, 7 of 15 ulcerative colitis patients had proctitis alone, and one had a "distal colitis". As well, the mean duration of disease before diagnosis (18.6 vs 12 weeks), and of steroid use (1.2 vs 0.5 weeks) before BMD, measurements are slightly longer in the Crohn's group, again suggesting that disease severity rather than diagnosis may be the important factor. Bernstein *et al.* in a study of 26 Crohn's disease and 23 ulcerative colitis patients, also found a greater prevalence of osteopenia among the former [80]. However, using stepwise discriminant analysis, the authors found that steroid use rather than disease type was the most important predictive factor of osteopenia.

A cross-sectional study of 51 Crohn's disease, 40 ulcerative colitis patients and 30 age and sex-matched controls by Ardizzone *et al.* found no significant difference in mean T-score values between patients with Crohn's or ulcerative colitis but did find that 37% of Crohn's and 18% of ulcerative colitis patients were osteoporotic based on WHO criteria [81]. Stepwise regression showed that in Crohn's disease, the femoral neck T-score was inversely related to disease duration and lumbar spine T-score was inversely related to age. Reffitt *et al.* also found that BMD improved with increasing duration of remission and found a benefit with azathioprine induced remission [82]. There were baseline differences in disease duration between the two groups. Schulte studied the rate of BMD change in 80 patients with IBD. The results indicated that the average annual rate of bone loss was small. There was a large range in BMD results in these patients, suggesting that certain subgroups may lose bone more quickly than others.

The study of metabolic bone disease in ulcerative colitis before and after restorative proctocolectomy also suggests that disease activity plays an important role, since BMD increases significantly with time after colectomy, with a mean annual increase of around 2% [83].

Fracture prevalence estimates in IBD from cross-sectional and prospective studies have been variable, with larger series reporting vertebral fractures in 7–22% [84] and nonvertebral fractures in 27% of patients, although these data may have been affected by referral bias. There have been three population-based studies of fracture risk in IBD. Bernstein *et al.* identified 6027 IBD patients through an administrative database in a Canadian population and matched them to 60,270 controls by age, sex and geographic residence [85]. The overall fracture rate was higher compared with controls with a 41% overall increased incidence of hip, spine, wrist and rib fractures among IBD patients (RR 1.41, 95% CI: 1.27–1.56). The incidence rate ratio was 1.59 (95% CI: 1.27–2.00) for hip fractures. There were no difference in fracture rates between males and females or between Crohn's and ulcerative colitis patients, except that males with ulcerative colitis had a higher fracture rate than females. Although the fracture risk of IBD patients was higher than controls, the increase was one patient per 100 patient years. Another North American study in Olmsted County, Minnesota assessed fracture risk in 238 Crohn's disease patients through a review of radiology reports and found that compared with age and sex-matched controls the overall risk ratio for any fracture was 0.9 (95% CI: 0.6–1.4), which was not statistically significant. The risk ratio for vertebral fracture was 2.2 (95% CI: 0.9–5.5), and the relative risk for an osteoporotic fracture was 1.4 (95% CI: 0.7–2.7), all statistically non-significant [86]. Age was the only significant predictor of fracture risk in a multivariate analysis and fracture risk was not increased in comparison with the general population except in the elderly patients. The findings were similar for the ulcerative colitis patients. Vestergaard and Mosekilde in a population-based study from hospital discharge data did not find an increase in fracture risk except for a small increase risk of fracture that required hospitalization in Crohn's disease patients [87]. The difference from fracture rates seen in ulcerative colitis patients was not statistically significant. A potential weakness of this study was the use of administrative databases which could result in the underreporting of fractures that do not require hospitalization. In addition, the diagnosis of Crohn's disease and ulcerative colitis was only validated in a small sample of patients.

A recent nested case-control study of 231,778 fracture cases from the UK General Practice Research Database demonstrated an increased risk of vertebral (OR 1.72; 95% CI: 1.13–2.61) and hip fracture (OR 1–59; 95% CI: 1.14–2.23) in patients with IBD. There was a greater risk of hip fracture seen in Crohn's disease patients compared with ulcerative colitis patients. This study also noted that only 13% of IBD patients who had already sustained a fracture were on osteoporosis treatment [88]. Corticosteroid use was associated with an increased risk of fracture and this association persisted after adjustment for disease severity (OR 1.10; 95% CI: 1.00–1.20). Limitations of this study included the method used to ascertain fractures and the fact that only clinically diagnosed fractures were included.

The literature suggests that there is a discrepancy between BMD findings and fracture risk in the IBD population and that the greatest risk is in elderly patients with IBD.

Treatment

Clements *et al.* in an uncontrolled two-year prospective study of HRT in 47 postmenopausal women with IBD (25 ulcerative colitis, 22 Crohn's disease), found that radial and spine BMD rose significantly over baseline with HRT [89]. **B4** The authors found no differences in the responses between patients with ulcerative colitis and Crohn's disease. Patients using corticosteroids also seemed to respond.

Vogelsang *et al.* randomized 75 Crohn's disease patients, without short bowel syndrome to either 1000 IU vitamin D_3 + calcium or placebo. The BMD of the forearm decreased in 80% of the control group compared to 50% of the treatment group at one year. BMD decreased less in calcium/vitamin D-treated patients (median decrease in BMD: treated 0.2%, interquartile range 3.8–(+14)%; control 7%, range 12.6–(+14)%; p < 0.005). **Ald** The correlation between the change in vitamin D and change in BMC was low (r = 0.19) [90]. Bernstein *et al.* [91] in a pilot study of 17 IBD patients with a history of steroid use (14 men, 10 Crohn's disease), assessed the efficacy of calcium supplementation (1000 mg/day) and vitamin D 250 IU on BMD by DXA. The authors found that the dose of prednisone in the year prior to the study inversely correlated with bone density at the hip, but not at the lumbar spine. There was no effect on bone density demonstrated after one year. **Ald** However, there is a significant risk of a type 2 error in this small study.

Robinson *et al.* [92] assessed the effect of low impact exercise in a randomized controlled trial. Although no statistically significant increase in BMD was observed in the exercise group, secondary analysis revealed that the number of exercise sessions correlated significantly with increased BMD at the hip and spine. **Ald**

Haderslev *et al.* assessed the impact of alendronate in Crohn's disease patients with osteopenia in a 12-month RCT. Alendronate increased the BMD of the lumbar spine by 5.5% compared with control over a one-year period. Fractures were not evaluated [93]. Bartram *et al.* similarly evaluated IV pamidronate + calcium/vitamin D compared to calcium/vitamin D alone in an RCT and found that while both groups showed improvement in BMD of the LS and hip, the improvement with pamidronate was statistically significantly higher (2.6% vs 1.6% at the LS) [94]. Another bisphoshonate, risedronate also appears to be effective at improving BMD at the hip and LS [95]. However, in another study of 154 Crohn's disease patients, Siffledeen *et al.* found that the addition of etidronate to calcium/vitamin D did not further improve BMD over that seen with calcium and vitamin D alone [96]. **Ald**

von Tirpitz *et al.* studied the effectiveness of NaF (75 mg SR) on 33 subjects with Crohn's disease in a 12-month RCT. The results indicated that NaF is effective at increasing mean spine Z-score (p = 0.02). In contrast, the control arm of calcium 1000 mg/day and vitamin D 1000 IU/day did not result in increases in spine BMD [97]. **Ald**

Biological therapies are now becoming commonplace for the treatment and maintenance of patients with IBD. The use of anti-TNF therapies appears to improve bone mineral density in IBD patients [98–101]. This effect may stem from several properties of these agents, such as: improvement in disease activity per se, reduction in inflammatory mediators, reduction in corticosteroid use, or a direct bone antire-sorptive effect. To study the relative effect of these factors, Pazianas *et al.* conducted a retrospective cohort study and found a greater improvement in BMD in IBD patients taking infliximab with a bisphosphonate compared to a bisphosphonate alone. This effect was inhibited by corticosteroid use. The authors did not find an independent effect of infliximab alone, suggesting that a primary effect on bone is likely not the main mode of action of this agent [102].

In summary, osteopenia is an important problem among patients with IBD, even at initial diagnosis. The risk appears to be greatest among those with the greatest disease activity and duration, and those treated with corticosteroids. It is difficult to distinguish the impact on bone density of corticosteroid use from that of disease activity, since these factors are linked. The risk of osteoporosis and facture in ulcerative colitis is similar to that seen in Crohn's disease and after proctocolectomy the bone density of ulcerative colitis patients increases. The risk for osteoporosis and fractures appears to be similar in males and females. Crohn's and ulcerative colitis patients seem to have comparable risks for fracture; although the overall rate for fracture is increased, the rate is affected by age.

There is evidence that IBD patients with low BMD benefit from a combination of vitamin D and calcium. HRT may be a less attractive option based on results from the Women's Health Initiative study and concerns about an unfavorable risk profile, including an increased risk of breast cancer. Existing studies have used surrogate outcome measures, such as BMD, and management has been frequently been based on results from postmenopausal osteoporosis treatment trials. Further studies are needed to assess the impact of bisphosphonates on the clinically important outcome of fracture in the IBD population. Current recommendations are that for individuals with T-scores < –2.5 or vertebral compression fractures, therapy should include calcium and vitamin D, in addition to bisphosphonates. **Ald** For those with T-scores between –2.5 and –1.0, therapy should include calcium, vitamin D and bisphosphonate therapy for patients on prolonged corticosteroid therapy. In patients with active Crohn's disease parenteral administration of a bisphosphonate such as pamidronate or zoledronic acid may be indicated. **C**

Celiac disease

Prevalence

Osteoporosis

Prevalence rates of osteoporosis in celiac disease vary depending on the population studied (adults vs children) and whether the disease has been treated. Lower BMD values have been noted in untreated populations, including those individuals who are asymptomatic at presentation. A number of cross-sectional studies have evaluated the prevalence of osteoporosis in (1) newly diagnosed celiac patients and (2) individuals treated with a gluten-free diet [103–110]. In general, studies in untreated celiac disease demonstrate diminished bone density. When compared with age-matched controls (Z-score of <–2 at the spine), the prevalence of osteopenia in untreated patients varied among studies from 15–40% [105, 108]. Serum PTH levels have been shown to correlate inversely with BMD [105, 109] and levels of 25(OH) D correlate positively with BMD in untreated celiac disease patients [109].

Fractures

Vasquez *et al.* estimated the incidence of fractures from a case-control study (ascertained fractures by interview) and found that 25% of patients had a history of previous fractures, compared with 8% of age and sex-matched controls (odds ratio (OR) 3.5; 95% CI: 1.8–7.2), with the majority of fractures occurring prior to diagnosis or in those individuals who were non-compliant [110]. The most common fracture was a wrist fracture and there was a trend to increased vertebral fractures. Vasquez studied patients from a malabsorption clinic and therefore this rate may not be representative of the general celiac population. Neither BMD or body mass index correlated with the presence of fractures, suggesting that there are other factors beside BMD, such as disease duration, that account for increased fracture risk.

Vestergaard and Mosekilde (2002) in Denmark in a retrospective cohort study examined hospital discharge abstracts for patients previously hospitalized with a diagnosis of celiac disease and did not detect a significant difference in fracture rates compared with controls [87]. Age was the only significant risk factor for fracture. There are potential sources of bias in using hospital-based discharge data including the fact that outpatient fracture diagnoses are not included. Thomason *et al.* (2003) in a case-control study in which fractures were ascertained using a questionnaire did not find an increased fracture risk in celiac disease patients compared with controls [111], and other small longitudinal studies have yielded similar findings [106, 112].

A recent systematic review and meta-analysis identified 60 potential studies of which eight met the inclusion criteria for the meta-analysis (e.g. outcome of fractures and controlled studies). The pooled prevalence of fractures in celiac disease patients was 8.7% (1819/20,955) compared to 6.1% (5955/96,777) for controls for a pooled odds ratio = 1.43; 95% CI: 1.15–1.78) although significant heterogeneity was observed (I^2 = 85.1%), as evidenced by poor overlapping of confidence intervals for individual studies [113]. Six of the eight studies showed a significant association between fractures and celiac disease.

The largest included study in the meta-analysis was a retrospective population based cohort study by Ludvigsson

et al. (2007) that used the Swedish National Registers to estimate the risk of hip and any fracture. They found that individuals with celiac disease were at increased risk of hip fracture (HR 2.1; 95% CI: 1.8–2.4) and for any type of fracture (HR 1.4; 95% CI: 1.3–1.5) [114]. Limitations include the inability to control for all potential confounding variables such as body mass index, smoking and the use of bisphosphonates or hormone replacement therapy. West *et al.* (2003) in another large retrospective cohort study in the UK also found a significant increase in fractures in celiac disease patients [115].

Further clarification of the risk of fracture in celiac disease with a large prospective cohort study with rigorous ascertainment of fractures would be helpful.

Pathogenesis

Reduced calcium absorption can result in hypersecretion of PTH, enhanced 1,25-dihydroxy vitamin D and decreased 25 hydroxy-vitamin D [116]. In addition, systemic inflammatory effects may result in bone loss via action of interleukin (IL)-1 and IL-6, the levels of which have been shown to correlate with BMD [117]. It is also thought that zinc deficiency may lead to reduced IGF-1 levels which in turn results in impaired bone metabolism and reduced bone mass [118]. It is not clear what proportion of individuals with celiac disease have osteomalacia, due to the lack of bone biopsy data, but many individuals are vitamin D deficient.

Treatment

Longitudinal studies of patients with celiac disease have demonstrated increases in BMD after starting on a gluten-free diet and the majority of the change occurs within the first year, particularly at the lumbar spine [119]. **B4** The average increase in lumbar spine BMD is approximately 5% within the initial year. A number of observational studies have shown that children will often normalize their BMD after a gluten-free diet [119–122]. **B4** Adults, however, may continue to have BMDs below average (Z-score of –1 at the spine) [106, 123]. Premenopausal females have shown a greater increase in BMD than postmenopausal females.

Valdimarsson *et al.* found that patients with secondary hyperparathyroidism at baseline did not increase their BMD to normal by three years in comparison to those who had a normal baseline PTH, and did achieve a normal BMD [105].

The goal of treatment should be to maintain normal serum 25(OH) D levels, with vitamin D supplements and higher doses may be required initially. Bone density scans should be recommended in newly diagnosed adult celiac patients after one year on a gluten-free diet. Initial evaluation should also include serum calcium, 25(OH)D and PTH levels. Additional osteoporosis therapies may be considered depending on the severity of bone loss.

Glucocorticoid-induced bone loss

Glucocorticoids are widely used in the treatment of inflammatory bowel disease, and are an important independent risk factor for bone loss. Observational studies have demonstrated an association between cumulative corticosteroid dose and increased bone loss, in multiple populations, but some prospective studies have failed to support this relationship, perhaps because of a beneficial effect of corticosteroids on disease activity [124].

Data from cross-sectional studies of patients on corticosteroids estimate that the incidence of fractures varies from 30% to 50% [84, 125]. In a study by Adinoff and Hollister, 11% of asthma patients on oral steroids for one year developed vertebral fractures [126]. In a case-control study, Cooper et al. (Van Staa et al. [127]) found that use of oral steroids resulted in an RR of 1.16 (CI: 1.47–1.76) for hip fracture and 2.6 (CI: 2.31–2.92) for vertebral fracture. A nested case-control study from the Study for Osteoporotic Fractures Cohort confirmed an increase incidence of hip fractures in patients on corticosteroids with an adjusted relative risk of hip fracture of 2.1 (95% CI: 1.0– 4.4) [128]. A meta-analysis of seven prospective cohort studies, found that previous GC use was associated with an RR of 2.63 of sustaining an osteoporotic fracture and 4.42 for hip fracture after adjusting for BMD [129]. The risk of fracture is increased at higher doses of corticosteroids.

There is evidence that the relationship between bone density may underestimate the risk of fracture in patients on corticosteroids, highlighting the importance of bone quality [130, 131]. Glucocorticoid-induced bone loss is greatest in the initial 6–12 months of treatment [132–134], and involves areas of the skeleton which have the greatest turnover, in particular, the lumbar spine, cortical rim of the vertebral body, ribs and proximal femur. Hahn et al. demonstrated that trabecular bone loss is greater than cortical bone loss in rheumatoid arthritis patients on prednisone [135]. Fracture risk increases within the first 3–6 months of glucocorticoid treatment [131].

Pathogenesis

The mechanism of corticosteroid-induced osteoporosis (CSOP) is multifactorial [139]. CSOP differs from postmenopausal osteoporosis in that bone formation is greatly decreased at a time of increased bone resorption. This imbalance between formation and resorption results in a reduction in the total amount of bone replaced in each remodeling cycle. Corticosteroids cause a reduction in bone formation by decreasing the production of osteoblasts and increasing the apoptosis of osteoblasts and osteocytes [140]. Corticosteroids also prolong the lifespan of mature osteoclasts, resulting in bone resorption [133]. Glucocorticoids also suppress the hypothalamic-pituitary-gonadal axis that leads to a functional hypogonadism and increased bone loss [141]. Finally, steroids cause loss of muscle mass, decrease the intestinal absorption of calcium and increase renal excretion of calcium.

One explanation for the rapid bone loss seen with corticosteroids could be related to the increase bone resorption that occurs secondary to the down-regulation of osteoprotegerin (OPG), an osteoblast-derived soluble decoy receptor. OPG blocks the interaction between RANK and RANK-L (receptor activator of nuclear factor κB ligand) that inhibits osteoclast formation and also increases expression of RANK-L by osteoblasts [142]. The result is a decrease in the OPG/RANK-L ratio leading to an increase in cancellous osteoclasts and rapid bone loss [143].

Prevention and treatment

A baseline bone density measurement is recommended for patients who are to remain on steroids for a prolonged period and in patients who are at risk of other types of osteoporosis, such as postmenopausal osteoporosis. The first principle of prevention is to minimize the dose of steroids. **C5** Maintenance of muscle mass through exercise is also beneficial. Supplemental calcium 1000–1500 mg/day and vitamin D 800 IU/day should be recommended.

A number of medications have been used for the prevention and treatment of CSOP. Tables 16.4–16.6 summarize the results of those controlled trials of prevention and treatment of CSOP, which had vertebral fractures as an endpoint. These tables show results according to intention to treat analysis. Efficacy results are indicated. Unfortunately, patients with IBD have been underrepresented in these trials. WMD (weighted mean difference) is the weighted mean average of the trials and the weight given to each study is the inverse of the variance. To calculate the WMD, the mean percentage change from baseline in the treatment and control groups was multiplied by the inverse of the associated variance.

Recent guidelines have been developed by consensus groups for the primary and secondary prevention of glucocorticoid-induced osteoporosis, based on evidence from recent clinical trials [130]. This group recommends that patients be considered for therapeutic intervention if the BMD T-score is below –1.5. Follow-up bone densitometry is recommended after one year and then every 1–3 years depending on the result.

Calcium and vitamin D

Calcium and vitamin D have been used to prevent losses that occur from decreased calcium absorption, increased renal excretion of calcium.

Table 16.4 Randomized trials of calcium/vitamin D for prevention and treatment of steroid-induced osteoporosis and fractures[a].

Study	Disease (no. of patients)	Placebo (M:F)	Treatment (M:F)	Intervention (duration)	Control	Lumbar BMD (% change)	Vertebral fractures RR (95% CI)
Sambrook et al. (1993) [136]	PMR/RA (63)	29 (7:22)	34 (7:27)	Calcitriol 0.5–1.0 micrograms (two years)	Calcium 1000 mg	−1.3	Efficacy: 0.43 (0.04 to 4.47)
Adachi et al. (1996) [137]	PMR/TA (62)	31	31	50,000 U vitamin D (three years)	Placebo	−0.7	ITT: 0.56 (0.24 to 1.32)
Dyckman et al. (1984) [138]	Rheumatic disease (23)	10 (1:9)	13 (3:10)	Calcium + 1,25 vitamin D (18 months)	Placebo + 500 mg calcium		Efficacy: 0.58 (0.17 to 2.01)

[a] Only studies in which vertebral fractures were included as an outcome measure have been listed.
ITT: intention to treat analysis; PMR: polymyalgia rheumatica; RA: rheumatoid arthritis; TA: temporal arteritis; RR: relative risk.

Table 16.5 Randomized trials of calcitonin for prevention and treatment of steroid-induced osteoporosis and fractures[a].

Study	Disease (no. of patients)	Placebo (M:F)	Treatment (M:F)	Dose (duration)	Control	Lumbar BMD (% change)	Vertebral fractures RR (95% CI)
Healey et al. (1996) [144]	PMR/TA (48)	23 (3:20)	25 (9:16)	100 IU 3/week SC (one year)	Calcium/vitamin D	−1.5	Efficacy: 0.74 (0.14 to 3.95)
Kotaniemi et al. (1996) [145]	RA/all women (63)	31	32	100 IU intranasal (one year)	Placebo + calcium	10.9	ITT: 0.32 (0.01 to 7.65)
Luengo et al. (1994) [146]	Asthma (44)	22 (3:19)	22 (3:19)	200 IU every 2 days intranasal (one year)	Placebo + calcium	0.6	ITT: 1.00 (0.15 to 0.48)
Sambrook et al. (1993) [136]	RA, PMR (58)	29 (7:22)	29 (6:23)	400 IU intranasal (two years)	Calcium	1.1	Efficacy: 1.00 (0.15 to 6.63)
Ringe et al. (1987) [147]	Lung disease (36)	18 (4:14)	18 (3:15)	100 IU every 2 days SC (six months)	Placebo + calcium		Efficacy: 0.14 (0.01 to 2.58)

[a] Only studies in which vertebral fractures were included as an outcome measure have been listed.
PBC: primary biliary cirrhosis; OLT: orthotopic liver transplantation; CAH: chronic active hepatitis; ALD: alcoholic liver disease; HA: hydroxyapatite; NaF: sodium fluoride; UDCA: ursodeoxycholic acid; DPA: dual photon absorptiometry; DXA: dual X-ray absorptiometry; PBA: photon beam absorptiometry; SPA: single photon absorptiometry; LS: lumbar spine; FN: femoral neck; 25-OH-D$_3$: 25-hydroxy-vitamin D$_3$; PO: per os; SC: subcutaneous; IM: intramuscular.
ITT: intention to treat analysis; PMR: polymyalgia rheumatica; RA: rheumatoid arthritis; TA: temporal arteritis; RR: relative risk.

Buckley conducted a two-year RCT with calcium (1000 mg/day) and vitamin D$_3$ (500 IU/day) in rheumatoid arthritis patients on steroids and found that the loss of BMD in the lumbar spine and trochanter was prevented [155]. **B4** Adachi et al. evaluated the efficacy of vitamin D (50,000 U per week) and 1000 mg calcium in patients on moderate to high dose corticosteroids and found that vitamin D and calcium prevented the early loss of bone but

did not seem to be beneficial in the long term [137]. A Cochrane meta-analysis found that calcium and vitamin D prevented bone loss at the lumbar spine with a pooled WMD of 2.6% (95% CI: 0.76–453) [156]. **A1a** Another meta-analysis by Amin et al. that examined all therapies concluded that vitamin D and calcium is more effective than placebo or calcium alone [157]. **A1a** Three trials using vitamin D and calcium have assessed vertebral frac-

Table 16.6 Randomized trials of bisphosphonates for prevention or treatment of steroid-induced osteoporosis and fractures[a].

Study	Disease (no. of patients)	Placebo (M:F)	Treatment (M:F)	Intervention (duration)	Control	LS BMD (% change)	Vertebral fractures RR (95% CI)
Worth et al. (1994) [148]	Asthma (33)	14 (3:11)	19 (9:10)	Etidronate 400 mg (six months)	Calcium	9.3	0.11 (0.01 to 1.94)
Adachi et al. (1997) [149]	PMR/TA (141)	74 (28:46)	67 (26:41)	Etidronate 400 mg (one year)	Placebo + calcium	3.8	0.58 (0.20 to 1.60) Men: 1.44 (0.35 to 5.81) Women: 0.15 (0.02 to 1.13)
Saag et al. (1998) [150]	RA/PMR/IBD/ asthma (477)	159 (52:107)	318 (89:229)	Alendronate 5 or 10 mg (48 weeks)	Placebo + calcium/ vitamin D	2.5	0.60 (0.19 to 1.94) Men: 1.18 (0.35 to 4.01) Women: 0.51 (0.14 to 1.83)
Boutsen et al. (1997) [151]	PMR/TA (32)	17	15	Pamidronate IV (one year)	Placebo	—	0.38 (0.02 to 8.57)
Roux et al. (1998) [152]	PMR/RA (117)	58	59	Etidronate 400 mg (one year)	Placebo + calcium	3.1	0.79 (0.22 to 2.78)
Reid et al. (2000) [153]	(290) RA, Asthma, PMR, TA	96 (36:60)	194	Risedronate 2.5; 5.0 mg	Calcium, vitamin D	2.7	0.33 (0.12 to 0.89) for 2.5 and 5 mg 5 mg dose 0.33 (0.09–1.17)
Cohen et al. (1999) [154]	RA/PMR/SLE/TA (228)	77 (25:52)	151 (52:99)	Risedronate 2.5 mg/5.0 mg	Calcium/vitamin D	4.4	Both doses 0.43 (0/16 to 1.15) 5 mg dose 0.33, (0.09 to 1.14)

[a] Only studies in which vertebral fractures were included as an outcome measure have been listed. PM: postmenopausal; IV: intravenous; PBC: primary biliary cirrhosis; OLT: orthotopic liver transplantation; CAH: chronic active hepatitis; ALD: alcoholic liver disease; HA: hydroxyapatite; NaF: sodium fluoride; UDCA: ursodeoxycholic acid; DPA: dual photon absorptiometry; DXA: dual X-ray absorptiometry; PBA: photon beam absorptiometry; SPA: single photon absorptiometry; LS: lumbar spine; FN: femoral neck; 25-OH-D_3: 25-hydroxy-vitamin D_3; PO: per os; SC: subcutaneous; IM: intramuscular.

ITT: intention to treat analysis; PMR: polymyalgia rheumatica; RA: rheumatoid arthritis; TA: temporal arteritis; RR: relative risk.

tures as an outcome (Table 16.4). Neither the individual trials nor a meta-analysis of the three trials demonstrated a statistically significant reduction in vertebral fractures (pooled relative risk 0.56; 95% CI: 0.24 to 1.32). **A1c** However, the number of patients included in these trials was small.

Antiresorptive agents

Since steroids increase bone resorption, antiresorptive agents such as bisphosphonates, calcitonin and hormone replacement have been used for the treatment and prevention of osteoporosis.

There have been six published RCTs of calcitonin (intranasal or subcutaneous) for prevention of osteoporosis in patients on corticosteroids with fracture data. These trials show a positive effect of calcitonin on lumbar spine bone

density at one year. However, no statistically significant reduction in fractures was demonstrated in the five trials in which this was analyzed (Table 16.5). Meta-analysis of these five trials did not demonstrate a significant reduction in fractures (pooled relative risk was 0.60; 95% CI: 0.24 to 1.46) [158]. **A1c**

HRT was compared to calcium supplementation in a two-year RCT in 200 patients with rheumatoid arthritis, of whom 41 were receiving corticosteroids [159]. BMD in the spine fell by 1.19% (95% CI: 2.29–0.09) in the control group, but increased in HRT-treated patients (2.22%; 95% CI: 0.72–3.72; p < 0.001). **A1a** Subgroup analysis of the steroid treated group also showed benefit of HRT treatment on spine BMD (3.75%; 95% CI: 0.72–6.78). There are no published data on fracture reduction with HRT in CSOP. Similarly, there is little evidence to support the use of testosterone in men on corticosteroids. A small RCT of 15 men with asthma on oral glucocorticoids demonstrated that monthly testosterone injections were effective in preventing bone loss [160]. **Ald**

Bisphosphonates have been used for the treatment and prevention of CSOP (Table 16.6). A Cochrane meta-analysis of 13 trials (n = 842) published in 2000 found that the weighted mean difference of percent change in lumbar spine BMD between bisphosphonates and placebo groups was 4.3% (95% CI: 2.7–5.9) at one year, using a random effects model [161]. There was significant heterogeneity between trials. In the Cochrane Review, the pooled RR from four studies that reported outcomes on vertebral fractures was 0.76 (95% CI: 0.4–1.5), a result that was not statistically significant.

Since the Cochrane Review there have been additional randomized trials with vertebral fractures as an endpoint (see Table 16.6) [150, 153, 154, 162]. The baseline characteristics (BMD, prevalent fractures) were different among these trials. The relative risk reduction for vertebral fractures in these trials ranged from 40% to 70%, although the upper limit of the 95% CI overlaps 1.0. **Ala** The individual trials did not reveal a statistically significant effect of bisphosphonates on vertebral fractures. However, if all seven prevention and treatment trials with bisphosphonates are pooled, the RR of vertebral fractures is 0.50 (95% CI: 0.30–0.80), consistent with an absolute risk reduction of 6.3%. A one-year extension study of the original alendronate trial demonstrated a significant reduction in morphometric vertebral fractures (ARR of 6.1%) [162]. There was no significant difference in non-vertebral fractures between bisphosphonates and calcium and vitamin D, although these trials were not powered to detect a difference in fractures. Kanis *et al.* in a systematic review compared the efficacy of different therapies for CSOP. A pooled analysis of risedronate, etidronate and alendronate demonstratated a significant reduction in vertebral fractures, RR 0.46 (95% CI: 0.28–0.77). For non-vertebral fractures the pooled estimate was 0.77 (9% CI: 0.39–1.51) [163].

Amin *et al.* conducted a metaregression of all therapies for CSOP, using lumbar spine BMD as the outcome and found that bisphosphonates were more effective than calcitonin, vitamin D or fluoride [164] (with an effect size of 1.03, 95%, CI: 0.85–1.17). The authors also found that the efficacy of bisphosphonates was enhanced with the concomitant use of vitamin D.

Other new agents such as strontium ranelate have proved antifracture efficacy in postmenopausal osteoporosis and may be useful for the treatment of CSOP.

Bone formation (anabolic) agents

Monosodium fluoride has been shown to increase BMD at the lumbar spine [165–167]. **Ald** However, efficacy of fluoride for vertebral fracture reduction has not been demonstrated for CSOP [165, 166]. Other anabolic agents include

injections of human PTH 1.34 (hPTH 1.34) fragment which stimulates osteoblastogenesis and inhibits osteoblast apoptosis. Lane *et al.* compared daily injections of synthetic hPTH 1-34 along with estrogens with estrogen therapy alone in 51 osteoporotic postmenopausal women receiving glucocorticoids for rheumatic diseases. These women had been taking HRT for more than one year and were randomized to receive either HRT and parathyroid hormone PTH 25 micrograms daily or HRT alone. All subjects received calcium and vitamin D. None of the patients had liver disease or IBD. The mean steroid dose was 8.0 + 3.8 mg for PTH with estrogen group and 9.5 + 4.5 for the estrogen alone group. At 12 months the mean difference in the lumbar spine was 9.8% favoring PTH and estrogen over estrogen alone. **Ald** There were no significant differences seen between treatment and control at the distal radius, femoral neck, trochanter and hip [168].

A second publication presented 24-month follow-up data after patients had discontinued medication at 12 months. The lumbar spine BMD was maintained at 24 months with a mean difference of 11.9%. The study was not powered to assess a difference in fractures [169].

The choice of corticosteroid may also influence the propensity for the development of CSOP. For example, in the subset of steroid naive patients with active ileocecal Crohn's disease, budesonide was associated with less bone loss then prednisolone. However, this effect was not seen in patients who had previously received steroids or those who were steroid dependent [170].

In a 36-month randomized trial Saag *et al.* compared daily human recombinant parathyroid hormone (1-34) or teriparatide 20 ug s/c (n = 214) to alendronate 10 mg daily (n = 214) in patients (ages 22 to 89 years) who had received glucocorticoids at a dose of 5 mg or more for at least three months (n = 428). Both groups received 1000 mg of calcium and 800 IU of vitamin D. The 18-month results were published in 2007. The majority of patients in this trial had a rheumatologic disorder with rheumatoid arthritis being the most common diagnosis. The median dose of glucocorticoids was 7.5 mg/day in the teriparatide group and 7.8 in the alendronate group. The majority of participants were taking glucocorticoids for more than one year. Mean lumbar spine BMD was −2.5 and −2.6 respectively. Loss to follow-up was a limitation of this trial, with over 40% of participants lost by 36 months. There was a significantly greater increase in lumbar spine BMD in the PTH 1-34 group compared to alendronate at 36 months (11 vs 5.3%, p < 0.001). Using the last observation carried forward the difference was 8.9 vs. 4.2%, p < 0.001. At 18 months, significantly fewer radiographic vertebral fractures occurred in the teriparatide group (1/171) compared to alendronate treated group (10/165, p = 0.004) although the incidence of non-vertebral fractures was not significantly different in both groups [171].

Proton pump inhibitors and fracture risk

Proton pump inhibitors (PPIs) are widely used in a variety of gastrointestinal disorders including peptic ulcer disease, gastroesophageal reflux disease (GERD) and non-ulcer dyspepsia. Their main mechanism of action is an irreversible inhibition of active acid secreting pumps on the luminal side of gastric parietal cells. These medications are relatively well tolerated with few side effects.

There is an emerging body of literature suggesting a possible link between chronic PPI therapy and increased fracture risk [172, 173]. *In vitro*, achlorhydria limits the dissolution of ionized calcium from its insoluble forms, a step important for its absorption in the gastrointestinal tract [174]. *In vivo* calcium malabsorption has been associated with hypochlorhydria [175]. However, there are conflicting data about the biologic plausibility of this hypothesis as the majority of calcium is absorbed in the non-acidic environment of the small bowel [175–177]. Furthermore, *in vitro*, PPIs have been shown to inhibit osteoclastic H^+-K^+-ATPase which may in fact reduce bone resorption [178].

Studies using large administrative databases from Denmark [172], the UK [173] and Canada[179] consistently found a small increase in risk of hip fracture from chronic PPI use, with adjusted odds ratios (AOR) ranging from 1.45 (95% CI: 1.28–1.65) [172] to 1.62 ((95% CI: 1.02–2.58) [179], (95% CI: 1.41–1.89)) [173]. Yang *et al.*, using the UK's General Practice Research Database [173], which included nearly 200,000 PPI users, found that the risk of hip fracture was significantly increased after as little as one year of PPI exposure (AOR 1.22; 95% CI: 1.15–1.30), increasing with duration of therapy and daily PPI dosage. The association was stronger in men than women. In a restricted analysis for chronic GERD sufferers, the risk was greatest with high dose long-term PPI therapy (AOR 3.49; 95% CI: 1.24–9.84) [173]. Targownik *et al.*, in a retrospective cohort of almost 16,000 PPI exposed subjects from Manitoba, found that the risk of hip fracture was significantly increased after at least five years of continuous PPI exposure (AOR 1.62; 95% CI: 1.02–2.59), and that the risk of any osteoporosis-related fracture increased after at least seven years of continuous PPI exposure (AOR 1.92; 95% CI: 1.16–3.18) [179]. In elderly patients, a study of the risk of admission to hospital for hip fracture within five years of onset of therapy with either warfarin, thyroid supplements, corticosteroids or PPIs, showed that corticosteroid-exposed patients had a significantly increased risk compared to those on PPIs (ARR 1.44; 95% CI: 1.21–1.70) [180]; by comparison, the warfarin and the thyroid replacement patients had adjusted risk ratios similar to those on PPIs (ARR 0.94; 95% CI: 0.81–1.09 and 1.02; 95% CI: 0.89–1.18 respectively) [180]. This suggests that if PPIs do have an adverse effect on fracture risk, this effect is small.

The risk of lowered BMD and fracture was studied in three prospective cohorts, two from the USA [181] and one from Europe [182]. After a mean follow up of 6.1 years, postmenopausal women chronically using omeprazole had a significant increase in risk of vertebral fracture (RR 3.10; 95% CI: 1.14–8.44 in the multivariate analysis); by comparison, the RR was 3.62 (95% CI: 1.63–8.08) in those with history of prior vertebral fracture and 2.38 (95% CI: 1.03–5.49) in those with lumbar spine T-score <–2.5 [182]. The Osteoporosis Fractures in Men Study (MrOS) and the Study of Osteoporotic Fractures (SOF) followed BMD and the incidence of non-vertebral fractures in 5755 men for an average of up to 5.6 years (MrOS) and 5339 women for an average of up to 7.6 years (SOF) [181]. When controlling for other risk factors for bone loss, chronic PPI use was not associated with any significant difference in change in total hip BMD, or of hip fracture risk. A small increase in the risk of non-vertebral fractures was seen in chronic female PPI users (relative hazard (RH) 1.34; 95% CI: 1.10–1.64) and among male PPI users who were not taking calcium supplements (RH 1.49; 95% CI: 1.04–2.14).

Multiple confounders can influence these observations, as chronic PPI users are more likely to harbour multiple risk factors for bone loss as well as increased fall risk. Such risk factors include: multiple co-morbidities; poor nutritional status; smoking and alcohol intake; and low BMI [183]. In addition, bone remodeling agents, corticosteroids and NSAIDs [181, 184] may cause dyspepsia, which in turn can lead to PPI use [185]. In the studies discussed above, controlling for confounding factors consistently lowered the magnitude of the risk associated with PPI use, sometimes by as much as 25% [179]. Moreover, a recent nested case-control study again using the UK's General Practice Research Database, but restricting the analysis to chronic PPI users with no other identifiable risk factor for fracture, did not find an increase risk of hip fracture with PPI use (RR 0.9; 95% CI: 07–1.1) [183].

In summary, current evidence suggests an association between chronic PPI use and osteoporosis-related fractures. There are multiple confounders of this association, which can falsely inflate the magnitude of the risk. If present, the absolute fracture risk in chronic PPI users is low, but may be clinically relevant in patients with multiple other risk factors for osteoporosis, especially if using high-dose, long-term PPIs.

Conclusion

Metabolic bone disease is an important problem in patients with liver disease and inflammatory bowel disease and the pathogenesis is multifactorial. Osteomalacia does not appear to be common in IBD and osteoporosis appears to be the major metabolic bone disorder in IBD, Crohn's disease and chronic liver disease. The use of corticosteroids in IBD and chronic liver disease is an important, but not a precisely defined contributing factor since it is difficult to distinguish corticosteroid use from disease activity. Few controlled trials have evaluated the efficacy of treatments in the absence of steroid therapy and the inflammatory cytokines that are involved in the immune response have been linked to increased bone resorption. In patients on corticosteroids, however, there is information from a number of RCTs about the efficacy of therapeutic agents in other patient populations.

Patients at particular risk for osteoporosis and fracture include: patients on glucocorticoids for IBD; those with endstage liver disease and liver transplant patients; post-menopausal women who may already be osteopenic; patients with Crohn's disease; and patients with low trauma fractures. In these individuals bone density measurement early in their treatment is recommended, although bone density does not exactly correlate with fracture risk in these populations. Minimization of steroid use and use of preventive agents such as calcium and vitamin D are indicated. In those individuals who are on corticosteroids (>3 months) (defined as daily dose ranges from 5–7.5 mg depending on guideline recommendation) or have a T-score below −2.0, although less stringent T-score cutoffs (e.g. −1.5) may be used on higher doses, or a fragility fracture, then bisphosphonates should be recommended.

While the evidence for prevention and treatment of steroid-induced osteoporosis is convincing, additional trials of interventions specifically for the bone disease associated with IBD and liver disease are needed. RCTs with fracture as the primary outcome may be difficult to conduct given the sample sizes required. Clarification of the risk of the fracture in patients with liver disease, IBD and celiac disease is required, with identification of high risk subgroups. Evidence-based guidelines of strategies to prevent osteoporosis in these populations are needed [186, 187] in addition to the development of better tools to predict the risk of fracture in individuals with IBD and celiac disease.

Additional research to clarify the association between PPI use and osteoporotic fractures is needed (e.g. prospective cohorts). Clinicians should assess the benefit-risk ratio for each patient and consider re-evaluating the need for long-term use in individuals at high risk of fracture or in patients who do not have a clear-cut indication for the use of PPIs.

References

1 Assessment of fracture risk and its application to screening for postmenopausal osteoporosis. World Health Organization Report No 843, 1994.

2 Center JR, Nguyen TV, Schneider D, Sambrook PN, Eisman JA. Mortality after all major types of osteoporotic fracture in men and women: An observational study. *Lancet* 1999; **353**(9156): 878–882.

3 Eastell R, Boyle IT, Compston J *et al.* Management of male osteoporosis: report of the UK Consensus Group. *QJM* 1998; **91**(2): 71–92.

4 Melton LJ 3rd, Atkinson EJ, O'Fallon WM, Wahner HW, Riggs BL. Long-term fracture prediction by bone mineral assessed at different skeletal sites. *J Bone Miner Res* 1993; **8**(10): 1227–1233.

5 Hui SL, Slemenda CW, Johnston CC Jr. Age and bone mass as predictors of fracture in a prospective study. *J Clin Invest* 1988; **81**(6): 1804–1809.

6 Marshall D, Johnell O, Wedel H. Meta-analysis of how well measures of bone mineral density predict occurrence of osteoporotic fractures. *BMJ* 1996; **312**(7041): 1254–1259.

7 Lunt M, Felsenberg D, Adams J *et al.* Population-based geographic variations in DXA bone density in Europe: the EVOS Study. European Vertebral Osteoporosis. *Osteoporos Int* 1997; **7**(3): 175–189.

8 Nguyen T, Sambrook P, Kelly P *et al.* Prediction of osteoporotic fractures by postural instability and bone density. *BMJ* 1993; **307**(6912): 1111–1115.

9 Compston JE. Hepatic osteodystrophy: Vitamin D metabolism in patients with liver disease. *Gut* 1986; **27**(9): 1073–1090.

10 Eastell R, Dickson ER, Hodgson SF *et al.* Rates of vertebral bone loss before and after liver transplantation in women with primary biliary cirrhosis. *Hepatology* 1991; **14**(2): 296–300.

11 Hay JE, Lindor KD, Wiesner RH, Dickson ER, Krom RA, LaRusso NF. The metabolic bone disease of primary sclerosing cholangitis. *Hepatology* 1991; **14**(2): 257–261.

12 Mobarhan SA, Russell RM, Recker RR, Posner DB, Iber FL, Miller P. Metabolic bone disease in alcoholic cirrhosis: A comparison of the effect of vitamin D2, 25-hydroxyvitamin D, or supportive treatment. *Hepatology* 1984; **4**(2): 266–273.

13 Chappard D, Plantard B, Fraisse H, Palle S, Alexandre C, Riffat G. Bone changes in alcoholic cirrhosis of the liver. A histomorphometric study. *Pathol Res Pract* 1989; **184**(5): 480–485.

14 Stellon AJ, Webb A, Compston JE. Bone histomorphometry and structure in corticosteroid treated chronic active hepatitis. *Gut* 1988; **29**(3): 378–84.

15 Angelopoulos NG, Goula AK, Papanikolaou G, Tolis G. Osteoporosis in HFE2 juvenile hemochromatosis. A case report and review of the literature. *Osteoporos Int* 2006; **17**(1): 150–155.

16 Guggenbuhl P, Deugnier Y, Boisdet JF *et al.* Bone mineral density in men with genetic hemochromatosis and HFE gene mutation. *Osteoporos Int* 2005; **16**(12): 1809–1814.

17 Chen CC, Wang SS, Jeng FS, Lee SD. Metabolic bone disease of liver cirrhosis: is it parallel to the clinical severity of cirrhosis? *J Gastroenterol Hepatol* 1996; **11**(5): 417–421.

18 Gallego-Rojo FJ, Gonzalez-Calvin JL, Munoz-Torres M, Mundi JL, Fernandez-Perez R, Rodrigo-Moreno D. Bone mineral density, serum insulin-like growth factor I, and bone turnover markers in viral cirrhosis. *Hepatology* 1998; **28**(3): 695–699.

19 Jablkowski M, Bialkowska J, Bartkowiak J *et al.* Evaluation of bone mineral density in women with chronic liver diseases

during perimenopausal period. *Pol Arch Med Wewn* 2006; **116**(4): 924–929.

20 Carey EJ, Balan V, Kremers WK, Hay JE. Osteopenia and osteoporosis in patients with end-stage liver disease caused by hepatitis C and alcoholic liver disease: Not just a cholestatic problem. *Liver Transpl* 2003; **9**(11): 1166–1173.

21 Porayko MK, Wiesner RH, Hay JE *et al.* Bone disease in liver transplant recipients: incidence, timing, and risk factors. *Transplant Proc* 1991; **23**(1 Pt 2): 1462–1465.

22 Park KM, Hay JE, Lee SG *et al.* Bone loss after orthotopic liver transplantation: FK 506 versus cyclosporine. *Transplant Proc* 1996; **28**(3): 1738–1740.

23 Diamond T, Stiel D, Lunzer M, Wilkinson M, Roche J, Posen S. Osteoporosis and skeletal fractures in chronic liver disease. *Gut* 1990; **31**(1): 82–87.

24 Mounach A, Ouzzif Z, Wariaghli G *et al.* Primary biliary cirrhosis and osteoporosis: a case-control study. *J Bone Miner Metab* 2008; **26**(4): 379–384.

25 Solaymani-Dodaran M, Card TR, Aithal GP, West J. Fracture risk in people with primary biliary cirrhosis: A population-based cohort study. *Gastroenterology* 2006; **131**(6): 1752–1757.

26 Diamond TH, Stiel D, Lunzer M, McDowall D, Eckstein RP, Posen S. Hepatic osteodystrophy. Static and dynamic bone histomorphometry and serum bone Gla-protein in 80 patients with chronic liver disease. *Gastroenterology* 1989; **96**(1): 213–221.

27 Guanabens N, Pares A, Ros I *et al.* Severity of cholestasis and advanced histological stage but not menopausal status are the major risk factors for osteoporosis in primary biliary cirrhosis. *J Hepatol* 2005; **42**(4): 573–577.

28 Benetti A, Crosignani A, Varenna M *et al.* Primary biliary cirrhosis is not an additional risk factor for bone loss in women receiving regular calcium and vitamin D supplementation: A controlled longitudinal study. *J Clin Gastroenterol* 2008; **42**(3): 306–311.

29 Boulton-Jones JR, Fenn RM, West J, Logan RF, Ryder SD. Fracture risk of women with primary biliary cirrhosis: No increase compared with general population controls. *Aliment Pharmacol Ther* 2004; **20**(5): 551–557.

30 Campbell MS, Lichtenstein GR, Rhim AD, Pazianas M, Faust T. Severity of liver disease does not predict osteopenia or low bone mineral density in primary sclerosing cholangitis. *Liver Int* 2005; **25**(2): 311–316.

31 Krawitt EL, Grundman MJ, Mawer EB. Absorption, hydroxylation, and excretion of vitamin D3 in primary biliary cirrhosis. *Lancet* 1977; **2**(8051): 1246–1249.

32 Davies M, Mawer EB, Klass HJ, Lumb GA, Berry JL, Warnes TW. Vitamin D deficiency, osteomalacia, and primary biliary cirrhosis. Response to orally administered vitamin D3. *Dig Dis Sci* 1983; **28**(2): 145–153.

33 Wagonfeld JB, Nemchausky BA, Bolt M, Horst JV, Boyer JL, Rosenberg IH. Comparison of vitamin D and 25-hydroxy-vitamin-D in the therapy of primary biliary cirrhosis. *Lancet* 1976; **2**(7982): 391–394.

34 Dibble JB, Sheridan P, Hampshire R, Hardy GJ, Losowsky MS. Osteomalacia, vitamin D deficiency and cholestasis in chronic liver disease. *Q J Med* 1982; **51**(201): 89–103.

35 Cuthbert JA, Pak CY, Zerwekh JE, Glass KD, Combes B. Bone disease in primary biliary cirrhosis: increased bone resorption and turnover in the absence of osteoporosis or osteomalacia. *Hepatology* 1984; **4**(1): 1–8.

36 Jung RT, Davie M, Siklos P, Chalmers TM, Hunter JO, Lawson DE. Vitamin D metabolism in acute and chronic cholestasis. *Gut* 1979; **20**(10): 840–847.

37 Hodgson SF, Dickson ER, Wahner HW, Johnson KA, Mann KG, Riggs BL. Bone loss and reduced osteoblast function in primary biliary cirrhosis. *Ann Intern Med* 1985; **103**(6 Pt 1): 855–860.

38 Maddrey WC. Bone disease in patients with primary biliary cirrhosis. *Prog Liver Dis* 1990; **9**: 537–554.

39 Stellon AJ, Webb A, Compston J, Williams R. Low bone turnover state in primary biliary cirrhosis. *Hepatology* 1987; **7**(1): 137–142.

40 Herlong HF, Recker RR, Maddrey WC. Bone disease in primary biliary cirrhosis: histologic features and response to 25-hydroxyvitamin D. *Gastroenterology* 1982; **83**(1 Pt 1): 103–108.

41 Peris P, Pares A, Guanabens N *et al.* Bone mass improves in alcoholics after 2 years of abstinence. *J Bone Miner Res* 1994; **9**(10): 1607–1612.

42 Mitchison HC, Bassendine MF, Malcolm AJ, Watson AJ, Record CO, James OF. A pilot, double-blind, controlled 1-year trial of prednisolone treatment in primary biliary cirrhosis: hepatic improvement but greater bone loss. *Hepatology* 1989; **10**(4): 420–429.

43 Compston JE, Horton LW, Thompson RP. Treatment of osteomalacia associated with primary biliary cirrhosis with parenteral vitamin D2 or oral 25-hydroxyvitamin D3. *Gut* 1979; **20**(2): 133–136.

44 Reed JS, Meredith SC, Nemchausky BA, Rosenberg IH, Boyer JL. Bone disease in primary biliary cirrhosis: reversal of osteomalacia with oral 25-hydroxyvitamin D. *Gastroenterology* 1980; **78**(3): 512–517.

45 Floreani A, Carderi I, Ferrara F *et al.* A 4-year treatment with clodronate plus calcium and vitamin D supplements does not improve bone mass in primary biliary cirrhosis. *Dig Liver Dis* 2007; **39**(6): 544–548.

46 Pereira SP, O'Donohue J, Moniz C *et al.* Transdermal hormone replacement therapy improves vertebral bone density in primary biliary cirrhosis: results of a 1-year controlled trial. *Aliment Pharmacol Ther* 2004; **19**(5): 563–570.

47 Floreani A, Zappala F, Fries W *et al.* A 3-year pilot study with 1,25-dihydroxyvitamin D, calcium, and calcitonin for severe osteodystrophy in primary biliary cirrhosis. *J Clin Gastroenterol* 1997; **24**(4): 239–244.

48 Riemens SC, Oostdijk A, van Doormaal JJ *et al.* Bone loss after liver transplantation is not prevented by cyclical etidronate, calcium and alphacalcidol. The Liver Transplant Group, Groningen. *Osteoporos Int* 1996; **6**(3): 213–218.

49 Neuhaus R, Lohmann R, Platz KP *et al.* Treatment of osteoporosis after liver transplantation. *Transplant Proc* 1995; **27**(1): 1226–1227.

50 Crippin JS, Jorgensen RA, Dickson ER, Lindor KD. Hepatic osteodystrophy in primary biliary cirrhosis: effects of medical treatment. *Am J Gastroenterol* 1994; **89**(1): 47–50.

51 Matloff DS, Kaplan MM, Neer RM, Goldberg MJ, Bitman W, Wolfe HJ. Osteoporosis in primary biliary cirrhosis: effects of 25-hydroxyvitamin D3 treatment. *Gastroenterology* 1982; **83**(1 Pt 1): 97–102.

52 Shiomi S, Masaki K, Habu D *et al*. Calcitriol for bone disease in patients with cirrhosis of the liver. *J Gastroenterol Hepatol* 1999; **14**(6): 547–552.

53 Epstein O, Kato Y, Dick R, Sherlock S. Vitamin D, hydroxyapatite, and calcium gluconate in treatment of cortical bone thinning in postmenopausal women with primary biliary cirrhosis. *Am J Clin Nutr* 1982; **36**(3): 426–430.

54 Boone RH, Cheung AM, Girlan LM, Heathcote EJ. Osteoporosis in primary biliary cirrhosis: a randomized trial of the efficacy and feasibility of estrogen/progestin. *Dig Dis Sci* 2006; **51**(6): 1103–1112.

55 Ormarsdottir S, Mallmin H, Naessen T *et al*. An open, randomized, controlled study of transdermal hormone replacement therapy on the rate of bone loss in primary biliary cirrhosis. *J Intern Med* 2004; **256**(1): 63–69.

56 Guanabens N, Pares A, Ros I *et al*. Alendronate is more effective than etidronate for increasing bone mass in osteopenic patients with primary biliary cirrhosis. *Am J Gastroenterol* 2003; **98**(10): 2268–2274.

57 Shiomi S, Nishiguchi S, Kurooka H *et al*. Cyclical etidronate for treatment of osteopenia in patients with cirrhosis of the liver. *Hepatol Res* 2002; **22**(2): 102–106.

58 Lindor KD, Jorgensen RA, Tiegs RD, Khosla S, Dickson ER. Etidronate for osteoporosis in primary biliary cirrhosis: a randomized trial. *J Hepatol* 2000; **33**(6): 878–882.

59 Guanabens N, Pares A, Monegal A *et al*. Etidronate versus fluoride for treatment of osteopenia in primary biliary cirrhosis: Preliminary results after 2 years. *Gastroenterology* 1997; **113**(1): 219–224.

60 Camisasca M, Crosignani A, Battezzati PM *et al*. Parenteral calcitonin for metabolic bone disease associated with primary biliary cirrhosis. *Hepatology* 1994; **20**(3): 633–637.

61 Wolfhagen FH, van Buuren HR, den Ouden JW *et al*. Cyclical etidronate in the prevention of bone loss in corticosteroid-treated primary biliary cirrhosis. A prospective, controlled pilot study. *J Hepatol* 1997; **26**(2): 325–330.

62 Guanabens N, Pares A, del Rio L *et al*. Sodium fluoride prevents bone loss in primary biliary cirrhosis. *J Hepatol* 1992; **15**(3): 345–349.

63 Lindor KD, Janes CH, Crippin JS, Jorgensen RA, Dickson ER. Bone disease in primary biliary cirrhosis: Does ursodeoxycholic acid make a difference? *Hepatology* 1995; **21**(2): 389–392.

64 Stellon A, Davies A, Webb A, Williams R. Microcrystalline hydroxyapatite compound in prevention of bone loss in corticosteroid-treated patients with chronic active hepatitis. *Postgrad Med J* 1985; **61**(719): 791–796.

65 Heijckmann AC, Huijberts MS, Schoon EJ *et al*. High prevalence of morphometric vertebral deformities in patients with inflammatory bowel disease. *Eur J Gastroenterol Hepatol* 2008; **20**(8): 740–747.

66 Abitbol V, Roux C, Chaussade S *et al*. Metabolic bone assessment in patients with inflammatory bowel disease. *Gastroenterology* 1995; **108**(2): 417–422.

67 Motley RJ, Clements D, Evans WD *et al*. A four-year longitudinal study of bone loss in patients with inflammatory bowel disease. *Bone Miner* 1993; **23**(2): 95–104.

68 Motley RJ, Crawley EO, Evans C, Rhodes J, Compston JE. Increased rate of spinal trabecular bone loss in patients with inflammatory bowel disease. *Gut* 1988; **29**(10): 1332–1336.

69 Ryde SJ, Clements D, Evans WD *et al*. Total body calcium in patients with inflammatory bowel disease: A longitudinal study. *Clin Sci* (Lond) 1991; **80**(4): 319–324.

70 Dinca M, Fries W, Luisetto G *et al*. Evolution of osteopenia in inflammatory bowel disease. *Am J Gastroenterol* 1999; **94**(5): 1292–1297.

71 Schulte C, Dignass AU, Mann K, Goebell H. Bone loss in patients with inflammatory bowel disease is less than expected: A follow-up study. *Scand J Gastroenterol* 1999; **34**(7): 696–702.

72 Roux C, Abitbol V, Chaussade S *et al*. Bone loss in patients with inflammatory bowel disease: a prospective study. *Osteoporos Int* 1995; **5**(3): 156–160.

73 Hela S, Nihel M, Faten L *et al*. Osteoporosis and Crohn's disease. *Joint Bone Spine* 2005; **72**(5): 403–407.

74 Bernstein CN, Leslie WD. The pathophysiology of bone disease in gastrointestinal disease. *Eur J Gastroenterol Hepatol* 2003; **15**(8): 857–864.

75 Andreassen H, Rungby J, Dahlerup JF, Mosekilde L. Inflammatory bowel disease and osteoporosis. *Scand J Gastroenterol* 1997; **32**(12): 1247–1255.

76 Hessov I, Mosekilde L, Melsen F *et al*. Osteopenia with normal vitamin D metabolites after small-bowel resection for Crohn's disease. *Scand J Gastroenterol* 1984; **19**(5): 691–696.

77 Croucher PI, Vedi S, Motley RJ, Garrahan NJ, Stanton MR, Compston JE. Reduced bone formation in patients with osteoporosis associated with inflammatory bowel disease. *Osteoporos Int* 1993; **3**(5): 236–241.

78 Ghosh S, Cowen S, Hannan WJ, Ferguson A. Low bone mineral density in Crohn's disease, but not in ulcerative colitis, at diagnosis. *Gastroenterology* 1994; **107**(4): 1031–1039.

79 Jahnsen J, Falch JA, Aadland E, Mowinckel P. Bone mineral density is reduced in patients with Crohn's disease but not in patients with ulcerative colitis: A population based study. *Gut* 1997; **40**(3): 313–319.

80 Bernstein CN, Seeger LL, Sayre JW, Anton PA, Artinian L, Shanahan F. Decreased bone density in inflammatory bowel disease is related to corticosteroid use and not disease diagnosis. *J Bone Miner Res* 1995; **10**(2): 250–256.

81 Ardizzone S, Bollani S, Bettica P, Bevilacqua M, Molteni P, Bianchi Porro G. Altered bone metabolism in inflammatory bowel disease: There is a difference between Crohn's disease and ulcerative colitis. *J Intern Med* 2000; **247**(1): 63–70.

82 Reffitt DM, Meenan J, Sanderson JD, Jugdaohsingh R, Powell JJ, Thompson RP. Bone density improves with disease remission in patients with inflammatory bowel disease. *Eur J Gastroenterol Hepatol* 2003; **15**(12): 1267–1273.

83 Clements D, Motley RJ, Evans WD *et al*. Longitudinal study of cortical bone loss in patients with inflammatory bowel disease. *Scand J Gastroenterol* 1992; **27**(12): 1055–1060.

84 Klaus J, Armbrecht G, Steinkamp M *et al*. High prevalence of osteoporotic vertebral fractures in patients with Crohn's disease. *Gut* 2002; **51**(5): 654–658.

85 Bernstein CN, Blanchard JF, Leslie W, Wajda A, Yu BN. The incidence of fracture among patients with inflammatory bowel disease. A population-based cohort study. *Ann Intern Med* 2000; **133**(10): 795–799.

86 Loftus EV Jr, Crowson CS, Sandborn WJ, Tremaine WJ, O'Fallon WM, Melton LJ 3rd. Long-term fracture risk in patients with

Crohn's disease: A population-based study in Olmsted County, Minnesota. *Gastroenterology* 2002; **123**(2): 468–475.

87 Vestergaard P, Mosekilde L. Fracture risk in patients with celiac disease, Crohn's disease, and ulcerative colitis: A nationwide follow-up study of 16,416 patients in Denmark. *Am J Epidemiol* 2002; **156**(1): 1–10.

88 van Staa TP, Cooper C, Brusse LS, Leufkens H, Javaid MK, Arden NK. Inflammatory bowel disease and the risk of fracture. *Gastroenterology* 2003; **125**(6): 1591–1597.

89 Clements D, Compston JE, Evans WD, Rhodes J. Hormone replacement therapy prevents bone loss in patients with inflammatory bowel disease. *Gut* 1993; **34**(11): 1543–1546.

90 Vogelsang H, Ferenci P, Resch H, Kiss A, Gangl A. Prevention of bone mineral loss in patients with Crohn's disease by long-term oral vitamin D supplementation. *Eur J Gastroenterol Hepatol* 1995; **7**(7): 609–614.

91 Bernstein CN, Seeger LL, Anton PA *et al.* A randomized, placebo-controlled trial of calcium supplementation for decreased bone density in corticosteroid-using patients with inflammatory bowel disease: A pilot study. *Aliment Pharmacol Ther* 1996; **10**(5): 777–786.

92 Robinson RJ, Iqbal SJ, Wolfe R, Patel K, Abrams K, Mayberry JF. The effect of rectally administered steroids on bone turnover: A comparative study. *Aliment Pharmacol Ther* 1998; **12**(3): 213–217.

93 Haderslev KV, Tjellesen L, Sorensen HA, Staun M. Alendronate increases lumbar spine bone mineral density in patients with Crohn's disease. *Gastroenterology* 2000; **119**(3): 639–646.

94 Bartram SA, Peaston RT, Rawlings DJ, Francis RM, Thompson NP. A randomized controlled trial of calcium with vitamin D, alone or in combination with intravenous pamidronate, for the treatment of low bone mineral density associated with Crohn's disease. *Aliment Pharmacol Ther* 2003; **18**(11–12): 1121–1127.

95 Henderson S, Hoffman N, Prince R. A double-blind placebo-controlled study of the effects of the bisphosphonate risedronate on bone mass in patients with inflammatory bowel disease. *Am J Gastroenterol* 2006; **101**(1): 119–123.

96 Siffledeen JS, Fedorak RN, Siminoski K *et al.* Randomized trial of etidronate plus calcium and vitamin D for treatment of low bone mineral density in Crohn's disease. *Clin Gastroenterol Hepatol* 2005; **3**(2): 122–132.

97 von Tirpitz C, Klaus J, Bruckel J *et al.* Increase of bone mineral density with sodium fluoride in patients with Crohn's disease. *Eur J Gastroenterol Hepatol* 2000; **12**(1): 19–24.

98 Bernstein M, Irwin S, Greenberg GR. Maintenance infliximab treatment is associated with improved bone mineral density in Crohn's disease. *Am J Gastroenterol* 2005; **100**(9): 2031–2035.

99 Abreu MT, Geller JL, Vasiliauskas EA *et al.* Treatment with infliximab is associated with increased markers of bone formation in patients with Crohn's disease. *J Clin Gastroenterol* 2006; **40**(1): 55–63.

100 Mauro M, Radovic V, Armstrong D. Improvement of lumbar bone mass after infliximab therapy in Crohn's disease patients. *Can J Gastroenterol* 2007; **21**(10): 637–642.

101 Ryan BM, Russel MG, Schurgers L *et al.* Effect of antitumour necrosis factor-alpha therapy on bone turnover in patients with active Crohn's disease: A prospective study. *Aliment Pharmacol Ther* 2004; **20**(8): 851–857.

102 Pazianas M, Rhim AD, Weinberg AM, Su C, Lichtenstein GR. The effect of anti-TNF-alpha therapy on spinal bone mineral density in patients with Crohn's disease. *Ann N Y Acad Sci* 2006; **1068**: 543–556.

103 Di Stefano M, Jorizzo RA, Veneto G, Cecchetti L, Gasbarrini G, Corazza GR. Bone mass and metabolism in dermatitis herpetiformis. *Dig Dis Sci* 1999; **44**(10): 2139–2143.

104 Valdimarsson T, Lofman O, Toss G, Strom M. Reversal of osteopenia with diet in adult coeliac disease. *Gut* 1996; **38**(3): 322–327.

105 Valdimarsson T, Toss G, Lofman O, Strom M. Three years' follow-up of bone density in adult coeliac disease: Significance of secondary hyperparathyroidism. *Scand J Gastroenterol* 2000; **35**(3): 274–280.

106 Bai JC, Gonzalez D, Mautalen C *et al.* Long-term effect of gluten restriction on bone mineral density of patients with coeliac disease. *Aliment Pharmacol Ther* 1997; **11**(1): 157–164.

107 Meyer D, Stavropolous S, Diamond B, Shane E, Green PH. Osteoporosis in a North American adult population with celiac disease. *Am J Gastroenterol* 2001; **96**(1): 112–119.

108 McFarlane XA, Bhalla AK, Robertson DA. Effect of a gluten free diet on osteopenia in adults with newly diagnosed coeliac disease. *Gut* 1996; **39**(2): 180–184.

109 Kemppainen T, Kroger H, Janatuinen E *et al.* Osteoporosis in adult patients with celiac disease. *Bone* 1999; **24**(3): 249–255.

110 Vasquez H, Mazure R, Gonzalez D *et al.* Risk of fractures in celiac disease patients: a cross-sectional, case-control study. *Am J Gastroenterol* 2000; **95**(1): 183–189.

111 Thomason K, West J, Logan RF, Coupland C, Holmes GK. Fracture experience of patients with coeliac disease: A population based survey. *Gut* 2003; **52**(4): 518–522.

112 Valdimarsson T, Toss G, Ross I, Lofman O, Strom M. Bone mineral density in coeliac disease. *Scand J Gastroenterol* 1994; **29**(5): 457–461.

113 Olmos M, Antelo M, Vazquez H, Smecuol E, Maurino E, Bai JC. Systematic review and meta-analysis of observational studies on the prevalence of fractures in coeliac disease. *Dig Liver Dis* 2008; **40**(1): 46–53.

114 Ludvigsson JF, Michaelsson K, Ekbom A, Montgomery SM. Coeliac disease and the risk of fractures – a general population-based cohort study. *Aliment Pharmacol Ther* 2007; **25**(3): 273–285.

115 West J, Logan RF, Card TR, Smith C, Hubbard R. Fracture risk in people with celiac disease: A population-based cohort study. *Gastroenterology* 2003; **125**(2): 429–436.

116 Selby PL, Davies M, Adams JE, Mawer EB. Bone loss in celiac disease is related to secondary hyperparathyroidism. *J Bone Miner Res* 1999; **14**(4): 652–657.

117 Fornari MC, Pedreira S, Niveloni S *et al.* Pre- and post-treatment serum levels of cytokines IL-1beta, IL-6, and IL-1 receptor antagonist in celiac disease. Are they related to the associated osteopenia? *Am J Gastroenterol* 1998; **93**(3): 413–418.

118 Jameson S. Coeliac disease, insulin-like growth factor, bone mineral density, and zinc. *Scand J Gastroenterol* 2000; **35**(8): 894–896.

119 Kemppainen T, Kroger H, Janatuinen E *et al.* Bone recovery after a gluten-free diet: A 5-year follow-up study. *Bone* 1999; **25**(3): 355–360.

120 Mora S, Barera G, Ricotti A, Weber G, Bianchi C, Chiumello G. Reversal of low bone density with a gluten-free diet in children and adolescents with celiac disease. *Am J Clin Nutr* 1998; **67**(3): 477–481.

121 Mora S, Weber G, Barera G *et al*. Effect of gluten-free diet on bone mineral content in growing patients with celiac disease. *Am J Clin Nutr* 1993; **57**(2): 224–228.

122 Tau C, Mautalen C, De Rosa S, Roca A, Valenzuela X. Bone mineral density in children with celiac disease. Effect of a Gluten-free diet. *Eur J Clin Nutr* 2006; **60**(3): 358–363.

123 Ciacci C, Maurelli L, Klain M *et al*. Effects of dietary treatment on bone mineral density in adults with celiac disease: Factors predicting response. *Am J Gastroenterol* 1997; **92**(6): 992–996.

124 Lane NE. An update on glucocorticoid-induced osteoporosis. *Rheum Dis Clin North Am* 2001; **27**(1): 235–253.

125 Lukert BP, Raisz LG. Glucocorticoid-induced osteoporosis: Pathogenesis and management. *Ann Intern Med* 1990; **112**(5): 352–364.

126 Adinoff AD, Hollister JR. Steroid-induced fractures and bone loss in patients with asthma. *N Engl J Med* 1983; **309**(5): 265–268.

127 Van Staa TP, Leufkens HG, Abenhaim L, Zhang B, Cooper C. Use of oral corticosteroids and risk of fractures. *J Bone Miner Res* 2000; **15**(6): 993–1000.

128 Baltzan MA, Suissa S, Bauer DC, Cummings SR. Hip fractures attributable to corticosteroid use. Study of Osteoporotic Fractures Group. *Lancet* 1999; **353**(9161): 1327.

129 Kanis JA, Johansson H, Oden A *et al*. A meta-analysis of prior corticosteroid use and fracture risk. *J Bone Miner Res* 2004; **19**(6): 893–899.

130 Eastell R, Reid DM, Compston J *et al*. A UK Consensus Group on management of glucocorticoid-induced osteoporosis: An update. *J Intern Med* 1998; **244**(4): 271–292.

131 Van Staa TP, Laan RF, Barton IP, Cohen S, Reid DM, Cooper C. Bone density threshold and other predictors of vertebral fracture in patients receiving oral glucocorticoid therapy. *Arthritis Rheum* 2003; **48**(11): 3224–3229.

132 Hahn BH, Mazzaferri EL. Glucocorticoid-induced osteoporosis. *Hosp Pract (Minneap)* 1995; **30**(8): 45–49, 52–53; discussion 53–56.

133 von Tirpitz C, Epp S, Klaus J *et al*. Effect of systemic glucocorticoid therapy on bone metabolism and the osteoprotegerin system in patients with active Crohn's disease. *Eur J Gastroenterol Hepatol* 2003; **15**(11): 1165–1170.

134 Tobias JH, Sasi MR, Greenwood R, Probert CS. Rapid hip bone loss in active Crohn's disease patients receiving short-term corticosteroid therapy. *Aliment Pharmacol Ther* 2004; **20**(9): 951–957.

135 Hahn TJ, Boisseau VC, Avioli LV. Effect of chronic corticosteroid administration on diaphyseal and metaphyseal bone mass. *J Clin Endocrinol Metab* 1974; **39**(2): 274–282.

136 Sambrook P, Birmingham J, Kelly P *et al*. Prevention of corticosteroid osteoporosis. A comparison of calcium, calcitriol, and calcitonin. *N Engl J Med* 1993; **328**(24): 1747–1752.

137 Adachi JD, Bensen WG, Bianchi F *et al*. Vitamin D and calcium in the prevention of corticosteroid induced osteoporosis: A 3 year followup. *J Rheumatol* 1996; **23**(6): 995–1000.

138 Dykman TR, Haralson KM, Gluck OS *et al*. Effect of oral 1,25-dihydroxyvitamin D and calcium on glucocorticoid-induced osteopenia in patients with rheumatic diseases. *Arthritis Rheum* 1984; **27**(12): 1336–1343.

139 Manolagas SC, Weinstein RS, Jilka RL, Parfitt AM. Parathyroid hormone and corticosteroid-induced osteoporosis. *Lancet* 1998; **352**(9144): 1940.

140 Manolagas SC, Weinstein RS. New developments in the pathogenesis and treatment of steroid-induced osteoporosis. *J Bone Miner Res* 1999; **14**(7): 1061–1066.

141 Sambrook PN. Corticosteroid induced osteoporosis. *J Rheumatol Suppl* 1996; **45**: 19–22.

142 Aubin JE, Bonnelye E. Osteoprotegerin and its ligand: A new paradigm for regulation of osteoclastogenesis and bone resorption. *Osteoporos Int* 2000; **11**(11): 905–913.

143 Manolagas SC. Corticosteroids and fractures: A close encounter of the third cell kind. *J Bone Miner Res* 2000; **15**(6): 1001–1005.

144 Healey JH, Paget SA, Williams-Russo P *et al*. A randomized controlled trial of salmon calcitonin to prevent bone loss in corticosteroid-treated temporal arteritis and polymyalgia rheumatica. *Calcif Tissue Int* 1996; **58**(2): 73–80.

145 Kotaniemi A, Piirainen H, Paimela L *et al*. Is continuous intranasal salmon calcitonin effective in treating axial bone loss in patients with active rheumatoid arthritis receiving low dose glucocorticoid therapy? *J Rheumatol* 1996; **23**(11): 1875–1879.

146 Luengo M, Pons F, Martinez de Osaba MJ, Picado C. Prevention of further bone mass loss by nasal calcitonin in patients on long term glucocorticoid therapy for asthma: A two year follow up study. *Thorax* 1994; **49**(11): 1099–1102.

147 Ringe JD, Welzel D. Salmon calcitonin in the therapy of corticoid-induced osteoporosis. *Eur J Clin Pharmacol* 1987; **33**(1): 35–39.

148 Worth H, Stammen D, Keck E. Therapy of steroid-induced bone loss in adult asthmatics with calcium, vitamin D, and a diphosphonate. *Am J Respir Crit Care Med* 1994; **150**(2): 394–397.

149 Adachi JD, Bensen WG, Brown J *et al*. Intermittent etidronate therapy to prevent corticosteroid-induced osteoporosis. *N Engl J Med* 1997; **337**(6): 382–387.

150 Saag KG, Emkey R, Schnitzer TJ *et al*. Alendronate for the prevention and treatment of glucocorticoid-induced osteoporosis. Glucocorticoid-Induced Osteoporosis Intervention Study Group. *N Engl J Med* 1998; **339**(5): 292–299.

151 Boutsen Y, Jamart J, Esselinckx W, Stoffel M, Devogelaer JP. Primary prevention of glucocorticoid-induced osteoporosis with intermittent intravenous pamidronate: A randomized trial. *Calcif Tissue Int* 1997; **61**(4): 266–271.

152 Roux C, Oriente P, Laan R *et al*. Randomized trial of effect of cyclical etidronate in the prevention of corticosteroid-induced bone loss. Ciblos Study Group. *J Clin Endocrinol Metab* 1998; **83**(4): 1128–1133.

153 Reid DM, Hughes RA, Laan RF *et al*. Efficacy and safety of daily risedronate in the treatment of corticosteroid-induced osteoporosis in men and women: A randomized trial. European Corticosteroid-Induced Osteoporosis Treatment Study. *J Bone Miner Res* 2000; **15**(6): 1006–1013.

154 Cohen S, Levy RM, Keller M *et al*. Risedronate therapy prevents corticosteroid-induced bone loss: A twelve-month, multicenter,

randomized, double-blind, placebo-controlled, parallel-group study. *Arthritis Rheum* 1999; **42**(11): 2309–2318.

155 Buckley LM, Leib ES, Cartularo KS, Vacek PM, Cooper SM. Calcium and vitamin D3 supplementation prevents bone loss in the spine secondary to low-dose corticosteroids in patients with rheumatoid arthritis. A randomized, double-blind, placebo-controlled trial. *Ann Intern Med* 1996; **125**(12): 961–968.

156 Homik J, Suarez-Almazor ME, Shea B, Cranney A, Wells GA, Tugwell P. Calcium and vitamin D for corticosteroid-induced osteoporosis. *Cochrane Database of Systematic Reviews* 1998, Issue 2. Art. No.: CD000952. DOI: 10.1002/14651858.CD000952.

157 Amin S, LaValley MP, Simms RW, Felson DT. The role of vitamin D in corticosteroid-induced osteoporosis: A meta-analytic approach. *Arthritis Rheum* 1999; **42**(8): 1740–1751.

158 Cranney A, Welch V, Adachi J, Homik J, Shea B, Suarez-Almazor ME, Tugwell P, Wells GA. Calcitonin for preventing and treating corticosteroid-induced osteoporosis. *Cochrane Database of Systematic Reviews* 2000, Issue 1. Art. No.: CD001983. DOI: 10.1002/14651858.CD001983.

159 Hall GM, Daniels M, Doyle DV, Spector TD. Effect of hormone replacement therapy on bone mass in rheumatoid arthritis patients treated with and without steroids. *Arthritis Rheum* 1994; **37**(10): 1499–1505.

160 Reid IR, Wattie DJ, Evans MC, Stapleton JP. Testosterone therapy in glucocorticoid-treated men. *Arch Intern Med* 1996; **156**(11): 1173–1177.

161 Homik J, Cranney A, Shea B, Tugwell P, Wells GA, Adachi J, Suarez-Almazor ME. Bisphosphonates for steroid induced osteoporosis. *Cochrane Database of Systematic Reviews* 1999, Issue 1. Art. No.: CD001347. DOI: 10.1002/14651858.CD001347.

162 Adachi JD, Saag KG, Delmas PD *et al*. Two-year effects of alendronate on bone mineral density and vertebral fracture in patients receiving glucocorticoids: A randomized, double-blind, placebo-controlled extension trial. *Arthritis Rheum* 2001; **44**(1): 202–211.

163 Kanis JA, Stevenson M, McCloskey EV, Davis S, Lloyd-Jones M. Glucocorticoid-induced osteoporosis: A systematic review and cost-utility analysis. *Health Technol Assess* 2007; **11**(7): iii–iv, ix–xi, 1–231.

164 Amin S, Lavalley MP, Simms RW, Felson DT. The comparative efficacy of drug therapies used for the management of corticosteroid-induced osteoporosis: A meta-regression. *J Bone Miner Res* 2002; **17**(8): 1512–1526.

165 Lems WF, Jacobs WG, Bijlsma JW *et al*. Effect of sodium fluoride on the prevention of corticosteroid-induced osteoporosis. *Osteoporos Int* 1997; **7**(6): 575–582.

166 Lippuner K, Haller B, Casez JP, Montandon A, Jaeger P. Effect of disodium monofluorophosphate, calcium and vitamin D supplementation on bone mineral density in patients chronically treated with glucocorticosteroids: A prospective, randomized, double-blind study. *Miner Electrolyte Metab* 1996; **22**(4): 207–213.

167 Guaydier-Souquieres G, Kotzki PO, Sabatier JP, Basse-Cathalinat B, Loeb G. In corticosteroid-treated respiratory diseases, monofluorophosphate increases lumbar bone density: A double-masked randomized study. *Osteoporos Int* 1996; **6**(2): 171–177.

168 Lane NE, Sanchez S, Modin GW, Genant HK, Pierini E, Arnaud CD. Parathyroid hormone treatment can reverse corticosteroid-induced osteoporosis. Results of a randomized controlled clinical trial. *J Clin Invest* 1998; **102**(8): 1627–1633.

169 Lane NE, Sanchez S, Modin GW, Genant HK, Pierini E, Arnaud CD. Bone mass continues to increase at the hip after parathyroid hormone treatment is discontinued in glucocorticoid-induced osteoporosis: Results of a randomized controlled clinical trial. *J Bone Miner Res* 2000; **15**(5): 944–951.

170 Schoon EJ, Bollani S, Mills PR *et al*. Bone mineral density in relation to efficacy and side effects of budesonide and prednisolone in Crohn's disease. *Clin Gastroenterol Hepatol* 2005; **3**(2): 113–121.

171 Saag KG, Shane E, Boonen S *et al*. Teriparatide or alendronate in glucocorticoid-induced osteoporosis. *N Engl J Med* 2007; **357**(20): 2028–2039.

172 Vestergaard P, Rejnmark L, Mosekilde L. Proton pump inhibitors, histamine H2 receptor antagonists, and other antacid medications and the risk of fracture. *Calcif Tissue Int* 2006; **79**(2): 76–83.

173 Yang YX, Lewis JD, Epstein S, Metz DC. Long-term proton pump inhibitor therapy and risk of hip fracture. *JAMA* 2006; **296**(24): 2947–2953.

174 Sheikh MS, Santa Ana CA, Nicar MJ, Schiller LR, Fordtran JS. Gastrointestinal absorption of calcium from milk and calcium salts. *N Engl J Med* 1987; **317**(9): 532–536.

175 O'Connell MB, Madden DM, Murray AM, Heaney RP, Kerzner LJ. Effects of proton pump inhibitors on calcium carbonate absorption in women: A randomized crossover trial. *Am J Med* 2005; **118**(7): 778–781.

176 Moayyedi P, Cranney A. Hip fracture and proton pump inhibitor therapy: balancing the evidence for benefit and harm. *Am J Gastroenterol* 2008; **103**(10): 2428–2431.

177 Serfaty-Lacrosniere C, Wood RJ, Voytko D *et al*. Hypochlorhydria from short-term omeprazole treatment does not inhibit intestinal absorption of calcium, phosphorus, magnesium or zinc from food in humans. *J Am Coll Nutr* 1995; **14**(4): 364–368.

178 Farina C, Gagliardi S. Selective inhibition of osteoclast vacuolar H+ – ATPase. *Curr Pharm Des* 2002; **8**(23): 2033–2048.

179 Targownik LE, Lix LM, Metge CJ, Prior HJ, Leung S, Leslie WD. Use of proton pump inhibitors and risk of osteoporosis-related fractures. *CMAJ* 2008; **179**(4): 319–3126.

180 Mamdani M, Upshur RE, Anderson G, Bartle BR, Laupacis A. Warfarin therapy and risk of hip fracture among elderly patients. *Pharmacotherapy* 2003; **23**(1): 1–4.

181 Yu EW, Blackwell T, Ensrud KE *et al*. Acid-suppressive medications and risk of bone loss and fracture in older adults. *Calcif Tissue Int* 2008; **83**(4): 251–259.

182 Roux C, Briot K, Gossec L *et al*. Increase in vertebral fracture risk in postmenopausal women using omeprazole. *Calcif Tissue Int* 2009; **84**(1): 13–19.

183 Kaye JA, Jick H. Proton pump inhibitor use and risk of hip fractures in patients without major risk factors. *Pharmacotherapy* 2008; **28**(8): 951–959.

184 Vestergaard P, Rejnmark L, Mosekilde L. Fracture risk associated with use of nonsteroidal anti-inflammatory drugs, acetylsalicylic acid, and acetaminophen and the effects of rheu-

matoid arthritis and osteoarthritis. *Calcif Tissue Int* 2006; **79**(2): 84–94.

185 Penning-van Beest FJ, Goettsch WG, Erkens JA, Herings RM. Determinants of persistence with bisphosphonates: A study in women with postmenopausal osteoporosis. *Clin Ther* 2006; **28**(2): 236–242.

186 Brown JP, Josse RG. 2002 clinical practice guidelines for the diagnosis and management of osteoporosis in Canada. *CMAJ* 2002; **167**(10 Suppl): S1–S34.

187 Bernstein CN, Leslie WD, Leboff MS. AGA technical review on osteoporosis in gastrointestinal diseases. *Gastroenterology* 2003; **124**(3): 795–841.

17 Colorectal cancer in ulcerative colitis: Surveillance

Paul Collins[1], Bret A Lashner[2] and Alastair JM Watson[1]

[1] School of Clinical Sciences, University of Liverpool, Liverpool, UK
[2] Center for Inflammatory Bowel Disease, Cleveland Clinic, Cleveland, USA

Epidemiological investigation

Many questions are posed by patients, clinicians and investigators regarding the recommended methods of cancer surveillance in ulcerative colitis. In the absence of scientific rigor conferred by randomized clinical trials, answers to these questions only can be inferred from observational studies. The evidence from cohort studies, case-control studies, and studies of diagnostic testing, coupled with surveillance theory and perceived patient preferences can be used to answer some of the more pressing questions and provide recommendations.

Cohort studies are epidemiological investigations that address specific natural history questions [1]. Groups of ulcerative colitis patients and controls are followed from the inception of disease until the development of specific outcomes, such as dysplasia or cancer, and incidence rates are compared between groups. Cohort studies, comparisons between patients with the designated outcome to those without the outcome, are particularly useful for quantifying cancer risk as well as for identifying risk factors for disease outcome [2–12]. For example, most recent cohort studies have found primary sclerosing cholangitis to be a risk factor for dysplasia or colorectal cancer in patients with ulcerative colitis (Table 17.1) [13–20]. However, incorrect conclusions related to prognosis can be made if cohort studies are carried out without careful attention to issues of bias and confounding variables. Standards have been published delineating the scientific requirements for the performance of valid cohort studies of cancer risk in ulcerative colitis. These include assembly of an inception cohort, blind assessment of objective outcomes, complete follow-up and a description of the referral pattern [1].

Case-control studies also can be used to examine etiological associations [21]. Patients with ulcerative colitis with cancer or dysplasia are compared with controls without neoplasia to test for differences in the odds of exposure to possible causative agents. Case-control studies are highly susceptible to bias and confounding variables. For a putative etiological factor to be considered valid it must be strong, consistent from study to study, occur before the effect, be biologically plausible and exhibit a dose–response relationship to the event of interest. As an example, case-control studies are best for identifying agents such as folic acid that may prevent the development of cancer or dysplasia [22–24].

Two case-control studies have shown that colonoscopic surveillance may be effective by identifying patients at high risk of developing cancer. Karlen and colleagues from Stockholm compared 40 ulcerative colitis patients who died from colorectal cancer with 102 ulcerative colitis controls [25]. Patients who had undergone a surveillance colonoscopy had a 71% decrease in risk of cancer mortality (odds ratio (OR) 0.29; 95% CI: 0.06–1.31). Having two or more examinations had an even greater beneficial effect (OR 0.22; 95% CI: 0.03–1.74). Similarly, Eaden *et al*. compared 102 patients with ulcerative colitis and colorectal cancer with an equal number of ulcerative colitis controls matched for age, sex and extent and duration of disease [26]. Surveillance colonoscopy was associated with a decreased risk of developing colorectal cancer (one to two examinations OR 0.22; 95% CI: 0.09–0.77; more than two examinations OR 0.42; 95% CI: 0.16–1.56).

Studies of diagnostic testing provide important insights into the optimization of parameters related to cancer surveillance [21, 27]. Studies comparing the sensitivity and specificity of different diagnostic tests can help choose the best test. Studies examining the sensitivity–specificity trade-off between different cut-points of the same test can help choose the optimal criterion for a positive test. Dysplasia in colonic biopsies is the best studied surveillance test for ulcerative colitis and has the best surveillance

Evidence-Based Gastroenterology and Hepatology, 3rd edition.
J. McDonald, A.K. Burroughs, B. Feagan, and M.B. Fennerty. © 2010
Blackwell Publishing Ltd

Table 17.1 Cohort studies of primary sclerosing cholangitis (PSC) as a risk factor for dysplasia or cancer in ulcerative colitis.

Study	Center	No. of patients	Dysplasia or cancer (%)	Relative risk (95% CI)
Broome *et al.* (1992) [13]	Huddinge	5 PSC 67 controls	4 (80) 8 (12)	6.7 (2.6 to 17.4)
Gurbuz *et al.* (1995) [14]	Baltimore	35 PSC	13 (37)	Increased
Broome *et al.* (1995) [15]	Huddinge	40 PSC 80 controls	16 (40) 10 (12)	3.2 (1.6 to 6.2)
Brentnall *et al.* (1996) [16]	Seattle	20 PSC 25 controls	9 (45) 406)	4.9 (1.4 to 17.7)
Loftus *et al.* (1996) [17]	Rochester	143 PSC	8 (6)	4.9 (0.1 to 27)
Marchesa *et al.* (1997) [18]	Cleveland	27 PSC 1185 controls	18 (67) 145 (12)	10.4 (4.1 to 26.1)
Shetty *et al.* (1999) [19]	Cleveland	132 PSC 196 controls	33 (25) 11 (16)	3.2 (1.4 to 7.3)
Lindberg *et al.* (2001) [20]	Huddinge	19 PSC 124 controls	12 (63) 31 (30)	3.1 (1.1 to 8.9)

program performance [28]. When evaluating biopsy specimens for dysplasia, the optimal criterion for a positive test is low grade dysplasia (a criterion with high sensitivity), rather than high grade dysplasia (a criterion with high specificity).

Axioms

Many accepted practices related to cancer surveillance in ulcerative colitis have not been studied, but are assumed to be valid. Indeed, there are certain axiomatic statements that must be true for surveillance to be at all accepted by patients and physicians.

(1) *The cancer risk is elevated in ulcerative colitis patients and is too high to ignore.* There have been many epidemiological studies investigating the cancer risk in ulcerative colitis [2–12, 29–33], mostly from northern Europe or North America, where the incidence of ulcerative colitis is high and accurate and complete databases exist. From these studies, it is reasonable to assume that the lifetime incidence of colorectal cancer in a patient with pan-ulcerative colitis is approximately 6%, since a risk of this magnitude has been established for the background risk in the American population [34], and the risk of cancer-related mortality is approximately 3%. These figures are too high to ignore, assuming that there is either effective surveil-

lance available or acceptable prophylactic treatment. Furthermore, in some countries like the USA, either prophylactic colectomy or cancer surveillance colonoscopy have become the standard of care for ulcerative colitis patients, especially those diagnosed at a young age. In older patients, especially those with severe comorbidity or disability, the case for surveillance is much less clear, since they may be more likely to die from other diseases and not be fit for proctocolectomy.

Newer studies report a lower risk of cancer than previously described. In a recent meta-analysis, Jess and colleagues calculate a lower risk of cancer than previously reported (standardised incidence ratio, 1.9; 95% CI: 1.4–5.2) [35]. More recent cohort studies report a risk of cancer less than this [29–31, 33, 36]. This apparent reduction in cancer risk may be due to the protective effect of adherence to a colonoscopic surveillance program in which colectomy is offered to those in whom dysplasia is detected. It may also reflect the use of mesalamine for which there is evidence of a protective effect against colorectal cancer in ulcerative colitis [37].

(2) *Most patients would rather not have prophylactic colectomy.* Colectomy prior to the development of dysplasia or cancer is sure to dramatically reduce, if not eliminate, the mortality from colorectal cancer [38]. The existence of cancer surveillance programs, whether or not they are effective, has convinced some patients that the excess cancer mortality risk with ulcerative colitis can be minimized, and that the minimized risk is preferred to the morbidity following proctocolectomy.

(3) *Patients would agree to proctocolectomy if the cancer risk is very high, as it is with a positive test from surveillance.* There is no point in performing surveillance colonoscopy if a patient will refuse to have a proctocolectomy for a positive test. Clinicians need to counsel patients carefully so they understand that surveillance is meant to identify the patients at very high cancer risk for proctocolectomy and allow the remaining patients to continue in the cancer surveillance program. From that approach, a majority of patients, those without dysplasia, will not have a colectomy recommended.

In an optimally performing program, all cancer deaths will be averted through colectomy on high risk patients, and no cancer deaths will occur among patients not having colectomy. There has been no perfectly performing surveillance program reported. Program performance is likely to improve following the development of a diagnostic test with better sensitivity and specificity than the presence or absence of dysplasia and/or with more frequent testing than is currently done.

Questions

Existing evidence can only partially answer some of the questions related to cancer surveillance in ulcerative colitis. Understanding the limits of this evidence and identifying priorities for future investigation could improve technical aspects of surveillance and, ultimately, decrease cancer-related mortality. Questions regarding expected outcomes, the method of surveillance, testing intervals and the criterion for a positive test will be addressed.

(1) *How effective will a surveillance program be for reducing cancer-related mortality?* Although there is no direct evidence for a survival benefit in patients undergoing surveillance, there is evidence that cancers tend to be detected at an earlier stage, and these patients have a correspondingly better prognosis [39]. However lead-time bias may contribute substantially to this apparent benefit.

The number of patients needed to be enrolled in a surveillance program who comply with all of its parameters (i.e. repeated testing with colectomy for a positive test) in order to avert one cancer death can be calculated using expected risk reductions. The number-needed-to-treat (NNT) is the inverse of the absolute risk reduction [21]. Assuming the cancer-related mortality in high risk patients is 3%, the NNT in a perfectly performing program in which colectomy for dysplasia is highly effective for prevention of death from cancer and results in the complete elimination of cancer-related mortality is 1/0.03 or 33. For an absolute

risk reduction from surveillance of 1% (i.e. 3% to 2%), the NNT is 100, and for an absolute risk reduction of 2% (i.e. 3% to 1%), the NNT is 50. It is reasonable to assume that surveillance will have some benefit and the NNT most likely will fall between 33 and 100. Therefore, for every 100 patients with pan-ulcerative colitis who are entered into and faithfully comply with the parameters of a surveillance program, between one and three cancer deaths will be averted.

(2) *What is the best testing method for cancer surveillance?* Using colonoscopy with multiple biopsies of the colon to detect dysplasia is the best and most accepted strategy employed for cancer surveillance in ulcerative colitis. Since dysplasia can be present focally, and not necessarily diffusely, biopsies must be taken throughout the colon. Histological interpretation can be problematic in the presence of inflammation and surveillance endoscopy is best performed when the disease is in remission. It is necessary to take at least 33 biopsies from around the colon to have a 90% sensitivity for the detection of dysplasia [40], but even the most intensive sampling protocols sample less than 0.05% of the colon. While it has not been studied, it seems to be a reasonable trade-off between sensitivity and cost/morbidity to sample the colon with four biopsies taken from each 10 cm colonic segment and of any raised or strictured lesions. **C5**

Intensive biopsy protocols, in which 33 or more biopsies are taken at each surveillance colonoscopy, have an impact on pathology services. Techniques to target biopsies to those sites likely to be harboring dysplasia would reduce this burden.

Dysplasia can be visualised at white light colonoscopy [41], which is able to detect prominent polypoid lesions. Careful mucosal inspection, even without chromoendoscopy will improve detection of dysplasia. The finding that there is a significant correlation between the mean duration of colonoscopy and detection rate of flat dysplasia seems intuitive [42].

Chromoendoscopy using indigo carmine or methylene blue highlights architectural abnormalities allowing flat or depressed dysplastic lesions to be seen with a related increase in diagnostic yield [43–47]. This was highlighted in the study by Rutter and colleagues in which one hundred patients with ulcerative colitis attending for surveillance colonoscopy underwent back-to-back colonoscopies with indigo carmine dye spraying at the second examination. No dysplasia was found in the 2904 random biopsies taken, whereas dye spraying and targeted biopsies revealed seven dysplastic lesions [48]. Combining chromoendoscopy with high magnification endoscopy allows the surface staining pattern to be analyzed. Kiesslich and colleagues have used this technique to differentiate between neoplastic and non-neoplastic tissue with a sensitivity and specificity of 93% [49].

Chromoendoscopy with targeted biopsies reduces the burden on the histopathologist while increasing the yield of surveillance colonoscopy. There is a trade-off in terms of increased procedural time, with examinations taking approximately 10 minutes longer in expert hands [49, 50]. Colonoscopists will require adequate training in this technique and guidelines exist to aid optimal performance [51].

The addition of endomicroscopy allows *in vivo* histology to analyse lesions identified by chromoendoscopy, which further increases the yield of intra-epithelial neoplasia as compared to chromoendoscopy alone [52]. The diagnostic yield for intraepithelial neoplasia was improved 4.75-fold using this technique [43].

Other emerging endoscopic technologies may aid in the visualisation of architectural abnormalities and distinguish neoplastic from non-neoplastic lesions (narrow band imaging, fluoroendoscopy, optical coherence tomography and confocal laser microscopy) [43, 53–56], but it remains to be seen to what extent these technologies will be utilized in daily practice.

A dysplasia-associated lesion or mass (DALM) correlates with a high risk for cancer and prophylactic colectomy can be advocated [57, 58]. On colonoscopic appearance, it can be difficult to distinguish a DALM from a sporadic adenomatous polyp. Although it has been suggested that such lesions may be safely removed provided surrounding flat mucosa shows no dysplasia, recurrent raised dysplastic lesions occur in half these patients [58–61]. If colectomy is deferred, intensive follow-up with 3–6 monthly colonoscopy is advised. **C5**

Problematical issues involve pseudopolyps and strictures. Pseudopolyps have been associated with double the risk of colorectal cancer [62, 63]. Multiple pseudopolyps cannot be adequately biopsied and could easily harbor dysplastic tissue. These patients need to be informed of the poor sensitivity of surveillance, and the benefits of prophylactic colectomy. **C5** Likewise, colonic strictures that do not allow passage of the colonoscope and adequate sampling could, and very often do, harbor dysplasia [64]. Once again, these patients should be considered for prophylactic colectomy since surveillance of these patients is insensitive. **C5**

Research is progressing in the area of alternatives to histological assessment of dysplasia as a surveillance strategy. Detection of acquired DNA changes in biopsy samples (aneuploidy, p53 and k-ras mutations) or glycosylation abnormalities (sialyl-Tn) may contribute to the sensitivity of surveillance [65]. DNA fingerprinting or fluorescent in situ hybridization has been used to demonstrate genomic instability in rectal biopsies as a marker of neoplasia in inflammatory bowel disease [66]. Analysis of DNA from stool samples allows analysis of DNA from more cells than pinch biopsies alone. Extraction of DNA from faecal samples and subsequent analysis for mutations associated

with sporadic colon cancer has been performed [67, 68], and it remains to be seen whether this non-invasive testing strategy will have a place in surveillance in ulcerative colitis.

Patients would be considered to have a positive test if either dysplasia or a genetic abnormality is present. Of course, improved sensitivity will be at the cost of specificity and result in increased numbers of false positives. The penalty for lowering specificity is high – a proctocolectomy in a patient who might not have developed cancer. These alternative tests would be acceptable for use in a surveillance program if the cost were relatively low, the availability high, the gain in sensitivity great and the loss of specificity minimal.

(3) *What is the best testing interval?* The more tests that are carried out in a lifetime, the higher the likelihood that dysplasia will be detected and treated prior to the development of cancer and that cancer-related mortality will be reduced. Of course, the more tests that are done, the higher will be the cost, morbidity and patient intolerance to colonoscopy. A balance between benefits and costs needs to be struck [69, 70].

While lesions could progress at different rates, the mean value for the time between the development of low grade dysplasia and cancer (lead time) is believed to be three years [71, 72]. Therefore, testing at intervals longer than three years should be discouraged, as the majority of patients who develop cancer would not have had an opportunity for dysplasia to be detected at surveillance examinations.

The risk of developing cancer or dysplasia increases with increasing duration of disease. The benefits of frequent testing (short interval) also increase with increasing duration of disease. It can be concluded that uniform testing intervals over a lifetime of disease is not an efficient way to allocate the performance of costly and invasive test procedures. A decision analysis suggests that efficient testing is characterized by decreasing the testing interval with increasing duration of disease [71]. One reasonable method, which certainly can be adjusted according to patient and physician preferences, specifies testing every 3 years for the first 20 years of disease, every 2 years for the next 10 years of disease, and yearly thereafter. **C5** Complications of colonoscopy are rare but can be serious or life-threatening. However, this approach would require at least 20 tests over a 40-year lifetime of disease, with most allocated in the later years when the risk is the highest and with the associated cumulative risk of multiple procedures. The risk of bleeding or perforation is less for diagnostic colonoscopy than for therapeutic colonoscopy (up to 0.35% and 2.3% respectively [73]).

(4) *What is the best criterion for a positive test?* The type of dysplastic lesion to be used as a criterion for a positive test is best determined by weighing the trade-off between

Table 17.2 Contingency table for calculating sensitivity and specificity of dysplasia for the diagnosis of cancer.

	Cancer	No Cancer
Dysplasia	a	b
No Dysplasia	c	d

Table 17.3 The sensitivity and specificity of dysplasia to diagnose colorectal cancer in ulcerative colitis patients stratified by degree of dysplasia.

Study center	Sensitivity (%)	Specificity (%)
University of Chicago (1985) [74]		
Any dysplasia	73	73
High grade dysplasia	50	91
Mayo Clinic (1992) [75]		
Any dysplasia	74	74
High grade dysplasia	32	98
St Mark's Hospital (1994) [76]		
Any dysplasia	74	—
High grade dysplasia	32	—
Mount Sinai (2000) [77]		
Any dysplasia	84	93
High grade dysplasia	61	95
Heidelberg (2001) [78]		
Any dysplasia	71	83
High-grade dysplasia	55	90

sensitivity and specificity. Sensitivity is defined as the proportion of patients with disease who are positive for the test in question. Likewise, specificity is defined as the proportion of patients without disease who are negative for the test in question. A standard 2×2 contingency table for n patients (n = a + b + c + d) is shown in Table 17.2.

In normally distributed populations, sensitivity (a / [a + c]) and specificity (d / [b + d]) are stable values that do not vary with prevalence of disease. Sensitivity and specificity will vary though, when the "cut-point" or the criterion for a positive test changes. For example, if the criterion for a positive test changes from high grade dysplasia to low grade dysplasia, the sensitivity will increase (more "a"s and less "c"s) and the specificity will decrease (more "b"s and less "d"s). As the criterion for a positive test changes, there is a trade-off between sensitivity and specificity – as one increases, the other decreases.

The sensitivity and specificity of screening for dysplasia to identify patients with asymptomatic cancer has been studied with remarkably consistent results. A blinded review from the University of Chicago of all regions in colectomy specimens in 22 ulcerative colitis patients with cancer identified dysplasia distant from the malignancy in 16 (73% sensitivity for any dysplasia) [74]. Eleven patients had high grade dysplasia (50% sensitivity for high grade dysplasia). In a comparable group of 22 ulcerative colitis patients without cancer, six had dysplasia (73% specificity for any dysplasia) and two had high grade dysplasia (91% specificity for high-grade dysplasia). Nearly identical results were found in a study from the Mayo Clinic, where one hundred colectomy specimens from patients with ulcerative colitis, 50 of whom had cancer, were studied [75]. The sensitivity for any dysplasia was 74% (37/50) and the sensitivity for high grade dysplasia was 32% (16/50). The specificity of any dysplasia was 74% (37/50) and the specificity of high grade dysplasia was 98% (49/50). Both studies acknowledged that only a small minority of patients were followed in cancer surveillance programs. In a study from St Mark's Hospital, London, principally of ulcerative colitis patients participating in surveillance programs, 37 of 50 colectomy specimens with cancer had dysplasia distant from the malignancy (74% sensitivity for any dysplasia) [76]. Sixteen of those patients had high grade dys-

plasia (32% sensitivity for high grade dysplasia). A large review from Mount Sinai Hospital in New York of 590 colectomy specimens from ulcerative colitis patients, 38 (6%) of whom had colorectal cancer, found that multifocal dysplasia was highly associated with cancer (OR 6.0; 95% CI: 2.5–14.4) [77]. Another large review from Heidelberg, Germany, of 595 colectomy specimens in ulcerative colitis patients, found that high grade dysplasia, low grade dysplasia and backwash ileitis were highly associated with colorectal cancer [78]. Collectively from these studies, both the sensitivity and specificity of testing for any dysplasia are at least 74% (Table 17.3). If high grade dysplasia were to be used as a criterion for a positive test, the sensitivity would fall to about 50% and the specificity would rise to greater than 90%.

Thomas and colleagues have described the risk of colon cancer in patients in whom low grade dysplasia was found [79]. The positive predictive value of low grade dysplasia was calculated to be 18% for the progression to any advanced lesion and 8% specifically for cancer [79]. When low grade dysplasia was the reason for colectomy, colorectal cancer was present in 26% of patients.

Definitions for sensitivity and specificity for surveillance are somewhat different from these definitions for screening. The endpoint of interest in the former situation is death from colon cancer in distinction to its detection alone. Over the course of the disease, patients in a surveillance program will have several colonoscopic examinations with biopsies for dysplasia or cancer. The sensitivity of a surveillance program may be regarded as the proportion of patients with cancer who are successfully treated with colectomy. Those who die from colorectal cancer are false negative patients (group "c" in Table 17.2) in whom surveillance has failed to prevent a cancer-related death. This definition of sensitivity represents a conservative value, since there are patients who had a colectomy for dysplasia in whom cancer would have developed if the colectomy had not been done. Since it is impossible to know which patients with dysplasia would have developed cancer, these patients are not included in the calculations of sensitivity. The specificity of a surveillance program is the proportion of patients who do not develop cancer and who do not have dysplasia detected. Since cancer is rare in a surveillance program, specificity is very well estimated by the proportion of patients in the surveillance program who do not develop dysplasia ([c + d] / n). For the purposes of this review, sensitivity of surveillance is defined as the proportion of patients with cancer who survive following colectomy, and specificity is defined as the proportion of patients without cancer who do not develop dysplasia. Using these definitions, estimates of sensitivity and specificity from 13 large surveillance programs are shown in Table 17.4 [80–92]. Specificity from surveillance is approximately 85%. The estimate of sensitivity is much less stable from study to study due to the low number of cancers in each program, but is for the most part over 50%.

If high grade dysplasia is used as the criterion for a positive test, specificity will increase. The trade-off between specificity and sensitivity is impossible to determine, since patients with low grade dysplasia often are not observed for the development of cancer; rather colectomy or more intensive surveillance is recommended. The increase in specificity with high grade dysplasia rather than low grade dysplasia as the criterion for a positive test is shown in Table 17.5. Specificity using high grade dysplasia as a criterion for a positive test is approximately 96%.

The optimal criterion for a positive test also depends on the consequences of false positive (group "b", Table 17.2) and false negative (group "c", Table 17.2) testing. Patients who have a false positive test have dysplasia but are not destined to develop malignancy. These are the patients who have proctocolectomy without truly needing one. Unfortunately, there is currently no way to predict which patients will fall into this false positive category. In the future, alternative markers of malignancy, such as the presence of p53 suppressor gene mutations, may help in determining which patient with dysplasia is a true positive patient (group "a") and which is a false positive patient (group "b"). Likewise, patients with false negative examinations die of cancer without having proctocolectomy recommended from the detection of dysplasia. In these patients, either the testing interval was too long or the

Table 17.4 The sensitivity and specificity of 13 large colorectal cancer surveillance programs for patients with ulcerative colitis.

Study center	No. of patients	Sensitivity	Specificity
University of Leeds (1980) [80]	43	2/2 (100%)	34/41 (83%)
Cleveland Clinic (1985) [81]	248	6/7 (86%)	194/241 (80%)
University of Chicago (1989) [82]	99	4/8 (50%)	73/91 (80%)
Karolinska Institute (1990) [83]	72	2/2 (100%)	54/70 (77%)
Lahey Clinic (1991) [84]	213	4/10 (40%)	171/203 (84%)
Helsinki University (1991) [85]	66	0/0	57/66 (86%)
Lennox Hill Hospital (1992) [86]	121	4/7 (57%)	91/114 (80%)
St Mark's Hospital (1994) [87]	284	13/17 (76%)	205/267 (77%)
Ornskoldsvik Hospital (1994) [88]	131	2/4 (50%)	103/127 (81%)
Tel Aviv Medical Center (1995) [89]	154	3/4 (75%)	141/150 (94%)
University of Bologna (1995) [90]	65	4/4 (100%)	58/61 (95%)
University of Tokyo (2003) [91]	217	5/5 (100%)	202/212 (95%)
St Marks' Hospital (2006) [92]	600	27/30 (90%)	521/570 (91%)

imperfect specificity of testing (mostly due to the focality of dysplasia) led to a false negative test. A further complicating factor is the recognition that low grade dysplasia has high rates of inter-observer variation even among expert histopathologists [93, 94]. While both false positive and false negative errors are difficult to accept, false negative errors are the more grievous and the category that should be minimized with the most vigor. Therefore, the criterion for a positive test should be the detection of any dysplasia, low grade or high grade, on any biopsy of any examination. Also, since the mortality rate of proctocolectomy is very low, less than 1%, the risk/benefit ratio of opting for surgery in patients with dysplasia against no surgery favors surgical management [95].

Table 17.5 Comparisons of specificity with low grade dysplasia or high grade dysplasia used as the criterion for a positive test in colorectal cancer surveillance from 13 large surveillance programs.

Study center	Specificity using low grade dysplasia as a cut-point	Specificity using high grade dysplasia as a cut-point
University of Leeds (1980) [80]	34/41 (83%)	40/41 (98%)
Cleveland Clinic (1985) [81]	194/241 (80%)	231/241 (96%)
University of Chicago (1989) [82]	73/91 (80%)	87/91 (96%)
Karolinska Institute (1990) [83]	54/70 (77%)	64/70 (91%)
Lahey Clinic (1991) [84]	171/203 (84%)	182/203 (90%)
Helsinki University (1991) [85]	57/66 (86%)	58/66 (88%)
Lennox Hill Hospital (1992) [86]	91/114 (80%)	114/114 (100%)
St Mark's Hospital (1994) [87]	205/267 (77%)	255/267 (96%)
Ornskoldsvik Hospital (1994) [88]	103/127 (81%)	123/127 (97%)
Tel Aviv Medical Center (1995) [89]	141/150 (94%)	144/150 (96%)
University of Bologna(1995) [90]	58/61 (95%)	61/61 (100%)
University of Tokyo (2003) [91]	202/212 (95%)	210/212 (99%)
St Marks' Hospital (2006) [92]	521/570 (91%)	558/570 (98%)

Chemoprevention

A reduced risk of colorectal cancer with mesalamine use in ulcerative colitis has been reported in a recent meta-analysis (OR 0.51; 95% CI: 0.38–0.69) [37]. Mesalamine has low toxicity. **B4** The number needed to treat (NNT) to prevent one death from colorectal cancer may be seven patients with 30 years of disease [96]. Ursodeoxycholic acid, an agent with similarly low toxicity, has been associated with a significantly reduced risk of dysplasia and colorectal cancer in patients with ulcerative colitis and primary sclerosing cholangitis (RR 0.26; p = 0.034) [97, 98]. It is interesting to note that use of statins was associated with a 94% risk reduction for the development of colorectal cancer in a subset analysis of patients in a case-control study of patients with colorectal cancer in Israel [99]. **B3**

Improving cancer surveillance programs in ulcerative colitis

Evidence-based recommendations can be made to improve and optimize cancer surveillance strategies using currently available techniques. Factors related to the disease, the test and the treatment can be optimized based on the above discussion.
• Preferentially test high risk patients, such as patients with pan-ulcerative colitis of at least eight years' duration and patients with primary sclerosing cholangitis, with colonoscopy and extensive biopsy. **C5**
• Patients with lower cancer risk, such as ulcerative colitis patients with left-sided disease, could begin cancer surveillance after 15 years of disease. **C5**
• The risk of cancer in colonic Crohn's disease is similar to that in ulcerative colitis of similar extent and duration [100] and should undergo similar surveillance strategy.
• The testing interval should shorten with increasing duration of disease to maximize the efficiency of a surveillance program. **C5**
• Chromoendoscopy with targeted biopsy of highlighted areas should be undertaken by appropriately trained endoscopists. Alternatively, two to four biopsies should be taken every 10 cm, with additional biopsies of any suspicious areas.

The natural history of the risk of cancer in IBD may well improve with the development of tools to enhance the detection of dysplasia at surveillance colonoscopy.

The criterion for a positive test should optimize sensitivity. A positive test is defined as the presence of any dysplasia on any biopsy on any examination. "Confirmatory" testing is unnecessary. A positive test places the patient at extremely high risk of dying from colorectal cancer and thus necessitates a strong recommendation for proctocolectomy.

References

1 Sackett DL, Whelan G. Cancer risk in ulcerative colitis: Scientific requirements for the study of prognosis. *Gastroenterology* 1980; **78**(6): 1632–1635.
2 Greenstein AJ, Sachar DB, Smith H *et al.* Cancer in universal and left-sided ulcerative colitis: Factors determining risk. *Gastroenterology* 1979; **77**(2): 290–294.

3 Brostrom O, Lofberg R, Nordenvall B, Ost A, Hellers G. The risk of colorectal cancer in ulcerative colitis. An epidemiologic study. *Scand J Gastroenterol* 1987; **22**(10): 1193–1199.

4 Gyde SN, Prior P, Allan RN, *et al.* Colorectal cancer in ulcerative colitis: A cohort study of primary referrals from three centres. *Gut* 1988; **29**(2): 206–217.

5 Gilat T, Fireman Z, Grossman A *et al.* Colorectal cancer in patients with ulcerative colitis. A population study in central Israel. *Gastroenterology* 1988; **94**(4): 870–877.

6 Lashner BA, Kane SV, Hanauer SB. Colon cancer surveillance in chronic ulcerative colitis: Historical cohort study. *Am J Gastroenterol* 1990; **85**(9): 1083–1087.

7 Lennard-Jones JE, Melville DM, Morson BC, Ritchie JK, Williams CB. Precancer and cancer in extensive ulcerative colitis: Findings among 401 patients over 22 years. *Gut* 1990; **31**(7): 800–806.

8 Ekbom A, Helmick C, Zack M, Adami HO. Ulcerative colitis and colorectal cancer. A population-based study. *N Engl J Med* 1990; **323**(18): 1228–1233.

9 Farmer RG, Easley KA, Rankin GB. Clinical patterns, natural history, and progression of ulcerative colitis. A long-term follow-up of 1116 patients. *Dig Dis Sci* 1993; **38**(6): 1137–1146.

10 Lashner BA, Provencher KS, Bozdech JM, Brzezinski A. Worsening risk for the development of dysplasia or cancer in patients with chronic ulcerative colitis. *Am J Gastroenterol* 1995; **90**(3): 377–380.

11 Wandall EP, Damkier P, Moller PF, Wilson B, Schaffalitzky de Muckadell OB. Survival and incidence of colorectal cancer in patients with ulcerative colitis in Funen county diagnosed between 1973 and 1993. *Scand J Gastroenterol* 2000; **35**(3): 312–317.

12 Ishibashi N, Hirota Y, Ikeda M, Hirohata T. Ulcerative colitis and colorectal cancer: A follow-up study in Fukuoka, Japan. *Int J Epidemiol* 1999; **28**(4): 609–613.

13 Broome U, Lindberg G, Lofberg R. Primary sclerosing cholangitis in ulcerative colitis – a risk factor for the development of dysplasia and DNA aneuploidy? *Gastroenterology* 1992; **102**(6): 1877–1880.

14 Gurbuz AK, Giardiello FM, Bayless TM. Colorectal neoplasia in patients with ulcerative colitis and primary sclerosing cholangitis. *Dis Colon Rectum* 1995; **38**(1): 37–41.

15 Broome U, Lofberg R, Veress B, Eriksson LS. Primary sclerosing cholangitis and ulcerative colitis: Evidence for increased neoplastic potential. *Hepatology* 1995; **22**(5): 1404–1408.

16 Brentnall TA, Haggitt RC, Rabinovitch PS *et al.* Risk and natural history of colonic neoplasia in patients with primary sclerosing cholangitis and ulcerative colitis. *Gastroenterology* 1996; **110**(2): 331–338.

17 Loftus EV, Jr., Sandborn WJ, Tremaine WJ, Mahoney DW, Zinsmeister AR, Offord KP *et al.* Risk of colorectal neoplasia in patients with primary sclerosing cholangitis. *Gastroenterology* 1996; **110**(2): 432–440.

18 Marchesa P, Lashner BA, Lavery IC, *et al.* The risk of cancer and dysplasia among ulcerative colitis patients with primary sclerosing cholangitis. *Am J Gastroenterol* 1997; **92**(8): 1285–1288.

19 Shetty K, Rybicki L, Brzezinski A, Carey WD, Lashner BA. The risk for cancer or dysplasia in ulcerative colitis patients with primary sclerosing cholangitis. *Am J Gastroenterol* 1999; **94**(6): 1643–1649.

20 Lindberg BU, Broome U, Persson B. Proximal colorectal dysplasia or cancer in ulcerative colitis. The impact of primary sclerosing cholangitis and sulfasalazine: Results from a 20-year surveillance study. *Dis Colon Rectum* 2001; **44**(1): 77–85.

21 Sackett DL, Hayes RB, Guyatt GH, Tugwell P. *Clinical Epidemiology: A Basic Science for Clinical Medicine*. 2nd edn. Little Brown, Boston, 1991.

22 Lashner BA, Heidenreich PA, Su GL, Kane SV, Hanauer SB. Effect of folate supplementation on the incidence of dysplasia and cancer in chronic ulcerative colitis. A case-control study. *Gastroenterology* 1989; **97**(2): 255–259.

23 Lashner BA. Red blood cell folate is associated with the development of dysplasia and cancer in ulcerative colitis. *J Cancer Res Clin Oncol* 1993; **119**(9): 549–554.

24 Lashner BA, Provencher KS, Seidner DL, Knesebeck A, Brzezinski A. The effect of folic acid supplementation on the risk for cancer or dysplasia in ulcerative colitis. *Gastroenterology* 1997; **112**(1): 29–32.

25 Karlen P, Kornfeld D, Brostrom O, Lofberg R, Persson PG, Ekbom A. Is colonoscopic surveillance reducing colorectal cancer mortality in ulcerative colitis? A population based case control study. *Gut* 1998; **42**(5): 711–714.

26 Eaden J, Abrams K, Ekbom A, Jackson E, Mayberry J. Colorectal cancer prevention in ulcerative colitis: A case-control study. *Aliment Pharmacol Ther* 2000; **14**(2): 145–153.

27 Cole P, Morrison AS. Basic issues in population screening for cancer. *J Natl Cancer Inst* 1980; **64**(5): 1263–1272.

28 Shapiro BD, Lashner BA. Cancer biology in ulcerative colitis and potential use in endoscopic surveillance. *Gastrointest Endosc Clin N Am* 1997; **7**(3): 453–468.

29 Jess T, Riis L, Vind I, *et al.* Changes in clinical characteristics, course, and prognosis of inflammatory bowel disease during the last 5 decades: A population-based study from Copenhagen, Denmark. *Inflamm Bowel Dis* 2007; **13**(4): 481–489.

30 Jess T, Loftus EV, Jr., Velayos FS *et al.* Risk of intestinal cancer in inflammatory bowel disease: A population-based study from olmsted county, Minnesota. *Gastroenterology* 2006; **130**(4): 1039–1046.

31 Winther KV, Jess T, Langholz E, Munkholm P, Binder V. Long-term risk of cancer in ulcerative colitis: A population-based cohort study from Copenhagen County. *Clin Gastroenterol Hepatol* 2004; **2**: 1088–1095.

32 Lakatos L, Mester G, Erdelyi Z *et al.* Risk factors for ulcerative colitis – associated colorectal cancer in a Hungarian cohort of patients with ulcerative colitis: Results of a population-based study. *Inflamm Bowel Dis* 2006; **12**(3): 205–211.

33 Rutter MD, Saunders BP, Wilkinson KH, *et al.* Thirty year analysis of a colonoscopic surveillance program for neoplasia in ulcerative colitis. *Gastroenterology* 2006; **130**: 1030–1038.

34 Byers T, Levin B, Rothenberger D, Dodd GD, Smith RA. American Cancer Society guidelines for screening and surveillance for early detection of colorectal polyps and cancer: Update 1997. American Cancer Society Detection and Treatment Advisory Group on Colorectal Cancer. *CA Cancer J Clin* 1997; **47**(3): 154–160.

35 Jess T, Gamborg M, Matzen P, Munkholm P, Sorensen TI. Increased risk of intestinal cancer in Crohn's disease: A meta-analysis of population-based cohort studies. *Am J Gastroenterol* 2005; **100**(12): 2724–2729.

36 Lakatos L, Mester G, Erdelyi Z, *et al.* Risk factors for ulcerative colitis-associated colorectal cancer in a Hungarian cohort of patients with ulcerative colitis: Results of a population-based study. *Inflamm Bowel Dis* 2006; **12**(3): 205–211.

37 Velayos FS, Terdiman JP, Walsh JM. Effect of 5-aminosalicylate use on colorectal cancer and dysplasia risk: A systematic review and metaanalysis of observational studies. *Am J Gastroenterol* 2005; **100**(6): 1345–1353.

38 Provenzale D, Kowdley KV, Arora S, Wong JB. Prophylactic colectomy or surveillance for chronic ulcerative colitis? A decision analysis. *Gastroenterology* 1995; **109**(4): 1188–1196.

39 Collins PD, Mpofu C, Watson AJ, Rhodes JM. Strategies for detecting colon cancer and/or dysplasia in patients with inflammatory bowel disease. *Cochrane Database of Systematic Reviews* 2006, Issue 2. Art. No.: CD000279. DOI: 10.1002/14651858. CD000279.pub3.

40 Fireman Z, Grossman A, Lilos P *et al.* Intestinal cancer in patients with Crohn's disease. A population study in central Israel. *Scand J Gastroenterol* 1989; **24**(3): 346–350.

41 Rutter MD, Saunders BP, Wilkinson KH, Kamm MA, Williams CB, Forbes A. Most dysplasia in ulcerative colitis is visible at colonoscopy. *Gastrointest Endosc* 2004; **60**: 334–339.

42 Toruner M, Harewood GC, Loftus EV, Jr. *et al.* Endoscopic factors in the diagnosis of colorectal dysplasia in chronic inflammatory bowel disease. *Inflamm Bowel Dis* 2005; **11**(5): 428–434.

43 Kiesslich R, Goetz M, Lammersdorf K, *et al.* Chromoscopy-guided endomicroscopy increases the diagnostic yield of intraepithelial neoplasia in ulcerative colitis. *Gastroenterology* 2007; **132**(3): 874–882.

44 Kiesslich R, Fritsch J, Holtmann M *et al.* Methylene blue-aided chromoendoscopy for the detection of intraepithelial neoplasia and colon cancer in ulcerative colitis. *Gastroenterology* 2003; **124**: 880–888.

45 Hurlstone DP, McAlindon ME, Sanders DS, Koegh R, Lobo AJ, Cross SS. Further validation of high-magnification chromoscopic-colonoscopy for the detection of intraepithelial neoplasia and colon cancer in ulcerative colitis. *Gastroenterology* 2004; **126**: 376–378.

46 Rutter MD, Saunders BP, Schofield G, Forbes A, Price AB, Talbot IC. Pancolonic indigo carmine dye spraying for the detection of dysplasia in ulcerative colitis. *Gut* 2004; **53**: 256–260.

47 Hurlstone DP, Sanders DS, Lobo AJ, McAlindon ME, Cross SS. Indigo carmine-assisted high-magnification chromoscopic colonoscopy for the detection and characterisation of intraepithelial neoplasia in ulcerative colitis: A prospective evaluation. *Endoscopy* 2005; **37**(12): 1186–1192.

48 Rutter MD, Saunders BP, Schofield G, Forbes A, Price AB, Talbot IC. Pancolonic indigo carmine dye spraying for the detection of dysplasia in ulcerative colitis. *Gut* 2004; **53**: 256–260.

49 Kiesslich R, Fritsch J, Holtmann M *et al.* Methylene blue-aided chromoendoscopy for the detection of intraepithelial neoplasia and colon cancer in ulcerative colitis. *Gastroenterology* 2003; **124**: 880–888.

50 Hurlstone DP, Sanders DS, McAlindon ME, Thomson M, Cross SS. High-magnification chromoscopic colonoscopy in ulcerative colitis: A valid tool for *in vivo* optical biopsy and assessment of disease extent. *Endoscopy* 2006; **38**(12): 1213–1217.

51 Kiesslich R, Neurath MF. Surveillance colonoscopy in ulcerative colitis: Magnifying chromoendoscopy in the spotlight. *Gut* 2004; **53**(2): 165–167.

52 Hurlstone DP, Kiesslich R, Thomson M, Atkinson R, Cross SS. Confocal chromoscopic endomicroscopy is superior to chromoscopy alone for the detection and characterisation of intraepithelial neoplasia in chronic ulcerative colitis. *Gut* 2008; **57**(2): 196–204.

53 East JE, Suzuki N, von HA, Saunders BP. Narrow band imaging with magnification for dysplasia detection and pit pattern assessment in ulcerative colitis surveillance: A case with multiple dysplasia associated lesions or masses. *Gut* 2006; **55**(10): 1432–1435.

54 Obrador A, Ginard D, Barranco L. Review article: Colorectal cancer surveillance in ulcerative colitis – what should we be doing? *Aliment Pharmacol Ther* 2006; **24**(Suppl 3): 56–63.

55 Messmann H, Endlicher E, Freunek G, Rummele P, Scholmerich J, Knuchel R. Fluorescence endoscopy for the detection of low and high grade dysplasia in ulcerative colitis using systemic or local 5-aminolaevulinic acid sensitisation. *Gut* 2003; **52**(7): 1003–1007.

56 Ochsenkuhn T, Tillack C, Stepp H *et al.* Low frequency of colorectal dysplasia in patients with long-standing inflammatory bowel disease colitis: Detection by fluorescence endoscopy. *Endoscopy* 2006; **38**(5): 477–482.

57 Blackstone MO, Riddell RH, Rogers BH, Levin B. Dysplasia-associated lesion or mass (DALM) detected by colonoscopy in long-standing ulcerative colitis: An indication for colectomy. *Gastroenterology* 1981; **80**(2): 366–374.

58 Engelsgjerd M, Farraye FA, Odze RD. Polypectomy may be adequate treatment for adenoma-like dysplastic lesions in chronic ulcerative colitis. *Gastroenterology* 1999; **117**: 1288–1294.

59 Rubin PH, Friedman S, Harpaz N *et al.* Colonoscopic polypectomy in chronic colitis: Conservative management after endoscopic resection of dysplastic polyps. *Gastroenterology* 1999; **117**: 1295–1300.

60 Rutter MD, Saunders BP, Wilkinson KH, Kamm MA, Williams CB, Forbes A. Most dysplasia in ulcerative colitis is visible at colonoscopy. *Gastrointest Endosc* 2004; **60**: 334–339.

61 Odze RD, Farraye FA, Hecht JL, Hornick JL. Long-term follow-up after polypectomy treatment for adenoma-like dysplastic lesions in ulcerative colitis. *Clin Gastroenterol Hepatol* 2004; **2**: 534–541.

62 Rutter M, Saunders B, Wilkinson K *et al.* Severity of inflammation is a risk factor for colorectal neoplasia in ulcerative colitis. *Gastroenterology* 2004; **126**(2): 451–459.

63 Velayos FS, Loftus EV, Jr., Jess T *et al.* Predictive and protective factors associated with colorectal cancer in ulcerative colitis: A case-control study. *Gastroenterology* 2006; **130**(7): 1941–1949.

64 Lashner BA, Turner BC, Bostwick DG, Frank PH, Hanauer SB. Dysplasia and cancer complicating strictures in ulcerative colitis. *Dig Dis Sci* 1990; **35**(3): 349–352.

65 Itzkowitz SH. Molecular biology of dysplasia and cancer in inflammatory bowel disease. *Gastroenterol Clin North Am* 2006; **35**(3): 553–571.

66 Brentnall TA. Molecular underpinnings of cancer in ulcerative colitis. *Curr Opin Gastroenterol* 2003; **19**(1): 64–68.

67 Ahlquist DA, Skoletsky JE, Boynton KA *et al*. Colorectal cancer screening by detection of altered human DNA in stool: Feasibility of a multitarget assay panel. *Gastroenterology* 2000; **119**(5): 1219–1227.

68 Tagore KS, Lawson MJ, Yucaitis JA *et al*. Sensitivity and specificity of a stool DNA multitarget assay panel for the detection of advanced colorectal neoplasia. *Clin Colorectal Cancer* 2003; **3**(1): 47–53.

69 Provenzale D, Onken J. Surveillance issues in inflammatory bowel disease: Ulcerative colitis. *J Clin Gastroenterol* 2001; **32**(2): 99–105.

70 Provenzale D, Wong JB, Onken JE, Lipscomb J. Performing a cost-effectiveness analysis: Surveillance of patients with ulcerative colitis. *Am J Gastroenterol* 1998; **93**(6): 872–880.

71 Lashner BA, Hanauer SB, Silverstein MD. Optimal timing of colonoscopy to screen for cancer in ulcerative colitis. *Ann Intern Med* 1988; **108**(2): 274–278.

72 Lashner BA, Shapiro BD, Husain A, Goldblum JR. Evaluation of the usefulness of testing for p53 mutations in colorectal cancer surveillance for ulcerative colitis. *Am J Gastroenterol* 1999; **94**(2): 456–462.

73 Dominitz JA, Eisen GM, Baron TH *et al*. Complications of colonoscopy. *Gastrointest Endosc* 2003; **57**(4): 441–445.

74 Ransohoff DF, Riddell RH, Levin B. Ulcerative colitis and colonic cancer. Problems in assessing the diagnostic usefulness of mucosal dysplasia. *Dis Colon Rectum* 1985; **28**(6): 383–388.

75 Taylor BA, Pemberton JH, Carpenter HA *et al*. Dysplasia in chronic ulcerative colitis: Implications for colonoscopic surveillance. *Dis Colon Rectum* 1992; **35**(10): 950–956.

76 Connell WR, Talbot IC, Harpaz N, Britto N, Wilkinson KH, Kamm MA *et al*. Clinicopathological characteristics of colorectal carcinoma complicating ulcerative colitis. *Gut* 1994; **35**(10): 1419–1423.

77 Gorfine SR, Bauer JJ, Harris MT, Kreel I. Dysplasia complicating chronic ulcerative colitis: Is immediate colectomy warranted? *Dis Colon Rectum* 2000; **43**(11): 1575–1581.

78 Heuschen UA, Hinz U, Allemeyer EH *et al*. Backwash ileitis is strongly associated with colorectal carcinoma in ulcerative colitis. *Gastroenterology* 2001; **120**(4): 841–847.

79 Thomas T, Abrams KA, Robinson RJ, Mayberry JF. Meta-analysis: Cancer risk of low-grade dysplasia in chronic ulcerative colitis. *Aliment Pharmacol Ther* 2007; **25**(6): 657–668.

80 Dickinson RJ, Dixon MF, Axon AT. Colonoscopy and the detection of dysplasia in patients with longstanding ulcerative colitis. *Lancet* 1980; **2**(8195 pt 1): 620–622.

81 Rosenstock E, Farmer RG, Petras R, Sivak MV, Jr., Rankin GB, Sullivan BH. Surveillance for colonic carcinoma in ulcerative colitis. *Gastroenterology* 1985; **89**(6): 1342–1346.

82 Lashner BA, Silverstein MD, Hanauer SB. Hazard rates for dysplasia and cancer in ulcerative colitis. Results from a surveillance program. *Dig Dis Sci* 1989; **34**(10): 1536–1541.

83 Lofberg R, Brostrom O, Karlen P, Tribukait B, Ost A. Colonoscopic surveillance in long-standing total ulcerative colitis – a 15-year follow-up study. *Gastroenterology* 1990; **99**(4): 1021–1031.

84 Nugent FW, Haggitt RC, Gilpin PA. Cancer surveillance in ulcerative colitis. *Gastroenterology* 1991; **100**(5 Pt 1): 1241–1248.

85 Leidenius M, Kellokumpu I, Husa A, Riihela M, Sipponen P. Dysplasia and carcinoma in longstanding ulcerative colitis: An endoscopic and histological surveillance programme. *Gut* 1991; **32**(12): 1521–1525.

86 Woolrich AJ, DaSilva MD, Korelitz BI. Surveillance in the routine management of ulcerative colitis: The predictive value of low-grade dysplasia. *Gastroenterology* 1992; **103**(2): 431–438.

87 Connell WR, Lennard-Jones JE, Williams CB, Talbot IC, Price AB, Wilkinson KH. Factors affecting the outcome of endoscopic surveillance for cancer in ulcerative colitis. *Gastroenterology* 1994; **107**(4): 934–944.

88 Jonsson B, Ahsgren L, Andersson LO, Stenling R, Rutegard J. Colorectal cancer surveillance in patients with ulcerative colitis. *Br J Surg* 1994; **81**(5): 689–691.

89 Rozen P, Baratz M, Fefer F, Gilat T. Low incidence of significant dysplasia in a successful endoscopic surveillance program of patients with ulcerative colitis. *Gastroenterology* 1995; **108**(5): 1361–1370.

90 Biasco G, Brandi G, Paganelli GM *et al*. Colorectal cancer in patients with ulcerative colitis. A prospective cohort study in Italy. *Cancer* 1995; **75**(8): 2045–2050.

91 Hata K, Watanabe T, Kazama S *et al*. Earlier surveillance colonoscopy programme improves survival in patients with ulcerative colitis associated colorectal cancer: Results of a 23-year surveillance programme in the Japanese population. *Br J Cancer* 2003; **89**: 1232–1236.

92 Rutter MD, Saunders BP, Wilkinson KH *et al*. Thirty Year Analysis of a Colonoscopic Surveillance program for Neoplasia in Ulcerative Colitis. *Gastroenterology* 2006; **130**: 1030–1038.

93 Melville DM, Jass JR, Morson BC *et al*. Observer study of the grading of dysplasia in ulcerative colitis: Comparison with clinical outcome. *Hum Pathol* 1989; **20**: 1008–1014.

94 Lim CH, Dixon MF, Vail A, Forman D, Lynch DA, Axon AT. Ten year follow up of ulcerative colitis patients with and without low grade dysplasia. *Gut* 2003; **52**(8): 1127–1132.

95 Fazio VW, Ziv Y, Church JM *et al*. Ileal pouch-anal anastomoses complications and function in 1005 patients. *Ann Surg* 1995; **222**(2): 120–127.

96 Munkholm P, Loftus EV, Jr., Reinacher-Schick A, Kornbluth A, Mittmann U, Esendal B. Prevention of colorectal cancer in inflammatory bowel disease: Value of screening and 5-aminosalicylates. *Digestion* 2006; **73**(1): 11–19.

97 Pardi DS, Loftus EV, Jr., Kremers WK, Keach J, Lindor KD. Ursodeoxycholic acid as a chemopreventive agent in patients with ulcerative colitis and primary sclerosing cholangitis. *Gastroenterology* 2003; **124**(4): 889–893.

98 Tung BY, Emond MJ, Haggitt RC *et al*. Ursodiol use is associated with lower prevalence of colonic neoplasia in patients with ulcerative colitis and primary sclerosing cholangitis. *Ann Intern Med* 2001; **134**: 89–95.

99 Poynter JN, Gruber SB, Higgins PD *et al*. Statins and the risk of colorectal cancer. *N Engl J Med* 2005; **352**(21): 2184–2192.

100 Choi PM, Zelig MP. Similarity of colorectal cancer in Crohn's disease and ulcerative colitis: Implications for carcinogenesis and prevention. *Gut* 1994; **35**(7): 950–954.

Colorectal cancer: Population screening and surveillance

Theodore R Levin[1] and Linda Rabeneck[2]

[1]The Permanente Medical Group, Inc., Walnut Creek, California, USA
[2]University of Toronto, Toronto, Canada

Rules of evidence and feasibility of evidence

The rules of evidence for evaluating studies of treatment interventions are well developed. The randomized controlled trial (RCT) is the scientific gold standard [1]. The prominence of RCT evidence is underscored in a comprehensive guideline that outlined five phases of biomarker development for the early detection of cancer, which described the final phase as "standard parallel-arm randomized clinical trial … with one arm consisting of subjects undergoing the screening protocol and the other arm consisting of unscreened subjects" [2]. However, large-scale RCTs are expensive to conduct and their results may not be available for many years. This is certainly the case for RCTs of colorectal cancer (CRC) screening if CRC mortality is the primary outcome. A good example is the UK Flexible Sigmoidoscopy Trial which compared flexible sigmoidoscopy as an intervention for CRC screening versus usual care, with CRC mortality as the primary outcome. After several years of work, during which the trial was designed, the protocol was developed, funding was obtained, patients were enrolled during 1996–1999. The baseline findings were published in 2002 [3]. The results for the primary outcome, CRC mortality, are not yet available in early 2010. Since the original conception of this trial, CRC screening technology has evolved considerably.

What to do when ideal evidence is lacking

The first US Multi-Society Task Force (USMSTF) guideline states that:

> The authors believe that it might be appropriate in the future to substitute a newer test for currently recommended ones if there is convincing evidence that the new test has: (1) comparable performance (e.g., sensitivity and specificity) in detecting cancers or adenomatous polyps at comparable stages; (2) is equally acceptable to patients; and (3) has comparable or lower complication rates and costs. Provided this is the case, the authors feel that it would not be necessary to submit each new technology to the original standard of proof, i.e. a RCT with death from CRC as the outcome measure [4].

A recently published framework for evaluating diagnostic tests refines this approach by clarifying that the cases detected by the new technology should represent a similar spectrum of disease, so that the evidence of effectiveness applies to these new cases as well as the cases detected by the older technology [5]. It also goes one step further, indicating a role for decision analytic modeling when the new test has both favorable and unfavorable attributes, such as improved sensitivity but reduced specificity. A good example of the use of decision analysis is the most recent US Preventive Services Task Force (USPSTF) recommendations for CRC screening [6], which used microsimulation modeling to help inform the recommendations. As noted by the authors "well-validated microsimulation models may be used to highlight the tradeoff between clinical benefit and resource utilization from different screening policies and inform decision making with standardized comparisons of net benefits and risks" [7]. As new tech-

Evidence-Based Gastroenterology and Hepatology, 3rd edition.
J. McDonald, A.K. Burroughs, B. Feagan, and M.B. Fennerty. © 2010
Blackwell Publishing Ltd

nologies arise that offer trade-offs in performance, acceptability to patients and costs, we have to acknowledge that RCTs with CRC mortality as the primary outcome will not be feasible, and we will need to agree on what constitutes adequate evidence.

Colorectal cancer: an ideal target for prevention and early detection through screening

Colorectal cancer is a common condition, with a pre-malignant lesion (the tubular adenoma) with a long dwell time, making it an ideal target for early detection and cancer prevention through screening. CRC is the second leading cause of cancer death in the USA and the third leading cause of cancer death among both men and women [8]. Over 148,000 people are diagnosed with colorectal cancer in the USA every year, and over 49,000 people die from it [8]. It is generally accepted that detection and removal of polyps at colonoscopy decreases colorectal cancer incidence. **B** The magnitude of that benefit is estimated to be between 76–90% [9]. There are data that show a gradual decline in CRC incidence in the USA since 1985 [10]. This incidence decline is greater for distal CRC than for proximal CRC. Possible explanations for this include: (1) earlier uptake of flexible sigmoidoscopy than colonoscopy for screening; (2) higher effectiveness of polypectomy for cancer prevention in the left than in the right colon due to colonoscopy technique or different polyp morphology; (3) biologic differences between distal and proximal cancers [11].

Screening for colorectal cancer is now widely recommended and screening programs are in place in many countries [12]. A number of randomized trials are also underway that evaluate flexible sigmoidoscopy compared with no screening [3, 13]. These data, coupled with evidence from the randomized trials of fecal occult blood testing [14–18], should provide ample evidence on the overall benefit of screening. As policy makers, clinicians and researchers launch their screening programs, they have to choose a test or strategy to implement, based on the trade-offs of operational demands, patient acceptance, capacity constraints and overall program cost. These decisions are often difficult and are often driven by political or economic issues.

Organized vs opportunistic screening

The International Agency for Research on Cancer (IARC) defines an organized screening program as one that has the following features: (1) an explicit policy with specified age categories, method and interval for screening; (2) a defined target population; (3) a management team respon-

sible for implementation; (4) a health care team for decisions and care; (5) a quality assurance structure; and (6) a method for identifying cancer occurrence in the population [19]. In contrast, opportunistic screening is done outside of an organized screening program, often delivered through fee-for-service reimbursement of physicians. Compared with opportunistic screening, organized screening focuses much greater attention on the quality of the screening process including follow-up of participants [20]. Thus, a key advantage of organized screening is that it provides greater protection against the harms of screening, including over-screening, poor quality and complications of screening, and poor follow-up of those who test positive [20].

A critical appraisal has assessed the evidence for organized cancer screening programs by systematically evaluating the published literature from 1966 to 2002 [21]. The authors reported that although there is a substantial body of literature on organized cancer screening programs, most studies are descriptive, and of those that are evaluative, the focus is on components of the programs, rather than the organized screening programs as a whole. For the relatively few studies that evaluated the effectiveness of organized versus opportunistic screening, most are from the Scandinavian countries and focus on cervix cancer screening. The authors concluded that there is limited evidence to directly support the effectiveness of organized cervix cancer screening and somewhat weaker evidence for other cancers. The promise of organized cancer screening programs is that they achieve better accessibility, quality, accountability and outcomes. In this way, benefits are maximized and harms are reduced. We need further research that compares organized versus opportunistic CRC screening to determine whether organized screening delivers on this promise.

Fecal occult blood testing

Fecal occult blood testing (FOBT) is the only colorectal cancer screening approach demonstrated to be effective in randomized controlled trials. Depending on whether the tests were done biennially or annually, and whether the tests were or were not rehydrated, fecal occult blood testing is associated with a 15–33% reduction in colorectal cancer mortality [14–16, 18], and a 17–20% reduction in colorectal cancer incidence [17]. The randomized trials that provided this evidence were all conducted with the originally available, standard guaiac FOBT (gFOBT), which is still widely used throughout the world. Fecal blood testing, offers the advantage of being non-invasive and convenient for patients. Tests can be sent through the mail directly to patients, samples are collected in the privacy of their homes and can be returned by mail to a central processing laboratory. All of these are advantages for population screening.

Since the publication of those landmark studies, many newer tests for fecal blood have been approved for clinical use. There is evidence demonstrating that fecal immuno-chemical tests (FIT) are more sensitive then standard guaiac tests (GT), such as Hemoccult [22]. There is also evidence from a randomized trial that they are associated with improved adherence to screening, perhaps because they have improved collection devices, and require fewer samples and no dietary restrictions [23]. There is also mounting evidence that FITs have better sensitivity than high sensitivity GTs such as Hemoccult II SENSA, with preserved specificity [24, 25]. Selected FITs offer the option of automated test reading, with resulting improved precision and reliability of the interpretation, and also the possibility to report a quantitative result, but with resultant trade-offs in sensitivity and specificity [26].

Expected sensitivity of FITs

The standard hemoglobin concentration in most studies of FITs has been 100 ng of hemoglobin per ml of stool. At this concentration, results have varied somewhat between settings and depend on the number of samples and the gold standard used to determine the true prevalence of cancer. All studies have evaluated a single application of the FIT, leaving to modeling and speculation about the benefits of screening that accrue to patients who continue to screen in an annual or biennial program of screening. In a preventive health appraisal population from Kaiser Permanente, Allison used the three samples of the HemeSelect FIT and reported that the sensitivity for cancer was 68.8% and specificity for cancer was 94.4% [22]; this study used two-year follow-up for clinical cancer incidence as the gold standard for the presence of cancer. In a large screening colonoscopy cohort from Japan, Morikawa *et al.* reported a sensitivity of 65.8% and specificity of 95.5%, using a single application of the Magstream 1000 test [27]. The highest cancer sensitivity reported to date was 81.8%, with a specificity of 98.1%, using the three samples of the FlexSure OBT FIT and a definition of cancer that was a based on a combination of flexible sigmoidoscopy evaluation for determination of the presence of left-sided colorectal cancers and two years of clinical follow-up for the presence of proximal colorectal cancers [24].

An explicit evaluation of varying the numbers of samples and the target concentration of hemoglobin was performed by Levi *et al.* in a high risk colonoscopy population [26]. Increasing the number of specimens increases the sensitivity for cancer detection from 64.7 to 82.4% to 88.2%, for one, two or three specimens. Specificity declines with the addition of each sample, from 94.3% to 91.9% to 89.7%. Lowering

the hemoglobin cutoff from 100 to 75, increases sensitivity by 0–6%, depending on the number of specimens and decreases specificity by 2% [26].

Studies that have directly compared the sensitive gFOBT (Hemoccult SENSA) to a FIT, in a population large enough to obtain precise point estimates of sensitivity and specificity have been difficult to evaluate. Each study used a different reference standard and a different population. Since the same criterion was applied to both tests in each study, they do provide some evidence of relative sensitivity and specificity. In the one study in which a standard GT (Hemoccult II) was used, both the sensitive gFOBT and the FIT showed improved sensitivity (37.1% for Hemoccult II vs 68.8% for the FIT vs 79.4% for SENSA). The major drawback with sensitive gFOBT has been its much lower specificity (94.4% for the FIT vs 86.7% for the gFOBT) [22].

At the current time, due to heterogeneity in the evidence, it is difficult to say that one FIT is clearly superior [28]. Sensitivity and specificity point estimates have varied across studies due to differences in populations and the criterion standard used to determine the true incidence of cancer. In most recent studies, however, the FIT has performed better than either standard GT or the increased sensitivity GT. In population screening practical considerations such as patient acceptance and reliability of results reporting, become nearly as important as pure test operating characteristics. This was recently demonstrated in Holland, where higher acceptance of FIT resulted in higher neoplasia detection [23]. In mass screening, the automated test processing available with the FIT offers an important advantage of improved test reliability and less risk of repetitive strain injury. The non-invasive, easily scaled option of the FIT is an important option for CRC screening applicable for most population screening programs.

Stool DNA

Tests for deoxyribonucleic acid (DNA) mutations in stool were first described in 1992 [29]. There are two pathways providing targets for fecal screening. Genomic instability is caused by oncogene and tumor suppressor gene mutations, believed to occur in a specific sequence as colonic epithelium progresses through the adenoma–carcinoma sequence [30]. Microsatellite instability may be inherited as mutations in specific genes or acquired through epigenetic DNA methylation, providing an alternative pathway to tumorigenesis, and another target for fecal screening [31]. The initial approach to fecal DNA testing was in the form of a multi-target assay panel, combining detection of mutations in chromosomal instability markers k-ras, p53 and APC with BAT-26 (a marker of microsatellite instability). A DNA integrity assay (long DNA) was added as a generalized marker of escape from apoptosis. The initial report demonstrated sensitivity of 93% for cancer and 87% for adenomas, with a specificity of 93% [32]. Other promising results were reported in several other small studies [33–36].

As evaluation of stool DNA moved from small, single center studies in high risk patients to large, multi-site clinical trials in average risk, asymptomatic screening subjects, sensitivity decreased. The sensitivity of the initial version of the stool DNA test, using 21 mutations in a range of markers (Version 1.0 or SDT-1) has been reported in larger studies to be between 25–52% for cancer and 18–20% for cancers plus advanced adenomas [37, 38]. This decrease in performance occurred for several reasons. The initially selected DNA mutations were not as commonly found among sporadic colorectal cancers and adenomas in a screening population compared to the high risk populations in the earlier studies. In addition, bacterial enzymes in stool digested the DNA during transport to a central testing site. The 21 marker panel is also very expensive to run, leading to a test that is too expensive to be clinically viable.

The testing panel has evolved to a more streamlined set of markers, primarily exploiting the hypermethylation of vimentin as a screening target, and a buffering system to preserve the long DNA marker during transport. In smaller, high risk patient populations, the newer assay (also known as Version 2.0) has demonstrated 86–88% sensitivity and 82–83% specificity for cancer [39, 40]. In the NCI funded screening study, the addition of a methylated vimentin based assay to a k-ras mutation assay combined with a scanning of cluster regions in APC, without the use of the buffer (SDT-2), was reported to be 58% sensitive for cancer alone, and 40% sensitive for cancer plus advanced adenomas [37]. Due to US FDA concerns, neither version 2.0 nor SDT-2 is available. A single marker test, based on hypermethylation of vimentin alone, is available from LabCorp. The performance of the current version of this test for screening patients is not known, and it has not been widely used.

Flexible sigmoidoscopy

Flexible sigmoidoscopy is an endoscopic procedure that examines approximately the lower half of the colon. It may be performed with a variety of endoscopic instruments, including a 60 to 70 cm version of a standard colonoscope, an upper endoscope, a standard pediatric colonoscope or a short (70 cm) pediatric colonoscope. It is typically performed without sedation and a more limited bowel preparation than is used for standard colonoscopy. Since sedation is not required, it can be performed in office based settings and by diverse examiners, including specially trained nurses or physician assistants [41].

Flexible sigmoidoscopy use in the USA has been decreasing in the recent decade. Approximately 2.8 million flexible sigmoidoscopies and 14.2 million colonoscopies were estimated to have been performed in 2002 [42]. Low reimbursement and a shortage of adequately trained examiners are two barriers to flexible sigmoidoscopy availability [43, 44]. In settings where reimbursement has not been a concern, and where nurse endoscopists have been employed, high rates of flexible sigmoidoscopy utilization have been achieved and it continues to be performed [45, 46].

The use of flexible sigmoidoscopy for colorectal cancer screening is supported by high quality case-control and cohort studies. **B2, 3** In general, flexible sigmoidoscopy appears to be associated with a 60% reduction in colorectal cancer mortality for the area of the colon within its reach, and this protective effect appears to persist for 10 years or more [47]. A small randomized trial demonstrated decreased colorectal cancer incidence in the sigmoidoscopy screened group compared to a non-screened control group, but not an overall mortality benefit from screening [48]. There was higher all-cause mortality in the screening group, perhaps due to unbalanced distribution of cardiac risk factors in the two groups, or due to changes in lifestyle behavior after screening [49]. There are four randomized controlled trials ongoing in the USA and Europe [3, 50–52], and results should be reported soon.

The evidence for the diagnostic accuracy of flexible sigmoidoscopy is primarily derived from colonoscopy studies. Flexible sigmoidoscopy is 60–70% as sensitive as colonoscopy for detection of advanced adenomas and cancers in the colon [53, 54]. However, this figure varies according to age, since proximal neoplasia becomes more common after age 65 [55]. Flexible sigmoidoscopy may also be less sensitive in women than in men [56], but the overall prevalence of advanced colonic neoplasia is lower in women than in men [57].

The key limitation in the evidence is the lack of any longitudinal head- to-head comparison of flexible sigmoidoscopy screening with other screening techniques, such as colonoscopy or fecal blood testing. The key question for screening policy is the incremental benefit of colonoscopy over flexible sigmoidoscopy, given the higher direct medical and indirect (patient) costs of colonoscopy and the higher risk of complications with colonoscopy. There is also a lack of evidence on how race, ethnicity, gender or other cultural factors affect patients' perceptions of the optimal screening test.

Several lines of evidence support the idea that the incremental benefit of colonoscopy is less than simply the difference in sensitivity for advanced adenomas between colonoscopy and flexible sigmoidoscopy. A key issue is the rate at which these advanced adenomas progress to invasive and life-threatening colorectal cancers. Proximal and distal colorectal cancers are, generally speaking, biologically different [11], and these biologic differences are known to affect the rate of progression through the adenoma–carcinoma sequence. Colonoscopy follow-up studies, including the National Polyp Study and the recent Manitoba Colonoscopy Study, have found that colorectal cancers that occur shortly after a colonoscopy with or without polypectomy are found disproportionately in the proximal colon [9, 58]. Therefore, published evidence suggests that most of the benefit of colonoscopy for cancer prevention through polyp detection and removal occurs in the distal colon, a region of the colon that is examined by flexible sigmoidoscopy. This feature decreases the risk-benefit advantage of colonoscopy over flexible sigmoidoscopy.

The chief advantage of flexible sigmoidoscopy is that it can be performed without sedation, by a variety of examiners in diverse settings. The absence of sedation is perceived by some patients as an advantage and by others as a disadvantage. The chief limitation of flexible sigmoidoscopy is that it does not examine the entire colon, but only the rectum, sigmoid and descending colon. The complications of flexible sigmoidoscopy include colonic perforation, even if no biopsy or polypectomy is performed, but this complication occurs in fewer than one in 20,000 examinations [3, 59].

The available published evidence supports performing flexible sigmoidoscopy screening at least every 10 years. More frequent examinations may be justified based on patient or provider preference, but there is no evidence to suggest that more frequent examinations will result in improved patient outcomes. Recent colorectal cancer screening guidelines have recommended a five-year interval between normal flexible sigmoidoscopies, while recommending a 10-year interval between colonoscopies [6, 60, 61]. The shorter interval is recommended for flexible sigmoidoscopy out of concern that it may be less sensitive than colonoscopy even in the area examined because of the differences in bowel preparation, the experience of the examiners performing the procedure and the effect that patient discomfort may have on depth of sigmoidoscope insertion and adequacy of mucosal inspection. **C5** The five-year interval also led to improved outcomes at acceptable cost in the USPSTF simulation modeling study [7]. In examinations where an experienced examiner feels comfortable that a well cleansed colon has been thoroughly examined, a 10-year interval between exams may be sufficient.

There may be considerable variation in adenoma detection at flexible sigmoidoscopy between different examiners [62, 63], and this variability may reduce the effectiveness of flexible sigmoidoscopy for colorectal cancer screening. Quality assurance is an important issue for flexible sigmoidoscopists, and has been reviewed in detail elsewhere [41]. Providers should be well trained, and should consider

exceeding the published ASGE standards for a minimum number of training examinations prior to performing sigmoidoscopy without supervision.

An incomplete flexible sigmoidoscopy, defined as a depth of insertion less than 40 cm, is associated with an increased risk for interval colorectal cancers in the time after a flexible sigmoidoscopy [55]. Incomplete examinations should be followed by alternative screening using a different method (annual fecal blood tests, double contrast barium enema or colonoscopy) if the examination was limited by angulation or patient discomfort, or if the colonic preparation was inadequate. **C5**

Ideally, providers performing flexible sigmoidoscopy should be skilled and comfortable taking biopsies, to allow the determination of whether small polyps are adenomas. The decision to follow up a flexible sigmoidoscopy with colonoscopy in patients with 1–2 adenomas smaller than 1 cm should be individualized based on provider and patient preferences, and concern about the risk of complications. In the absence of biopsies, referring all patients with polyps larger than 5 mm for colonoscopy is a reasonably effective management strategy [64]. **C5**

Flexible sigmoidoscopy is an effective, affordable and safe option for colorectal cancer screening. A shortage of adequately trained examiners and low reimbursement has limited its use. For providers who have been able to implement large-scale flexible sigmoidoscopy programs, it has been a feasible and safe test for screening. There are four randomized trials of this intervention currently ongoing, and we should learn significantly more about the performance of this test when the results of these are available.

Radiologic screening

Double contrast barium enema

Double contrast barium enema (DCBE) is endorsed for CRC screening in the current joint guideline from the American Cancer Society, the US Multi-Society Task Force on Colorectal Cancer and the American College of Radiology (ACS/USMSTF/ACR) [60, 61], but not in the current USPSTF guideline [6].

There are no RCTs with CRC mortality as the outcome that have evaluated DCBE for CRC screening. Few studies have compared DCBE with colonoscopy for the rate of dection of polyps in asymptomatic individuals. In the National Polyp Study (NPS), after prior adenoma removal 580 persons underwent 862 paired colonoscopy and DCBE examinations during surveillance. DCBE detected 48% of adenomas >1 cm [65]. Several studies have estimated the sensitivity of DCBE for CRC detection. In a UK national audit of 5454 CRC patients, a sensitivity of 85.9% for CRC detection was reported [66]. In a US study of 485 CRC patients seen at 20 central Indiana hospitals a sensitivity of 85.2% for CRC detection was reported [67]. In a population-based Ontario study of 13,849 persons with CRC who had a prior DCBE, the sensitivity was 77.6% [68]. The range of reported values may be in part due to differences in study populations, study design and methods. However, taken together these findings indicate that the sensitivity of DCBE for the detection of large adenomas and CRC is lower than is the case for colonoscopy or CTC. Given the emergence of CT colonography (CTC) for CRC screening, the role of DCBE will likely continue to diminish.

CT colonography (CTC) or virtual colonoscopy (VC)

CTC for CRC screening is endorsed by the ACS/USMSTF/ACR guideline [60, 61] but not the USPSTF [6]. The evidence to support CTC for CRC screening is indirect, as there are no RCTs that have evaluated the impact of CTC on CRC incidence or CRC mortality. The evidence for CTC is from cross-sectional studies that compare CTC and colonoscopy for the detection of colorectal neoplasia.

Two US studies have compared CTC with colonoscopy screening in asymptomatic adults. Pickhardt *et al.*, in a study of 1233 asymptomatic adults enrolled at three medical centers, reported 94% sensitivity and 96% specificity for detecting adenomas ≥1 cm [69]. The ACRIN study enrolled 2531 asymptomatic adults at 15 centers [70]. ACRIN reported 90% sensitivity and 86% specificity for detecting adenomas ≥1 cm and cancers. The sensitivity and specificity for smaller lesions was lower. In both studies barium and oral contrast tagging and 3D detectors were used. Whether the results of CTC detection for large adenomas can be generalized to community settings is unclear.

Several additional issues regarding CTC remain unresolved. First, the sensitivity and specificity of CTC for lesions <6 mm is low. Some have advocated a policy of not reporting these small lesions, although this is contentious. If these small lesions are reported when detected at CTC, the question is whether these individuals should be advised to undergo colonoscopy, or whether surveillance CTC is appropriate, and if so, at what interval [71]? Second, there is a risk of cancer associated with radiation exposure [72]. Third, there is lack of consensus regarding the reporting of extracolonic lesions detected at CTC and the management of these patients [73, 74]. Taken together, these issues, coupled with the lack of information of CTC performance in community settings, led the USPSTF to exclude CTC from its recommendations [6].

A US cost-effectiveness model that compared clinical and economic outcomes of CTC versus colonoscopy screening reported that even with similar performance, colonoscopy was preferred over CTC unless CTC were to cost significantly less than colonoscopy [75]. Similar findings were reported in a Canadian cost-effectiveness study [76].

Notwithstanding these unresolved issues, based on the endorsement of CTC by the ACS/USMSTF/ACR guideline, CTC screening is likely to increase in the USA and Canada. This is especially true if payers provide physician reimbursement for CTC screening.

A key operational issue with CTC is that if an abnormality is detected and colonoscopy is advised, the patient usually has to repeat the colon preparation and return for colonoscopy on a subsequent day. This will likely present a barrier to patient adherence. Optimizing CTC for CRC screening will likely mean integrating it with an expedited same-day colonoscopy service.

Colonoscopy screening

Evidence

Colonoscopy is endorsed for CRC screening by the ACS/USMSTF/ACR [60, 61] and the USPSTF [6]. The evidence to support this recommendation is indirect as there are no RCTs that have evaluated the impact of screening colonoscopy on CRC mortality. Nonetheless, the body of evidence to support screening colonoscopy is substantial [60, 61]. The evidence includes the role of colonoscopy in the three landmark RCTs that established the evidence for gFOBT screening, as well as the mortality reduction observed in case-control studies of flexible sigmoidosccopy [47]. An additional source of evidence is the National Polyp Study (NPS), a cohort study that demonstrated that patients with adenomas who underwent a baseline clearing colonoscopy had a 76 to 90% reduction in CRC incidence compared with the CRC incidence reported in three reference populations [9]. **B2** Subsequent studies have reported CRC incidence reductions that are smaller in magnitude than that observed in the NPS. For example, a study that combined data from three US adenoma chemoprevention trials, in which patients were followed after undergoing a clearing colonoscopy, reported a three-fold higher incidence of CRC compared with the NPS [77].

We lack evidence concerning the relative effectiveness and incremental benefit of colonoscopy compared with other less invasive screening tests, such as flexible sigmoidoscopy. Recent evidence indicates that in usual clinical practice, colonoscopy is less effective for lesions in the proximal colon. A population-based cohort study of 39,375 individuals of all ages from Manitoba demonstrated that negative colonoscopy was associated with a standardized incidence ratio (SIR) for CRC of 0.28 (95% CI: 0.09–0.65) at 10 years. In that study, the proportion of incident CRCs in the proximal colon was higher in the negative colonoscopy cohort than in the Manitoba population, 47% vs 28%, respectively (p < 0.001) [58]. In an Ontario study of 110,402 individuals with a negative complete colonoscopy, there was a sustained reduction in incident CRC overall and incident distal CRC for up to 14 years following the procedure. In the proximal colon, however, the reduction in incidence differed in magnitude and timing, and was observed in about half of the 14 follow-up years, and for the most part occurred after seven years of follow-up [78]. **B4** An Ontario case-control study reported that colonoscopy was associated with decreased CRC mortality, but this association was primarily due to lower mortality from left-sided cancers [79]. **B3** The estimates of the association of colonoscopy with lower mortality from left-sided CRC are similar to those case-control studies of sigmoidoscopy [47]. Two other studies showed that colonoscopy effectiveness differs for right and left-sided CRC [80, 81]. These case-control studies found that colonoscopy was associated with a much lower incidence of left-sided CRC relative to proximal cancers. **B3** Taken together, these studies provide consistent evidence that colonoscopy is less effective in the right colon.

There are several possible explanations for this finding. One possibility is the unique molecular characteristics that have been observed in proximal lesions. Proximal and distal lesions display differences in gene expression and tumor phenotype [11]. Another possibility is the different morphological characteristics of proximal lesions. For example, flat lesions, which may be more readily missed at colonoscopy, may be more common in the proximal colon [82]. Furthermore, the reduced effectiveness of colonoscopy in the proximal colon may be related to aspects of colonoscopy quality, such as inadequate bowel preparation or failed cecal intubation [83]. Future research should be directed at disentangling the relative contributions of tumor biology and colonoscopy quality in explaining these results. Regardless of their explanation, these results highlight an important limitation of colonoscopy in usual clinical practice.

Quality

Recently, colonoscopy quality has received considerable attention [84–86]. Proposed intraprocedure quality indicators for screening colonoscopy and their targets include: cecal intubation rates >95%; adenoma detection rates >25% for men and >15% for women 50 years and older; mean colonoscope withdrawal times >6 minutes in normal colonoscopies. Standardized colonoscopy reporting systems [87] and public reporting by individual endoscopists have been proposed to facilitate quality improvement [88]. Evidence

to support these indicators includes reports of highly variable adenoma detection rates among endoscopists in practice and an association between higher detection rates and longer colonoscope withdrawal times [89]. Clearly, withdrawal time is a proxy for careful technique. In one large institution, increasing withdrawal time alone had no effect on polyp detection [90]. The colonoscopy quality program in the UK focuses on adenoma detection rates rather than withdrawal time (personal communication: Roland Valori, September 2008).

Tandem colonoscopy studies [91] and studies of CTC followed by colonoscopy [92] report colonoscopy miss rates for adenomas >1 cm of 6–12%. In addition, the colonoscopy miss rate for CRC is about 5%. Evidence to support this estimate includes a retrospective study at 20 Indiana hospitals that reported 47 (5%) of 941 CRC patients who had a colonoscopy within three years prior to their diagnosis of CRC had a reportedly normal colonoscopy [67]. An Ontario population-based cohort study of 12,487 persons with CRC reported a CRC miss rate of 2–6%, depending on cancer site, with right-sided CRC associated with higher (6%) miss rates [93].

A recent study of 1819 (largely) male veterans reported a 9.4% prevalence of non-polypoid (flat and depressed) colorectal neoplasia [94]. The investigators used indigo carmine dye to spray the mucosa to assist in the detection of these lesions at colonoscopy. The implications of this study for usual clinical practice are unclear. Whether this rather high prevalence is generalizable to other populations, whether missing such lesions contributes to missed CRCs, and whether advanced colonoscopy techniques will be required to detect these lesions remain unresolved.

The rates of colonoscopy-associated bleeding, perforation and death have been reported in two population-based studies that used information from administrative databases with validation using chart review. A US study evaluated 16,318 individuals 40 years of age and older who underwent outpatient colonoscopy at Kaiser Permanente of Northern California between January 1994 and July 2002. The rates of colonoscopy-related bleeding and perforation within 30 days following the procedure were 3.2/1000 and 0.9/1000 respectively, and the risk of death was 0.06/1000 or approximately 1/16,000 [95]. A Canadian study evaluated 97,091 persons 50 to 75 years of age who had an outpatient colonoscopy during 2002–2003 [96]. The rates of colonoscopy-related bleeding and perforation requiring hospital admission were 1.64/1000 and 0.85/1000 respectively, and the risk of death was 0.074/1000 or approximately 1/14,000. In both studies older age and having a polypectomy were associated with increased risk of bleeding or perforation. Given the central role of polypectomy in CRC prevention and its strong association with bleeding and perforation, best practice in terms of polypectomy technique needs to be defined [97]. Although colonoscopy-related bleeding and perforation have received the most attention, these do not account for all serious complications of colonoscopy. We currently lack estimates of the risks of other important complications of colonoscopy, such as cardiovascular events, in usual clinical practice.

Costs

The direct cost per patient for a single episode of screening using colonoscopy exceeds the cost for FOBT. In addition, the indirect costs, including time off work for the screened subject and any accompanying caregiver, travel, and out of pocket expenses (e.g. for bowel preparation) are substantial and account for one-third of the total cost of the colonoscopy [98]. The burden of indirect costs may lead to reduced uptake of screening colonoscopy. In addition, the estimated additional cost in the USA of CRC care (screening, diagnosis, complications, treatment) with widespread screening colonoscopy at 75% compliance, was an additional $3.8 billion per year [99].

Capacity

A US simulation study evaluated capacity to provided CRC screening for the 41.8 million US adults who had not been screened in 2002 [100]. The results indicate that sufficient capacity for population screening exists only for FOBT. A screening colonoscopy program would require 10 years to screen the unscreened population because the demand would exceed supply [100]. This result has also been reported by others [101]. These findings provide a strong stimulus for screening approaches that focus constrained colonoscopy resources on those most likely to benefit.

Patient acceptance

Screening colonoscopy requires a motivated patient, given the need for bowel preparation and conscious sedation, as well as the time involved, including time off work. Studies of patient preferences for CRC screening show no consistent preference among screening tests [102–104]. Not all patients will choose to undergo screening colonoscopy when provided with alternatives.

Implementing screening

Cost effectiveness

CRC screening is not only effective, but also cost-effective. In 2002, the USPSTF performed a systematic review of the cost-effectiveness of CRC screening (using gFOBT; FS; gFOBT and FS; DCBE; or colonoscopy) and reported that

compared with no screening, cost-effectiveness ratios for screening with any of these methods were between $10,000 and $25,000 per life-year saved [105]. No particular screening strategy was consistently found to have the best incremental cost-effectiveness ratio. A more recent cost-effectiveness study incorporated new information on costs and test performance of the stool-based CRC tests (gFOBT, FIT, fDNA) and compared these tests with colonoscopy [106]. All three stool-based tests were cost-effective, with gFOBT and FIT preferred if adherence to yearly testing is high, whereas FIT was preferred if adherence is poor. Importantly, the authors note that as the costs of care of patients with colorectal cancer increases because of the use of costly biologic agents, screening with inexpensive gFOBT and FIT may actually be cost saving. A recent decision analysis assessed life-years gained and colonoscopy requirements for several CRC screening strategies [7]. This analysis was done to inform the USPSTF recommendation. CRC screening with colonoscopy every 10 years, annual screening with a sensitive FOBT, or flexible sigmoidoscopy every five years with a midinterval FOBT, for persons age 50 to 75 years, provided similar gains in life-years assuming perfect adherence.

Practical considerations

Although the cost per life-year saved for CRC screening compared with no screening is comparable to other interventions that are currently endorsed, such as breast cancer screening with mammography in women 50 years and older, this is only one aspect to consider in deciding whether to move forward with implementing population-based screening. In an organized screening program funding must be allocated to run the program. In addition, social marketing and health care provider campaigns are needed. Laboratory services and colonoscopy capacity must be in place, as well as treatment capacity. Clear referral pathways must be established. Finally, there must be quality assurance and monitoring and reporting systems [19].

In jurisdictions with publicly funded health care systems, a jurisdiction-wide policy must be in place that defines the target age group, the screening test to be implemented, and the testing interval. In Canada, Ontario was the first province to implement a population-based CRC screening program. In 1999, Cancer Care Ontario (CCO), the provincial agency responsible for cancer, convened an expert panel to develop recommendations for an organized CRC screening program in Ontario. The panel recommended a province-wide gFOBT-based CRC screening program for average-risk individuals 50 to 74 years of age (Ontario Expert Panel on Colorectal Cancer. Colorectal cancer screening: final report of the Ontario Expert Panel. Toronto, Ontario: CCO; 1999.) In 2002, this recommendation was echoed at the national level by a committee convened by Health Canada (National Committee on Colorectal Cancer Screening, Recommendations for population-based colorectal cancer screening, Ottawa, Canada: Public Health Agency of Canada; 2002). A one-year pilot study to evaluate recruitment strategies for gFOBT screening was funded by the Ontario Ministry of Health and Long-Term Care (MOHLTC) in June 2003 (CCO: Ontario FOBT Project Steering Committee. Ontario FOBT project: final report (monograph on the Internet). Toronto, Ontario: CCO; 2006 Mar (cited 2007 Apr 05). Available from: http://cancercare.on.ca/documents/OntarioFOBTProject-FinalReport.pdf). In June 2005 CCO submitted a proposal to the MOHLTC for a provincial population-based CRC screening program. Based on the existing evidence for effectiveness and cost-effectiveness, coupled with the provincial and national consensus on CRC screening policy, and taking into account findings from the Ontario Pilot, the MOHLTC announced funding for the program in January 2007. Implementation began in April 2007. In March 2008 the MOHLTC and Cancer Care Ontario announced the public launch of the program, called ColonCancerCheck. ColonCancerCheck involves gFOBT for average risk individuals and colonoscopy for those at increased risk because of a family history of one or more first-degree relatives with CRC.

Operational challenges are multiple. Stakeholder engagement is crucial, particularly among physicians and their professional societies. This is especially the case when there is skepticism about the choice of screening test and program model. Laboratory professionals must be engaged and committed to quality assurance. In Ontario, CCO developed evidence-based FOBT standards to guide laboratory processing and kit performance [107]. CCO also developed colonoscopy standards [108] to set forth endoscopist, institution and performance standards for colonoscopy. For example, the standards state that endoscopists are required to perform at least 200 colonoscopies per year. Contracts with the laboratories set forth requirements for processing gFOBT kits, quality assurance and reporting to the Program. Funding was provided to 71 public hospitals to deliver additional colonoscopies to support the Program. The contracts with the public hospitals set forth requirements for monthly reporting to the Program of volumes, wait times and performance. The IM/IT system to support monitoring and reporting requirements, as well as letters of invitation to the target population and letters of recall for those with a negative gFOBT is under development.

In the USA, quality report cards for health plans, such as the Healthcare Effectiveness Data and Information Set (HEDIS), provide impetus for health insurers to compete on quality. Using published guidelines as a basis for setting specification, a hybrid of claims data and chart review is used to measure screening rates. Northern California Kaiser Permanente reported that screening rates increased from 37% to 53% between 2005 and 2008, with a rate over 65% expected in 2009. The increase in screening rates has required an unprecedented investment in colonoscopy capacity and organized screening.

Comparing guidelines

In 2008 two high profile, influential US organizations have published colorectal cancer screening guidelines: the American Cancer Society, US Multi-Society Task Force on Colorectal Cancer and American College of Radiology (ACS/USMSTF/ACR) [60, 61], and the US Preventive Services Task Force (USPSTF) (Table 18.1) [6]. The authors took somewhat different approaches, and this resulted in some differences in emphasis and recommendations [109]. The USPSTF undertook a formal, systematic, in-depth evidence review [28], and used simulation modeling when the evidence base was not sufficient to guide recommendations [7]. The ACS/MSTF/ACR process was more driven by expert opinion, when the evidence base was lacking. As a result, the USPSTF is more conservative in its recommendations, emphasizing the balance of risks and harms of screening. In the end, the guidelines are similar with several key differences.

Both guidelines, summarized in Table 18.1 emphasize a menu of options, recognizing that existing evidence and modeling studies do not support one clearly preferred

Table 18.1 Comparison of guidelines for screening persons at average risk for colorectal cancer.

Screening method or variable	ACS-MSTF Recommendation	USPSTF Recommendation
Standard guaiac FOBT (gFOBT)	No	Annually
High sensitivity FOBT (gFOBT or FIT)	Annually	Annually
Flexible sigmoidoscopy alone	Every five years	Every five years
Double contrast barium enema	Every five years	Not recommended
CT colonography	Every five years	Not recommended
Colonoscopy	Every 10 years	Every 10 years
Stool DNA tests	Interval Uncertain	Not recommended
Age to begin screening	50	50
Age to end screening	Not stated	75

screening approach. Both guidelines recommend fecal occult blood testing, done annually in average risk patients. The ACS/MSTF/ACR makes a clear statement in favor of high sensitivity fecal blood tests, either gFOBT or FIT. Both guidelines recommend flexible sigmoidoscopy every five years, and the USPSTF model demonstrates an advantage of the five-year interval over the 10-year interval [7]. Both guidelines recommend colonoscopy every 10 years. The USPSTF explicitly rejects VC, citing inadequate information about the harms of radiation exposure and the problem of extracolonic findings as reasons to be cautious about VC. The ACS/MSTF/ACR included VC, as a screening option to be done every five years, citing the diagnostic accuracy studies demonstrating sensitivity approaching that of colonoscopy for larger polyps. Barium enema and stool DNA are both options on the ACS/MSTF/ACR guideline, but the USPSTF has excluded them due to a lack of evidence supporting their use.

Two other differences between the guidelines bear mentioning, and reflect the process differences between the two groups. The ACS/MSTF/ACR guideline came out with a strong statement in favor of tests that prevent cancer through the early detection and removal of adenomas, including flexible sigmoidoscopy, colonoscopy, virtual colonoscopy and double contrast barium enema [60, 61]. The USPSTF made no such distinction, taking a more firm evidence-based approach. The only evidence for the cancer prevention benefit of colonoscopy comes from the National Polyp Study [9]. A major limitation of that study was the lack of a concurrent control group [110]. In addition, the USPSTF made a firm statement about the age to begin and end screening for CRC screening, based on its simulation model, recommending discontinuing screening after age 75 in people who have had prior screening, or 85 for all patients [6]. Relying on the consensus of expert opinion, the ACS/MSTF/ACR guideline did not comment on a stopping age for screening.

How should the practicing physician handle the discrepancy between guidelines and the challenges with the implementation of a menu of screening options? The best approach is one that is organized, consistent and evidence-based. It is most effective for a group of physicians to decide together on an approach that will work for their setting, based on achievable capacity, patient acceptance, and the balance of risks and benefits. Once that approach has been agreed upon, efforts should be made to ensure that all eligible members of the target population receive the invitation to be screened, and that barriers to patient acceptance are removed, through the development of reminders, tracking systems and ease of appointments. It matters less which test is performed, since there is no clearly dominant strategy. The key issue is that patients receive regular screening at appropriate intervals and with adequate quality control.

References

1 Fletcher RH. Evaluation of interventions. *J Clin Epidemiol* 2002; **55**: 1183–1190.

2 Sullivan Pepe M, Etzioni R, Feng Z et al. Phases of biomarker development for early detection of cancer. *JNCI* 2001; **93**: 1054–1061.

3 UK Flexible Sigmoidoscopy Screening Trial Investigators. Single flexible sigmoidoscopy screening to prevent colorectal cancer: Baseline findings of a UK multicentre randomised trial. *Lancet* 2002 (13 Apr); **359**(9314): 1291–1300.

4 Winawer SJ, Fletcher RH, Miller L et al. Colorectal cancer screening: Clinical guidelines and rationale. *Gastroenterology* 1997 (Feb); **112**(2): 594–642.

5 Lord SJ, Irwig L, Simes RJ. When is measuring sensitivity and specificity sufficient to evaluate a diagnostic test, and when do we need randomized trials? *Annals of Internal Medicine* 2006 (6 Jun); **144**(11): 850–855.

6 US Preventive Services Task Force. Screening for Colorectal Cancer: US Preventive Services Task Force Recommendation Statement. *Annals of Internal Medicine* 2008 (4 Nov); **149**(9): 627–637.

7 Zauber AG, Lansdorp-Vogelaar I, Knudsen AB, Wilschut J, van Ballegooijen M, Kuntz KM. Evaluating test strategies for colorectal cancer screening: A decision analysis for the US Preventive Services Task Force. *Annals of Internal Medicine* 2008 (4 Nov); **149**(9): 659–669.

8 Jemal A, Siegel R, Ward E et al. Cancer Statistics, 2008. *CA: A Cancer Journal for Clinicians* 2008 (1 March); **58**(2): 71–96.

9 Winawer SJ, Zauber AG, Ho MN et al. Prevention of colorectal cancer by colonoscopic polypectomy. The National Polyp Study Workgroup. *The New England Journal of Medicine* 1993 (30 Dec); **329**(27): 1977–1981.

10 Ries L, Melbert D, Krapcho M. *SEER Cancer Statistics Review, 1975–2004*. National Cancer Institute. Bethesda, MD, 2007.

11 Lindblom A. Different mechanisms in the tumorigenesis of proximal and distal colon cancers. *Curr Opin Oncol* 2001; **13**(1): 63–69.

12 Benson VS, Patnick J, Davies AK, Nadel MR, Smith RA, Atkin WS. Colorectal cancer screening: A comparison of 35 initiatives in 17 countries. *International Journal of Cancer* 2008 (15 Mar); **122**(6): 1357–1367.

13 Prorok PC, Andriole GL, Bresalier RS et al. Design of the prostate, lung, colorectal and ovarian (PLCO) cancer screening trial. *Controlled clinical trials*. 2000 (Dec); **21**(6 Suppl): 273S–309S.

14 Hardcastle JD, Chamberlain JO, Robinson MH et al. Randomised controlled trial of faecal-occult-blood screening for colorectal cancer. *Lancet* 1996; **348**(9040): 1472–1477.

15 Kronborg O, Fenger C, Olsen J, Jorgensen OD, Sondergaard O. Randomised study of screening for colorectal cancer with faecal-occult- blood test. *Lancet* 1996; **348**(9040): 1467–1471.

16 Mandel JS, Bond JH, Church TR et al. Reducing mortality from colorectal cancer by screening for fecal occult blood. Minnesota Colon Cancer Control Study. *The New England Journal of Medicine* 1993; **328**(19): 1365–1371.

17 Mandel JS, Church TR, Bond JH et al. The effect of fecal occult-blood screening on the incidence of colorectal cancer. *The New England Journal of Medicine* 2000; **343**(22): 1603–1607.

18 Mandel JS, Church TR, Ederer F, Bond JH. Colorectal cancer mortality: Effectiveness of biennial screening for fecal occult blood. *J Natl Cancer Inst* 1999; **91**(5): 434–437.

19 International Agency for Research on Cancer. Cervix Cancer Screening. *IARC Handbook of Cancer Prevention* 2005; **10**: 117–162.

20 Miles A, Cockburn J, Smith RA, Wardle J. A perspective from countries using organized screening programs. *Cancer* 2004 (1 Sep); **101**(5 Suppl): 1201–1213.

21 Madlensky L, Goel V, Polzer J, Ashbury FD. Assessing the evidence for organised cancer screening programmes. *Eur J Cancer* 2003 (Aug); **39**(12): 1648–1653.

22 Allison JE, Tekawa IS, Ransom LJ, Adrain AL. A comparison of fecal occult-blood tests for colorectal-cancer screening. *The New England Journal of Medicine* 1996 (18 Jan); **334**(3): 155–159.

23 van Rossum LG, van Rijn AF, Laheij RJ *et al*. Random comparison of guaiac and immunochemical fecal occult blood tests for colorectal cancer in a screening population. *Gastroenterology* 2008; **135**(1): 82–90.

24 Allison JE, Sakoda LC, Levin TR *et al*. Screening for colorectal neoplasms with new fecal occult blood tests: Update on performance characteristics. *J Natl Cancer Inst* 2007 (3 Oct); **99**(19): 1462–1470.

25 Smith A, Young GP, Cole SR, Bampton P. Comparison of a brush-sampling fecal immunochemical test for hemoglobin with a sensitive guaiac-based fecal occult blood test in detection of colorectal neoplasia. *Cancer* 2006 (1 Nov); **107**(9): 2152–2159.

26 Levi Z, Rozen P, Hazazi R *et al*. A quantitative immunochemical fecal occult blood test for colorectal neoplasia. *Annals of Internal Medicine* 2007 (20 Feb); **146**(4): 244–255.

27 Morikawa T, Kato J, Yamaji Y, Wada R, Mitsushima T, Shiratori Y. A comparison of the immunochemical fecal occult blood test and total colonoscopy in the asymptomatic population. *Gastroenterology* 2005 (Aug); **129**(2): 422–428.

28 Whitlock EP, Lin JS, Liles E, Beil TL, Fu R. Screening for colorectal cancer: A targeted, updated systematic review for the US Preventive Services Task Force. *Annals of Internal Medicine* 2008 (4 Nov); **149**(9): 638–658.

29 Sidransky D, Tokino T, Hamilton SR *et al*. Identification of ras oncogene mutations in the stool of patients with curable colorectal tumors. *Science* 1992 (3 Apr); **256**(5053): 102–105.

30 Fearon ER, Vogelstein B. A genetic model for colorectal tumorigenesis. *Cell* 1990 (1 Jun); **61**(5): 759–767.

31 Grady WM, Carethers JM. Genomic and epigenetic instability in colorectal cancer pathogenesis. *Gastroenterology* 2008 (Oct); **135**(4): 1079–1099.

32 Ahlquist DA, Skoletsky JE, Boynton KA *et al*. Colorectal cancer screening by detection of altered human DNA in stool: Feasibility of a multitarget assay panel. *Gastroenterology* 2000 (Nov); **119**(5): 1219–1227.

33 Dong SM, Traverso G, Johnson C *et al*. Detecting colorectal cancer in stool with the use of multiple genetic targets. *J Natl Cancer Inst* 2001 (6 Jun); **93**(11): 858–865.

34 Tagore KS, Lawson MJ, Yucaitis JA *et al*. Sensitivity and specificity of a stool DNA multitarget assay panel for the detection of advanced colorectal neoplasia. *Clinical Colorectal Cancer* 2003 (May); **3**(1): 47–53.

35 Traverso G, Shuber A, Levin B *et al*. Detection of APC mutations in fecal DNA from patients with colorectal tumors. *The New England Journal of Medicine* 2002 (31 Jan); **346**(5): 311–320.

36 Traverso G, Shuber A, Olsson L *et al*. Detection of proximal colorectal cancers through analysis of faecal DNA. *Lancet* 2002 (2 Feb); **359**(9304): 403–404.

37 Ahlquist DA, Sargent DJ, Loprinzi CL *et al*. Stool DNA and Occult Blood Testing for Screen Detection of Colorectal Neoplasia. *Annals of Internal Medicine* 2008 (7 Oct); **149**(7): 441–450.

38 Imperiale TF, Ransohoff DF, Itzkowitz SH, Turnbull BA, Ross ME. Fecal DNA versus fecal occult blood for colorectal-cancer screening in an average-risk population. *The New England Journal of Medicine* 2004 (23 Dec); **351**(26): 2704–2714.

39 Itzkowitz S, Brand R, Jandorf L *et al*. A simplified, noninvasive stool DNA test for colorectal cancer detection. *Am J Gastroenterology* 2008 (Nov); **103**(11): 2862–2870.

40 Itzkowitz SH, Jandorf L, Brand R *et al*. Improved fecal DNA test for colorectal cancer screening. *Clin Gastroenterol Hepatol* 2007 (Jan); **5**(1): 111–117.

41 Levin TR, Farraye FA, Schoen RE *et al*. Quality in the technical performance of screening flexible sigmoidoscopy: Recommendations of an international multi-society task group. *Gut* 2005 (Jun); **54**(6): 807–813.

42 Seeff LC, Richards TB, Shapiro JA *et al*. How many endoscopies are performed for colorectal cancer screening? Results from CDC's survey of endoscopic capacity. *Gastroenterology* 2004 (Dec); **127**(6): 1670–1677.

43 Lewis JD, Asch DA. Barriers to office-based screening sigmoidoscopy: Does reimbursement cover costs? *Annals of Internal Medicine* 1999 (16 Mar); **130**(6): 525–530.

44 Tangka FK, Molinari NA, Chattopadhyay SK, Seeff LC. Market for colorectal cancer screening by endoscopy in the United States. *Am J Prev Med* 2005 (Jul); **29**(1): 54–60.

45 Palitz AM, Selby JV, Grossman S *et al*. *The Colon Cancer Prevention Program (CoCaP): Rationale, Implementation, and Preliminary Results*. HMO practice/HMO Group. 1997 (Mar); **11**(1): 5–12.

46 Shapero TF, Hoover J, Paszat LF *et al*. Colorectal cancer screening with nurse-performed flexible sigmoidoscopy: Results from a Canadian community-based program. *Gastrointestinal Endoscopy* 2007 (Apr); **65**(4): 640–645.

47 Selby JV, Friedman GD, Quesenberry CP, Jr, Weiss NS. A case-control study of screening sigmoidoscopy and mortality from colorectal cancer. *The New England Journal of Medicine* 1992 (5 Mar); **326**(10): 653–657.

48 Thiis-Evensen E, Hoff GS, Sauar J, Langmark F, Majak BM, Vatn MH. Population-based surveillance by colonoscopy: Effect on the incidence of colorectal cancer. Telemark Polyp Study I. *Scand J Gastroenterol* 1999 (Apr); **34**(4): 414–420.

49 Hoff G, Thiis-Evensen E, Grotmol T, Sauar J, Vatn MH, Moen IE. Do undesirable effects of screening affect all-cause mortality in flexible sigmoidoscopy programmes? Experience from the Telemark Polyp Study 1983–1996. *Eur J Cancer Prev* 2001 (Apr); **10**(2): 131–137.

50 Segnan N, Senore C, Andreoni B *et al*. Baseline findings of the Italian multicenter randomized controlled trial of "once-only sigmoidoscopy" – SCORE. *J Natl Cancer Inst* 2002 (4 Dec); **94**(23): 1763–1772.

51 Weissfeld JL, Schoen RE, Pinsky PF *et al*. Flexible sigmoidoscopy in the PLCO cancer screening trial: Results from the base-

line screening examination of a randomized trial. *J Natl Cancer Inst* 2005 (6 Jul); **97**(13): 989–997.

52 Gondal G, Grotmol T, Hofstad B, Bretthauer M, Eide TJ, Hoff G. The Norwegian Colorectal Cancer Prevention (NORCCAP) screening study: Baseline findings and implementations for clinical work-up in age groups 50–64 years. *Scand J Gastroenterol* 2003 (Jun); **38**(6): 635–642.

53 Lieberman DA, Weiss DG, Bond JH, Ahnen DJ, Garewal H, Chejfec G. Use of colonoscopy to screen asymptomatic adults for colorectal cancer. Veterans Affairs Cooperative Study Group 380. *The New England Journal of Medicine* 2000 (20 Jul); **343**(3): 162–168.

54 Imperiale TF, Wagner DR, Lin CY, Larkin GN, Rogge JD, Ransohoff DF. Risk of advanced proximal neoplasms in asymptomatic adults according to the distal colorectal findings. *The New England Journal of Medicine* 2000 (20 Jul); **343**(3): 169–174.

55 Doria-Rose VP, Newcomb PA, Levin TR. Incomplete screening flexible sigmoidoscopy associated with female sex, age, and increased risk of colorectal cancer. *Gut* 2005 (Sep); **54**(9): 1273–1278.

56 Schoenfeld P, Cash B, Flood A *et al.* Colonoscopic screening of average-risk women for colorectal neoplasia. *The New England Journal of Medicine* 2005 (19 May); **352**(20): 2061–2068.

57 Regula J, Rupinski M, Kraszewska E *et al.* Colonoscopy in colorectal-cancer screening for detection of advanced neoplasia. *The New England Journal of Medicine* 2006 (2 Nov); **355**(18): 1863–1872.

58 Singh H, Turner D, Xue L, Targownik LE, Bernstein CN. Risk of developing colorectal cancer following a negative colonoscopy examination: Evidence for a 10-year interval between colonoscopies. *Jama* 2006 (24 May); **295**(20): 2366–2373.

59 Levin TR, Conell C, Shapiro JA, Chazan SG, Nadel MR, Selby JV. Complications of screening flexible sigmoidoscopy. *Gastroenterology* 2002 (Dec); **123**(6): 1786–1792.

60 Levin B, Lieberman DA, McFarland B *et al.* Screening and surveillance for the early detection of colorectal cancer and adenomatous polyps, 2008: A joint guideline from the American Cancer Society, the US Multi-Society Task Force on Colorectal Cancer, and the American College of Radiology. *Gastroenterology* 2008 (May); **134**(5): 1570–1595.

61 Levin B, Lieberman DA, McFarland B *et al.* Screening and surveillance for the early detection of colorectal cancer and adenomatous polyps, 2008: A joint guideline from the American Cancer Society, the US Multi-Society Task Force on Colorectal Cancer, and the American College of Radiology. *CA: A Cancer Journal for Clinicians* 2008 (May-Jun); **58**(3): 130–160.

62 Atkin W, Rogers P, Cardwell C *et al.* Wide variation in adenoma detection rates at screening flexible sigmoidoscopy. *Gastroenterology* 2004 May; **1247–26**(5): 11256.

63 Pinsky PF, Schoen RE, Weissfeld JL, Kramer B, Hayes RB, Yokochi L. Variability in flexible sigmoidoscopy performance among examiners in a screening trial. *Clin Gastroenterol Hepatol* 2005 (Aug); **3**(8): 792–797.

64 Schoen RE, Weissfeld JL, Pinsky PF, Riley T. Yield of advanced adenoma and cancer based on polyp size detected at screening flexible sigmoidoscopy. *Gastroenterology* 2006 (Dec); **131**(6): 1683–1689.

65 Winawer SJ, Stewart ET, Zauber AG *et al.* A comparison of colonoscopy and double-contrast barium enema for surveillance after polypectomy. National Polyp Study Work Group. *The New England Journal of Medicine* 2000 (15 Jun); **342**(24): 1766–1772.

66 Tawn DJ, Squire CJ, Mohammed MA, Adam EJ. National audit of the sensitivity of double-contrast barium enema for colorectal carcinoma, using control charts. For the Royal College of Radiologists Clinical Radiology Audit Sub-Committee. *Clinical radiology* 2005 (May); **60**(5): 558–564.

67 Rex DK, Rahmani EY, Haseman JH, Lemmel GT, Kaster S, Buckley JS. Relative sensitivity of colonoscopy and barium enema for detection of colorectal cancer in clinical practice. *Gastroenterology* 1997 (Jan); **112**(1): 17–23.

68 Toma J, Paszat LF, Gunraj N, Rabeneck L. Rates of new or missed colorectal cancer after barium enema and their risk factors: A population-based study. *The American Journal of Gastroenterology* 2008; **103**(12): 3142–3148.

69 Pickhardt PJ, Choi JR, Hwang I *et al.* Computed tomographic virtual colonoscopy to screen for colorectal neoplasia in asymptomatic adults. *The New England Journal of Medicine* 2003 (4 Dec); **349**(23): 2191–2200.

70 Johnson CD, Chen MH, Toledano AY *et al.* Accuracy of CT colonography for detection of large adenomas and cancers. *The New England Journal of Medicine* 2008 (18 Sep); **359**(12): 1207–1217.

71 Rex DK, Ransohoff DF, Achkar E. Debate: Colonoscopy is justified for any polyp discovered during computed tomographic colonography. *The American Journal of Gastroenterology* 2005; **100**: 1903–1908.

72 Brenner DJ, Hall EJ. Computed tomography – an increasing source of radiation exposure. *The New England Journal of Medicine* 2007 (29 Nov); **357**(22): 2277–2284.

73 Edwards JT, Wood CJ, Mendelson RM, Forbes GM. Extracolonic findings at virtual colonoscopy: Implications for screening programs. *The American Journal of Gastroenterology* 2001 (Oct); **96**(10): 3009–3012.

74 Fletcher RH, Pignone M. Extracolonic findings with computed tomographic colonography: Asset or liability? *Archives of Internal Medicine* 2008 (14 Apr); **168**(7): 685–686.

75 Ladabaum U, Song K, Fendrick AM. Colorectal neoplasia screening with virtual colonoscopy: When, at what cost, and with what national impact? *Clin Gastroenterol Hepatol* 2004 (Jul); **2**(7): 554–563.

76 Heitman SJ, Manns BJ, Hilsden RJ, Fong A, Dean S, Romagnuolo J. Cost-effectiveness of computerized tomographic colonography versus colonoscopy for colorectal cancer screening. *CMAJ* 2005 (11 Oct); **173**(8): 877–881.

77 Robertson DJ, Greenberg ER, Beach M *et al.* Colorectal cancer in patients under close colonoscopic surveillance. *Gastroenterology* 2005 (Jul); **129**(1): 34–41.

78 Lakoff J, Paszat LF, Saskin R, Rabeneck L. Risk of developing proximal versus distal colorectal cancer after a negative colonoscopy: A population-based study. *Clin Gastroenterol Hepatol* 2008 (Oct); **6**(10): 1117–1121, quiz 064.

79 Baxter NN, Goldwasser MA, Paszat LF, Saskin R, Urbach DR, Rabeneck L. Association of colonoscopy and death from colorectal cancer: A population-based, case-control study. *Annals of Internal Medicine.* 2009 **150**: 1–8.

80 Singh G, Mannalithara A, Wang HJ, Graham DJ, Gerson LB, Triadafilopoulos G. Is protection against colorectal cancer good

enough: A comparison between sigmoidoscopy and colonoscopy in the general population. *Gastroenterology* 2007; **132**(Suppl 2): A81.

81 Brenner H, Chang-Claude J, Seiler CM, Sturmer T, Hoffmeister M. Potential for colorectal cancer prevention of sigmoidoscopy versus colonoscopy: Population-based case control study. *Cancer Epidemiol Biomarkers Prev* 2007 (Mar); **16**(3): 494–499.

82 East JE, Suzuki N, Stavrinidis M, Guenther T, Thomas HJW, Saunders BP. Narrow band imaging for colonoscopic surveillance in hereditary non-polyposis colorectal cancer. *Gut* 2008 (1 Jan); **57**(1): 65–70.

83 Rex DK, Eid E. Considerations regarding the present and future roles of colonoscopy in colorectal cancer prevention. *Clin Gastroenterol Hepatol* 2008 (May); **6**(5): 506–514.

84 Rex DK, Bond JH, Winawer S *et al.* Quality in the technical performance of colonoscopy and the continuous quality improvement process for colonoscopy: Recommendations of the US Multi-Society Task Force on Colorectal Cancer. *The American Journal of Gastroenterology* 2002 (Jun); **97**(6): 1296–1308.

85 Rex DK, Petrini JL, Baron TH *et al.* Quality indicators for colonoscopy. *The American Journal of Gastroenterology* 2006 (Apr); **101**(4): 873–885.

86 Rex DK, Petrini JL, Baron TH *et al.* Quality indicators for colonoscopy. *Gastrointestinal Endoscopy* 2006 (Apr); **63**(4 Suppl): S16–S28.

87 Lieberman D, Nadel M, Smith RA *et al.* Standardized colonoscopy reporting and data system: Report of the Quality Assurance Task Group of the National Colorectal Cancer Roundtable. *Gastrointestinal Endoscopy* 2007 (May); **65**(6): 757–766.

88 Cotton PB, Connor P, McGee D *et al.* Colonoscopy: Practice variation among 69 hospital-based endoscopists. *Gastrointestinal Endoscopy* 2003 (Mar); **57**(3): 352–357.

89 Barclay RL, Vicari JJ, Doughty AS, Johanson JF, Greenlaw RL. Colonoscopic withdrawal times and adenoma detection during screening colonoscopy. *The New England Journal of Medicine.* 2006 (14 Dec); **355**(24): 2533–2541.

90 Sawhney MS, Cury MS, Neeman N *et al.* Effect of institution-wide policy of colonoscopy withdrawal time >=7 minutes on polyp detection. *Gastroenterology* 2008 (Dec); **135**(6): 1892–1898.

91 Rex DK, Cutler CS, Lemmel GT *et al.* Colonoscopic miss rates of adenomas determined by back-to-back colonoscopies. *Gastroenterology* 1997 (Jan); **112**(1): 24–28.

92 Pickhardt PJ, Nugent PA, Mysliwiec PA, Choi JR, Schindler WR. Location of adenomas missed by optical colonoscopy. *Annals of Internal Medicine* 2004 (7 Sep); **141**(5): 352–359.

93 Bressler G, Paszat LF, Chen Z *et al.* Rate of new or missed colorectal cancers after colonoscopy and their risk factors: A population-based analysis. *Gastroenterology* 2007; **132**: 96–102.

94 Soetikno RM, Kaltenbach T, Rouse RV *et al.* Prevalence of non-polypoid (flat and depressed) colorectal neoplasms in asymptomatic and symptomatic adults. *Jama* 2008 (5 Mar); **299**(9): 1027–1035.

95 Levin TR, Zhao W, Conell C *et al.* Complications of colonoscopy in an integrated health care delivery system. *Annals of Internal Medicine* 2006 (19 Dec); **145**(12): 880–886.

96 Rabeneck L, Paszat LF, Hilsden RJ *et al.* Bleeding and perforation after outpatient colonoscopy and their risk factors in usual clinical practice. *Gastroenterology* 2008 (Dec); **135**(6): 1899–1906 e1.

97 Rex DK. Have we defined best colonoscopic polypectomy practice in the United States? *Clin Gastroenterol Hepatol* 2007 (Jun); **5**(6): 674–677.

98 Heitman SJ, Au F, Manns BJ, McGregor SE, Hilsden RJ. Nonmedical costs of colorectal cancer screening with the fecal occult blood test and colonoscopy. *Clin Gastroenterol Hepatol* 2008 (Aug); **6**(8): 912–927 e1.

99 Ladabaum U, Song K. Projected national impact of colorectal cancer screening on clinical and economic outcomes and health services demand. *Gastroenterology* 2005 (Oct); **129**(4): 1151–1162.

100 Seeff LC, Manninen DL, Dong FB *et al.* Is there endoscopic capacity to provide colorectal cancer screening to the unscreened population in the United States? *Gastroenterology* 2004 (Dec); **127**(6): 1661–1669.

101 Vijan S, Inadomi J, Hayward RA, Hofer TP, Fendrick AM. Projections of demand and capacity for colonoscopy related to increasing rates of colorectal cancer screening in the United States. *Aliment Pharmacol Ther* 2004 (1 Sep); **20**(5): 507–515.

102 DeBourcy AC, Lichtenberger S, Felton S, Butterfield KT, Ahnen DJ, Denberg TD. Community-based preferences for stool cards versus colonoscopy in colorectal cancer screening. *J Gen Intern Med* 2008 (Feb); **23**(2): 169–174.

103 Hawley ST, Volk RJ, Krishnamurthy P, Jibaja-Weiss M, Vernon SW, Kneuper S. Preferences for colorectal cancer screening among racially/ethnically diverse primary care patients. *Medical Care* 2008 (Sep); **46**(9 Suppl 1): S10–S16.

104 Schroy PC, 3rd, Lal S, Glick JT, Robinson PA, Zamor P, Heeren TC. Patient preferences for colorectal cancer screening: How does stool DNA testing fare? *The American Journal of Managed Care.* 2007 (Jul); **13**(7): 393–400.

105 Pignone M, Saha S, Hoerger T, Mandelblatt J. Cost-effectiveness analyses of colorectal cancer screening: A systematic review for the US Preventive Services Task Force. *Annals of Internal Medicine* 2002 (16 Jul); **137**(2): 96–104.

106 Parekh M, Fendrick AM, Ladabaum U. As tests evolve and costs of cancer care rise: Reappraising stool-based screening for colorectal neoplasia. *Aliment Pharmacol Ther* 2008 (Apr); **27**(8): 697–712.

107 Rabeneck L, Zwaal C, Goodman JH, Mai V, Zamkanei M. Cancer Care Ontario guaiac fecal occult blood test (FOBT) laboratory standards: Evidentiary base and recommendations. *Clinical Biochemistry* 2008 (Nov); **41**(16–17): 1289–1305.

108 Rabeneck L, Rumble RB, Axler J *et al.* Cancer Care Ontario Colonoscopy Standards: Standards and evidentiary base. *Canadian journal of Gastroenterology* 2007 (Nov); **21**(Suppl D): 5D–24D.

109 Pignone M, Sox HC. Screening guidelines for colorectal cancer: A twice-told tale. *Annals of Internal Medicine* 2008 (4 Nov); **149**(9): 680–682.

110 Ransohoff DF. How much does colonoscopy reduce colon cancer mortality? *Annals of Internal Medicine* 2009 **150**: 50–52.

19 Prevention and treatment of travelers' diarrhea

Herbert L DuPont

Center for Infectious Disease, University of Texas Health Science Center at Houston, School of Public Health *and* Internal Medical Service, St. Luke's Episcopal Hospital, Department of Medicine, Baylor College of Medicine, Houston, USA

Background

The first studies of travelers' diarrhea were carried out in the 1950s and 1960s by Kean and colleagues [1]. Kean's research team found that antibiotic drugs would successfully prevent TD during high-risk travel. Despite more than 50 years of research aimed at defining the cause and source of the causative agents we have seen no reduction in frequency of TD among persons venturing into tropical and semi-tropical areas from industrialized countries [1–3]. Following studies defining the importance of bacterial enteropathogens in TD, it was shown that antibacterial drugs could shorten the illness [4]. Recent studies have provided evidence that TD not only produces a full day of disability when it occurs but an important number of affected persons develop chronic functional bowel disease as a complication of TD.

This review looks at the available scientific evidence supporting the use of drugs and vaccines to prevent TD and therapies, new and old, aimed at shortening the duration of illness when it develops.

Epidemiology of travelers' diarrhea

The world can be divided into three regions depending upon the rate of TD among visitors from industrialized countries (Figure 19.1). The high-risk regions of the world for TD are Latin America, Africa and Southern Asia, the moderate-risk regions are certain Caribbean islands (e.g. Jamaica), the Middle East, China, Thailand and Russia and the low-risk areas are the United States, Canada, north-

western Europe, Japan, New Zealand and Australia. The rate of diarrhea when people from low-risk areas visit the three regions are 40% [5, 6], 8–15% [6, 7] and ~4% [6], respectively. The 4% for groups moving from one low-risk area to another, is approximately the same as is seen when people from a high-risk area visits a low-risk region [8, 9]. Why diarrhea develops among people traveling to low-risk areas probably relates to multiple factors, including eating all meals at public restaurants with its increased risks of enteric infection compared with self-preparation of meals in homes [10], increased stress leading to autonomic intestinal motility alterations [11], and possibly excessive alcohol ingestion in a subset of travelers [12].

Etiology of travelers' diarrhea

Studies in the 1970s identified enerotoxigenic *Escherichia coli* (ETEC) as the principal cause of TD [13–16]. In the last two decades enteroaggregative *E. coli* (EAEC) [17] and a variety of other bacteria [18] have been shown to be important causes of TD. The diarrheagenic *E. coli* (ETEC and EAEC) cause a majority of the diarrhea in Latin America [3, 18, 19] and Africa [20, 21]. While ETEC and EAEC are important causes of TD in Asia [18, 22, 23] other bacteria are important, including *Shigella*, *Campylobacter*, *Salmonella* and *Aeromonas* spp. [18, 22, 24–26]. The fact that invasive enteropathogens are relatively more important causes of TD in Asia influences recommendations on self-treatment for travel to these countries. Noroviruses explain between 10%–20% of cases of TD [27].

Evidence-base evaluation

Guidelines used to establish the evidence base for evaluating evidence of efficacy of drugs and vaccines are outlined in Table 19.1.

Evidence-Based Gastroenterology and Hepatology, 3rd edition. J. McDonald, A.K. Burroughs, B. Feagan, and M.B. Fennerty. © 2010 Blackwell Publishing Ltd

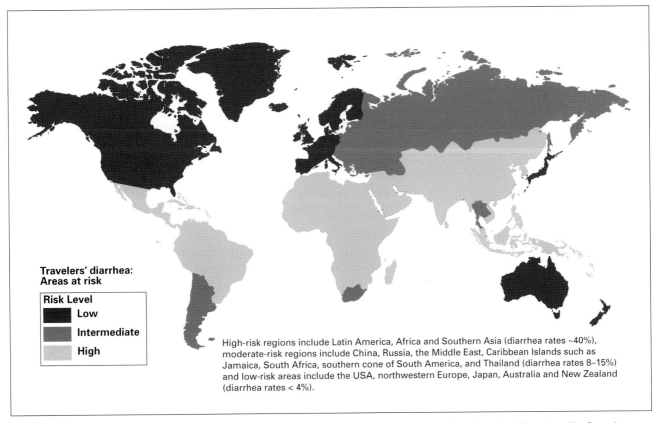

Travelers' diarrhea: Areas at risk

Risk Level
- Low
- Intermediate
- High

High-risk regions include Latin America, Africa and Southern Asia (diarrhea rates ~40%), moderate-risk regions include China, Russia, the Middle East, Caribbean Islands such as Jamaica, South Africa, southern cone of South America, and Thailand (diarrhea rates 8–15%) and low-risk areas include the USA, northwestern Europe, Japan, Australia and New Zealand (diarrhea rates < 4%).

Figure 19.1 World map showing variation in risk of acquiring travelers' diarrhea among international visitors from low-risk regions. The figure is reprinted with permission from *Aliment Pharmacol Ther* [95].

Table 19.1 Grading of clinical evidence in the chemoprevention and chemotherapy of travelers' diarrhea [80].

Category	Grade	Definition
Strength of evidence	A	Good evidence to support a recommendation for use
	B	Moderate evidence to support a recommendation for use
	C	Poor evidence to support a recommendation
	D	Moderate evidence to support a recommendation against use
	E	Good evidence to support a recommendation against use
Quality of evidence	I	Evidence from ≥1 properly randomized, controlled trial
	II	Evidence from ≥1 well-designed clinical trial without randomization, from case-controlled analysis of cohort study
	III	Consensus evidence, evidence from one authority or reports of expert committees

Prevention of travelers' diarrhea

Given the high risk of acquiring TD and the importance of bacterial enteropathogens it is easy to see why there is such an active interest in preventing the illness through chemo or immune-prophylaxis.

Historical considerations

The first evidence that bacterial enteropathogens were responsible for TD was provided by Kean and colleagues, showing the value of antibiotics in preventing the disease [1]. Prophylactic use of antibiotics during international travel in the 1950s was widely practiced. A study carried out in 1957 demonstrated that more than 35% of persons returning to the USA from Mexico were taking prophylactic antibiotics to prevent diarrhea during their trip [28]. During the 1968 Olympic Games in Mexico City, the British team credited taking multiple doses of oral sulfonamides and oral streptomycin for keeping them well during competition; the American. and Australian teams had higher rates of diarrhea, probably because they relied upon a single daily dose of sulfonamide for protection [29].

Bradley and David Sack from Johns Hopkins then demonstrated the value of doxycycline in preventing TD [30, 31] until resistance to the drug prevented further evaluation [32]. In the 1980s studies were conducted showing the effectiveness of liquid [33] or tablet formulation [34] of bismuth subsalicylate (BSS) in preventing TD. BSS was safely given to the trial participants, with only darkening of stools and tongues from harmless bismuth sulfide, and mild tinnitus, presumably from the absorbed salicylate, as adverse effects. The drug was more effective when it was taken in a total dose of 2.1 g/d in four equally divided doses than when it was taken in a similar daily dose on a twice a day regimen, or in half of this dose four times a day [35].

Trimethoprim/sulfamethoxazole was shown to prevent TD in studies carried out in the 1980s [36]. Also, in the 1980s and 1990s, a number of trials established the value of the fluoroquinolones in preventing TD [37–40]. General use of antibiotics for chemoprophylaxis during travel was largely stopped by a Consensus Development Conference held at the National Institutes of Health in 1985 [41], because of concern about adverse effects, and the stimulation of resistance by widespread use of systemically absorbed antibiotics and also because of the difficulty in identifying appropriate recipients of preventive drugs.

The concept became of interest once more with the availability of non-absorbed (<0.4%) rifaximin. This antibacterial preparation had no obvious safety issues, as seen in the clinical trials, and the non-absorbed nature of the drug reduced the concerns about systemic side effects and development of resistance among extra-intestinal bacteria. Rifaximin was shown to be effective in preventing TD in two studies in Mexico, in 2003 [3] and 2005 [42]. A third trial was carried out in Thailand, but the frequency of TD was too low to permit evaluation of the efficacy of the drug (Steffen R, unpublished data).

Immunoprophylaxis

After World War II it was found that rates of diarrhea in people became lower as they lived in high risk areas [43]. This immunity was shown to occur over several months in American students attending classes in Mexico [2]. The natural immunity that developed in these students was associated with reduced rates of ETEC diarrhea [14, 44]. Not surprisingly the first successful TD vaccine was directed toward prevention of ETEC. The first licensed vaccine, developed by the Swedish Biological Laboratories, consisted of a combination of whole cell *Vibrio cholerae* strains together with a recombinant form of the binding subunit of cholera toxin. The vaccine Dukoral provided short-term protection against ETEC [45] because of the similarity of the binding subunit of cholera toxin with the

binding subunit of heat labile enterotoxin (LT) of ETEC. This vaccine was shown to prevent TD [46] and is presently available commercially as an ETEC and cholera vaccine throughout Europe and Canada.

Following studies demonstrated the feasibility of developing a brisk IgG antibody response to transcutaneously administered ETEC LT [47] when a randomized, placebo-controlled trial was carried out in which the antigen or placebo was administered twice by skin patch to approximately 200 adults before travel to Mexico and Guatemala [48]. In this trial, the observed rates of moderate to severe diarrhea were: placebo 21%, LT patch, 5%, p = 0.007. A larger phase III study was planned for 2009.

Effectiveness of chemoprophylaxis and immunoprophylaxis in the prevention of TD

In Table 19.2 the strength of evidence for the various preventive drugs and vaccines is provided. BSS, fluoroquinolones and rifaximin are labeled as A1 to indicate the existence of good evidence for efficacy in preventing TD, with at least one well designed randomized controlled clinical trial having been performed.

Current practice and recommendations

In Figure 19.2, an algorithm is provided that outlines one approach to identifying persons who might be candidates for chemoprophylaxis during high-risk travel. If persons stay in better hotels, eat at hotel restaurants and exercise care on what foods and beverages are consumed, the need to use active prevention methods is lessened. Chemoprophylaxis is appropriate to offer to persons with underlying medical conditions that may be complicated by a diarrheal illness [5, 49], persons for whom an 8–10 hour illness could jeopardize the purpose of an important trip such as athletes during competition, politicians and business travelers with important meetings, musicians and certain tourists with a carefully planned itinerary [49], persons who have experienced a previous bout of TD, suggesting the presence of a genetic susceptibility [50–52], and other travelers who request a preventive medication [49]. The preferred drug is rifaximin used in a dose of one 200 mg tablet with the major daily meal(s). Taking two tablets a day with the two major meals is recommended to help deal with compliance concerns [3]. If only one dose a day is taken and it is missed, protection cannot be assured. In the second trial carried out in Mexico, a single dose of 600 mg/day was given with the first meal of the day [42]. BSS is a less convenient and slightly less effective alternative to rifaximin.

Table 19.2 Evidence base of chemoprophylaxis in travelers' diarrhea (preventive drugs are given daily while in high-risk region).

Therapeutic agent (dose for preparations with good quality of evidence)	Strength of evidence	Quality of evidence	Comments (references)
Bismuth subsalicylate (BSS) (2–262 mg tablets chewed well with meals and at bedtime, eight tablets or 2.1 g/d)	A	I	Turns stools and tongue black (from bismuth sulfide salt which is harmless); can lead to important levels of serum salicylate [81]; must be taken 4 times/d; is inexpensive; should not be used in people with IBD or AIDS or for prolonged time periods as bismuth may be absorbed from an abnormal mucosa [82–84].
Doxycycline and TMP/SMX	D	III	Worldwide resistance to these drugs makes them ineffective currently.
Fluoroquinolone (ciprofloxacin 750 mg or levofloxacin 500 mg once a day)	A	I	Effective [37–40]; being absorbed will have side effects, for example insomnia, headache, *Candida* vaginitis [85]; may cause resistance among extra-intestinal bacteria [86] and *Clostridium difficile* colitis [73].
Rifaximin (200 mg once or twice a day with major meals, or 600 mg once a day with major meal)	A	I	Safest preparation available; provides high degree of protection [3, 42]; of uncertain value in preventing the broad range of invasive bacteria although active against *Shigella* [57]; lack of absorption (<0.4%) should prevent development of resistance among extra-intestinal flora.
Azithromycin	C	III	Optimal therapy for dysenteric illness, not recommended for chemoprophylaxis.
Lactobacillus GG (2 x 10^9 bacteria/day in a single daily capsule)	B	I	Minimal level of protection provided (~ 40%) in one clinical trial [87].
Saccharomyces boulardii (500 mg twice a day)	C	I	Moderate level of protection in one study group, ineffective in others [88].
Whole cell (*V. cholerae*), binding subunit of cholera toxin ETEC vaccine (Dukoral) (two doses by mouth taken one week apart before travel)	B	I	Provides short-term protection against LT-ETEC [45] and possibly other forms of TD [46].
Transcutaneous heat labile enterotoxin (LT) ETEC vaccine (two skin patches are applied and left in place for six hours 2–3 weeks before travel)	B	I	Provides protection of uncertain duration against LT-ETEC and possibly other causes of TD [48].

TMP/SMX: trimethoprim/sulfamethoxazole; IBD: inflammatory bowel disease; AIDS: acquired immune deficiency syndrome.

The primary objective of chemoprophylaxis is to prevent the disability associated with TD, which averages approximately 24 hours per illness [53, 54]. An unproven benefit of chemoprophylaxis is prevention of the chronic functional bowel syndromes, including IBS secondary to TD, which occur in approximately 10% of persons who experience diarrhea during international travel [55, 56].

Future research in prevention of travelers' diarrhea

A fundamental question in the prevention of TD remains. Can careful attention to food and beverage intake, focusing on consumption of only the safest items, lower the risk of TD? This is largely an unstudied area that needs innovative research approaches. A second question is: does rifaximin taken for chemoprophylaxis during high-risk travel prevent infection and diarrhea caused by invasive bacteria including *Campylobacter*, *Shigella* and *Salmonella*? Rifaximin prevented shigellosis and *Shigella* dysentery when adult volunteers were challenged with a virulent strain of *Shigella* [57]. Preventing invasive forms of TD should be a far easier task than treating an invasive enteric infection once the organisms have extensively penetrated the mucosa. The third question concerning prevention is whether chemoprophylaxis prevents the occurrence of post-infectious IBS. With the frequency of occurrence approaching 10% of TD

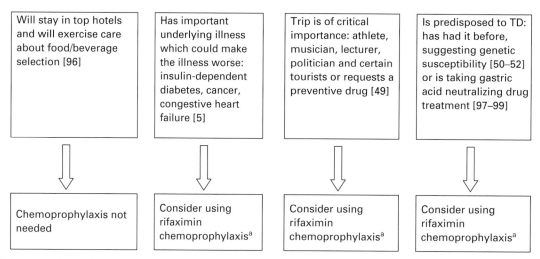

Figure 19.2 Recommendations for chemoprophylaxis based on characteristics of future traveler.
[a] 200 mg once or twice a day with major meals or 600 mg in a single dose with the first daily meal while out of town; alternative drug bismuth subsalicylate 2–262 mg tablets with meals and at bedtime (eight tablets/d or 2.1 g/d).

cases, prevention of IBS should be studied in future clinical trials.

Treatment of travelers' diarrhea

Symptomatic therapy

Drugs in this class are designed to reduce the number of unformed stools passed, allowing the traveler to better cope with illness symptoms. The drugs are not designed to cure this form of bacterial infection, and in many treated people the symptoms will continue, although improved, until antibacterial therapy is given. The first drug shown to have value in treatment of TD is bismuth subsalicylate (BSS) [58], which reduced the number of stools passed by 50% compared with placebo treatment. BSS exerts its antidiarrheal effect through the drug's salicylate moiety [59]. Loperamide was more effective than BSS in a randomized controlled trial, reducing the number of stools passed in TD by 60% [60]. Loperamide decreases diarrhea by slowing the intraluminal column, giving more opportunity for the gut to absorb water and electrolytes [61]. The drug also has direct antisecretory effects [62].

Antimicrobial therapy

Antimicrobial therapy is the mainstay of treatment of TD and is aimed at illness cure. Symptomatic treatments characteristically require rescue medication with antibacterial therapy to stop diarrhea [60, 63]. Trimethoprim/sulfamethoxazole was the first antibiotic shown to effectively reduce the duration of diarrhea. When TMP/SMX resist-

ance became widespread [64] other drugs were evaluated. The fluoroquinolones were found to be highly active in treating TD [23, 65–68]. Rifaximin, a poorly absorbed (<0.4%) antibacterial drug has been shown to be as effective as fluoroquinolones for overall TD [23, 69], while the drug is less effective against invasive pathogens as a group [23]. Azithromycin has been shown to effectively treat TD due to non-invasive [70] and invasive [26, 71] pathogens. The fluoroquinolones have adverse effects, including Achilles tendon rupture [72], for which a "black box warning" has been issued by the US FDA, and the occurrence of *Clostridium difficile* infection [73] due to near depletion of colonic flora caused by this class of drugs [37]. Azithromycin in the dose recommended commonly causes nausea [26]. The safest antibiotic treatment appears to be rifaximin, which has been as safe as the placebo control in each one of the clinical trials so far conducted.

Combination therapy

Where loperamide has rapid onset of action and effectively controls the number of stools passed, antibiotics have slow onset of action but are employed to cure the infection and stop the diarrhea. The drugs can be given together, obtaining additive benefits [63, 74, 75].

Evidence-based review of travelers' diarrhea treatment

All persons planning trips to developing regions should arm themselves with antidiarrheal drugs to employ if they develop diarrhea (see Table 19.3). The drugs for which

Table 19.3 Evidence-base of chemotherapeutic agents in the travelers' diarrhea therapy.

Chemotherapeutic agent	Strength of evidence	Quality of evidence	Comments
Bismuth subsalicylate (BSS) (2–262 mg tablets chewed well or 30 ml of liquid preparation each 30 minutes for up to eight doses 2.1 g/d)	A	I	BSS is an effective treatment of TD leading to reduction in number of stools passes [58]. Turns stools and tongue black (from bismuth sulfide salt which is harmless); can lead to important levels of serum salicylate [81], taken four times a day, is inexpensive but should not be used in persons with advanced GI disease such as IBD or AIDS as bismuth may be absorbed from an abnormal mucosa [82–84].
Kaolin/pectin or attipulgite	C	I	Binds to water, making stools more formed without other apparent value [89].
Loperamide (4 mg initially followed by 2 mg after each unformed stools passed not to exceed 8 mg/d for ≤48 hours)	A	I	Most effective symptomatic drug in TD, can be used with antibiotics for maximum value, produces post-treatment constipation [60, 90].
Diphenoxylate hydrochloride with atropine (Lomotil) (2 tablets four times a day for ≤48 hours)	A	I	Effective, contains atropine which may produce cholinergic side effects without antidiarrheal properties [91], causes central opiate effects in with respiratory depression in children taking overdose [92].
TMP/SMX[a]	D	III	While earlier found to be safe and effective, current levels of resistance lower the drug's value [64].
Fluoroquinolones + (750 mg cipro or 500 mg levo once, can repeat next two mornings with incomplete response)	A	I	Effective in most cases, shortens diarrhea quickly, *Campylobacter* resistance strains [26, 93] and occurrence of post-treatment CDAD [73] remain problems; ciprofloxacin should have the lowest price as it has become a generic preparation in USA.
Rifaximin (200 mg three times a day for three days)	A	I	Safest drug, effective for therapy of non-invasive/inflammatory enteric pathogens due to diarrheagenic *E. coli* strains [23, 69, 94].
Azithromycin (1000 mg in single dose)	A	I	Effectively treats all bacterial causes of TD, treatment of choice for high fever and dysentery (passage of grossly bloody stools) [26, 70].

[a] trimethoprim/sulfamethoxazole; + ciprofloxacin (cipro), levofloxacin (levo); CDAD: *Clostridium difficile* associated diarrhea.

there is strong and quality evidence to support their use in the treatment of TD include BSS, loperamide, fluoroquinolones, rifaximin and azithromcyin.

Current practice and recommendations

In Figure 19.3 four treatment options are provided, along with a perspective on their specific usage. Option 1 is for travel medicine clinics to use as a routine, or for general travelers not likely to appreciate important clinical features of their illness. Option 2 is for the seasoned or insightful traveler who wants to tailor treatment to the specific syndrome experienced. For travel to Latin America or Africa where ETEC and EAEC are the principal pathogens, any one of the three principal TD antibiotics can be employed routinely, including fluoroquinolones, rifaximin or azithromycin. In the algorithm, option 2 requires that travelers make a distinction between their condition that is associated with passage of watery stools without fever versus a febrile and/or dysenteric illness. If fever (oral temperature >39.4°C) or if grossly bloody stools are passed the preferred drug is azithromycin in a single 1000 mg dose [26, 76]. This syndrome occurs in approximately 1–5% of TD cases developing in Latin America or Africa and at a slightly higher rate among travelers with diarrhea acquired in Southern Asia [20, 77, 78]. For travel to Southern Asia, where invasive pathogens are more common, the azithromycin option is relatively more important. Option 1 for travel to Southern Asia includes use of azithromycin for treatment of all cases of TD.

For the workhorse of TD treatment regardless of destination, rifaximin should be the standard drug for cases of watery diarrhea without fever or dysentery. This recommendation is based on the safety of the drug, which resembles the placebo controls in all studies so far conducted, and efficacy in the treatment of uncomplicated TD that is equivalent to that observed with the absorbed antibacterial

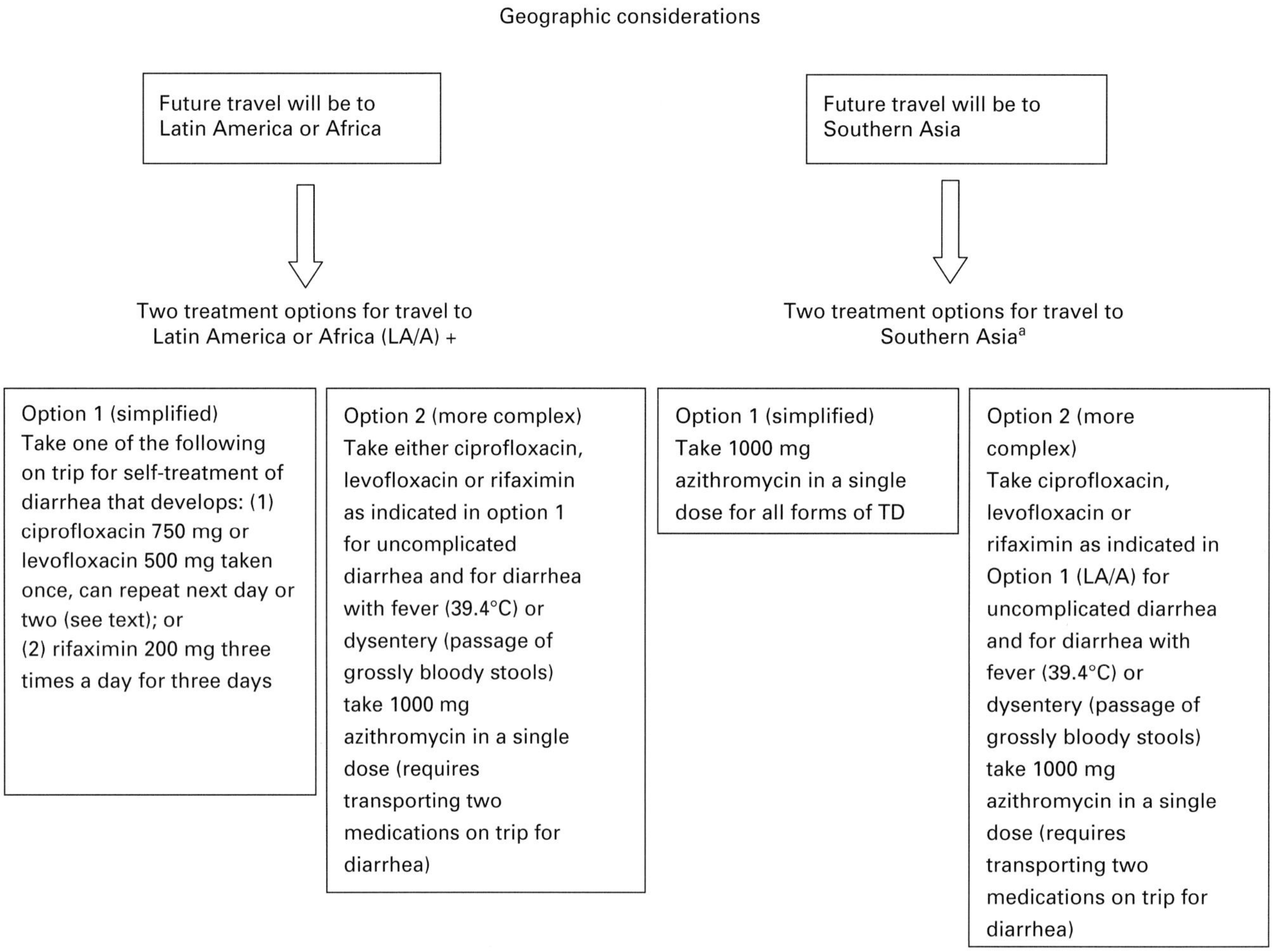

Geographic considerations

Future travel will be to
Latin America or Africa

Future travel will be to
Southern Asia

Two treatment options for travel to
Latin America or Africa (LA/A) +

Two treatment options for travel to
Southern Asia[a]

Option 1 (simplified)
Take one of the following
on trip for self-treatment of
diarrhea that develops: (1)
ciprofloxacin 750 mg or
levofloxacin 500 mg taken
once, can repeat next day or
two (see text); or
(2) rifaximin 200 mg three
times a day for three days

Option 2 (more complex)
Take either ciprofloxacin,
levofloxacin or rifaximin
as indicated in option 1
for uncomplicated
diarrhea and for diarrhea
with fever (39.4°C) or
dysentery (passage of
grossly bloody stools)
take 1000 mg
azithromycin in a single
dose (requires
transporting two
medications on trip for
diarrhea)

Option 1 (simplified)
Take 1000 mg
azithromycin in a single
dose for all forms of TD

Option 2 (more
complex)
Take ciprofloxacin,
levofloxacin or
rifaximin as indicated in
Option 1 (LA/A) for
uncomplicated diarrhea
and for diarrhea with
fever (39.4°C) or
dysentery (passage of
grossly bloody stools)
take 1000 mg
azithromycin in a single
dose (requires
transporting two
medications on trip for
diarrhea)

Figure 19.3 Recommendations for self-therapy of travelers' diarrhea based on geographic considerations and clinical features of illness (Option 1 in the various regions lists the drugs in order of their development for TD therapy; Option 2 is for the more sophisticated traveler).
+ The major pathogens causing travelers' diarrhea in Latin America and Africa are the diarrheagenic *E. coli*: enterotoxigenic *E. coli* (ETEC) and enteroaggregative *E. coli* (EAEC). These organisms respond to all antibiotics listed in Options 1 and 2.
[a] While ETEC and EAEC remain the major pathogens for travel to Southern Asia, invasive pathogens are more important for travel to this region of the world, which are best treated by azithromycin (fluoroquinolone resistance among *Campylobacter* isolates is common and rifaximin shows reduced effectiveness in diarrhea caused by invasive pathogens).

drugs. The drug preserves colonic flora [3, 79] while fluoro-quinolones deplete flora [37] and predispose to *C. difficile* diarrhea and colitis [73]. When rifaximin is used for chemo-prophylaxis, azithromycin is recommended for break-through diarrhea [76]. The traveler can save unused drugs for future trips to high-risk areas if not needed during the current travels and before reaching the drug expiration date.

Future research for treatment of travelers' diarrhea

The most important question about therapeutic recommen-dations in TD relates to resistance patterns of the important enteropathogens causing disease in the region being visited. Antimicrobial susceptibility patterns should be monitored for ciprofloxacin, levofloxacin, rifaximin, azi-thromycin and new antibiotics being developed for enteric bacterial infection. We also need to know more about safety of the available drugs. For example, will widespread use of the fluoroquinolones lead to important occurrence of fluoroquinolone resistance among extra-intestinal patho-gens, including *Streptococcus pneumonia*, and will this class of drugs encourage the overgrowth of *C. difficile* in a clini-cally important number of treated subjects?

Further research is needed to know the importance of TD to the development of PI-IBS and to the overall pool of IBS disease suffered by general populations. The natural history of PI-IBS needs further study to better understand prognosis, pathogenesis and prevention. Randomized trials are needed to determine if very early antimicrobial therapy, initiated with the first symptom, including passage of the first unformed stool, significantly reduces the occurrence of PI-IB.

Conclusions

For the foreseeable future, persons venturing into developing regions of Latin America, selected Caribbean islands, Africa and Southern Asia are at risk for TD. Education about the usually safe and often unsafe foods should be undertaken in all cases, although the value of dietary restrictions for prevention of enteric disease during high-risk travel is uncertain. To help determine whether chemoprophylaxis should be employed prior to travel, travelers should be screened for underlying illness, for the importance of the planned trip and for probable enhanced host susceptibility to diarrhea. The standard preventive drug for those falling into the recommended criteria is rifaximin. All travelers should be provided with curative treatment of TD that may develop. The mainstay of therapy is one of three antibacterial drugs: a fluoroquinolone, rifaximin or azithromycin. Azithromycin, while not recommended for all cases of TD, should be used preferentially for TD associated with fever or passage of grossly bloody stools. When rifaximin is used for chemoprophylaxis, azithromycin is the recommended backup drug for treatment of breakthrough diarrhea.

Acknowledgments

Dr. DuPont has received honoraria for speaking for the following companies: Salix Pharmaceuticals; McNeil Consumer Healthcare; and IOMAI Corporation and has received grants through the University of Texas to support research from: Salix Pharmaceuticals; IOMAI Corporation and Optimer Pharmaceuticals.

References

1 Kean BH. The Diarrhea of Travelers to Mexico. Summary of Five-Year Study. *Ann Intern Med* 1963 (Nov); **59**: 605–614.

2 DuPont HL, Haynes GA, Pickering LK, Tjoa W, Sullivan P, Olarte J. Diarrhea of travelers to Mexico. Relative susceptibility of United States and Latin American students attending a Mexican University. *Am J Epidemiol* 1977 (Jan); **105**(1): 37–41.

3 DuPont HL, Jiang ZD, Okhuysen PC *et al.* A randomized, double-blind, placebo-controlled trial of rifaximin to prevent travelers' diarrhea. *Ann Intern Med* 2005 (17 May); **142**(10): 805–812.

4 DuPont HL, Reves RR, Galindo E, Sullivan PS, Wood LV, Mendiola JG. Treatment of travelers' diarrhea with trimetho-prim/sulfamethoxazole and with trimethoprim alone. *N Engl J Med* 1982 (30 Sep); **307**(14): 841–844.

5 DuPont HL, Ericsson CD. Prevention and treatment of traveler's diarrhea. *N Engl J Med* 1993 (24 Jun); **328**(25): 1821–1827.

6 Steffen R. Epidemiologic studies of travelers' diarrhea, severe gastrointestinal infections, and cholera. *Rev Infect Dis* 1986 (May-Jun); **8**(Suppl 2): S122–S130.

7 Steffen R, Collard F, Tornieporth N *et al.* Epidemiology, etiology, and impact of traveler's diarrhea in Jamaica. *Jama* 1999 (3 Mar); **281**(9): 811–817.

8 Dandoy S. The diarrhea of travelers: Incidence in foreign students in the United States. *Calif Med* 1966 (Jun); **104**(6): 458–462.

9 Ryder RW, Wells J, Gangarosa EJ. A study of travelers' diarrhea in foreign visitors to the United States. *J Infect Dis* 1977; **136**: 605–607.

10 Jones TF, Angulo FJ. Eating in restaurants: A risk factor for food-borne disease? *Clin Infect Dis* 2006 (15 Nov); **43**(10): 1324–1328.

11 Gareau MG, Silva MA, Perdue MH. Pathophysiological mechanisms of stress-induced intestinal damage. *Curr Mol Med* 2008 (Jun); **8**(4): 274–281.

12 Huang DB, Sanchez AP, Triana E, Jiang ZD, DuPont HL, Ericsson CD. United States male students who heavily consume alcohol in Mexico are at greater risk of travelers' diarrhea than their female counterparts. *J Travel Med* 2004 (May-Jun); **11**(3): 143–145.

13 DuPont HL, Formal SB, Hornick RB *et al.* Pathogenesis of Escherichia coli diarrhea. *N Engl J Med* 1971 (1 Jul); **285**(1): 1–9.

14 DuPont HL, Olarte J, Evans DG, Pickering LK, Galindo E, Evans DJ. Comparative susceptibility of Latin American and United States students to enteric pathogens. *N Engl J Med* 1976 (30 Dec); **295**(27): 1520–1521.

15 Gorbach SL, Kean BH, Evans DG, Evans DJ, Jr., Bessudo D. Travelers' diarrhea and toxigenic *Escherichia coli*. *N Engl J Med* 1975 (1 May); **292**(18): 933–936.

16 Merson MH, Morris GK, Sack DA *et al.* Travelers' diarrhea in Mexico. A prospective study of physicians and family members attending a congress. *N Engl J Med* 1976 (10 Jun); **294**(24): 1299–1305.

17 Adachi JA, Jiang ZD, Mathewson JJ *et al.* Enteroaggregative *Escherichia coli* as a major etiologic agent in traveler's diarrhea in 3 regions of the world. *Clin Infect Dis* 2001 (15 Jun); **32**(12): 1706–1709.

18 Jiang ZD, Lowe B, Verenkar MP *et al.* Prevalence of enteric pathogens among international travelers with diarrhea acquired in Kenya (Mombasa), India (Goa), or Jamaica (Montego Bay). *J Infect Dis* 2002 (15 Feb); **185**(4): 497–502.

19 Sack DA, Shimko J, Torres O *et al.* Randomised, double-blind, safety and efficacy of a killed oral vaccine for enterotoxigenic *E. Coli* diarrhoea of travellers to Guatemala and Mexico. *Vaccine* 2007 (30 May); **25**(22): 4392–4400.

20 Haberberger RL, Jr., Mikhail IA, Burans JP *et al.* Travelers' diarrhea among United States military personnel during joint American-Egyptian armed forces exercises in Cairo, Egypt. *Mil Med* 1991 (Jan); **156**(1): 27–30.

21 Taylor DN, Sanchez JL, Candler W, Thornton S, McQueen C, Echeverria P. Treatment of travelers' diarrhea: Ciprofloxacin plus loperamide compared with ciprofloxacin alone. A placebo-controlled, randomized trial. *Ann Intern Med* 1991 (1 May); **114**(9): 731–734.

22 Echeverria P, Sack RB, Blacklow NR, Bodhidatta P, Rowe B, McFarland A. Prophylactic doxycycline for travelers' diarrhea in Thailand. Further supportive evidence of *Aeromonas hydrophila* as an enteric pathogen. *Am J Epidemiol* 1984 (Dec); **120**(6): 912–921.

23 Taylor DN, Bourgeois AL, Ericsson CD *et al.* A randomized, double-blind, multicenter study of rifaximin compared with placebo and with ciprofloxacin in the treatment of travelers' diarrhea. *Am J Trop Med Hyg* 2006 (Jun); **74**(6): 1060–1066.

24 Black RE. Epidemiology of travelers' diarrhea and relative importance of various pathogens. *Rev Infect Dis* 1990 (Jan–Feb); **12**(Suppl 1): S73–S79.

25 Jiang ZD, DuPont HL. Rifaximin: *In vitro* and *in vivo* antibacterial activity – a review. *Chemotherapy* 2005; **51**(Suppl 1): 67–72.

26 Tribble DR, Sanders JW, Pang LW *et al.* Traveler's diarrhea in Thailand: Randomized, double-blind trial comparing single-dose and 3-day azithromycin-based regimens with a 3-day levofloxacin regimen. *Clin Infect Dis* 2007 (1 Feb); **44**(3): 338–346.

27 Ko G, Garcia C, Jiang ZD *et al.* Noroviruses as a cause of traveler's diarrhea among students from the United States visiting Mexico. *J Clin Microbiol* 2005 (Dec); **43**(12): 6126–6129.

28 Kean BH, Waters S. The diarrhea of travelers. I. Incidence in travelers returning to the United States from Mexico. *AMA Arch Ind Health* 1958 (Aug); **18**(2): 148–150.

29 Owen JR. Diarrhoea at the Olympics. *Br Med J* 1968 (7 Dec); **4**(631): 645.

30 Sack DA, Kaminsky DC, Sack RB *et al.* Prophylactic doxycycline for travelers' diarrhea. Results of a prospective double-blind study of Peace Corps volunteers in Kenya. *N Engl J Med* 1978 (6 Apr); **298**(14): 758–763.

31 Sack RB, Froehlich JL, Zulich AW *et al.* Prophylactic doxycycline for travelers' diarrhea: Results of a prospective double-blind study of Peace Corps volunteers in Morocco. *Gastroenterology* 1979 (Jun); **76**(6): 1368–1373.

32 Sack RB, Santosham M, Froehlich JL, Medina C, Orskov F, Orskov I. Doxycycline prophylaxis of travelers' diarrhea in Honduras, an area where resistance to doxycycline is common among enterotoxigenic *Escherichia coli. Am J Trop Med Hyg* 1984 (May); **33**(3): 460–466.

33 DuPont HL, Sullivan P, Evans DG *et al.* Prevention of traveler's diarrhea (emporiatric enteritis). Prophylactic administration of subsalicylate bismuth). *Jama* 1980 (18 Jan); **243**(3): 237–241.

34 DuPont HL, Ericsson CD, Johnson PC, Bitsura JA, DuPont MW, de la Cabada FJ. Prevention of travelers' diarrhea by the tablet formulation of bismuth subsalicylate. *Jama* 1987 (13 Mar); **257**(10): 1347–1350.

35 Steffen R, DuPont HL, Heusser R *et al.* Prevention of traveler's diarrhea by the tablet form of bismuth subsalicylate. *Antimicrob Agents Chemother* 1986 (Apr); **29**(4): 625–627.

36 DuPont HL, Galindo E, Evans DG, Cabada FJ, Sullivan P, Evans DJ, Jr. Prevention of travelers' diarrhea with trimethoprim-sulfamethoxazole and trimethoprim alone. *Gastroenterology* 1983 (Jan); **84**(1): 75–80.

37 Johnson PC, Ericsson CD, Morgan DR, DuPont HL, Cabada FJ. Lack of emergence of resistant fecal flora during successful prophylaxis of traveler's diarrhea with norfloxacin. *Antimicrob Agents Chemother* 1986 (Nov); **30**(5): 671–674.

38 Rademaker CM, Hoepelman IM, Wolfhagen MJ, Beumer H, Rozenberg-Arska M, Verhoef J. Results of a double-blind pla-

cebo-controlled study using ciprofloxacin for prevention of travelers' diarrhea. *Eur J Clin Microbiol Infect Dis* 1989 (Aug); **8**(8): 690–694.

39 Scott DA, Haberberger RL, Thornton SA, Hyams KC. Norfloxacin for the prophylaxis of travelers' diarrhea in US military personnel. *Am J Trop Med Hyg* 1990 (Mar); **42**(2): 160–164.

40 Wistrom J, Norrby SR, Burman LG, Lundholm R, Jellheden B, Englund G. Norfloxacin versus placebo for prophylaxis against travellers' diarrhoea. *J Antimicrob Chemother* 1987 (Nov); **20**(4): 563–574.

41 Gorbach S, Edelman, R. Travelers' diarrhea: National Institutes of Health Consensus Development Conference 1986; **8**(Suppl 2): S109–S233.

42 DuPont HL, Ericsson CD, Jiang ZD *et al.* Prevention of travelers' diarrhea with rifaximin: A phase 3, randomized, double-blind, placebo-controlled trial in US students in Mexico. American College of Gastroenterology Annual Meeting (Abstract). Las Vegas (20–25 Oct 2006); Abstract number 516 (Page 259 abstract book).

43 Bulmer E. A survey of tropical diseases as seen in the Middle East. *Trans R Soc Trop Med Hyg* 1944; **37**: 225–242.

44 Brown MR, DuPont HL, Sullivan PS. Effect of duration of exposure on diarrhea due to enterotoxigenic *Escherichia coli* in travelers from the United States to Mexico. *J Infect Dis* 1982 (Apr); **145**(4): 582.

45 Clemens JD, Sack DA, Harris JR *et al.* Cross-protection by B subunit-whole cell cholera vaccine against diarrhea associated with heat-labile toxin-producing enterotoxigenic *Escherichia coli*: Results of a large-scale field trial. *J Infect Dis* 1988 (Aug); **158**(2): 372–377.

46 Peltola H, Siitonen A, Kyronseppa H *et al.* Prevention of travellers' diarrhoea by oral B-subunit/whole-cell cholera vaccine. *Lancet* 1991 (23 Nov); **338**(8778): 1285–1289.

47 Glenn GM, Flyer DC, Ellingsworth LR *et al.* Transcutaneous immunization with heat-labile enterotoxin: Development of a needle-free vaccine patch. *Expert Rev Vaccines* 2007 (Oct); **6**(5): 809–819.

48 Frech SA, DuPont HL, Bourgeois AL *et al.* Use of a patch containing heat-labile toxin from *Escherichia coli* against travellers' diarrhoea: A phase II, randomised, double-blind, placebo-controlled field trial. *Lancet* 2008 (14 Jun); **371**(9629): 2019–2025.

49 Gorbach SL. How to hit the runs for fifty million travelers at risk. *Ann Intern Med* 2005 (17 May); **142**(10): 861–862.

50 Flores J, DuPont HL, Lee SA *et al.* Influence of host interleukin-10 polymorphisms on development of traveler's diarrhea due to heat-labile enterotoxin-producing *escherichia coli* in travelers from the United States who are visiting Mexico. *Clin Vaccine Immunol* 2008 (Aug); **15**(8): 1194–1198.

51 Jiang ZD, Okhuysen PC, Guo DC *et al.* Genetic susceptibility to enteroaggregative *Escherichia coli* diarrhea: Polymorphism in the interleukin-8 promotor region. *J Infect Dis* 2003 (15 Aug); **188**(4): 506–511.

52 Mohamed JA, DuPont HL, Jiang ZD *et al.* A novel single-nucleotide polymorphism in the lactoferrin gene is associated with susceptibility to diarrhea in North American travelers to Mexico. *Clin Infect Dis* 2007 (1 Apr); **44**(7): 945–952.

53 Steffen R, Tornieporth N, Clemens SA *et al.* Epidemiology of travelers' diarrhea: Details of a global survey. *J Travel Med* 2004 (Jul–Aug); **11**(4): 231–237.

54 von Sonnenburg F, Tornieporth N, Waiyaki P *et al.* Risk and aetiology of diarrhoea at various tourist destinations. *Lancet* 2000 (8 Jul); **356**(9224): 133–134.

55 Okhuysen PC, Jiang ZD, Carlin L, Forbes C, DuPont HL. Post-diarrhea chronic intestinal symptoms and irritable bowel syndrome in North American travelers to Mexico. *Am J Gastroenterol* 2004 (Sep); **99**(9): 1774–1778.

56 Stermer E, Lubezky A, Potasman I, Paster E, Lavy A. Is traveler's diarrhea a significant risk factor for the development of irritable bowel syndrome? A prospective study. *Clin Infect Dis* 2006 (1 Oct); **43**(7): 898–901.

57 Taylor DN, McKenzie R, Durbin A *et al.* Rifaximin, a nonabsorbed oral antibiotic, prevents shigellosis after experimental challenge. *Clin Infect Dis* 2006 (1 May); **42**(9): 1283–1288.

58 DuPont HL, Sullivan P, Pickering LK, Haynes G, Ackerman PB. Symptomatic treatment of diarrhea with bismuth subsalicylate among students attending a Mexican university. *Gastroenterology* 1977 (Oct); **73**(4 Pt 1): 715–718.

59 Powell DW, Tapper EJ, Morris SM. Aspirin-stimulated intestinal electrolyte transport in rabbit ileum *in vitro*. *Gastroenterology* 1979 (Jun); **76**(6): 1429–1437.

60 Johnson PC, Ericsson CD, DuPont HL, Morgan DR, Bitsura JA, Wood LV. Comparison of loperamide with bismuth subsalicylate for the treatment of acute travelers' diarrhea. *JAMA* 1986 (14 Feb); **255**(6): 757–760.

61 Schiller LR, Santa Ana CA, Morawski SG, Fordtran JS. Mechanism of the antidiarrheal effect of loperamide. *Gastroenterology* 1984 (Jun); **86**(6): 1475–1480.

62 Epple HJ, Fromm M, Riecken EO, Schulzke JD. Antisecretory effect of loperamide in colon epithelial cells by inhibition of basolateral K+ conductance. *Scand J Gastroenterol* 2001 (Jul); **36**(7): 731–737.

63 DuPont HL, Jiang ZD, Belkind-Gerson J *et al.* Treatment of travelers' diarrhea: Randomized trial comparing rifaximin, rifaximin plus loperamide, and loperamide alone. *Clin Gastroenterol Hepatol* 2007 (Apr); **5**(4): 451–456.

64 Gomi H, Jiang ZD, Adachi JA *et al. In vitro* antimicrobial susceptibility testing of bacterial enteropathogens causing traveler's diarrhea in four geographic regions. *Antimicrob Agents Chemother* 2001 (Jan); **45**(1): 212–216.

65 DuPont HL, Ericsson CD, Mathewson JJ, DuPont MW. Five versus three days of ofloxacin therapy for traveler's diarrhea: A placebo-controlled study. *Antimicrob Agents Chemother* 1992 (Jan); **36**(1): 87–91.

66 Mattila L, Peltola H, Siitonen A, Kyronseppa H, Simula I, Kataja M. Short-term treatment of traveler's diarrhea with norfloxacin: A double-blind, placebo-controlled study during two seasons. *Clin Infect Dis* 1993 (Oct); **17**(4): 779–782.

67 Salam I, Katelaris P, Leigh-Smith S, Farthing MJ. Randomised trial of single-dose ciprofloxacin for travellers' diarrhoea. *Lancet* 1994 (3 Dec); **344**(8936): 1537–1539.

68 Wistrom J, Jertborn M, Hedstrom SA *et al.* Short-term self-treatment of travellers' diarrhoea with norfloxacin: a placebo-controlled study. *J Antimicrob Chemother* 1989 (Jun); **23**(6): 905–913.

69 DuPont HL, Jiang ZD, Ericsson CD *et al.* Rifaximin versus ciprofloxacin for the treatment of traveler's diarrhea: A randomized, double-blind clinical trial. *Clin Infect Dis* 2001 (1 Dec); **33**(11): 1807–1815.

70 Adachi JA, Ericsson CD, Jiang ZD *et al.* Azithromycin found to be comparable to levofloxacin for the treatment of US travelers with acute diarrhea acquired in Mexico. *Clin Infect Dis* 2003 (1 Nov); **37**(9): 1165–1171.

71 Kuschner RA, Trofa AF, Thomas RJ *et al.* Use of azithromycin for the treatment of *Campylobacter enteritis* in travelers to Thailand, an area where ciprofloxacin resistance is prevalent. *Clin Infect Dis* 1995 (Sep); **21**(3): 536–541.

72 Akali AU, Niranjan NS. Management of bilateral Achilles tendon rupture associated with ciprofloxacin: A review and case presentation. *J Plast Reconstr Aesthet Surg* 2008 (Jul); **61**(7): 830–834.

73 Norman F, Perez-Molina J, de Ayala P, Jimenez B, Navarro M, Lopez-Velez R. *Clostridium difficile*-associated diarrhea after antibiotic treatment for traveler's diarrhea. *Clin Infect Dis* 2008; **46**: 1060–1063.

74 Ericsson CD, DuPont HL, Mathewson JJ. Single Dose Ofloxacin plus Loperamide Compared with Single Dose or Three Days of Ofloxacin in the Treatment of Traveler's Diarrhea. *J Travel Med* 1997 (1 Mar); **4**(1): 3–7.

75 Ericsson CD, DuPont HL, Mathewson JJ. Optimal dosing of ofloxacin with loperamide in the treatment of non-dysenteric travelers' diarrhea. *J Travel Med* 2001 (Jul–Aug); **8**(4): 207–209.

76 DuPont HL. Azithromycin for the self-treatment of traveler's diarrhea. *Clin Infect Dis* 2007 (1 Feb); **44**(3): 347–349.

77 Ericsson CD, Patterson TF, DuPont HL. Clinical presentation as a guide to therapy for travelers' diarrhea. *Am J Med Sci* 1987 (Aug); **294**(2): 91–96.

78 Mattila L. Clinical features and duration of traveler's diarrhea in relation to its etiology. *Clin Infect Dis* 1994 (Oct); **19**(4): 728–734.

79 DuPont HL, Jiang ZD. Influence of rifaximin treatment on the susceptibility of intestinal Gram-negative flora and enterococci. *Clin Microbiol Infect* 2004 (Dec); **10**(11): 1009–1011.

80 Gross PA, Barrett TL, Dellinger EP, Krause PJ *et al.* Purpose of quality standards for infectious diseases.Infectious Diseases Society of America. *Clin Infect Dis* 1994 (Mar); **18**(3): 421.

81 Pickering LK, Feldman S, Ericsson CD, Cleary TG. Absorption of salicylate and bismuth from a bismuth subsalicylate – containing compound (Pepto-Bismol). *J Pediatr* 1981 (Oct); **99**(4): 654–656.

82 Gordon MF, Abrams RI, Rubin DB, Barr WB, Correa DD. Bismuth subsalicylate toxicity as a cause of prolonged encephalopathy with myoclonus. *Mov Disord* 1995 (Mar); **10**(2): 220–222.

83 Hasking GJ, Duggan JM. Encephalopathy from bismuth subsalicylate. *Med J Aust* 1982 (21 Aug); **2**(4): 167.

84 Mendelowitz PC, Hoffman RS, Weber S. Bismuth absorption and myoclonic encephalopathy during bismuth subsalicylate therapy. *Ann Intern Med* 1990 (15 Jan); **112**(2): 140–141.

85 Mehlhorn AJ, Brown DA. Safety concerns with fluoroquinolones. *Ann Pharmacother* 2007 (Nov); **41**(11): 1859–1866.

86 Fuller JD, Low DE. A review of Streptococcus pneumoniae infection treatment failures associated with fluoroquinolone resistance. *Clin Infect Dis* 2005 (1 Jul); **41**(1): 118–121.

87 Hilton E, Kolakowski P, Singer C, Smith M. Efficacy of Lactobacillus GG as a Diarrheal Preventive in Travelers. *J Travel Med* 1997 (1 Mar); **4**(1): 41–43.

88 Kollaritsch H, Holst H, Grobara P, Wiedermann G. Prevention of traveler's diarrhea with Saccharomyces boulardii. Results of a placebo controlled double-blind study. *Fortschr Med* 1993 (30 Mar); **111**(9): 152–156.

89 Portnoy BL, DuPont HL, Pruitt D, Abdo JA, Rodriguez JT. Antidiarrheal agents in the treatment of acute diarrhea in children. *JAMA* 1976 (16 Aug); **236**(7): 844–846.

90 DuPont HL, Flores Sanchez J, Ericsson CD *et al.* Comparative efficacy of loperamide hydrochloride and bismuth subsalicylate in the management of acute diarrhea. *Am J Med* 1990 (20 Jun); **88**(6A): 15S-19S.

91 Reves R, Bass P, DuPont HL, Sullivan P, Mendiola J. Failure to demonstrate effectiveness of an anticholinergic drug in the symptomatic treatment of acute travelers' diarrhea. *J Clin Gastroenterol* 1983 (Jun); **5**(3): 223–227.

92 Ahmad SR. Lomotil overdose. *Pediatrics* 1992 (May); **89**(5 Pt 1): 980–981.

93 Kassenborg HD, Smith KE, Vugia DJ *et al.* Fluoroquinolone-resistant Campylobacter infections: Eating poultry outside of the home and foreign travel are risk factors. *Clin Infect Dis* 2004 (15 Apr); **38**(Suppl 3): S279–S284.

94 Steffen R, Sack DA, Riopel L *et al.* Therapy of travelers' diarrhea with rifaximin on various continents. *Am J Gastroenterol* 2003 (May); **98**(5): 1073–1078.

95 DuPont HL. Systematic review: Prevention of travellers' diarrhoea. *Aliment Pharmacol Ther* 2008 (May); **27**(9): 741–751.

96 Kozicki M, Steffen R, Schar M. 'Boil it, cook it, peel it or forget it': does this rule prevent travellers' diarrhoea? *Int J Epidemiol* 1985 (Mar); **14**(1): 169–172.

97 Nalin DR, Levine RJ, Levine MM *et al.* Cholera, non-vibrio cholera, and stomach acid. *Lancet* 1978 (21 Oct); **2**(8095): 856–859.

98 Sack GH, Jr., Pierce NF, Hennessey KN, Mitra RC, Sack RB, Mazumder DN. Gastric acidity in cholera and noncholera diarrhoea. *Bull World Health Organ* 1972; **47**(1): 31–36.

99 Van Loon FP, Clemens JD, Shahrier M *et al.* Low gastric acid as a risk factor for cholera transmission: Application of a new non-invasive gastric acid field test. *J Clin Epidemiol* 1990; **43**(12): 1361–1367.

Clostridium difficile associated disease: Diagnosis and treatment

Lynne V McFarland[1] *and Christina M Surawicz*[2]

[1] Department of Medicinal Chemistry, School of Pharmacy, University of Washington, Washington, USA
[2] Department of Gastroenterology, Harborview Medical Center, Washington, USA

Introduction

The occurrence of large outbreaks of severe *Clostridium difficile* disease in Canada refocused attention on this interesting pathogen. The availability of newer techniques for strain typing and rapid diagnostic assays has increased the detection of emergent strains of "hypervirulent" types of *C. difficile*. The incidence of severe cases of *C. difficile* disease and the spread into populations once considered at low risk for *C. difficile* disease (peripartum women and non-health care associated cases) is described. Recently, a decreasing response rate to metronidazole therapy has increased the interest in investigational treatments. Evidence for effective treatment for initial episodes of *C. difficile* disease still favors metronidazole, but there is evidence that the more effective treatment for severe *C. difficile* disease is vancomycin. Investigational treatments for recurrent *C. difficile* disease have expanded to toxin absorbents, rifamycin-class antibiotics, probiotics and immunoglobulin preparations. Preventive strategies include *C. difficile* vaccines and enhanced infection control programs.

Clostridium difficile-associated disease (CDAD) has been studied since the first outbreaks of hospital-based CDAD cases were described in the early 1980s [1, 2]. Although formidable work has been accomplished on the epidemiology, clinical diagnosis and control of hospital outbreaks, CDAD continues to persist as a leading cause of nosocomial gastrointestinal illness [3–5]. Outbreaks of an emergent strain, BI/NAP1/027, caused large outbreaks of severe CDAD with high rates of mortality in Canada during 2003–2005 [6]. Other forms of CDAD that are now recognized include recurrent CDAD, toxic megacolon and *C. difficile*-associated septicemia [7–11]. Little is known about these forms of CDAD (toxin megacolon, septicemia, brain empyema) other than that they occur sporadically and may cause significant clinical problems for patients and challenges for health care providers [12].

Vancomycin or metronidazole are typically used for the treatment of the first episode of CDAD. However, approximately 10–24% of patients with an episode of CDAD have at least one recurrence after the first antibiotic treatment is discontinued. Some of these patients develop a form of the disease known as recurrent CDAD that is characterized by recurrent episodes over several years despite treatment [13–16]. Since 2003, rates of metronidazole failure and recurrence rates have increased, casting doubts about the effectiveness of this antibiotic for CDAD [17]. In addition, vancomycin is now considered to be more effective in severe cases of CDAD [18].

The objective of this chapter is to describe the epidemiology, diagnosis and evidence-based treatment strategies for treatment and prevention of primary and recurrent CDAD.

Diagnosis

Unlike most diseases, a simple laboratory assay is not definitive for the diagnosis of CDAD. The presence of *Clostridium difficile* (either a culture or positive toxin assay) must be accompanied by an appropriate clinical presentation (usually diarrhea), and other etiologies of diarrhea must be excluded [19]. The requirement for a combination of laboratory results and an appropriate clinical presentation is due to the occurrence of the asymptomatic carrier state in some patients who have a positive laboratory test for *C. difficile*, but no clinical symptoms. On the other hand, some patients with symptomatic disease may have negative laboratory tests for stool toxins.

The cell cytotoxin assay is considered to be the "gold standard" for diagnosis, but stool culture has the advan-

Evidence-Based Gastroenterology and Hepatology, 3rd edition.
J. McDonald, A.K. Burroughs, B. Feagan, and M.B. Fennerty. © 2010
Blackwell Publishing Ltd

tage of detecting one-third more cases than cell cytotoxin assay. However, these two methods have lost favor in current practice [20, 21]. Currently, 79–95% of hospitals use rapid enzyme-immunoassays (EIA) to diagnose CDAD [22, 23]. These EIA kits have the advantages of rapid turnover (usually within one day) and high specificity (94–100%), but exhibit somewhat lower sensitivity (88–93%) [24, 25]. Newer types of tests using DNA probes for *C. difficile* toxin genes are promising. Direct stool PCR assays are rapid (<4 hours) and have better sensitivities than EIA. Peterson *et al.* tested 1368 stool samples and reported that PCR has 93.3% sensitivity and 97.4% specificity when compared to culture [19]. In an effort to combine rapid turn-around time and high sensitivities, a number of algorithms have been proposed. Most of these combine a screening step with rapid EIA for glutamate dehydrogenase (GDH), *C. difficile* antigen assay with a confirmatory assay for those who are GDH positive (either the cell cytotoxicity assay or an EIA for toxin A or B). A three-step algorithm consisting of (1) GDH screening, (2) a stool cytotoxin confirmation for positive GDH and (3) a toxigenic isolate assay from stool culture for all samples negative for stool cytotoxin was tested on 439 diarrheal stools. The sensitivity of this approach was 87%. The third step (stool culture and assaying isolates for toxin production) resulted in the detection of 33% more cases than were found using only the first two steps [20]. Balancing costs with the need for rapid diagnosis and high sensitivity for CDAD is paramount and continues to be challenging.

Clinical presentation

Diarrhea due to CDAD has been defined as a change in bowel habits with at least three loose or watery bowel movements per day for at least two consecutive days or greater than eight loose or watery stools within 48 hours [26, 27]. The symptoms of CDAD can also include fever, nausea and abdominal cramping or pain [28].

The incubation period after acquisition of *Clostridium difficile* is usually one week or less, but can be up to as long as eight weeks after exposure to antibiotics [13, 29]. Asymptomatic carriers may also become symptomatic after exposure to antibiotics.

In 2005, a prospective observational study in 88 Quebec hospitals yielded 478 isolates of *C. difficile* with 61 different PFGE profiles. Severe disease was 2.3 times more frequent when both binary toxin genes and tcdC deletion were present. "Severe CDAD" was defined as being the cause or a contributing factor to 30-day mortality, or to the requirement for colectomy or admission to an intensive care unit [30].

Approximately 3–8% of CDAD patients develop "fulminant CDAD", in which the clinical course is complicated by perforation, severe ileus with toxic megacolon, hypotension requiring vasopressors or refractory septicemia. A significant number of these patients require emergency colectomy [31].

Complications

Complications of recurrent CDAD in one study included repeated hospitalizations for cases of severe recurrences (3 hospitalizations of 100 patients), development of toxic megacolon (0.5 of 100), septicemia (0.5 of 100) and *C. difficile*-associated arthritis (0.5 of 100) [14].

During the outbreaks in Canada, complicated cases of CDAD (elevated fever, leukocytosis, shock, ICU admission, requirement for colectomy) increased from 7% to 18%. It was postulated that the emergent BI/NAP10/27 strain was responsible [32]. Other strain types of CDAD are also associated with severe disease, but not with the hyperproduction of toxins.

Costs

Studies of patients with CDAD have shown that the cost of medical care associated with CDAD cases may range from $2000 to $6000 per patient [28, 33, 34]. Recurrent CDAD has a higher impact on the medical care system. The impact is reflected in high costs of medical care, readmissions to hospital for severe recurrent episodes, and complications (toxic megacolon, septicemia, arthritis). In one study of 209 patients with recurrent CDAD, the total lifetime cost for direct medical expenses (including all prior episodes, enrollment episodes and subsequent recurrences) averaged $10,970 per person [14]. The average cost of diagnosis and treatment for episodes other than the enrollment episode was $3103 per patient. These costs do not include lost time from work, costs of complications, additional clinic visits or any indirect costs. In one prospective study, the average length of stay for a hospitalization due to a CDAD recurrence was 8.8 ± 8.6 days (ranging from 3 to 26 days) [14]. Other studies have documented that CDAD extends hospital stays for hospitalized patients from 4 to 36 days [28, 34–36]. In a study of 1034 CDAD cases in Massachusetts during 2000, the average cost ranged from $10,212–13,675/patient, projecting a national (US) cost of CDAD of $3.2 billion/year [37].

Epidemiology

Incidence/prevalence

The prevalence of CDAD ranges from 0.15% to 10% in hospitalized patients during non-outbreak situations and may increase from 16% to 29% during hospital outbreaks of CDAD [4, 38–40]. The rates of CDAD have been increasing globally over the years. In the USA, CDAD rates have doubled between 2001 and 2005 to 301,200 cases [41]. The prevalence of community acquired CDAD is typically much lower than health care associated CDAD but has increased from 7.7–12 per 100,000 person-years during the years from 1994 to 2000 [42, 43] to 22 per 100,000 in 2004 [44]. Community acquired cases may have a different clinical profile, because infection is not acquired at a health care setting and most (45–60%) are not associated with recent antibiotic use [21, 45, 46]. The rate of community acquired CDAD may be underestimated if patients with atypical risk factor profiles and no history of a recent health care admission are not assayed for *C. difficile*.

Health care associated outbreaks

Documented outbreaks due to this organism are reported in hospitals and long-term care facilities around the world with increasing frequency [4, 47, 48].

A variety of patient populations has been shown to be susceptible to nosocomial CDAD. Outbreaks or nosocomial acquisition have occurred in patients in general medicine wards [4], surgical wards [49, 50], long-term care facilities [51], in elderly patients [52, 53], in pediatric patients [54, 55], patients who are immunocompromised either by HIV infection [48, 56], by cancer [57, 58], or by transplantation [59] and, less commonly, in new mothers [60, 61].

Strain typing techniques have been a valuable tool in tracking the routes of transmission during hospital outbreaks and in documenting those hospitals that may harbor both endemic strains and epidemic strains of *Clostridium difficile* [4, 62, 63]. Strain typing of isolates from hospitalized patients has also shown that half of clinical recurrences may be re-infections with a different strain of *Clostridium difficile*, adding support to the importance of nosocomial acquisition of new strains [15, 64].

The BI/NAP1/027 strain was associated with the Canadian outbreaks during 2003–2005. This strain is of toxinotype III (presence of binary toxin CDT) and contains dysfunctioning tcdC gene. A single nucleotide deletion at position 117 resulted in a stop codon for the tcdC gene, thus inactivating the down-regulation of tcdA and tcdB [65]. Strains with the tcdC deletion have been found to produce 16 times more Toxin A and 23 times more Toxin B than other *C. difficile* strains [66]. Another novel characteristic of this strain is that it is resistant to gatifloxacin and moxifloxacin. Older isolates (pre-2002) of BI/NAP1/027 were not resistant to fluoroquinolones [67]. As fluoroquinolones became commonly prescribed, the development of antibiotic resistance in health care associated strains of CDAD was a focus of clinical concern. Since the Canadian outbreaks, several outbreaks of the BI/NAP1/027 strain have been reported. Biller *et al.* reported that an outbreak in a hospital in Pennsylvania occurred after a formulary change

from levofloxacin to moxifloxacin and did not resolve after levofloxacin was reinstated. This outbreak was associated with the emergent strain [68]. A prospective study in Canada that collected *C. difficile* isolates from 88 hospitals in Quebec continued to find the persistence of the BI/NAP1/027 strain (57% were positive) after the outbreaks subsided [30]. In the USA, as of November 2007, 38 states have found BI/NAP1/027 in their hospital populations [69]. In contrast to studies reporting severe CDAD associated with BI/NAP1/027 isolates, a study at the Veterans' Administration (VA) Medical Center in Cleveland, Ohio, found 68 asymptomatic carriers of *C. difficile* and 13 (37%) were NAP1 isolates [70]. Tracking this emergent strain of *C. difficile* has documented how easily global transmission of this organism is achieved.

Transmission

Transmission within the hospital has been shown to be largely due to horizontal transmission via environmental surface contamination, hand carriage by hospital personnel and infected roommates [4, 39, 62, 71]. In a cohort of 3500 patients, a multivariate analysis found that physical proximity to a patient with CDAD significantly increased the risk of CDAD (RR = 1.86; 95% CI: 1.06–3.28) [71]. New admissions who are *Clostridium difficile* positive have been shown to be a source of infection for susceptible patients [72]. In a prospective cohort study of 428 patients admitted to one general medicine ward, a multivariate model documented that the risk of nosocomial acquisition of *Clostridium difficile* was significantly higher after exposure to an infected roommate (RR 1.73; 95% CI: 1.15–2.55) [4]. Environmental surfaces are uniformly positive for *C. difficile* if a CDAD patient is in the room, compared to only 33% positivity if no CDAD patient is present (100%) [69].

Risk factors

Risk factors for primary CDAD usually involve factors in one of three general areas: (1) factors that disrupt normal colonic flora, such as broad-spectrum antibiotics or surgery, (2) host factors, such as age, gender, diet, immune status, concurrent medical conditions or diseases, such as cancer, transplantation, other gastrointestinal conditions, or co-infection with other enteric pathogens and (3) exposure to the organism, usually through admission to a hospital with endemic *Clostridium difficile* or admission when an outbreak is occurring.

The normal colonic microflora has been shown to be protective of colonization by *Clostridium difficile* through a multifocal mechanism known as colonization resistance. This complex interaction of the intestinal microflora produces a wide variety of protective effects that may include spatial interference, attachment inhibition, production of bacteriocins, production of toxin degrading proteases and stimulation of immunoglobulins that act as a barrier to the colonization of newly introduced pathogens [73]. Factors that disrupt this colonization resistance, such as exposure to antibiotics, surgery or medications, have been shown in epidemiologic studies to increase the risk of CDAD. Exposure to broad spectrum antibiotics has the highest risk associated with CDAD, but narrow spectrum antibiotics have also been implicated. Neither the dose nor the total duration of antibiotic therapy seems to be correlated with higher risk of developing CDAD in some studies [5, 28, 35, 48, 49, 51, 52, 53, 71]. Gastrointestinal surgery or manipulation, or nasogastric tube feeding have also been shown to be significant risk factors for CDAD in epidemiologic studies [35, 51, 74, 75].

Host factors that have been shown to be significant risk factors for CDAD include increasing age [14, 16, 28, 52], female gender [28, 49], serious underlying illness and the presence of other concurrent diseases [51, 52, 60]. Prolonged hospitalization has also been shown to increase the risk of *Clostridium difficile* acquisition [76].

Since many of these risk factors for CDAD are correlated, multivariate analysis is appropriate to provide an assessment of the independent risks associated with these factors. Most multivariate analyses have provided evidence that advanced age, antibiotic use, co-morbidities and longer hospital stays are independently predictive of CDAD [21, 77–79]. Using multivariate analysis of data from 37 hospitalized patients with cytotoxin positive CDAD and 37 hospital controls Brown reported that age greater than 65 yrs (OR 14.1; 95% CI: 1.4, 141), stay in an intensive care unit (OR 39.2; 95% CI: 2.2, 713), gastrointestinal procedures (OR 23.2; 95% CI: 2.1, 255) and over ten days of antibiotics (OR 16.1; 95% CI: 2.2, 117) were significant risk factors for CDAD [75]. Nelson *et al.* studied 33 hospitalized patients with CDAD and 32 controls and showed that the use of second or third-generation cephalosporin was a significant risk factor (OR 8.3; CI 95%: 1.4 to 48.9), as was the use of two or more antibiotics (OR 18.7; 95 % CI: 4.1–85.8) [80]. McFarland *et al.* studied 428 patients admitted to a general medicine ward and found five risk factors for CDAD using age and severity of co-morbidity-adjusted multivariate analysis severe underlying disease (RR = 5.18; 95% CI: 1.2, 22.2), cephalosporin use for at least one week (RR = 2.1; 95% CI: 1.1, 3.8), penicillin use for two weeks (RR = 3.4; 95% CI: 1.5, 7.9) and use of gastrointestinal stimulants (RR = 3.1; 95% CI: 1.7,5.6), enemas (RR = 3.3: 95% CI 1: 5, 7.0) or stool softeners (RR = 1.7; 95% CI: 1.02, 3.0) [35]. Dubberke *et al.* studied 382 CDAD cases and 35,704 controls admitted to a St Louis Missouri hospital from January 2003 to December 2003. Multivariate analysis revealed the following risk factors: age over 45 years (adjusted odds ratio = 2.3), CDAD colonization pressure (adjusted odds ratio = 4.0) and antibiotic use (cephalosporins and fluoro-

quinolones) and third-generation cephalosporin use (over seven days' use) had an aOR = 9.2, 95% CI: 5.9–14.5) and over one week use of fluoroquinolones had an aOR = 2 .5, 95% CI: 1.8–3.5) [81]. CDAD colonization pressure is an indicator of how long an affected patient was exposed to another patient infected with *C. difficile*.

Recurrent disease

Prospective studies of risk factors for recurrent CDAD may help to define this subset of highly susceptible patients who have a tendency to develop the recurrent form of CDAD. The risk factors for recurrent CDAD have been reported to be slightly different from risk factors found for primary CDAD or risk factors for nosocomial CDAD [9, 26, 35, 75, 80, 82, 83]. In a prospective cohort study of 209 patients with recurrent CDAD, logistic regression revealed two significant independent risk factors for CDAD recurrence: increased age and a lower quality of health index at enrollment (X^2 = 9.03, p = 0.01) [14]. Patients who experienced recurrent disease were older (64.8 ± 1.65 years) than patients who did not (54.6 ± 19.6 years) and also exhibited a lower quality of health index (42.9 ± 17.8) compared to patients who did not experience recurrent disease (50.3 ± 18.5). The estimates of risk for CDAD recurrence were as follows: age (odds ratio (OR), 1.04; 95% CI: 1.01, 1.08) and a lower mean quality of health index (OR 0.96; 95% CI: 0.93, 0.99). There were no significant interactions observed in the analysis. No other risk factor was significant, including gender, number of prior episodes, type or dose of standard antibiotic, dose or duration of inciting antibiotic, days of follow-up, number of medications or prior surgeries, allergies, severity of enrollment episode, study center, or type of patient (inpatient or outpatient).

In another study comparing 34 patients with recurrent CDAD and 33 patients with non-recurrent CDAD, the risk factors for subsequent recurrences included a higher number of prior episodes (RR = 3.87, 95% CI: 1.12, 13.34), spring onset of initial episode (RR = 7.73; 95% CI: 1.07, 55.89) and the use of additional antibiotics (RR = 2.97; 95% CI: 1.11, 7.93) [9]. Do *et al.* analyzed 13 patients with recurrent CDAD and 46 patients with an initial episode of CDAD in a case-control study [84]. Risk factors for recurrent CDAD in this very small study included a history of chronic renal insufficiency and white blood cell count over 15,000/mm^3.

Tal *et al.* performed a case-control study to compare 43 patients with recurrent CDAD to 38 patients with initial CDAD at a subacute geriatric department over a period of 18 months [82]. Risk factors for recurrent CDAD included fecal incontinence (OR = 2.75; 95% CI: 1.05, 7.54), longer duration of fever from admission until first episode of CDAD (OR = 1.11; 95% CI: 1.02, 1.25) and H$_2$-antagonist exposure (OR = 1.03; 95% CI: 1.14, 7.29). Given the small numbers of patients studied and the rather low values for these observed odds ratios, these results provide only very limited evidence.

Treatment for the initial episode

If possible, the inciting antibiotic should be discontinued. Fluid support (oral or intravenous) may be needed. Anti-peristaltic or opiate drugs should be avoided on the basis of physiologiocal considerations rather than clinical evidence. There is no proven role for treatment of asymptomatic carriers [85]. If the index of suspicion for CDAD is high, it is recommended that empiric therapy should be initiated, rather than waiting for confirmatory stool tests, although there is no good evidence on this point.

Antibiotic treatments

Given the number and variety of clinical trials of antibiotics to treat CDAD, a 1997 meta-analysis proved to be valuable in assessing the efficacy of the various antibiotics. Of nine trials with suitable methodology to permit inclusion in the systematic review, only two were placebo controlled. Six other trials compared vancomycin to other antibiotics (fusidic acid, bacitracin and teicoplanin,). No single antibiotic was shown to be more effective than any other [86].

Vancomycin

Several trials have demonstrated the efficacy of oral vancomycin for therapy of initial CDAD, given orally at doses of 500–1225 mg four times a day for 7–14 days (Table 20.1) [18, 27, 87–98]. Wenisch *et al.* performed a randomized, controlled trial of four antibiotic regimens [93]. One hundred and nineteen patients with *Clostridium difficile* toxin positive diarrhea were randomized to receive a 10-day course of one of the four antibiotic regimens: metronidazole (1.5 g/d), vancomycin (1.5 g/d), fusidic acid (1.5 g/d), or teicoplanin (800 mg/d) and followed for initial resolution of symptoms ("cure") and for occurrence of a relapse within 30 days of antibiotic discontinuation ("relapse"). The four groups were comparable in terms of age, sex and previous antibiotic exposure. The initial cure rate was not significantly different among the treatment groups and ranged from 93–96%. The observed recurrence rates were: metronidazole 16%, vancomycin 16%, teicoplanin 7% and fusidic acid 28%. The difference between teicoplanin and fusidic acid groups was statistically significant (p = 0.04). There were no reported adverse reactions to any of the four antibiotics. **A1c**

Several studies have shown equal efficacy for metronidazole and vancomycin [88, 93], Teasley *et al.* [88] reported a randomized, controlled trial in which 94 patients with CDAD were randomized to vancomycin (2 g/d for 10 days) or metronidazole 1 g/d for 10 days). The initial response rates (vancomycin 100%, metronidazole 95%) and recurrence rates (vancomycin 5%, metronidazole 11.5%) were not significantly different. **A1c** Olson *et al.* reported a case series of 908 patients in a 10-year surveillance study of *Clostridium difficile* at the Minneapolis VA Medical Center [99]. The initial response rates to metronidazole and vancomycin in a variety of dosage regimens were, respectively, 98 and 99%. **B4** When the relative odds of treatment failure or subsequent *Clostridium difficile* recurrence are used to evaluate the different antibiotics available to treat initial episodes of CDAD, vancomycin and metronidazole appear to have equal efficacies (Table 20.2).

In a randomized, controlled trial in which 46 patients were randomized to receive vancomycin at high dose (2 grams/day) or lower dose (500 mg/day) both groups responded with a mean of four days of diarrhea after initiation of therapy and nearly uniform resolution of diarrhea by a week of therapy [91]. Given the expense of vancomycin therapy, these data support the use of the lower dose regimen. **A1d**

As seen in Table 20.1, vancomycin cures rates are high, with failure rates ranging from 1–16%. Relapse rates after vancomycin have been fairly stable over the years. Vancomycin appears to be superior to metronidazole for cases of *severe* CDAD. If patients have severe CDAD (diarrhea with leukocytosis, fever >38.5°C, PMC or toxic shock), and the intestines are functioning and not obstructed, vancomycin is more effective than metronidazole (97% vs 76%, respectively, p = 0.002) [18]. **A1c** Vancomycin is also associated with more rapid recovery and less total cost of health care. A retrospective review of 32,325 cases of CDAD, revealed that patients treated with vancomycin exhibited shorter hospital stays (vancomycin 11.5 days, metronidazole 12.8 days, p < 0.001), and the mortality rate was also lower (vancomycin 6.8%, metronidazole 7.9%, p = 0.02). **B4** The estimated costs of hospital care were $14,718 for vancomycin treated patients and $16,953 for the metronidazole group (p < 0.001) [100]. At a Cleveland Veterans' Administration hospital, in a small two-month observational study of 52 patients with CDAD, 18 patients were treated with vancomycin and 34 with metronidazole for at least six days [101]. Similar rates of treatment failure (persistent diarrhea at the end of treatment) were seen in patients treated with vancomycin: 1/18 (16%) and metronidazole: 4/34 (12%). Similar rates of CDAD recurrences were also observed: 2 (11%) patients receiving vancomycin and 4 (12%) receiving metronidazole. Although there was no significant difference between the treatments for cure rate and recurrence rate, it appeared that diarrhea resolved more rapidly and a greater proportion of patients' stools became negative for *C. difficile* on the fifth day of treatment in vancomycin treated patients. **B4**

Table 20.1 Randomized, controlled trials of treatments for patients with initial *Clostridium difficile* associated disease (CDAD).

Treatment	Daily dose (mg/d)	Duration (days)	No.	Initial cure (%)	Recurrence (%)	Reference
Antibiotics						
Vancomycin vs placebo	500	5	12	92	0[a]	Keighley *et al.* 1978 [87]
	500	5	9	22	44	
Vancomycin vs metronidazole	2000	10	52	100	11	Teasley *et al.* 1983 [88]
	1000	10	42	95	5 ns	
Bacitracin vs vancomycin	800,000 U	10	21	76	24	Young *et al.* 1985 [89]
	500	10	21	86	29 ns	
Bacitracin vs vancomycin	100,000 U	10	15	80	33	Dudley *et al.* 1986 [90]
	2000	10	15	93	20 ns	
Vancomycin vs vancomycin	500	10	24	100	21	Fekety *et al.* 1989 [91]
	2000	10	22	100	18 ns	
Teicoplanin vs vancomycin	200	10	26	96	8[a]	DeLalla *et al.* 1992 [92]
	2000	10	20	100	20	
Teicoplanin vs fusidic acid vs vancomycin	800	10	28	96	7[a]	Wenisch *et al.* 1996 [93]
vs metronidazole	1500	10	29	93	28	
	1500	10	31	94	16 ns	
	1500	10	31	94	16 ns	
Ramoplanin vs mamoplanin vs vancomycin	400 mg	10	28	79	23	Pullman *et al.* 2004 [94]
	800 mg	10	29	86	20	
	500 mg	10	29	86	20	
Rifampin ± metronidazole vs	600	10	19	63	42	Lagrotteria *et al.* 2006
metronidazole	1500					[95]
	1500	10	20	65	38 ns	
Vancomycin vs metronidazole	500	10	71	97	7	Zar *et al.* 2007 [18]
	1000	10	79	84	14 ns	
Other						
Tolevamer vs Tolevamer vs vancomycin	3000	10	30	nr	13	Louie *et al.* 2006 [96]
	6000	10	39	nr	13	
	500	10	56	nr	18 ns	
Fusidic acid vs metronidazole	750	7	59	83	27	Wullt *et al.* 2004 [97]
	600	7	55	93	29 ns	
S. boulardii adjunct vs placebo adjunct	1000	28	31	nr	19	McFarland *et al.* 1994
	1000	28	33	nr	24[a]	[27]
L. rhamnosus GG adjunct vs placebo	nr	21	6	nr	0%	Pochapin *et al.* 2000 [98]
adjunct	nr	21	10	nr	30%	

[a] $p < 0.05$.

Abbreviations: nr: not reported; ns: not significant; adjunct: in addition to standard antibiotics (vancomycin or metronidazole).

Ten metronidazole treated patients had their treatment changed to vancomycin due to lack of response, but only four completed an entire 10-day course of metronidazole, a factor that may bias these results.

While intravenous vancomycin has little efficacy, use of vancomycin enemas is an alternative when the oral route is not feasible, e.g. in patients with paralytic ileus. However, there are no controlled trials demonstrating efficacy of this approach. Even the case series that suggest benefit are small. A recent series of nine hospitalized patients with severe *C. difficile* colitis showed response to adjunctive intracolonic therapy in eight (89%) [102]. Previously pub-

Table 20.2 Randomized, controlled trials of treatments for patients with recurrent *Clostridium difficile* associated disease (CDAD).

Treatment	Daily dose (mg or organisms/day)	No.	Duration (days)	Recurred (%)	Reference
Antibiotics					
Vancomycin vs vancomycin vs metronidazole	2000	14	10	50%	Surawicz *et al.* 2000 [116]
	500	38	10	44.7%, ns	
	1000	26	10	50%, ns	
Vancomycin vs metronidazole	800	65	11	43%	McFarland *et al.* 1994 [27]
	1200	37	12	32%, ns	
Vancomycin taper vs vancomycin pulse vs vancomycin	2000 to 500	21	29	31%[a]	McFarland *et al.* 2002 [117]
	250	Q3D for 18 d	7	14%[a]	
	1000–1500	10	14	71%	
Probiotic adjuncts					
Vancomycin and *S. boulardii* vs placebo	2000		10		Surawicz *et al.* 2000 [116]
	1000	18	28	16.7[a]	
	1000	14	28	50	
Standard antibiotic and *S. boulardii* vs placebo	1784[b]		20[b]		McFarland *et al.* 1994 [27]
	1000	26	28	35[a]	
	1000	34	28	65	
Standard antibiotic and *L. rhamnosus* GG vs placebo	varied				Pochapin *et al.* 2000 [98]
	nr	5	21	80%, ns	
	nr	4	21	50	
Standard antibiotic and *L. rhamnosus* GG vs placebo	varied				Lawrence *et al.* 2005 [118]
	8×10^{10}	8	Nr	37.5%, ns	
	0	7	nr	14.3%	
Absorbents					
Tolevamer vs Tolevamer vs vancomycin	3000	11	10	36%, ns	Louie *et al.* 2006 [96]
	6000	12	10	0	
	500	15	10	27%, ns	

[a] p < 0.05
[b] dose or day varied, mean reported
Abbreviations: bid: twice a day; qid: four times a day; Q3D: once every three days; ns: not significant.

lished data suggested an overall efficacy of 83% (from 24 prior cases). There are insufficient data on which to make a recommendation for this form of therapy.

Metronidazole

Oral metronidazole has been used for treatment of initial CDAD, and several clinical practice guidelines suggest that it should be first- line therapy. Recommended treatment is 250–500 mg orally four times a day for 7–14 days. Studies have shown a good response rate (>95%) [88, 93]. **A1c**

Metronidazole cure rates generally range between 76–90%, but the failure rate has increased from <16% pre-2003 to over 35% since 2004. In addition, the recurrence rate has also increased from ~20% pre-2003 to up to 47% since 2004. In 845 patients treated with metronidazole in Quebec during the 2003–2004 outbreaks, 26% failed initial treatment and 47.2% recurred within 60 days of treatment [17]. **B4** One proposed explanation of a higher rate of metronidazole treatment failure is that metronidazole resistance may have developed. However, metronidazole resistance is infrequent in *C. difficile* isolates. Of 415 *C. difficile* isolates from patients in Spain, only 6% of isolates were resistant to metronidazole and 3% exhibited reduced susceptibility to vancomycin [103].

Another area of debate is the route of administration. Oral antibiotic treatment is preferred, but some patients have an ileus or toxic colon precluding the oral route. Observational evidence from case reports suggests that intravenous metronidazole is effective. In a series of 10 patients with *C. difficile* colitis given intravenous therapy a good response was observed in nine [104]. There are no controlled trials evaluating the efficacy of intravenous metronidazole.

Investigational treatments

As shown in Table 20.1, due to the occurrence of treatment failures and of recurrent disease , new interventions are under investigation. Tinidazole has been tested and found to be safe in phase 2 trials, but phase 3 trials are needed to demonstrate efficacy [105].

Absorbents

Another approach is the administration of an agent that may bind *C. difficile* toxins within the intestinal lumen. In a phase 2 randomized double-blind trial, tolevamer in doses of 3 or 6g/d) was compared to vancomycin (500mg/d) for 10 days in patients with initial or recurrent CDAD [96]. For patients with initial CDAD, the rates of recurrence were not significantly different by treatment group: 4/30 (13%) in the 3g tolevamer group, 5/39 (13%) in the 6g tolevamer group and 10/56 (18%) in the vancomycin group. **A1d** Phase 3 trials were recently completed, but the results have not yet been published.

Bacitracin

Bacitracin is an orally administered non-absorbable antibiotic, that is characterized by an unpleasant taste and is relatively expensive. Two uncontrolled studies in 1980 showed response to therapy in small numbers of patients (two and four patients each) [106, 107]. More recently a double-blind randomized, controlled trial compared bacitracin (80,000 units daily) with vancomycin (500mg daily) in 42 patients. Clinical response (decreased diarrhea at four days) was similar in the two groups. **A1d** However, the bacitracin treated patient had higher rates of persistent *C. difficile* positive cultures in the stools [89]. The authors recommended bacitracin as a first-line alternative to vancomycin, A second randomized, controlled trial in 24 patients also showed similar efficacy of bacitracin and vancomycin, although vancomycin was more effective in clearing *C. difficile* and toxin from the stool [90]. A randomized trial com-

paring metronidazole and bacitracin would be important and has not been performed.

Fusidic acid

Fusidic acid is considered to be an L-selectin blocker that inhibits leukocyte extravasation into inflamed sites [108]. In a small randomized trial in which 40 patients were randomized to one of four oral agents: fusidic acid, metronidazole, vancomycin and teicoplanin the response rates were similar for all four groups (93–96%). The authors recommend metronidazole because of its lower costs, reserving other drugs for patients who do not tolerate or respond to metronidazole [93]. A randomized, controlled trial in 131 patients with initial episodes of CDAD comparing fusidic acid (750mg/d) and metronidazole (1200mg/d) for seven days showed no statistically significant difference in clinical cure rate [97]. **A1d**

A phase 3 trial with patients randomized to fusidic acid (n = 59) or metronidazole (n = 55) for seven days found equivalent rates of cure and recurrences. **A1d** Resistance to fusidic acid was found in 1% of colonic isolates obtained from pre-treatment patients and from 11/20 (55%) of isolates in those patients who remained culture positive after treatment with fusidic acid [109].

Probiotics

Probiotics are defined as live microorganisms that confer a health benefit on the host when administered in adequate amounts [110]. Probiotics have no proven role in treatment of initial CDAD. In a placebo controlled randomized trial of a probiotic mixture for the prevention of antibiotic-associated diarrhea, a secondary outcome was the prevention of CDAD [111]. Patients were randomized to receive either a probiotic mixture of *Lactobacillus casei*, *Lactobacillus bulgaricus* and *Streptococcus thermophilus* (Actimel drink) at a dose of 2.2×10^8 cfu/day or a placebo drink for the duration of antibiotic therapy plus one additional week. Of the 113 subjects completing the trial, 0/56 (0%) developed CDAD in the probiotic group compared to 9/53 (17%) in the placebo group, p < 0.05. **A1c** The estimated cost of preventing one case of CDAD with probiotic was $120.00. Currently, several probiotics are under development for CDAD including *Lactobacillus acidophilus*, *Saccharomyces boulardii* and a non-toxigenic strain of *Clostridium difficile*.

Ramoplanin

This antibiotic targets bacterial DNA-dependent RNA polymerase and inhibits cell wall synthesis. In a phase 2 open-label trial of 86 CDAD patients were treated with 10 days of either ramoplanin (200mg bid or 400mg bid) or vancomycin (125 mg qid) [94]. The rates of cure were similar in all groups: 83% and 85% for patients receiving 200 mg or 400 mg of ramoplanin and 86% for patients receiving vancomycin. **A1d**

Rifampin

In a phase 2 study of Rifampin 39 patients were randomized to receive either metronidazole 500 mg tid or metronidazole plus rifampin 300 mg bid for 10 days. The recurrence rates were similar by day 40 (38% and 42% respectively) [95]. **A1d**

Teicoplanin

De Lalla *et al.* reported a randomized, controlled trial in which 46 patients with CDAD received either teicoplanin (200 mg) or vancomycin 2 g daily for 10 days [92]. The initial cure rates for teicoplanin and vancomycin were 96% and 100%, and the recurrence rates were 7.7% and 20%. These differences were not statistically significant. However, teicoplanin appeared to be significantly more protective against recurrent disease than fusidic acid (RR = 0.19; 95% CI: 0.04 to 0.99) (Table 20.1) [93]. **A1d**

Tiacumicin B

Tiacumicin B (also known as OPT-80 and PAR-101) is a macrocyclic antibiomicrobial that targets RNA polymerase. Early phase 1 studies showed it was well tolerated in healthy volunteers at doses up to 450 mg/day [112]. In a phase 2 dose ranging study in 49 patients with mild to moderate CDAD [105] the cure rates were similar in patients receiving 100 mg (86 %), 200 mg (87%) or 400 mg (100%). The recurrence rates for these treatments were also similar: 8%, 0% and 6%. Phase 3 trials are in progress.

Treatment for recurrent CDAD

Most patients (76–98%) with their first episode of CDAD are cured after treatment with either vancomycin or metronidazole [9, 99]. However, a proportion of patients develop recurrent episodes of CDAD that may last for years, despite antibiotic treatment [9, 60]. Once a second episode of CDAD occurs, 60% of patients continue to experience subsequent episodes and are considered to have an especially difficult form of CDAD, designated "recurrent CDAD" [9, 60]. Treatment of recurrent CDAD has traditionally relied upon antibiotics (usually vancomycin or metronidazole), toxin binding resins, fecal enemas and the use of biotherapeutic agents [13, 26, 27, 113–115].

Vancomycin or metronidazole treatments

There are a limited number of randomized trials comparing antibiotic treatments in patients with recurrent CDAD (in which patients with an initial episode have been specifically excluded) (Table 20.2) [27, 96, 98, 116–118]. Most trials have been in patients with initial disease, or have not specifically included or excluded patients with prior CDAD episodes. In a randomized, double-blind, placebo-controlled trial of an investigational probiotic treatment patients with recurrent CDAD were randomized to receive 10 days of either high dose vancomycin (2 g/d), low dose vancomycin (500 mg/d) or metronidazole (1 g/d) plus either the probiotic or a placebo. In the three antibiotic treatment groups that received the probiotic placebo the observed recurrence rates were similar: high dose vancomycin 50%, low dose vancomycin 45% and metronidazole 50%. An earlier double-blind, placebo-controlled trial compared the efficacy of these antibiotics in various doses with a placebo in 102 patients. [27]. The observed recurrence rates of 43% for vancomycin-treated patients and 32% for metronidazole-treated patients were not significantly different. **A1a**

A series of 163 patients with recurrent CDAD who were followed prospectively documented the rate of CDAD recurrences over a two-month period in patients who were treated with a variety of strategies using either vancomycin or metronidazole [117]. Of the 125 patients treated with a variety of doses and durations of vancomycin, 46% subsequently developed recurrent CDAD. This recurrence rate was not significantly different from the rate of 42% in the 38 patients treated with metronidazole (p > 0.05). **B4**

Similar rates of recurrence following therapy with vancomycin and metronidazole are seen despite the differences in the pharmacokinetics of these agents in the intestine. In the healthy intestine, metronidazole is rapidly absorbed from the feces, and the concentration within the lumen of the gut is low. Once an acute episode of CDAD occurs, high concentrations of metronidazole have been documented in the infected intestine [119]. Vancomycin is bacteriostatic on *Clostridium difficile* organisms, thus allowing the persistence of vegetative cells of *Clostridium difficile* and the rapid increase in *Clostridium difficile* after discontinuation [120]. The time required for spore germination, *C. difficile* overgrowth and acute toxigenic symptoms may be extremely short (usually 3–5 days) once the treatment antibiotics have been discontinued. In one long-term follow-up study 97% of recurrences were observed within four weeks of stopping antibiotics (median of seven days) [14]. The short time between the end of antibiotic therapy and the recurrence of symptoms was confirmed by two other studies of patients with recurrent CDAD [9, 99]. Delayed onsets of new episodes (four to eight weeks later) reported in some studies may be due to the exposure to exogenous spores or germination of asymptomatic carriage of *Clostridium difficile* during the time when the normal colonic flora has not yet recovered. A previous study has shown that antibiotics may disrupt the normal flora for up to six weeks after discontinuation [121]. Continuation or restarting inciting antibiotics after successful treatments has been shown to increase the risk of recurrence [122].

Thus, the efficacy of treatment for recurrent CDAD may be influenced by the presence of residual *Clostridium difficile* spores in the intestinal tract and the interval over which the intestine is susceptible to *Clostridium difficile* overgrowth. Short duration antibiotic treatments may be effective in initially resolving the symptoms of diarrhea, but may be ineffective during the "window of susceptibility", i.e. the interval during which the intestinal microflora needs to be re-established in order to resist the overgrowth of *Clostridium difficile* and recurrence of disease. Several strategies have been tested, including providing extended protection by tapering the dose or providing "pulsed" doses of antibiotics, use of biotherapeutic agents ("beneficial microbes") or restoration of intestinal microflora using fecal infusions of bacteria or normal stool contents.

Vancomycin taper/pulse

There have been two studies of patients with recurrent CDAD treated with either tapering or pulsed dosing of vancomycin. In an observational study of 163 patients with recurrent CDAD who were treated with a variety of strategies that included either vancomycin or metronidazole and followed for two months the overall recurrence rates for all patients receiving the two antibiotics were not significantly different [117]. **B4** Vancomycin tapering and vancomycin pulsed dosing were shown to be effective for reducing the frequency of recurrences. The recurrence rate for 14 patients treated with vancomycin in doses between 1 and 1.5 g/d for 10 days was 71% compared to a rate of 31% in 29 patients treated with a tapering dose of vancomycin (over a mean of 21 days), and there was only one recurrence in seven patients treated with a pulsed dosing of vancomycin (125–500 mg pulse every three days over a mean of 18 days). Although these patients were studied using standardized protocols this was not a randomized trial and the results are suggestive, but not definitive.

Tedesco *et al.* reported an uncontrolled study of 22 patients who had recurrent CDAD and were treated with a tapering dose of vancomycin for 21 days (500 mg/d for one week, 250 mg/d for the second week, 125 mg/d for the third week, and 125 mg on alternate days for a fourth week) and a pulse dose (125 mg every third day for 21 days). There were no recurrences, but the results of this uncontrolled study do not constitute definitive evidence [123]. **B4**

Adjunctive intracolonic vancomycin appeared to be beneficial in a case series of nine patients (three of whom had recurrent CDAD) but the results have not been confirmed in a randomized trial [102].

Other investigational treatments

In contrast to patients with initial CDAD, no randomized, controlled trials of teicoplanin, bacitracin, or rifampin have been performed for patients with recurrent CDAD.

Absorbents

Another approach that has been investigated in a phase 2 randomized double-blind trial is administration of an agent that may bind *C. difficile* toxins within the intestinal lumen. Tolevamer in doses of 3 or 6 g/d was compared to vancomycin 500 mg/d for 10 days in patients with initial or recurrent CDAD. In patients with recurrent CDAD, the rates of recurrence were: 4/11 in the 3 g tolevamer group, 0/12 in the 6 g tolevamer group and 4/15 in the vancomycin group [96]. These differences were not statistically significant, but this small study lacked power to demonstrate true differences in efficacy of these regimens, should they exist.

Ion exchange resins

Although *in vivo* studies of two resins, cholestyramine and colestipol, demonstrated binding of cytotoxin (as well as some binding of vancomycin), and cholestyramine delayed death in the hamster model of clindamycin-induced cecitis [124] trials of ion exchange materials to bind toxins in humans have produced negative results. Colestipol was compared to placebo in a randomized, controlled trial in 38 patients with postoperative diarrhea. There was no difference in fecal excretion of *C. difficile* toxin, and treatment with ion exchange resins currently is not recommended [125]. **A1d** The study, however, lacks adequate power to show true differences between the treatment groups, should they exist.

Probiotics

A meta-analysis of six randomized, controlled trials using probiotics combined with one of the two standard antibiotics to treat CDAD found that probiotics significantly reduced the risk of CDAD (combined RR = 0.59; 95% CI: 0.41, 0.85; $p = 0.005$) [126]. **A1c** Although a variety of probiotic strains have been tested, most studies were not large randomized, controlled trials. It is important to note that the term "probiotic" covers a wide variety of bacterial and yeast strains, and clinical efficacy may be linked to a specific strain. For example, not all Lactobacilli strains are equally effective probiotics for specific diseases. When considering efficacy of probiotics for any disease, it is important to link the clinical evidence with specific strains.

Saccharomyces boulardii

There have been two double-blind randomized, controlled trials for the use of *Saccharomyces boulardii* and antibiotics for patients with recurrent CDAD (Table 20.2). In a trial in 168 patients with recurrent CDAD, standard antibiotics were combined with *Saccharomyces boulardii* or placebo [116]. Three antibiotic regimens were used for 10 days: vancomycin in doses of 2 g or 500 mg/d or metronidazole 1 g/d. At the end of the 10-day period either *Saccharomyces boulardii* or placebo (1 g/d for 28 days) were added to the antibiotic regimen. The patients were followed for two months for subsequent *Clostridium difficile* recurrences. A significant decrease in recurrences was observed only in patients treated with the high dose vancomycin and *Saccharomyces boulardii* treatment (16.7%) compared with patients who received high dose vancomycin and placebo (50%, p = 0.05). **A1c** No significant reductions in recurrence rates in either the low dose vancomycin or metronidazole treatment groups, were observed in *Saccharomyces boulardii* treated patients, compared to placebo controls. No serious adverse effects were noted in any of these patients.

An earlier study had also indicated the efficacy of the combination treatment using a standard antibiotic (vancomycin or metronidazole) and *Saccharomyces boulardii* for patients with CDAD [27]. In this trial patients who received vancomycin or metronidazole in doses determined by the physician were randomized to receive either *Saccharomyces boulardii* (1 g/d) or placebo for 28 days. All patients were followed for two months for subsequent recurrences. Approximately half of the enrolled patients were experiencing their first episode and half had recurrent CDAD. In the 60 patients with recurrent CDAD the recurrence rate in patients who received *Saccharomyces boulardii* was 35% compared to 65% for patients in the placebo group (p = 0.04). **A1d** In this small study vancomycin was not shown to be more effective than metronidazole, regardless of the dose or duration of treatment.

Lactobacillus rhamnosus GG

Lactobacillus GG is another probiotic that has been reported to reduce CDAD recurrences in several case series and case reports [113, 127, 128]. A small randomized trial comparing *L. rhamnosus* GG (8×10^{10} organisms/day) to placebo as an adjunctive to standard antibiotic therapy with vancomycin or metronidazole was terminated due to poor enrollment. The observed recurrence rates were 3/8 and 1/7 in the *Lactobacillus* and placebo groups [118].

Fecal biotherapy

In an effort to replace the microflora disrupted by recurrent CDAD and antibiotic treatments, fecal enemas of normal stool contents have been administered to patients with recurrent CDAD [129–133]. However, no randomized, placebo-controlled trials have been performed. In the case reports describing the use of fecal enemas in a total of 87 patients with recurrent CDAD, 77 (89%) of the patients responded to fecal biotherapy [134]. **B4**

Immunoglobulin

The use of immunoglobulin for patients with recurrent CDAD has been reported in the literature in small case series or case reports [135–137]. A phase 2 study of 79 patients who had toxin positive CDAD compared results in 18 patients given standard antibiotics and IV IgG treatment (200–300 mg/kg/d) with 61 controls who received standard antibiotics only. No significant differences in mortality (three died in each group) or colectomy (three in each group) were observed [138]. **B4**

Whey protein made from cows immunized with *C. difficile* is also being tested. In a phase 2 trial 77 CDAD patients were given anti-*C. difficile* whey protein concentrate in a dose of 5 g tid for 14 days after 10 days of treatment with vancomycin. No adverse effects were observed. Four of 63 (6.3%) patients experienced relapse within 46 days of completing this treatment [139]. Phase 3 trials are in progress. Another investigational approach is the use of a targeted immunoglobulin product specifically directed against *C. difficile* toxin. The safety and kinetics of neutralizing human monoclonal antibody against *C. difficile* toxin A is under study. In a phase 2 dose ranging study in 30 CDAD patients no serious adverse effects were noted [140]. Phase 3 trials are in progress.

Treatment of asymptomatic carriers

Asymptomatic carriers of *Clostridium difficile* have been shown to be a source of new nosocomial cases of CDAD. In order to control the spread of *Clostridium difficile*, a policy of treating asymptomatic carriers has been tested by several investigators. However, treatment of asymptomatic carriers has not been found to reduce the incidence of CDAD and has not been shown to reduce the frequency of nosocomial outbreaks [141]. Bender *et al.* demonstrated that treatment of carriers with metronidazole was ineffective in reducing the incidence of new CDAD cases at a chronic care facility [142]. Delmee *et al.* were able to reduce the CDAD frequency in patients on a leukemia unit from 16.6% to 3.6% after all patients with *Clostridium difficile* were treated with vancomycin [143]. However, this study was not randomized and both symptomatic and asymptomatic

Clostridium difficile cases were treated. Johnson *et al.* treated 30 asymptomatic carriers of *Clostridium difficile* in a randomized, placebo-controlled trial with either vancomycin (1 g/d), metronidazole (1 g/d), or placebo [85]. Although vancomycin significantly reduced *Clostridium difficile* carriage at the end of the 10 days of treatment (10%) compared to either metronidazole (70%, p = 0.02) or placebo (80%, p = 0.005), the recurrence rate at the end of the two-month follow-up period was significantly higher (67%) in the vancomycin group compared to the placebo group (11%, p < 0.05). **A1d** Although there are small randomized, placebo-controlled trials demonstrating the effectiveness of treating asymptomatic carriers, the overall evidence is not sufficiently strong to support a recommendation for the use of this intervention.

Prevention

Infection control

The importance of infection control practices for the prevention and control of nosocomial infections of CDAD and recurrent CDAD has been well documented [13, 26]. Studies documenting that 48–56% of clinical recurrences are new infections with a different strain of *Clostridium difficile* also add support to the importance of disrupting the nosocomial acquisition of new strains of *Clostridium difficile* in the hospital environment [15, 64, 144].

The most important intervention for prevention of CDAD is the interruption of the horizontal transmission of *Clostridium difficile*. Five aspects of infection control practices have been investigated: (1) environmental disinfection of contaminated surfaces or fomites, and medical equipment or use of disposable instruments, (2) reducing hand carriage by hospital care personnel, (3) isolation or cohorting of infected patients, (4) treatment of asymptomatic carriers and (5) multi-disciplinary approach using a combination of the above. None of these infection control practices has been evaluated in randomized, controlled trials, but most have been evaluated in the hospital environment using a defined intervention and have compared infection rates before and after the introduction of the intervention or have compared the results between a ward in which the intervention was introduced with those in a control ward in which the new intervention was not used.

Another strategy under investigation is vaccination of newly admitted patients at health care facilities using a vaccine against the toxins of *C. difficile*. One such vaccine, developed by Acambis, is currently under investigation in phase 3 trials. A small phase 2 study in 30 subjects showed that this vaccine was not associated with any serious adverse effects [145].

Environmental disinfectants

Contamination of environmental surfaces by *Clostridium difficile* and its spores presents an extremely challenging problem for hospitals. The spores of *Clostridium difficile* can persist on surfaces or fomites for months and are not susceptible to normal room cleaning agents, and patients who are carriers of *Clostridium difficile* shed the spores onto a wide variety of hospital surfaces [4, 26, 146–148] Several reviews have presented evidence that the use of environmental cleaning and an effective disinfectant has resulted in lower rates of health care associated CDAD [26, 149]. Mayfield *et al.* changed the type of room disinfectant used (to 1:10 hypochlorite solution) in rooms with 4252 bone marrow transplant patients and studied the incidence of CDAD [150]. The incidence of CDAD was 8.6 cases/1000 patient days before the intervention was introduced and decreased significantly to 3.3 cases/1000 patient days, (hazard ratio 0.37; 95% CI: 0.19–0.74). No similar decrease in the incidence of CDAD was noted for control wards where the new disinfectant was not tested. **B2** Struelens *et al.* found that the frequency of environmental positive isolation of *Clostridium difficile* fell significantly from 13% to 3% (p = 0.04) after daily room disinfection was used (0.03% glutaraldehyde and 0.04% formaldehyde solution), along with a concurrent decrease in the incidence of CDAD cases [151]. Kaatz *et al.* used a phosphate buffered hypochlorite solution to disinfect hospital room surfaces during an outbreak of CDAD. The isolation rate for *Clostridium difficile* was 31.4% before and 0.6% after the hypochlorite disinfectant was introduced, and the outbreak ceased [152]. McMullen *et al.* compared room disinfection protocols in two intensive care units with high endemic rates of *C. difficile* [153]. The unit that followed a protocol using hypochlorite solution disinfection in all rooms within the unit (regardless of the location of a CDAD patient) exhibited a decline from 16.6/1000 to 2.8/1000 patient-days. However, the unit that only disinfected rooms with an infected CDAD patient also showed a significant decrease in CDAD rates from 10.4/1000 to 2.2/1000 patient days. The important conclusion is that hypochlorite disinfection appears to be effective, even when it is used only in rooms in which CDAD cases are located. **B2**

Disinfection of medical equipment

Medical equipment that is used for patients infected with CDAD may become a source of new infections if not properly cleaned. Fiberoptic endoscopes have been shown to be a source of *Clostridium difficile*, but two studies found that exposure to 2% alkaline glutaraldehyde for five minutes resulted in 99% killing of *Clostridium difficile* on the surfaces [154, 155]. However, neither of these studies used a control group and they were not designed to document if the disinfection procedure resulted in fewer clinical cases of CDAD. Brooks *et al.* studied whether the replacement of electronic rectal thermometers, of which 21% had tested positive for *Clostridium difficile*, with single-use disposable thermometers resulted in lower rates of CDAD [156]. The incidence of *Clostridium difficile*-associated diarrhea decreased from 2.71/1000 patient days to 1.76/1000 patient days (p < 0.05) after the introduction of disposable thermometers at the acute care hospital. A significant reduction of CDAD casea was also observed by Brooks *et al.* at a skilled nursing facility. Although this study was not a randomized trial, the pre and post-intervention measures were carried out using the same testing procedures and at the same institutions. **B4**

Hand washing and disinfection

Nosocomial *Clostridium difficile* is frequently transmitted to other patients via the hands of hospital care personnel and visitors [4, 99]. Efforts to disrupt this method of transmission have included handwashing with disinfectants instead of non-disinfectant soaps, training programs on the importance of proper handwashing techniques, and the use of disposable gloves. In one prospective study, handwashing with 4% chlorhexidine gluconate resulted in a significantly lower isolation frequency of *Clostridium difficile* on the hand surfaces of tested hospital personnel (14%, p = 0.002) compared to an isolation rate of 88% when non-disinfectant soap was used [4]. Currently, newer enteric precaution policies have included the use of vinyl disposable gloves. Three studies have documented that the use of gloves reduces the rate of *Clostridium difficile* isolation on the hands of health care personnel. In a study of 42 health care workers (doctors, nurses, physical therapists), the use of disposable gloves during the care of infected CDAD patients significantly reduced the rate of isolation of the hand carriage of *Clostridium difficile* from 58% prior to the use of gloves to 0% after the introduction of the requirement for wearing gloves (p = 0.04) [4]. **B2** Johnson *et al.* tested the effectiveness of an educational program involving the use of disposable gloves on two wards assigned to the program and compared the results to two control wards [157]. The incidence of CDAD decreased from 7.7/1000 patient discharges before the program was started to 1.5/1000 during the six-month intervention (p = 0.01). No significant decreases in CDAD were noted on the two control wards. **B2** Bettin *et al.* seeded 10 volunteers with *Clostridium difficile* and found that *Clostridium difficile* counts were significantly lower on gloved hands compared to bare hands, regardless of the type of handwashing agent used [158]. However, the effectiveness of limiting nosocomial spread of *Clostridium difficile* by handwashing or use of gloves as the sole control policy has not been tested in randomized, controlled trials.

Alcohol-based gels are effective for methicillin-resistant Staphylococcal elimination, but are not effective against spores of *C. difficile* [159, 160].

Isolation or cohorting practices

Both asymptomatic and symptomatic infected patients increase the risk of nosocomial spread of *Clostridium difficile*. One control policy that has been investigated is the isolation of patients from the pool of susceptible uninfected patients in private rooms, or by "cohorting" patients who are infected with *Clostridium difficile* (or putting patients who are infected with *Clostridium difficile* in the same room). Boone *et al.* tested a new re-admission policy for patients who had been *Clostridium difficile* positive during a previous hospital stay [161]. These patients were screened for *Clostridium difficile* toxin shortly before or on admission and if positive, they were placed in isolation. The attack rate decreased from 13.3/1000 admissions before the policy was introduced to 8.7/1000. **B2** Another observational study of 428 patients admitted to a general medicine ward found that the *Clostridium difficile* acquisition rate tended to be higher in patients in double rooms (17/100) than in single rooms (7/100). **B4** However, it should be noted that these studies were not randomized, controlled trials. Most studies attempting to reduce the transmission of *Clostridium difficile* use the policy of private rooms or "cohorting", but only as part of a multi-disciplinary approach rather than as an independent control policy.

Antibiotic stewardship

Antibiotic stewardship programs are multi-disciplinary programs involving physicians, microbiologists, pharmacists and infection control practitioners, set protocols for prior authorization and concurrent review and feedback on antibiotic use. Health care systems, clinicians and patients need to be proactive in collaborative efforts. Valiquette *et al.* implemented an antimicrobial stewardship program during the Canadian outbreaks of 2005–2006 and decreased the use of target antibiotics by 54%, with a concurrent reduction in CDAD infection of 60% [162]. **B4** Increased infection control practices by themselves (2003–2004) did not appear to decrease CDAD rates.

Antibiotic restriction programs may also be effective in reducing CDAD rates. Three separate studies at Veterans' Affairs hospitals documented control of epidemics by restriction of clindamycin use. The first study from Tucson identified a five-fold increase in *C. difficile*, over half of which was associated with a single strain. Antibiotic use was analyzed and the introduction of a restriction on use of clindamycin was accompanied by a decrease in infection rates [38]. **B4** A second study at another VA medical center showed a prompt reduction in the frequency of CDAD cases following introduction of a restricted clindamycin use policy. Although some more expensive antibiotics were used, net cost savings were realized, and isolates showed a return of clindamycin susceptibility [163]. A third study documented a decrease in CDAD following removal of several antibiotics from the hospital formulary [164]. **B4**

CDAD rates in an elderly care unit decreased following introduction of a restrictive antibiotic policy that specifically targeted cefuroxine use, substituting penicillin, trimethoprim and gentamycin for broad spectrum cephalosporins [165]. **B4**

Introduction of a restriction policy for injectable third-generation cephalosporins for elderly medical patients resulted in a significant reduction of CDAD cases from 4.5% of 2157 admissions before the policy to 2.2% of 2037 admissions during the antibiotic restriction policy [166]. **B2** No decrease in CDAD cases was observed in other wards used as controls.

Multi-disciplinary practices

Integrated, interdisciplinary infection control programs involving educational programs (handwashing, use of gloves, enteric precaution procedures), environmental disinfection and aggressive surveillance are effective in reducing CDAD rates. **B4** Struelens *et al.* demonstrated a significant reduction in new CDAD cases from 1.5 to 0.3 cases per 1000 discharges (p < 0.05) after introduction of a control program consisting of intensive screening for *Clostridium difficile*, early enteric isolation precautions, rapid treatment of CDAD cases with vancomycin and room disinfection [151]. **B2** Brown *et al.* reported control practices including rapid patient isolation, treatment of CDAD cases and antibiotic restriction resulted in a decline of CDAD incidence from 2.2 % to 0.7% [75]. Bundled infection control programs (increased hand washing programs, environmental disinfection, antibiotic stewardship) have resulted in significant reductions of CDAD rates [159, 167–169], but randomized, controlled trials have not been published. Several reviews have presented evidence that the use of multi-disciplinary infection control programs have resulted in lower rates of nosocomial CDAD [26, 76, 149].

Summary

Clostridium difficile-associated diarrhea (CDAD) is an important cause of nosocomial outbreaks of gastrointestinal disease. Despite years of research regarding the pathogenesis and nosocomial transmission of this organism,

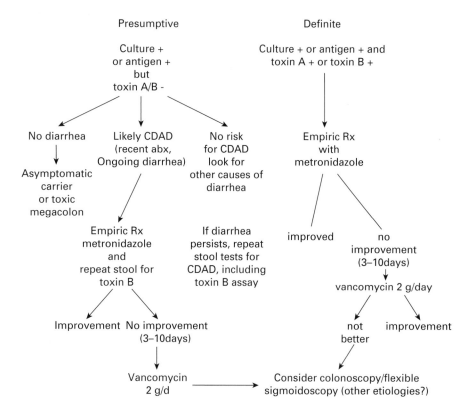

Figure 20.1 Management of an initial episode of *Clostridium difficile*-associated diarrhea.
Abbreviations: CDAD: *Clostridium difficile* associated diarrhea; PMC: pseudomembranous colitis.

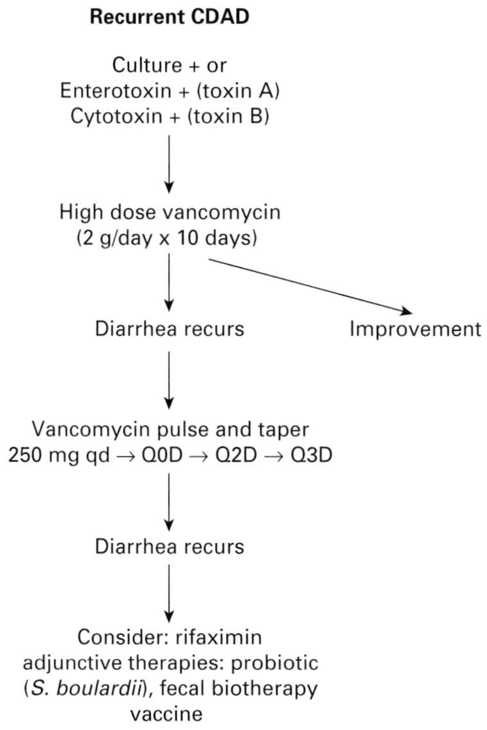

Recurrent CDAD

Culture + or
Enterotoxin + (toxin A)
Cytotoxin + (toxin B)

↓

High dose vancomycin
(2 g/day x 10 days)

↓

Diarrhea recurs   Improvement

↓

Vancomycin pulse and taper
250 mg qd → Q0D → Q2D → Q3D

↓

Diarrhea recurs

↓

Consider: rifaximin
adjunctive therapies: probiotic
(*S. boulardii*), fecal biotherapy
vaccine

Figure 20.2 Management of recurrent *Clostridium difficile*-associated disease.
Abbreviations: CDAD: *Clostridium difficile* associated diarrhea; QOD: every other day; Q2D: once every two days; Q3D: once every third day.

hospital outbreaks continue to occur. The management of patients with recurrent CDAD is appropriately focused more on efforts to clear the toxins of *Clostridium difficile* and restore the normal microbial flora. The treatment for this disease is complicated by the high frequency of asymptomatic carriers. Although these individuals contribute to spread of the disease, they should not be treated with antibiotics. Treatment strategies for the disease are dependent upon the individual patient's history of CDAD. Patients with an initial episode of CDAD may be treated equally well with either vancomycin 500 mg/day or metronidazole 1000–1500 mg/day (Figure 20.1), but the optimal management strategy has not been established in well-designed, randomized, controlled trials. Patients who develop the recurrent form of the disease may have a more difficult course, and the treatment choice is even less clear (Figure 20.2). Antibiotic treatment alone for recurrent CDAD may not be the optimal approach, since relapse remains a common problem, although prolonged vancomycin taper and pulsed doses demonstrate promise (Figure 20.2). There is evidence that combination therapy using vancomycin and a probiotic is also an effective treatment. More research is needed to investigate the value of other types of probiotics for recurrent CDAD and of other types of antibiotics for initial CDAD.

Acknowledgement

VA Disclaimer: the views expressed in this article are those of the author and do not represent the views of the Department of Veterans' Affairs.

References

1 Burdon DW. *Clostridium difficile*: The epidemiology and prevention of hospital-acquired infection. *Infection* 1982; **10**: 203–204.

2 Wüst J, Sullivan NM, Hardegger U, Wilkins TD. Investigation of an outbreak of antibiotic-associated colitis by various typing methods. *J Clin Microbiol* 1982; **16**: 1096–1101.

3 Tabaqchali S, O'Farrell S, Holland D, Silman R. Typing scheme for *Clostridium difficile*: Its application in clinical and epidemiological studies. *Lancet* 1984; **I**: 935–938.

4 McFarland LV, Mulligan ME, Kwok RYY, Stamm WE. Nosocomial acquisition of *Clostridium difficile* infection. *N Engl J Med* 1989; **320**: 204–210.

5 Shek FW, Stacey BSF, Rendell J, Hellier MD, Hanson PJV. The risk of *Clostridium difficile*: The effect of length of stay, patient age and antibiotic use. *J Hosp Infect* 2000; **45**: 235–237.

6 Pepin J, Valiquette L, Cossette B. Mortality attributable to nosocomial *Clostridium difficile*-associated disease during an epidemic caused by a hypervirulent strain in Quebec. *CMAJ* 2005; **173**(9): 1037–1042.

7 Feldman RJ, Kallich M, Weinstein MP. Bacteremia due to *Clostridium difficile*: Case report and review of extraintestinal *C difficile* infections. *Clin Infect Dis* 1995; **20**: 1560–1562.

8 Lowenkron SE, Waxner J, Khullar P, Ilowite JS, Niederman MS, Fein AM. *Clostridium difficile* infection as a cause of severe sepsis. *Intensive Care Med* 1996; **22**: 990–994.

9 Fekety R, McFarland LV, Surawicz CM, Greenberg RN, Elmer GW, Mulligan ME. Recurrent *Clostridium difficile* diarrhea: Characteristics of and risk factors for patients enrolled in a prospective, randomized, double-blinded trial. *Clin Infect Dis* 1997; **24**: 324–333.

10 Qualman SJ, Petric M, Karmali MA, Smith CR, Hamilton SR. *Clostridium difficile* invasion and toxin circulation in fatal pediatric pseudomembranous colitis. *Am J Clin Pathol* 1990; **94**: 410–416.

11 Walley T, Milson D. Loperamide related toxic megacolon in *Clostridium difficile* colitis (letter). *Postgrad Med J* 1990; **66**: 582.

12 Gravisse J, Bernaud G, Hanau-Bercot B, Raskine L, Riahi J, Gaillard JL, Sandon-Le-Pors MJ. *Clostridium difficile* brain empyema after prolonged intestinal carriage. *J Clin Microbiol* 2003; **41**: 509–511.

13 Fekety R. Guidelines for the diagnosis and management of *Clostridium difficile*-associated diarrhea and colitis. *Am J Gastroenterol* 1997; **92**: 739–750.

14 McFarland LV, Surawicz CM, Rubin M, Fekety R, Elmer GW, Greenberg RN. Recurrent *Clostridium difficile* disease: Epidemiology and clinical characteristics. *Infect Control Hosp Epidemiol* 1999; **20**: 43–50.

15 Barbut F, Richard A, Hamadi K, Chomette V, Burghoffer B, Petit JC. Epidemiology of recurrences or reinfections of

Clostridium difficile-associated diarrhea. *J Clin Microbiol* 2000; **38**: 2386–2388.

16 Kyne L, Merry C, O'Connell B, Kelly A, Keane C, O'Neill D. Factors associated with prolonged symptoms and severe disese due to *Clostridium difficile*. *Age and Ageing* 1999; **28**: 107–113.

17 Pepin J, Alary ME, Valiquette L, Raiche E, Ruel J, Fulop K, Godin D, Bourassa C. Increasing risk of relapse after treatment of *Clostridium difficile* colitis in Québec. *Can Clin Infect Dis* 2005; **40**: 1591–1597.

18 Zar FA, Bakkanagari SR, Moorthi KM, Davis MB. A comparison of vancomycin and metronidazole for the treatment of *Clostridium difficile*-associated diarrhea, stratified by disease severity. *Clin Infect Dis* 2007; **45**: 302–307.

19 Petersen LR, Manson RU, Paule SM *et al.* Detection of toxigenic *Clostridium difficile* in stool samples by real-time polymerase chain reaction for the diagnosis of *C. difficile* – associated diarrhea. *Clin Infect Dis* 2007; **45**: 1152–1160.

20 Reller ME, Lema CA, Perl TM *et al.* Yield of stool culture with isolate toxin testing versus a two-step algorithm including stool toxin testing for detection of toxigenic *Clostridium difficile*. *J Clin Microbiol* 2007; **45**: 3601–3605.

21 McFarland LV, Clarridge JE, Beneda HW, Raugi GR. Fluoroquinolone use and risk factors for *Clostridium difficile* disease within a Veterans Administration Health Care System. *Clin Infect Dis* 2007; **45**(9): 1141–1151.

22 Barbut F, Delmée M, Brazier JS *et al.*; ESCMID Study Group on Clostridium difficile (ESGCD). A European survey of diagnostic methods and testing protocols for *Clostridium difficile*. *Clin Microbiol Infect* 2003; **9**(10): 989–996.

23 McDonald LC. Trends in antimicrobial resistance in health care-associated pathogens and effect on treatment. *Clin Infect Dis* 2006; **42**(Suppl 2): S65–S71.

24 Rüssmann H, Panthel K, Bader RC, Schmitt C, Schaumann R. Evaluation of three rapid assays for detection of *Clostridium difficile* toxin A and toxin B in stool specimens. *Eur J Clin Microbiol Infect Dis* 2007; **26**(2): 115–119.

25 Toyokawa M, Ueda A, Nishi I *et al.* Usefulness of immunological detection of both toxin A and toxin B in stool samples for rapid diagnosis of *Clostridium difficile* – associated diarrhea. *Kansenshogaku Zasshi* 2007; **81**(1): 33–38.

26 Gerding DN, Johnson S, Peterson LR, Mulligan ME, Silva J Jr. *Clostridium difficile*-associated diarrhea and colitis. *Infect Control Hosp Epidemiol* 1995; **16**: 459–477.

27 McFarland LV, Surawicz CM, Greenberg RN *et al.* A randomized placebo-controlled trial of *Saccharomyces boulardii* in combination with standard antibiotics for *Clostridium difficile* disease. *JAMA* 1994; **271**: 1913–1918.

28 Al-Eidan FA, McElnay JC, Scott MG, Kearney MP. *Clostridium difficile*-associated diarrhea in hospitalised patients. *J Clin Pharm Therapeu* 2000; **25**: 101–109.

29 Chang HT, Krezolek D, Jojhnson S, Parada JP, Evans CT, Gerding DN. Onset of symptoms and time to diagnosis of *Clostridium difficile*-associated disease following discharge from an acute care hospital. *Infect Control Hosp Epidemiol* 2007; **28**(8): 926–931.

30 Hubert B, Baron A, Le Quere JM, Renard CM. A portrait of the geographic dissemination of the *Clostridium difficile* North American pulsed-field type 1 strain and the epidemiology of C.

difficile-associated disease in Québec. *Clin Infect Dis* 2007; **44**(2): 238–244.

31 Koss K, Clark MA, Sanders DS *et al.* The outcome of surgery in fulminant *Clostridium difficile* colitis. *Colorectal Dis* 2006; **8**: 149–154.

32 Pepin J, Valiquette L, Alary ME *et al.* Clostridium difficile–associated diarrhea in a region of Québec from 1991 to 2003: A changing pattern of disease severity. *CMAJ* 2004; **171**: 466–472.

33 Kofsky P, Rosen L, Reed J, Tolmie M, Ufberg D. *Clostridium difficile* – a common and costly colitis. *Dis Colon Rectum* 1991; **34**: 244–248.

34 Kyne L, Sougioultzis S, McFarland LV, Kelly CP. Underlying disease severity as a major risk factor for nosocomial *Clostridium difficile* diarrhea. *Infect Control Hosp Epidemiol* 2002; **23**: 653–659.

35 McFarland LV, Surawicz CM, Stamm WE. Risk factors for *Clostridium difficile* carriage and *C difficile*-associated diarrhea in a cohort of hospitalized patients. *J Infect Dis* 1990; **162**: 678–684.

36 Eriksson S, Aronsson B. Medical implications of nosocomial infection with *Clostridium difficile*. *Scand J Infect Dis* 1989; **21**: 733–734.

37 O'Brien JA, Lahue BJ, Caro JJ, Davidson DM. The emerging infectious challenge of *Clostridium difficile*-associated disease in Massachusetts hospitals: clinical and economic consequences. *Infect Control Hosp Epidemiol* 2007; **28**(11): 1219–1227.

38 Pear SM, Williamson TH, Bettin KM, Gerding DN, Galgiani JN. Decrease in nosocomial *Clostridium difficile*-associated diarrhea by restricting clindamycin use. *Ann Intern Med* 1994; **120**: 272–277.

39 Samore MH, Venkataraman L, DeGirolami PC, Arbeit R, Karchmer A. Clinical and molecular epidemiology of sporadic and clustered cases of nosocomial *Clostridium difficile* diarrhea. *Am J Med* 1996; **100**: 32–40.

40 Barbut F, Corthier G, Charpak Y *et al.* Prevalence and pathogenicity of *Clostridium difficile* in hospitalized patients. A French multicenter study. *Arch Intern Med* 1996; **156**: 1449–1454.

41 Elixhauser A, Jhung M. *Clostridium difficile*-associated disease in US Hospitals, 1993–2005. Agency for Healthcare Research and Quality, Statistical brief no. 50 April 2008. www.hcup-us.ahrq.gov/reports/statbriefs/Sb50.pdf

42 Hirschhorn LR, Trnka Y, Onderdonk A, Lee M-LT, Platt R. Epidemiology of community-acquired *Clostridium difficile*-associated diarrhea. *J Infect Dis* 1994; **169**: 127–133.

43 Levy DG, Stergachis A, McFarland LV *et al.* Antibiotics and *Clostridium difficile* diarrhea in the ambulatory care setting. *Clin Therapeut* 2000; **22**: 91–102.

44 Dial S, Delaney JA, Barkun AN, Suissa S. Use of gastric acid-suppressive agents and the risk of community-acquired *Clostridium difficile*-associated disease. *JAMA* 2005; **294**(23): 2989–2995.

45 Dial S, Delaney JA, Schneider V, Suissa S. Proton pump inhibitor use and risk of community-acquired *Clostridium difficile*-associated disease defined by prescription for oral vancomycin therapy. *CMAJ* 2006 (26 Sep); **175**(7): 745–748.

46 Bauer MP, Goorhuis A, Koster T *et al.* Community-onset *Clostridium difficile*-associated diarrhoea not associated with

antibiotic usage-two case reports with review of the changing epidemiology of *Clostridium difficile*-associated diarrhoea. *Neth J Med* 2008; **66**(5): 207–211.

47 Kato H, Kato N, Watanabe K *et al.* Analysis of *Clostridium difficile* isolates from nosocomial outbreaks at three hospitals in diverse areas of Japan. *J Clin Microbiol* 2001; **39**: 1391–1395.

48 Mody LR, Smith SM, Dever LL. *Clostridium difficile*-associated diarrhea in a VA Medical Center: Clustering of cases, association with antibiotic usage and impact on HIV-infected patients. *Infect Control Hosp Epidemiol* 2001; **22**: 42–45.

49 Crabtree TD, Pelletier SJ, Gleason TG, Pruett TL, Sawyer RG. Clinical characteristics and antibiotic utilization in surgical patients with *Clostridium difficile*-associated diarrhea. *Amer Surg* 2000; **66**: 507–512.

50 Bradbury AW and Barrett S. Surgical aspects of *Clostridium difficile* colitis. *Brit J Surg* 1997; **84**: 150–159.

51 Simor AE, Yake SL, Tsimidis K. Infection due to *Clostridium difficile* among elderly residents of a long-term-care facility. *Clin Infect Dis* 1993; **17**: 672–678.

52 Dharmarajan TS, Sipalay M, Shyamsundar R, Norkus EP, Pitchumoni CS. Co-morbidity, not age predicts adverse outcome in *Clostridium difficile* colitis. *World J Gastroenter* 2000; **6**: 198–201.

53 Settle CD, Wilcox MH, Fawley N, Corrado OK, Hawkey PM. Prospective study of the risk of *Clostridium difficile* diarrhea in elderly patients following treatment with cefotaxime or piperacillin-tazobactam. *Aliment Pharmacol Ther* 1998; **12**: 1217–1223.

54 Langley JM, LeBlanc JC, Hanakowski M, Goloubeva O. The role of *Clostridium difficile* and viruses as causes of nosocomial diarrhea in children. *Infect Control Hosp Epidemiol* 2002; **23**: 660–664.

55 McFarland LV, Brandmarker SA, Guandalini S. Pediatric *Clostridium difficile*: A phantom menace or clinical reality? *J Ped Gastroenterol Nutrition* 2000; **31**: 220–231.

56 Pulvirenti J, Gerding DN, Nathan C *et al.* Difference in the incidence of *Clostridium difficile* among patients infected with human immunodeficiency virus admitted to a public hospital and a private hospital. *Infect Control Hosp Epidemiol* 2002; **23**: 641–647.

57 Gorschluter M, Glasmacher A, Hahn C *et al. Clostridium difficile* infection in patients with neutropenia. *Clin Infect Dis* 2001; **33**: 786–791.

58 Bilgrami S, Feingold JM, Dorsky D *et al.* Incidence and outcome of *Clostridium difficile* infection following autologous peripheral blood stem cell transplantation. *Bone Marrow Transplant* 1999; **23**: 1039–1042.

59 Chakrabarti S, Lees A, Jones SG, Milligan DW. *Clostridium difficile* infection in allogeneic stem cell transplant recipients is associated with severe graft-versus-host disease and non-relapse mortality. *Bone Marrow Transplant* 2000; **26**: 871–876.

60 McFarland LV, Surawicz CM, Greenberg RN *et al.* Possible role of cross-transmission between neonates and mothers with recurrent *Clostridium difficile* infections. *Am J Infect Control* 1999; **27**: 301–303.

61 Rouphael NG, O'Donnell JA, Bhatnagar J *et al. Clostridium difficile*-associated diarrhea: An emerging threat to pregnant women. *Am J Obstet Gynecol* 2008; **198**(6): 635.e1–6.

62 Cohen SH, Tang YJ, Rahmani D, Silva J. Persistence of an endemic (toxigenic) isolate of *Clostridium difficile* in the environment of a general medicine ward. *Clin Infect Dis* 2000: **30**: 952–954.

63 Mekonen ET, Gerding DN, Sambot SP, Pottinger JM *et al.* Predominance of a single restriction endonuclease analysis group with intrahospital subgroup diversity among *Clostridium difficile* isolates at two Chicago hospitals. *Infect Control Hosp Epidemiol* 2002; **23**: 648–652.

64 Johnson S, Adelmann A, Clabots CR, Peterson LR, Gerding DN. Recurrences of *Clostridium difficile* diarrhea not caused by the original infecting organism. *J Infect Dis* 1989; **159**: 340–341.

65 Curry SR, Marsh JW, Muto CA, O'Leary MM, Pasculle AW, Harrison LH. TcdC genotypes associated with severe TcdC truncation in an epidemic clone and other strains of *Clostridium difficile*. *J Clin Microbiol* 2007; **45**(1): 215–221.

66 Warny M, Pepin J, Fang A *et al.* Toxin production by an emerging strain of *Clostridium difficile* associated with outbreaks of severe disease in North America and Europe. *Lancet* 2005; **366**(9491): 1079–1084.

67 McDonald LC, Killgore GE, Thompson A *et al.* An epidemic, toxin gene–variant strain of *Clostridium difficile*. *N Engl J Med* 2005; **353**: 2433–2441.

68 Biller P, Shank B, Lind L *et al.* Moxifloxacin therapy as a risk factor for *Clostridium difficile*–associated disease during an outbreak: Attempts to control a new epidemic strain. *Infect Control Hosp Epidemiol* 2007; **28**(2): 198–201.

69 Dubberke EF, Reske KA, Noble-Wang J *et al.* Prevalence of *C. difficile* environmental contamination and strain variability in multiple health care facilities. *Am J Infect Control* 2007; **35**(5): 315–318.

70 Riggs MM, Sethi AK, Zabarsky TF *et al.* Asymptomatic carriers are a potential source for transmission of epidemic and nonepidemic *Clostridium difficile* strains among long-term care facility residents. *Clin Infect Dis* 2007; **45**(8): 992–998.

71 Chang VT, Nelson K. The role of physical proximity in nosocomial diarrhea. *Clin Infect Diseases* 2000; **31**: 717–722.

72 Clabots CR, Johnson S, Olson MM, Peterson LR, Gerding DN. Acquisition of *Clostridium difficile* by hospitalized patients: Evidence for colonized new admissions as a source of infection. *J Infect Dis* 1992; **166**: 561–567.

73 McFarland LV. Normal Flora: Diversity and Functions. *Microbial Ecology in Health and Disease* 2000; **12**(4): 193–207.

74 Bliss DZ, Johnson S, Savik K, Clabots CR, Willard K, Gerding DN. Acquisition of *Clostridium difficile* and *Clostridium difficile*-associated diarrhea in hospitalized patients receiving tube feeding. *Ann Intern Med* 1998; **129**: 1012–1019.

75 Brown EB, Talbot GH, Axelrod P, Provencher M, Hoegg C. Risk factors for *Clostridium difficile* toxin-associated diarrhea. *Infect Control Hosp Epidemiol* 1990; **11**: 283–290.

76 Johnson S, Gerding DN. *Clostridium difficile* -associated diarrhea. *Clin Infect Dis* 1998; **26**: 1027–1036.

77 Beaulieu M, Williamson D, Pichette G, Lachaine J. Risk of *Clostridium difficile*-associated disease among patients receiving proton-pump inhibitors in a Quebec medical intensive care unit. *Infect Control Hosp Epidemiol* 2007; **28**(11): 1305–1307.

78 Peled N, Pitlik S, Samra Z, Kazakov A, Bloch Y, Bishara J. Predicting *Clostridium difficile* toxin in hospitalized patients with antibiotic-associated diarrhea. *Infect Control Hosp Epidemiol* 2007; **28**(4): 377–381.

79 Manian FA, Aradhyula S, Greisnauer S *et al*. Is it *Clostridium difficile* infection or something else? A case-control study of 352 hospitalized patients with new-onset diarrhea. *South Med J* 2007; **100**(8): 782–786.

80 Nelson DE, Auerbach SB, Baltch AL *et al*. Epidemic *Clostridium difficile*-associated diarrhea: Role of second- and third-generation cephalosporins. *Infect Control Hosp Epidemiol* 1994; **15**: 88–94.

81 Dubberke EF, Reske KA, Yan Y, Olsen MA, McDonald LC, Fraser VJ. *Clostridium difficile*-associated disease in a setting of endemicity: Identification of novel risk factors. *Clin Infect Dis* 2007: **45**: 1543–1549.

82 Tal S, Gurevich A, Guller V, Gurevich I, Berger D, Levi S. Risk factors for recurrence of *Clostridium difficile*-associated diarrhea in the elderly. *Scan J Infect Dis* 2002; **34**: 594–597.

83 Zimmerman RK. Risk factors for *Clostridium difficile* cytotoxin-positive diarrhea after control for horizontal transmission. *Infect Control Hosp Epidemiol* 1991; **12**: 96–100.

84 Do AN, Fridkin SK, Yechouron S *et al*. Risk factors for early recurrent *Clostridium difficile*-associated disease. *Clin Infect Dis* 1998; **26**: 954–959.

85 Johnson S, Homann SR, Bettin KM, Quick JN, Clabots CR, Peterson LR, Gerding DN. Treatment of asymptomatic *Clostridium difficile* carriers (fecal excretors) with vancomycin or metrodindazole. A randomized, placebo-controlled trial. *Ann Infect Med* 1992; **15**: 297–302.

86 Zimmermann MJ, Bak A, Sutherland LR. Review article: Treatment of *Clostridium difficile* infection. *Aliment Pharmacol Ther* 1997; **11**: 1003–1012.

87 Keighley MR, Burdon DW, Arabi Y *et al*. Randomised controlled trial of vancomycin for pseudomembranous colitis and postoperative diarrhoea. *Br Med J* 1978 Dec 16; **2**(6153): 1667–1669.

88 Teasley DG, Gerding DN, Olson MM *et al*. Prospective randomised trial of metronidazole versus vancomycin for *Clostridium difficile*-associated diarrhoea and colitis. *Lancet* 1983; **ii**: 1043–1046.

89 Young GP, Ward PB, Bayley N *et al*. Antibiotic-associated colitis due to *Clostridium difficile*: Double-blind comparison of vancomycin with bacitracin. *Gastroenteorlogy* 1985; **89**: 1038–1045.

90 Dudley MN, McLaughlin JC, Carrington G, Frick J, Nightingale CH, Quintiliani R. Oral bacitracin vs vancomycin therapy for *Clostridium difficile*-associated diarrhea. A randomized double-blind trial. *Arch Intern Med* 1986; **146**: 1101–1104.

91 Fekety R, Silva J, Kauffman C, Buggy B, Deery HG. Treatment of antibiotic-associated *Clostridium difficile* colitis with oral vancomycin: Comparison of two dosage regimens. *Am J Med* 1989; **86**: 15–19.

92 De Lalla F, Nicolin R, Rinaldi E *et al*. Prospective study of oral teicoplanin versus oral vancomycin for therapy of pseudomembranous colitis and *C. difficile*-associated diarrhea. *Antimicrob Agents Chemother* 1992; **36**: 2192–2196.

93 Wenisch C, Parschalk B, Hasenhündl M, Hirschl AM, Graninger W. Comparison of vancomycin, teicoplanin, metronidazole, and fusidic acid for the treatment of *Clostridium difficile*-associated diarrhea. *Clin Infect Dis* 1996; **22**: 813–818.

94 Pullman J, Prieto J, Leach TS. Ramoplanin vs. vancomycin in the treatment of *Clostridium difficile* diarrhea: A phase II study

(abstract). Presented at: 44th Interscience Conference on Antimicrobial Agents and Chemotherapy. DC, USA, October 30–November 2, 2004.

95 Lagrotteria D, Holmes S, Smiega M, Smaill F, Lee C. Prospective, randomized inpatient study of oral metronidazole versus oral metronidazole and rifampin for treatment of primary episode of *Clostridium difficile*-associated diarrhea. *Clin Infect Dis* 2006; **43**: 547–552.

96 Louie TJ, Peppe J, Watt CK *et al*. Tolevamer, a novel nonantibiotic polymer, compared with vancomycin in the treatment of mild to moderately severe *Clostridium difficile* associated diarrhea. *Clin Infect Dis* 2006; **43**: 411–420.

97 Wullt M, Odenholt I. A double-blind randomized controlled trial of fusidic acid and metronidazole for treatment of an initial episode of *Clostridium difficile*-associated dharrhoea. *J Antimicrob Chemother* 2004; **54**: 211–216.

98 Pochapin M. The effect of probiotics on *Clostridium difficile* diarrhea. *Am J Gastroenterol* 2000; **95**(S1): S11–13.

99 Olson MM, Shanholtzer CJ, Lee JT Jr, Gerding DN. Ten years of prospective *Clostridium difficile*-associated disease surveillance and treatment at the Minneapolis VA Medical Center, 1982–1991. *Infect Control Hosp Epidemiol* 1994; **15**: 371–81.

100 Bartlett JG. The case for vancomycin as the preferred drug for treatment of *Clostridium difficile* infection. *Clin Infect Dis* 2008; **46**(10): 1489–1492.

101 Al-Nassir WN, Sethi AK, Nerandzic MM *et al*. Comparison of clinical and microbiological response to treatment of *Clostridium difficile*-associated disease with metronidazole and vancomycin. *Clin Infect Dis* 2008; **47**(1): 56–62.

102 Apisarnthanarak A, Razavi B, Mundy LM. Adjunctive intracolonic vancomycin for severe *Clostridium difficile* colitis: Case series and review of the literature. *Clin Infect Dis* 2002; **35**: 90–96.

103 Pelaez T, Alcála R, Alonso M *et al*. Reassessment of *Clostridium difficile* susceptibility to metronidazole and vancomycin. *Antimicrob Agents Chemother* 2002; **46**: 1647–1650.

104 Friedenberg F, Fernandez A, Kaul V, Niami P, Levine GM. Intravenous metronidazole for the treatment of *Clostridium difficile* colitis. *Diseases Colon & Rectum* 2001; **44**: 1176–1180.

105 Johnson AP. Drug evaluation: OPT-80, a narrow spectrum macrocyclic antibiotic. *Curr Opin Invest Drugs* 2007; **8**: 168–173.

106 Tedesco FJ. Bacitracin therapy in antibiotic-associated pseudomembranous colitis. *Dig Dis Sci* 1980; **10**: 783–784.

107 Chang TW, Gorbach SL, Bartlett JG, Saginur R. Bacitracin treatment of antibiotic-associated colitis and diarrhea caused by *Clostridium difficile* toxin. *Gastroenterology* 1980; **78**: 1584–1586.

108 Barreto ARF, Cavalcante IC, Castro MV *et al*. Fucoidin prevents *Clostridium difficile* toxin-A-induced ileal enteritis in mice. *Dig Dis Sci* 2008; **53**(4): 990–996.

109 Norén T, Wullt M, Akerlund T *et al*. Frequent emergence of resistance in *Clostridium difficile* during treatment of *C. difficile*-associated diarrhea with fusidic acid. *Antimicrob Agents Chemother* 2006; **50**(9): 3028–3032.

110 Hoffman FA, Heimbach JT, Sanders ME, Hibberd PL. Executive summary: Scientific and regulatory challenges of development of probiotics as foods and drugs. *Clin Infect Dis* 2008 Feb 1; **46**(Suppl 2): S53–S57. PMID: 18181723.

111 Hickson M, D'Souza AL, Muthu N *et al*. Use of probiotic Lactobacillus preparation to prevent diarrhoea associated with

antibiotics: Randomised double-blind placebo controlled trial. *BMJ* 2007 (14 Jul); **335**(7610): 80.

112 Shue YK, Sears PS, Shangle S, Walsh RB, Lee C, Gorbach SL, Okumu F, Preston RA. Safety, tolerance, and pharmacokinetic studies of OPT-80 in healthy volunteers following single and multiple oral doses. *Antimicrob Agents Chemother* 2008 (Apr); **52**(4): 1391–1395.

113 Biller JA, Katz AJ, Flores AF, Buie TM, Gorbach SL. Treatment of recurrent *Clostridium difficile* colitis with *Lactobacillus* GG. *J Pediatr Gastroenterol Nutr* 1995; **21**: 224–226.

114 Surawicz CM, McFarland LV, Elmer G, Chinn J. Treatment of recurrent *Clostridium difficile* colitis with vancomycin and *Saccharomyces boulardii*. *Am J Gastroenterol* 1989; **84**: 1285–1287.

115 Ariano RE, Zhanel GG, Harding GKM. The role of anion-exchange resins in the treatment of antibiotic-associated pseudomembranous colitis. *Can Med Assoc J* 1990; **142**: 1049–1051.

116 Surawicz CM, McFarland LV, Greenberg RN *et al*. The search for a better treatment for recurrent *Clostridium difficile* disease: Use of high-dose vancomycin combined with Saccharomyces boulardii. *Clin Infect Dis* 2000; **31**: 1012–1017.

117 McFarland LV, Elmer GW, Surawicz CM. Breaking the Cycle: Treatment strategies for 163 cases of recurrent *Clostridium difficile* disease. *Am J Gastroenterol* 2002; **97**: 1769–1775.

118 Lawrence SJ, Puzniak LA, Shadel BN, Gillespie KN, Kollef MH, Mundy LM. *Clostridium difficile* in the intensive care unit: Epidemiology, costs, and colonization pressure. *Infect Control Hosp Epidemiol* 2007 Feb; **28**(2): 123–130.

119 Bolton RP, Culsaw MA. Fecal metronidazole concentrations during oral and intravenous therapy for antibiotic-associated colitis due to *Clostridium difficile*. *Gut* 1986; **27**: 1169–1172.

120 Levett PN. Time-dependent killing of *Clostridium difficile* by metronidazole and vancomycin. *J Antimicro Chemother* 1991; **27**: 55–62.

121 Larson HE, Borriello SP. Quantitative study of antibiotic-induced susceptibility to *Clostridium difficile* enterocecitis in hamsters. *Antimicrob Agents Chemother* 1990; **34**: 1348–1353.

122 Nair S, Yadav D, Corpuz M, Pitchumoni CS. *Clostridium difficile* colitis: Factors influencing treatment failure and relapse-a prospective evaluation. *Amer J Gastroenterol* 1998; **93**: 1873–1876.

123 Tedesco FJ, Gordon D, Fortson WC. Approach to patients with multiple relapses of Antibiotic-associated pseudomembranous colitis. *Am J Gastroenterol* 1985; **80**: 867–868.

124 Taylor NS, Bartlett JG. Binding of *Clostridium difficile* cytotoxin and vancomycin by anion-exchange resins. *J Infect Dis* 1980; **141**: 92–97.

125 Mogg GA, George RH, Youngs D, Johnson M, Thompson H, Burdon DW, Keighley MR. Randomized controlled trial of colestipol in antibiotic-associated colitis. *Br J Surg* 1982 (Mar); **69**(3): 137–139.

126 McFarland LV. Meta-analysis of probiotics for prevention of antibiotic associated diarrhea and treatment of *Clostridium difficile* disease. *Am J Gastroenterol* 2006; **101**: 812–822.

127 Bennett RG, Gorbach SL, Goldin R, Chang T. Treatment of relapsing *Clostridium difficile* diarrhea with Lactobacillus GG. *Nutr Today* 1996; **31**: S35–S38.

128 Gorbach SL, Chang T, Goldin B. Successful teatment of relapsing *Clostridium difficile* colitis with Lactobacillus GG. *The Lancet* 1987; **2**: 1519.

129 Aas J, Gessert CE, Bakken JS. Recurrent *Clostridium difficile* colitis: Case series involving 18 patients treated with donor stool administered via a nasogastric tube. *Clin Infect Dis* 2003; **36**: 580–585.

130 Bowden TA, Mansberger AR, Lykins LE. Pseudomembraneous enterocolitis: Mechanism for restoring floral homeostasis. *Am Surg* 1981; **47**: 178–183.

131 Persky SE, Brandt LJ. Treatment of recurrent *Clostridium difficile*-associated diarrhea by administration of donated stool directly through a colonoscope. *Am J Gastroenterol* 2000; **95**: 3283–3285.

132 Schwan A, Sjolin S, Trottestam U, Aronsson B. Relapsing *Clostridium difficile* enterocolitis cured by rectal infusion of normal faeces. *Scan J Infect Dis* 1984; **16**: 211–215.

133 Tvede M, Rask-Madsen J. Bacteriotherapy for chronic relapsing *Clostridium difficile* diarrhoea in six patients. *Lancet* 1989; **i**: 1156–1160.

134 Mc Farland LV. Renewed interest in a difficult disease: Clostridium difficile infestions – epidemiology and current treatment strategies. *Curr Opinion Gastroenterology* 2009; **25**: 24–35.

135 Beales ILP. Intravenous immunoglobulin for recurrent *Clostridium difficile* diarrhoea. *Gut* 2002; **51**: 455–458.

136 Hassett J, Meyers S, McFarland LV, Mulligan ME. Recurrent *Clostridium difficile* infection in a patient with selective IgG1 deficiency treated with intravenous immune globulin and *Saccharomyces boulardii*. *Clin Infect Diseases* 1995; **20**: S266–S268.

137 Leung DY, Kelly CP, Boguniewicz M, Pothoulakis C, LaMont JT, Flores A. Treatment with intravenously administered gamma globulin of chronic relapsing colitis inducted by *Clostridium difficile* toxin. *J Pediatr* 1991; **118**: 633–637.

138 Juang P, Skledar SJ, Zgheib NK *et al*. Clinical outcomes of intravenous immune globulin in severe *Clostridium difficile*-associated diarrhea. *Am J Infect Control* 2007; **35**: 131–137.

139 Young KW, Munro IC, Taylor SL *et al*. The safety of whey protein concentrate derived from the milk of cows immunized against *Clostridium difficile*. *Regul Toxicol Pharmacol* 2007; **47**: 317–326.

140 Taylor CP, Tummala S, Molrine D *et al*. Open-label, dose escalation phase I study in healthy volunteers to evaluate the safety and pharmacokinetics of a human monoclonal antibody to *Clostridium difficile* toxin A. *Vaccine* 2008 May 7, epub.

141 Kerr RB, McLaughlin DI, Sonnenberg LW. Control of *Clostridium difficile* colitis outbreak by treating asymptomatic carriers with metronidazole. *Am J Infect Control* 1990; **18**: 332–323.

142 Bender BS, Bennett RG, Laughon B *et al*. Is *Clostridium difficile* endemic in chronic-care facilities? *Lancet* 1986; **2**: 11.

143 Delmee M, Vandercam B, Avesani V, Michaux JL. Epidemiology and prevention of *Clostridium difficile* infections in a leukemia unit. *Eur J Clin Microbiol* 1987; **6**: 623–627.

144 Wilcox MH. Treatment of *Clostridium difficile* infection. *J Antimicrob Chemother* 1998; **41**(Suppl C): 41–46.

145 Kotloff KL, Wasserman SS, Losonsky GA *et al*. Safety and immunogenicity of increasing doses of a *Clostridium difficile* toxoid vaccine administered to healthy adults. *Infect Immun* 2001; **69**: 988–995.

146 Mulligan ME, Rolfe RD, Finegold SM, George WL. Contamination of a hospital environment by *Clostridium difficile*. *Curr Microbiol* 1979; **3**: 173–175.

147 Malamou-Ladas H, Farrell SO, Nash JO, Tabaqchali S. Isolation of *Clostridium difficile* from patients and the environment of hospital wards. *J Clin Path* 1983; **6**: 88–92.

148 Fekety R, Kim KH, Brown D, Batts DH, Cudmore M, Silva J. Epidemiology of antibiotic-associated colitis: Isolation of *Clostridium difficile* from the hospital environment. *Am Med* 1981; **70**: 906–908.

149 McFarland LV, Beneda HW, Clarridge JE, Raugi GJ. Implications of the changing face of *Clostridium difficile* disease for health care practitioners. *Am J Infect Control* 2007; **35**: 237–253.

150 Mayfield JL, Leet T, Miller J, Mundy LM. Environmental control to reduce transmission of *Clostridium difficile*. *Clin Infect Dis* 2000; **31**: 995–1000.

151 Struelens MJ, Maas A, Nonhoff C *et al.* Control of nosocomial transmission of *Clostridium difficile* based on sporadic case surveillance. *Am J Med* 1991; **91**(Suppl 3B): 138–144.

152 Kaatz GW, Gitlin SD, Schaberg DR, Wilson KH, Kauffman CA, Seo SM, Fekety R. Acquisition of *Clostridium difficile* from the hospital environment. *Am J Epidemiol* 1988; **127**: 1289–1294.

153 McMullen KM, Zack J, Coopersmith CM, Kollef M, Dubberke E, Warren DK. Use of hypochlorite solution to decrease rates of *Clostridium difficile*-associated diarrhea. *Infect Cont Hosp Epidemiol* 2007; **28**(2): 205–207.

154 Hughes CE, Gebhard RL, Peterson LR, Gerding DN. Efficacy of routine fiberoptic endoscope cleaning and disinfection for killing *Clostridium difficile*. *Gastrointest Endo* 1986; **32**: 7–9.

155 Rutala WA, Gergen MF, Weber DJ. Inactivation of *Clostridium difficile* spores by disinfectants. *Infect Control Hopsp Epidemiol* 1993; **14**: 36–39.

156 Brooks SE, Veal RO, Kramer M, Dore L, Schupf N, Adachi M. Reduction in the incidence of *Clostridium difficile*-associated diarrhea in an acute care hospital and a skilled nursing facility following replacement of electronic thermometers with single-use disposables. *Infect Control Hosp Epidemiol* 1992; **13**: 98–103.

157 Johnson S, Clabots CR, Linn FV, Olson MM, Peterson LR, Gerding DN. Nosocomial *Clostridium difficile* colonisation and disease. *Lancet* 1990 Jul 14; **336**(8707): 97–100.

158 Bettin K, Clabots C, Methie P, Willard K, Gerding DN. Effectiveness of liquid soap vs chlorhexidine gluconate for the removal of *Clostridium difficile* from bare hands and gloved hands. *Infec Control Hosp Epidemiol* 1994; **15**: 697–702.

159 Muto CA, Blank MK, Marsh JW *et al.* Control of an outbreak of infection with the hypervirulent *Clostridium difficile* BI strain in a University hospital using a comprehensive "bundle" approach. *Clin Infect Dis* 2007; **45**: 1266–1273.

160 Boyce JM, Ligi C, Kohan C, Dumigan D, Havill NL. Lack of association between the increased incidence of *Clostridium difficile*-associated disease and the increasing use of alcohol-based hand rubs. *Infect Control Hosp Epidemiol* 2006; **27**: 479–483.

161 Boone N, Eagan JA, Gillern P, Armstrong D, Sepkovitz KA. Evaluation of an interdisciplinary re-isolation policy for patients with previous *Clostridium difficile* diarrhea. *Am J Infect Control* 1998; **26**: 584–587.

162 Valiquette L, Cossette B, Garant MP, Diab H, Pepin J. Impact of a reduction in the use of high-risk antibiotics on the course of an epidemic of *Clostridium difficile*-associated disease cause by the hypervirulent NAP1/027 Strain. *Clin Infect Dis* 2007; **45**: S112–S121.

163 Climo MW, Israel DS, Wong ES, Williams D, Courdon P, Markowitz SM. Hospital-wide restriction of clindamycin: Effect on the incidence of *Clostridium difficile*-associated diarrhea and cost. *Ann Intern Med* 1998; **128**: 989–995.

164 Ho M, Yang D, Wyle FA, Mulligan ME. Increased incidence of *Clostridium difficile*-associated diarrhea following decreased restriction of antibiotic use. *Clin Infect Dis* 1996; Suppl **1**: S102–S106.

165 McNulty C, Logan M, Donald IP, Ennis D, Taylor D, Baldwin RN *et al.* Successful control of *Clostridium difficile* infection in an elderly care unit through use of a restrictive antibiotic policy. *J Antimicrob Chemother* 1997; **40**: 707–711.

166 Ludlam H, Brown N, Sule O, Redpath C, Coni N, Owen G. An antibiotic policy associated with reduced risk of *Clostridium difficile*-associated diarrhea. *Age and Ageing* 1999; **28**: 578–580.

167 Drudy D, Harnedy N, Fanning S, Hannan M, Kyne L. Emergence and control of fluoroquinolone-resistant, toxin A-negative, toxin B-positive *Clostridium difficile*. *Infect Control Hosp Epidemiol* 2007; **28**(8): 932–940.

168 Cherifi S, Delmee M, Van Broeck J, Beyer I, Byl B, Mascart G. Management of an outbreak of *Clostridium difficile*-associated disease among geriatric patients. *Infect Control Hosp Epidemiol* 2006 (Nov); **27**(11): 1200–1205.

169 Whitaker J, Brown S, Vidal S *et al.* Designing a protocol that eliminates *Clostridium difficile*: A collaborative venture. *Am J Infect Control* 2007; **35**: 310–314.

21 Irritable bowel syndrome

Alexander C Ford[1], Paul Moayyedi[2] and Nicholas J Talley[3]

[1] Department of Gastroenterology, St James's University Hospital, Leeds, UK
[2] Gastroenterology Division, McMaster University Medical Centre, Hamilton, Canada
[3] Department of Medicine, The Mayo Clinic Jacksonville, USA

Definition of irritable bowel syndrome

Irritable bowel syndrome (IBS) is a chronic functional disorder of the lower gastrointestinal (GI) tract characterized by abdominal pain or discomfort and disordered bowel habit [1]. Sufferers often report coexistent symptoms such as bloating, passage of mucus per rectum and a sensation of incomplete evacuation. In the last 30 years several symptom-based diagnostic criteria have been developed in an attempt to allow physicians to make a positive diagnosis of IBS without the need for recourse to invasive investigations of the GI tract to exclude organic disease. These include the Manning criteria, the Kruis scoring system, and the Rome criteria (Table 21.1).

The Manning criteria were first described in 1978 [2], when it was observed that individuals with an ultimate diagnosis of IBS following normal investigations of the lower GI tract were more likely to report certain individual symptom items than those who were found to have organic disease. These were lower abdominal pain relieved by defecation, a change in the frequency or form of stool associated with the onset of abdominal pain, patient-reported visible distension, the passage of mucus per rectum and a sensation of incomplete evacuation. The original authors did not recommend or validate a specific number of these criteria that should be used as a cutoff to diagnose IBS, but three or more are most often used in clinical practice.

The Kruis scoring system is a statistical model [3], and is used to predict the likelihood of a patient having IBS. It includes a combination of symptoms reported by the patient, signs recorded by the physician and laboratory tests (full blood count and erythrocyte sedimentation rate). A score of 44 or more is used as the cutoff to define the presence of IBS. The model is complex and this may explain why it is little used, both in everyday clinical practice and in epidemiological surveys of the condition.

The Rome criteria were first proposed in 1990 [4]. These require the presence of abdominal pain or discomfort, which may or may not be relieved by defecation, in combination with either a change in the frequency or form of stool. The rationale for the development of these criteria was to allow a more reliable diagnosis of IBS to be reached, aid the development of specific therapies, reduce the ordering of unnecessary diagnostic tests, and help standardize the selection of patients for clinical trials of potential therapies for the condition [5]. From a research perspective, the Rome criteria have become increasingly important over the last 10 years, and have been revised in 1999 [6], and 2006 [1], to produce the Rome II and Rome III criteria. Whilst the process involved in developing and revising these criteria has been rigorous it has, for the most part, been based on literature review in order to allow a panel of experts to reach a consensus opinion, rather than on the results of well-designed prospective validation studies. The Rome criteria now allow the subclassification of individuals with IBS according to the predominant abnormality of stool pattern experienced: constipation; diarrhea; or those who have a mixed bowel pattern (previously termed alternating).

Prevalence and incidence of irritable bowel syndrome

Irritable bowel syndrome is sufficiently common that between 3% and 22% of the general population report symptoms compatible with IBS in cross-sectional surveys [7–15]. The variability in reported prevalence is partly explained by the use of the various diagnostic criteria used to define IBS. Community based studies demonstrate a consistently higher prevalence when the Manning criteria are used than when the Rome criteria are utilized [7–9, 16].

Evidence-Based Gastroenterology and Hepatology, 3rd edition.
J. McDonald, A.K. Burroughs, B. Feagan, and M.B. Fennerty. © 2010
Blackwell Publishing Ltd

Table 21.1 Existing symptom-based diagnostic criteria and scoring systems for the diagnosis of irritable bowel syndrome.

Diagnostic criteria or model	Year described	Symptoms, signs, and laboratory investigations included in criteria or scoring system	Symptom duration required
Manning [2]	1978	Abdominal pain relieved by defecation Looser or more frequent stools with onset of pain Mucus per rectum Feeling of incomplete evacuation Patient-reported visible abdominal distension	No
Kruis [3]	1984	**Symptoms (reported by the patient):** Abdominal pain, flatulence, or bowel irregularity Description of abdominal pain as "burning, cutting, very strong, terrible, feeling of pressure, dull, boring, or 'not so bad'" Alternating constipation and diarrhea **Signs (recorded by the physician):** Abnormal physical findings and/or history pathognomonic for any diagnosis other than IBS Elevated erythrocyte sedimentation rate Elevated white cell count Anemia A history suggestive of blood in the stools	>2 years
Rome I [4]	1990	Abdominal pain or discomfort relieved with defecation, or associated with a change in stool frequency or consistency, *plus* two or more of the following on at least 25% of occasions or days: Altered stool frequency Altered stool form Altered stool passage Passage of mucus Bloating or distension	≥3 months
Rome II [6]	1999	Abdominal discomfort or pain that has two of three features: Relieved with defecation Onset associated with a change in frequency of stool Onset associated with a change in form of stool	≥12 weeks (need not be consecutive) in last one year
Rome III [1]	2006	Recurrent abdominal pain or discomfort ≥3 days per month in the last three months associated with two or more of: Improvement with defecation Onset associated with a change in frequency of stool Onset associated with a change in form of stool	Symptom onset ≥6 months prior to diagnosis

This difference may exist because the latter criteria are more restrictive and require minimum symptom duration of three months. The prevalence may also vary according to the demographics of the population under study. Irritable bowel syndrome is commoner in females [17, 18], and younger individuals [9, 19, 20] while the evidence for an effect of socioeconomic status on prevalence of IBS is conflicting [15, 21, 22]. The prevalence of IBS appears to be comparable among Western nations and those of the developing world and the Far East [9, 13, 23, 24], although there are fewer data available from the latter regions.

The prevalence of IBS is reported to remain relatively stable over short periods of time [11, 25, 26], with the resolution of symptoms in some individuals matched by the onset of new symptoms in others. However, individuals readily change their subgroup, as defined by predominant stool pattern [27]. Over longer time-frames an increase in prevalence of IBS has been reported after 7 and 10 years of follow-up [28, 29]. The incidence of IBS is poorly reported. In a longitudinal study conducted in Sweden the three-month incidence was 0.2% [25]. A medical records review of a random sample of residents of Olmsted County, Minnesota, estimated that the incidence of clinically diagnosed IBS was 2 per 1000 adults per year [30]. Since many people with IBS do not seek health care, the true incidence may well be higher. In a more recent study, conducted in almost 4000 individuals from a UK population based sample, the incidence was 1.5% per year during a 10-year period of follow-up [29].

Irritable bowel syndrome and health services

Individuals with IBS are more likely to consume health care resources than those without GI symptoms [31]. Up to 80% of sufferers may consult their primary care physician as a result of symptoms [32, 33]. Factors that drive this choice are poorly understood, but symptom frequency and severity, fear of serious underlying illness, poor quality of life, and other coexisting functional GI diseases have all been shown to predict consultation behaviour [13–15, 32–35]. It has been estimated that IBS accounts for at least 3% of all consultations in primary care [35]. Of those who do consult a primary care physician, the majority are diagnosed and managed in primary care [36], but a significant proportion will be referred for a specialist opinion at some point [9, 10, 15, 33, 35].

The condition accounts for up to 25% of a gastroenterologist's time in the outpatient department [37], and medical treatment is considered to be unsatisfactory, with patients with IBS representing a significant financial burden to health services. Despite the recommendations made by various medical organisations for a diagnosis of IBS to be made on clinical grounds alone [38–41], rather than following attempts to exclude all possible organic pathology by exhaustive investigation, many patients with symptoms suggestive of IBS will undergo colonic investigation, performed presumably in an attempt to reassure both the patient and the physician due to the potential uncertainty that may surround the diagnosis [42], or incur other medical costs [31, 35]. The annual cost of drug therapy for IBS has been estimated at $80 million in the USA [43]. In addition, patients with IBS are more likely to undergo unnecessary surgical procedures, with cholecystectomy, appendicectomy and hysterectomy rates two to three-fold higher than those observed in controls without IBS [44].

A recent systematic review of 18 studies from the UK and USA examined direct and indirect costs to the health service arising from IBS [45]. The authors estimated that IBS accounted for direct costs of between $348 and $8750 per patient per year, indirect costs of between $355 and $3344 per patient per year, and between 8.5 and 21.6 days of IBS-related sickness absence per patient per year.

Pathogenesis of irritable bowel syndrome

There is no known structural, anatomical, or physiological abnormality that accounts for the symptoms that IBS suf-

ferers experience, and it seems unlikely that a single unifying mechanism explains them. It is more plausible that a combination of factors contributes to the abdominal pain and disturbance in bowel habit. Several proposed etiologies are discussed below.

Evidence for genetic susceptibility

Irritable bowel syndrome aggregates within families. Relatives of a patient with IBS are almost three times more likely to report symptoms compatible with IBS than relatives of the patient's spouse [46]. Whether this is due to genetic susceptibility, shared childhood environment, or learned illness-behaviour is unclear. Twin studies demonstrate that there is a greater concordance of IBS in monozygotic versus dizygotic twins [47, 48]. However, having a parent with IBS was a stronger predictor than having a twin with IBS [48]. There is also evidence that children with a parent with IBS are more likely to report GI symptoms and have GI symptom-related absence from school [49]. There have been studies of various candidate genes [50, 51], but the results are conflicting, and their clinical significance is debatable.

Evidence for disturbed gastrointestinal motility

Disturbances in GI motility are thought to play a role in IBS. Previous studies have demonstrated evidence of delayed gastric emptying [52], abnormalities in small bowel and colonic transit time [53], and an increase in colonic motility in response to meal ingestion in IBS [54]. However, these abnormalities are not always reproducible, cannot be used to aid diagnosis, and vary from patient to patient. Some of this variability may be related to the predominant stool pattern experienced by the patient, but as this pattern does not exhibit great stability during follow-up [27], it is conceivable that the disturbances themselves change with time.

Evidence for visceral hypersensitivity and abnormalities of central pain processing

Abdominal pain in IBS is proposed to be related to visceral hypersensitivity, due to abnormal sensitisation of the peripheral and central nervous system. The cause of this sensitisation is unknown, but IBS sufferers report lower thresholds of pain during colonic, rectal and foregut stimulation [55, 56], with radiation to extra-abdominal sites. In addition, patients demonstrate enhanced activation of regions in the brain that are required for central pain processing in functional magnetic resonance imaging studies conducted during gut stimulation compared to controls [57, 58].

Evidence for a post-infectious etiology and altered gut flora

There are numerous studies reporting an increase in symptoms that meet diagnostic criteria for IBS in individuals who have been exposed to an acute gastroenteritis of either bacterial or viral origin [59–61]. The development of post-infective IBS in one study was more likely to occur with younger age, female gender, and certain features of the initial acute illness, including bloody stools, abdominal pain and prolonged diarrhea [59]. Biopsies from the colon and terminal ileum of patients with post-infectious IBS demonstrate an increased inflammatory cell infiltrate [62], and when intestinal permeability is measured in these subjects it is increased compared to that of healthy individuals [63], which may allow luminal gut bacteria to activate an immune response in the GI mucosa, thereby leading to chronic low-grade inflammation in a subset [64].

The existence of post-infectious IBS has led to an increased interest in possible abnormalities in gut flora as a cause for the condition. Some investigators have reported altered gut flora in subjects with IBS compared to healthy controls [65], and others have reported a higher prevalence of small intestinal bacterial overgrowth in IBS patients than controls, as demonstrated by lactulose and glucose hydrogen breath testing [66, 67], as well as an improvement in symptoms after therapy with non-absorbable antibiotics [68].

Making a diagnosis of irritable bowel syndrome

The assessment of a patient with suspected IBS should begin with a structured history to assess whether the individual's symptoms are compatible with the diagnosis. In a patient presenting with lower GI symptoms it is important to elicit the presence of alarm (red flag) symptoms such as weight loss, diarrhea and rectal bleeding as, if these are present, they are thought to predict colorectal cancer and therefore require urgent lower GI investigation, though their diagnostic utility in this situation is suboptimal [69]. Physical examination, including digital rectal examination, is unlikely to confirm the diagnosis of IBS, but should be conducted in order to exclude other organic causes of lower GI symptoms and, if normal, may reassure both the physician and patient.

Utility of a physician's diagnosis

As all the current available symptom-based diagnostic criteria for IBS have been developed by gastroenterologists in secondary or tertiary care, their generalisability to patients presenting to a primary care physician is debatable. A con-sensus panel reported that existing criteria were insufficiently broad for use in primary care [70], and a recent survey demonstrated that few physicians in primary care were familiar with these criteria, or used them to make a diagnosis of IBS, yet could still diagnose the condition with confidence using a pragmatic approach [71]. Guidelines for the management of IBS in primary care still advocate the use of diagnostic criteria [40, 72]. Unfortunately, there are no published studies reporting on the utility of a physician's opinion in making a diagnosis of IBS.

Utility of individual lower gastrointestinal symptoms

The prevalence of symptoms such as lower abdominal pain, mucus per rectum, incomplete evacuation, looser or more frequent stools at the onset of abdominal pain, patient-reported visible distension and pain relieved by defecation has been reported in individuals with IBS compared to individuals without the syndrome [2–3,73–76]. Unfortunately, nocturnal diarrhea, a symptom that is often used by physicians when taking a clinical history, as an indicator of organic disease, was not studied. Since none of the other lower GI symptoms has good sensitivity or specificity for making the diagnosis of IBS [77], combinations of symptoms, in the form of symptom based diagnostic criteria, have been recommended as a means of reaching a clinical diagnosis.

Utility of symptom based diagnostic criteria

Utility of the Manning criteria
The Manning criteria have been validated prospectively in three subsequent studies since their original description in 1978 [75, 76, 78]. Therefore in total they have been validated in over 500 patients. They performed best in the original validation study [2], but also performed well in a study conducted in secondary care in Turkey [78]. However, they performed poorly in the two other studies in India [76] and Korea [75]. A recent systematic review of pooled data from these four studies assessed the utility of the Manning criteria in predicting a diagnosis of IBS [77]. The presence of three or more of the Manning criteria appeared to increase the likelihood of IBS almost three-fold, while if only two or fewer criteria were present the likelihood of the diagnosis was reduced by over 70%.

Utility of the Kruis scoring system
The utility of the Kruis scoring system has also been examined prospectively in three studies published since the original report in 1984 [73, 78, 79]. When data were pooled from all four studies [77], containing almost 1200 patients, a Kruis score of 44 or more increased the likelihood of IBS eight-fold, whilst a score less than 44 reduced the likeli-

hood of the diagnosis by 70%. Whilst the Kruis score appears to have good utility in confirming a diagnosis of IBS, it is probably too complex to be used in routine clinical practice. In addition, one of the items it collects, "a history pathognomonic for any diagnosis other than IBS", and the fact that symptom duration is required to be in excess of two years, probably account for its higher utility than the Manning criteria, which do not require minimum symptom duration.

Utility of the Rome criteria

Only one study has validated the Rome I criteria in a tertiary care setting in the UK [80]. The Rome I criteria had a sensitivity of 71%, a specificity of 85%, and their presence in a patient made a diagnosis of IBS four times more likely [77]. The Rome III criteria were validated in questionnaire form prior to their publication in two studies, using a group of patients with functional GI disorders as well as population controls, and were reported to have sensitivity of 71% and specificity of 88% for the diagnosis of IBS, as well as good test-retest reliability [81]. However, there have been no published studies that have validated either the Rome II or Rome III criteria prospectively, so their utility is relatively unknown. Given that the Rome I criteria were first described almost 20 years ago, and the Rome II criteria 10 years ago, the lack of validation is disappointing, particularly as these have become the gold standard, in research terms, for making a clinical diagnosis of IBS.

Role of investigations in excluding organic disease in patients meeting diagnostic criteria for irritable bowel syndrome

Patients with IBS may have a degree of symptom overlap with individuals with organic diseases. Thyroid disease, celiac disease, inflammatory bowel disease, microscopic colitis, lactose intolerance, small intestinal bacterial overgrowth and even colorectal cancer, in the absence of alarm symptoms, may all present with similar symptoms. As we have discussed, current diagnostic criteria are not infallible, so there may be some value to performing a limited number of clinical investigations in individuals with suspected IBS in order to exclude organic diseases that may present in a similar manner. There have been numerous studies conducted in subjects meeting diagnostic criteria for IBS that have examined the role of applying various diagnostic tests, and which report the prevalence of organic disease in these individuals (Table 21.2). The available evidence is summarized below.

Role of lower gastrointestinal investigations in irritable bowel syndrome

Five studies have reported findings following lower GI investigation in patients with IBS defined according to various diagnostic criteria [79, 82–85]. Three of these utilized complete colonic investigation in over 600 patients, two with either full colonoscopy, or barium enema in combination with flexible sigmoidoscopy [83, 85], and one with either full colonoscopy or barium enema alone [79]. Only seven patients (1.1%) had an organic explanation for their symptoms, such as inflammatory bowel disease or colorectal cancer, after complete colonic investigation. One study used complete colonic investigation in patients aged over 50, and flexible sigmoidoscopy alone in the under 50s [84]. The study included 306 patients with IBS, according to the Rome I criteria, and only four (1.3%) had organic disease after investigation. Finally, one study used flexible sigmoidoscopy with routine rectal biopsy in 89 IBS patients [82]. None of these patients had organic disease diagnosed following this. This observation is in contrast to a series of patients diagnosed with microscopic colitis between 1985 and 2001 from Olmsted County, Minnesota, 40% to 55% of whom reported symptoms that met the Rome or Manning criteria, and one-third had been previously labeled as having IBS [86]. It appears, therefore, that colonic investigation has a very low yield in patients presenting with symptoms that are highly suggestive of IBS in the absence of alarm features.

Role of celiac antibodies and distal duodenal biopsy in irritable bowel syndrome

Several case-control studies have examined the role of testing for celiac disease in patients meeting diagnostic criteria for IBS, but the results are conflicting. Studies from the UK and Iran have demonstrated an increased prevalence of positive celiac serology and biopsy-proven celiac disease in individuals with IBS [87–89], as defined using the Rome II criteria, compared to controls, but data from studies conducted in the USA and Turkey do not support this association [90–92]. Of the available current guidelines for the management of IBS, only those from the National Institute of Health and Clinical Excellence in the UK, which are written from a primary care perspective, recommend routinely screening for celiac disease, using serology, in patients with suspected IBS [40].

A recent systematic review and meta-analysis has examined this issue [93]. Pooled prevalence of positive IgA-class anti-gliadin antibodies was 4% in subjects meeting diagnostic criteria for IBS in seven studies. Six were case-control studies, and the odds of a positive test in cases was three-fold that of controls. Pooled prevalence of positive anti-endomysial antibodies or tissue transglutaminase was 1.6% in subjects meeting diagnostic criteria for IBS in 13 studies. Seven of these were case-control studies, with an odds ratio of almost 3 for a positive test in those meeting diagnostic criteria for IBS. The pooled prevalence of biopsy-proven celiac disease, following positive serology of any type, was 4% in seven studies. Five of these were case-

Table 21.2 Yield of investigations in subjects meeting diagnostic criteria for irritable bowel syndrome.

Investigation used	Number of studies	Number of subjects meeting diagnostic criteria for IBS	Number with organic disease after investigation applied (%)
Complete colonic imaging	3	636	7 (1.1)
Complete colonic imaging for 50 years and over, flexible sigmoidoscopy for under 50s	1	306	4 (1.3)
Flexible sigmoidoscopy and rectal biopsy	1	89	0 (0)
IgA-class antigliadin antibodies	7	1104	36 (3.3)
Anti-endomysial or tissue transglutaminase antibodies	13	2021	41 (2.0)
Celiac serology of any type followed by distal duodenal biopsy if positive	7	1464	62 (4.2)
Lactose hydrogen breath testing	7	2149	756 (35)
Lactulose hydrogen breath testing	4	612	379 (62)
Glucose hydrogen breath testing	2	208	75 (36)
Jejunal aspirate and culture	1	162	7 (4.3)
Full blood count	2	496	1 (0.2)
C-reactive protein/erythrocyte sedimentation rate	1	300	3 (1)
Thyroid function tests	5	2160	91 (4.2)
Stool ova, cysts and parasites	2	1324	19 (1.4)
Barium meal and follow-through	1	114	1 (0.9)
Abdominal ultrasound scan	1	125	22 (18)

control studies, and the odds of biopsy-proven celiac disease in cases meeting diagnostic criteria for IBS was over four-fold that of controls. The odds of biopsy-proven celiac disease were not significantly different in those with constipation-predominant, diarrhea-predominant, or mixed bowel pattern, suggesting that screening for celiac disease should not be reserved for individuals with diarrhea-predominant IBS.

The pooled prevalence of biopsy-proven celiac disease in individuals meeting diagnostic criteria for IBS was estimated to be between 2% and 7% [93]. The true prevalence may be higher in these studies for several reasons. First, only individuals with positive serology were offered duodenal biopsy. Second, studies did not screen these individuals for IgA deficiency, which can lead to false negative serological tests. Third, a recent report has demonstrated that the sensitivity of serology is substantially lower in individuals who do not have total villous atrophy on duodenal biopsy [94]. Economic modelling studies suggest that if the prevalence of celiac disease in subjects meeting diagnostic criteria for IBS were between 5% and 8% then screen-

ing using serology, with duodenal biopsy for those testing positive, could be cost-effective depending on the willingness to pay, with a cost per quality adjusted life year gained of $5000 [95, 96]. These data indicate that testing for celiac disease in patients with suspected IBS may be a worthwhile strategy.

Role of testing for lactose intolerance in irritable bowel syndrome

Seven studies have screened IBS patients for lactose intolerance using lactose hydrogen breath testing [83, 84, 97–101]. Two studies conducted in Italy reported a prevalence of lactose intolerance in excess of 60% among those meeting diagnostic criteria for IBS [97, 100], but in the majority of studies the prevalence was around 25%, although in one study it was only 4% [101]. Of these seven studies, three were case-control studies [97, 98, 101], two of which used healthy controls from the general population [97, 101], and the third used healthy volunteers from among hospital staff [98]. Again results were conflicting, with one study suggesting a five-fold increase in lactose intolerance in IBS subjects compared to controls, one study showing no difference in prevalence between the two, and the third a more modest increase in prevalence in cases with IBS. The data to support the role of lactose hydrogen breath testing in IBS are therefore conflicting, and at present no recommendation for the routine exclusion of lactose intolerance can be made.

Role of testing for small intestinal bacterial overgrowth in irritable bowel syndrome

Small intestinal bacterial overgrowth has been proposed as a possible etiological factor in IBS. Lactulose and glucose hydrogen breath tests, and jejunal aspirate and culture, have been utilized in suspected IBS patients. Three studies have demonstrated a positive lactulose hydrogen breath test in 50–80% of patients with IBS defined according to the Rome I or II criteria [67, 102, 103], whilst the prevalence of a positive glucose hydrogen breath test has been reported to be between 30% and 40% in patients defined by Rome II criteria [66, 104]. These studies have caused considerable interest, and as a result of their findings antibiotics, such as rifaximin, have been used for the treatment of IBS [68]. However, a Swedish case-control study has reported that the prevalence of small intestinal bacterial overgrowth, following jejunal aspirate and culture, is no higher in subjects meeting the Rome II criteria for IBS than in healthy controls from the general population [105]. Only 7 (4%) of 162 IBS patients had a positive culture compared to 1 (4%) of 26 controls. These data are supported by a large case-control study conducted recently in the USA [106], in which the prevalence of a positive lactulose hydrogen breath test was equally high between IBS patients defined by Rome II criteria and healthy controls, suggesting that the high rates of positive breath testing may not be specific to individuals with IBS.

Role of blood tests in irritable bowel syndrome

Several studies have reported on the yield of certain blood tests in suspected IBS patients [83, 84, 87, 107, 108]. Two of these reported on the utility of a full blood count [83, 87], but only one patient had an organic explanation for their symptoms, biopsy-proven celiac disease, after applying the test. Five studies have utilized thyroid function tests in IBS [83, 84, 87, 107, 108]. When data from these studies are combined, 91 (4.2%) of 1860 IBS patients had abnormal thyroid function. One study performed C-reactive protein and erythrocyte sedimentation rate in 300 IBS patients, only three of whom had organic disease after applying the tests [87]. A panel of blood tests, often performed when patients with IBS are first seen in the outpatient clinic, therefore has a low yield in detecting organic disease in this situation. However, it would appear that the routine checking of thyroid function in subjects meeting diagnostic criteria for IBS is a reasonable strategy.

Role of stool examination

Two studies, which used the Rome I criteria and the International Congress definition of IBS [83, 84], tested stool for ova, cysts and parasites in over 1300 patients with suspected IBS. Of these, only 19 (1.4%) had a positive result. In one study none of the subjects meeting diagnostic criteria for IBS patients had a positive test.

Role of other abdominal investigations

Only one study has reported on the utility of abdominal ultrasound scan in 125 individuals with Rome I IBS [109]. Of these subjects, 22 (18%) had abnormal ultrasound findings, 6 (5%) of whom had gallstones. However, the detection of gallstones did not lead to a revision of the diagnosis of IBS in any of the included patients. One study used barium meal and follow-through in 114 patients meeting Rome I criteria for IBS [107]. Only one patient was found to have Crohn's disease after investigation. These limited data do not support the routine use of either of these investigations in the diagnostic workup of patients with suspected IBS.

Summary

There remains some uncertainty surrounding the diagnosis of IBS for both the patient and clinician. Despite the fact that many physicians, particularly those in primary care, are either unaware of or do not use current recommended diagnostic criteria for IBS, there is no evidence that IBS can be reliably diagnosed using a physician's opinion. Individual symptom items from the clinical history are unsatisfactory. Of the current symptom-based diagnostic criteria, the Manning criteria perform only modestly well overall, and less well in the two of the three prospective studies conducted since the original validation was performed. There are few data to support the use of the Rome I criteria, and no studies have validated the Rome II or III criteria, which is disappointing given that the latter are the current gold standard for the diagnosis of IBS. The best evidence appears to exist for the Kruis scoring system, although this system is probably too unwieldy for everyday use. Either further well-designed studies are required to validate current diagnostic criteria, or more accurate ways of diagnosing IBS without the need for investigation need to be developed.

In terms of investigating individuals with symptoms suggestive of IBS, there is limited evidence for a routine panel of blood tests, and more invasive investigations such as colonoscopy, breath testing, or barium studies appear to either have a very low yield, or have limited discriminatory value between IBS patients and normal individuals. In addition, the vast majority of studies have been conducted in secondary care settings, where the yield of organic disease is likely to be higher, and the findings should not be extrapolated to patients presenting to a primary care physician with symptoms suggestive of IBS. Current evidence does suggest, however, that screening all individuals with suspected IBS for thyroid dysfunction and celiac disease, with distal duodenal biopsy in those with positive serology, is a worthwhile strategy.

Treatment of irritable bowel syndrome

As IBS is a prevalent condition, with a chronic, relapsing and remitting course physicians need to have effective therapies available to them in order to drive down the costs of consultation and investigation in sufferers. Unfortunately, many of the traditional therapies, when studied in randomized controlled trials (RCTs), have shown variable efficacy in terms of their effect on resolution or cure of symptoms and follow-up in many cases has been limited to two or three months. In addition, newer agents such as the 5-hydroxytryptamine (5-HT) receptor agonists and antagonists, which showed initial promise, have been withdrawn due to concerns over their safety profile, though some of these are now available on a restricted use basis. Data from individual RCTs of various therapies are conflicting in many cases, and systematic reviews and meta-analyses do not always produce consistent evidence of benefit [110–117]. However, recently a number of systematic reviews and meta-analyses have been completed as part of the update of the American College of Gastroenterology's monograph on IBS [118], and have demonstrated some clinically useful results.

Efficacy of fiber in irritable bowel syndrome

Traditionally, patients with IBS were told to increase the amount of fiber in their diet, due to potentially beneficial effects on intestinal transit time [119]. However, evidence for any benefit on global IBS symptoms from individual placebo-controlled trials has been conflicting [120–123], although many of these studies are small and may have lacked sufficient power to detect a significant benefit, should one exist. Previous systematic reviews have also disagreed on whether fiber has any therapeutic effect [110, 114, 117], and current guidelines for the management of IBS make varying recommendations concerning the role of fiber [38–41]. The use of insoluble fiber, such as bran, is generally discouraged due to concerns that it may exacerbate symptoms, particularly pain and bloating.

A recent systematic review and meta-analysis identified 12 placebo-controlled trials of fiber in IBS [124]. The main results of the meta analysis are shown in Figure 21.1. Overall, there appeared to be a modest benefit of fiber supplementation in IBS, with a number needed to treat (NNT) of 11. However, this effect was limited to ispaghula, a

soluble fiber, with a number needed to treat of 6. Insoluble fiber did not lead to any improvement in symptoms of IBS, though there was no convincing evidence that it worsened symptoms when data were pooled. Adverse events were very rare.

Unfortunately, the method of concealment of allocation was not reported in any of the trials, which may have led to an overestimation of the efficacy of fiber in IBS [125]. In addition, none of the trials adhered to the recommendations of the Rome committee for the design of trials of therapies for the functional GI disorders [126], most having been designed and conducted before these were published. Despite the methodological limitations of many of these RCTs, ispaghula is cheap and available over the counter, so it is probably a worthwhile first-line agent in patients with constipation-predominant IBS. **A1c**

Efficacy of antispasmodics and peppermint oil in irritable bowel syndrome

The pain, discomfort and altered bowel habit that IBS sufferers report may result from a combination of altered GI motility, smooth muscle spasm, visceral hypersensitivity and abnormalities of central pain processing [54, 56, 127]. Smooth muscle relaxants could therefore ameliorate some of the symptoms of IBS. Numerous antispasmodic agents have been studied, but the existing RCTs have produced disparate results [128–131]. Peppermint oil may also have antispasmodic properties [132]. In contrast to antispasmodics, the available RCT evidence for peppermint oil shows definite benefit [133–136].

A systematic review and meta-analysis identified 22 placebo-controlled trials of various antispasmodics in IBS [124], and demonstrated an overall benefit with active therapy, with NNT = 5 (Figure 21.2). There were significantly more adverse events in participants randomized to antispasmodics, though the majority consisted of dry mouth, dizziness, and blurred vision, and none were serious. When subgroup analyses were conducted according to the type of antispasmodic used, it became apparent that many of the antispasmodics that are most commonly used in clinical practice, such as mebeverine, alverine and dicycloverine had little or no evidence of efficacy in IBS. The best evidence, in terms of the number of patients studied, appeared to exist for otilonium (435 patients) and hyoscine (426 patients), with NNT = 5 and 4 respectively. **A1a** When data were pooled for the four RCTs of peppermint oil in a systematic review, there was evidence of a clear benefit, NNT = 3 (Figure 21.3) [124]. **A1a** Adverse events with peppermint oil were very rare, and not more frequent than were observed with placebo.

Again, the majority of these studies predated the Rome recommendations for RCTs of therapies for IBS [126], and none reported the method of concealment of allocation, so

Review: Efficacy of fibre, antispasmodics, and peppermint oil irritable bowel syndrorne: systernatic review and meta-analysis
Comparsion: 01 Fibre
Outcome: 01 Global IBS symptoms or abdominal pain unimproved or persistent after therapy

Study or sub-category	Treatment n/N	Control n/N	RR (random) 95% CI	Weight %	RR (random) 95% CI
01 Bran					
Soltoft 1976	17/32	12/27		6.19	1.20 (0.70, 2.04)
Manning 1977	7/14	7/12		3.65	0.86 (0.42, 1.74)
Kruis 1986	29/40	28/40		17.86	1.04 (0.78, 1.37)
Lucey 1987	3/14	4/14		1.13	0.75 (0.20, 2.75)
Rees 2005	6/14	7/14		2.91	0.86 (0.39, 1.91)
Subtotal (95% CI)	**114**	**107**		**31.75**	**1.02 (0.62, 1.27)**
Total events: 62 (treatment), 58 (control)					
Test for Heterogeneity: Chi^2 = 0.99, df = 4 (p = 0.91), I^2 = 0%					
Test for overall effect: Z = 0.16 (p = 0.88)					
02 Ispaghula					
Ritchie 1979	7/12	12/12		7.50	0.58 (0.36, 0.94)
Longstreth 1981	17/37	16/40		6.56	1.15 (0.69, 1.92)
Arthurs 1983	11/40	14/38		4.26	0.75 (0.39, 1.43)
Nigam 1984	13/21	21/21		13.54	0.62 (0.44, 0.87)
Prior 1987	33/40	37/40		32.59	0.89 (0.75, 1.05)
Jalihal 1990	2/11	3/9		0.80	0.55 (0.11, 2.59)
Subtotal (95% CI)	**161**	**160**		**65.24**	**0.78 (0.63, 0.96)**
Total events: 83 (treatment), 103 (control)					
Test for Heterogeneity: Chi^2 = 7.63, df = 5 (p = 0.18), I^2 = 34.4%					
Test for overall effect: Z = 2.31 (p = 0.02)					
03 Fibre (unspecified)					
Fowlie 1992	10/25	7/24		3.00	1.37 (0.62, 3.01)
Subtotal (95% CI)	**25**	**24**		**3.00**	**1.37 (0.62, 3.01)**
Total events: 10 (treatment), 7 (control)					
Test for Heterogeneity: not applicable					
Test for overall effect: Z = 0.79 (p = 0.43)					
Total (95% CI)	**300**	**291**		**100**	**0.87 (0.76, 1.00)**
Total events: 155(treatment), 168 (control)					
Test for Heterogeneity: Chi^2 = 12.82, df = 11 (p = 0.31), I^2 = 14.2%					
Test for overall effect: Z = 1.93 (p = 0.05)					

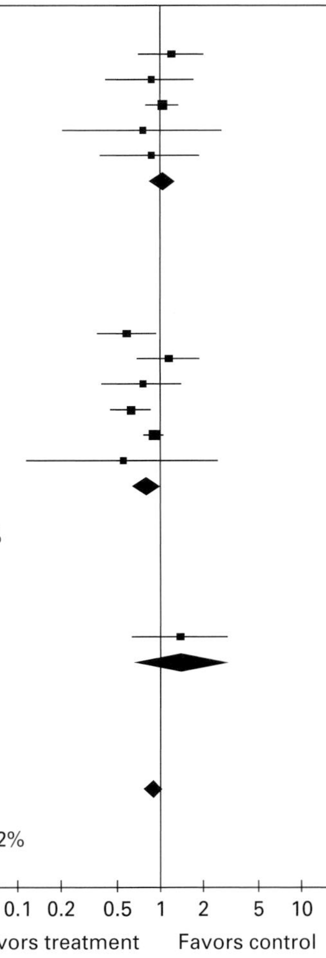

0.1   0.2   0.5   1   2   5   10

Favors treatment   Favors control

Figure 21.1 Forest plot of randomized controlled trials of fiber versus placebo or low fiber diet in irritable bowel syndrome.
Ford AC, Talley NJ, Spiegel BMR *et al.* Effect of fiber, antispasmodics, and peppermint oil in irritable bowel syndrome: Systematic review and meta-analysis. *Br Med J* 2008; **337**: a2313.

the number needed to treat may well be higher. The rationale for the efficacy of these drugs in IBS is speculative. Diarrhea-predominant IBS patients have a reduced colon diameter and accelerated small bowel transit on magnetic resonance imaging [137], so it may be that antispasmodics have their beneficial action via a combination of reduced colonic contraction and transit time, which may in turn lead to reduced pain and stool frequency. Peppermint oil has been shown to have antagonistic effects on the calcium channel [132], and may bring about smooth muscle relaxation, and therefore reduced contractility and pain.

As with ispaghula, antispasmodics and peppermint oil are cheap, and the latter is available over the counter. These therapies should probably be used as first-line interven-

tions for diarrhea-predominant IBS, although most of the trials predated the creation of these diagnostic subgroups, eliminating the possibility of analysis according to predominant stool pattern. **A1a** These agents may also benefit individuals whose predominant symptoms are either pain or bloating. Of the available antispasmodics, the strongest evidence base exists for hyoscine.

Efficacy of antidepressants in irritable bowel syndrome

Patients with IBS demonstrate visceral hypersensitivity [56, 127], and exhibit lower pain thresholds to balloon distension of the rectum than normal individuals [56].

Figure 21.2 Forest plot of randomized controlled trials of antispasmodics versus placebo in irritable bowel syndrome.

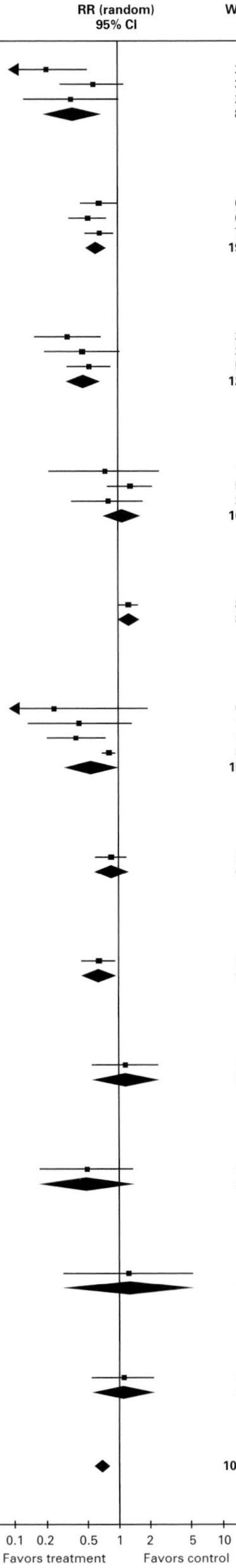

Review: Efficacy of fibre, antispasmodics, and peppermint oil irritable bowel syndrorne: systernatic review and meta-analysis
Comparsion: 03 Peppermint oil
Outcome: 01 Global IBS symptoms or abdominal pain unimproved or persistent after therapy

Study or sub-category	Treatment n/N	Control n/N	RR (random) 95% CI	Weight %	RR (random) 95% CI
Lech 1988	10/23	18/24		23.82	0.58 (0.34, 0.98)
Liu 1997	14/55	34/55		25.33	0.41 (0.25, 0.68)
Capanni 2005	18/91	56/87		29.58	0.31 (0.20, 0.48)
Cappello 2007	10/28	19/29		21.27	0.55 (0.31, 0.96)
Total (95% CI)	**197**	**195**		**100.00**	**0.43 (0.32, 0.59)**

Total events: 52 (treatment), 127 (control)
Test for heterogeneity: Chi^2 = 4.36, df = 3 (p = 0.23), I^2 = 31.1%
Test for overall effect: Z = 5.39 (p < 0.00001)

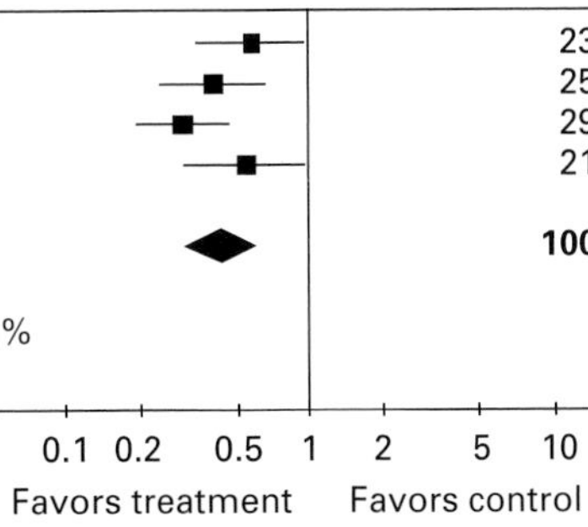

0.1 0.2   0.5   1   2   5   10
Favors treatment   Favors control

Figure 21.3 Forest plot of randomized controlled trials of peppermint oil versus placebo in irritable bowel syndrome.

Antidepressants are often used to treat chronic pain, due to their modulatory effects on pain perception, and previous systematic reviews have demonstrated their efficacy in this situation [138, 139]. For these reasons, it has been postulated that tricyclic antidepressants (TCADs) or serotonin re-uptake inhibitors (SSRIs) may be beneficial in IBS, but existing data from both RCTs [140–143], and systematic reviews and meta-analyses are conflicting [113, 114, 117]. Therefore, recommendations made in IBS management guidelines are equivocal [38–41].

There has been a recent systematic review and meta-analysis identifying 13 RCTs of antidepressant therapy in IBS, reporting a number needed to treat with antidepressants of four [144]. It appeared that both TCADs and SSRIs were effective, with NNT = 4 (Figure 21.4). **A1a** Adverse events were commoner in those receiving active therapy, though this difference was not statistically significant, and none were serious.

Trials of antidepressant therapy were generally of higher quality than those of fiber, antispasmodics and peppermint oil. Imipramine has been shown to prolong orocecal transit time, whilst paroxetine reduces it [145]. It could be hypothesized, therefore, that TCADs will work better in diarrhea-predominant IBS and SSRIs in patients with the constipation-predominant pattern. **C5** Unfortunately, the majority of trials did not report data according to predominant stool pattern reported by the patient, so it was not possible to examine this issue in the systematic review. An alternative explanation for the beneficial effect of antidepressants in IBS is the treatment of coexistent depression. However, improvements in IBS symptoms did not correlate with depression scores in the included RCTs that reported these data, as is also the case for their effects in neuropathic pain [139].

As the RCTs identified in the systematic review used several different TCADs and SSRIs, it is difficult to know if this is a true class effect, or whether the benefit is limited to specific drugs within these groups. Individual trials that demonstrated the greatest benefit of TCADs over placebo used amitriptyline, trimipramine and imipramine [142, 146, 147], whilst for SSRIs RCTs using fluoxetine, citalopram and paroxetine all demonstrated a greater efficacy than placebo [141, 143, 148]. It would therefore seem reasonable to use a TCAD, such as amitryptiline, in subjects with diarrhea-predominant IBS who do not respond to antispasmodics or peppermint oil, or an SSRI, such as citalopram, in constipation-predominant patients who have failed therapy with ispaghula. **C5**

Efficacy of probiotics in irritable bowel syndrome

The role of altered gut flora in IBS is controversial [149], but there are studies that have demonstrated changes in intestinal microbiota in IBS patients compared to controls [65]. In addition, there have been many reports of new onset of symptoms compatible with IBS following acute bacterial and viral gastroenteritis [61]. Probiotics, which are live, or attenuated bacteria, or bacterial products that are beneficial to the host, have the potential to alter gut flora and have been shown to reduce the risk of antibiotic-associated diarrhea [150], and traveller's diarrhea [151], and to reduce the duration of acute illness in acute gastroenteritis [152]. They may have a beneficial effect on symptoms of IBS through a similar mechanism of action.

The effect of probiotics on IBS has been the subject of numerous RCTs, but results have been conflicting. A systematic review and meta-analysis identified 10 RCTs reporting dichotomous outcome data, and 15 RCTs reporting the effect of probiotics on overall IBS symptom scores [153]. The NNT for probiotics to improve or cure one patient's IBS symptoms was four, though there was statisti-

Review: Efficacy of antidepressants and psychological therapies in irritable bowel syndrome: systematic
review and meta-analysis
Comparsion: 01 Antidepressants
Outcome: 01 Global IBS symptoms or abdominal pain unimproved or persistent after therapy

Study or subcategory	Treatment n/N	Control n/N	RR (random) 95% CI	Weight %	RR (random) 95% CI
01 Tricyclic antidepressants					
Heefner 1978	10/22	12/22		5.94	0.83 (0.46, 1.51)
Myren 1982	5/30	10/31		2.66	0.52 (0.20, 1.33)
Nigam 1984	14/21	21/21		14.74	0.67 (0.49, 0.90)
Boerner 1988	16/42	19/41		7.63	0.82 (0.50, 1.36)
Bergmann 1991	5/19	14/16		3.82	0.30 (0.14, 0.65)
Vij 1991	14/25	20/25		10.67	0.70 (0.47, 1.04)
Drossman 2003	60/115	36/57		16.77	0.83 (0.63, 1.08)
Talley 2008	0/18	5/16		0.33	0.08 (0.00, 1.36)
Vahedi 2008	8/27	16/27		5.02	0.50 (0.26, 0.97)
Subtotal (95% CI)	**319**	**256**		**67.56**	**0.68 (0.56, 0.83)**
Total events: 132 (treatment), 153 (control)					
Test for heterogeneity: Chi² = 10.94, df = 8 (p = 0.21), I² = 26.9%					
Test for overall effect: Z = 3.86 (p = 0.0001)					
02 Selective serotonin re-uptake inhibitors					
Kuiken 2003	9/19	12/21		5.85	0.83 (0.45, 1.51)
Tabas 2004	25/44	36/46		14.90	0.73 (0.54, 0.98)
Vahedi 2005	6/22	19/22		4.52	0.32 (0.16, 0.64)
Tack 2006	5/11	11/12		4.90	0.50 (0.25, 0.97)
Talley 2008	5/17	5/16		2.27	0.94 (0.33, 2.65)
Subtotal (95% CI)	**113**	**117**		**32.44**	**0.62 (0.45, 0.87)**
Total events: 50 (treatment), 83 (control)					
Test for heterogeneity: Chi² = 6.46, df = 4 (p = 0.17), I² = 38.1%					
Test for overall effect: Z = 2.74 (p = 0.006)					
Total (95% CI)	**435**	**373**		**100.00**	**0.66 (0.57, 0.78)**
Total events: 182 (treatment), 236 (control)					
Test for heterogeneity: Chi² = 17.66, df = 13 (p = 0.17), I² = 26.4%					
Test for overall effect: Z = 4.95 (p < 0.00001)					

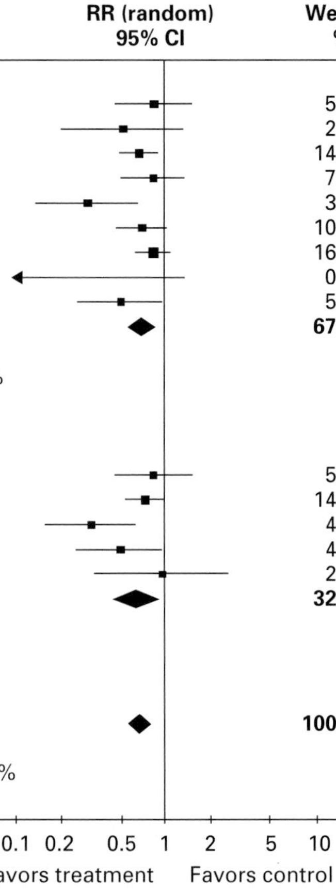

0.1 0.2 0.5 1 2 5 10
Favors treatment   Favors control

Figure 21.4 Forest plot of randomized controlled trials of antidepressants versus placebo in irritable bowel syndrome.
Ford AC, Talley NJ, Schoenfeld PS, *et al.* Efficacy of antidepressants and psychological therapies in irritable bowel syndrome: systematic review and meta-analysis. *Gut* 2009; **58**: 367–378.

cally significant heterogeneity, possibly associated with the clinical heterogeneity inherent in the use of many different probiotics in these studies. Global IBS symptom scores were also reduced by a significantly greater amount with probiotics than with placebo, symptom scores for abdominal pain were significantly reduced, and there was a trend towards a reduction in bloating scores. When subgroup analyses were conducted to examine the effect on symptom status according to the probiotic preparation used, there were no significant differences detected between *Lactobacillus*, *Bifidobacterium*, *Streptococcus* and combinations of probiotics. When effect on symptom scores was assessed, it appeared that combinations of probiotics had the greatest effect, followed by *Bifidobacterium*, with *Lactobacillus* having no effect.

How probiotics may exert their effects on patients with IBS is unclear, but animal models have demonstrated attenuation of post-infective intestinal dysmotility and improve-ments in visceral hypersensitivity with probiotics [154–156]. Certain strains of probiotics have demonstrated the ability to induce the expression of cannabinoid and opioid receptors on intestinal cells [157], and to reduce circulating levels of cytokines [158]. These properties may explain possible benefits in IBS, by leading to a reduction in both visceral hypersensitivity and inflammation.

It would appear from the available evidence that probiotics are more effective than placebo in IBS. They may be of use as second-line interventions in individuals with particularly troublesome abdominal pain and bloating. **A1c**

Efficacy of psychological therapies in irritable bowel syndrome

Subjects with IBS are more likely to report a low quality of life [159–161], and have a higher prevalence of mood disorder, anxiety and neuroticism than patients with organic disease or healthy controls [162]. Studies of IBS patients consulting in tertiary care settings have shown that a significant proportion have an underlying psychiatric illness [163, 164]. Even individuals who do not consult a physician with symptoms have higher levels of depression than normal subjects [165, 166]. Psychological interventions, such as cognitive behavioural therapy (CBT) [167, 168], relaxation therapy [169, 170], dynamic psychotherapy [171, 172] and multi-component psychological therapy [173, 174] have all been used in IBS. A previous systematic review identified 17 studies [175], 10 of which provided extractable dichotomous data, and reported an NNT of two for these interventions to improve or cure one patient's symptoms. However, there were less than 200 patients in total included in these ten studies, and nine of these were published by the same group of researchers, meaning that the validity of the findings of this review are questionable.

A more recent systematic review and meta-analysis published in 2008 identified 20 RCTs of psychological therapies in almost 1300 IBS patients [144]. The results are shown in Figure 21.5. When data from all studies were pooled the NNT was four, but there was significant heterogeneity between studies and evidence of publication bias, suggesting that this may be an overestimate of the treatment effect. In addition, there were nine studies emanating from the same centre, and when these were excluded from the analysis, the treatment effect was lower, but still statistically significant.

There appeared to be a beneficial effect of CBT, hypnotherapy, multi-component psychological therapy, and dynamic psychotherapy, but no effect was demonstrated for relaxation therapy or stress management. The largest number of trials studied CBT, and it may be that this modality has the greatest efficacy, but when the three RCTs originating from the same centre were excluded from the analysis the effect of CBT on IBS symptoms in the remaining four trials was no longer statistically significant. These interventions are time-consuming and expensive, and may not be cost-effective as an initial management strategy for IBS. As a result, they should be reserved for individuals who are unresponsive to, or intolerant of, more conventional therapies. **A1d**

Efficacy of 5-HT$_3$ antagonists and 5-HT$_4$ agonists in irritable bowel syndrome

Abnormal levels of 5-hydroxytryptamine have been demonstrated in individuals with IBS, and this plays an important role in GI motility and sensation [176]. Pharmaceutical agents that act on this receptor have therefore been developed as a potential treatment for IBS. Alosetron, a 5-HT$_3$ antagonist, and tegaserod, a 5-HT$_4$ agonist, showed initial promise for the treatment of diarrhea and constipation-predominant IBS respectively, particularly in females [177–

180]. Unfortunately, both of these drugs demonstrated serious adverse effects during subsequent routine clinical use, with alosetron causing a number of cases of ischaemic colitis and severe constipation [181], and tegaserod being associated with an excess of cardiac and cerebrovascular ischaemic events [182]. As a result, both were withdrawn by the manufacturers, though alosetron is now available on a restricted use basis. Other agents that act on the 5-HT receptor that have been studied in IBS include cisapride, which is also only available on a restricted basis due to concerns about cardiovascular adverse effects.

Systematic reviews and meta-analyses conducted as part of the American College of Gastroenterology's monograph on IBS have studied the efficacy of all available 5-HT$_3$ antagonists and 5-HT$_4$ agonists [183]. Both alosetron and cilansetron were more effective than placebo in IBS, with numbers needed to treat of eight and six respectively [183]. Tegaserod was also more effective than placebo in 11 RCTs, with a number needed to treat of 10 [183]. Neither cisapride or renzapride appeared to have any benefit over placebo in IBS.

The NNTs for these agents are higher than those for ispaghula, antispasmodics, peppermint oil, antidepressants and psychological therapies. However, this may be due, in part, to the much higher quality of RCTs of 5-HT$_3$ antagonists and 5-HT$_4$ agonists [184], and adherance to the Rome committee recommendations for the design of treatment trials for functional GI disorders [126]. Due to their adverse safety profile, these drugs cannot be recommended as first-line therapies for the management of IBS and, where available, should probably be held in reserve for patients non-responsive to first-line therapies. **A1a**

Efficacy of lubiprostone in irritable bowel syndrome

Lubiprostone is a prostaglandin E$_1$ derivative that activates a specific chloride channel in the GI tract, causing increased fluid secretion, and thereby improving GI transit. The drug has been used in chronic idiopathic constipation, and has been shown to be effective, leading to a significant improvement in patient-reported spontaneous bowel movements [185]. Recent trials have demonstrated both a statistically significant improvement in mean abdominal pain scores in patients with constipation-predominant IBS randomized to 12 weeks of lubiprostone compared with placebo [186]. A significant improvement in global symptoms [187], in terms of the responder rates, using an a priori definition based on the number of weeks during the trial that the treatment was deemed to be effective by the patient was also observed. Individual symptoms including abdominal pain or discomfort, stool consistency, straining and severity of constipation were all significantly improved with lubiprostone compared with placebo [187]. The only

Review: Efficacy of antidepressants and psychological therapies in irritable bowel syndrome: systernatic
review and meta-analysis
Comparsion: 02 Psychological therapies
Outcome: 01 Global IBS symptoms or abdominal pain unimproved or persistent after therapy

Study or sub-category	Treatment n/N	Control n/N	RR (random) 95% CI	Weight %	RR (random) 95% CI
01 Cognitive behavioral therapy					
Greene 1994	2/10	9/10		1.44	0.22 (0.06, 0.78)
Payne 1995	3/12	9/10		2.06	0.28 (0.10, 0.76)
Vollmer 1998	11/24	9/10		4.88	0.51 (0.31, 0.82)
Boyce 2003	27/35	25/34		6.81	1.05 (0.80, 1.38)
Drossman 2003	51/112	36/57		6.69	0.72 (0.54, 0.96)
Tkachuk 2003	0/14	6/14		0.34	0.08 (0.00, 1.25)
Kennedy 2005	24/72	36/77		5.56	0.71 (0.48, 1.07)
Subtotal (95% CI)	**279**	**212**		**27.78**	**0.60 (0.42, 0.87)**
Total events: 118 (treatment), 130 (control)					
Test for heterogeneity: Chi² = 20.48, df = 6 (p = 0.002), I² = 70.7%					
Test for overall effect: Z = 2.68 (p = 0.007)					
02 Hypnotherapy					
Galovski 1998	3/6	6/6		2.83	0.50 (0.22, 1.11)
Simren 2004	4/14	9/14		2.35	0.44 (0.18, 1.11)
Subtotal (95% CI)	**20**	**20**		**5.18**	**0.48 (0.26, 0.87)**
Total events: 7 (treatment), 15 (control)					
Test for heterogeneity: Chi² = 0.04, df = 1 (p = 0.84), I² = 0%					
Test for overall effect: Z = 2.42 (p = 0.02)					
03 Multi-component psychological therapy					
Blanchard 1992a	4/10	8/10		2.74	0.50 (0.22, 1.14)
Neff 1987	4/10	8/9		2.86	0.45 (0.20, 0.99)
Blanchard 1992b	22/38	29/39		6.27	0.78 (0.56, 1.08)
Heitkemper 2004	25/48	35/47		6.36	0.70 (0.51, 0.96)
Subtotal (95% CI)	**106**	**105**		**18.23**	**0.69 (0.56, 0.86)**
Total events: 55 (treatment), 80 (control)					
Test for heterogeneity: Chi² = 2.26, df = 3 (p = 0.52), I² = 0%					
Test for overall effect: Z = 3.39 (p = 0.0007)					
04 Dynamic psychotherapy					
Guthrie 1991	20/53	39/49		5.84	0.47 (0.33, 0.69)
Creed 2003	41/85	56/86		6.82	0.74 (0.57, 0.97)
Subtotal (95% CI)	**138**	**135**		**12.66**	**0.60 (0.39, 0.93)**
Total events: 61 (treatment), 95 (control)					
Test for heterogeneity: Chi² = 3.62, df = 1 (p = 0.06), I² = 72.4%					
Test for overall effect: Z = 2.26 (p = 0.02)					
05 Relaxation training or therapy					
Lynch 1989	4/11	10/10		2.92	0.36 (0.17, 0.79)
Blanchard 1993	10/14	8/9		5.57	0.80 (0.54, 1.20)
Keefer 2001	3/7	7/8		2.43	0.49 (0.20, 1.20)
Boyce 2003	31/36	25/34		7.08	1.17 (0.92, 1.49)
van der Veek 2007	46/54	50/51		7.98	0.87 (0.77, 0.98)
Subtotal (95% CI)	**122**	**112**		**25.97**	**0.82 (0.63, 0.93)**
Total events: 94 (treatment), 100 (control)					
Test for heterogeneity: Chi² = 12.56, df = 4 (p = 0.01), I² = 68.2%					
Test for overall effect: Z = 1.39 (p = 0.16)					
06 Self-administered cognitive behavioral therapy					
Sanders 2007	16/17	10/11		7.24	1.04 (0.83, 1.29)
Subtotal (95% CI)	**17**	**11**		**7.24**	**1.04 (0.83, 1.29)**
Total events: 16 (treatment), 10 (control)					
Test for heterogeneity: not applicable					
Test for overall effect: Z = 0.31 (p = 0.76)					
07 Stress management					
Shaw 1991	5/18	14/17		2.94	0.34 (0.16, 0.73)
Subtotal (95% CI)	**18**	**17**		**2.94**	**0.34 (0.16, 0.73)**
Total events: 5 (treatment), 14 (control)					
Test for heterogeneity: not applicable					
Test for overall effect: Z = 2.74 (p = 0.006)					
Total (95% CI)	**700**	**612**		**100.00**	**0.67 (0.57, 0.79)**
Total events: 356 (treatment), 444 (control)					
Test for heterogeneity: Chi² = 77.58, df = 21 (p < 0.00001), I² = 72.9%					
Test for overall effect: Z = 4.72 (p < 0.00001)					

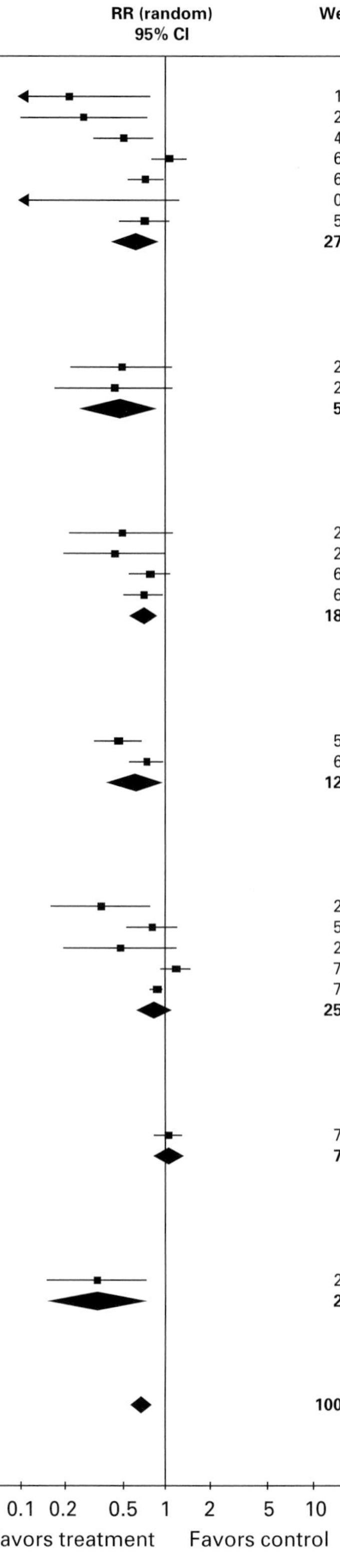

0.1 0.2   0.5   1   2   5   10

Favors treatment   Favors control

Figure 21.5 Forest plot of randomized controlled trials of psychological therapies versus control therapy or a physician's "usual management" in irritable bowel syndrome.

adverse events occurring more frequently in those receiving lubiprostone were diarrhea and nausea, particularly with higher doses [186, 187]. In an open-label extension of one of these trials, patients originally randomized to either lubiprostone or placebo were treated with the drug for a further 36 weeks [188]. Initial response rates were 15% with lubiprostone and 8% with placebo at 12 weeks, and these increased to 37% and 31% respectively at week 48. There were no serious adverse events in over 450 patients treated, suggesting that longer term treatment is both effective and safe. In another trial, patients receiving lubiprostone were randomized after 12 weeks of therapy to either a further four weeks of treatment, or four weeks of placebo [189]. The response rates at week 16 were 38% with lubiprostone compared to 40% with placebo, indicating a possible sustained effect of the initial 12 weeks of therapy on symptoms. The drug has recently been approved for the treatment of constipation-predominant IBS in women in some jurisdictions, but not in others. **A1a** Additional data from other RCTs may establish lubiprostone's true efficacy and place in the treatment of IBS.

Efficacy of anti-diarrheals in irritable bowel syndrome

In individuals with diarrhea-predominant or alternating IBS there may be a role for anti-diarrheal agents, such as loperamide. These drugs are relatively safe, and are often available over the counter, but unfortunately there are few data to support their routine use in IBS patients. There have been only two placebo-controlled trials conducted in Scandinavia [190, 191], which when pooled contain fewer than 50 patients. Stool consistency and frequency improved in a greater proportion of individuals randomized to loperamide than placebo in both trials, but in terms of this translating into an improvement in other symptoms of IBS the results were conflicting. One study demonstrated a clear improvement in abdominal pain with loperamide after 13 weeks of therapy [191], but the second showed no beneficial effect on global IBS symptoms [190]. There are insufficient data to make any clear recommendations for the use of loperamide in IBS at the present time, but the drug class does improve diarrhea. **A1d**

Efficacy of an exclusion diet in irritable bowel syndrome

Some individuals with IBS believe that they have food allergy or intolerance and therefore the exclusion of certain foods from the diet may have a beneficial effect in these individuals. In a UK study of over 100 subjects with IBS, IgG4 titres were significantly higher in IBS cases compared to controls for wheat, beef, lamb and pork [192], and symptoms improved significantly among sufferers following the exclusion of some of these items [193]. Celiac disease may be more prevalent in patients with symptoms suggestive of IBS, and these individuals may respond to a gluten-free diet [88, 89]. There is now limited evidence that a gluten-free diet will alleviate symptoms in some IBS patients who do not have histological evidence of celiac disease [194]. As mentioned in the previous section, there is little convincing evidence that lactose intolerance is any commoner in IBS sufferers, though if an individual feels that their symptoms are made worse by dairy products a trial of withdrawal of these from the diet may be worthwhile. A systematic review of exclusion diets in individuals with IBS suggested that symptoms improved in a subset of patients [195], but the majority of these studies were non-randomized. As there are limited data from high quality studies to support a role for exclusion diets in the management of IBS these should not be used as a first-line therapy.

Summary

Insoluble fiber such as wheat bran appears to have no benefit in IBS, but does not exacerbate symptoms, whilst soluble fiber in the form of ispaghula is beneficial and should be considered first line in constipation-predominant patients. Antispasmodics, particularly hyoscine, and peppermint oil are also effective in IBS, and should be used first line in diarrhea-predominant patients and those whose main complaints are pain and bloating. Anti-diarrheal agents, such as loperamide, improve stool form and frequency in IBS patients, but there is no clear evidence that this translates into a beneficial effect on either pain or global IBS symptoms. Antidepressants should be considered second line, in patients failing these therapies: TCADs for patients with the diarrhea-predominant pattern; and SSRIs for constipation-predominant IBS. Probiotics may also be considered second line in those with particularly troublesome pain and bloating. Psychological interventions, alosetron and lubiprostone should be considered for individuals who are non-responsive to first and second-line therapies, though psychological interventions are likely to be expensive and time-consuming to administer, alosetron has potentially serious side effects, and there are relatively few published data for lubiprostone. Exclusion diets do not have any high-quality evidence to support their use, but may still be helpful in a minority of challenging patients. A suggested treatment algorithm for patients with IBS, according to predominant symptom, is provided in Table 21.3.

Prognosis of irritable bowel syndrome

Individuals with IBS suffer from a chronic relapsing and remitting medical disorder. Longitudinal studies have

Table 21.3 Suggested order of medical therapies for irritable bowel syndrome according to predominant symptom.

Predominant symptom	First line	NNT	Strength of recommendation and quality of evidence	Second line	NNT	Strength of recommendation and quality of evidence	Third line	NNT	Strength of recommendation and quality of evidence
Pain and bloating	Antispasmodics (preferably hyoscine), peppermint oil	5 4 3	A1a A1a	Probiotics	4	A1c	Psychological therapies	4	A1d
Constipation	Ispaghula	6	A1c	SSRIs	4	A1c	Lubiprostone (where approved)	13	A1a
Diarrhea	Antispasmodics (preferably hyoscine), peppermint oil, loperamide (for diarrhea only)	5 4 3	A1a A1a A1a A1d	TCADs	4	A1a	Alosetron	8	A1a

examined the natural history of the condition. It appears that up to two-thirds of those reporting symptoms compatible with IBS in such surveys continue to experience symptoms over prolonged periods of follow-up [28, 29]. As these studies did not administer questionnaires to individuals at several points in time it is difficult to know whether symptoms were present continuously. This would seem unlikely, given that functional GI symptoms tend to fluctuate, with individuals developing symptoms compatible with other functional GI disorders, such as dyspepsia and reflux, during prolonged periods of follow-up [28, 196, 197]. Evidence of the degree of fluctuation in IBS is conflicting, however, with a seven-year follow-up study from Sweden suggesting that IBS was the most stable of all the functional GI disorders [28], whilst a study with 10 years of follow-up conducted in the UK demonstrated the opposite [197], with only 20% of individuals still meeting diagnostic criteria for IBS at 10 years. Even among those who do remain symptomatic, the predominant stool pattern experienced is reported to change in up to three-quarters of individuals [27]. Thus, individuals with IBS may need to be reassessed intermittently, and their current treatment reviewed.

Despite potential uncertainty surrounding the diagnosis of IBS it is unlikely to be revised during future follow-up. In a cohort of 112 IBS patients at the Mayo Clinic, less than 10% developed a subsequent organic GI disease, after a median length of follow-up of almost 30 years, and in almost all cases this was felt to be unrelated to their original presentation with symptoms that were compatible with IBS [198]. In another study from the USA, individuals meeting diagnostic criteria for IBS were followed up

between 10 and 13 years later [199]. Almost 50% had undergone a repeat structural evaluation of the lower GI tract in the intervening years, but this had not led to a diagnosis of organic disease in any of the subjects.

As there is no single pathophysiological abnormality that explains all the symptoms of IBS, there is no specific target for medical therapies. Treatment for the condition is largely directed toward relieving symptoms. This situation may be viewed as unsatisfactory, particularly from the patient's perspective, but there is now evidence from systematic reviews and meta-analyses of randomized controlled trials that many of the interventions that have been used traditionally in IBS are effective, despite earlier reports to the contrary, and newer agents continue to be developed.

References

1 Longstreth GF, Thompson WG, Chey WD *et al.* Functional bowel disorders. *Gastroenterology* 2006; **130**: 1480–1491.

2 Manning AP, Thompson WG, Heaton KW *et al.* Towards positive diagnosis of the irritable bowel. *Br Med J* 1978; **277**: 653–654.

3 Kruis W, Thieme CH, Weinzierl M *et al.* A diagnostic score for the irritable bowel syndrome. Its value in the exclusion of organic disease. *Gastroenterology* 1984; **87**: 1–7.

4 Drossman DA, Thompson WG, Talley NJ. Identification of subgroups of functional gastrointestinal disorders. *Gastroenterology Intl* 1990; **3**: 159–172.

5 Drossman DA. The functional gastrointestinal disorders and the Rome II process. *Gut* 1999; **45**(supp II): II1–II5.

6 Thompson WG, Longstreth GF, Drossman DA *et al.* Functional bowel disorders and functional abdominal pain. *Gut* 1999; **45**(suppl II): II43–II47.

7 Agreus L, Talley NJ, Svardsudd K *et al.* Identifying dyspepsia and irritable bowel syndrome: The value of pain or discomfort, and bowel habit descriptors. *Scand J Gastroenterol* 2000; **35**: 142–151.

8 Hillila MT, Farkkila MA. Prevalence of irritable bowel syndrome according to different diagnostic criteria in a non-selected adult population. *Aliment Pharmacol Ther* 2004; **20**: 339–345.

9 Hungin APS, Whorwell PJ, Tack J *et al.* The prevalence, patterns and impact of irritable bowel syndrome: An international survey of 40 000 subjects. *Aliment Pharmacol Ther* 2003; **17**: 643–650.

10 Jones R, Lydeard S. Irritable bowel syndrome in the general population. *Br Med J* 1992; **304**: 87–90.

11 Mearin F, Baro E, Roset M *et al.* Clinical patterns over time in irritable bowel syndrome: Symptom instability and severity variability. *Am J Gastroenterol* 2004; **99**: 113–121.

12 Saito YA, Locke GR, Talley NJ *et al.* A comparison of the Rome and Manning criteria for case identification in epidemiological investigations of irritable bowel syndrome. *Am J Gastroenterol* 2000; **95**: 2816–2824.

13 Talley NJ, Zinsmeister AR, Van Dyke C *et al.* Epidemiology of colonic symptoms and the irritable bowel syndrome. *Gastroenterology* 1991; **101**: 927–934.

14 Talley NJ, Zinsmeister AR, Melton III LJ. Irritable bowel syndrome in a community: Symptom subgroups, risk factors, and health care utilization. *Am J Epidemiol* 1995; **142**: 76–83.

15 Wilson S, Roberts L, Roalfe A *et al.* Prevalence of irritable bowel syndrome: A community survey. *Br J Gen Pract* 2004; **54**: 495–502.

16 Mearin F, Badia X, Balboa A *et al.* Irritable bowel syndrome prevalence varies enormously depending on the employed diagnostic criteria: Comparison of Rome II versus previous criteria in a general population. *Scand J Gastroenterol* 2001; **36**: 1155–1161.

17 Sperber AD, Shvartzman P, Friger M *et al.* Unexpectedly low prevalence rates of IBS among adult Israeli Jews. *Neurogastroenterol Motil* 2005; **17**: 207–211.

18 Thompson WG, Irvine EJ, Pare P *et al.* Functional gastrointestinal disorders in Canada: First population-based survey using Rome II criteria with suggestions for improving the questionnaire. *Dig Dis Sci* 2002; **47**: 225–235.

19 Lau EM, Chan FK, Ziea ET *et al.* Epidemiology of irritable bowel syndrome in Chinese. *Dig Dis Sci* 2002; **47**: 2621–2624.

20 Hungin AP, Chang L, Locke GR *et al.* Irritable bowel syndrome in the United States: Prevalence, symptom patterns and impact. *Aliment Pharmacol Ther* 2005; **21**: 1365–1375.

21 Howell S, Talley NJ, Quine S *et al.* The irritable bowel syndrome has origins in the childhood socioeconomic environment. *Am J Gastroenterol* 2004; **99**: 1572–1578.

22 Minocha A, Chad W, Do W *et al.* Racial differences in epidemiology of irritable bowel syndrome alone, un-investigated dyspepsia alone, and "overlap syndrome" among African Americans compared to Caucasians: A population-based study. *Dig Dis Sci* 2006; **51**: 218–226.

23 Gwee KA, Wee S, Wong ML *et al.* The prevalence, symptom characteristics, and impact of irritable bowel syndrome in an Asian urban community. *Am J Gastroenterol* 2004; **99**: 924–931.

24 Lule GN, Amayo EO. Irritable bowel syndrome in Kenyans. *East Afr Med J* 2002; **79**: 360–363.

25 Agreus L, Svardsudd K, Nyren O *et al.* Irritable bowel syndrome and dyspepsia in the general population: Overlap and lack of stability over time. *Gastroenterology* 1995; **109**: 671–680.

26 Williams RE, Black CL, Kim HY *et al.* Stability of irritable bowel syndrome using a Rome II-based classification. *Aliment Pharmacol Ther* 2006; **23**: 197–205.

27 Drossman DA, Morris CB, Hu Y *et al.* A prospective assessment of bowel habit in irritable bowel syndrome in women: Defining an alternator. *Gastroenterology* 2005; **128**: 580–589.

28 Agreus L, Svardsudd K, Talley NJ *et al.* Natural history of gastroesophageal reflux disease and functional abdominal disorders. *Am J Gastroenterol* 2001; **96**: 2905–2914.

29 Ford AC, Forman D, Bailey AG *et al.* Irritable bowel syndrome: A 10-year natural history of symptoms, and factors that influence consultation behavior. *Am J Gastroenterol* 2008; **103**: 1229–1239.

30 Locke III GR, Yawn BP, Wollan PC *et al.* Incidence of a clinical diagnosis of the irritable bowel syndrome in a United States population. *Aliment Pharmacol Ther* 2004; **19**: 1025–1031.

31 Talley NJ, Gabriel SE, Harmsen WS *et al.* Medical costs in community subjects with irritable bowel syndrome. *Gastroenterology* 1995; **109**: 1736–1741.

32 Koloski NA, Talley NJ, Boyce PM. Epidemiology and health care seeking in the functional GI disorders: A population-based study. *Am J Gastroenterol* 2002; **97**: 2290–2209.

33 Koloski NA, Talley NJ, Huskic SS *et al.* Predictors of conventional and alternative health care seeking for irritable bowel syndrome and functional dyspepsia. *Aliment Pharmacol Ther* 2003; **17**: 841–851.

34 Talley NJ, Boyce PM, Jones M. Predictors of health care seeking for irritable bowel syndrome: A population based study. *Gut* 1997; **41**: 394–398.

35 Thompson WG, Heaton KW, Smyth GT *et al.* Irritable bowel syndrome in general practice: Prevalence, characteristics, and referral. *Gut* 2000; **46**: 78–82.

36 Yawn BP, Locke III GR, Lydick E *et al.* Diagnosis and care of irritable bowel syndrome in a community-based population. *Am J Manag Care* 2001; **7**: 585–592.

37 Harvey RF, Salih SY, Read AE. Organic and functional disorders in 2000 gastroenterology outpatients. *Lancet* 1983; **321**: 632–634.

38 American College of Gastroenterology Functional Gastrointestinal Disorders Task Force. Evidence-based position statement on the management of irritable bowel syndrome in North America. *Am J Gastroenterol* 2002; **97**(suppl 2): S2–S5.

39 Drossman DA, Camilleri M, Mayer EA *et al.* AGA technical review on irritable bowel syndrome. *Gastroenterology* 2002; **123**: 2108–2131.

40 National Institute for Health and Clinical Excellence. Irritable bowel syndrome in adults: Diagnosis and management of irritable bowel syndrome in primary care. 2008. Published online at http://www.nice.org.uk/nicemedia/pdf/CG061NICEGuidelinepdf 2008.

41 Spiller R, Aziz Q, Creed FEA *et al*. Guidelines on the irritable bowel syndrome: Mechanisms and practical management. *Gut* 2007; **56**: 1770–1798.

42 May C, Allison G, Chapple A *et al*. Framing the doctor-patient relationship in chronic illness: A comparative study of general practitioners' accounts. *Sociol Health Illn* 2004; **26**: 135–158.

43 Sandler RS, Everhart JE, Donowitz M *et al*. The burden of selected digestive diseases in the United States. *Gastroenterology* 2002; **122**: 1500–1511.

44 Longstreth GF, Yao JF. Irritable bowel syndrome and surgery: A multivariate analysis. *Gastroenterology* 2004; **126**: 1665–1673.

45 Maxion-Bergemann S, Thielecke F, Abel F *et al*. Costs of irritable bowel syndrome in the UK and US. *Pharmacoeconomics* 2006; **24**: 21–37.

46 Kalantar JS, Locke GR, Zinsmeister AR *et al*. Familial aggregation of irritable bowel syndrome: A prospective study. *Gut* 2003; **52**: 1703–1707.

47 Bengtson MB, Ronning T, Vatn MH *et al*. Irritable bowel syndrome in twins: Genes and environment. *Gut* 2006; **55**: 1754–1759.

48 Levy RL, Jones KR, Whitehead WE *et al*. Irritable bowel syndrome in twins: Heredity and social learning both contribute to etiology. *Gastroenterology* 2001; **121**: 799–804.

49 Levy RL, Whitehead WE, Walker LS *et al*. Increased somatic complaints and health-care utilization in children: Effects of parent IBS status and parent response to gastrointestinal symptoms. *Am J Gastroenterol* 2004; **99**: 2442–2451.

50 Pata C, Erdal E, Yazc K *et al*. Association of the -1438G/A and 102T/C polymorphism of the 5-Ht2A receptor gene with irritable bowel syndrome 5-Ht2A gene polymorphism in irritable bowel syndrome. *J Clin Gastroenterol* 2004; **38**: 561–566.

51 Grudell AB, Camilleri M, Carlson P *et al*. An exploratory study of the association of adrenergic and serotonergic genotype and gastrointestinal motor functions. *Neurogastroenterol Motil* 2008; **20**: 213–219.

52 Stanghellini V, Tosetti C, Barbara G *et al*. Dyspeptic symptoms and gastric emptying in the irritable bowel syndrome. *Am J Gastroenterol* 2002; **97**: 2738–2743.

53 Cann PA, Read NW, Brown C *et al*. Irritable bowel syndrome: Relationship of disorders in the transit of a single solid meal to symptom patterns. *Gut* 1983; **24**: 405–411.

54 McKee DP, Quigley EM. Intestinal motility in irritable bowel syndrome: Is IBS a motility disorder? Part 1. Definition of IBS and colonic motility. *Dig Dis Sci* 1993; **38**: 1761–1762.

55 Moriarty KJ, Dawson AM. Functional abdominal pain: Further evidence that whole gut is affected. *Br Med J* 1982; **284**: 1670–1672.

56 Trimble KC, Farouk R, Pryde A *et al*. Heightened visceral sensation in functional gastrointestinal disease is not site-specific. Evidence for a generalized disorder of gut sensitivity. *Dig Dis Sci* 1995; **40**: 1607–1613.

57 Mertz H, Morgan V, Tanner G *et al*. Regional cerebral activation in irritable bowel syndrome and control subjects with painful and nonpainful rectal distention. *Gastroenterology* 2000; **118**: 842–848.

58 Bonaz B, Baciu M, Papillon E *et al*. Central processing of rectal pain in patients with irritable bowel syndrome: An fMRI study. *Am J Gastroenterol* 2002; **97**: 654–661.

59 Marshall JK, Thabane M, Garg AX *et al*. Incidence and epidemiology of irritable bowel syndrome after a large waterborne outbreak of bacterial dysentery. *Gastroenterology* 2006; **131**: 445–450.

60 Marshall JK, Thabane M, Borgaonkar MR *et al*. Postinfectious irritable bowel syndrome after a food-borne outbreak of gastroenteritis attributed to a viral pathogen. *Clin Gastroenterol Hepatol* 2007; **5**: 457–460.

61 Thabane M, Kottachchi D, Marshall JK. Systematic review and meta-analysis: Incidence and prognosis of post-infectious irritable bowel syndrome. *Aliment Pharmacol Ther* 2007; **26**: 535–544.

62 Wang LH, Fang XC, Pan GZ. Bacillary dysentery as a causative factor of irritable bowel syndrome and its pathogenesis. *Gut* 2004; **53**: 1096–1101.

63 Marshall JK, Thabane M, Garg AX *et al*. Intestinal permeability in patients with irritable bowel syndrome after a waterborne outbreak of acute gastroenteritis in Walkerton, Ontario. *Aliment Pharmacol Ther* 2004; **20**: 1317–1322.

64 Chadwick V, Chen W, Shu D *et al*. Activation of the mucosal immune system in irritable bowel syndrome. *Gastroenterology* 2002; **122**: 1778–1783.

65 Kassinen A, Krogius-Kurikka L, Makivuokko H *et al*. The fecal microbiota of irritable bowel syndrome patients differs significantly from that of healthy subjects. *Gastroenterology* 2007; **133**: 24–33.

66 Lupascu A, Gabrielli M, Lauritano EC *et al*. Hydrogen glucose breath test to detect small intestinal bacterial overgrowth: A prevalence case-control study in irritable bowel syndrome. *Aliment Pharmacol Ther* 2005; **22**: 1157–1160.

67 Parodi A, Greco A, Savarino E *et al*. May breath test be useful in diagnosis of IBS patients? An Italian study. *Gastroenterology* 2007; **132**(suppl 1): A192.

68 Pimentel M, Park S, Mirocha J *et al*. The effect of a nonabsorbed oral antibiotic (rifaximin) on the symptoms of the irritable bowel syndrome: A randomized trial. *Ann Intern Med* 2006; **145**: 557–563.

69 Ford AC, Veldhuyzen Van Zanten SJO, Rodgers CC *et al*. Diagnostic utility of alarm features for colorectal cancer: Systematic review and meta-analysis. *Gut* 2008; **57**: 1545–1553.

70 Rubin G, de Wit N, Meineche-Schmidt V *et al*. The diagnosis of IBS in primary care: Consensus development using nominal group technique. *Fam Pract* 2006; **23**: 687–692.

71 Thompson WG, Heaton KW, Smyth GT *et al*. Irritable bowel syndrome: The view from general practice. *Eur J Gastroenterol Hepatol* 1997; **9**: 689–692.

72 Paterson WG, Thompson WG, Vanner SJ *et al*. Recommendations for the management of irritable bowel syndrome in family practice. IBS Consensus Conference Participants. *CMAJ* 1999; **161**: 154–160.

73 Frigerio G, Beretta A, Orsenigo G *et al*. Irritable bowel syndrome. Still far from a positive diagnosis. *Dig Dis Sci* 1992; **37**: 164–167.

74 Hammer J, Eslick GD, Howell SC *et al*. Diagnostic yield of alarm features in irritable bowel syndrome and functional dyspepsia. *Gut* 2004; **53**: 666–672.

75 Jeong H, Lee HR, Yoo BC *et al*. Manning criteria in irritable bowel syndrome: Its diagnostic significance. *Korean J Intern Med* 1993; **8**: 34–39.

76 Rao KP, Gupta S, Jain AK *et al*. Evaluation of Manning's criteria in the diagnosis of irritable bowel syndrome. *J Assoc Physicians India* 1993; **41**: 357–363.

77 Ford AC, Talley NJ, Veldhuyzen Van Zanten SJ *et al*. Will the history and physical examination help establish that irritable bowel syndrome is causing this patient's lower gastrointestinal tract symptoms? *JAMA* 2008; **300**: 1793–1805.

78 Dogan UB, Unal S. Kruis scoring system and Manning's criteria in diagnosis of irritable bowel syndrome: Is it better to use combined? *Acta Gastroenterol Belg* 1996; **59**: 225–228.

79 Bellentani S, Baldoni P, Petrella S *et al*. A simple score for the identification of patients at high risk of organic diseases of the colon in the family doctor consulting room. *Fam Pract* 1990; **7**: 307–312.

80 Tibble JA, Sigthorsson G, Foster R *et al*. Use of surrogate markers of inflammation and Rome criteria to distinguish organic from nonorganic intestinal disease. *Gastroenterology* 2002; **123**: 450–460.

81 Whitehead WE, and the Validation Working Team Committee in association with the Rome Questionnaire Committee. (2006) Development and validation of the Rome III diagnostic questionnaire. In: Drossman DA, eds. *Rome III: The functional gastrointestinal disorders*, 3rd edn. Degnon Associates Inc, Virginia 2006: 835–853.

82 MacIntosh DG, Thompson WG, Patel DG *et al*. Is rectal biopsy necessary in irritable bowel syndrome? *Am J Gastroenterol* 1992; **87**: 1407–1409.

83 Tolliver BA, Herrera JL, DiPalma JA. Evaluation of patients who meet clinical criteria for irritable bowel syndrome. *Am J Gastroenterol* 1994; **89**: 176–178.

84 Hamm LR, Sorrells SC, Harding JP *et al*. Additional investigations fail to alter the diagnosis of irritable bowel syndrome in subjects fulfilling the Rome criteria. *Am J Gastroenterol* 1999; **94**: 1279–1282.

85 Ameen VZ, Patterson MH, Colopy MW *et al*. Confirmation of presumptive diagnosis of irritable bowel syndrome utilizing Rome II criteria and simple laboratory screening tests with diagnostic GI evaluation. *Gastroenterology* 2001; **120**(suppl 1): A635.

86 Limsui D, Pardi DS, Camilleri M *et al*. Symptomatic overlap between irritable bowel syndrome and microscopic colitis. *Inflamm Bowel Dis* 2007; **13**: 175–181.

87 Sanders DS, Carter MJ, Hurlstone DP *et al*. Association of adult celiac disease with irritable bowel syndrome: A case-control study in patients fulfilling ROME II criteria referred to secondary care. *Lancet* 2001; **358**: 1504–1508.

88 Sanders DS, Patel D, Stephenson TJ *et al*. A primary care cross-sectional study of undiagnosed celiac disease. *Eur J Gastroenterol Hepatol* 2003; **15**: 407–413.

89 Shahbazkhani B, Forootan M, Merat S *et al*. Celiac disease presenting with symptoms of irritable bowel syndrome. *Aliment Pharmacol Ther* 2003; **18**: 231–235.

90 Agreus L, Svardsudd K, Tibblin G *et al*. Endomysium antibodies are superior to gliadin antibodies in screening for celiac disease in patients presenting supposed functional gastrointestinal symptoms. *Scand J Gastroenterol* 2000; **18**: 105–110.

91 Chey WD, Nojkov B, Saad RJ *et al*. Screening for celiac sprue in patients with suspected irritable bowel syndrome: Results from a prospective US multi-center trial. *Gastroenterology* 2007; **132**(suppl 1): A147.

92 Locke GR, III, Murray JA, Zinsmeister AR *et al*. Celiac disease serology in irritable bowel syndrome and dyspepsia: A population-based case-control study. *Mayo Clin Proc* 2004; **79**: 476–482.

93 Ford AC, Chey WD, Talley NJ *et al*. Utility of diagnostic tests for celiac disease in irritable bowel syndrome: Systematic review and meta-analysis. *Arch Intern Med* 2009; **169**: 651–658.

94 Abrams JA, Brar P, Diamond B *et al*. Utility in clinical practice of immunoglobulin A anti-tissue transglutaminase antibody for the diagnosis of celiac disease. *Clin Gastroenterol Hepatol* 2006; **4**: 726–730.

95 Mein SM, Ladabaum U. Serological testing for celiac disease in patients with symptoms of irritable bowel syndrome: A cost-effectiveness analysis. *Aliment Pharmacol Ther* 2004; **19**: 1199–1210.

96 Spiegel BMR, DeRosa VP, Gralnek IM *et al*. Testing for celiac sprue in irritable bowel syndrome with predominant diarrhea: A cost-effectiveness analysis. *Gastroenterology* 2004; **126**: 1721–1732.

97 Sciarretta G, Giacobazzi G, Verri A *et al*. Hydrogen breath test quantification and clinical correlation of lactose malabsorption in adult irritable bowel syndrome and ulcerative colitis. *Dig Dis Sci* 1984; **29**: 1098–1104.

98 Bohmer CJM, Tuynman HA. The clinical relevance of lactose malabsorption in irritable bowel syndrome. *Eur J Gastroenterol Hepatol* 1996; **8**: 1013–1016.

99 Parker TJ, Woolner JT, Prevost AT *et al*. Irritable bowel syndrome: Is the search for lactose intolerance justified? *Eur J Gastroenterol Hepatol* 2001; **13**: 219–225.

100 Vernia P, Di Camillo M, Marinaro V. Lactose malabsorption, irritable bowel syndrome and self-reported milk intolerance. *Dig Liver Dis* 2001; **33**: 234–239.

101 Farup PG, Monsbakken KW, Vandvik PO. Lactose malabsorption in a population with irritable bowel syndrome: Prevalence and symptoms. A case-control study. *Scand J Gastroenterol* 2004; **39**: 645–649.

102 Pimentel M, Chow EJ, Lin HC. Eradication of small intestinal bacterial overgrowth reduces symptoms of irritable bowel syndrome. *Am J Gastroenterol* 2000; **95**: 3503–3506.

103 Nucera G, Gabrielli M, Lupascu A *et al*. Abnormal breath tests to lactose, fructose and sorbitol in irritable bowel syndrome may be explained by small intestinal bacterial overgrowth. *Aliment Pharmacol Ther* 2005; **21**: 1391–1395.

104 McCallum R, Schultz C, Sostarich S. Evaluating the role of small intestinal bacterial overgrowth in diarrhea predominant irritable bowel syndrome patients utilizing the glucose breath test. *Gastroenterology* 2005; **128**(suppl 2): A460.

105 Posserud I, Stotzer P-O, Bjornsson ES *et al*. Small intestinal bacterial overgrowth in patients with irritable bowel syndrome. *Gut* 2007; **56**: 802–808.

106 Bratten JR, Spanier J, Jones MP. Lactulose breath testing does not discriminate patients with irritable bowel syndrome from healthy controls. *Am J Gastroenterol* 2008; **103**: 958–963.

107 Banerjee R, Choung OW, Gupta R *et al*. Rome I criteria are more sensitive than Rome II for diagnosis of irritable bowel syndrome in Indian patients. *Indian J Gastroenterol* 2005; **24**: 164–166.

108 Cash BD, Kim CH, Lee DH *et al*. Yield of diagnostic testing in patients with suspected irritable bowel syndrome: A prospec-

tive, US multi-center trial. *Gastroenterology* 2007; **132**(suppl 1): A678.

109 Francis CY, Duffy JN, Whorwell PJ *et al.* Does routine abdominal ultrasound enhance diagnostic accuracy in irritable bowel syndrome? *Am J Gastroenterol* 1996; **91**: 1348–1350.

110 Bijkerk CJ, Muris JWM, Knottnerus JA *et al.* Systematic review: The role of different types of fiber in the treatment of irritable bowel syndrome. *Aliment Pharmacol Ther* 2004; **19**: 245–251.

111 Cremonini F, Delgado-Aros S, Camilleri M. Efficacy of alosetron in irritable bowel syndrome: A meta-analysis of randomized controlled trials. *Neurogastroenterol Motil* 2003; **15**: 79–86.

112 Evans BW, Clark WK, Moore DJ, Whorwell PJ. Tegaserod for the treatment of irritable bowel syndrome and chronic constipation. *Cochrane Database of Systematic Reviews* 2007, Issue 4. Art. No.: CD003960. DOI: 10.1002/14651858.CD003960.pub3.

113 Jackson JL, O'Malley PG, Tomkins G *et al.* Treatment of functional gastrointestinal disorders with antidepressant medications: A meta-analysis. *Am J Med* 2000; **108**: 65–72.

114 Lesbros-Pantoflickova D, Michetti P, Fried M *et al.* Meta-analysis: The treatment of irritable bowel syndrome. *Aliment Pharmacol Ther* 2004; **20**: 1253–1269.

115 Pittler MH, Ernst E. Peppermint oil for irritable bowel syndrome: A critical review and meta-analysis. *Am J Gastroenterol* 1998; **93**: 1131–1135.

116 Poynard T, Regimbeau C, Benhamou Y. Meta-analysis of smooth muscle relaxants in the treatment of irritable bowel syndrome. *Aliment Pharmacol Ther* 2001; **15**: 355–361.

117 Quartero AO, Meiniche-Schmidt V, Muris J, Rubin G, de Wit N. Bulking agents, antispasmodic and antidepressant medication for the treatment of irritable bowel syndrome. *Cochrane Database of Systematic Reviews* 2005, Issue 2. Art. No.: CD003460. DOI: 10.1002/14651858.CD003460.pub2.

118 American College of Gastroenterology Task Force. An evidence based review of the management of irritable bowel syndrome. *Am J Gastroenterol* 2009; **104**(suppl I): S1–S35.

119 Harvey RF, Pomare EW, Heaton KW. Effects of increased dietary fibre on intestinal transit. *Lancet* 1973; **301**: 1278–1280.

120 Longstreth GF, Fox DD, Youkeles L *et al.* Psyllium therapy in the irritable bowel syndrome: A double-blind trial. *Ann Intern Med* 1981; **95**: 53–56.

121 Nigam P, Kapoor KK, Rastog CK *et al.* Different therapeutic regimens in irritable bowel syndrome. *J Assoc Physicians India* 1984; **32**: 1041–1044.

122 Ritchie JA, Truelove SC. Treatment of irritable bowel syndrome with lorazepam, hyoscine butylbromide, and ispaghula husk. *Br Med J* 1979; **278**: 376–378.

123 Soltoft J, Krag B, Gudmand-Hoyer E *et al.* A double-blind trial of the effect of wheat bran on symptoms of irritable bowel syndrome. *Lancet* 1976; **307**: 270–272.

124 Ford AC, Talley NJ, Spiegel BMR *et al.* Effect of fibre, antispasmodics and peppermint oil in irritable bowel syndrome: Systematic review and meta-analysis. *Br Med J* 2008; **337**: 1388–1392.

125 Juni P, Altman DG, Egger M. Assessing the quality of controlled clinical trials. *Br Med J* 2001; **323**: 42–46.

126 Veldhuyzen Van Zanten SJ, Talley NJ, Bytzer P *et al.* Design of treatment trials for functional gastrointestinal disorders. *Gut* 1999; **45**(suppl II): II69–II77.

127 Aziz Q, Thompson DG, Ng VW *et al.* Cortical processing of human somatic and visceral sensation. *J Neurosci* 2000; **20**: 2657–2663.

128 Fielding JF. Double blind trial of trimebutine in the irritable bowel syndrome. *Ir Med J* 1980; **73**: 377–379.

129 Glende M, Morselli-Labate AM, Battaglia G *et al.* Extended analysis of a double blind, placebo-controlled, 15-week study with otilinium bromide in irritable bowel syndrome. *Eur J Gastroenterol Hepatol* 2002; **14**: 1331–1338.

130 Kruis W, Weinzierl M, Schussler P *et al.* Comparison of the therapeutic effects of wheat bran and placebo in patients with the irritable bowel syndrome. *Digestion* 1986; **34**: 196–201.

131 Page JG, Dirnberger GM. Treatment of the irritable bowel syndrome with Bentyl (dicyclomine hydrochloride). *J Clin Gastroenterol* 1981; **3**: 153–156.

132 Hills JM, Aaronson PI. The mechanism of action of peppermint oil on gastrointestinal smooth muscle. *Gastroenterology* 1991; **101**: 55–65.

133 Capanni M, Surrenti E, Biagini M *et al.* Efficacy of peppermint oil in the treatment of irritable bowel syndrome: A randomized, controlled trial. *Gazz Med Ital* 2005; **164**: 119–126.

134 Cappello G, Spezzaferro M, Grossi L *et al.* Peppermint oil (Mintoil) in the treatment of irritable bowel syndrome: A prospective double blind placebo-controlled randomized trial. *Dig Liver Dis* 2007; **39**: 530–536.

135 Lech Y, Olesen KM, Hey H *et al.* Treatment of irritable bowel syndrome with peppermint oil. A double-blind investigation with a placebo. *Ugeskr Laeger* 1988; **150**: 2388–2389.

136 Liu J-H, Chen G-H, Yeh H-Z *et al.* Enteric-coated peppermint-oil capsules in the treatment of irritable bowel syndrome: A prospective, randomized trial. *J Gastroenterol* 1997; **32**: 765–768.

137 Marciani L, Foley S, Hoad CL *et al.* Accelerated small bowel transit and contracted transverse colon in diarrhea-predominant irritable bowel syndrome (IBS-D): Novel insights from magnetic resonance imaging (MRI). *Gastroenterology* 2007; **132**(suppl 1): A141.

138 McQuay HJ, Tramer M, Nye BA *et al.* A systematic review of antidepressants in neuropathic pain. *Pain* 1996; **68**: 217–227.

139 Saarto T, Wiffen PJ. Antidepressants for neuropathic pain. *Cochrane Database of Systematic Reviews* 2007, Issue 4. Art. No.: CD005454. DOI: 10.1002/14651858.CD005454.pub2.

140 Heefner JD, Wilder RM, Wilson ID. Irritable colon and depression. *Psychosomatics* 1978; **19**: 540–547.

141 Tack J, Broekaert D, Fischler B *et al.* A controlled crossover study of the selective serotonin reuptake inhibitor citalopram in irritable bowel syndrome. *Gut* 2006; **55**: 1095–1103.

142 Talley NJ, Kellow JE, Boyce P *et al.* Antidepressant therapy (imipramine and citalopram) for irritable bowel syndrome: A double-blind, randomized, placebo-controlled trial. *Dig Dis Sci* 2008; **53**: 108–115.

143 Vahedi H, Merat S, Rashidioon A *et al.* The effect of fluoxetine in patients with pain and constipation-predominant irritable bowel syndrome: A double-blind randomized-controlled study. *Aliment Pharmacol Ther* 2005; **22**: 381–385.

144 Ford AC, Talley NJ, Schoenfeld PS *et al.* Efficacy of antidepressants and psychological therapies in irritable bowel syndrome: Systematic review and meta-analysis. *Gut* 2009; **58**: 367–378.

145 Gorard DA, Libby GW, Farthing MJ. Influence of antidepressants on whole gut orocaecal transit times in health and irritable bowel syndrome. *Aliment Pharmacol Ther* 1994; **8**: 159–166.

146 Bergmann M, Heddergott A, Schlosser T. Die therapie des colon irritabile mit trimipramin (Herphonal) – Eine kontrollierte studie. *Z Klin Med* 1991; **46**: 1621–1628.

147 Vahedi H, Merat S, Momtahen S *et al.* Clinical trial: The effect of amitriptyline in patients with diarrhea-predominant irritable bowel syndrome. *Aliment Pharmacol Ther* 2008; **27**: 678–684.

148 Tabas G, Beaves M, Wang J *et al.* Paroxetine to treat irritable bowel syndrome not responding to high fiber diet: A double-blind placebo-controlled trial. *Am J Gastroenterol* 2004; **99**: 914–920.

149 Shanahan F. Irritable bowel syndrome: Shifting the focus towards the gut microbiota. *Gastroenterology* 2007; **133**: 340–342.

150 Colombel JF, Cortot A, Neut C *et al.* Yoghurt with *Bifidobacterium* reduces erythromycin induced gastrointestinal effects. *Lancet* 1987; **330**: 43–44.

151 Katelaris PH, Salam I, Farthing MJ. *Lactobacilli* to prevent traveller's diarrhea. *N Engl J Med* 1995; **333**: 1360–1361.

152 Allen SJ, Okoko B, Martinez EG, Gregorio GV, Dans LF. Probiotics for treating infectious diarrhea. *Cochrane Database of Systematic Reviews* 2003, Issue 4. Art. No.: CD003048. DOI: 10.1002/14651858.CD003048.pub2.

153 Moayyedi P, Ford AC, Brandt LJ *et al.* The efficacy of probiotics in the therapy of irritable bowel syndrome: A systematic review. *Gut* 2008 (published online 17 Dec) doi:10.1136/Gut.2008.167270.

154 Verdu EF, Bercik P, Bergonzelli GE *et al. Lactobacillus paracasei* normalizes muscle hypercontractility in a murine model of postinfective gut dysfunction. *Gastroenterology* 2004; **127**: 826–837.

155 Verdu EF, Bercik P, Verma-Gandhu M *et al.* Specific probiotic therapy attenuates antibiotic induced visceral hypersensitivity in mice. *Gut* 2006; **55**: 182–190.

156 Kamiya T, Wang L, Forsythe P *et al.* Inhibitory effects of *Lactobacillus* reuteri on visceral pain induced by colorectal distension in Sprague-Dawley rats. *Gut* 2006; **55**: 191–196.

157 Rousseaux C, Thuru X, Gelot A *et al. Lactobacillus acidophilus* modulates intestinal pain and induces opioid and cannabinoid receptors. *Nat Med* 2007; **13**: 35–37.

158 O'Mahony L, McCarthy J, Kelly P *et al. Lactobacillus* and *bifidobacterium* in irritable bowel syndrome: Symptom responses and and relationship to cytokine profiles. *Gastroenterology* 2005; **128**: 541–551.

159 Hahn BA, Kirchdoerfer LJ, Fullerton S *et al.* Patient perceived severity of irritable bowel syndrome in relation to symptoms, health resource utilization and quality of life. *Aliment Pharmacol Ther* 1997; **11**: 553–559.

160 Halder SLS, Locke GR, Talley NJ *et al.* Impact of functional gastrointestinal disorders on health-related quality of life: A population-based case-control study. *Aliment Pharmacol Ther* 2004; **19**: 233–242.

161 Koloski NA, Talley NJ, Boyce PM. The impact of functional gastrointestinal disorders on quality of life. *Am J Gastroenterol* 2000; **95**: 67–71.

162 Henningsen P, Zimmermann T, Sattel H. Medically unexplained physical symptoms, anxiety and depression: A meta-analytic review. *Psychosom Med* 2003; **65**: 528–533.

163 Solmaz M, Kavuk I, Sayar K. Psychological factors in the irritable bowel syndrome. *Eur J Med Res* 2003; **8**: 549–556.

164 Sykes MA, Blanchard EB, Lackner J *et al.* Psychopathology in irritable bowel syndrome: Support for a psychophysiological model. *J Behav Med* 2003; **26**: 361–372.

165 Osterberg E, Blomquist L, Krakau I *et al.* A population study on irritable bowel syndrome and mental health. *Scand J Gastroenterol* 2000; **35**: 264–268.

166 Whitehead WE, Palsson O, Jones KR. Systematic review of the comorbidity of irritable bowel syndrome with other disorders: What are the causes and implications? *Gastroenterology* 2002; **122**: 1140–1156.

167 Drossman DA, Toner BB, Whitehead WE *et al.* Cognitive-behavioral therapy versus education and desipramine versus placebo for moderate to severe functional bowel disorders. *Gastroenterology* 2003; **125**: 19–31.

168 Kennedy T, Jones R, Darnley S *et al.* Cognitive behaviour therapy in addition to antispasmodic treatment for irritable bowel syndrome in primary care: Randomised controlled trial. *Br Med J* 2005; **331**: 435–437.

169 Boyce PM, Talley NJ, Balaam B *et al.* A randomized controlled trial of cognitive behavior therapy, relaxation training, and routine clinical care for the irritable bowel syndrome. *Am J Gastroenterol* 2003; **98**: 2209–2218.

170 van der Veek PPJ, van Rood YR, Masclee AAM. Clinical trial: Short- and long-term benefit of relaxation training for irritable bowel syndrome. *Aliment Pharmacol Ther* 2007; **26**: 943–952.

171 Creed F, Fernandes L, Guthrie E *et al.* The cost-effectiveness of psychotherapy and paroxetine for severe irritable bowel syndrome. *Gastroenterology* 2003; **124**: 303–317.

172 Guthrie E, Creed F, Dawson D *et al.* A controlled trial of psychological treatment for the irritable bowel syndrome. *Gastroenterology* 1991; **100**: 450–457.

173 Heitkemper M, Jarrett ME, Levy RL *et al.* Self-management for women with irritable bowel syndrome. *Clin Gastroenterol Hepatol* 2004; **2**: 585–596.

174 Neff DF, Blanchard EB. A multi-component treatment for irritable bowel syndrome. *Behav Ther* 1987; **18**: 70–83.

175 Lackner JM, Mesmer C, Morley S *et al.* Psychological treatments for irritable bowel syndrome: A systematic review and meta-analysis. *J Consult Clin Psychol* 2004; **72**: 1100–1113.

176 Atkinson W, Lockhart S, Whorwell PJ *et al.* Altered 5-hydroxytryptamine signaling in patients with constipation-and diarrhea-predominant irritable bowel syndrome. *Gastroenterology* 2006; **130**: 34–43.

177 Bardhan KD, Bodemar G, Geldof H *et al.* A double-blind, randomized, placebo-controlled dose-ranging study to evaluate the efficacy of alosetron in the treatment of irritable bowel syndrome. *Aliment Pharmacol Ther* 2000; **14**: 23–34.

178 Camilleri M, Mayer EA, Drossman DA *et al.* Improvement in pain and bowel function in female irritable bowel patients with alosetron, a 5-HT3 receptor antagonist. *Aliment Pharmacol Ther* 1999; **13**: 1149–1159.

179 Kellow J, Lee OY, Chang FY *et al.* An Asia-Pacific, double-blind, placebo-controlled, randomised study to evaluate the efficacy, safety, and tolerability of tegaserod in patients with irritable bowel syndrome. *Gut* 2003; **52**: 671–676.

180 Muller-Lissner SA, Fumagalli I, Bardhan KD *et al.* Tegaserod, a 5-HT4 receptor partial agonist, relieves symptoms in irritable

bowel syndrome patients with abdominal pain, bloating and constipation. *Aliment Pharmacol Ther* 2001; **15**: 1655–1666.

181 Anonymous. Glaxo Wellcome withdraws irritable bowel syndrome medication. *FDA Consum* 2001; **35**: 3.

182 FDA public health advisory: Tegaserod maleate (marketed as Zelnorm). 2007. Published online at http://www.fda.gov/cder/drug/advisory/tegaserod.htm

183 Ford AC, Brandt LJ, Young C, Chey WD, Foxx-Orenstein AE, Moayyedi P. Efficacy of 5-HT$_3$ antagonists and 5-HT$_4$ agonists in irritable bowel syndrome: Systematic review and meta-analysis. *Am J Gastroenterol* 2009;**104**:1831–1843

184 Jadad AR, Moore RA, Carroll D *et al.* Assessing the quality of reports of randomized clinical trials: Is blinding necessary? *Control Clin Trials* 1996; **17**: 1–12.

185 Johanson JF, Ueno R. Lubiprostone, a locally acting chloride channel activator, in adult patients with chronic constipation: A double-blind, placebo-controlled, dose-ranging study to evaluate efficacy and safety. *Aliment Pharmacol Ther* 2007; **25**: 1351–1361.

186 Johanson JF, Drossman DA, Panas R *et al.* Clinical trial: Phase 2 study of lubiprostone for irritable bowel syndrome with constipation. *Aliment Pharmacol Ther* 2008; **27**: 685–696.

187 Drossman DA, Chey WD, Panas R *et al.* Lubiprostone significantly improves symptom relief rates in adults with irritable bowel syndrome and constipation (IBS-C): Data from two twelve-week, randomized, placebo-controlled,double-blind trials. *Gastroenterology* 2007; **132**: 2586–2587.

188 Drossman DA, Chey WD, Johanson JF, *et al.* Clinical trial: Lubiprostone in patients with constipation-associated irritable bowel syndrome – results of two randomized, placebo-controlled studies. *Aliment Pharmacol Ther* 2009; **29**: 329–341.

189 Chey WD, Saad RJ, Panas RM *et al.* Discontinuation of lubiprostone treatment for irritable bowel syndrome with constipation is not associated with symptom increase or recurrence: Results from a randomized withdrawal study. *Gastroenterology* 2008; **134**(suppl 1): A401.

190 Hovdenak N. Loperamide treatment of the irritable bowel syndrome. *Scand J Gastroenterol* 1987; **130**: 81–84.

191 Lavo B, Stenstam M, Nielsen A-L. Loperamide in treatment of irritable bowel syndrome – A double-blind placebo controlled study. *Scand J Gastroenterol* 1987; **130**: 77–80.

192 Zar S, Benson MJ, Kumar D. Food-specific serum IgG4 and IgE titers to common food antigens in irritable bowel syndrome. *Am J Gastroenterol* 2005; **100**: 1550–1557.

193 Zar S, Mincher L, Benson MJ *et al.* Food-specific IgG4 antibody-guided exclusion diet improves symptoms and rectal compliance in irritable bowel syndrome. *Scand J Gastroenterol* 2005; **40**: 800–807.

194 Wahnschaffe U, Schulzke JD, Zeitz M *et al.* Predictors of clinical response to gluten-free diet in patients diagnosed with diarrhea-predominant irritable bowel syndrome. *Clin Gastroenterol Hepatol* 2007; **5**: 844–850.

195 Park MI, Camilleri M. Is there a role of food allergy in irritable bowel syndrome and functional dyspepsia? A systematic review. *Neurogastroenterol Motil* 2006; **18**: 595–607.

196 Halder SLS, Locke III GR, Schleck CD *et al.* Natural history of functional gastrointestinal disorders: A 12-year longitudinal population-based study. *Gastroenterology* 2007; **133**: 799–807.

197 Ford AC, Forman D, Bailey AG *et al.* Fluctuation of gastrointestinal symptoms in the community: A 10-year longitudinal follow-up study. *Aliment Pharmacol Ther* 2008; **28**: 1013–1020.

198 Owens DM, Nelson DK, Talley NJ. The irritable bowel syndrome: Long-term prognosis and the physician-patient interaction. *Ann Intern Med* 1995; **122**: 107–112.

199 Adeniji OA, Barnett CB, Di Palma JA. Durability of the diagnosis of irritable bowel syndrome based on clinical criteria. *Dig Dis Sci* 2004; **49**: 572–574.

22 Ogilvie's syndrome

Michael D Saunders

Digestive Diseases Center, University of Washington School of Medicine, Washington, USA

Introduction

Acute colonic pseudo-obstruction (ACPO), also referred to as Ogilvie's syndrome [1], is a clinical condition with symptoms, signs and radiographic appearance of acute large bowel obstruction without a mechanical cause. ACPO occurs most often in hospitalized or institutionalized patients with serious underlying medical and surgical conditions. ACPO is an important cause of morbidity and mortality. The mortality rate is estimated at 40% when ischemia or perforation occurs [2]. Early detection and prompt appropriate management are critical to minimizing morbidity and mortality.

Pathogenesis

The pathogenesis of ACPO is not completely understood but likely results from an alteration in the autonomic regulation of colonic motor function [3]. Colonic pseudo-obstruction was first described in 1948 by Sir Heneage Ogilvie, who reported two patients with chronic colonic dilation associated with malignant infiltration of the celiac plexus [4]. Ogilvie attributed the syndrome to sympathetic deprivation. A better understanding of the autonomic nervous system in the gut has modified this hypothesis. The parasympathetic nervous system increases contractility, whereas the sympathetic nerves decrease motility [3]. An imbalance in autonomic innervation, produced by a variety of factors, leads to excessive parasympathetic suppression or sympathetic stimulation. The result is colonic atony and pseudo-obstruction.

Evidence-Based Gastroenterology and Hepatology, 3rd edition.
J. McDonald, A.K. Burroughs, B. Feagan, and M.B. Fennerty. © 2010
Blackwell Publishing Ltd

Multiple predisposing factors or conditions have been associated with ACPO (Table 22.1). In a large retrospective series of 400 patients, the most common predisposing conditions were non-operative trauma (11.3%), infections (10%) and cardiac disease (10%) [2]. Cesarean section and hip surgery were the most common surgical procedures, with the onset of the syndrome occurring postoperatively at an average of 4.5 days. In another retrospective analysis of 48 patients, the spine or retroperitoneum had been traumatized or manipulated in 52% [4]. Over half the patients were receiving narcotics, and electrolyte abnormalities were present in approximately two-thirds. Thus, multiple metabolic, pharmacologic, or traumatic factors appear to alter the autonomic regulation of colonic function, resulting in pseudo-obstruction.

Clinical features

The exact incidence of ACPO is unknown. In the retrospective series of patients undergoing orthopedic procedures reported by Norwood and colleagues [5], the incidence of ACPO was 1.3%, 1.19%, and 0.65% following hip replacement, spinal operations and knee replacement respectively. ACPO most often affects those in late middle age (mean of 60 years of age), with a slight male predominance (60%) [2]. ACPO occurs almost exclusively in hospitalized or institutionalized patients with serious underlying medical and surgical conditions. Abdominal distention usually develops over three to seven days but can occur as rapidly as over a 24 to 48-hour period [2]. In surgical patients, symptoms and signs develop at a mean of five days postoperatively.

The clinical features of ACPO include abdominal distension, abdominal pain (80%), and nausea and/or vomiting (60%) [2]. Passage of flatus or stool is reported in up to 40% of patients. There is no significant difference in symptoms of patients with ischemic or perforated bowel, except for a

Table 22.1 Predisposing conditions associated with acute colonic pseudo-obstruction – an analysis of 400 cases[a].

Condition	No. of patients	Proportion (%)
Trauma (non-operative)	45	11.3
Infection (pneumonia, sepsis most common)	40	10.0
Cardiac (myocardial infarction, heart failure)	40	10.0
Obstetrics/gynecology	39	9.8
Abdominal/pelvic surgery	37	9.3
Neurologic	37	9.3
Orthopedic surgery	29	7.3
Miscellaneous medical conditions (metabolic, cancer, respiratory failure, renal failure)	128	32
Miscellaneous surgical conditions (urologic, thoracic, neurosurgery)	47	11.8

[a] Associated conditions in approximately 400 patients, reported by Vanek and Al-Salti [2]. Some patients had more than one associated condition.

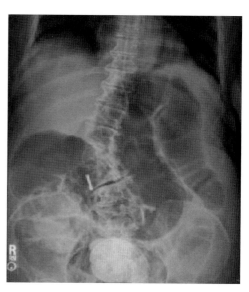

Figure 22.1 Abdominal radiographs of a patient with acute colonic pseudo-obstruction. The plain abdominal film shows marked dilatation, especially of the right colon. In addition, moderate small bowel dilatation is present.

BOX 22.1 Supportive therapy for acute colonic pseudo-obstruction

- Nil per os
- Correct fluid and electrolyte imbalances
- Nasogastric tube suction
- Rectal tube to gravity drainage
- Limit offending medications (especially narcotics)
- Frequent position changes, ambulate if possible

higher incidence of fever [2]. On examination, the abdomen is tympanitic and bowel sounds are typically present. Fever, marked abdominal tenderness and leukocytosis are more common in patients with ischemia or perforation but also occur in those who have not developed these complications [2].

The diagnosis of ACPO is confirmed by plain abdominal radiographs, which show varying degrees of colonic dilatation (Figure 22.1). Air fluid levels and dilatation can also be seen in the small bowel. Typically, the right colon and cecum show the most marked distension, and cutoffs at the splenic flexure are common. This distribution of colonic dilation may be caused by the different origins of the proximal and distal parasympathetic nerve supply to the colon [3]. A water soluble contrast enema or computed tomography (CT) scan should be obtained to exclude mechanical obstruction if gas and distension are not present throughout all colonic segments including the rectum and sigmoid colon.

Keys to management of ACPO include (1) early recognition and diagnosis, (2) evaluation to exclude mechanical obstruction or other causes of pseudo-obstruction (such as *Clostridium difficile* colitis [6], (3) assessment for signs of ischemia or perforation which would warrant urgent surgi-cal intervention, and (4) initiation of appropriate treatment measures.

Management

Treatment options for ACPO include appropriate supportive measures, medical therapy, colonoscopic decompression, and surgery. Despite extensive literature documenting the clinical features of ACPO, there are very few randomized controlled clinical trials on the treatment of this condition, and most evidence for efficacy of treatments comes from uncontrolled studies.

Supportive therapy

Supportive therapy (Box 22.1) should be instituted in all patients as it appears to be successful as the primary treatment in the majority of patients [7]. **B4** Patients are given nothing by mouth. Intravenous fluids are administered and electrolyte imbalances are corrected. Nasogastric suction is provided to limit swallowed air from contributing further to colonic distension. A rectal tube should be inserted and attached to gravity drainage. Medications that can adversely affect colonic motility, such as opiates, anticholinergics and calcium channel antagonists are discontinued if possible. Ambulation and mobilization of patients are encouraged. The knee-chest position with hips held high has been advocated as aiding in evacuation of colonic gas [8]. None of these supportive measures has been studied in a randomized trial. **C5**

The reported success of supportive management is variable, with pooled rates from several retrospective series of approximately 85% [7, 9–13]. In these combined series, 111 patients were treated conservatively, of which 95 (86%) had resolution of the pseudo-obstruction. **B4** Sloyer *et al.* reported outcomes of 25 cancer patients with ACPO (mostly non-gastrointestinal malignancies) [7]. The mean cecal diameter was 11.7 cm (range 9–18 cm). Of the 24 patients treated conservatively, 23 (96%) improved by clinical and radiologic criteria with the median time to improvement of 1.6 days (mean 3 days). There were no perforations or ACPO-related deaths. The authors concluded that early endoscopic or surgical decompression is not necessary in patients with ACPO. **B4** In another recent retrospective series of 151 patients reported by Loftus *et al.*, 117 (77%) had spontaneous resolution of ACPO with conservative treatment [14]. **B4** These studies demonstrate that the initial management of ACPO should be directed towards eliminating or reducing the factors known to contribute to the problem.

Patient outcome

The clinical dilemma facing the clinician caring for a patient with ACPO is whether to treat the patient with conservative measures and close observation versus proceeding with medical or endoscopic decompression of the dilated colon. The outcome of patients with ACPO is determined by multiple factors. The severity of the underlying illness appears to exert the greatest influence on patient outcome. ACPO often afflicts debilitated patients, which explains the significant morbidity and mortality even with successful treatment of the colonic dilatation. Other factors that appear to influence outcome are increasing age, maximal cecal diameter, delay in decompression and status of the bowel [2]. The risk of spontaneous colon perforation in ACPO is low but clearly exists. Rex reviewed all available reports in the literature and estimated the risk of spontaneous perforation to be approximately 3% [15]. The mortality rate in ACPO is approximately 40% when ischemia or perforation are present, compared with 15% in patients with viable bowel [2]. Retrospective analyses of patients with ACPO [2, 13] have attempted to identify clinical factors that

predict which patients are more likely to have complications such as ischemia or perforation. The risk of colonic perforation has been reported to increase with cecal diameter greater than 12 cm and when distension has been present for more than six days [13]. In the large series reported by Vanek and Al-Salti, no cases of perforation were seen when the cecal diameter was less than 12 cm [2]. However, at diameters greater than 12 cm, there was no clear relationship between risk of ischemia or perforation and the size of the cecum. The duration and progression of colonic distension may be more important. Johnson and Rice reported a mean duration of distension of six days in patients who perforated compared with two days in those who did not [13]. A two-fold increase in mortality occurs when cecal diameter is greater than 14 cm and a five-fold increase when delay in decompression is greater than seven days [2]. Thus, the decision to intervene with medical therapy, colonoscopy or surgery is dictated by the patient's clinical status. On the basis of the limited available evidence patients with marked cecal distension (>10 cm) of significant duration (>3–4 days) and those not improving after 24–48 hours of supportive therapy are considered to be candidates for further intervention. **B4** In the absence of signs of ischemia or perforation, medical therapy with neostigmine should be considered the initial therapy of choice.

Medical therapy

Neostigmine

The only randomized controlled trial of an intervention for ACPO involves the use of neostigmine [16]. Neostigmine, a reversible acetylcholinesterase inhibitor, indirectly stimulates muscarinic receptors, thereby enhancing colonic motor activity, inducing colonic propulsion and accelerated transit [17]. The rationale for using neostigmine stems from the imbalance in autonomic regulation of colonic function that is proposed to occur in ACPO. Neostigmine was first used for manipulation of the autonomic innervation to the gastrointestinal tract by Neely and Catchpole over 30 years ago in studies on small bowel paralytic ileus [18]. Neostigmine, administered intravenously, has a rapid onset (1–20 minutes) and short duration (1–2 hours) of action [19]. The elimination half-life averages 80 minutes, but is more prolonged in patients with renal insufficiency [20].

A randomized double-blind, placebo-controlled trial evaluated neostigmine in patients with ACPO with a cecal diameter of >10 cm and no response to 24 hours of conservative therapy [16]. Exclusion criteria were suspected ischemia or perforation, pregnancy, severe active bronchospasm, cardiac arrhythmias and renal failure. Patients were randomized to receive neostigmine, 2 mg, or saline by intravenous infusion over 3–5 minutes. The primary endpoint was the clinical response to infusion, defined as a prompt reduction in abdominal distension by physical examination. Secondary endpoints included the change in measurements of colonic diameter on radiographs and abdominal girth. Patients not responding within three hours to initial infusion were eligible for open label neostigmine. A clinical response was observed in 10 of 11 patients (91%) randomized to receive neostigmine compared to 0 of 10 receiving placebo. **A1d** The median time to response was four minutes. Median reduction in cecal diameter (5 cm vs 2 cm) and abdominal girth (7 cm vs 1 cm) were significantly reduced in neostigmine-treated patients. Open-label neostigmine was administered to eight patients who failed to respond to the initial infusion (seven placebo, one neostigmine), and all had prompt decompression. Of the 18 patients who received neostigmine, either initially or during open-label treatment, 17 (94%) had a clinical response. The recurrence rate of colonic distension after neostigmine decompression was low (11%). The most common adverse effects observed with neostigmine were mild abdominal cramping and excessive salivation. Symptomatic bradycardia requiring atropine occurred in 2 of 19 patients.

Neostigmine was also evaluated in a double-blinded, placebo-controlled trial involving 24 critically ill, ventilated patients with ileus (defined as absence of stools for three days) [21]. No details of the extent and duration of colonic distention were provided. Neostigmine was administered as a continuous infusion (0.4 mg/hour for 24 hours). Of the 13 patients receiving neostigmine, 11 passed stools, whereas none of the placebo treated patients passed stools (p < 0.001). No acute serious adverse events occurred, but three patients had ischemic colonic complications 7 to 10 days after treatment.

There are also several uncontrolled observational studies supporting the use of neostigmine in this condition [14, 22–27]. Collectively, rapid decompression of colonic distension was observed in 88% of patients with a recurrence rate of 7% (Table 22.2). **B4** In the case series reported by Mehta and colleagues [28], a response to neostigmine was more likely in the postoperative setting (11 of 15 patients (73%) versus one of four patients (25%), p = 0.07), and less likely in those with electrolyte imbalance or receiving antimotility agents (3 of 15 (20%) versus 4 of 4, p = 0.003). This study suggests that it may be important to correct electrolyte abnormalities and to limit potentially exacerbating medications.

Repeated infusions or more prolonged treatment with neostigmine have not been evaluated fully. There have been reports of patients with ACPO receiving repeated infusions and prolonged treatment with resolution [29]. This experience suggests that cautious repeated infusions can be successful and merits further study in patients with persistent or recurrent pseudo-obstruction.

Table 22.2 Neostigmine for colonic decompression in patients with acute colonic pseudo-obstruction.

Study	No. of patients	Design	Dose	Decompression	Recurrence
Ponec et al. (1999) [16]	21 (neostigmine 11, placebo 10)	RCT; (OL in non-responders)	2.0 mg IV over 3–5 min	Neostigmine 10/11 in RCT; 17/18 total; placebo 0/10	2
Hutchinson and Griffiths (1992) [22]	11	OL	2.5 mg IV in one min.	8/11	0
Stephenson et al. (1995) [23]	12	OL	2.5 mg IV over 1–3 min.	12/12 (two patients required two doses)	1
Turegano-Fuentes et al. (1997) [24]	16	OL	2.5 mg IV over 60 min	12/16	0
Trevisani et al. (2000) [25]	28	OL	2.5 mg IV over 3 min	26/28	0
Paran et al. (2001) [26]	11	OL	2.5 mg IV over 60 min	10/11 (two patients required two doses)	0
Abeyta et al. (2001) [27]	8	Retrospective	2.0 mg IV	6/8 (two patients required two doses)	0
Loftus et al. (2002) [14]	18	Retrospective	2.0 mg IV	16/18	5

RCT: randomized controlled trial; OL: open-label trial; IV: intravenous.

The cost of neostigmine is minimal, with a 2 mg ampoule for parenteral use costing only US$3 [16]. The cost to the patient after storage and handling fees are included is approximately US$15.

Although neostigmine was associated with a favorable safety profile in the reported clinical trials, caution should be used when administering the medication. Neostigmine should be administered with the patient kept supine in bed with continuous electrocardiographic monitoring, physician assessment and measurement of vital signs for 15–30 minutes following administration [16]. Contraindications to its use include mechanical bowel obstruction, presence of ischemia or perforation, pregnancy, uncontrolled cardiac arrhythmias, severe active bronchospasm and renal insufficiency.

Thus, neostigmine appears to be an effective, safe and inexpensive method of colonic decompression in ACPO. The published data support its use as the initial therapy of choice for patients not responding to conservative therapy if there are no contraindications to its use. **A1d**, **B4** In patients with only a partial response or recurrence after an initial infusion, a repeated dose is reasonable and often successful. If the patient fails to respond after two doses, proceeding with colonoscopic decompression is advised.

Other medications

Administration of polyethylene glycol electrolyte solution (PEG) in patients who have ACPO after initial resolution may decrease the recurrence rate of colonic dilation. Sgouros and colleagues [30] evaluated PEG in a randomized, controlled trial in ACPO patients who had initial resolution of colonic dilation. The study enrolled 30 patients with cecal diameter 10 cm or greater that had resolution of the colonic dilation with either neostigmine (22 patients) or endoscopic decompression (eight patients). Patients then were randomized to receive daily PEG 29.5 g or placebo. Recurrence was defined as a cecal diameter of 8 cm or greater with a concomitant 10% increase after the initial successful decompression. Five (33%) patients in the placebo group had recurrent cecal dilation compared with none in the PEG group (p = 0.04). **A1d** Therapy with PEG resulted in a significant increase in stool and flatus output, decrease in colonic distention on radiographic measurements and improvement in abdominal girth [30].

There are few data on strategies to prevent the development of ACPO. A recent double-blind, randomized, placebo-controlled trial evaluated whether lactulose or PEG were effective in promoting defecation in critically ill patients, whether either of the two is superior, and whether the use of enteral laxatives is related to clinical outcome [31]. Three hundred and eight consecutive patients with multiple organ failure in whom defecation did not occur on the third day of admission to the ICU were included. Defecation occurred during the study period in a larger proportion of patients receiving either laxative: (placebo 31%, PEG 74% and lactulose 69%, p = 0.001). ACPO occurred in 4.1% of patients in the placebo group, 5.5% of patients in the lactulose group and 1.0% of patients in the polyethylene glycol group. Thus, it appears that the use of PEG in critically ill patients to promote defecaton may prevent the development of ACPO, and that its use following a pseudo-obstruction episode decreases the recurrence rate. **A1c**

There are only anecdotal reports using other prokinetic agents in ACPO, and their use for the treatment of this condition cannot be recommended. Erythromycin, a motilin receptor agonist, has been reported to be successful in treating patients in a few case reports [32, 33]. Armstrong *et al.* reported decompression in two patients with ACPO with oral erythromycin (500 mg four times daily) for 10 days [32]. In another report, one patient had resolution of ACPO after three days of intravenous erythromycin therapy [33]. Cisapride, a partial 5-HT$_4$-receptor agonist, has also been employed with some success in patients with ACPO [34]. However, this agent is no longer available for use in the USA and Canada due to class III arrhythmogenic properties. Lubiprostone, a novel chloride 2 channel activator approved for the treatment of constipation [35], has not been studied in pseudo-obstruction.

Endoscopic decompression

Colonoscopic decompression may be required in patients with persistent, marked colonic dilatation that has failed to respond to supportive therapy and neostigmine, or when neostigmine is contraindicated. There is no well-defined standard of care regarding the use of colonoscopy in ACPO [8]. Colonoscopic decompression appears to be beneficial in ACPO, but it is associated with a greater risk of complications, is not completely effective and can be followed by recurrence [36]. **B4** Colonoscopy is done to prevent bowel ischemia and perforation. It should not be done if these complications have already developed.

Colonoscopy in ACPO is a technically difficult procedure and should be carried out by experts. Oral laxatives and bowel preparations should not be administered prior to colonoscopy [37]. Air insufflation should be minimized and the entire colon need not be examined. Prolonged attempts at cecal intubation are not necessary because reaching the hepatic flexure usually appears to be effective. Gas should be aspirated and the viability of the mucosa assessed during slow withdrawal of the endoscope. A tube for decompression should be placed in the right colon with the aid of a guidewire and fluoroscopic guidance. Commercially available, single use, over-the-wire colon decompression tubes are available. The guidewires for these kits are quite flexible (0.035 inches (0.89 mm)) and must be watched under fluoroscopy during advancement

Table 22.3 Observational studies of colonoscopic decompression in acute colonic pseudo-obstruction.

Study	No. of patients	Successful initial decompression (%)	Overall colonoscopic success (%)	Complications
Nivatvongs et al. (1982) [38]	22	68	73	<1% (no perforations)
Strodel et al. (1983) [39]	44	61	73	2% (1 perforation)
Bode et al. (1984) [40]	22	68	77	4.5% (1 perforation)
Jetmore et al. (1992) [4]	45	84	36	<1% (no perforations)
Geller et al. (1996) [41]	41	95	88	2% (2 perforations)

and endoscopic withdrawal to minimize the formation of loops and ensure placement into the right colon.

The efficacy of colonoscopic decompression has not been established in randomized trials. Successful colonoscopic decompression has been reported in several case series that included hundreds of patients [4, 38–41]. **B4** Table 22.3 summarizes the larger reported series of colonoscopic decompression in ACPO. Rex reviewed the available literature of patients with ACPO treated with colonoscopy [36]. Successful initial decompression, determined by a reduction in radiographically measured cecal diameter was observed in 69% of 292 patients. Forty percent of patients treated without decompression tube placement had at least one recurrence, requiring an additional colonoscopy. Thus, an initial decompression colonoscopy without tube placement can be considered to be definitive therapy for less than 50% of patients [36]. To improve the therapeutic benefit, decompression tube placement at the time of colonoscopy is strongly recommended. The value of decompression tubes has not been evaluated in controlled trials, but anecdotal evidence suggests that they may lower the recurrence rate. In the series reported by Geller et al., the overall clinical success of colonoscopic decompression was 88%. However, in procedures where a decompression tube was not placed the clinical success was poor (25%) [41].

Surgical therapy

Surgical management is reserved for patients with signs of colonic ischemia or perforation, or for those who fail endoscopic and pharmacologic treatment. Surgical intervention is associated with significant morbidity and mortality, probably related to the severity of the underlying medical conditions in this group of patients. In the large retrospective series reported by Vanek and Al-Salti, 179 patients underwent surgery for ACPO with resulting morbidity and mortality rates of 30% and 6% respectively [2]. **B4** The type of surgery depends on the status of the bowel. Without perforated or ischemic bowel, cecostomy is the procedure of choice because the success rate is high, morbidity is relatively low and the procedure can be carried out under local anesthesia [2]. Alternatively, percutaneous cecostomy through a combined endoscopic-radiologic approach can be considered in high surgical risk patients [42–44]. **C5** In cases of ischemic or perforated bowel, segmental or subtotal colonic resection is indicated, with either exteriorization or primary anastomosis.

Clinical guidelines

An evidence-based guideline for the treatment of ACPO was recently published by the American Society for Gastrointestinal Endoscopy [8]. The guidelines recommend conservative therapy as the initial preferred management, based on observational studies only. Potentially contributory metabolic, infectious and pharmacologic factors should be identified and corrected. Active intervention is indicated for patients at risk of perforation and/or failing conservative therapy. Neostigmine is effective for the majority of patients. **A1a**, **B4** Colonic decompression is the initial invasive procedure of choice for patients who fail neostigmine therapy or for whom this drug is contraindicated. **B4** Surgical decompression should be reserved for patients with peritonitis or perforation and for those who fail endoscopic and medical therapy. **B4** A proposed algorithm for the management of ACPO is detailed in Figure 22.2.

Summary

ACPO is a syndrome of massive dilatation of the colon without mechanical obstruction that results from an imbalance in the autonomic control of the colon. Evaluation involves exclusion of mechanical obstruction and assessing for signs of ischemia or perforation. Appropriate management includes supportive measures and selective use of neostigmine and colonoscopic decompression. Neostigmine is the only therapy for ACPO proved to be efficacious in a randomized controlled trial. Patient outcome is determined by the severity of the predisposing illness, patient age,

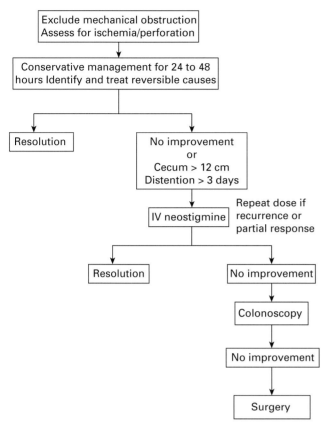

Figure 22.2 Algorithm for suggested management for acute colonic pseudo-obstruction.
IV: intravenous.

maximal cecal diameter, duration of colonic distension and viability of the bowel. Of these factors affecting outcome, the latter three are amenable to intervention. Thus, early recognition and management are critical to minimizing morbidity and mortality.

References

1 Ogilvie WH. Large intestine colic due to sympathetic deprivation: A new clinical syndrome. *BMJ* 1948; **2**: 671–673.

2 Vanek VW, Al-Salti M. Acute pseudo-obstruction of the colon (Ogilvie's syndrome). An analysis of 400 cases. *Dis Colon Rectum* 1986; **29**: 203–210.

3 Dorudi S, Berry AR, Kettlewell MGW. Acute colonic pseudo-obstruction. *Br J Surg* 1992; **79**: 99–103.

4 Jetmore AB, Timmcke AE, Gathright Jr BJ *et al.* Ogilvie's syndrome: Colonoscopic decompression and analysis of predisposing factors. *Dis Colon Rectum* 1992; **35**: 1135–1142.

5 Norwood MG, Lykostratis H, Garcea G *et al.* Acute colonic pseudo-obstruction following major orthopedic surgery. *Colorectal Dis* 2005; **7**: 496–499.

6 Sheikh RA, Yasmeen S, Pauly MP *et al.* Pseudomembranous colitis without diarrhea presenting clinically as acute intestinal pseudo-obstruction. *J Gastroenterol* 2001; **36**: 629–632.

7 Sloyer AF, Panella VS, Demas BE *et al.* Ogilvie's syndrome. Successful management without colonoscopy. *Dig Dis Sci* 1988; **33**: 1391–1396.

8 Eisen GM, Baron TH, Dominitiz JA *et al.* Acute colonic pseudo-obstruction. *Gastrointest Endosc* 2002; **56**: 789–-792.

9 Wandeo H, Mathewson C, Conolly B. Pseudo-obstruction of the colon. *Surg Gynecol Obstet* 1971; **133**: 44.

10 Meyers MA. Colonic ileus. *Gastrointest Radiol* 1977; **2**: 37–40.

11 Bachulis BL, Smith PE. Pseudo-obstruction of the colon. *Am J Surg* 1978; **136**: 66–72.

12 Baker DA, Morin ME, Tan A *et al.* Colonic ileus: Indication for prompt decompression. *JAMA* 1979; **241**: 2633–2634.

13 Johnson CD, Rice RP. The radiographic evaluation of gross cecal distention. *Am J Radiol* 1985; **145**: 1211–1217.

14 Loftus CG, Harewood GC, Baron TH. Assessment of predictors of response to neostigmine for acute colonic pseudo-obstruction. *Am J Gastroenterol* 2002; **97**: 3118–3122.

15 Rex DK. Acute colonic pseudo-obstruction (Ogilvie's syndrome). *Gastroenterology* 1994; **2**: 223–228.

16 Ponec RJ, Saunders MD, Kimmey MB. Neostigmine for the treatment of acute colonic pseudo-obstruction. *N Engl J Med* 1999; **341**: 137–141.

17 Law NM, Bharucha AE, Undale AS *et al.* Cholinergic stimulation enhances colonic motor activity, transit, and sensation in humans. *Am J Physiol Gastrointest Liver Physiol* 2001; **281**: G1228–1237.

18 Neely J, Catchpole B. Ileus: The restoration of alimentary tract motility by pharmacologic means. *Br J Surg* 1971; **58**: 21–28.

19 Aquilonius SM, Hartvig P. Clinical pharmacokinetics of cholinesterase inhibitors. *Clin Pharmacokinet* 1986; **11**: 236–249.

20 Cronnelly R, Stanski DR, Miller RD *et al.* Renal function and the pharmacokinetics of neostigmine in anesthetized man. *Anesthesiology* 1979; **51**: 222–226.

21 van der Spoel JI, Oudemans-van StraatenHM, Stoutenbeck CP *et al.* Neostigmine resolves critical illness-related colonic ileus in intensive care patients with multiple organ failure a prospective, double-blind, placebo-controlled trial. *Intensive Care Med* 2001; **27**: 822–827.

22 Hutchinson R, Griffiths C. Acute colonic pseudo-obstruction: A pharmacologic approach. *Ann R Coll Surg Engl* 1992; **74**: 364–367.

23 Stephenson BM, Morgan AR, Salaman JR *et al.* Ogilvie's syndrome: A new approach to an old problem. *Dis Colon Rectum* 1995; **38**: 424–427.

24 Turegano-Fuentes F, Munoz-Jimenez F, Del Valle-Hernandez E *et al.* Early resolution of Ogilvie's syndrome with intravenous neostigmine. A simple, effective treatment. *Dis Colon Rectum* 1997; **40**: 1353–1357.

25 Trevisani GT, Hyman NH, Church JM. Neostigmine: Safe and effective treatment for acute colonic pseudo-obstruction. *Dis Colon Rectum* 2000; **43**: 599–603.

26 Paran H, Silverberg D, Mayo A *et al.* Treatment of acute colonic pseudo-obstruction with neostigmine. *J Am Coll Surg* 2000; **190**: 315–318.

27 Abeyta BJ, Albrecht RM, Schermer CR. Retrospective study of neostigmine for the treatment of acute colonic pseudo-obstruction. *Am Surg* 2001; **67**: 265–268.

28 Mehta R, John A, Nair P *et al.* Factors predicting successful outcome following neostigmine therapy in acute colonic pseudo-

obstruction: A prospective study. *J Gastroenterol Hepatol* 2006; **21**: 459–461.

29 Cherta I, Forne M, Quintana S *et al.* Prolonged treatment with neostigmine for resolution of acute colonic pseudo-obstruction. *Aliment Pharmacol Ther* 2006; **23**: 1678–1679.

30 Sgouros SN, Vlachogiannakos J, Vassilliadis K *et al.* Effect of polyethylene glycol electrolyte- balanced solution on patients with acute colonic pseudo-obstruction after resolution of colonic dilation: A prospective, randomized, placebo controlled trial. *Gut* 2006; **55**: 638–642.

31 van der Spoel JI, Oudemans-van Straaten HM, Kuiper MA *et al.* Laxation of critically ill patients with lactulose or polyethylene glycol: A two-center randomized, double-blind, placebo-controlled trial. *Critical Care Medicine* 2007; **35**: 2726–2731.

32 Armstrong DN, Ballantyne GH, Modlin IM. Erythromycin for reflex ileus in Ogilvie's syndrome. *Lancet* 1991; **337**: 378.

33 Bonacini M, Smith CJ, Pritchard T. Erythromycin as therapy for acute colonic pseudo-obstruction (Ogilvie's syndrome). *J Clin Gastroenterol* 1991; **13**: 475–476.

34 MacColl C, MacCannell KL, Baylis B *et al.* Treatment of acute colonic pseudo-obstruction (Ogilvie's syndrome) with cisapride. *Gastroenterology* 1990; **98**: 773–776.

35 Johanson JF, Morton D, Geenen J, Ueno R. Multicenter, 4-week, double-blind, randomized, placebo-controlled trial of lubiprostone, a locally-acting type-2 chloride channel activator, in patients with chronic constipation. *Am J Gastroenterol* 2008 Jan; **103**(1): 170–177.

36 Rex DK. Colonoscopy and acute colonic pseudo-obstruction. *Gastrointest Endosc Clin North Am* 1997; **7**: 499–508.

37 Saunders MD, Cappell MS. Endoscopic management of acute colonic pseudo-obstruction. *Endoscopy* 2005; **37**: 760–763.

38 Nivatvongs S, Vermeulen FD, Fang DT. Colonoscopic decompression of acute pseudo-obstruction of the colon. *Ann Surg* 1982; **196**: 598–600.

39 Strodel WE, Nostrant TT, Eckhauser FE *et al.* Therapeutic and diagnostic colonoscopy in non-obstructive colonic dilatation. *Ann Surg* 1983; **19**: 416–421.

40 Bode WE, Beart RW, Spencer RJ *et al.* Colonoscopic decompression for acute pseudo-obstruction of the colon (Ogilvie's syndrome): Report of 22 cases and review of the literature. *Am J Surg* 1984; **147**: 243–245.

41 Geller A, Petersen BT, Gostout CJ. Endoscopic decompression for acute colonic pseudo-obstruction. *Gastrointest Endosc* 1996; **44**: 144–150.

42 van Sonnenberg E, Varney RR, Casola G *et al.* Percutaneous cecostomy for Ogilvie's syndrome: Laboratory observations and clinical experience. *Radiology* 1990; **175**: 679–682.

43 Chevallier P, Marcy PY, Francois E *et al.* Controlled transperitoneal percutaneous cecostomy as a therapeutic alternative to the endoscopic decompression for Ogilvie's syndrome. *Am J Gastroenterol* 2002; **97**: 471–474.

44 Baraza W, Brown S, McAlindon M, Hurlstone P. Prospective analysis of percutaneous endoscopic colostomy at a tertiary referral centre. *Br J Surg* 2007; **94**: 1415–1420.

23 Gallstone disease

Laura VanderBeek[1], Calvin HL Law[2] and Véd R Tandan[3]

[1] McMaster University, Hamilton, Ontario, Canada
[2] Hepatobiliary, Pancreatic and Gastrointestinal Surgery, Department of Health Policy, Management and Evaluation, University of Toronto *and* Institute for Clinical Evaluative Sciences, Toronto, Ontario, Canada
[3] Department of Surgery, St Joseph's Healthcare Hamilton, McMaster University, Hamilton, Ontario, Canada

Introduction

Surgical therapy for gallstones can be associated with morbidity and mortality, which has led to debate on its use, especially in asymptomatic and mildly symptomatic patients. Advancements in minimally invasive and endoscopic techniques make it imperative to understand the current evidence concerning the benefits and risks of surgical therapy for gallstone disease and its complications.

Elective cholecystectomy

Asymptomatic cholelithiasis in the general population

As abdominal ultrasound has become a routine investigation for abdominal symptoms, asymptomatic cholelithiasis is being diagnosed more frequently. Management of uncomplicated gallstones poses a dilemma as there are no controlled trials comparing prophylactic surgery with expectant management in asymptomatic patients with cholelithiasis. However, a number of cohort studies have been done to assess the probability of developing biliary pain and biliary complications in asymptomatic persons with gallstones.

Through the 1980s, a series of cohort studies were conducted by Gracie and Ransohoff [1], McSherry *et al.* [2], and Freidman *et al.* [3,4]. Gracie's study had complete follow-up on 123 people for 11–24 years. The cumulative probability of the development of biliary pain was 10% at five years, 15% at ten years, and 18% at twenty years. However, the fact that 89% of the study population were white American

males, and all were faculty members of the University of Michigan, limits the generalizability of this study. McSherry's study retrospectively identified 135 patients with asymptomatic cholelithiasis who were subscribers to the Health Insurance Plan of Greater New York, a mainly middle-income population of diverse ethnic origin. Over a mean follow-up of 46 months, 10.4% of patients developed symptoms, yielding a 2.7% annual rate of developing symptoms. Similarly, Friedman followed 123 ethnically diverse patients with asymptomatic gallstones in the Kaiser Permanente Medical Care Program (San Francisco) for 16–25 years. There was a 3–4% annual rate of biliary events in the initial ten years, and a 1–2% annual rate in the following ten years. At five years, 18% of patients had developed biliary symptoms. One death was attributable to cholangitis secondary to gallstones. A more detailed explanation of Gracie's data revealed that three patients eventually experienced biliary complications (2.4% of the population), but all of these had presented with pain before the complication. In McSherry's study, 10% of the population eventually developed symptoms and 71% of these patients had biliary colic as their only indication for elective cholecystectomy. Although the remaining patients had biliary complications prior to surgery (3% of the study population), it is unclear if they presented with pain first. Overall these studies yield an estimate of an annual rate of 1–2% of symptom development, and provide evidence that 90% of patients will present with pain prior to developing a biliary complication. Only 10% of patients will present with a biliary complication as the first manifestation of their biliary tract disease [4].

The Group for Epidemiology and Prevention of Cholelithiasis (GREPCO) in Italy prospectively followed 118 patients with asymptomatic cholelithiasis [5]. The cumulative probability of developing biliary colic was 12% at two years, 17% at four years and 26% at ten years. The cumulative probability of biliary complications was 3% at ten years. One patient died of gallbladder carcinoma. This represents a higher rate of symptoms, but not a higher rate

Evidence-Based Gastroenterology and Hepatology, 3rd edition.
J. McDonald, A.K. Burroughs, B. Feagan, and M.B. Fennerty. © 2010
Blackwell Publishing Ltd

of complications than the studies from the 1980s. This study also showed that 74% of patients remained asymptomatic at ten years.

Ransohoff et al. performed a decision analysis on data first published by Gracie [1, 6, 7]. Using cholecystectomy mortality figures up to 1983, they found prophylactic cholecystectomy slightly decreased survival. The economic analysis did not favor prophylactic cholecystectomy. Although the models were constructed using data prior to laparoscopic cholecystectomies, the new approach is unlikely to alter the results.

Considering the current evidence, expectant management rather than prophylactic cholecystectomy is indicated for the typical patient with asymptomatic gallstones. However, certain populations who are more at risk for complications of gallstone disease should be considered separately.

Asymptomatic cholelithiasis in diabetic patients

More liberal thresholds for elective cholecystectomy in asymptomatic diabetic patients have been suggested [8], based on early evidence suggesting a higher incidence of gallstone disease and biliary complications, and poorer outcomes for emergency surgery for biliary complications. Only Grade B evidence is available, which supports expectant management of asymptomatic cholelithiasis in this population rather than a more aggressive approach.

Chapman reviewed 308 diabetic patients and 318 non-diabetic controls [9]. The incidence of cholelithiasis was higher in the diabetic population (32.7% vs 20.8%, p < 0.001). However, when the data were subjected to multivariate analysis, diabetes did not correlate strongly with the incidence of cholelithiasis, except in a subgroup of females with non-insulin dependent diabetes.

Del Favero prospectively studied the natural history of cholelithiasis in diabetes by following a cohort of 47 diabetic patients with asymptomatic cholelithiasis [10]. After five years, five patients presented with pain as their first symptom, one patient presented with cholecystitis and another patient presented with jaundice. The percentage of initially asymptomatic non-insulin dependent diabetic patients who went on to develop symptoms (14.9%) or complications (4.2%) compares favorably with the data available from studies of the general population.

Higher complication rates with emergency surgery for biliary complications in diabetic patients have been observed. Hickman et al. studied 72 diabetic patients who underwent cholecystectomy for cholecystitis and matched them for age, sex and date of operation with 72 non-diabetic patients [11]. Morbidity for the diabetic patients was 38.9% compared with 20.8% in the non-diabetic population. Mortality in the diabetic population was 4.2%, compared with zero in the control population and was

attributed to sepsis. The septic complication rate was higher in the diabetic (19.4%) than in the non-diabetic group (6.9%). This higher rate was maintained whether the diabetic patients had concurrent medical illness or not.

Landau et al. (1992) analyzed 566 cholecystectomies performed in the presence of acute cholecystitis [12]. Of these patients, 123 had diabetes mellitus and 433 did not have diabetes. The diabetic patients were found to have a higher rate of infected bile, gangrenous changes and perforation of the GB, in comparison with non-diabetic patients. Also, the morbidity rate of surgery for acute cholecystitis was significantly higher (21% vs 9%) in diabetic patients. Sandler used logistic regression when analyzing 126 diabetic patients and 855 non-diabetic patients with cholecystectomy and found diabetics have an increased morbidity primarily because they are older and have other medical problems [13]. Diabetes itself was not statistically significant for associated increased morbidity.

The natural history of asymptomatic cholelithiasis in diabetic patients appears to be similar to that in the general population. Asymptomatic cholelithiasis in diabetics should be managed expectantly and preventative surgery should not be recommended routinely. However, once symptoms develop early laparoscopic cholecystectomy is recommended to prevent complications.

Asymptomatic cholelithiasis and the risk of cancer

Autopsy data have provided evidence that more than 80% of patients with gallbladder cancer have concomitant cholelithiasis. Maringhini et al. followed 2583 patients with known gallstones [14]. Only five patients (0.2%) developed gallbladder carcinoma. Ransohoff et al. reviewed 1000 patients with silent gallstones for a total of 7000 patient years and no patients developed gallbladder cancer [6]. The GREPCO in Italy followed up 118 patients with asymptomatic gallstones for ten years and only one patient developed and died of gallbladder cancer [5].

The incidence of gallbladder cancer varies widely in different populations, even in the presence of gallstone disease. Lowenfels et al. reported a case-control study of 131 patients with gallbladder carcinoma and 2399 patients without gallbladder carcinoma [15]. The 20-year cumulative risk for gallbladder cancer ranged from 0.13% in black males to 1.5% in native American females. The authors calculated that 769 cholecystectomies were required to prevent one gallbladder cancer in a low-risk population. However, only 67 cholecystectomies would be necessary to prevent one gallbladder malignancy in a high-risk population. **B3**

Hsing et al. conducted a population-based study from Shanghai of 627 patients with biliary tract cancers, 368 being gallbladder cancer [16]. Gallbladder cancer risk was higher among subjects with both gallstones and self-reported cholecystitis, with an OR of 34.4. The OR associated with gallstones and gallbladder cancer was 23.8.

Patients with gallstones greater than 3 cm may be at risk for the development of gallbladder carcinoma. In 1983 Diehl reported this in a case-control study and the study by Lowenfels confirmed this observation in 1989 [17, 18]. These studies provided evidence for a nine to ten-fold increase in relative risk of developing gallbladder carcinoma for patients with stones greater than 3 cm in diameter compared to patients with stones less than 1 cm in diameter. Srikanth *et al.* found that one-half of gallbladders with a wall thickness >3 mm on US are likely to have xanthogranulomatous cholecystitis, and the risk of the patient having a gallbladder cancer is higher (3.3%) [19].

Grade B evidence supports the view that the risk of developing gallbladder cancer may be higher in patients with cholelithiasis. However, the increased risk appears to be insufficient to support a recommendation for prophylactic cholecystectomy. Although some subsets of the population (especially native American females) and patients with stones greater than 3 cm or gallbladder wall thickness >3 mm may be at sufficient risk to justify prophylactic cholecystectomy, further evidence would be needed to support a firm recommendation. **B3, B4**

Porcelain gallbladder and risk of gallbladder cancer

Early case reports and small series initially indicated a correlation between porcelain gallbladder and carcinoma, which guided a recommendation for surgical therapy. However, more relevant information has only recently been published. A retrospective assessment by Towfigh *et al.* [20] examined 10,741 gallbladder specimens. Only 15 (0.14%) were porcelain gallbladders. All porcelain gallbladder specimens demonstrated chronic cholecystitis and partial calcification of the gallbladder wall and nine had cholelithiasis (60%). During this same period, 88 (0.82%) patients developed gallbladder cancer, none of whom showed calcification of the gallbladder wall. From these data, the authors challenged the link between porcelain gallbladder and gallbladder cancer. However, further insight may be gained from a study by Stephen and Berger [21]. This study reported data on 25,900 gallbladder specimens, of which 150 cases of gallbladder cancer and 44 cases of porcelain gallbladder (defined as the presence of wall calcifications) were identified. This study demonstrated that there are two types of wall calcification – diffuse intramural calcification and selective mucosal calcification. Gallbladder cancer was found in 7% of cases with selective mucosal calcification, but no case of gallbladder cancer was identified in the specimens with diffuse intramural calcification. Thus, conflicting data in the past may be attribut-

able to misclassification. However, in the preoperative setting, it may be difficult to distinguish these types of calcifications with standard imaging modalities. As a result, the authors still recommend cholecystectomy for patients with porcelain gallbladder, especially in those where there is incomplete calcification of the gallbladder wall. **CS**

Symptomatic cholelithiasis

Grade B evidence supports the current approach to patients with symptomatic cholelithiasis. Patients with uncomplicated biliary colic should be offered surgery as an option to controlling symptoms. Patients with complications of cholelithiasis should have surgery to prevent further complications. The previously discussed natural history studies of McSherry *et al.* and Friedman *et al.* included a group of patients with symptomatic cholelithiasis [2, 3]. Additional data are also available from the National Cooperative Gallstone Study (NCGS) [22, 23]. McSherry followed 556 patients with symptomatic cholelithiasis [2]. During an average follow-up of 83 months, 169 (30%) patients reported worsening or continued severe symptoms, nine (1.6%) patients developed jaundice, and 47 (8.5%) patients developed cholecystitis. These data indicate a 4.3% annual rate of worsening or persistently severe symptoms and a 1.5% annual rate of biliary complications arising from symptomatic cholelithiasis. Friedman followed 298 patients with mild or non-specific symptoms and cholelithiasis for 16–25 years [3, 4]. The annual rate of developing cholecystitis or jaundice was 1%.

The NCGS was designed as a double-blind, randomized controlled trial of chenodiol [22, 23]. The group of patients who had received placebo provided another opportunity to study the natural history of symptomatic cholelithiasis. Seventy-seven patients presented with worsening symptoms of biliary colic or prolonged biliary pain during two years of follow-up. Seven patients "required cholecystectomy" during the follow-up, which represents a 34% annual incidence of "requiring a cholecystectomy". The patients with symptomatic cholelithiasis in these studies did not suffer any greater mortality during the follow-up period than was experienced by patients in the asymptomatic population.

The rate of complications secondary to symptomatic cholelithiasis appears to be higher than that in patients with asymptomatic cholelithiasis. Recurrent or worsening symptoms may develop but there is no increased mortality from observation, at least in the short term. Therefore, "the subjective experience of the patient should be the principal determinant of whether and when the procedure should be performed". Early surgical treatment is indicated once cholelithiasis is complicated by acute cholecystitis, choledocholithiasis, or cholangitis.

Elective laparoscopic versus open cholecystectomy

Laparoscopic cholecystectomy is now considered standard of care for elective cholecystectomy. This approach has been "accepted" despite the lack of any evidence from a randomized controlled trial comparing standard open cholecystectomy and standard laparoscopic cholecystectomy. There is a lack of convincing evidence of decreases in length of stay, recovery time or economics (hospital or societal). However, the general acceptance of laparoscopic cholecystectomy as the standard of care, as well as public demand for minimally invasive surgery, will prevent a future randomized controlled trial that may definitively answer these questions. Nonetheless, laparoscopic cholecystectomy has had a significant impact on the management of gallstone disease, as evidenced by increasing rates

of elective cholecystectomy since its introduction in the 1980s [24, 25].

Evidence from five randomized controlled trials comparing elective laparoscopic cholecystectomy and minilaparotomy cholecystectomy is available [26–30] (Table 23.1). **A1c** There is no statistically significant difference in the incidence of biliary tract injuries, although in a study by McMahon *et al.* the only major biliary injury occurred in the laparoscopic group [27]. Quality of life data were obtained by both Barkun *et al.* and McMahon *et al.* [26, 27]. The laparoscopic group experienced a faster improvement in quality of life, but the two treatment groups were equal in this respect at three months. Similarly, there was better satisfaction with scarring in the laparoscopic group, but both groups were equally satisfied with their result at three months. The data from Majeed revealed no difference in time off work or time to return to full activity [29]. A cost minimization economic analysis was carried out by

Table 23.1 Randomized controlled trials of laparoscopic cholecystectomy (LC) and mini-cholecystectomy (MC).

		Study				
		Barkun *et al.* [26]	McMahon *et al.* [27]	McGinn *et al.* [28]	Majeed *et al.* [29]	Keus *et al.* [30]
No. of patients	LC	37	151	155	100	105
	MC	25	148	155	100	118
Operative time (minutes)	LC	85.9	57[a]	74[a]	69.2[a]	71.9[a]
	MC	73.1	71[a]	50	45.4[a]	60.4[a]
Conversion to standard open cholecystectomy	LC	1 (3%)	15 (10%)	20 (13%)	20 (20%)	14 (11.7%)
	MC	0 (0%)	14 (10%)	6 (4%)	22 (22%)	22 (16.1%)
Time to oral intake	LC	1.1 days[a]	N/A	N/A	24.7 hrs	N/A
	MC	1.7 days[a]	N/A	N/A	22.4 hrs	N/A
Hospital stay (days)	LC	3[a]	2[a]	2[b]	3	2.4
	MC	4[a]	4[a]	3[b]	3	3.1
Non-biliary complications	LC	1 (3%)	30 (20%)[b]	12 (7.7%)[a]	11 (11%)	20 (19%)
	MC	1 (4%)	26 (17%)[c]	2 (1.3%)[a]	14 (14%)	10 (8.5%)
Biliary complications	LC	0 (0%)	5 (3%)[d]	1 (0.6%)	1 (1%)	1 (1%)
	MC	1 (4%)	3 (2%)[d]	2 (1.3%)	0 (0%)	3 (2.5%)
Mortality	LC	0 (0%)	0 (0%)	1 (0.6%)	0 (0%)	0 (0%)
	MC	0 (0%)	1 (0.7%)	0 (0%)	1 (1%)[e]	0 (0%)

N/A, data not available.

[a] Indicates differences reached statistical significance.

[b] This difference was statistically significant but did not include patients who were converted to standard cholecystectomy. If included, there was no statistically significant difference in length of hospital stay.

[c] Total complications.

[d] This included 1 (0.7%) major biliary injury in the LC group and no major biliary injuries in the MC group.

[e] Histology revealed a carcinoma of the gallbladder and ultrasound at three months showed multiple liver metastases and the patient died two months later.

McMahon [27]. Laparoscopic cholecystectomy was more costly after considering both perioperative and hospitalization costs (£1486 compared with £1090, p < 0.001). Keus *et al.* found no significant difference in complications, but there was a significantly shorter operative time in the small-incision technique (mean 60.4 min.) compared to the laparoscopic cholecystectomy (mean 71.9 min.) [30].

Further data comparing laparoscopic to open cholecystectomy are available from the meta-analysis of Shea *et al.* of the outcomes of 78,747 patients undergoing laparoscopic cholecystectomy and 12,973 patients undergoing open cholecystectomy [31]. Mortality rates were lower for laparoscopic cholecystectomy than for open cholecystectomy, while common bile duct injury was higher for laparoscopic cholecystectomy than for open cholecystectomy. The data for common bile duct injury were re-analyzed by group-level logistic regressions to identify the differences in rates among the studies. A pattern of infrequent common duct injury in early studies, an increased incidence in studies initiated in early 1990, followed by a subsequent decrease in rate was revealed. However, the data were quite variable in terms of reporting of results and length of follow-up. The authors conceded, "there are still some considerable uncertainties that need to be addressed by better-designed studies and more complete reporting".

Considering the current evidence, in the elective setting, laparoscopic cholecystectomy appears to be as safe as open cholecystectomy and may provide short-term improvement in quality of life. **A1a, C** There is a lack of convincing evidence of decreases in length of stay, recovery time or economics (hospital or societal). However, the general acceptance of laparoscopic cholecystectomy as the standard of care as well as public demand for minimally invasive surgery will prevent a future randomized controlled trial that may definitively answer these questions.

Further issues in elective laparoscopic cholecystectomy

With the advent of the laparoscopic cholecystectomy, there has been a move towards ambulatory surgery. Grade A evidence from two randomized trials which compared outpatient to inpatient laparoscopic cholecystectomy are available [32, 33]. Exclusion criteria included American Society of Anesthesiologists (ASA) III/IV, patients less than 18 and more than 70 years old, lack of a capable caregiver at home and complicated cholelithiasis (common bile duct stones or acute cholecystitis). The degree of pain, readmission and complication rates were the same in both groups. Late complications such as bile leaks became evident several days later and there was no benefit from 24-hour admission. Keulemans *et al.* found that 92% of the outpatients preferred outpatient care to clinical observa-

tion [33]. Of the 504 planned outpatient laparoscopic cholecystectomies, Bueno Lledo *et al.* found that 88.8% were discharged the same day [34]. Fifty-one patients required overnight stays (10.1%), most of them for "social" causes, and five patients required 1–2 day admission for intraoperative and postoperative complications. Six patients (1.1%) required readmission. In summary, outpatient laparoscopic cholecystectomy is a safe and feasible option for selected patients (defined by the exclusion criteria in the randomized trials). **A1c**

There are two randomized trials comparing three-port versus four-port laparoscopic cholesyctectomy [35, 36]. In both studies there was no significant difference in operative time or complications. The main advantages of the three-port technique are that it causes less pain and leaves fewer scars. Again, this technique was carried out by expert hands and may not be generalized to all surgeons.

Acute cholecystitis

Acute cholecystitis, inflammation secondary to obstruction of the cystic duct, is the most common complication of cholelithiasis. Laparoscopic cholecystectomy has become the treatment of choice for acute cholecystitis and there is now little controversy concerning the use of laparoscopic versus open cholecystectomy. Controversy remains over the timing of cholecystectomy.

In the pre-laparoscopic era, the question of early versus delayed cholecystectomy was heavily debated. Evidence from five randomized trials carried out in the 1970s and 1980s is available [37–41]. **A1c** These studies demonstrated that cholecystectomy could be carried out in the acute stage with shorter hospital stay, decreased mortality and fewer operative complications (Table 23.2).

The introduction of laparoscopic cholecystectomy caused a movement to return to delayed cholecystectomy for acute cholecystitis. This movement arose because laparoscopic cholecystectomy was considered to be associated with more complications and an increased risk of common bile duct injuries than interval laparoscopic cholecystectomy after the resolution of the acute episode. Grade A evidence from six randomized controlled trials on early versus delayed laparoscopic cholecystectomy is available (Table 23.3) [42–47]. Once again, the data show that early cholecystectomy, even if carried out with the laparoscopic approach, is safer and better for patients in terms of shorter illness and hospital stay, compared with delayed surgery.

Evidence regarding laparoscopic versus open cholecystectomy for acute cholecystitis is available from two randomized trials [48, 49]. **A1c** The results are summarized in Table 23.4. The laparoscopic approach did not increase mortality or morbidity compared with the open approach

Table 23.2 Randomized controlled trials comparing early versus delayed open cholecystectomy for acute cholecystitis.

		Study			
		McArthur *et al.* [37]	Lahtinen *et al.* [38][a]	van der Linden *et al.* [39][a]	Jarvinen and Hastbacka [40]
No. of patients	Early	15	47	70	80
	Delayed	13	44	58	75
Operative time (minutes)	Early	N/A	76.7	N/A[b]	93
	Delayed	N/A	98.0	N/A[b]	85
Hospital stay (days)	Early	13.1	13.0	10.1	10.7
	Delayed	24.2	25.0	10.9 + 8[c]	18.2
Biliary complications	Early	1 (6.7%)	1 (2.1%)	0	3 (3.8%)
	Delayed	0	3 (6.8%)	0	2 (2.7%)
Non-biliary complications	Early	3 (20%)	12 (25.5%)	10 (14.3%)	11 (13.8%)
	Delayed	5 (38.4%)	16 (36.4%)	2 (3.4%)	13 (17.3%)
Mortality	Early	0	0	0	0
	Delayed	0	4 (9.1%)	0	1 (1.3%)
Failure of delayed treatment[d]		3 (23.1%)	7 (15.9%)	0	10 (13.3%)

N/A, data not available.

[a] Also showed decreased insurance payments (for time off work) for the patients treated with early cholecystectomy.

[b] No average or mean time for surgery was given but the distributions of operative times were similar.

[c] The mean stay for initial conservative management was 10.9 days followed by a mean stay of 8.0 days at the time of the delayed cholecystectomy.

[d] Patients randomized to conservative treatment initially who failed and required urgent cholecystectomy.

Table 23.3 Randomized controlled trials comparing early versus delayed laparoscopic cholecystectomy for acute cholecystitis.

		Study				
		Lo *et al.* [42]	Lai *et al.* [43]	Kolla *et al.* [44]	Johansson *et al.* [45]	Serralta *et al.* [46]
No. of patients	Early	45	53	20	74	82
	Delayed	41	51	20	71[a]	87
Operative time (minutes)	Early	135[b]	122.8[b]	104	98	75[b]
	Delayed	105[b]	106.6[b]	93	100	93[b]
Conversion	Early	5 (11%)	(21%)	5 (25%)	23 (31%)	2 (2%)[b]
	Delayed	9 (23%)	(24%)	5 (25%)	20 (29%)	15 (17%)[b]
Hospital stay (days)	Early	6[b]	7.6[b]	4.1[b]	5[b]	6[b]
	Delayed	11[b]	11.6[b]	10.1[b]	8[b]	13[b]
Biliary complications	Early	1 (2.2%)	1 (%)	2 (10%)	6 (8%)	1 (1%)
	Delayed	3 (7.3%)	0 (0%)	0	1 (1%)	1 (1%)
Non-biliary complications	Early	5 (11.1%)	4 (8%)	2 (10%)	7 (9%)	9 (11%)
	Delayed	9 (22.0%)	3 (8%)	3 (15%)	6 (9%)	12 (14%)
Mortality	Early	0	0	0	0	0
	Delayed	0	0	0	0	0
Failure of delayed treatment[c]		8 (19.5%)	8 (16%)	0	18 (26%)	8 (9%)

[a] Two patients refused surgery and were excluded.

[b] Indicates differences reached statistical significance.

[c] Patients randomized to conservative treatment initially who failed and required urgent cholecystectomy.

Table 23.4 Randomized controlled trials comparing open (OC) versus laparoscopic (LC) cholecystectomy for acute cholecystitis.

		Study	
		Kiviluoto *et al.* [48]	Lujan *et al.* [49]
No. of patients	OC	31	110
	LC	32	114
Operative time (minutes)	OC	99.8	77
	LC	108.2	88
Conversion	LC (only)	5 (16%)	17 (15%)
Hospital stay (days)	OC	6	8.1
	LC	4	3.3
Biliary complications	OC	0	1 (0.9%)
	LC	0	4 (3.5%)[a]
Non-biliary complications	OC	7 (minor) (23%) 6 (major) (19%)	28 (25.5%)
	LC	1 (minor) (3%)	14 (12.3%)
Mortality	OC	0	0
	LC	0	0

[a] Two out of four were retained common bile duct stones.

and offered the benefit of shorter hospital stay. Both studies found that the rate of conversion to the open procedure was slightly higher than the average observed in elective cholecystectomy series.

A retrospective study of 202 consecutive laparoscopic cholecystectomy patients compared complications and conversion rates when performed in the acute (<72 hrs), intermediate (between 72 hrs and 5 weeks) or delayed (>5 weeks) settings [50]. There was no significant difference in conversion rates (11–20%) or complication rates (7–16%) between the three groups and it was concluded that cholecystectomy can be performed safely during initial hospitalization regardless of symptom duration. Considering the current evidence, acute cholecystitis should be treated with early laparoscopic cholecystectomy (within the first 96 hours of symptoms).

Cholecystectomy via NOTES

Natural orifice transluminal endoscopic surgery (NOTES) is a new technique that can be used to perform cholecystectomies through a transvaginal approach. The first human case was reported on 13 March 2007 by Zorron on a 43-year-old female with biliary colic [51]. Since then, Zornig reports 20 patients who have had transvaginal cholecystectomies with no intra- or postoperative compli-

cations [52]. Another three females of varying BMIs have successfully undergone cholecystectomy using the NOTES technique with no postoperative complications [53]. Also, there was a case report of a morbidly obese female with a BMI of 35.8 who had a cholecystectomy via transvaginal NOTES approach with no postoperative analgesic use and no postoperative complications [54]. Transvaginal endoscopic cholecystectomies may in the future provide a safe surgical technique for women of varying BMIs with less visible scars and less postoperative pain, but it is currently still under investigation and further research is required before its use is widely accepted.

Gallstone pancreatitis

Early endoscopic retrograde cholangiopancreatography

Evidence from three randomized controlled trials on early endoscopic retrograde cholangiopancreatography (ERCP) with stone extraction versus conservative therapy as a treatment for biliary pancreatitis is available [55–57]. **A1c** In patients with severe pancreatitis or with evidence of biliary obstruction or cholangitis, early ERCP within 72 hours of presentation probably decreases morbidity and mortality rates. In patients without these criteria, early ERCP has no benefit and may in fact increase morbidity and mortality. Therefore, patients must be carefully selected for early ERCP. (See Chapter 24 for further discussion.)

Preoperative endoscopic retrograde cholangiopancreatography versus cholecystectomy with cholangiogram

Gallstone pancreatitis is considered to be an indication for imaging the biliary tree with either ERCP or intraoperative cholangiogram (IOC). In order to determine if ductal evaluation is always necessary before or during cholecystectomy for biliary pancreatitis, Ito *et al.* examined 148 patients undergoing cholecystectomy for biliary pancreatitis [58]. Only those patients at low risk for choledocholithiasis were included (normal or decreasing liver function tests and no ductal dilation on non-invasive preoperative imaging). The choice to perform IOC was based on the preference of the operating surgeon. Twenty-seven patients underwent IOC and 121 patients did not undergo IOC. There was no difference in recurrent pancreatitis, cholangitis and asymptomatic elevation of liver function tests three months after discharge. This study suggests that direct ductal evaluation can be omitted safely in patients with low risk of choledocholithiasis.

Seven observational studies, two with controls, have assessed the optimal approach to imaging the biliary tree following an attack of gallstone pancreatitis [59–65]. Gallstone pancreatitis does not appear to be a strong predictor of CBD stones without evidence of a dilated CBD, persistently abnormal alkaline phosphatase or bilirubin, or evidence of cholangitis. Patients with these features may be considered for preoperative ERCP. **C5** In one retrospective study, the incidence of procedure-induced pancreatitis was 19% in the ERCP group and 6% in the surgical/IOC group [59]. The other retrospective study demonstrated similar results with pancreatic-biliary complications in 24% of the ERCP group and 6% of the surgical/IOC group [65]. The data suggest that preoperative ERCP may in fact increase overall morbidity compared with cholecystectomy with IOC, further supporting the approach of selective ERCP in this group of patients. **C5**

Timing of surgery with gallstone pancreatitis

A number of studies have evaluated early versus delayed cholecystectomy in patients with gallstone pancreatitis. Burch *et al.* evaluated patients who underwent surgery after recovering from acute pancreatitis either during the same hospital admission or following discharge and scheduled elective surgery [66]. Although surgical complication rates were the same in both groups, total hospital stay was significantly longer in the delayed surgery group (14 vs 17 days, p = 0.01). Furthermore, in the delayed group only 60% returned for surgery, and 29% of the original cohort required emergency treatment for recurrent pancreatitis or biliary disease before elective surgery. Kelly *et al.* randomized patients to early (less than 48 hours) and delayed (more than 48 hours) surgery [67]. With early surgery the morbidity and mortality rates were 30.1% and 15.1%, as compared with 5.1 and 2.4% in the delayed group (p < 0.005). **A1c** When patients were stratified for disease severity based on Ranson's criteria, the differences in morbidity and mortality rates between early and delayed surgery were not statistically significant in patients with three or fewer Ranson's criteria. In patients with severe pancreatitis (more than three Ranson's criteria), the differences remained significant.

A retrospective review identified 164 patients with gallstone pancreatitis: 90 patients were discharged for readmission cholecystectomy and 74 patients had the cholecystectomy before discharge [68]. The patients in the discharged group waited on average 40+/−69 days versus 8+/−10 days in the group which remained in hospital (mean+/−SD). Of those patients who were discharged 20% (18 of 90) xperienced an adverse event requiring readmission while awaiting their cholecystectomy: three had recurrent pancreatitis, ten had recurrent pain, and five developed acute cholecystitis.

Grade B/C evidence has recently been published examining the issue of whether cholecystectomy is even neces-

sary after successful ERCP with endoscopic sphincterotomy (ES) and clearance of bile duct stones [69, 70]. Kaw *et al.* followed patients prospectively to compare outcome after laparoscopic cholecystectomy and ERCP with ES or ERCP and ES alone for an average of 33 and 34 months respectively [69]. During follow-up, there was no significant difference in biliary complications or procedure-related complications. They concluded that laparoscopic cholecystectomy should only be attempted in patients with overt biliary symptoms and not for the prevention of gallstone pancreatitis. Kwon *et al.* found that only 4.8% of patients required a cholecystectomy for biliary complications at an average of 18.4 months following ERCP and ES [70]. This issue should be examined further by randomized controlled trials, but at this point there is no clear evidence that biliary complications can be completely avoided by ERCP and ES alone. In addition, these data conflict with Grade A evidence from studies looking at CBD stones (see below).

Based on these data, it is recommended that patients with acute severe gallstone pancreatitis undergo cholecystectomy following resolution of the acute episode but during the initial hospital stay. Patients with mild to moderate pancreatitis (three or fewer Ranson's criteria) can be considered for early laparoscopic cholecystectomy. **A1c, C5**

Choledocholithiasis

Once CBD stones have been identified, the standard of care is to remove them, since stones left in the CBD may cause subsequent biliary complications including obstructive jaundice, pancreatitis and cholangitis.

See Chapter 24 for further discussion.

The surgical method for identifying CBD stones is operative cholangiography. However, the choice of routine versus selective cholangiography remains somewhat controversial [71–73]. Flum *et al.* performed a retrospective nationwide cohort analysis of 1,570,361 patients undergoing cholecystectomy from 1 January 1992, to 31 December 1999 [73]. There were 7911 common bile duct injuries (0.5%) with 2380 (0.39%) occurring in the 613,706 patients undergoing cholecystectomy with IOC and 5531 (0.58%) occurring in the 956,655 patients undergoing cholecystectomy without IOC (unadjusted relative risk, 1.49). After controlling for patient-level factors and surgeon-level factors, the risk of common bile duct injury was increased when IOC was not used (adjusted relative risk, 1.71). In a review of 2043 patients undergoing routine laparoscopic operative cholangiography, the incidence of unsuspected CBD stones was 2.8% [71]. Only 0.30% of patients not undergoing operative cholangiography ever became symptomatic. In order to better use resources, other studies have attempted to determine criteria for selective operative cholangiography. Borjeson *et al.* proposed criteria that included: normal liver function tests, CBD diameter <10 mm and no history of gallstone pancreatitis or jaundice [72]. One hundred and fifty-five patients who met these criteria were followed prospectively after laparoscopic cholecystectomy for a mean follow-up of 26 months. No patients had retained CBD stones during the follow-up period. Although none of these data provides Grade A evidence, the literature suggests that selective operative cholangiography is justified.

Once CBD stones are identified, there are three approaches to the management: open common bile duct exploration (OCBDE), ERCP and sphincterotomy, and laparoscopic common bile duct exploration (LCBDE).

Five randomized trials (Grade A) have compared OCBDE with ERCP in the management of CBD stones [74–78]. In the two smaller trials with 52 and 34 patients respectively, no differences in morbidity or mortality were seen [75, 76]. OCBDE was more successful at clearing stones than ERCP in one study (88% vs 65%) [75]. The two larger studies, with 228 and 120 patients respectively, demonstrated statistically significant increases in morbidity with ERCP, with the latter study also showing an increase in mortality with ERCP [74,77]. **A1c** The fifth study (n = 83) also demonstrated a trend to increased morbidity with ERCP, but the difference was not statistically significant [78].

Evidence from three randomized trials comparing LCBDE and ERCP showed no difference in morbidity and mortality between the two approaches [79–81]. **A1c** One trial demonstrated a statistically significant decrease in hospital stay for LCBDE (1 day vs 3–5 days) and another demonstrated a similar trend that was not statistically significant [80, 81]. It should be noted that the rates of complications with ERCP in these studies were relatively high (11–28%). More recent studies demonstrate a much lower complication rate. Masci *et al.* reported a series of 2444 ERCPs where the rate of complications was only 4.95% (pancreatitis in 1.8%, hemorrhage in 1.13%, cholangitis in 0.57%, perforation in 0.57% and death in 0.12%) [82]. Morino *et al.* found that the laparoendoscopic rendezvous technique allows a higher rate of clearance of common bile duct stones (95.6% vs 80%), shorter hospital stay (4.3 vs 8.0 days) and a reduction in costs compared to ERCP with ES followed by laparoscopic cholecystectomy with no significant difference in morbidity and mortality [83]. Grade A evidence regarding timing of surgery for choledocholithiasis following ERCP is available in the randomized trial reported by Boerma *et al.* [84]. These authors randomized 120 patients who underwent ERCP and stone extraction with proven gallbladder stones to a "wait and see" policy or to laparoscopic cholecystectomy after ERCP. In the wait and see group, 47% had recurrent biliary symptoms compared with 2% of laparoscopic cholecystectomy patients (relative risk 22.42, 95% CI: 3.16–159.14, p < 0.0001). The conversion rate to open surgery in patients allocated to

"wait and see" was 55% compared with 23% in the laparoscopic group (p = 0.0104). Also, morbidity appeared to be increased in the "wait and see" group, although the difference was not statistically significant (32% vs 14%, p = 0.1048), and length of stay was longer in the "wait and see" group (9 vs 7 days). **A1c**

Conflicting data with respect to the outcomes observed in these studies may be explained in part by variation in operator expertise. LCBDE and ERCP are highly operator-dependent techniques with a steep learning curve. The approach to CBD stones should be individualized and based on the type of expertise available at each institution.

References

1 Gracie WA, Ransohoff DF. The natural history of silent gallstones: the innocent gallstone is not a myth. *N Engl J Med* 1982; **307**: 790–800.

2 McSherry CK, Ferstenberg H, Calhoun WF *et al.* The natural history of diagnosed gallstone disease in symptomatic and asymptomatic patients. *Ann Surg* 1985; **202**: 59–63.

3 Friedman GD, Raviola CA, Fireman B. Prognosis of gallstones with mild or no symptoms: 25 years of follow up in a health maintenance organization. *J Clin Epidemiol* 1989; **42**: 127–136.

4 Friedman GD. Natural history of asymptomatic and symptomatic gallstones. *Am J Surg* 1993; **165**: 399–404.

5 Attili AF, De Santis A, Capri R *et al.* The natural history of gallstones; the GREPCO experience. The GREPCO Group. *Hepatology* 1995; **21**: 655–660.

6 Ransohoff DF, Gracie WA. Treatment of gallstones. *Ann Intern Med* 1993; **119**: 606–619.

7 Ransohoff DF, Gracie WA, Wolfenson LB *et al.* Prophylactic cholecystectomy or expectant management for silent gallstone? A decision analysis to assess survival. *Ann Intern Med* 1983; **99**: 199–204.

8 Gibney EJ. Asymptomatic gallstones. *Br J Surg* 1990; **77**: 368–372.

9 Chapman BA, Wilson IR, Frampton CM *et al.* Prevalence of gallbladder disease in diabetes mellitus. *Dig Dis Sci* 1996; **41**: 2222–2228.

10 Del Favero G, Meggiato CA, Volpi A *et al.* Natural history of gallstones in non-insulin dependent diabetes mellitus. A prospective 5-year follow up. *Dig Dis Sci* 1994; **39**: 1704–1707.

11 Hickman MS, Schwesinger WH, Page CP. Acute cholecystitis in the diabetic. A case-control study of outcome. *Arch Surg* 1988; **123**: 409–411.

12 Landau O, Deutsch AA, Kott I *et al.* The risk of cholecystectomy for acute cholecystitis in diabetic patients. *Hepatogastroenterology* 1992; **39**: 437–438.

13 Sandler RS, Maule WF, Baltus ME. Factors associated with postoperative complications in diabetics after biliary tract surgery. *Gastroenterology* 1986; **91**: 1157–1162.

14 Maringhini A, Moreau JA, Melton LJ *et al.* Gallstones, gallbladder cancer and other gastrointestinal malignancies; an epidemiologic

study in Rochester, Minnesota. *Ann Intern Med* 1987; **107**: 30–35.

15 Lowenfels AB, Lindstron CG, Conway MJ *et al.* Gallstones and risk of gallbladder cancer. *J Natl Cancer Inst* 1985; **75**: 77–80.

16 Hsing AW, Gao Y-T, Han T-Q *et al.* Gallstones and the risk of biliary tract cancer: a population-based study in China. *British Journal of Cancer* 2007; **97**: 1577–1582.

17 Diehl AK. Gallstone size and the risk of gallbladder cancer. *JAMA* 1983; **250**: 2323–2326.

18 Lowenfels AB, Walker AM, Althaus DP *et al.* Gallstone growth, size, and risk of gallbladder cancer: an interracial study. *Int J Epidemio* 1989; **18**: 50–54.

19 Srikanth G, Kumar A, Khare R *et al.* Should laparoscopic cholecystectomy be performed in patients with thick walled gall bladder? *J HPB Surg* 2004; **11**: 40–44.

20 Towfigh S, McFadden DW, Cortina GR *et al.* Porcelain gallbladder is not associated with gallbladder carcinoma. *Am Surg* 2001; **67**: 7–10.

21 Stephen AE, Berger DL. Carcinoma in the porcelain gallbladder: a relationship revisited. *Surgery* 2001; **129**: 699–703.

22 Thistle JL, Cleary PA, Lachin JM *et al.* The natural history of cholelithiaisis: the National Cooperative Gallstone Study. *Ann Intern Med* 1984; **101**: 171–175.

23 Way LW. The National Cooperative Gallstone study and chenodiol. *Gastroenterology* 1983; **84**: 648–651.

24 Wetter LA, Way LW. Surgical therapy of gallstone disease. *Gastroenterol Clin North Am* 1991; **20**: 157–169.

25 Steinle EW, VanderMolen RL, Silbergleit A *et al.* Impact of laparoscopic cholecystectomy on indications for surgical treatment of gallstones. *Surg Endosc* 1997; **11**: 933–935.

26 Barkun JS, Barkum AN, Sampalis JS *et al.* Randomised controlled trial of laparoscopic versus mini cholecystectomy. *Lancet* 1992; **340**: 116–119.

27 McMahon AJ, Russell, IT, Baxter JN. Laparoscopic versus minilaparotomy cholecystectomy: a randomised trial. *Lancet* 1994; **343**: 135–138.

28 McGinn FP, Miles AJ, Ulgalow M *et al.* Randomized trial of laparoscopic cholecystectomy and mini-cholecystectomy. *Br J Surg* 1995; **82**: 1347–1377.

29 Majeed AW, Troy G, Nicholl JP *et al.* Randomised, prospective, single blind comparison of laparscopic versus small incision cholecystectomy. *Lancet* 1996: **347**; 989–994.

30 Keus F, Werner J, Gooszen H *et al.* Randomized clinical trial of small-incision and laparoscopic cholecystectomy in patients with symptomatic cholecystolithiasis. *Arch Surg* 2008; **14**: 371–377.

31 Shea JA, Healey MJ, Berlin JA *et al.* Mortality and complications associated with laparoscopic cholecystectomy. A meta-analysis. *Ann Surg* 1996; **224**: 690–720.

32 Curet MJ, Contreras M, Weber DM *et al.* Laparoscopic cholecystectomy: outpatient versus inpatient management. *Surg Endosc* 2002; **16**: 453–457.

33 Keulemans Y, Eshuis J, de Haes H, de Wit LT, Gouma DJ. Laparoscopic cholecystectomy: day-care versus clinical observation. *Ann Surg* 1998; **228**: 734–740.

34 Bueno Lledó J, Planells Roig M, Arnau Bertomeu C *et al.* Outpatient laparoscopic cholecystectomy: a new gold standard for cholecystectomy. *Rev Esp Enferm Dig* 2006; **98**: 14–24.

35 Kumar M, Agrawal CS, Gupta RK. Three-port versus standard four-port laparoscopic cholecystectomy: a randomized control-

led clinical trial in a community-based teaching hospital in eastern Nepal. *JSLS* 2007; **11**: 358–362.

36 Trichak S. Three-port vs standard four-port laparoscopic cholecystectomy. *Surg Endosc* 2003; **17**: 1434–1436.

37 McArthur P, Cuschieri A, Sells RA *et al.* Controlled clinical trial comparing early with interval cholecystectomy for acute cholecystitis. *Br J Surg* 1975; **62**: 850–852.

38 Lahtinen J, Alhava EM, Aukee S. Acute cholecystitis treated by early and delayed surgery. A controlled clinical trial. *Scand J Gastroenterol* 1978; **13**: 673–678.

39 van der Linden W, Sunzel H. Early versus delayed operation for acute cholecystitis. A controlled clinical trial. *Am J Surg* 1970; **120**: 7–13.

40 Jarvinen HJ, Hastbacka J. Early cholecystectomy for acute cholecystitis: a prospective randomized study. *Ann Surg* 1980; **191**: 501–505.

41 Norrby S, Herlin P, Holmin T *et al.* Early or delayed cholecystectomy in acute cholecystitis? A clinical trial. *Br J Surg* 1983; **70**: 163–165.

42 Lo CM, Liu Cl, Fan ST *et al.* Prospective randomized study of early versus delayed laparoscopic cholecystectomy for acute cholecystitis. *Ann Surg* 1998; **227**: 461–467.

43 Lai PB, Kwong KH, Leung KL *et al.* Randomized trial of early versus delayed laparoscopic cholecystectomy for acute cholecystitis. *Br J Surg* 1998; **85**: 764–767.

44 Kolla SB, Aggarwal S, Kumar A *et al.* Early vs delayed laparoscopic cholecystectomy for acute cholecystitis. *Surg Endosc* 2004; **18**: 1323–1327.

45 Johansson M, Thune A, Blomqvist A *et al.* Management of acute cholecystitis in the laparoscopic era: results of a prospective, randomized clinical trial. *J Gastrointest Surg* 2003; **7**: 642–645.

46 Serralta AS, Bueno JL, Planells MR, Rodero DR. Prospective evaluation of emergency versus delayed laparoscopic cholecystectomy for early cholecystitis. *Surg Laparosc Endosc Percutan Tech* 2003; **13**: 71–75.

47 Chandler CF, Lane JS, Ferguson P, Thompson JE, Ashley SW Prospective evaluation of early versus delayed laparoscopic cholecystectomy for treatment of acute cholecystitis. *Am Surg* 2000; **66**: 896–900.

48 Kiviluoto T, Siren J, Luukkonen P *et al.* Randomised trial of laparoscopic versus open cholecystectomy for acute and gangrenous cholecystitis. *Lancet* 1998; **351**: 321–325.

49 Lujan JA, Parilla P, Robles R *et al.* Laparoscopic cholecystectomy vs open cholecystectomy in the treatment of acute cholecystitis: a prospective study. *Arch Surg* 1998; **133**: 173–175.

50 Lee AY, Carter JJ, Hochberg MS *et al.* The timing of surgery for cholecystitis: a review of 202 consecutive patients at a large municipal hospital. *The American Journal of Surgery* 2008; **195**: 467–470.

51 Zorrón R, Filgueiras M, Maggioni LC *et al.* NOTES transvaginal cholecystectomy: report of the first case. *Surg Innov* 2007; **14**: 279–283.

52 Zornig C, Mofid H, Emmermann A *et al.* Scarless cholecystectomy with combined transvaginal and transumbilical approach in a series of 20 patients. *Surg Endosc* 2008; **22**: 1427–1429.

53 Forgione A, Maggioni D, Sansonna F *et al.* Transvaginal endoscopic cholecystectomy in human beings: preliminary results. *J Laparoendosc Adv Surg Tech A* 2008; **18**: 345–351.

54 Decarli L, Zorron R, Branco A *et al.* Natural orifice translumenal endoscopic surgery (NOTES) transvaginal cholecystectomy in a morbidly obese patient. *Obes Surg* 2008; **18**: 886–889.

55 Neoptolemos JP, Carr-Locke DL, London NJ *et al.* Controlled trial of urgent endoscopic retrograde cholangiopancreatography and endoscopic spincterotomy versus conservative treatment for acute pancreatitis due to gallstones. *Lancet* 1988; **2**: 979–983.

56 Fan ST, Lai EC, Mok FP *et al.* Early treatment of acute biliary pancreatitis by endoscopic papillotomy. *N Engl J Med* 1993; **328**: 228–232.

57 Folsch UR, Nitsche R, Ludtke R *et al.* Early ERCP and papillotomy compared with conservative treatment for acute biliary pancreatitis. The German Study Group on Acute Biliary Pancreatitis. *N Engl Med* 1997; **336**: 237–242.

58 Ito K, Ito H, Tavakkolizadeh A *et al.* Is ductal evaluation always necessary before or during surgery for biliary pancreatitis? *American Journal of Surgery* 2008; **195**: 463–466.

59 Sees DW, Martin RR. Comparison of preoperative endoscopic retrograde cholangiopancreatography and laparoscopic cholecystectomy with operative management of gallstone pancreatitis. *Am J Surg* 1997; **174**: 719–722.

60 Lin G, Halevy A, Girtler O, Gold-Deutch R, Zisman A, Scapa E. The role of endoscopic retrograde cholangiopancreatography in management of patients recovering from acute biliary pancreatitis in the laparoscopic era. *Surg Endosc* 1997; **11**: 371–375.

61 Robertson GS, Jagger C, Johnson PR *et al.* Selection criteria for preoperative endoscopic retrograde cholangiopancreatography in the laparoscopic era. *Arch Surg* 1996; **131**: 89–94.

62 Scapa E. To do or not to do an endoscopic retrograde cholangiopancreatography in acute biliary pancreatitis? *Surg Laparosc Endosc* 1995; **5**: 453–454.

63 de Virgilio C, Verbin C, Chang L, Linder S, Stabile BE, Klein S. Gallstone pancreatitis. The role of preoperative endoscopic retrograde cholangiopancreatography. *Arch Surg* 1994; **129**: 909–912.

64 Leitman IM, Fisher ML, McKinley MJ *et al.* The evaluation and management of known or suspected stones of the common bile duct in the era of minimal access surgery. *Surg Gynecol Obstet* 1993; **176**: 527–533.

65 Srinathan SK, Barkun JS, Mehta SN, Meakins JL, Barkun AN. Evolving management of mild-to-moderate gallstone pancreatitis. *J Gastrointest Surg* 1998; **2**: 385–390.

66 Burch JM, Feliciano DV, Mattox KL, Jordan GL Jr. Gallstone pancreatitis. The question of time. *Arch Surg* 1990; **125**: 853–859.

67 Kelly TR, Wagner DS, Kelly TR, Wagner DS. Gallstone pancreatitis: a prospective randomized trial of the timing of surgery. *Surgery* 1988; **104**: 600–605.

68 McCullough L, Sutherland F, Preshaw R, Kim S. Gallstone pancreatitis: does discharge and readmission for cholecystectomy affect outcome? *HPB (Oxford)* 2003; **5**: 96–99.

69 Kaw M, Al-Antably Y, Kaw P. Management of gallstone pancreatitis: cholecystectomy or FRCP and endoscopic sphincterotomy. *Gastrointest Endosc* 2002; **56**: 61–65.

70 Kwon SK, Lee BS, Kim NJ *et al.* Is cholecystectomy necessary after FRCP for bile duct stones in patients with gallbladder in situ? *Korean J Intern Med* 2001; **16**: 254–259.

71 Snow LL, Weinstein LS, Hannon JK *et al.* Evaluation of operative cholangiography in 2043 patients undergoing laparoscopic cholecystectomy. A case for the selective operative cholangiogram. *Surg Endosc* 2001; **15**: 14–20.

72 Borjeson J, Liu SK, Jones S, Matolo NM. Selective intraoperative cholangiography during laparoscopic cholecystectomy: how selective? *Am Surg* 2000; **66**: 616–618.

73 Flum DR, Dellinger EP, Cheadle A *et al.* Bile duct injury during cholecystectomy. *JAMA* 2003; **289**: 1639–1644.

74 Neoptolemos JP, Carr-Locke DL, Fossard DP. Prospective randomised study of preoperative endoscopic sphincterotomy versus surgery alone for common bile duct stones. *BMJ* (Clin Res Ed) 1987; **294**: 470–474.

75 Stain SC, Cohen H, Tsuishoysha M, Donovan AJ. Choledocholithiasis. Endoscopic sphincterotomy or common bile duct exploration. *Ann Surg* 1991; **213**: 627–633.

76 Stiegmann GV, Goff JS, Mansour A, Pearlman N, Reveille RM, Norton L. Precholecystectomy endoscopic cholangiography and stone removal is not superior to cholecystectomy, cholangiography, and common duct exploration. *Am J Surg* 1992; **163**: 227–230.

77 Suc B, Escat J, Cherqui D *et al.* Surgery vs endoscopy as primary treatment in symptomatic patients with suspected common bile duct stones: a multicenter randomized trial. French Associations for Surgical Research. *Arch Surg* 1998; **133**: 702–708.

78 Hammarstrom LE, Holmin T, Stridbeck H, Ihse I. Long-term follow up of a prospective randomized study of endoscopic versus surgical treatment of bile duct calculi in patients with gallbladder in situ. *Br J Surg* 1995; **82**: 1516–1521.

79 Sgourakis G, Karaliotas K. Laparoscopic common bile duct exploration and cholecystectomy versus endoscopic stone extraction and laparoscopic cholecystectomy for choledocholithiasis. A prospective randomized study. *Minerva Chir* 2002; **57**: 467–474.

80 Rhodes M, Sussman L, Cohen L, Lewis MP. Randomised trial of laparoscopic exploration of common bile duct versus postoperative endoscopic retrograde cholangiography for common bile duct stones. *Lancet* 1998; **351**: 159–161.

81 Cuschieri A, Croce E, Faggioni A *et al.* SAES ductal stone study. Preliminary findings of multi-center prospective randomized trial comparing two-stage vs single-stage management. *Surg Endosc* 1996; **10**: 1130–1135.

82 Masci E, Toti G, Mariani A *et al.* Complications of diagnostic and therapeutic ERCP: a prospective multicenter study. *Am J Gastroenterol* 2001; **96**: 417–423.

83 Morino M, Baracchi F, Miglietta C *et al.* Preoperative endoscopic sphincterotomy versus laparoendoscopic rendezvous in patients with gallbladder and bile duct stones. *Ann Surg* 2006; **244**: 889–896.

84 Boerma D, Rauws EAJ, Keulemans YCA *et al.* Wait-and-see policy or laparoscopic cholecystectomy after endoscopic spincterotomy for bile duct stones: a randomized trial. *Lancet* 2002; **360**: 761–765.

24 Acute pancreatitis

Colin D Johnson and Hassan Elberm

Department of Surgery, Southampton University Hospitals, Southampton, UK

Acute pancreatitis is a growing clinical problem with an emergency presentation. While many cases resolve spontaneously, some patients become severely ill, requiring intensive care and support of failing organ systems. The incidence of acute pancreatitis has increased in the UK [1], USA [2], Japan [3] and in many other countries [4, 5]. This may be due to changes in gallstone incidence, related to rising rates of obesity, and to changes in alcohol consumption [6, 7], but the evidence to confirm these associations is lacking.

This chapter reviews the current evidence to underpin the assessment and management of patients with acute pancreatitis. These topics have been extensively reviewed over the last decade. There have been many national and international guidelines that have carefully reviewed the published evidence, from the UK, USA [8, 9], Japan [3], and from the World Association of Gastroenterology [10]. The 1998 UK guidelines [11] were updated on the basis of new evidence in 2005 [12], and these two documents provide a clear summary of the evidence available at that time. They should be read together, as the full evidence base was not repeated in the revision. The main recommendations in those guidelines are reproduced in Table 24.1, and the relevant ones are repeated at the head of each section below. The present chapter will focus on the additional evidence that has been acquired since that time. In each section, we take the current UK guidelines as a starting point, and comment on the background to the recommendations before outlining any necessary amendments to the advice based on new evidence.

To prepare the present chapter, the MEDLINE database for the years 2004–2008 was searched for articles with title words "acute pancreatitis" and each section heading

reviewed. Randomized trials, systematic reviews and meta-analyses, and review articles of special interest were read and summarised. A formal meta-analysis was not conducted. In addition, reliance is placed on the international guidelines noted above that were prepared on the basis of critical reviews of the field. Finally, the Cochrane Library was reviewed to identify all Cochrane Reviews related to acute pancreatitis.

Definition of acute pancreatitis

In 1998, the UK Guidelines [11] defined acute pancreatitis as:

> An acute inflammatory process of the pancreas, with variable involvement of other regional tissues or remote organ systems. Severe acute pancreatitis is associated with organ failure and/or local complications such as necrosis (with infection), pseudocyst or abscess. Most often this is an expression of the development of pancreatic necrosis, although patients with oedematous pancreatitis may manifest clinical features of a severe attack. Mild acute pancreatitis is associated with minimal organ dysfunction and an uneventful recovery. The predominant pathological feature is interstitial oedema of the gland.

Pathological changes of acute inflammation are followed by resolution in the majority of cases (mild pancreatitis, edematous pancreatitis). Almost all patients with mild pancreatitis recover without specific intervention. Severe acute pancreatitis is characterized by the presence of local or systemic complications, and by varying degrees of parenchymal damage (necrosis, apoptosis) which may be followed by some acinar regeneration or by fibrosis. Severe pancreatitis may be fatal in 14–25% of cases, with overall mortality rates for acute pancreatitis usually in the range 2.1–7.8% [3]. A recent population based study from the

Evidence-Based Gastroenterology and Hepatology, 3rd edition.
J. McDonald, A.K. Burroughs, B. Feagan, and M.B. Fennerty. © 2010
Blackwell Publishing Ltd

Table 24.1 Recommendations published in UK National Guidelines in 1998 [11] and 2005 [12]. Headings in italics are reviewed in this chapter, to incorporate new evidence.

Heading	Recommendations for management of acute pancreatitis	Date	Grade
Initial assessment			
Diagnosis	Although amylase is widely available and provides acceptable accuracy of diagnosis, where lipase is available it is preferred for the diagnosis of acute pancreatitis.	2005	A
	The correct diagnosis of acute pancreatitis should be made within 48 hours of admission. Although this may strain support and diagnostic facilities, the risk of missing an alternative life-threatening intra-abdominal catastrophe demands full investigation.	1998	C
	Where doubt exists, imaging may be useful for diagnosis: ultrasonography is often unhelpful and pancreatic imaging by contrast enhanced CT provides good evidence for the presence or absence of pancreatitis.	2005	C
Etiology	The etiology of acute pancreatitis should be determined in at least 80% of cases and no more than 20% should be classified as idiopathic.	2005	B
Severity	The definitions of severity, as proposed in the Atlanta criteria, should be used. However, organ failure present within the first week, which resolves within 48 hours, should not be considered an indicator of a severe attack.	2005	B
	Severity stratification should be made in all patients within 48 hours. It is recommended that all patients should be assessed by the Glasgow score and CRP. The APACHE II score is equally accurate, and may be used for initial assessment; it should be used for ongoing monitoring in severe cases.[a]	1998	B
	Available prognostic features which predict complications in acute pancreatitis are clinical impression of severity, obesity, or APACHE II > 8 in the first 24 hours of admission, and C reactive protein levels >150 mg/l, Glasgow score 3 or more, or persisting organ failure after 48 hours in hospital.[a]	2005	B
Use of CT	Patients with persisting organ failure, signs of sepsis, or deterioration in clinical status 6–10 days after admission will require CT.	2005	B
Management			
Organization of care	All cases of severe acute pancreatitis should be managed in an HDU or ITU setting with full monitoring and systems support.	1998	B
	Every hospital that receives acute admissions should have a single nominated clinical team to manage all patients with acute pancreatitis.	2005	C
	Management in, or referral to, a specialist unit is necessary for patients with >30% necrosis or with other complications.	2005	B
Antibiotics	The evidence for antibiotic prophylaxis against infection of pancreatic necrosis is conflicting and difficult to interpret. At present there is no consensus on this issue.[a]	2005	C
	If antibiotic prophylaxis is used, it should be given for a maximum of 14 days.	2005	B
	Further studies are needed.[a]	2005	C
	A German trial which compared ciprofloxacin-metronidazole and placebo is the only double-blind, placebo-controlled trial published to date. The results do not support the use of prophylactic antibiotics. This study was stopped after interim analysis of 76 patients with necrosis showed no differences in the primary outcomes of infected necrosis, systemic complications and mortality rates.[a]	2005	C
Enteral nutrition	The evidence is not conclusive to support the use of enteral nutrition in all patients with severe acute pancreatitis. However, if nutritional support is required, the enteral route should be used if that can be tolerated.	2005	A
	The nasogastric route for feeding can be used as it appears to be effective in 80% of cases.	2005	B
Management of gallstones	All patients with biliary pancreatitis should undergo definitive management of gall stones during the same hospital admission, unless a clear plan has been made for definitive treatment within the next two weeks.	2005	C
Early endoscopic sphincterotomy	Patients with signs of cholangitis require endoscopic sphincterotomy or duct drainage by stenting to ensure relief of biliary obstruction.	2005	A
	Urgent therapeutic ERCP should be performed in patients with acute pancreatitis of suspected or proven gall stone etiology who satisfy the criteria for predicted or actual severe pancreatitis, or when there is cholangitis, jaundice, or a dilated common bile duct.[a]	2005	B
	All patients undergoing early ERCP for severe gall stone pancreatitis require endoscopic sphincterotomy whether or not stones are found in the bile duct.	2005	C

Table 24.1 Continued

Heading	Recommendations for management of acute pancreatitis	Date	Grade
Intervention for necrosis	All patients with persistent symptoms and greater than 30% pancreatic necrosis, and those with smaller areas of necrosis and clinical suspicion of sepsis, should undergo image guided FNA to obtain material for culture 7–14 days after the onset of the pancreatitis.	2005	B
	Patients with infected necrosis will require intervention to completely debride all cavities containing necrotic material.	2005	B
	The choice of surgical technique for necrosectomy, and subsequent postoperative management depends on individual features and locally available expertise.	2005	B

CT: computed tomography.

Grade indicates a recommendation based on: A, at least one randomised controlled trial as part of evidence of overall good quality and consistency; B, clinical studies without randomisation; C, expert consensus.

[a] Indicates recommendations that should be reconsidered in light of new evidence.

USA indicates that overall mortality from acute pancreatitis is falling and is now less than 2% [13].

Diagnosis

Although amylase is widely available and provides acceptable accuracy of diagnosis, where lipase is available it is preferred for the diagnosis of acute pancreatitis. Lipase is more specific and more sensitive than amylase. Amylase levels generally rise within a few hours after the onset of the symptoms and return to normal values within 3–5 days. However, serum lipase concentrations remain high for a longer period of time than do amylase concentrations, which gives slightly greater sensitivity for lipase than for amylase in patients with delayed presentation [14].

The correct diagnosis of acute pancreatitis should be made within 48 hours of admission. Although this may strain support and diagnostic facilities, the risk of missing an alternative life-threatening intra-abdominal catastrophe demands full investigation. Where doubt exists, imaging may be useful for diagnosis: ultrasonography is often unhelpful and pancreatic imaging by contrast enhanced CT provides good evidence for the presence or absence of pancreatitis.

Clinical diagnosis is usually straightforward, but overlap may exist with the clinical presentation of perforated viscus or gangrenous bowel. These serious alternative diagnoses may require urgent intervention and in case of doubt they must be excluded, usually by CT. It has been known for many years that contrast-enhanced CT shortly after admission has 87–90% sensitivity and 90–92% specificity to confirm the diagnosis of pancreatitis [15–17].

The presence of two of three diagnostic features (typical abdominal pain, elevated concentrations of serum amylase, or lipase above three times the upper limit of normal, and the presence of inflammatory changes in and around the pancreas on abdominal CT) confirms the diagnosis. These cutoffs for lipase and amylase are widely accepted [18], but the World Association Guidelines [10] point out that:

Pancreatic enzymes are released into the circulation during an acute attack. Levels peak early and decline over 3–4 days. An important concept derives from this: the diagnosis of acute pancreatitis should not rely on arbitrary limits of values three or four times greater than normal, but values should be interpreted in light of the time since the onset of abdominal pain.

Severe acute pancreatitis

In 1992, our understanding of acute pancreatitis was greatly improved by a consensus conference that took place in Atlanta [19]. This conference defined the terminology of acute pancreatitis and its complications, and has been the basis for much progress in improved management. However, some problems with terminology and definitions have been noted in the Atlanta document. Currently, the International Association of Pancreatology is attempting to revise these definitions by international consensus, focusing on the diagnosis and imaging of severe acute pancreatitis during two distinct phases: the first week (early phase characterized by Systemic Inflammatory Response Syndrome, SIRS, and organ failure), and a later phase characterized by depressed immune response and local complications, especially pancreatic and peripancreatic necrosis. This consensus, led by Doctors Michael Sarr and Peter Banks, aims to collate the views of numerous pancreatic specialists around the world and to present an evidence base to shape clinical practice for the next decade.

Definition of severe pancreatitis

The definitions of severity, as proposed in the Atlanta criteria, should be used. However, organ failure present within the first week, which resolves within 48 hours, should not be considered an indicator of a severe attack (UK Guidelines 2005).

The Atlanta criteria [19] for severe pancreatitis remain widely accepted. In this definition, severe acute pancreatitis is characterized by the presence of any systemic or local complication. Other criteria of severe disease accepted by the Atlanta conference include the presence of a high Ranson or APACHE-II score (which are markers for systemic complications). The Atlanta criteria represent the first attempt to define cutoff values for organ failure in acute pancreatitis (Table 24.2). This was a useful step to clarify thinking about systemic complications, but it has become clear that the crossing of a threshold for organ failure is an inadequate definition for severe acute pancreatitis.

It is now understood that organ failure in acute pancreatitis is preceded by a phase of activation of the Systemic Inflammatory Response syndrome (SIRS) [20, 21]. The presence of SIRS is clinical evidence of inflammation (Table 24.3), and indicates high risk of progression to complications, but SIRS may resolve without consequence. However, the presence of SIRS in patients on admission to hospital is associated with increased risk of organ failure and death [21]. If SIRS persists for more than 48 hours beyond admission to hospital, the mortality rate rises to more than 20% [21], and the patient should be regarded as having severe pancreatitis (Figure 24.1).

Since the beginning of this century, it has become clear that the crucial feature of severity in relation to systemic complications during the first week of acute pancreatitis is the duration of organ failure, and that organ failure which resolves during the first week is associated with a very low mortality rate [22]. We showed in a national sample from 78 hospitals [23] that persistence of organ failure for more than 48 hours during the first week of the attack is associated with a 35% risk of fatal outcome. These patients also have a high risk of local complications. Others have confirmed this observation [21, 24, 25], and it is now established that persistent organ failure (>48 hours) during the first week of illness is part of the definition of severe acute pancreatitis.

The severity of early organ failure has also been shown by some authors [26, 27] to be associated with high risk of fatal outcome, but the interaction between severity and duration of organ failure has not been clarified.

Three organ systems are usually sufficient to assess organ failure: respiratory, cardiovascular and renal. In our study of 290 patients with predicted severe acute pancreatitis, these organs were always involved in patients with persistent organ failure, and only 3 of 71 patients with transient organ failure did not have one of these systems affected [23]. Organ failure is easily defined in accordance with the Marshall scoring system [28] as a score ≥2 for at least one of respiratory, renal or cardiovascular function

Table 24.2 Atlanta criteria for severe acute pancreatitis (16).

Criteria for severe acute pancreatitis – presence of one or more of the following:
(1) Ranson score during the first 48 hours, 3 or more
(2) APACHE II score at any time, 8 or more
(3) Presence of one or more organ failures
(4) Presence of one or more local complications

Organ failures include:
(1) Shock: systolic blood pressure,less than 90 mm Hg
(2) Pulmonary insufficiency: PaO2 on room air, 60 mm Hg or lower
(3) Renal failure: serum creatinine, >2 mg/dL after fluid replacement

(4) gastrointestinal bleeding:	blood loss	more than 500 mL/24 hours
(5) coagulopathy:	thrombocytopenia	fibrin split products in
	hypofibrinogenemia	plasma
(6) severe hypocalcemia:	calcium	7.5 mg/dL or lower

Local complications include
(1) pancreatic necrosis
(2) pancreatic abscess
(3) pancreatic pseudocyst

Table 24.3 Definition of SIRS [17]. Severe pancreatitis is diagnosed if SIRS criteria persist for >48 hours.

SIRS is defined by the presence of two or more of the following:	
pulse	>90 beats/min
rectal temperature	<36°C or >38°C
white blood count	<4000 or >12,000 per mm³
respirations	>20/min
or PCO₂	<32 mmHg

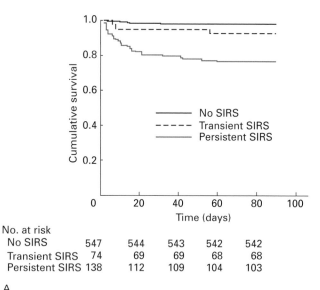

No. at risk

No SIRS	547	544	543	542	542
Transient SIRS	74	69	69	68	68
Persistent SIRS	138	112	109	104	103

A

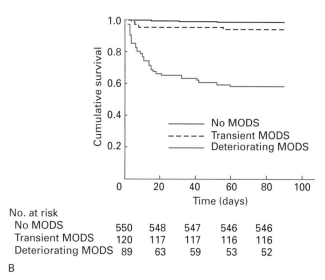

No. at risk

No MODS	550	548	547	546	546
Transient MODS	120	117	117	116	116
Deteriorating MODS	89	63	59	53	52

B

Figure 24.1 SIRS and organ failure in the first week are associated with high risk of fatal outcome (reproduced from Mofidi *et al.* [21]).

(Table 24.4). The full Marshall score (which includes the Glasgow coma score and platelet count) and the SOFA scoring system, which takes account of inotropic and respiratory support for patients managed in a critical care unit [29], may also be used for assessment of more severely ill patients with multiple organ/system failure. All these scores can be determined at presentation and daily to create a record of the presence and the severity of organ failure during the first week.

Prediction of severity

Severity stratification should be made in all patients within 48 hours. It is recommended that all patients should be assessed by the Glasgow score and CRP. The APACHE II score is equally accurate, and may be used for initial assessment; it should be used for ongoing monitoring in severe cases.

Available prognostic features which predict complications in acute pancreatitis are clinical impression of severity, obesity, or APACHE II >8 in the first 24 hours of admission, and C-reactive protein levels >150 mg/l, Glasgow score 3 or more, or persisting organ failure after 48 hours in hospital.

These recommendations are still relevant, but a new simple scoring system has been reported (see below).

The management of acute pancreatitis is supportive; mild attacks resolve without specific measures other than ensuring adequate analgesia, oxygenation and circulating volume. For many years it has been believed that early identification of patients with severe disease would be advantageous, leading to early institution of aggressive support for failing systems and early transfer to an appropriate critical care facility. This approach led to many reports of various tests and scoring systems designed to predict severe disease. As noted above, we now identify such patients by the presence of specific clinical markers of severity, especially the presence of persistent SIRS, or persistent organ failure. However, the observation of high risk predictive scores (e.g. Ranson, Glasgow, APACHE II) or high levels of confirmed markers or risk factors of severe disease (C-reactive protein >150 mg/l [10, 30], BMI > 30 [12, 31]) may help focus clinical attention on potentially ill patients.

Clinical markers of severity and predictive scores

Table 24.5 summarizes features that predict a severe attack of acute pancreatitis and that are available shortly after admission to hospital. Age is an independent risk factor, and age >70 years is associated with 17% mortality risk [32]. Obesity is a risk factor for complications and death

Table 24.4 Criteria from the Marshall Scoring System [25] which define organ failure and measure its severity. Any value scoring 2 or more indicates an organ failure; the total score is a marker of the severity of organ failure.

Organ system	Score				
	0	1	2	3	4
Respiratory (PO2/FIO2)	>400	301–400	201–300	101–200	≤101
Renal					
(serum creatinine, μmol/l)	≤134	134–169	170–310	311–439	>439
(serum creatinine, mg/dl)	<1.4	1.4–1.8	1.9–3.6	3.6–4.9	>4.9
Cardiovascular (systolic blood pressure, mmHg)	>90	<90 Fluid responsive	<90 Not fluid responsive	<90, pH < 7.3	<90, pH < 7.2

For non-ventilated patients, the FiO$_2$ can be estimated:

Supplemental Oxygen (L/min)	FiO$_2$
Room air	21%
2	25%
4	30%
6–8	40%
9–10	50%

Table 24.5 Features that predict a severe attack, that are present within 48 hours of admission to hospital. Modified from reference 12.

Initial assessment	Clinical impression of severity
	Body mass index > 30
	Pleural effusion on chest radiograph
	APACHE II score > 8
24 h after admission	Clinical impression of severity
	APACHE II score > 8
	Glasgow score 3 or more
	Persisting organ failure, especially if multiple
	C reactive protein > 150 mg/l
48 h after admission	Clinical impression of severity
	Glasgow score 3 or more
	C reactive protein > 150 mg/l
	Persisting organ failure for 48 h
	Multiple or progressive organ failure

[31]. The mechanism of this increased risk is unclear, but it seems that obesity is associated with an increased inflammatory response [33, 34]. Other proposed mechanisms include greater risk of respiratory complications and the presence of poorly perfused fat in and around the pancreas, increasing the risk of pancreatic and peripancreatic necrosis.

Objective parameters should be used to support the clinical examination in the first 24 hours of admission, as clinical examination is specific, but it is not sensitive when used alone [12]. The APACHE II score is widely used as a predictor of severity, and for monitoring progress early in the illness. The Atlanta criteria selected a cutoff score of 8 or more to define severe disease. This cutoff in the first 24 hours identifies almost all patients who will develop a complication. In a meta-analysis of three well-documented series comprising 627 cases (20% severe), Larvin [35] found no deaths in patients with initial APACHE II score below 10. A score of 10 or 11 was very unlikely to lead to death, but scores of 12 or more had a mortality rate over 20%, increasing with higher initial scores (Figure 24.2).

Recently, the Early Warning Score (EWS), based on routine nursing observations, and widely used to monitor the clinical condition of ill patients, has been proposed as a simple means of identifying high risk patients [36, 37]. The EWS also responds to the dynamic nature of the illness: deterioration of scores is associated with a worse outcome [36]. The ability of this system to predict severe pancreatitis has been compared with APACHE II scores, modified organ dysfunction scores, Glasgow scores, CT severity index and Ranson criteria for 181 admissions with acute

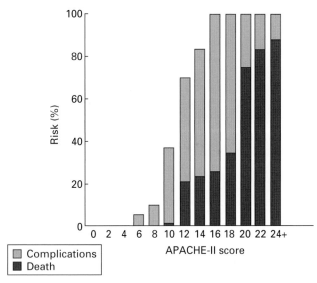

Figure 24.2 Percentage risk of death or complications associated with different initial APACHE-II scores (reproduced from Larvin [35]).

pancreatitis. Scores were calculated daily for the first three days. The APACHE II and EWS performed best in receiver operating curve analysis, with similar areas under the curve (APACHE II 0.876, 0.892 and 0.911; EWS 0.827, 0.910 and 0.934, on days 1, 2 and 3 respectively). These findings suggest that the simple and easily assessed EWS could be used at the bedside to monitor progress and identify severe acute pancreatitis soon after admission to the hospital. In particular, EWS reflects the dynamic nature of the illness in the same way as SIRS and organ failure. This simple clinical observation should permit reliable identification of patients at risk of complicated or fatal course in any hospital setting. Importantly, improvement in the EWS (or other scores discussed above) is reassuring that the patient is likely to recover without complications.

A large population based survey [13] has developed and validated a predictive system for severe acute pancreatitis based on easily obtained features present at the time of admission to hospital. The authors reviewed records of 17,992 patients for features associated with severe disease, that were present within 24 hours of admission. They identified five independent predictors: blood urea nitrogen >25 mg/dL (>8.93 mmol/L), impaired mental state, SIRS, age > 60 years and pleural effusion on chest X-ray (acronym BISAP score). Allocation of one point for each feature gives a simple BISAP score, which identifies low risk patients with low score, and high risk groups with a >10% risk of death for scores of 4, and >20% risk of death for scores of 5. The strength of this report is that the predictive ability of the scores was confirmed in a new sample of patient records, comprising over 18,000 patients treated in the years 2004–2005. The development and validation cohorts had mortality rates of 1.9% and 1.28% respectively, which

suggests that this study used "real world" data including all cases of mild disease in the contributing hospitals. The BISAP score promises to simplify the assessment of acute pancreatitis, particularly by the rapid identification of the large majority of patients who are at low risk of complications and death.

Laboratory markers

Plasma C-reactive protein is accurate, but delayed in its response, not peaking until 72–96 hours into the illness. A value >150 mg/l identifies patients at risk of pancreatic necrosis and potentially fatal outcome [12]. There is some evidence that serum or urine concentrations of the trypsinogen activation peptide (TAP) [38–41] and urine anionic trypsinogen 2 [42–44] might be useful to predict severity, although to date only the trypsinogen 2 test is available as a rapid bedside test.

Another promising early marker of severity is procalcitonin (PCT). Despite some contrary views (based on relatively small numbers) [45, 46], there is considerable evidence that PCT is a useful early marker of severe disease, and especially of pancreatic necrosis, or infected necrosis. A meta-analysis of the early evidence [47] reviewed nine reports. There was considerable variation of methodological quality. Considering only high quality reports, the sensitivity and specificity of PCT in the first 24 hours in hospital to predict severe disease were 82% and 89%, with an area under the curve value of 94%, indicating very good discrimination. The meta-analysis indicated that PCT may be especially useful for the identification of patients at risk of infected necrosis.

Two further studies support these findings. Rau has long advocated using this marker, and her latest publication [48] provides more evidence from a study of 104 patients in five European centers enrolled within 96 hours of symptom onset. Initial PCT concentrations were significantly elevated in patients with pancreatic infections and associated multi-organ dysfunction syndrome (MODS), all of whom required surgery (n = 10), and in non-survivors (n = 8). PCT levels were only moderately increased in seven patients with pancreatic infections in the absence of MODS, all of whom were managed non-operatively without mortality. A PCT value of 3.5 ng/ml or higher on two consecutive days had a sensitivity and specificity of 93% and 88% for the assessment of infected necrosis with MODS or non-survival. This prediction was possible on the third and fourth day after onset of symptoms with a sensitivity and specificity of 79% and 93% for PCT 3.8 ng/ml or higher. Another study of 40 patients (11 severe) supports these findings [49]. There is now strong evidence that early estimation of procalcitonin can identify patients at risk of infected necrosis or death, and the test may be repeated to improve the detection of these most severe cases.

Role of CT in acute pancreatitis

During the first week

As noted above, at the time of admission to hospital CT may be required if the diagnosis is in doubt: this may arise with delayed presentation, for example when the plasma enzyme levels have fallen below the diagnostic threshold. Sometimes CT may be helpful to exclude other diagnoses, such as perforation or gangrene of bowel. There is no evidence that early CT is helpful in the management of confirmed acute pancreatitis. Indeed, the UK guidelines [12] recommend that the first scan be delayed until 6–10 days after onset of symptoms. Arguments against early CT in all cases of pancreatitis are that early CT with intravenous contrast has the potential risk of worsening the renal impairment, and that an early CT may underestimate the full extent of pancreatic necrosis, which may evolve for at least four days after the onset. Most importantly, CT is unlikely to change management decisions in the first week. At this stage, treatment is supportive, and surgical or other intervention is avoided, and CT does not affect clinical decision-making.

Early CT may be used to assess the severity of the illness if this is required, for example to stratify patients in treatment trials. Balthazar and colleagues [50] proposed the CT severity index (Table 24.6) based on the grade of inflammation and the extent of pancreatic necrosis determined by enhancement. The sum of these two scores is used to calculate the severity index.

After the first week

Patients with persisting organ failure, signs of sepsis, or deterioration in clinical status 6–10 days after admission will require CT. CT is usually performed after 6–10 days in patients with persistent SIRS or organ failure to assess local complications such as fluid collections and necrosis [12, 50]. There is some evidence that MRI identifies necrosis and fluid collections better than does CT [51], although the practical difficulty of ensuring MR compatible equipment attached to a patient with organ failure may be a problem in some settings.

The Atlanta criteria are not clear on the distinction between fluid collections, pseudocyst and necrosis. The current international consensus revision of the Atlanta criteria mentioned above is likely to advocate the use of contrast enhanced CT for the characterisation of morphological changes in and around the pancreas, after the first week of the illness, and will probably recognise a number of local complications, namely pancreatic and peripancreatic necrosis, acute peripancreatic collections within four weeks from onset of symptoms, and pseudocyst and walled off

Table 24.6 Computed tomography (CT) grading of severity.

Computed tomography (CT) grading of severity	Score
CT grade	
(A) Normal pancreas	0
(B) Oedematous pancreatitis	1
(C) B plus mild extrapancreatic changes	2
(D) Severe extrapancreatic changes including one fluid collection	3
(E) Multiple or extensive extrapancreatic collections	4
Pancreatic necrosis (extent)	
None	0
Up to one third	2
Between one third and one half	4
More than half	6
CT severity index = CT grade + necrosis score	
Observed rates of complications and death related to CTSI score	Complications
0–3	8%
4–6	35%
7–10	92%
	Deaths
0–3	3%
4–6	6%
7–10	17%

Modified from the World Association guidelines [10] and based on Balthazar and colleagues [47].

pancreatic necrosis more than four weeks from onset. The extent of pancreatic necrosis on CT is useful information, because this is related directly to the risk of local and systemic complications [52, 53].

CT is unreliable for the discrimination of pseudocyst from necrosis. The Santorini consensus conference [30] recommended that either ultrasound or magnetic resonance imaging (MRI) should be used to differentiate between fluid and necrotic tissue. In practice, it is wise to consider all localized collections following necrotising pancreatitis to be pancreatic or peripancreatic necrosis until proved otherwise.

Organization of care

All cases of severe acute pancreatitis should be managed in an HDU or ITU setting with full monitoring and systems support. Every hospital that receives acute admissions should have a single nominated clinical team to manage all patients with acute pancreatitis. Management in, or referral to, a specialist unit is necessary for patients with >3 0% necrosis or with other complications.

It seems self-evident that the care of these potentially difficult and seriously ill patients should be concentrated in the hands of interested clinicians with appropriate expertise. **C5**

Initial management and resuscitation

Early fluid resuscitation and oxygen supplementation are simple measures that seem likely to be helpful in early resolution of organ failure [54]. Whether these interventions significantly reduce the mortality rate is not known, but it seems sensible to provide simple circulatory and respiratory support designed to achieve rapid resolution of organ failure. **C5** This approach may break the cycle of hypotension and hypoxaemia that can sustain and provoke more organ system failures. The fluid replacement with a mix of crystalloid and colloid solutions should aim to maintain good urine output (0.5 ml/kg) and can be monitored by central venous pressure reading in selected patients. Oxygenation ideally should maintain the arterial saturation above 95%. Oxygen saturations lower than this are associated with significant hypoxaemia [55].

Prophylactic antibiotics

The evidence for antibiotic prophylaxis against infection of pancreatic necrosis is conflicting and difficult to interpret. At present there is no consensus on this issue.

If antibiotic prophylaxis is used, it should be given for a maximum of 14 days. Further studies are needed.

It is pleasing to note that we now have evidence to resolve this issue, outlined below.

Since infected pancreatic necrosis is associated with high mortality rates (40%) and it is one of the leading causes of death in acute pancreatitis, many trials have been done to establish the role of prophylactic antibiotics in reducing the mortality rate and other infective and non-infective complications. The trials discussed up to 2005 had shown benefit for prophylaxis, but there were concerns that the improvements in outcome were seen for different endpoints in different studies. The guidelines quoted above should be re-evaluated in light of the publication of more high quality evidence. An interesting analysis [56] has shown an inverse relationship between the quality of studies and the observed effect, i.e. as study quality improves, the differences in outcome diminish.

In discussing the available evidence, the UK guidelines noted:

A German trial [57] which compared ciprofloxacin-metronidazole and placebo is the only double blind placebo controlled trial published to date. The results do not support the use of prophylactic antibiotics. This study was stopped after interim analysis of 76 patients with necrosis showed no differences in the primary outcomes of infected necrosis, systemic complications, and mortality rates.

A Cochrane Review [58] evaluated all the randomized trials with placebo controls, published up to July 2006. The conclusion of this review was that:

Antibiotic prophylaxis appeared to be associated with significantly decreased mortality but not infected pancreatic necrosis. Beta lactam antibiotics were associated with significantly decreased mortality and infected pancreatic necrosis, but quinolone plus imidazole regimens were not.

The review includes a trial from Finland [59] which compared cefuroxime with placebo, and demonstrated a difference in mortality. The validity of these data has been questioned, because only patients with alcohol related pancreatitis were included, and because the excess deaths in the placebo group all occurred in the first week of the illness, before any effect on infection of necrosis could be expected. The Cochrane Review also noted that there were variations in methodological quality and treatment regimens in the trials reviewed. More reliable data were awaited.

A subsequent meta-analysis of prophylactic antibiotic use in acute necrotizing pancreatitis [60] assessed whether intravenous prophylactic antibiotic use reduces infected necrosis and death in acute necrotizing pancreatitis. Six randomized controlled trials were analyzed, including the five analyzed for preparation of the UK Guidelines, and an additional trial published only in abstract form [61]. Primary outcome measures were infected necrosis and death. Secondary outcome measures were non-pancreatic infections, surgical intervention and length of hospital stay. Prophylactic antibiotic use was not associated with a statistically significant reduction in infected necrosis (RR = 0.77; 95% CI: 0.54–1.12; p = 0.173), mortality (RR = 0.78; 95 CI: 0.44–1.39; p = 0.404), non-pancreatic infections (RR = 0.71; 95% CI: 0.32–1.58; p = 0.402) or surgical intervention (RR = 0.78; 95% CI: 0.55–1.11; p = 0.167).

A double-blind randomized trial of meropenem versus placebo, published in May 2007, is probably the definitive study [62]. This trial was performed in 32 centers within North America and Europe and included one hundred patients with clinically severe, confirmed necrotizing pancreatitis who were randomized within five days of the onset of symptoms to receive Meropenem (1 g intravenously every eight hours) or placebo for 7 to 21 days. The trial was well designed, with entry criteria (>30% necrosis) that selected patients at greatest risk of infection. The sample size calculation indicated that approximately 120 subjects per group (240 subjects in all) would be required to detect a reduction of pancreatic infection rates by meropenem compared with placebo from 40% to 20% with 90% power and a 5% two-sided significance level. The trial included appropriate secondary endpoints (need for surgery, death). Recruitment was slow, because patients with >30% necrosis are relatively rare. (It is widely agreed that antibiotics should not be given to patients without necrosis, as they are very unlikely to develop pancreatic infections.) The trial was closed early, when it was clear that pancreatic infection rates overall (15%) were lower than expected. Pancreatic or peripancreatic infections developed in 18% (9 of 50) of patients in the meropenem group compared with 12% (6 of 50) in the placebo group. Despite the early closure, this RCT of antibiotic prophylaxis recruited more patients with pancreatic necrosis than any previous trial and it seems improbable that recruitment of a further 140 patients to achieve the initial target would have shown a different outcome. The results of this trial showed no statistically significant advantage for early use of meropenem for prevention of pancreatic or peripancreatic infection, requirement for surgical intervention, or death (Table 24.7).

Further evidence of lack of effect is presented in a single-centre, double-blind RCT of ciprofloxacin in patients with confirmed necrosis [63]. Although this trial included only 41 patients, it produced no evidence of benefit, consistent with the result of the larger trials discussed above.

The weight of evidence has shifted since preparation of the UK Guidelines Revision to favor the position that prophylactic antibiotics, prescribed early in the illness to prevent subsequent infection of necrotic tissue, confer no benefit and should not be part of the treatment plan. **A1c** There is no evidence of benefit in several recent well-designed RCTs, and the unnecessary use of antibiotics has

well-known adverse consequences, notably related to hospital acquired infection. However, it is not easy to define the need for antibiotics on purely clinical grounds. Patients with severe acute pancreatitis are likely to have signs of SIRS; this should not be taken as evidence of infection. In the early stages of the illness antibiotics should be used only when there is proof of infection from a positive culture.

Nutrition in acute pancreatitis patients

The evidence is not conclusive to support the use of enteral nutrition in all patients with severe acute pancreatitis. However, if nutritional support is required the enteral route should be used if tolerated. **A1d** The nasogastric route for feeding can be used as it appears to be effective in 80% of cases. **B4** We have found no additional evidence that requires a change to this advice.

In mild, acute pancreatitis there is no benefit from passage of a nasogastric tube [64, 65]. These patients can be allowed to drink small volumes of fluids as tolerated from the outset. A full oral diet can be restarted in most patients after a few days, when the pain has settled [66].

In severe disease, enteral feeding may be beneficial for two reasons. First, it may help to reduce the risks of complications when started early in the disease; second, in established, severe pancreatitis nutritional supplements will be required and the enteral route is preferred. Most studies have assumed that the enteral feeding solution should be delivered beyond the duodenum, by means of a nasojejunal tube. However, this placement is often unnecessary [67, 68]. **A1d** About 80% of patients with severe disease tolerate early enteral feeding by nasogastric tube, and this route is simpler and cheaper to establish. Nasojejunal feeding should be reserved for those patients in whom nasogastric feeding is unsuccessful because of failure of gastric emptying.

Prevention of complications

Enteral feeding is believed to be superior to parenteral nutrition in most critical care conditions. Reasons advanced to support this belief include the suggestion that enteral nutrition may maintain splanchnic protein synthesis and help to maintain normal gut mucosal function, including the mucosal barrier. This helps to reduce bacterial translocation, which may be the main driver for organ failure and sepsis. **C5** Although there were fears that enteral feeding might exacerbate acute pancreatitis because of the stimulatory effect of luminal nutrients on pancreatic enzyme synthesis, this adverse effect has not been found in practice, perhaps because pancreatic enzyme synthesis is inhibited immediately after onset of pancreatitis [69]. Data from

Table 24.7 Outcomes in the trial [59] of Meropenem versus placebo in the prevention of infection in severe acute pancreatitis. No differences were observed.

	Pancreatic or peripancreatic infections	Requirement of surgical intervention	Mortality
Meropenem group	18% (9 of 50)	26% (13 of 50)	20% (10 of 50)
Placebo group	12% (6 of 50)	20% (10 of 50)	18% (9 of 50)
P value	0.401	0.476	0.799

patients with acute pancreatitis show lower rate of secretions compared to healthy individuals, and this rate is inversely related to the severity of the pancreatitis [70].

In any attempt to prevent complications of pancreatitis, it is logical that enteral feeding should be started early in the course of the disease. Few RCTs have been performed to specifically address this point. In the first small trial 38 patients with severe pancreatitis were randomized to receive either enteral or parenteral nutrition [71]. Significantly fewer infected complications occurred in the enteral feeding group. Windsor *et al.* [72] and Gupta *et al.* [73] investigated markers of the inflammatory response in patients offered enteral or parenteral nutrition. Both studies showed less activation of inflammation with enteral feeding. The superiority of early enteral compared to parenteral nutrition has been confirmed in a meta-analysis [74] of eleven trials. **A1c** This meta-analysis showed benefit in terms of lower infection rates for enteral feeding started within 48 hours of admission, but no difference between the two routes if feeding was started later than this. It is possible that the results of these trials are due to stimulation of inflammation and increased septic complications in patients given parenteral feeding, rather than to a specific benefit of enteral feeding. In a small RCT which compared early enteral nutrition with no nutritional support in 27 patients, Powell *et al.* [75] found no difference in clinical outcomes or in immune markers, but this trial probably lacked adequate power.

Nutritional support

Concerning the requirement for nutritional support in patients with severe disease, there is conclusive evidence that the outcome is better and the cost is lower if the enteral rather than the parenteral route is used. Several RCTs and two meta-analyses have demonstrated improved infection rates and glucose control with enteral compared to parenteral nutrition [71, 76–79]. **A1c** Enteral nutrition is the cheaper option, and has become the new "gold standard" for nutritional support in acute pancreatitis.

"Immune-enhanced nutrition"

The type of feeding solution used may influence outcome, by providing a beneficial stimulus to the immune system, and perhaps by specific effects that enhance gut mucosal function. So-called "immune-enhanced nutrition" has been used in a variety of situations, but has not been shown to be superior to routine feeding solutions in acute pancreatitis. Although Hegazi [80] favored the use of immune-enhanced solutions, largely on the basis of experimental data, McClave performed a systematic review [77] that included assessment of the value of specific supplements added to EN, such as arginine, glutamine, omega-3 poly-unsaturated fatty acids and probiotics. The analysis indicated that these agents may be associated with a positive impact on patient outcome in acute pancreatitis, compared with EN alone, but the studies are too few to support strong treatment recommendations.

The case of probiotic bacteria is of interest, because several small studies have shown benefit from enteral nutrition supplemented with various *Lactobacillus* species, often with added dietary fiber [81–83]. However, when tested in a large multicentre study, the probiotic group suffered an excess of deaths, largely due to bowel perforation, usually at the cecum [84]. This well-designed, double-blind trial included 298 patients with severe pancreatitis (APACHE II 8 or more) randomly allocated within 72 hours of onset to receive either a multispecies probiotic preparation (n = 153) or placebo (n = 145), administered enterally twice daily for 28 days. The groups were well matched. There was no difference in infective complications (probiotic 46 (30%), placebo 41 (28%)), but 24 (16%) of the probiotic group died, compared with nine (6%) of the controls. There were nine cases of bowel ischemia in the trial, of which eight were fatal, and all occurred in the probiotic group. This well designed RCT did not confirm the treatment benefit suggested by earlier smaller studies, in patients with severe acute pancreatitis. **A1a**

Management of gallstones causing pancreatitis

All patients with biliary pancreatitis should undergo definitive management of gallstones during the same hospital admission, unless a clear plan has been made for definitive treatment within the next two weeks.

It is essential to deal promptly with gallstones, to prevent a further attack of pancreatitis. A recurrence of pancreatitis may occur at any time, and reports from health care systems in which early cholecystectomy is not universally available confirm the risk of fatal recurrence while awaiting treatment. **B4** Definitive treatment is usually by laparoscopic cholecystectomy with intra-operative cholangiography, carried out as soon as symptoms of pain and anorexia have resolved. Some experts prefer a pre-operative cholangiogram obtained by MRCP. Cholecystectomy is usually achieved within 4–7 days of onset of symptoms. At this time, cholangiography will demonstrate bile duct stones in fewer than 10% of these patients (Figure 24.3) [85]. Bile duct stones may be dealt with by laparoscopic bile duct exploration, or by ERCP and sphincterotomy. Approximately 90% of patients will have a normal bile duct at this time. They need no intervention on the bile duct and avoid the risks associated with endoscopic sphincterotomy. The endoscopic approach carries a well-recognised risk of 5–10% of exacerbation of the pancreatitis and of sphincterotomy

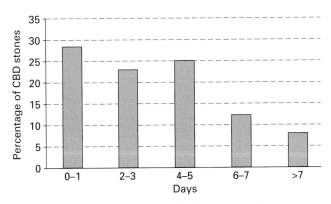

Figure 24.3 Prevalence of gallstones within the common bile duct at the time of cholangiography (days after onset of symptoms) (reproduced from De Waele *et al.* [85]).

bleeding. However, pancreatic duct stenting may reduce the risk of pancreatitis. Endoscopic sphincteroromy may be appropriate in patients in whom there is co-morbidity, which increases the risks of general anaesthesia for chole-cystectomy. **C5** In particular, elderly patients without pre-existing symptoms of cholelithiasis may be appropriate for endoscopic sphincterotomy, with conservative management of the gall bladder stones unless further symptoms arise. **C5**

In acute necrotizing pancreatitis, when surgery is indicated, cholecystectomy should always be done at the time of necrosectomy, if that can be achieved safely. **C5** Patients with severe disease who do not undergo surgery should also have the definitive management of their gallstones planned and carried out before discharge from hospital, although there may be circumstances in which a short delay is acceptable, for example to allow combined management of the stones and a pseudocyst. In any case, management of the gallstones must be integrated into the care plan for each individual.

The role of early ERCP in severe biliary pancreatitis

Patients with signs of cholangitis require endoscopic sphincterotomy or duct drainage by stenting to ensure relief of biliary obstruction. Urgent therapeutic ERCP should be performed in patients with acute pancreatitis of suspected or proven gallstone etiology who satisfy the criteria for predicted or actual severe pancreatitis, or when there is cholangitis, jaundice, or a dilated common bile duct. All patients undergoing early ERCP for severe gall-stone pancreatitis require endoscopic sphincterotomy whether or not stones are found in the bile duct. The indications for early ERCP now seem clearer.

Gallstone related pancreatitis is diagnosed when pancreatitis occurs and there are gallstones in the gall bladder, and

in the absence of any other known reason. The mechanism is related to the passage of a gallstone through the ampulla, with temporary obstruction of flow of pancreatic juice, and possible reflux of bile into the pancreatic duct. ERCP and endoscopic sphincterotomy (ES) prevents further damage by releasing stones form the bile duct, and by preventing further obstruction of, or reflux into, the pancreatic duct. Thus, early ES has been proposed as a preventive measure, to reduce complications. Clearly, there can be no rationale for using early ES in this way in mild disease, where the risk if complications is low, or in non-biliary pancreatitis, where there are no stones to pass through the ampulla. There is general agreement in published guidelines and in one large RCT that in pancreatitis associated with cholangitis, early ES can bring about a marked improvement in the patient's condition and should be performed as soon as practicable, ideally within 24 hours [8, 10–12, 86].

If ERC is attempted in patients with pancreatitis, ES should always be performed to minimize the risk of procedure induced cholangitis. This has been recommended on the basis of an RCT published only in abstract form [87], expert opinion and critical analysis of RCT data. A further preliminary report from Katowice [88] has described a randomized comparison of ERCP with or without ES, in patients with acute biliary pancreatitis who had ERCP within 12 hours of admission, but who had no evidence of cholangitis, biliary obstruction or bile duct stones. The complication rate was higher than expected in patients who did not have a sphincterotomy, especially in patients with mild pancreatitis. This result supports the view that if ERCP is undertaken early in acute pancreatitis, ES should be performed. **A1d**

The first two reported trials of early ERCP +/− ES found a significant reduction in the complication rate in severe biliary pancreatitis [89, 90], but subsequently a debate arose whether early ERCP is appropriate, driven by the results of a large RCT performed in Germany [86], which did not show benefit in a group of patients with mild or severe pancreatitis in whom cholangitis had been excluded. This study included patients with mild disease and sphincterotomy was not performed routinely after cholangiography, making it difficult to interpret the results. A Cochrane Review [91] of these three trials pooled data from 172 patients with severe biliary pancreatitis. The reduction in mortality was not statistically significant, but complications were much less likely after early ERCP (OR 0.27; 95% CI: 0.14–0.53) [91].

Two further studies have helped to clarify the indications for early ERCP. Acosta [92] studied 61 patients with gallstone pancreatitis who had evidence of biliary obstruction but no signs of cholangitis, in whom the obstruction persisted for 24 hours. Patients were randomized to early ERCP or to ERCP in the recovery phase; ES was performed only if there was evidence of obstruction. There were no deaths in this series, but immediate complications (which are likely to be systemic complications) were reduced from 26% to 3% in the early ERCP group. **A1d** There is no comment on the incidence of organ failure in this study, and this study is too small to enable firm conclusions to be drawn. However, the focus on patients with persistence of signs of obstruction is appropriate: there seems little point in early ES if a patient has passed a stone and if signs of systemic disturbance are resolving. **C5**

Oria [93] randomized 103 patients with a dilated bile duct or raised bilirubin, but without evidence of cholangitis, to undergo ES within 72 hours of onset of symptoms, or to standard management without endoscopy. They found no difference in the incidence of organ failure or local complications in the two groups. A crucial unanswered question in considering these trials is the definition of cholangitis. If the presence of SIRS together with biliary obstruction is taken to indicate likely cholangitis, then all patients with severe disease by currently understood definitions are likely to have been excluded.

A recent meta-analysis [94] concluded that there is no benefit from early sphincterotomy in severe gallstone pancreatitis, in the absence of signs of cholangitis. There was no difference in outcome in the treated and control patients in the three trials selected for analysis [86, 90, 93]. This analysis must be questioned, as the inclusion criteria used are puzzling. Two trials were excluded from analysis. The study of Fan et al. [89] was excluded on the grounds that all patients with pancreatitis were included, despite the fact that the outcomes for patients with severe pancreatitis and with gallstones are clearly presented in the report. There was a clear reduction in complications in these patients. This trial had been included in the Cochrane Review cited above [88]. The second trial [92] excluded by Petrov et al. examined the interesting question of the value of ES in patients who had failed to improve in the first 24 hours of admission. In other words, the investigators did not intervene in patients who did not meet current criteria for severity. Again, this trial showed benefit for early ES in appropriately selected patients. Finally, Petrov et al. did include the German study [86] which has been discussed above. This trial is flawed by the inclusion of patients with mild disease, and by the fact that sphincterotomy was not performed routinely. This trial did not support the use of early ES. Thus, the meta-analysis of Petrov et al. excluded two trials supportive of early ES and included a flawed trial that failed to support this approach, and the conclusions cannot be accepted.

A new study is consistent with these observations. Patients enrolled in the PROPATRIA trial [84] were randomly allocated to receive probiotics or not in association with enteral feeding. As noted above, the trial intervention did not produce any benefit. The trial data have been secondarily analyzed to throw light on the role of ERCP/ES,

which was used at the discretion of the responsible clinician. All patients had predicted severe pancreatitis and half had cholestasis (bilirubin > 40 micromol/l and or CBD > 8 mm). Differences in baseline features were taken into account in the recent preliminary report [95]. Of 78 patients with cholestasis, 56 had early ERCP/ES, with significant reduction in overall complications and the frequency of necrosis affecting more than 30% of the pancreas. Early ERCP/ES (n = 29) had no effect on complication rates in the 75 patients without evidence of cholestasis. **A1d**

Early (<72 hours of admission) ERCP/ES can be restricted to patients with *severe* acute pancreatitis, especially those with persistent SIRS or organ failure, who have *gallstones*, and who have signs of *cholestasis*. If signs of biliary obstruction, organ failure or SIRS resolve, ES may be deferred. If the bile duct is cannulated, a sphincterotomy should be performed.

Intervention for necrosis

All patients with persistent symptoms and greater than 30% pancreatic necrosis, and those with smaller areas of necrosis and clinical suspicion of sepsis, should undergo image guided fine needle aspiration to obtain material for culture 7–14 days after the onset of the pancreatitis. Patients with infected necrosis will require intervention to completely debride all cavities containing necrotic material. The choice of surgical technique for necrosectomy, and subsequent postoperative management depends on individual features and locally available expertise.

It is widely accepted that infected necrosis requires intervention, and that sterile necrosis can be managed expectantly in the majority of cases [10, 12]. The range of techniques advocated for the management of infected necrosis attests to our lack of knowledge and the difficulty of formulating a simple treatment policy in the face of a complex and variable disease. The crucial information required to determine the choice of antibiotic and the need for intervention, that is the presence or absence of infection and the sensitivities of the infecting organism(s), is usually provided by culture of fine needle aspirates from the necrotic material. Fine needle aspiration is safe and reliable in experienced hands [96, 97]. In a survey of European practice [98] most respondents regularly use fine needle aspiration and, of these, the large majority (131 of 174) use the culture results to determine the need for surgery. **C5** Sometimes aspiration may be omitted, if it is clear from imaging that the patient requires intervention. For example, the presence of gas bubbles in the necrotic cavity is convincing evidence of infection.

Several surgical approaches have been advocated for dealing with infected necrosis. It is difficult to compare different series and different techniques because of variations in the criteria for selection of patients for treatment. Most guidelines provide recommendations about indications for surgical intervention, but have avoided definitive statements about choice of technique [10, 12]. A small RCT that compared debridement and drainage with debridement and postoperative irrigation, was abandoned because of the poor outcome in the irrigation group [99]. Complete operative debridement of necrotic material by open exploration of all the cavities and blunt dissection or separation of the necrosis is currently the standard approach [100]. There are reports of transperitoneal laparoscopic access to achieve complete debridement [101–104]. Other minimally invasive approaches that are being evaluated include percutaneous debridement, using an image-guided drain track for access [105–116], endoscopic debridement with endoscopic ultrasound guidance [117–123], video-assisted retroperitoneal dissection using a limited posterior incision [124], and non-operative management with targeted antibiotic therapy and percutaneous drainage [125]. Non-operative management may be possible for some patients, but not all respond, and a high proportion go to surgery. Percutaneous necrosectomy is successful in many cases, especially if the necrosis affects mainly the body and tail, but may require multiple treatment sessions, whereas open necrosectomy can achieve complete debridement in one intervention, at the cost of greater morbidity. The newer transgastric and retroperitoneal techniques appear to offer alternative access routes, but are suitable only for patients with an appropriately placed necrotic cavity. Complex and extensive necrosis may need more extensive access, or a combination of approaches. Mortality rates are similar with all these techniques. The conclusion to be drawn from this range of options is that they are complementary rather than competing, and that different situations may be treated by different techniques. **C5** In each center treating pancreatic necrosis, there should be the skills to provide percutaneous drainage, some kind of minimally invasive necrosectomy, and open surgical debridement.

There is growing consensus that delay before operation is advantageous. One RCT showed lower mortality with operation after day 12, compared with operation in the first few days [126]. **A1d** Numerous series report acceptable mortality rates (15–25%) in patients operated for infected necrosis more than two or three weeks from onset. If operation is planned, it is best delayed until after three weeks of the illness if at all possible. At this stage, the cavity is usually demarcated, and the necrotic material is easier to separate from viable tissue than at earlier operation. The optimum period of delay has not been defined, but most patients with infected necrosis will show systemic signs of infection, and will be sufficiently stable for operative intervention, 3–5 weeks after onset. There seems little advantage in delay beyond five weeks in the large majority of patients. **C5**

Abdominal compartment syndrome

Acute pancreatitis is associated with inflammatory oedema of the pancreas and peripancreatic tissues. There may be accumulation of large volumes of fluid in the peritoneal cavity and the bowel may become distended by oedema and ileus. This can lead to raised intra-abdominal pressure. Organ failure occurs in the abdominal compartment syndrome (ACS) as a result of impaired ventilation (pressure on the diaphragm), hypotension (reduced venous return) and renal failure (increased filtration pressure required). ACS is well recognised in critically ill patients and is best treated by surgical decompression [127–129]. ACS is increasingly recognized as a mechanism of organ failure in acute pancreatitis.

In 2005, Gecalter [130] de Waele [131] and Wong [132] described a total of five cases of ACS in severe pancreatitis with apparent improvement after decompression. Other case reports have suggested similar outcomes [133–136]. Standard surgical management is upper abdominal laparostomy; a less invasive approach by subcutaneous fasciotomy has been proposed [136]. Several case series have indicated the value of surgical decompression, but there are no randomized trials reported. Early experience was reviewed in 2007 [137]. A further seven case series, including a total of 351 patients with severe acute pancreatitis, report consistently that raised intra-abdominal pressure correlates well with increasing severity of pancreatitis, worse organ failure, and with fatal outcome [138–144]. One report showed a correlation of abdominal pressure with CT severity index [142], and it has been suggested that raised intra-abdominal pressure in the first week of illness may predict outcome in terms of organ failure and death [141]. Chen [138] and Albahrani [139] both reported clear improvement in clinical condition in most patients after abdominal decompression. **B4** Although a randomized trial would be difficult to perform, further observational data comparing outcomes in patients who were decompressed with those in similar patients who did not undergo decompression are needed to confirm these observations.

Acknowledgement

Hassan Elberm is the recipient of a Fellowship from the Government of Syria.

References

1 Goldacre MJ, Roberts SE. Hospital admission for acute pancreatitis in an English population, 1963–1998: Database study of incidence and mortality. *BMJ* 2004; **328**(7454): 1466–1469.

2 Lowenfels AB, Sullivan T, Fiorianti J *et al.* The epidemiology and impact of pancreatic diseases in the United States. *Curr Gastroenterol Rep* 2005; **7**(2): 90–95.

3 Sekimoto M, Takada T, Kawarada Y *et al.* JPN Guidelines for the management of acute pancreatitis: Epidemiology, etiology, natural history, and outcome predictors in acute pancreatitis. *J Hepatobiliary Pancreat Surg* 2006; **13**(1): 10–24.

4 Yadav D, Lowenfels AB. Trends in the epidemiology of the first attack of acute pancreatitis: A systematic review. *Pancreas* 2006; **33**(4): 323–330.

5 Spanier BW, Dijkgraaf MG, Bruno MJ. Epidemiology, aetiology and outcome of acute and chronic pancreatitis: An update. *Best Pract Res Clin Gastroenterol* 2008; **22**(1): 45–63.

6 O'Farrell A, Allwright S, Toomey D *et al.* Hospital admission for acute pancreatitis in the Irish population, 1997–2004: Could the increase be due to an increase in alcohol-related pancreatitis? *J Public Health (Oxf)* 2007; **29**(4): 398–404.

7 Frey CF, Zhou H, Harvey DJ *et al.* The incidence and case-fatality rates of acute biliary, alcoholic, and idiopathic pancreatitis in California, 1994–2001. *Pancreas* 2006; **33**(4): 336–344.

8 Banks PA. Practice guidelines in acute pancreatitis. *Am J Gastroenterol* 1997; **92**(3): 377–386.

9 Banks PA, Freeman ML. Practice guidelines in acute pancreatitis. *Am J Gastroenterol* 2006; **101**(10): 2379–2400.

10 Toouli J, Brooke-Smith M, Bassi C *et al.* Guidelines for the management of acute pancreatitis. *J Gastroenterol Hepatol* 2002; **17**(Suppl): S15–S39.

11 United Kingdom guidelines for the management of acute pancreatitis. British Society of Gastroenterology. *Gut* 1998; **42** (Suppl 2): S1–13.

12 UK guidelines for the management of acute pancreatitis: First revision. *Gut* 2005; **54** (Suppl 3): iii1–iii9.

13 Wu BU, Johannes RS, Sun X *et al.* The early prediction of mortality in acute pancreatitis: A large population-based study. *Gut* 2008; **57**(12): 1698–1703.

14 Sternby B, O'Brien JF, Zinsmeister AR *et al.* What is the best biochemical test to diagnose acute pancreatitis? A prospective clinical study. *Mayo Clin Proc* 1996; **71**(12): 1138–1144.

15 Balthazar EJ. CT diagnosis and staging of acute pancreatitis. *Radiol Clin North Am* 1989; **27**(1): 19–37.

16 Block S, Maier W, Bittner R *et al.* Identification of pancreas necrosis in severe acute pancreatitis: Imaging procedures versus clinical staging. *Gut* 1986; **27**(9): 1035–1042.

17 Kivisaari L, Somer K, Standertskjold-Nordenstam CG *et al.* Early detection of acute fulminant pancreatitis by contrast-enhanced computed tomography. *Scand J Gastroenterol* 1983; **18**(1): 39–41.

18 Frossard JL, Steer ML, Pastor CM. Acute pancreatitis. *Lancet* 2008; **371**(9607): 143–152.

19 Bradley EL, III. A clinically based classification system for acute pancreatitis. Summary of the International Symposium on Acute Pancreatitis, Atlanta, Ga, September 11 through 13, 1992. *Arch Surg* 1993; **128**(5): 586–590.

20 Bone RC. Immunologic dissonance: A continuing evolution in our understanding of the systemic inflammatory response syndrome (SIRS) and the multiple organ dysfunction syndrome (MODS). *Ann Intern Med* 1996; **125**(8): 680–687.

21 Mofidi R, Duff MD, Wigmore SJ *et al.* Association between early systemic inflammatory response, severity of multiorgan dys-

function and death in acute pancreatitis. *Br J Surg* 2006; **93**(6): 738–744.

22 Buter A, Imrie CW, Carter CR *et al.* Dynamic nature of early organ dysfunction determines outcome in acute pancreatitis. *Br J Surg* 2002; **89**(3): 298–302.

23 Johnson CD, Abu-Hilal M. Persistent organ failure during the first week as a marker of fatal outcome in acute pancreatitis. *Gut* 2004; **53**(9): 1340–1304.

24 Lytras D, Manes K, Triantopoulou C *et al.* Persistent early organ failure: Defining the high-risk group of patients with severe acute pancreatitis? *Pancreas* 2008; **36**(3): 249–254.

25 Shaheen MA, Akhtar AJ. Organ failure associated with acute pancreatitis in African-American and Hispanic patients. *J Natl Med Assoc* 2007; **99**(12): 1402–1406.

26 Rau BM, Bothe A, Kron M *et al.* Role of early multisystem organ failure as major risk factor for pancreatic infections and death in severe acute pancreatitis. *Clin Gastroenterol Hepatol* 2006; **4**(8): 1053–1061.

27 Poves P, I, Fabregat PJ, Garcia Borobia FJ *et al.* Early onset of organ failure is the best predictor of mortality in acute pancreatitis. *Rev Esp Enferm Dig* 2004; **96**(10): 705–709.

28 Marshall JC, Cook DJ, Christou NV *et al.* Multiple organ dysfunction score: A reliable descriptor of a complex clinical outcome. *Crit Care Med* 1995; **23**(10): 1638–1652.

29 Halonen KI, Pettila V, Leppaniemi AK *et al.* Multiple organ dysfunction associated with severe acute pancreatitis. *Crit Care Med* 2002; **30**(6): 1274–1279.

30 Dervenis C, Johnson CD, Bassi C *et al.* Diagnosis, objective assessment of severity, and management of acute pancreatitis. Santorini consensus conference. *Int J Pancreatol* 1999; **25**(3): 195–210.

31 Martinez J, Johnson CD, Sanchez-Paya J *et al.* Obesity is a definitive risk factor of severity and mortality in acute pancreatitis: An updated meta-analysis. *Pancreatology* 2006; **6**(3): 206–209.

32 McKay CJ, Evans S, Sinclair M *et al.* High early mortality rate from acute pancreatitis in Scotland, 1984–1995. *Br J Surg* 1999; **86**(10): 1302–1305.

33 Sempere L, Martinez J, de ME *et al.* Obesity and fat distribution imply a greater systemic inflammatory response and a worse prognosis in acute pancreatitis. *Pancreatology* 2008; **8**(3): 257–264.

34 Papachristou GI, Papachristou DJ, Avula H *et al.* Obesity increases the severity of acute pancreatitis: Performance of APACHE-O score and correlation with the inflammatory response. *Pancreatology* 2006; **6**(4): 279–285.

35 Larvin M. (1998) Assessment of Clinical Severity and Prognosis. In: Beger HG, Warshaw AL, Buchler MW *et al.*, eds. *The Pancreas.* Blackwell Science, Oxford, 1998: 489–502.

36 Garcea G, Jackson B, Pattenden CJ *et al.* Progression of early warning scores (EWS) in patients with acute pancreatitis: A re-evaluation of a retrospective cohort of patients. *Postgrad Med J* 2008; **84**(991): 271–275.

37 Garcea G, Jackson B, Pattenden CJ *et al.* Early warning scores predict outcome in acute pancreatitis. *J Gastrointest Surg* 2006; **10**(7): 1008–1015.

38 Johnson CD, Lempinen M, Imrie CW *et al.* Urinary trypsinogen activation peptide as a marker of severe acute pancreatitis. *Br J Surg* 2004; **91**(8): 1027–1033.

39 Kemppainen E, Mayer J, Puolakkainen P *et al.* Plasma trypsinogen activation peptide in patients with acute pancreatitis. *Br J Surg* 2001; **88**(5): 679–80.

40 Neoptolemos JP, Kemppainen EA, Mayer JM *et al.* Early prediction of severity in acute pancreatitis by urinary trypsinogen activation peptide: A multicentre study. *Lancet* 2000; **355**(9219): 1955–1960.

41 Tenner S, Fernandez-del Castillo C, Warshaw A *et al.* Urinary trypsinogen activation peptide (TAP) predicts severity in patients with acute pancreatitis. *Int J Pancreatol* 1997; **21**(2): 105–110.

42 Lempinen M, Stenman UH, Finne P *et al.* Trypsinogen-2 and trypsinogen activation peptide (TAP) in urine of patients with acute pancreatitis. *J Surg Res* 2003; **111**(2): 267–273.

43 Kylanpaa-Back ML, Kemppainen E, Puolakkainen P *et al.* Comparison of urine trypsinogen-2 test strip with serum lipase in the diagnosis of acute pancreatitis. *Hepatogastroenterology* 2002; **49**(46): 1130–1134.

44 Lempinen M, Kylanpaa-Back ML, Stenman UH *et al.* Predicting the severity of acute pancreatitis by rapid measurement of trypsinogen-2 in urine. *Clin Chem* 2001; **47**(12): 2103–2107.

45 Modrau IS, Floyd AK, Thorlacius-Ussing O. The clinical value of procalcitonin in early assessment of acute pancreatitis. *Am J Gastroenterol* 2005; **100**(7): 1593–1597.

46 Frasquet J, Saez J, Trigo C *et al.* Early measurement of procalcitonin does not predict severity in patients with acute pancreatitis. *Br J Surg* 2003; **90**(9): 1129–1130.

47 Purkayastha S, Chow A, Athanasiou T *et al.* Does serum procalcitonin have a role in evaluating the severity of acute pancreatitis? A question revisited. *World J Surg* 2006; **30**(9): 1713–1721.

48 Rau BM, Kemppainen EA, Gumbs AA *et al.* Early assessment of pancreatic infections and overall prognosis in severe acute pancreatitis by procalcitonin (PCT): A prospective international multicenter study. *Ann Surg* 2007; **245**(5): 745–754.

49 Gurda-Duda A, Kusnierz-Cabala B, Nowak W *et al.* Assessment of the prognostic value of certain acute-phase proteins and procalcitonin in the prognosis of acute pancreatitis. *Pancreas* 2008; **37**(4): 449–453.

50 Balthazar EJ. Acute pancreatitis: Assessment of severity with clinical and CT evaluation. *Radiology* 2002; **223**(3): 603–613.

51 Matos C, Bali MA, Delhaye M *et al.* Magnetic resonance imaging in the detection of pancreatitis and pancreatic neoplasms. *Best Pract Res Clin Gastroenterol* 2006; **20**(1): 157–178.

52 Buchler MW, Gloor B, Muller CA *et al.* Acute necrotizing pancreatitis: treatment strategy according to the status of infection. *Ann Surg* 2000; **232**(5): 619–626.

53 Uhl W, Roggo A, Kirschstein T *et al.* Influence of contrast-enhanced computed tomography on course and outcome in patients with acute pancreatitis. *Pancreas* 2002; **24**(2): 191–197.

54 Brown A, Baillargeon JD, Hughes MD *et al.* Can fluid resuscitation prevent pancreatic necrosis in severe acute pancreatitis? *Pancreatology* 2002; **2**(2): 104–107.

55 Chiappini F, Fuso L, Pistelli R. Accuracy of a pulse oximeter in the measurement of the oxyhaemoglobin saturation. *Eur Respir J* 1998; **11**(3): 716–719.

56 de Vries AC, Besselink MG, Buskens E *et al.* Randomized controlled trials of antibiotic prophylaxis in severe acute pancreatitis: Relationship between methodological quality and outcome. *Pancreatology* 2007; **7**(5–6): 531–538.

57 Isenmann R, Runzi M, Kron M *et al.* Prophylactic antibiotic treatment in patients with predicted severe acute pancreatitis: A placebo-controlled, double-blind trial. *Gastroenterology* 2004; **126**(4): 997–1004.

58 Villatoro E, Bassi C, Larvin M. Antibiotic therapy for prophylaxis against infection of pancreatic necrosis in acute pancreatitis. *Cochrane Database of Systematic Reviews* 2006, Issue 4. Art. No.: CD002941. DOI: 10.1002/14651858.CD002941.pub2.

59 Sainio V, Kemppainen E, Puolakkainen P *et al.* Early antibiotic treatment in acute necrotising pancreatitis. *Lancet* 1995; **346**(8976): 663–667.

60 Mazaki T, Ishii Y, Takayama T. Meta-analysis of prophylactic antibiotic use in acute necrotizing pancreatitis. *Br J Surg* 2006; **93**(6): 674–684.

61 Spicak J, Hejtmankova S, Cech P *et al.* Antibiotic prophylaxis in large pancreatic necrosis: Multicenter randomized trial with ciprofloxacin and metronidazole or meropenem. *Gastroenterology* 2004; **126**(suppl 2): A229.

62 Dellinger EP, Tellado JM, Soto NE *et al.* Early antibiotic treatment for severe acute necrotizing pancreatitis: A randomized, double-blind, placebo-controlled study. *Ann Surg* 2007; **245**(5): 674-6-83.

63 Garcia-Barrasa A, Borobia FG, Pallares R *et al.* A double-blind, placebo-controlled trial of ciprofloxacin prophylaxis in patients with acute necrotizing pancreatitis. *J Gastrointest Surg* 2008; **13**: 768–774

64 Naeije R, Salingret E, Clumeck N *et al.* Is nasogastric suction necessary in acute pancreatitis? *Br Med J* 1978; **2**(6138): 659–660.

65 Sarr MG, Sanfey H, Cameron JL. Prospective, randomized trial of nasogastric suction in patients with acute pancreatitis. *Surgery* 1986; **100**(3): 500–504.

66 Levy P, Heresbach D, Pariente EA *et al.* Frequency and risk factors of recurrent pain during refeeding in patients with acute pancreatitis: A multivariate multicentre prospective study of 116 patients. *Gut* 1997; **40**(2): 262–266.

67 Eatock FC, Brombacher GD, Steven A *et al.* Nasogastric feeding in severe acute pancreatitis may be practical and safe. *Int J Pancreatol* 2000; **28**(1): 23–29.

68 Kumar A, Singh N, Prakash S *et al.* Early enteral nutrition in severe acute pancreatitis: A prospective randomized controlled trial comparing nasojejunal and nasogastric routes. *J Clin Gastroenterol* 2006; **40**(5): 431–434.

69 Iovanna JL, Keim V, Michel R *et al.* Pancreatic gene expression is altered during acute experimental pancreatitis in the rat. *Am J Physiol* 1991; **261**(3 Pt 1): G485–G489.

70 O'Keefe SJ, Lee RB, Li J *et al.* Trypsin secretion and turnover in patients with acute pancreatitis. *Am J Physiol Gastrointest Liver Physiol* 2005; **289**(2): G181–G187.

71 Kalfarentzos F, Kehagias J, Mead N *et al.* Enteral nutrition is superior to parenteral nutrition in severe acute pancreatitis: Results of a randomized prospective trial. *Br J Surg* 1997; **84**(12): 1665–1659.

72 Windsor AC, Kanwar S, Li AG *et al.* Compared with parenteral nutrition, enteral feeding attenuates the acute phase response and improves disease severity in acute pancreatitis. *Gut* 1998; **42**(3): 431–435.

73 Gupta R, Patel K, Calder PC *et al.* A randomized clinical trial to assess the effect of total enteral and total parenteral nutritional

support on metabolic, inflammatory and oxidative markers in patients with predicted severe acute pancreatitis (APACHE II > or = 6). *Pancreatology* 2003; **3**(5): 406–413.

74 Petrov MS, Pylypchuk RD, Uchugina AF. A systematic review on the timing of artificial nutrition in acute pancreatitis. *Br J Nutr* 2008; **101**: 787–793.

75 Powell JJ, Murchison JT, Fearon KC *et al*. Randomized controlled trial of the effect of early enteral nutrition on markers of the inflammatory response in predicted severe acute pancreatitis. *Br J Surg* 2000; **87**(10): 1375–1381.

76 Abou-Assi S, Craig K, O'Keefe SJ. Hypocaloric jejunal feeding is better than total parenteral nutrition in acute pancreatitis: Results of a randomized comparative study. *Am J Gastroenterol* 2002; **97**(9): 2255–2262.

77 McClave SA, Chang WK, Dhaliwal R *et al*. Nutrition support in acute pancreatitis: A systematic review of the literature. *JPEN J Parenter Enteral Nutr* 2006; **30**(2): 143–156.

78 Petrov MS, van Santvoort HC, Besselink MG *et al*. Enteral nutrition and the risk of mortality and infectious complications in patients with severe acute pancreatitis: A meta-analysis of randomized trials. *Arch Surg* 2008; **143**(11): 1111–1117.

79 Marik PE, Zaloga GP. Meta-analysis of parenteral nutrition versus enteral nutrition in patients with acute pancreatitis. *BMJ* 2004; **328**(7453): 1407.

80 Hegazi RA, O'Keefe SJ. Nutritional immunomodulation of acute pancreatitis. *Curr Gastroenterol Rep* 2007; **9**(2): 99–106.

81 Karakan T, Ergun M, Dogan I *et al*. Comparison of early enteral nutrition in severe acute pancreatitis with prebiotic fiber supplementation versus standard enteral solution: A prospective randomized double-blind study. *World J Gastroenterol* 2007; **13**(19): 2733–2737.

82 Olah A, Belagyi T, Issekutz A *et al*. Randomized clinical trial of specific lactobacillus and fibre supplement to early enteral nutrition in patients with acute pancreatitis. *Br J Surg* 2002; **89**(9): 1103–1107.

83 Qin HL, Zheng JJ, Tong DN *et al*. Effect of Lactobacillus plantarum enteral feeding on the gut permeability and septic complications in the patients with acute pancreatitis. *Eur J Clin Nutr* 2008; **62**(7): 923–930.

84 Besselink MG, van Santvoort HC, Buskens E *et al*. Probiotic prophylaxis in predicted severe acute pancreatitis: A randomized, double-blind, placebo-controlled trial. *Lancet* 2008; **371**(9613): 651–659.

85 De Waele E, Op de Beeck B, De Waele B *et al*. Magnetic resonance cholangiopancreatography in the preoperative assessment of patients with biliary pancreatitis. *Pancreatology* 2007; **7**(4): 347–351.

86 Folsch UR, Nitsche R, Ludtke R *et al*. Early ERCP and papillotomy compared with conservative treatment for acute biliary pancreatitis. The German Study Group on Acute Biliary Pancreatitis. *N Engl J Med* 1997; **336**(4): 237–242.

87 Nowak A, Nowakowska-Dulawa E, Marek TA. Final results of the prospective, randomized, controlled study on endoscopic sphincterotomy versus conventional management in acute biliary pancreatitis. *Gastroenterology* 1995; **108**: A380.

88 Nowakowska-Dulawa E, Nowak A, Marek TA *et al*. Urgent endoscopic sphincterotomy in patients with acute biliary pancreatitis without common bile duct stones. *Pancreatology* 2008; **8**: 348.

89 Fan ST, Lai EC, Mok FP *et al*. Early treatment of acute biliary pancreatitis by endoscopic papillotomy. *N Engl J Med* 1993; **328**(4): 228–232.

90 Neoptolemos JP, Carr-Locke DL, London NJ *et al*. Controlled trial of urgent endoscopic retrograde cholangiopancreatography and endoscopic sphincterotomy versus conservative treatment for acute pancreatitis due to gallstones. *Lancet* 1988; **2**(8618): 979–983.

91 Ayub K, Slavin J, Imada R. Endoscopic retrograde cholangiopancreatography in gallstone-associated acute pancreatitis. *Cochrane Database of Systematic Reviews* 2004, Issue 3. Art. No.: CD003630. DOI: 10.1002/14651858.CD003630.pub2.

92 Acosta JM, Katkhouda N, Debian KA *et al*. Early ductal decompression versus conservative management for gallstone pancreatitis with ampullary obstruction: A prospective randomized clinical trial. *Ann Surg* 2006; **243**(1): 33–40.

93 Oria A, Cimmino D, Ocampo C *et al*. Early endoscopic intervention versus early conservative management in patients with acute gallstone pancreatitis and biliopancreatic obstruction: A randomized clinical trial. *Ann Surg* 2007; **245**(1): 10–17.

94 Petrov MS, van Santvoort HC, Besselink MG *et al*. Early endoscopic retrograde cholangiopancreatography versus conservative management in acute biliary pancreatitis without cholangitis: A meta-analysis of randomized trials. *Ann Surg* 2008; **247**(2): 250–257.

95 van Santvoort HC, Besselink MG, de Vries AC *et al*. Early ERCP is only beneficial in predicted severe acute biliary pancreatitis in presence of cholestasis. *Pancreatology* 2008; **8**: 337.

96 Rau B, Steinbach G, Baumgart K *et al*. The clinical value of procalcitonin in the prediction of infected necrois in acute pancreatitis. *Intensive Care Med* 2000; **26** (Suppl 2): S159–S164.

97 Pezzilli R, Uomo G, Zerbi A *et al*. Diagnosis and treatment of acute pancreatitis: The position statement of the Italian Association for the study of the pancreas. *Dig Liver Dis* 2008; **40**(10): 803–808.

98 King NK, Siriwardena AK. European survey of surgical strategies for the management of severe acute pancreatitis. *Am J Gastroenterol* 2004; **99**(4): 719–728.

99 Teerenhovi O, Nordback I, Eskola J. High volume lesser sac lavage in acute necrotizing pancreatitis. *Br J Surg* 1989; **76**(4): 370–373.

100 Berzin TM, Mortele KJ, Banks PA. The management of suspected pancreatic sepsis. *Gastroenterol Clin North Am* 2006; **35**(2): 393–407.

101 Owera AM, Ammori BJ. Laparoscopic endogastric and transgastric cystgastrostomy and pancreatic necrosectomy. *Hepatogastroenterology* 2008; **55**(81): 262–265.

102 Parekh D. Laparoscopic-assisted pancreatic necrosectomy: A new surgical option for treatment of severe necrotizing pancreatitis. *Arch Surg* 2006; **141**(9): 895–902.

103 Adamson GD, Cuschieri A. Multimedia article. Laparoscopic infracolic necrosectomy for infected pancreatic necrosis. *Surg Endosc* 2003; **17**(10): 1675.

104 Hamad GG, Broderick TJ. Laparoscopic pancreatic necrosectomy. *J Laparoendosc Adv Surg Tech A* 2000; **10**(2): 115–118.

105 Carter CR, McKay CJ, Imrie CW. Percutaneous necrosectomy and sinus tract endoscopy in the management of infected pan-

creatic necrosis: An initial experience. *Ann Surg* 2000; **232**(2): 175–180.

106 Zuber-Jerger I, Zorger N, Kullmann F. Minimal invasive necrosectomy in severe pancreatitis. *Clin Gastroenterol Hepatol* 2007; **5**(11): e45.

107 Windsor JA. Minimally invasive pancreatic necrosectomy. *Br J Surg* 2007; **94**(2): 132–133.

108 Shelat VG, Diddapur RK. Minimally invasive retroperitoneal pancreatic necrosectomy in necrotising pancreatitis. *Singapore Med J* 2007; **48**(8): e220–e223.

109 Risse O, Auguste T, Delannoy P *et al*. Percutaneous video-assisted necrosectomy for infected pancreatic necrosis. *Gastroenterol Clin Biol* 2004; **28**(10 Pt 1): 868–871.

110 Loveday BP, Mittal A, Phillips A *et al*. Minimally invasive management of pancreatic abscess, pseudocyst, and necrosis: A systematic review of current guidelines. *World J Surg* 2008; **32**(11): 2383–2394.

111 Horvath KD, Kao LS, Wherry KL *et al*. A technique for laparoscopic-assisted percutaneous drainage of infected pancreatic necrosis and pancreatic abscess. *Surg Endosc* 2001; **15**(10): 1221–1225.

112 Endlicher E, Volk M, Feuerbach S *et al*. Long-term follow-up of patients with necrotizing pancreatitis treated by percutaneous necrosectomy. *Hepatogastroenterology* 2003; **50**(54): 2225–2258.

113 Connor S, Ghaneh P, Raraty M *et al*. Minimally invasive retroperitoneal pancreatic necrosectomy. *Dig Surg* 2003; **20**(4): 270–277.

114 Cheung MT, Ho CN, Siu KW *et al*. Percutaneous drainage and necrosectomy in the management of pancreatic necrosis. *ANZ J Surg* 2005; **75**(4): 204–207.

115 Bucher P, Pugin F, Morel P. Minimally invasive necrosectomy for infected necrotizing pancreatitis. *Pancreas* 2008; **36**(2): 113–119.

116 Bruennler T, Langgartner J, Lang S *et al*. Percutaneous necrosectomy in patients with acute, necrotizing pancreatitis. *Eur Radiol* 2008; **18**(8): 1604–1610.

117 Hocke M, Will U, Gottschalk P *et al*. Transgastral retroperitoneal endoscopy in septic patients with pancreatic necrosis or infected pancreatic pseudocysts. *Z Gastroenterol* 2008; **46**(12): 1363–1368.

118 Mathew A, Biswas A, Meitz KP. Endoscopic necrosectomy as primary treatment for infected peripancreatic fluid collections (with video). *Gastrointest Endosc* 2008; **68**(4): 776–782.

119 Antillon MR, Bechtold ML, Bartalos CR *et al*. Transgastric endoscopic necrosectomy with temporary metallic esophageal stent placement for the treatment of infected pancreatic necrosis (with video). *Gastrointest Endosc* 2009; **69**: 178–180.

120 Schrover IM, Weusten BL, Besselink MG *et al*. EUS-guided endoscopic transgastric necrosectomy in patients with infected necrosis in acute pancreatitis. *Pancreatology* 2008; **8**(3): 271–276.

121 Voermans RP, Veldkamp MC, Rauws EA *et al*. Endoscopic transmural debridement of symptomatic organized pancreatic necrosis (with videos). *Gastrointest Endosc* 2007; **66**(5): 909–916.

122 Papachristou GI, Takahashi N, Chahal P *et al*. Peroral endoscopic drainage/debridement of walled-off pancreatic necrosis. *Ann Surg* 2007; **245**(6): 943–951.

123 Charnley RM, Lochan R, Gray H *et al*. Endoscopic necrosectomy as primary therapy in the management of infected pancreatic necrosis. *Endoscopy* 2006; **38**(9): 925–928.

124 Besselink MG, van Santvoort HC, Nieuwenhuijs VB *et al*. Minimally invasive "step-up approach" versus maximal necrosectomy in patients with acute necrotising pancreatitis (PANTER trial): Design and rationale of a randomized controlled multicenter trial [ISRCTN38327949]. *BMC Surg* 2006; **6**: 6.

125 Runzi M, Niebel W, Goebell H *et al*. Severe acute pancreatitis: Nonsurgical treatment of infected necroses. *Pancreas* 2005; **30**(3): 195–199.

126 Mier J, Leon EL, Castillo A *et al*. Early versus late necrosectomy in severe necrotizing pancreatitis. *Am J Surg* 1997; **173**(2): 71–75.

127 Hunter JD. Abdominal compartment syndrome: An underdiagnosed contributory factor to morbidity and mortality in the critically ill. *Postgrad Med J* 2008; **84**(992): 293–298.

128 An G, West MA. Abdominal compartment syndrome: A concise clinical review. *Crit Care Med* 2008; **36**(4): 1304–1310.

129 Schein M, Wittmann DH, Aprahamian CC *et al*. The abdominal compartment syndrome: The physiological and clinical consequences of elevated intra-abdominal pressure. *J Am Coll Surg* 1995; **180**(6): 745–753.

130 Gecelter G, Fahoum B, Gardezi S *et al*. Abdominal compartment syndrome in severe acute pancreatitis: An indication for a decompressing laparotomy? *Dig Surg* 2002; **19**(5): 402–404.

131 De Waele JJ, Hesse UJ. Life saving abdominal decompression in a patient with severe acute pancreatitis. *Acta Chir Belg* 2005; **105**(1): 96–98.

132 Wong K, Summerhays CF. Abdominal compartment syndrome: A new indication for operative intervention in severe acute pancreatitis. *Int J Clin Pract* 2005; **59**(12): 1479–1481.

133 Jonsson M, Linder S, Soderlund C. Life-saving decompression in abdominal compartment syndrome and severe acute pancreatitis. *Lakartidningen* 2008; **105**(40): 2770–2771.

134 Siebig S, Iesalnieks I, Bruennler T *et al*. Recovery from respiratory failure after decompression laparotomy for severe acute pancreatitis. *World J Gastroenterol* 2008; **14**(35): 5467–5470.

135 Leppaniemi A, Mentula P, Hienonen P *et al*. Transverse laparostomy is feasible and effective in the treatment of abdominal compartment syndrome in severe acute pancreatitis. *World J Emerg Surg* 2008; **3**: 6.

136 Leppaniemi AK, Hienonen PA, Siren JE *et al*. Treatment of abdominal compartment syndrome with subcutaneous anterior abdominal fasciotomy in severe acute pancreatitis. *World J Surg* 2006; **30**(10): 1922–1924.

137 Leppaniemi A, Johansson K, De Waele JJ. Abdominal compartment syndrome and acute pancreatitis. *Acta Clin Belg Suppl* 2007; **1**: 131–135.

138 Chen H, Li F, Sun JB *et al*. Abdominal compartment syndrome in patients with severe acute pancreatitis in early stage. *World J Gastroenterol* 2008; **14**(22): 3541–3548.

139 Al-Bahrani AZ, Abid GH, Holt A *et al*. Clinical relevance of intra-abdominal hypertension in patients with severe acute pancreatitis. *Pancreas* 2008; **36**(1): 39–43.

140 Pupelis G, Plaudis H, Snippe K *et al*. Increased intra-abdominal pressure: Is it of any consequence in severe acute pancreatitis? *HPB (Oxford)* 2006; **8**(3): 227–232.

141 Zhang WF, Ni YL, Cai L *et al.* Intra-abdominal pressure monitoring in predicting outcome of patients with severe acute pancreatitis. *Hepatobiliary Pancreat Dis Int* 2007; **6**(4): 420–423.

142 Rosas JM, Soto SN, Aracil JS *et al.* Intra-abdominal pressure as a marker of severity in acute pancreatitis. *Surgery* 2007; **141**(2): 173–178.

143 Keskinen P, Leppaniemi A, Pettila V *et al.* Intra-abdominal pressure in severe acute pancreatitis. *World J Emerg Surg* 2007; **2**: 2.

144 Tao J, Wang C, Chen L *et al.* Diagnosis and management of severe acute pancreatitis complicated with abdominal compartment syndrome. *J Huazhong Univ Sci Technolog Med Sci* 2003; **23**(4): 399–402.

25 Obesity management: Considerations for the gastroenterologist

Leah Gramlich[1], Marilyn Zeman[1] and Arya M Sharma[2]

[1] Division of Gastroenterology, Royal Alexandra Hospital, University of Alberta, Edmonton, Canada
[2] Division of Endocrinology, University of Alberta, Edmonton, Canada

Introduction

Obesity is one of the most prevalent health problems in the Western world [1]. Obesity increases the risk of medical illness and premature death [2] and imposes an enormous economic burden on the health care system [3]. Obesity is also associated with a reduced quality of life, resulting from substantial limitations and restrictions in activities of daily living [4]. Obese individuals are less likely to obtain insurance, employment or promotion or to enjoy personal relationships [5]. Prevention and treatment of obesity is now widely recognized as an important priority for most health care systems.

Obesity is best defined as the accumulation of excess body fat that threatens or affects an individual's mental, physical or economic well-being. At a population level, the body-mass index (BMI) has been widely used to characterize and define obesity. In individuals, however, it is a rather poor measure of health or well-being [6]. Furthermore, current anthropometric definitions of obesity have been challenged with regard to their sensitivity and specificity to determine cardiometabolic risk across ethnic groups. Therefore, in addition to BMI other measures that better characterize fat distribution (waist circumference, waist-to-hip ratio) have been recommended [7], but have yet to be widely used in clinical practice.

Background

Assessing obesity

Obesity, or the accumulation of excess body fat, is best described as a "sign" of a derangement in energy balance (as edema is a "sign" of fluid retention). Given that energy balance is affected by a wide range of sociocultural, psychological, biological and iatrogenic factors, it is important in each case to determine the root cause of the derangement in energy balance. Derangements can occur in energy intake (e.g. homeostatic or hedonic hyperphagia), energy metabolism (e.g. hypothyroidism, beta-blockers) or energy expenditure (exercise or non-exercise thermogenesis). Work up of the obese patient must include assessment of all components of energy balance [7].

In assessing obesity it is also helpful to remember that overeating (hyperphagia), when present, in itself is not a diagnosis or a "root cause". Rather, increased food intake has to be interpreted as a perturbation of ingestive behavior that may have multiple causes [8]. These can range from simply overeating at meals in response to hunger precipitated from meal skipping or irregular eating (homeostatic hyperphagia), to emotional overeating, binge-eating disorder, or reward-seeking behaviors not unlike other addictions (hedonic hyperphagia). Asking a hyperphagic obese individual simply to eat less without attempting to determine the underlying problem or help develop specific alternative coping strategies is rarely effective or sustainable.

As with ingestive behavior, physical activity levels are also determined by a wide range of sociocultural, psychological, physical and economic factors [9]. Lack of time is probably the most common factor implicated in lack of exercise. However, as with emotional overeating, lack of motivation and low energy levels can be a sign of an underlying depression, sleep disorder, obstructive sleep apnea or vital exhaustion. Physical limitations to increasing physical activity may include back pain, osteoarthritis, trauma or plantar fasciitis. Again, determining the "root cause" of inactivity is important to determine the most likely line of treatment and approach to behavior change.

Assessing barriers

Long-term efficacy and effectiveness of obesity treatments is notoriously poor. This may in part be attributable to the

Evidence-Based Gastroenterology and Hepatology, 3rd edition.
J. McDonald, A.K. Burroughs, B. Feagan, and M.B. Fennerty. © 2010
Blackwell Publishing Ltd

substantial barriers that undermine long-term obesity management strategies [10]. These can include lack of recognition of obesity as a chronic condition, low socioeconomic status, time constraints, "intimate saboteurs" and a wide range of co-morbidities, including mental health, sleep disorders, chronic pain and musculoskeletal, cardiovascular, respiratory, digestive and endocrine diseases. Furthermore, medications used to treat some of these disorders may further undermine weight-loss efforts. Lack of specific obesity training of health professionals, attitudes and beliefs, as well as insurance coverage and availability of obesity treatments can likewise pose important barriers. Health professionals need to take care to identify, acknowledge and address these barriers where possible to increase patient success, compliance and adherence to treatments. Failure to do so may further undermine the sense of failure, low self-esteem and self-efficacy already common among obese individuals. Addressing treatment barriers can therefore save resources and increase the prospect of long-term success.

Managing expectations

Patients and health care providers generally have exaggerated expectations of what is possible in obesity management [11]. Current studies show that lifestyle management alone is generally associated with a mean weight loss of about 3–5% that can be maintained over 3–5 years [12]. Adding pharmacotherapy to lifestyle management can help achieve 5–15% weight loss, but the vast majority of patients will likely discontinue treatment and regain most of the weight within 3–5 years (Figures 25.1 and 25.2) [13]. Thus, as with other pharmacological treatments for chronic diseases, the importance of long-term adherence to anti-obesity medications cannot be overemphasized. The best long-term results are currently reported for surgical treatment of obesity, with an average sustained weight loss of 20–30% of initial body weight [14]. However, to achieve and sustain this degree of weight loss, surgical patients have to make substantial changes to their lifestyles, without which, a significant proportion of surgical patients will regain weight and/or develop nutritional deficiencies.

In this context, it is important to remember that even a 5% weight loss can produce dramatic improvements in cardiometabolic risk factors and even quality of life measures [15]. The benefits of even modest weight loss should therefore not be underestimated. Given the natural progression of obesity, even helping patients to maintain their current weight may be deemed successful obesity management.

It is not uncommon for a patient to be asked to lose an unreasonable amount of weight before undergoing an elective diagnostic or therapeutic procedure (e.g. joint replacement). The providers are often unaware that their request

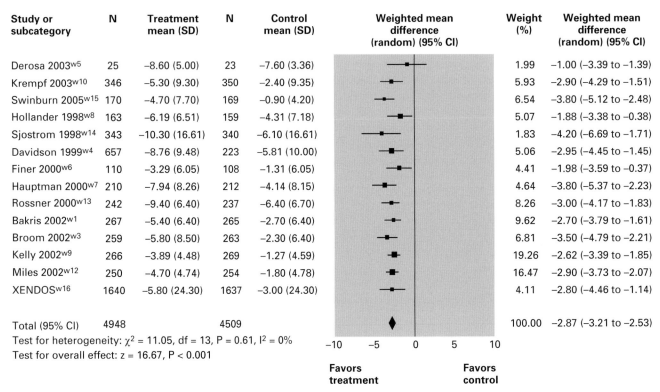

Study or subcategory	N	Treatment mean (SD)	N	Control mean (SD)	Weighted mean difference (random) (95% CI)	Weight (%)	Weighted mean difference (random) (95% CI)
Derosa 2003[w5]	25	−8.60 (5.00)	23	−7.60 (3.36)		1.99	−1.00 (−3.39 to −1.39)
Krempf 2003[w10]	346	−5.30 (9.30)	350	−2.40 (9.35)		5.93	−2.90 (−4.29 to −1.51)
Swinburn 2005[w15]	170	−4.70 (7.70)	169	−0.90 (4.20)		6.54	−3.80 (−5.12 to −2.48)
Hollander 1998[w8]	163	−6.19 (6.51)	159	−4.31 (7.18)		5.07	−1.88 (−3.38 to −0.38)
Sjostrom 1998[w14]	343	−10.30 (16.61)	340	−6.10 (16.61)		1.83	−4.20 (−6.69 to −1.71)
Davidson 1999[w4]	657	−8.76 (9.48)	223	−5.81 (10.00)		5.06	−2.95 (−4.45 to −1.45)
Finer 2000[w6]	110	−3.29 (6.05)	108	−1.31 (6.05)		4.41	−1.98 (−3.59 to −0.37)
Hauptman 2000[w7]	210	−7.94 (8.26)	212	−4.14 (8.15)		4.64	−3.80 (−5.37 to −2.23)
Rossner 2000[w13]	242	−9.40 (6.40)	237	−6.40 (6.70)		8.26	−3.00 (−4.17 to −1.83)
Bakris 2002[w1]	267	−5.40 (6.40)	265	−2.70 (6.40)		9.62	−2.70 (−3.79 to −1.61)
Broom 2002[w3]	259	−5.80 (8.50)	263	−2.30 (6.40)		6.81	−3.50 (−4.79 to −2.21)
Kelly 2002[w9]	266	−3.89 (4.48)	269	−1.27 (4.59)		19.26	−2.62 (−3.39 to −1.85)
Miles 2002[w12]	250	−4.70 (4.74)	254	−1.80 (4.78)		16.47	−2.90 (−3.73 to −2.07)
XENDOS[w16]	1640	−5.80 (24.30)	1637	−3.00 (24.30)		4.11	−2.80 (−4.46 to −1.14)
Total (95% CI)	4948		4509			100.00	−2.87 (−3.21 to −2.53)

Test for heterogeneity: $\chi^2 = 11.05$, df = 13, P = 0.61, $I^2 = 0\%$
Test for overall effect: z = 16.67, P < 0.001

Favors treatment — Favors control

Figure 25.1 Placebo subtracted weight reduction (kg) with orlistat [17].

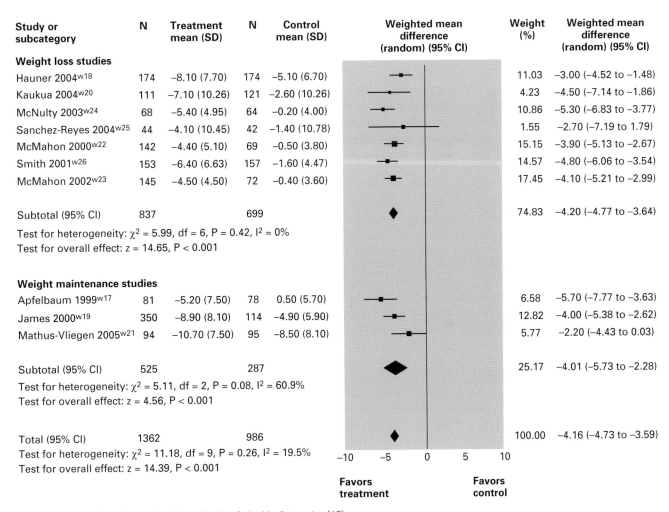

Study or subcategory	N	Treatment mean (SD)	N	Control mean (SD)	Weight (%)	Weighted mean difference (random) (95% CI)
Weight loss studies						
Hauner 2004[w18]	174	−8.10 (7.70)	174	−5.10 (6.70)	11.03	−3.00 (−4.52 to −1.48)
Kaukua 2004[w20]	111	−7.10 (10.26)	121	−2.60 (10.26)	4.23	−4.50 (−7.14 to −1.86)
McNulty 2003[w24]	68	−5.40 (4.95)	64	−0.20 (4.00)	10.86	−5.30 (−6.83 to −3.77)
Sanchez-Reyes 2004[w25]	44	−4.10 (10.45)	42	−1.40 (10.78)	1.55	−2.70 (−7.19 to 1.79)
McMahon 2000[w22]	142	−4.40 (5.10)	69	−0.50 (3.80)	15.15	−3.90 (−5.13 to −2.67)
Smith 2001[w26]	153	−6.40 (6.63)	157	−1.60 (4.47)	14.57	−4.80 (−6.06 to −3.54)
McMahon 2002[w23]	145	−4.50 (4.50)	72	−0.40 (3.60)	17.45	−4.10 (−5.21 to −2.99)
Subtotal (95% CI)	837		699		74.83	−4.20 (−4.77 to −3.64)

Test for heterogeneity: $\chi^2 = 5.99$, df = 6, P = 0.42, $I^2 = 0\%$
Test for overall effect: z = 14.65, P < 0.001

Study or subcategory	N	Treatment mean (SD)	N	Control mean (SD)	Weight (%)	Weighted mean difference (random) (95% CI)
Weight maintenance studies						
Apfelbaum 1999[w17]	81	−5.20 (7.50)	78	0.50 (5.70)	6.58	−5.70 (−7.77 to −3.63)
James 2000[w19]	350	−8.90 (8.10)	114	−4.90 (5.90)	12.82	−4.00 (−5.38 to −2.62)
Mathus-Vliegen 2005[w21]	94	−10.70 (7.50)	95	−8.50 (8.10)	5.77	−2.20 (−4.43 to 0.03)
Subtotal (95% CI)	525		287		25.17	−4.01 (−5.73 to −2.28)

Test for heterogeneity: $\chi^2 = 5.11$, df = 2, P = 0.08, $I^2 = 60.9\%$
Test for overall effect: z = 4.56, P < 0.001

Total (95% CI)	1362		986		100.00	−4.16 (−4.73 to −3.59)

Test for heterogeneity: $\chi^2 = 11.18$, df = 9, P = 0.26, $I^2 = 19.5\%$
Test for overall effect: z = 14.39, P < 0.001

−10 −5 0 5 10

Favors treatment   Favors control

Figure 25.2 Placebo subtracted weight reduction (kg) with sibutramine [17].

for weight loss is unreasonable. For example, even a 20 lb weight loss requires a total energy deficit of 70,000 Kcal. Using the recommended daily energy deficit of 500 Kcal, this would take a patient at least 20 weeks to achieve. However, safely achieving a daily energy deficit of 500 Kcal can be a challenge for sedentary individuals, who may often not need much more than 1500–2000 Kcal to sustain their weight. Thus, reducing energy intake to around 1000–1500 Kcal to achieve the recommended weight loss and still maintain a healthy nutritious balanced diet will pose a major challenge even for the most highly motivated patient. Without professional help, recommendations to lose an unrealistic amount of weight will not only substantially delay the elective procedure, but also increase the patient's sense of frustration and failure and risk promoting nutritional deficiencies.

Approach to treatment

Given the chronic progressive nature of obesity, obesity management has to be approached with the same persever-

ance and diligence as the management of other chronic diseases [7]. All behavioral, medical or surgical interventions have to be continued beyond the weight-loss phase to prevent weight regain. Therefore, in a given patient, any intervention aimed at weight loss has to be reasonably sustainable in the long term to avoid recidivism or weight regain.

A wide range of behavioral interventions has been shown to be successful in the long term. These include self-monitoring with food journals and pedometers, regular weighing and regular provider contact [7]. Patients with emotional and binge-eating disorder may benefit from cognitive behavioral therapy [16]. Failure to identify and manage binge-eating appropriately is associated with virtually 100% recidivism. Overall the long-term, weight-loss benefit of behavioral intervention is rather modest. In a recent multicentre study that randomized 1029 participants, who had lost an average of 8.5 kg through lifestyle change over six months, to various strategies for weight-loss maintenance (personal contact, unlimited access to an interactive technology-based intervention, or self-directed control) over 30 months, resulted in weight loss ranging between 2.9 to 4.2 kg at the end of the study [12]. **A1**

Pharmacological treatment for obesity should be considered in all patients who need to achieve a 5–10% weight loss [7]. In Canada and the USA there are currently two compounds licensed for the long-term treatment of obesity: orlistat, a gastrointestinal lipase inhibitor that reduces digestion and absorption of fat by around 30% [17] and sibutramine, a serotonin and norepinephrine reuptake inhibitor that increases satiety and may have modest effects on thermogenesis. Major adverse effects of orlistat include steatorrhea and oily rectal discharge. Use of sibutramine can be associated with xerostomia, constipation, hyperhydrosis, insomnia, palpitation and, in rare cases, an increase in blood pressure [17]. Both compounds have been shown to significantly increase weight loss when added to moderately caloric-restrictive diets. More importantly, continuation of pharmacotherapy is associated with a more significant reduction in weight regain than behavioral treatment alone. Therefore, long-term use of these agents in patients who respond to and tolerate these drugs is recommended. Despite documented effects on obesity-related morbidity, it should be noted that thus far, there is no evidence that behavioral or pharmacological therapy of obesity reduces overall or obesity-related mortality. **A1a**

Bariatric surgery is currently the most effective long-term treatment of severe obesity and has been shown to dramatically reduce the risk for co-morbidities including cardiovascular disease, type II diabetes, obstructive sleep apnea and certain cancers, and the risk for overall mortality alone (by up to 30%). Thus, for example, the recent Swedish Obesity Study was a prospective case control study comparing 2010 surgical to 2037 non-surgical matched controls [14]. During an average of 10.9 years of follow-up (follow-up rate, 99.9%) there were 129 deaths in the control group and 101 deaths in the surgery group (hazard ratio adjusted for sex, age, and risk factors was 0.71; p = 0.01). The most common causes of death were myocardial infarction (control group, 25 subjects; surgery group, 13 subjects) and cancer (control group, 47; surgery group, 29). These benefits were seen with average weight loss after 10 years of 25% (gastric bypass), 16% (vertical-banded gastroplasty) and 14% (gastric banding). Currently, the most common surgical procedures are laparoscopic adjustable gastric banding (LABG) and laparoscopic Roux-en-Y gastric bypass (RYGB) surgery. While overall complication rates at experienced centers are low (1–2%), surgical complications are even lower with LABG. However, weight loss with this procedure is less pronounced and is more dependent on patient compliance than is the case for RYGB. Other surgical approaches including sleeve gastrectomies and endoluminal approaches are currently under investigation.

Given the complexity of obesity management, interventions are best provided by an interdisciplinary team of nurses, psychologists, physiotherapists, dieticians, social workers, occupational therapists, physicians and surgeons. In light of the widespread bias and discrimination of health professionals against obese clients, bariatric personnel should undergo sensitivity training [5].

Currently there is no cure for obesity – only long-term treatments that require ongoing support and follow-up of all patients to ensure adherence and reduce recidivism. Therefore, it is important to make every effort possible to prevent the development of this chronic and debilitating condition.

The role of the gastrointestinal tract in ingestive behavior

Appetite is regulated by a complex interaction between central and peripheral signals that affect both the sensation of hunger and how an individual responds to food. While older models suggested that hypoglycemia stimulates food intake and post-prandial hyperglycemia activates the satiety centre of the brain [18], in the last decade a much more complex system has emerged that involves a multitude of neuropeptide and neurotransmitter systems, the enteroendocrine system and peripheral signals derived from adipose tissue (e.g. leptin).

The response to food ingestion is traditionally considered to occur in three phases. The cephalic phase is characterized by the secretion of saliva, gastric acid and pancreatic enzymes that is triggered by visual and olfactory stimulation. Relaxation of the sphincter of Oddi and the gastric fundus, and increased contractions of the gall bladder occur [19]. This cephalic phase is followed by the gastric phase, which involves relaxation of the proximal stomach. This is caused by the activation of inhibitory neurons on the gastric wall (accommodation). Finally, the intestinal or post-ingestion phase is characterized by a combination of duodenal, intestinal and colonic responses that may also play a role in satiety.

A multitude of enteroendocrine hormones or peptides play a role in regulating food intake by activating nearby extrinsic sensory fibers (vagal and spinal) or via the bloodstream (Table 25.1) [20]. They generally have a short half-life, interact with other hormones and they can modulate the sensitivity of the vagal response. Through activation of the vagus nerve or through direct neural stimulation, these peptides stimulate the hypothalamus, which then integrates these signals. The main site of integration is the arcuate nucleus of the hypothalamus (ARC). Two major sub-populations of neurons in the ARC are implicated in the regulation of feeding; cocaine and amphetamine related transcript (CART) and pro-opiomelanocortin (POMC)

Table 25.1 Role of enteroendocrine hormones and peptides in regulation of food intake.

Hormone	Effect on hunger	Stimulus for secretion	Location secreted	Effect
Ghrelin	↑	Cephalic phase	A-X like cells of the oxyntic glands (stomach)	• Enhances NPY/AgRP and inhibits POMC pathways. • Endogenous ligand for growth hormone secretagogue receptors. • Controls secretion of ACTH, prolactin, and plays a role in glucose and lipid metabolism. • Increases gastric mobility, gastric acid secretion and insulin secretion.
Cholecystokinin (CCK)	↓	Nutrients (especially lipids and proteins)	I-cells of the duodenum and ileal	• Enduces satiety and reduces meal intake through vagus nerve stimulation. • Inhibitory effect on gastric motility.
Glucagon-like peptide-1 (GLP-1)	↓	Nutrients (especially lipids and proteins)	L-cells of the distal small intestine	• Enhances the glucose-induced stimulation of insulin synthesis and secretion, while suppressing glucagon secretion. • Delays gastric acid secretion and emptying.
Peptide YY (3-36) (PYY$_{3-36}$)	↓	Nutrients (proportional to caloric intake)	L-cells of the distal small intestine	• Thought to act at the level of the hypothalamus; however, exact mechanism unclear.
Oxyntomodulin	↓	Nutrients (proportional to caloric intake)	L-cells of the distal small intestine	• Inhibits gastric acid secretion and gastric emptying. • In animals, found to increases gastric somatostatin release, potentiates the effects of PYY and found to inhibit insulin secretion. • Thought to work through GLP-1 receptor stimulation
Leptin	↓	Short chain fatty acids	Adipose tissue	• Low leptin activates anabolic and inhibits catabolic circuits. • Enhances NPY/AGRP while blocking POMC/CART release.
Pancreatic polypeptide (PP)	↓	Nutrients (proportional to caloric intake)	Pancreas	• Thought to act at level of hypothalamus and brainstem to decrease intake. • Effect unclear as PP injected directly into the brain increases food intake in rats. • May potentially affect gastric emptying.
Insulin	↓	Glucose	Pancreas	• Centrally, insulin reduces feeding by activating POMC. • Insulin also increases AgRP synthesis, which would increase hunger.

inhibit food intake, whereas neuropeptide Y (NPY) and agouti-related protein (AgRP) stimulate it. Both influence how the hypothalamus signals pituitary hormone secretion and appetite [21]. The neurophysiological pathways involved in triggering hunger and satiety are complex and beyond the scope of this chapter.

In the stomach, neural sensors perceive changes in the tension, stretch and volume of the stomach wall and outputs from these mechanoreceptors are relayed to the brain via the vagus and spinal sensory nerves [20] to the nucleus tractus solitarius (caudal brainstem) and then to the hypothalamus. Gastric distension induces a feeling of satiety [22]. Persistent delayed gastric emptying is known to decrease food intake, and artificial distension of the proximal stomach with a water-filled balloon has been found to reduce oral intake [23, 24]. On the other hand, the stomach is also the source of ghrelin, the only enteric hormone so far known to promote hunger and food intake.

In contrast, there are a number of enteric satiety signals, the best studied of which include cholecystokinin (CCK), glucagon-like peptide-1 (GLP-1) and peptide YY (PYY) [21]. Parental administration of CCK induces satiety in animals and humans [25, 26, 27], an effect that is eradicated by vagotomy. CCK also delays gastric emptying [28] resulting in gastric distension. Due to its short duration of action, attempts to utilize CCK as a treatment for obesity have failed. PYY, another satiety hormone released from the colon, also inhibits fasting small bowel motility and gastric emptying [29]. Parenteral PPY injection decreases food intake in normal and obese humans [30], potentially via a central mechanism. Exogenous GLP-1 has been found to decrease food intake [31], only when administered at doses much higher than those physiologically achieved after a normal meal [32].

Gastrointestinal symptoms and disease in the obese patient

Gastro-esophageal reflux disease (GERD)

Obesity is a significant risk factor for GERD. Obese individuals are more than twice as likely as non-obese individuals to admit to a history of GERD or symptomatic heartburn [33] [34]. The prevalence of GERD ranges from 8–26% in individuals with obesity [35] [36]. Similarly, endoscopically diagnosed erosive esophagitis is also more common in individuals with an increased BMI, with an odds ratio (OR) of 1.76 [37]. Several mechanisms have been described to explain this correlation. An increased intra-abdominal and resulting increase in intragastric pressure can precipitate reflux into the esophagus or hiatus hernia [38]. In addition, derangements of esophageal motility, including hypertensive contractions (nutcracker esophagus) or disordered contractions (non-specific motility disorder), decreased lower esophageal sphincter pressure, inappropriate lower esophageal relaxation, a sliding hiatus hernia and delayed gastric emptying have also been implicated (see motility section below) [39]. Finally, diet, refluxate composition and an increased incidence of *Helicobacter pylori* may also play significant roles in increasing the incidence of GERD in obese individuals.

Several (but not all) studies suggest that weight loss is associated with decreased esophageal acid exposure and an improvement in GERD symptoms [40]. The lack of symptomatic improvement in many patients following weight loss may be attributed to the persistence of a hiatus hernia [41]. Modifications in dietary composition may be more effective than an actual change in weight [42, 43]. Symptomatic improvement following bariatric surgery is likely secondary to both weight loss and a change in the anatomy of the gastrointestinal (GI) tract. Roux-en-Y consistently results in a favorable response as an anti-reflux procedure, with a significant improvement in reflux symptoms and a decrease in the use of GERD medication noted postoperatively. Adjustable gastric banding may not be a suitable option in obese individuals with symptomatic GERD, unless combined with anti-reflux surgery, since banding can precipitate the reflux of gastric contents into the esophagus from the small gastric reservoir [44].

Acute pancreatitis

Severe hypertriglyceridemia, not uncommon in overweight and obese individuals, is a rare but well recognized cause of acute pancreatitis [45]. Increased BMI is, however, considered to be a risk factor for a worse outcome in patients with acute pancreatitis [46, 47]. In a recent meta-analysis severe acute pancreatitis was more frequent in obese patients (BMI ≥ 30 kg/m^2) (OR 2.6), who also tended to develop more systemic (OR 2.0) and local complications (OR 4.3). Local complications from the greater accumulation of peripancreatic fat included fat necrosis, with necrosis becoming a nidus for infection [46]. This is particularly problematic in obese individuals with hyperinsulinemia and insulin resistance [48]. Obesity is also associated with respiratory, renal and circulatory compromise as well as an increased incidence of death [49]. In light of these observations, adding an obesity score (BMI ≥ 26 kg/m^2) to the APACHE II (Acute Physiology and Chronic Health Evaluation) score has been recommended to improve its predictive value for overweight and obese patients [50, 51]. Thus, the composite APACHE-O (APACHE-II plus obesity) score >8 has greater predictive accuracy than the APACHE-II score, with a sensitivity of 82%, specificity of 86%, positive predictive value (PPV) of 74% and a negative predictive value of 91% (NPV) in predicting morbidity and mortality [50].

Gallstone disease and cholecystitis

Both obesity and rapid weight loss are associated with an increased risk of gallstone disease, particularly in women. Risk appears highest when obesity begins in late adolescence [52] or if obesity is truncal [53]. The three major factors important in the development of gallstones include gall bladder dysmotilty, cholesterol hypersaturation of bile (i.e. a higher concentration of cholesterol to bile or phospholipids), and cholesterol nucleation. Obese patients have an increased biliary secretion of cholesterol from the liver, which leads to the formation of bile supersaturated with cholesterol and the precipitation of cholesterol microcrystals [54]. Both diabetes mellitus and insulin resistance are known to be confounding factors with respect to the association of obesity and gallstone disease [55]. Increased hepatic cholesterol synthesis and diets high in calories and refined carbohydrates, but low in fiber, also increase the risk. There is contradictory evidence, however, on the specific role of total fat intake [56]. There has been no correlation found between serum cholesterol level and a predisposition to gallstone formation [57].

Impaired gall bladder emptying or gall bladder stasis, and further cholesterol saturation, as would occur in individuals who lose weight rapidly with restricted dieting or following bariatric surgery, also precipitates stone formation [58]. Low calorie and low fat diets affect biliary lipid composition with increases in the hepatic uptake of cholesterol and hepatic cholesterol synthesis [59]. Weight loss is clearly associated with the development of gallstones, especially in women [51]. In several studies, approximately 11–28% of obese patients who severely restricted their dietary intake [60–62], and 27–43% of patients who underwent bariatric surgery developed gallstones within a period of 1–5 months [63, 64]. Routine concomitant chole-cystectomy with bariatric surgery has been suggested, but remains controversial. The rate of weight loss also influences gallstone development. As gallstone formation appears particularly high when weight loss is more than 1.5 kg per week [65], preventive strategies have been suggested. These include controlling the rate of weight loss, administration of ursodeoxycholic acid to decrease cholesterol saturation, limiting between meal fasting time and maintaining a small amount of fat in the diet [66].

Ursodeoxycholic acid has been shown in several small studies to reduce gallstone formation post-bariatric surgery. These studies are difficult to compare as they used different doses of ursodeoxycholic acid (i.e. 500 [67] to 1000 [68] mg/day), for different lengths of time (i.e. 3 [68] to 24 [67] months). The presence of gallstone formation is based upon different diagnostic imaging modalities. Miller [68], in the longest study to date, found that after 24 months the incidence of finding gallstones by ultrasound or CT scan was 8% in 76 patients treated with 250 mg ursodeoxycholic acid bid for six months postoperatively versus 30% in 76 patients treated with placebo. The true incidence of symptomatic cholecystitis in unknown. Miller [68] reported that 4.7% of patients in the ursodeoxycholic group and 12% in the placebo group underwent postoperative cholecystectomy for symptomatic gallstone disease. Though adverse effects of ursodeoxycholic acid are minor (nausea, constipation), and were not found to be significantly different in the treatment and placebo groups [68], ursodeoxycholic acid is relatively expensive and the pills are large, making passage through a small gastric reservoir difficult. Postoperative prophylactic treatment with ursodoxycholic acid at this time is not routinely recommended.

Diverticular disease and diverticulitis

The relationship between diverticular disease and obesity remains unclear. Obese patients are more likely than patients of normal body weight to present with diverticulitis and diverticular perforations. This association has been particularly noted in younger individuals [69, 70], in whom the diagnosis may be missed [71]. In one retrospective case series, individuals diagnosed with recurrent diverticulitis or diverticular perforations were significantly more likely to be obese [72]. Obesity has also been identified as a significant risk factor for mortality following elective sigmoid resection done specifically for diverticular complications.

Cancer

Several mechanisms have been proposed to explain the increased risk of malignancy in obese individuals. These include the insulin and insulin-like growth factor axis, the role of sex steroids and the influence of adipokines. Hyperinsulinemia or insulin resistance reduces insulin-like growth factor (IGF) binding protein, which increases free IGF-1 levels. Both insulin and IGF-1 are associated with increased cell growth and proliferation and both may promote neoplastic cell growth [73]. Hyperinsulinemia also reduces sex hormone-binding globulin, which leads to increased estrogen and androgen levels. These hormones have been shown to be involved in the regulation of cell differentiation, proliferation and apoptosis, and to selectively enhance the growth of preneoplastic and neoplastic cells [74]. Increased serum leptin, an adipocyte-derived hormone is considered to be an obesity signal, which acts centrally as a catabolic agent to regulate body weight. *In vitro* leptin has been found to stimulate cancer cells derived from the colon and esophagus [75, 76]. Obesity is also thought to be involved in the immunologic or inflammatory response as described above. Increased levels of cytokines and adipokines, such as adiponectin [77] and transforming growth factor beta [78], may contribute to cell growth and differentiation. A large prospective cohort study assessing cancer mortality in over 900,000 Americans determined that the death rate from all cancers (GI and non-GI) was 52% higher in obese men and 62% higher in obese women compared to men and women of normal body weight. The authors suggested that more than 90,000 deaths per year from cancer could be avoided by maintaining a BMI less than 25 kg/m^2 throughout life. The strongest association between obesity and gastrointestinal cancer risk has been demonstrated for esophageal, gall bladder, pancreas, liver and colorectal cancers [79]. A recent systematic review and meta-analysis found GI malignancies to be more prevalent in obese individuals, with a 5 kg/m^2 increase in BMI leading to an increased risk for gall bladder (RR = 1.59), esophageal (RR = 1.51) and colon adenocarcinomas (RR = 1.09) in women, and esophageal (RR = 1.52) and colon (RR = 1.24) adenocarcinomas in men [80]. For colon cancer, the association was significantly stronger in men than in women, an observation that gives credence to the finding that estrogen plus progestin may be protective against colon cancer formation [81].

Barrett's esophagus and esophageal adenocarcinoma

Both GERD and high BMI are considered risk factors for esophageal adenocarinoma. In a recent meta-analysis, individuals with a BMI > 25 kg/m^2 had an OR of 1.52 for esophageal adenocarcinoma compared to an OR of 2.78 in individuals with a BMI > 30 kg/m^2 [37]. Whether or not this risk is directly mediated by obesity remains unclear. It appears that the risk for Barrett's esphagus, the precursor to esophageal adenocarcinoma, may be entirely mediated through the increased risk of GERD in obese individuals [82]. Nevertheless, recent studies have suggested that adipokines like adiponectin and leptin [83] may be directly associated with Barrett's metaplasia. Whether or not weight loss results in a decreased risk of esophageal adenocarcinoma is not known.

Proximal gastric adenocarcinoma/cancer of the gastric cardia

The difficulty in endoscopically differentiating proximal gastric adenocarcinoma from distal esophageal adenocarcinoma complicates risk factor assessment. Several studies have confirmed that obesity is a significant independent risk factor for the development of proximal gastric adenocarcinoma [84–88] but not gastric non-cardiac adenocarcinoma [84, 85, 88]. In a large study of over 500,000 US patients, a BMI > 35 kg/m² was found to be a significant risk factor for esophageal and gastric cardia adenocarcinoma, with a hazard ratio of 2.27 and 2.46 respectively [84]. The association between these two cancers is unclear, as GERD was found to be a significant risk factor for the development of esophageal adenocarcinoma (see above esophageal adenocarcinoma section) but not for proximal gastric cancers [84, 88].

Pancreatic cancer

The only universally accepted risk factors for the development of pancreatic cancer are smoking and family history [89]. Data regarding any association with obesity and pancreatc cancer risk are based largely on case-control studies and may be biased by high fatality rates. The RR of obesity as a risk factor for pancreatic cancer was reported to range between 1.2 and 3.0. A recent meta-analysis of six case-control and eight cohort studies found a weak RR of 1.19 for men with a BMI > 30 kg/m² compared to individuals with a BMI < 22 kg/m², but not for women [90]. Not all studies corrected for the significant confounders of smoking and diabetes.

Much like the mechanism by which non-alcoholic steatosis leads to liver fibrosis and cirrhosis [91], it has been suggested that non-alcoholic fatty pancreas disease may lead to non-alcoholic steatopancreatitis, which can progress to pancreatic fibrosis and dysfunction (chronic pancreatitis), and eventually pancreatic cancer. The adipose-derived cytokines, IL-1 beta and TNF- alpha are thought to promote this progression [92].

Hepatocellular cancer (HCC)

The relative risk of mortality from primary HCC is 1.68 times higher among women and 4.52 times higher for men, with a baseline BMI ≥ 35 kg/m² compared to a BMI of 18.5–24.9 kg/m² [79]. In men, HCC had the highest obesity-related relative risk of all cancers. Hepatocellular cancer is a well-recognized complication of cirrhosis, and non-alcoholic fatty liver disease associated with obesity and the metabolic syndrome is a known cause of cirrhosis. A study,

by Nair *et al.* [93] of nearly 20,000 US patients found obesity to be an independent risk factor for HCC. However, on multivariate analysis, obesity was only found to be a significant risk factor in patients with either alcoholic or cryptogenic cirrhosis. This association was not found in patients with other causes of liver cirrhosis such as hepatitis C viral (HCV) infection. Similarly, diabetes mellitus has been suggested to be a risk factor for HCC development [94, 95], though obesity is a significant confounding variable. A recent study in nearly 1500 patients with chronic HCV cirrhosis followed for a mean of six years found that being overweight or obese were significant independent risk factors for HCC development, with a hazard ratio of 1.86 and 3.10 respectively [96]. Obesity, diabetes mellitus and hyperlipidemia are conditions known to have a synergistic effect on the progression of liver fibrosis in patients infected with HCV [97]. It is difficult to know whether fatty infiltration worsens HCV progression itself or whether non-alcoholic fatty liver disease is a potential secondary cause of liver cirrhosis in obese individuals.

Cholangiocarcinoma

Studying the risk factors associated with the development of cholangiocarcinoma is hindered by the fact that it is such a rare disease, and that only 10% of cases are associated with a recognized risk factor [98]. Obesity has been suggested to be a potential risk factor in some studies [99, 100] but not in others [101]. As with other cancers, studies are limited by the presence of confounding variables. Specifically, gallstone disease is a recognized risk factor for the development of cholangiocarcinoma, and obesity is a recognized risk factor for the development of gallstones [102].

Colorectal adenocarcinoma

A recent meta-analysis of 31 prospective studies performed between 1966 and 2007 found that a five-unit increase in BMI was associated with a 30% increased risk of colon cancer in men and a 12% increased risk in women [103]. BMI was a significant risk factor for the development of proximal colon cancer in men, and with distal colon cancer in both sexes. Rectal cancer was significantly related to BMI in men but not in women. Abdominal obesity showed a stronger relationship than overall obesity [103]. The reason for the apparent sex difference in the association between colon cancer rates and obesity is unclear. While obesity imposes a greater risk of colon cancer for men of all ages, the risk has been reported to be higher in premenopausal than in postmenopausal women [104]. Although, increased estrogen levels and insulin resistance in premenopausal women have been suggested to contribute [105], this would not explain why colon cancer risk is higher in men than in women [80] or why exogenous estrogen in the form of hormone replacement therapy may be protective [81].

Confounding factors for all studies related to cancer, but specifically to colon cancer, include the influence of exercise and diet. Physical activity is associated with lower rates of colon cancer [106]. The theoretical explanation for this is that physical activity increases colonic motility [107]. Dietary factors which have been associated with an increased risk of colon cancer include the high consumption of red meat, low consumption of fresh fruits and vegetables, low-fiber diets and diets low in certain vitamins and minerals including calcium and folate [108]. These diets may be more common in overweight individuals.

Gastrointestinal dysmotility

Alterations in gastrointestinal motility have been recognized in obese individuals, resulting in a variety of symptoms, most notably reflux, nausea, diarrhea and bloating.

Esophageal dysmotility

In the esophagus, transient lower esophageal sphincter (LES) relaxation and decreased esophageal clearance capacity may contribute to GERD [109]. Studies on esophageal dysmotility and obesity, however, have produced inconsistent results [110, 111]. Other pathophysiological factors that may contribute to the higher incidence of GERD in overweight and obese individuals include increased esophageal acid sensitivity [112] and the presence of a hiatal hernia. Koppman et al. [113] evaluated 116 obese individuals who presented for esophageal assessment by manometry prior to laparoscopic gastric banding, regardless of any dyspepsia or dysphagia history. An abnormal motility pattern was found in 41% of these patients, of whom 23% were diagnosed with non-specific esophageal motility disorders, 11% with nutcracker esophagus, 3% with isolated hypertensive LES, 3% with isolated hypotensive LES, 1% with esophageal spasm and 1% with achalasia. Interestingly, only one patient with abnormal esophageal motility had a history of non-cardiac chest pain. This observation is contrary to what one would expect given the relationship between obesity and GERD. One explanation for the apparent lack of GERD symptoms in this study is that patients with morbid obesity may have a depressed autonomic nervous system and may lack sensory perception through the vagus nerve. In addition, only 3% had evidence of an isolated hypotensive LES. Other studies have suggested a higher incidence of hypotensive LES in obesity, with a prevalence ranging from 14–69% [114–116] and with potential worsening of reflux following adjustable gastric banding [116]. There was no mention in Koppman's study of the number of transient LES relaxations, which has been suggested to be the most significant abnormality causing GERD in this population, through frequent overeating [109].

Gastric dysmotility

The relationship between obesity and gastric motility, as assessed by gastric emptying studies, has been contradictory [109]. In general, it is suggested that obese individuals have a larger gastric capacity and accelerated solid food gastric emptying [117]. Rapid emptying may reduce the negative feedback satiety signal and trigger hunger [118]. Myoelectrical studies suggest that individuals with morbid obesity have a decreased gastric slow wave frequency and an increased frequency of dysgastria in both the fasting and fed state, which would explain any increased gastric emptying [119]. No difference in either the gastric emptying of liquids or in gastric accommodation has been found in the obese [118]. Gastric electrical stimulation studies performed so far only in dogs have suggested that this intervention may become a viable therapeutic option to promote weight loss in the future [120].

Gall bladder dysmotility

Although decreased gall bladder motility has been implicated as a risk factor for the more frequent prevalence of gall bladder disease in obese individuals, the findings from motility studies have been inconsistent [121]. Insulin resistance [122] and hyperinsulinemia, which may decrease gall bladder sensitivity to cholecystokinin, and thus gall bladder contractions, may also play a role [123].

Small and large bowel dysmotility

While small and large bowel motility in obese individuals remain to be studied [118], no differences were found between obese and normal weight individuals in intestinal transit time as measured by hydrogen breath test [124].

Functional GI symptoms

Obesity and its relationship to upper GI symptoms, specifically GERD and dyspepsia, are well studied (see GERD section). In clinical practice, however, it has been well recognized that many obese patients appear to have gastrointestinal (GI) complaints for which no etiology can be found. Functional GI disorders are thought to be secondary to an initial inflammatory insult on the GI tract that affects visceral sensitivity and/or motility. The proinflammatory effects of obesity are only now being recognized. Functional GI disease may be related to unrecognized changes in GI motility affecting GI function, or to a relative difference in the levels of some GI peptides induced by altered food habits or binge eating [125] and their endocrine or neurological effects. Four studies have addressed the relationship between obesity and GI symptoms [126–129]. The largest, a cross-sectional survey study, done in Olmsted County, evaluated the association of self-reported GI symptoms with BMI in nearly 2000 individuals [126]. Four symptoms were found to be significantly more prominent in overweight and obese individuals: vomiting, upper abdominal pain, bloating and diarrhea. Similar results, with some variation, were found in the other three studies to date [127–129]. A linear increase in prevalence across BMI categories was not observed for any of the symptoms, though an incremental increase in OR across categories was found for diarrhea (overweight OR 1.0, class I OR 1.7, class II OR 2.7 and class III OR 2.8). An impressive 40.7% of individuals with class II obesity complained of diarrhea. However, 17.1% of patients with a normal weight also listed this as a GI complaint [126]. The authors suggested that the increased frequency of diarrhea may be secondary to changes in GI motility, such as increased gastric emptying, or decreased intestinal or colonic transit time, which have been reported in some studies (see motility section) in overweight individuals, or to the altered intestinal secretory response induced by the direct endocrine effects of some gut released adipokines [126]. Concomitant diabetes mellitus and the use of anti-obesity medications may be significant confounding variables [126]. In type II diabetics, diarrhea but not abdominal pain is associated with BMI independent of glycemic control, suggesting a causal link between diarrhea and obesity independent of any effect of diabetes on GI function [130].

The Olmsted study [126] also found that upper but not lower abdominal pain is significantly associated with BMI. The association between obesity and irritable bowel syndrome is unclear. Two studies evaluating this relationship have found contradictory results [125, 131]. Despite this contradiction, individuals with abdominal pain have been found to have a significant improvement in their symptoms following laparoscopic Roux-en-Y gastric bypass (LRNY) [132].

Bariatric surgery – a primer for the gastroenterologist

Bariatric surgical procedures reduce caloric intake and/ or nutrient absorption by modifying the anatomy of the gastrointestinal tract [133]. Expected results include a durable and significant weight loss of 24% of total weight after two years and 16% at 10 years (Figure 25.3) [134], with a remarkable reduction in obesity-related co-morbidities

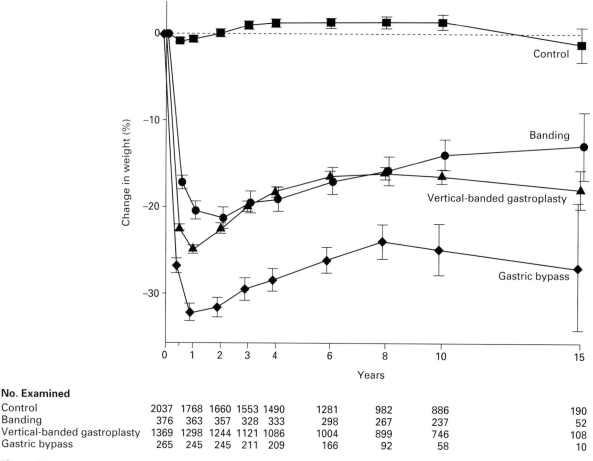

No. Examined

Control	2037	1768	1660	1553	1490	1281	982	886		190
Banding		376	363	357	328	333	298	267	237	52
Vertical-banded gastroplasty	1369	1298	1244	1121	1086	1004	899	746		108
Gastric bypass	265	245	245	211	209	166	92	58		10

Figure 25.3 Mean per cent weight change during a 15-year period in the control group and the surgery group, according to the method of bariatric surgery.

and mortality. In addition, with the advent of laparoscopic surgery, complications have been dramatically reduced [135, 136]. In 2001, the NIH consensus statement identified bariatric surgery as the only long-term treatment for morbidly obese individuals (BMI > 40 kg/m^2) [137]. More recently, there has been a dramatic increase in the frequency of bariatric surgical procedures in the USA and worldwide [138, 139]. As a result, the practicing gastroenterologist must be familiar with the common bariatric surgical procedures, their complications and the implications for endoscopy.

Surgical approaches to obesity

Bariatric surgery reduces nutrient intake and/or absorption by restrictive and/or malabsorptive modification of the gastrointestinal tract. Please see Figure 25.4 [133].

Restrictive procedures create an anatomically smaller proximal stomach (10–20 ml), resulting in early satiety and reduced oral intake. Procedures include gastric stapling gastroplasty, vertical banded gastroplasty (VBG)) and the placement, most commonly laparascopically, of a synthetic, inflatable band around the stomach to create a narrow outlet (LAGB) (Figure 25.4a). These techniques rely on foreign material (silicone or mesh) to maintain a narrow stoma to restrict the passage of food into the stomach. The size of the stomal outlet is typically 10–12 mm. Another recently developed procedure is the "sleeve gastrectomy" (Figure 25.4b), in which resection of much of the gastric body leaves a narrow tube of stomach in continuity with duodenum. While VBG is now largely considered to be obsolete, the use of LAGB is increasing because of its simplicity, ease of implementation, maintenance of intestinal continuity and reversibility [138]. The device can be manipulated in outpatient settings by altering the volume in the band, hence impacting the degree to which the stomal outlet is compromised.

Malabsorptive procedures (Figure 25.4c, d) include the Roux-en-Y gastric bypass (RYGB) in which the small intestine is divided at mid-jejunum and the distal portion is anastamosed to the stomach (often in combination with a restrictive gastrectomy, leaving a small residual gastric pouch to which the intestine is connected). The distal portion of stomach and proximal small bowel (bilio-pancreatic limb) are anastamosed end-to-side further down the jejunum. Although this length can vary (depending upon the amount of malabsorption that is desired) up to 150 cm, it is usually 60–75 cm. The degree of nutrient malabsorption is proportional to the length of the roux limb and inversely proportional to the length of the "common channel" – the portion of bowel remaining where pancreaticobiliary secretions and food come together. Another, less common malabsorptive procedure is the biliopancreatic diversion (BPD), often accompanied by a duodenal switch,

with restriction in the form of a sleeve gastrectomy. This procedure results in a relatively larger pouch and a greater predisposition to malabsorption (common channel of 50–100 cm).

The anatomic implications of bariatric surgery are of significant interest to the gastroenterologist and endoscopist. It is vital to understand the type of surgery that was undertaken, the expected results of this surgery, and the interpretation of patient symptoms and to implement and evaluate a treatment strategy in light of this understanding.

Complications of bariatric surgery

The complications of bariatric surgery are the topic of several recent review articles [140–142]. In individuals who have undergone Roux-en-Y gastric bypass, complications relate to the anastamosis and to bowel manipulation, and include mortality (0.2%), leaks (2.3%), staple line disruption (1.5%), marginal ulcers (2.5%), strictures (9.9%), bowel obstruction (3.3%), hernias (2.4%) and wound infections (3.4%). Following LAGB, complications relate to band malposition and/or malfunction and include mortality (0.14%), band slippage (5.5%), pouch enlargement (5.5%), obstruction/stenosis (1.9%), band erosion (2.7%), hardware infection (1.2%), hardware leak (3.6%), severe esophageal dilation (3.0%) and esophageal or gastric perforation (1.2%) [141].

Gastrointestinal symptoms and complications

Post-bariatric surgery patients will present in a number of different ways. Early complications occur within two months of the surgical procedure and are usually managed by the surgeon. In this population, because of large abdominal girth, physical findings may not correlate with postoperative complications, and there should be a low threshold for ordering contrast radiologic studies or computed tomograms. Later complications are more likely to require investigation by a gastroenterologist, and patients may present with various ill-defined symptoms, including abdominal pain, nausea and vomiting, abnormal, insufficient or excessive degrees of weight loss, diarrhea and gastrointestinal bleeding (Table 25.2).

Abdominal pain in the post-bariatric surgery patient may simply be due to the effects of rapid food consumption in the setting of a relatively fixed outlet. In patients with RYGB, pain may be related to stomal ulceration or stenosis or from an internal hernia. Biliary tract disease including cholelithiasis and choledocholithiasis occurs in up to 20% of patients in the setting of obesity and rapid weight loss and must be considered in the differential diagnosis. In individuals with RYGB, accessing the biliary tree is problematic and deserves special consideration, as does consideration for cholecystectomy in patients with gallstones at

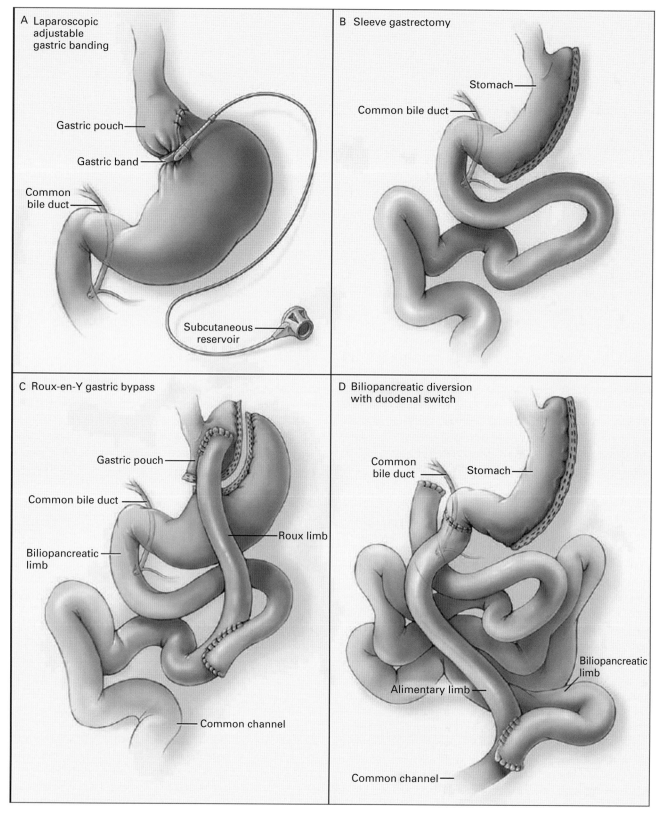

Figure 25.4 Common surgical procedures for weight loss. Restrictive operations for the treatment of morbid obesity and its coexisting conditions, popular today particularly because of laparoscopic surgical approaches, include adjustable gastric banding (LAGB) (a) and vertical (sleeve) gastrectomy (b). Roux-en Y gastric bypass (RYGB) (c), a procedure that combines restriction and malabsorption, is considered by many to be the gold standard because of its high level of effectiveness and its durability. More extreme malabsorption accompanies biliopancreatic diversion procedures, commonly performed with a duodenal switch (BPD-DS) (d), in which a short, distal, common-channel length of small intestine severely limits caloric absorption. This procedure also includes a sleeve gastrectomy.

Table 25.2 Diagnostic considerations after bariatric surgery.

Gastrointestinal symptom	Risk by procedure	Luminal considerations	Hepatobiliary considerations
Abdominal pain	RYGB	Stomal ulceration, stenosis, hernia, adhesions, band erosion	Gallstones
Vomiting	LABG, RYGB	Stenosis, ulceration, functional	Bile reflux
Insufficient weight change	LAGB	Dehiscence, diet, fistulae, pouch enlargement	
Excessive weight change	RYGB, BPD	Obstruction, bacterial overgrowth, neoplasm	
Diarrhea	RYGB, BPD	Dumping, bile salt diarrhea, bacterial overgrowth, IBS, diet	Bile salt diarrhea
GI bleeding	RYGB	Ulceration, gastric remnant, NSAIDS	

the time of bariatric surgery, although this approach is somewhat controversial [143–145]. Post-LAGB, the differential diagnosis includes band erosion or migration. Nausea and vomiting may be seen in any of these patients, but is more common post-LAGB, and an excessively tight band must be ruled out. Pre-existing esophageal and gastric motility disorders and functional upper gastrointestinal disorders may also play a role in the genesis of these symptoms. Insufficient weight loss (less than 50% of excess weight) is seen in 15% of patients. This lack of efficacy may be due to dietary indiscretion (high calorie liquids and snacks), insufficient activity or surgical result. Surgical considerations include enlarged pouch, deflation of band, a long common channel and dehiscence of the staple line. Excessive weight loss is less common after LAGB and more common after BPD or duodenal switch, because of the malabsorptive implications of these surgeries. Undernutrition in these individuals may be difficult to recognize. Other considerations include stomal stenosis or ulceration leading to obstruction. Eating disorders may also play a role in patients with excessive weight loss post-bariatric surgery, and history pertaining to this problem must be pursued. Diarrhea in the post-bariatric surgery patient may simply be a reflection of malabsorption and maldigestion expected from intestinal bypass, or it may be due to bile salt diarrhea or dumping. Dumping syndrome symptoms of flushing, lightheadedness, fatigue and postprandial diarrhea may occur following intake of sugars and can be seen in 5–10% of patients. Bacterial overgrowth in the bypassed intestinal limb may also contribute to the development of secretory diarrhea and may also be associated with symptoms of bloating and flatulence. Gastrointestinal bleeding may occur from stomal ulceration in both RYGB and BPD patients and may be exacerbated by concomitant use of NSAIDS or steroids. It is important to identify the site of bleeding endoscopically and to recognize that ulceration at the distal intestinal anastamosis and in the gastric remnant may not be accessible endoscopically using standard techniques.

In the evaluation of patients post-bariatric surgery who have GI complaints, radiologic imaging modalities including contrast studies to assess the possibility of leakage or perforation, computed tomography to detect herniation, bowel obstruction or fluid collections, and ultrasound to aid visualization of the hepatobiliary system are appropriate.

Nutritional complications

Medical professionals caring for bariatric surgery patients must be aware of the potential risk of nutritional deficiencies that are common in these patients and of strategies to prevent and treat nutrient deficiencies.

It is recognized that management of post-operative nutrition begins pre-operatively with nutritional status assessment, education and reinforcement of principles associated with long-term weight loss. This topic has recently been reviewed [146, 147]. Prior to bariatric surgery, micronutrient deficiencies that have been documented include vitamin D (60–80%), B-complex vitamins (important for carbohydrate metabolism), iron (50%), zinc, selenium and the antioxidant vitamins A, E and C.

The risk of micronutrient depletion is greatest in patients with surgical interventions affecting digestion and absorption of nutrients (RYGB, BPD). These procedures can result in either primary or secondary nutrient deficiency. BPD is thought to cause weight loss through both protein (25%) and fat (75%) malabsorption. This has implications for (mal) absorption of micronutrients, including vitamins A, D, E, K and zinc. The decrease in transit time associated with intestinal bypass can also result in the secondary malabsorption of nutrients bypassing the duodenum and jejunum. Malabsorption can also be due to limited contact with the intestinal mucosa secondary to a short common channel. Inadequate dietary intake in these patients may also result in nutrient deficiencies. This is particularly relevant for iron, calcium, vitamin B12, thiamine and folate. Purely restrictive procedures such as LAGB usually result in micronutrient deficiencies due to changes in dietary intake (Table 25.3).

Vitamins and minerals are factors and cofactors in many biologic processes that regulate body size, including appetite, hunger, nutrient absorption, metabolic rate, thyroid

Table 25.3 Nutrient deficiencies and suggested treatments after bariatric surgery[46].

Nutrient	Preoperative deficiency	Postoperative deficiency	Screening	Symptom of deficiency	Suggested treatment: AGB	Suggested treatment: RYGB	Suggested treatment: BPD/DS
Iron	9–16%	20–49%	ferritin	anemia	MVM* May require extra Fe	MVM bid +18–27 mg/d elemental Fe	MVM bid + 18–27 mg elemental Fe
Vitamin B12	10–13%	12–33%	Serum B12, methylmalonic acid	Megaloblastic anemia, neuropathy, delusions, hallucinations	MVM	MVM + 1000 ug/mo or 350–500 ug po/d	MVM
Folate	Uncommon	Uncommon	RBC folate	Megaloblastic anemia, neurologic symptoms	MVM, B-complex	MVM	MVM
Vitamin B1 (Thiamine)	15–29%	Rare but can occur	Serum thiamine	Wernike-Korsakoff syndrome	MVM, thiamine 50->100 mg/d (consider parenteral repletion with WKS)	MVM	MVM
Vitamin A	Uncommon (>7%)	Common (50%) with BPD, may occur with RYGB/LAGB	Plasma retinol	Ocular findings, night blindness	MVM	MVM	MVM + 10,000 IU/d vitamin A
Vitamin D	Common (60–70%)	Common, prevalence unknown	25(OH) D	Osteoporosis, associated risks of malignancy, autoimmune disease	MVM, 400–800 IU/d	MVM	MVM + 2000 IU/d vitamin D
Vitamin E	Uncommon	Uncommon	Plasma alpha tocopherol		MVM	MVM	MVM
Vitamin K	Variable	Uncommon	INR		MVM	MVM	MVM + 300 ug/d vitamin K
Zinc	Uncommon but increased risk with obesity	Common with BPD after one year, may occur with RYGB	Plasma zinc	Change taste acuity	MVM	MVM	MVM
Protein	Uncommon	Rare but can occur	Serum albumin, total protein				
Calcium	Common	Common	Bone density, PTH	Osteoporosis	1500 mg/d	1500 mg/d	1500 mg/d

and adrenal function, energy storage, glucose homeostatsis and others. Micronutrient repletion is vital for maximal weight loss and weight loss maintenance. Although obtaining micronutrients from food is the most desirable way to ensure adequacy of minerals and vitamins, for patients with severe obesity, multivitamin and mineral supplementation (MVM) is essential for repleting micronutrients before and after surgery. Table 25.3 identifies the prevalence of micronutrient deficiencies before and after bariatric surgery. Various algorithms have been designed to help the bariatric surgery team proactively address the potential for micronutrient deficiency and support the use of standard MVMs. Strategies must target the maintenance of stores as well as the repletion of losses and take into account the time course of development following a given bariatric surgery procedure.

Considerations in endoscopy

Endoscopy units providing care to the bariatric surgery patient need to be properly equipped for the care of these patients, commensurate with standards for a bariatric center of excellence. This equipment includes stretchers designed to support weights in excess of 350 lbs and physiologic monitoring equipment for larger individuals. Conscious sedation in patients with morbid obesity may be complicated due to the high prevalence of obstructive sleep apnea and increased risk for desaturation [148, 149]. Increased BMI has also been recognized as an independent risk factor predictive of difficult colonoscopy [150].

The role of endoscopy in the bariatric surgery patient has recently been reviewed by the American Society for Gastrointestinal Endoscopy [151]. The value of routine endoscopy before bariatric surgery in the patient without symptoms is controversial but is recommended in some guidelines [152]. Considerations for the endoscopist include the presence of a large hiatus hernia, which represents a relative contraindication to LAGB because of increased risk of band slippage. In patients undergoing RYGB and BPD/DS, because the surgery renders the distal stomach and/or duodenum inaccessible by a standard upper endoscope, the threshold for performing a pre-operative endoscopic evaluation of the upper GI tract is lower than for other surgeries. *Helicobacter pylori* infection is present in 30–40% of patients scheduled for bariatric surgery and may be associated with abnormal endoscopy and risk for marginal ulcers postoperatively. Pre-operative testing in these patients may be useful.

In the postoperative patient, endoscopy may be performed because of the symptoms discussed previously. The endoscopist should be aware of which operative procedure was performed and of findings on pre-procedural imaging studies. The choice of endoscope will depend on the indication and on the need for intubation of the excluded limb or on the need for therapeutic intervention (e.g. ERCP). In the early postoperative patient, insufflation may have potentially detrimental effects, and the endoscopist should first consider contrast radiography studies. After a RYGB, endoscopic findings should include a normal esophagus and gastroesophageal junction, a variably sized gastric pouch and a gastrojejunal stoma with a width of 10–12 mm in diameter. There may be a short blind limb

visible alongside of the efferent jejunal limb. The distal or excluded stomach cannot be visualized in the absence of a fistula. A VBG produces a pouch similar to the appearance of a RYGB with a 10–12 mm stoma and once this is traversed, the distal stomach and duodenum can be seen. LAGB produces a variable amount of extrinsic circumferential compression on the proximal stomach, evident at endoscopy. The endoscopist should note the length of the pouch and should evaluate the possibility of band erosion into the gastric wall.

Morbid obesity is a risk factor for gallstone formation, and rapid weight loss is an independent and potentially compounding risk factor. Whereas an ERCP can usually be performed after LAGB, an ERCP in an individual who has undergone RYGB represents a significant technical challenge. Factors influencing success in this group include endoscopic skill, jejunal loop length and afferent loop length. When standard endoscopy is not possible, laparascopically assisted transgastric ERCP has been employed [153, 154]. Alternative diagnostic modalities such as magnetic resonance cholangiopancreatography (MRCP) and therapeutic modalities such as percutaneous trans-hepatic intervention should also be considered. Both prophylactic cholecystectomy and the administration of ursodiol in these patients have been shown to reduce the incidence and complications of gallstones [155, 156]. **A1d**

Endoscopic treatments for obesity

Current endoscopic devices used for the treatment of obesity are space occupying balloons placed endoscopically into the stomach to promote weight loss. In a recent review of 30 studies, of which 18 were prospective including 5 randomized trials – and 12 were retrospective case studies, only one of three sham controlled studies found a significantly higher weight loss with the gastric balloon. In non-randomized studies, the average weight loss was 17.8 kg, with resolution or improvement in co-morbidities in 52–100% of patients. Complications from these devices include gastric perforation (0.2%) and obstruction (0.2%) and intolerance necessitating removal (2.5%) [157]. These devices are not approved for use in the USA and the best indications for this intervention remain to be defined.

Natural orifice translumenal endoscopic surgery (NOTES), using a hybrid of endoscopic and laparoscopic approaches, is increasingly described in patients with morbid obesity or with complications from bariatric surgery. Although not ready for "prime time", surgeons and endoscopists together are devising approaches to care of the bariatric surgery patient, and there is a large potential for development in this field [158].

References

1 World Health Organization. *Obesity: Preventing and Managing the Global Epidemic (WHO Technical Report Series no. 894)*. World Health Organization, Geneva, 2000.

2 Kopelman PG. Obesity as a medical problem. *Nature* 2000; **404**: 635–643.

3 Katzmarzyk PT, Janseen I. The economic costs associated with physical inactivity and obesity in Canada: An update. *Can J Appl Physiol* 2004; **29**: 90–115.

4 Visscher TLS, Rissanen A, Seidell JC *et al*. Obesity and unhealthy life-years in adult Finns: An empirical approach. *Archives of Internal Medicine* 2004; **164**(13): 1413–1420.

5 Puhl R, Brownell KD. Bias, discrimination, and obesity. *Obes Res* 2001; **9**: 788–805.

6 Kragelund C, Omland T. A farewell to body-mass index? *Lancet* 2005; **366**: 1589–1591.

7 Lau DC, Douketis JD, Morrison K *et al*. 2006 Canadian clinical practice guidelines on management and prevention of obesity in adults and children. *CMAJ* 2007; **176**: S1–13.

8 Blundell JE, Finlayson G. Is susceptibility to weight gain characterized by homeostatic or hedonic risk factors for overconsumption? *Physiol Behav* 2004; **82**: 21–25.

9 Sherwood NE, Jeffery RW. The behavioral determinants of exercise: Implications for physical activity interventions. *Annu Rev Nutr* 2000; **20**: 21–44.

10 Mauro M, Taylor V, Wharton S, Sharma AM. Barriers to obesity treatment. *Eur J Intern Med* 2008; **19**: 173–180.

11 Dalle Grave R, Calugi S, Magri F, Cuzzolaro M, Dall'aglio E, Lucchin L, Melchionda N, Marchesini G; QUOVADIS Study Group. Weight loss expectations in obese patients seeking treatment at medical centers. *Obes Res* 2004; **12**: 2005–2012.s.

12 Svetkey LP, Stevens VJ, Brantley PJ *et al*. Weight Loss Maintenance Collaborative Research Group. Comparison of strategies for sustaining weight loss: The weight loss maintenance randomized controlled trial. *JAMA* 2008; **299**: 1139–1148.

13 Padwal R, Kezouh A, Levine M, Etminan M. Long-term persistence with orlistat and sibutramine in a population-based cohort. *Int J Obes* 2007; **31**: 1567–1570.

14 Sjostrom L, Narbro K, Sjostrom CD *et al*. Swedish Obese Subjects Study. Effects of bariatric surgery on mortality in Swedish obese subjects. *N Engl J Med* 2007; **357**: 741–752.

15 Pi-Sunyer FX. A review of long term studies evaluating the efficacy of weight loss in ameliorating disorders associated with obesity. *Clin Ther* 1996; **18**: 1006–1035.

16 Dingemans AE, Bruna MJ, Furth EF. Binge eating disorder: A review. *Int J Obes* 2002; **26**: 299–307.

17 Rucker D, Padwal R, Li SK, Curioni C, Lau DC. Long term pharmacotherapy for obesity and overweight: Updated meta-analysis. *BMJ* 2007; **335**: 1194–1199.

18 Mayer J, Thoma DJ. Regulation of food intake and obesity. *Science* 1967; **156**: 328–337.

19 Cuomo R, Sarnelli G. Food intake and gastrointestinal motility. A complex interplay. *Nutr Metab Cardiovasc Dis* 2004; **14**: 173–179.

20 Cummings DE, Overduin J. Gastrointestinal regulation of food intake. *J Clin Invest* 2007; **117**: 13–23.

21 Chaudhri OB, Salem V, Murphy KG, Bloom SR. Gastrointestinal Satiety Signals. *Ann Rev Physiol* 2008; **70**: 239–255.

22 Camilleri M. Integrated upper gastrointestinal response to food intake. *Gastr* 2006; **131**: 640–658.

23 Xing J, Chen JD. Alterations of gastrointestinal motility in obesity. *Obes Res* 2004; **12**: 1723–1732.

24 Little TJ, Horowitz M, Feinle-Bisset C. Modulation by high-fat diets of gastrointestinal function and hormones associated with the regulation of energy intake: Implications for the pathophysiology of obesity. *Am J Clin Nutr* 2007; **86**: 531–541.

25 Kissileff HR, Pi-Sunyer X, Thornton J, Smith GP. C-terminal octapeptide of cholecytokinin decreases food intake in man. *Am J Clin Nutr* 1981; **34**: 154–160.

26 Ballinger A, McLoughlin L, Medback S, Clark M. Cholecytokinin is a satiety hormone in humans at physiological post-pradial concentrations. *Clin Sci* 1995; **89**: 375–381.

27 Lieverse RJ, Jansen JB, Masclee AA, Amers CB. Satiety effects of a physiological dose of cholecytokinin in humans. *Gut* 1995; **36**: 176–179.

28 Reubi JC, Waser B, Läderach U *et al*. Localization of cholecytokinin A and cholecystokinin B-gastrin receptors in the human stomach. *Gastroenterology* 1997; **112**: 1197–1205.

29 Savage AP, Adrian TE, Carolan G, Chatterjee VK, Bloom SR. Effects of peptide YY (PYY) on mouth to cecum intestinal transit time and on the rate of gastric emptying in healthy volunteers. *Gut* 1987; **28**: 166–170.

30 Batterham RL, Cohen MA, Ellis SM *et al*. Inhibition of food intake in obese subjects by peptide YY 3-36. *NEJM* 2003; **349**: 941–948.

31 Gutzwiller JP, Goke B, Drewe J *et al*. (1999) Glucagon-Like Peptide- 1 a potent regulator of food intake on humans. *Gut* **44**; 81–86.

32 Flint A, Raban A, Ersboll AK *et al*. The effect of physiological levels of Glucagon-Like Peptide 1 on appetite, gastric emptying, energy and substrate metabolism in obesity. *J Obes Relat Metab Disord* 2001; **25**: 781–792.

33 Nocon M, Labenz J, Willich SN. Lifestyle factors and symptoms of gastroesophageal reflux – a population based study. *Aliment Pharmacol Ther* 2006; **23**: 169–174.

34 Iovino P, Angrisani L, Galloro G *et al*. Proximal stomach function in obesity with normal or abnormal esophageal acid exposure. *Neurogastroenterol Motil* 2006; **18**: 425–432.

35 El-Serag HB, Graham DY, Satia JA, Rabeneck L. Obesity is an independent risk factor for GERD symptoms and erosive esophagitis. *Am J Gastroenterol* 2005; **100**: 1243–1250.

36 Rey E, Moreno-Elola-Olaso C, Artalejo FR, Locke GR, DiazRubio M. Association between weight gain and symptoms of gastroesophegal reflux in the general population. *Am J Gastro* 2006; **101**: 229–233.

37 Hampel H, Abraham N, El-Serag HB. Meta-analysis: Obesity and the risk for gastroesophageal reflux disease and its complications. *Ann Internal Med* 2005; **143**: 199–211.

38 De Vries DR, Van Herwaarden MA, Smout AJ *et al*. Gastroesophageal pressure gradients in gastroesophageal reflux disease: Relations with hiatus hernia, body mass index and esophageal acid exposure. *Am J Gastroenterol* 2008; **103**(6): 1349–1354.

39 Sise A, Friendenberg FK. A comprehensive review of gastro-esophageal reflux disease and obesity. *Obesity review* 2008; **9**: 194–203.

40 Kaltenbach T, Crockett S, Gerson LB. Are lifestyle measures effective in patients with gastroesophageal reflux disease? An evidence-based approach. *Arch Intern Med* 2006; **166**: 965–971.

41 Barak N, Ehrenpreis ED, Harrison JR, Sitrin MD. Gastroesophageal reflux disease in obesity: Pathophysiological and therapeutic considerations. *Obe Rev* 2002; **3**: 9–15.

42 Austin GL, Thiny MT, Westman EC, Yancy WS, Shaheen NJ. A very low-carbohydrate diet improves gastroesophageal reflux and its symptoms. *Dig Dis Sci* 2006; **51**: 1307–1312.

43 Fox M, Barr C, Nolan S, Lomer M, Anggiansah A, Wong T. The effects of dietary fat and calorie density on esophageal acid exposure and reflux symptoms. *Clin Gastroenterol Hepatol* 2007; **5**: 439–444.

44 Di Francesco V, Baggio E, Mastromauro M *et al.* Obesity and gastroesophageal acid reflux: Physiopathological mechanisms and role of bariatric surgery. *Obe Surg* 2004; **14**: 1095–1102.

45 Linare CL, Pelletier AL, Czernichow S *et al.* Acute pancreatitis in a cohort of 129 patients referred for severe hypertriglyceridia. *Pancreas* 2008; **37**(1): 13–20.

46 Funnell IC, Bornman PC, Weakly SP, Terblanche J, Marks IN. Obesity: An important prognostic factor in acute pancreatitis. *Br J Surg* 1993; **80**(4): 484–486.

47 Papachristou GI, Papachristou DJ, Avula H, Slivka A, Whitcomb DC. Obesity increases the severity of acute pancreatitis: Performance of APACHE-O score and correlation with inflammatory response. *Pancreatology* 2006; **6**(4): 275–285.

48 Toyama MT, Lewis MPN, Kusske AM *et al.* Ischemia-reperfusion mechanisms in acute pancreatitis. *Scan J Gastroenterol* 1996; **31**(Suppl): 20–23, 219.

49 Porter KA, Banks PA. Obesity as a predictor of severity in acute pancreatitis. *Int J Pancreatol* 1991; **10**(3–4): 247–252.

50 Johnson CD, Toh SK, Campbell MJ. Combination of APACHE-II score and an obesity score (APAHE-O) for the prediction of severe acute pancreatitis. *Pancreatology* 2004; **4**(1): 1–6.

51 Toh SKC, Walters J, Johnson CD. Apache-O a new predictor of severity in acute pancreatitis. *Gastro* 1996; **110**: A437.

52 Sahi T, Puffenbarger RS, Hseih C *et al.* Body mass index, cigarette smoking and other characteristics as predictors of self-reported, physician-diagnosed gallbladder disease in male college alumni. *Am J Epidemiol* 1998; **147**: 644–651.

53 Tsai C-J, Leitzmann MF, Willett WC *et al.* Prospective study of abdominal adiposity and gallstones in US men. *Am J Clin Nutr* 2002; **40**: 937–943.

54 Apstein MD, Carey MC. Pathogenesis of cholesterol gallstones: A parsimonious hypothesis. *Eur J Clin Invest* 1996; **26**: 343–352.

55 Diehl AK. Cholelithiasis and the insulin resistance syndrome. *Hepatology* 2000; **31** 528–530.

56 Mendez-Sanchez N, Zamora-Valdes D, Chavez-Tapia NC, Uribe M. Role of diet in cholesterol gallstone formation. *Clinica Chimica Acta* 2007; **376**: 1–8.

57 Thijs C, Knipschild P, Brombacher P. Serum lipids and gallstones: A case-control study. *Gastro* 1990; **99**: 843–849.

58 Inoue K, Fuchigami A, Higashide S *et al.* Gallbladder sludgy and stone formation in relation to contractile function after gastrectomy: A prospective study. *Ann Surg* 1992; **215**: 19–26.

59 Schlierf G, Schellenberg B, Stiehl A, Czygan P, Oster P. Bilary cholesterol saturation and weight reduction – effects of fasting and low calorie diet. *Digestion* 1981; **21**: 44–49.

60 Yang H, Petersen GM, Roth MP, Schonfield LJ, Marks JW. Risk factors for gallstone formation during rapid loss of weight. *Dig Dis Sci* 1992; **37**: 912–918.

61 Broomfield PH, Chopra R, Sheinbaum RC *et al.* Effects of ursodeoxycholic acid and aspirin on the formation of lithogenic bile and gallstones during loss of weight. *N Engl J Med* 1988; **319**: 1567–1572.

62 Liddle RA, Goldstein RB, Saxton J. Gallstone formation during weight reduction dieting. *Arch Intern Med* 1988; **149**: 1750–1753.

63 Shiffman ML, Sugerman HJ, Kellum JM, Brewer WH, Moore EW. Gallstone formation after rapid weight loss: A prospective study in patients undergoing gastric bypass surgery for treatment of morbid obesity. *Am J Gastroenterol* 1991; **86**: 1000–1005.

64 Wattchow DA. Prevalence and treatment of gallstones after gastric bypass surgery for morbid obese. *Br J Med* 1983; **286**: 763–764.

65 Weinsier RL, Wilson LJ, Lee J. Medically safe rate of weight loss for the treatment of obesity: A guideline based on risk of gallstone formation. *Am J Med* 1995; **98**: 115–117.

66 Erlinger S. Gallstones in obesity and weight loss. *Eur J Gastro Hepatol* 2000; **12**(12): 1347–1352.

67 Worobetz LJ, Inglis FG, Shaffer EA. The effect of ursodeoxycholic acid therapy on gallstone formation in the morbidly obese during rapid weight loss. *Am J Gastro* 1993; **88**(10): 1705–1710.

68 Miller K, Hell E, Lang B, Lengauer E. Gallstone formation prophylaxis after gastric restrictive procedures for weight loss: A randomized double-blind placebo-controlled trial. *Ann Surg* 2003; **238**(5): 697–702.

69 Konvolinka, CW. Acute diverticulitis under age forty. *Am J Surg* 1994; **167**: 562–565.

70 Zaidi E, Daly B. CT and Clinical Features of Acute Diverticulitis in an Urban US Population: Rising Frequency in Young, Obese Adults. *AJR* 2006; **187**: 689–694.

71 Schauer PR, Ramos R, Ghiata AA, Sirinek KR. Virulent diverticular disease in young obese men. *Am J Surg* 1992; **164**(5): 443–446.

72 Dobbins C, DeFontgalland D, Duthie G, Wattchow DA. The relationship of obesity to the complications of diverticular disease. *Colorectal Dis* 2006; **8**(1): 37–40.

73 Furstenberger G and Senn H. Insulin-like growth factors and cancer. *Lancet Obcol* 2002; **3**: 298–302.

74 Bianchini F, Kaaks R and Vainio H. Overweight, obesity and cancer risk. *Lancet Oncol* 2002; **3**: 565–574.

75 Somasundar P, Riggs D, Jackson B *et al.* Leptin stimulates esophageal adenocarcinoma growth by nonapoptotic mechanisms. *Am J Surg* 2003; **186**: 575–578.

76 Somasundar P, Yu AK, Vona-Davis L, McFadden DW. Differential effects of leptin on cancer *in vitro. J Surg Res* 2003; **113**: 50–55.

77 Brakenhielm E, Veitonmaki N, Cao R *et al.* Adiponectin-induced antiangiogenesis and antitumour activity involve caspase-mediated endothelial cell apoptosis. *Proc Natl Acad USA* 2004; **101**: 2476–2481.

78 Raju J, McCarthy B and Bird RP. Steady state levels of transforming growth factor beta 1 and beta 2 mRNA and protein expression are elevated in colonic tumours *in vivo* irrespective of dietary lipids intervention. *Int J Cancer* 2002; **100**: 635–641.

79 Calle EE, Rodriguez C, Walker-Thurmond K and Thun MJ. Overweight, obesity, and mortality from cancer in a prospectively studied cohort of US adults. *NEJM* 2003; **348**: 1625–1638.

80 Renehan AG, Tyson M, Egger M, Heller RF, Zwahlen M. Body-mass index and incidence of cancer: A systematic review and meta-analysis of prospective observational studies. *Lancet* 2008; **371**: 569–578.

81 Chlebowski RT, Wactawski-Wende J, Ritenbaugh C *et al.* for the Women's Health Initiative Investigators. Estrogen plus Progestin and Colorectal Cancer in Postmenopausal Women. *NEJM* 2004; **350**: 991–1004.

82 Cook MS, Greenwood DC, Hardie LJ, Wild CP, Forman D. A systematic review and meta-analysis of the risk of increasing adiposity on Barrett's esophagus. *Amer J Gastro* 2008; **103**: 292–300.

83 Kendall BJ, Macdonald GA, Hayward NK *et al.* Leptin and the risk of Barrett's esophagus. *Gut* 2008; **57**(4): 448–454.

84 Abnet CC, Freedman ND, Hollenbeck AR, Fraumeni JF Jr, Leitzmann M, Schatzkin A. A prospective study of BMI and risk of esophageal and gastric adenocarcinoma. *Eur J Cancer* 2008; **44**(3): 465–471.

85 Wu AH, Wan P, Berstein L. A multiethnic population-based study of smoking, alcohol and body size and risk of adenocarcinomas of the stomach and esophagus. *Cancer Causes Control* 2001; **12**(8): 721–732.

86 Lagergren J, Bergstrom R, Nyren O. Association between body mass and adenocarcinoma of the esophagus and gastric cardia. *Ann Intern Med* 1999; **130**: 883–890.

87 Vaughan TL, Davis S, Kristal A, Thomas DB. Obesity, alcohol, and tobacco as risk factors for cancers of the esophagus and gastric cardia: Adenocarcinoma versus squamous cell carcinoma. *Can Epidemiol Biomarkers Prev* 1995; **87**: 104–109.

88 Lindblad M, Rodriguez LA, Lagergren J. Body mass, tobacco and alcohol and risk of esophageal, gastric cardia, and gastric non-cardia adenocarcinoma among men and women in a nested case-control study. *Cancer Causes Control* 2005; **16**(3): 285–294.

89 Gumbs A. Obesity, Pancreatitis, and Pancreatic Cancer. *Obes Surg* 2008; **18**(9): 1183–1187.

90 Berrington de Gonzalez A, Sweetland S, Spencer E. A meta-analysis of obesity and the risk of pancreatic cancer. *Brit J Cancer* 2003; **89**: 519–523.

91 Pitt. Hepato-pancreato-biliary fat: The good, the bad and the ugly. *HPB* 2007; **9**: 92–97.

92 Mathur A, Marine M, Lu D, Swartz-Basile DA, Saxena R, Zyromski NJ, Pitt HA. Nonalcoholic fatty pancreas disease. *HPB* 2007; **9**(4): 312–318.

93 Nair S, Mason A, Eason J, Loss G, Perrillo RP. Is obesity an independent risk factor for hepatocellular carcinoma in cirrhosis? *Hepatology* 2002; **36**: 150–155.

94 Adami HO, Chow WH, Nyren O *et al.* Excess risk of primary liver cancer in patients with diabetes mellitus. *J Natl Cancer Inst* 1996; **89**: 317–318.

95 Wideroff L, Gridley G, Mellemkjaer L *et al.* Cancer incidence in a population based cohort of patients hospitalized with diabetes mellitus in Denmark. *J Natl Cancer Inst* 1997; **89**: 1360–1365.

96 Ohki T, Tateishi R, Sato T, Masuzaki R. Obesity is an independent risk factor for hepatocellular carcinoma development in chronic hepatitis C patients. *Clin Gastroenterology Hepatol* 2008; **6**(4): 459–464.

97 Kita Y, Mizukoshi E, Takamura T *et al.* Impact of diabetes mellitus on prognosis of patients infected with hepatitis C virus. *Metabolism* 2007; **56**(12): 1682–1688.

98 Lazaridis KN, Gores GJ. Cholangiocarcinoma. *Gastroenterology* 2005; **128**: 1655–1667.

99 Oh SW, Yoon YS, Shin SA. Effects of excess weight on cancer incidences depending on cancer sites and histologic findings among men: Korean national health insurance corporation study. *J Clin Oncol* 2005; **23**: 4742–4745.

100 Chow WH, McLaughlin JK, Menck HR, Mack TM. Risk factors for extrahepatic bile duct cancers: Los Angeles County, California (USA). *Cancer Causes Control* 1994; **5**: 267–272.

101 Welzel TM, Mellemkjaer L, Gloria G *et al.* Risk factors for intrahepatic cholangiocarcinoma in a low-risk population: A nationwide case-control study. *Int J Cancer* 2006; **120**: 638–641.

102 Ahrens W, Timmer A, Vyberg M *et al.* Risk Factors for extrahepatic biliary tract carcinoma in men: Medical conditions and lifestyle. *Eur J Gastroenterol Hepatol* 2007; **19**: 623–630.

103 Larsson SC and Wolk A. Obesity and colon and rectal cancer risk: A meta-analysis of prospective studies. *Am J Clin Nutr* 2007; **86**: 556–865.

104 Fressa EE, Wachtel MS, Chiriva-Internati M. Influence of obesity on the risk of developing colon cancer. *Gut* 2006; **55**: 285–291.

105 Giovannucci E. Obesity, gender, and colon cancer. *Gut* 2002; **51**: 147.

106 Samad AKA, Taylor RS, Marshall T *et al.* A meta-analysis of the association of physical activity with reduced risk of colorectal cancer. *Colorecatl Dis* 2005; **7**: 204–213.

107 Bingham SA, Cummings JH. Effect of exercise and physical fitness on large intestinal function. *Gastroenterology* 1989; **97**: 1389–1399.

108 El-Serag. Obesity and disease of the esophagus and colon. *Gastroenterol Clin N Am* 2005; **34**: 63–82.

109 Gallagher TK, Geoghegan JG, Baird AW, Winter DC. Implications of altered gastrointestinal motility in obesity. *Obesity Surgery* 2007; **17**: 1399–1407.

110 O'Brien TF Jr. Lower esophageal sphincter pressure (LESP) and esophageal function in obese humans. *J Clin Gastroenterol* 1980; **2**: 145–148.

111 Zacchi P, Mearin F, Humbert P, Formiguera X, Malagelada JR. Effect of obesity on gastroesophageal resistance to flow in man. *Dig Dis Sci* 1991; **36**: 1473–1480.

112 Mercer CD, Wren SF, DaCosta LR *et al.* Lower esophageal sphincter pressure and gastroesophageal pressure gradients in excessively obese patients. *J Med* 1987; **18**: 135–146.

113 Koppman JS, Poggi L, Szomstein S, Ukleja A, Botoman R, Rosenthal R. Esophageal motility disorders in the morbidly obese population. *Surg Endosc* 2007; **21**: 761–764.

114 Jaffin B, Knoeplmacher P, Greenstein R. High prevalence of asymptomatic esophageal motility disorders among morbidly obese patients. *Obes Surg* 1999; **9**: 390–395.

115 Greenstein RJ, Nissan A, Jaffin B. Esophageal anatomy and function in laparoscopic gastric restrictive bariatric surgery: Implications for patient selection. *Obes Surg* 1989; **8**: 199–206.

116 Merrouche M, Sabete M, Jouet P *et al.* Gastro-esophageal reflux and esophageal motility disorders in morbidly obese patients before and after bariatric surgery. *Obes Surg* 2007; **17**: 894–900.

117 Tosetti C, Corinaldesi R, Stanghellini V *et al.* Gastric emptying of solids in morbid obesity. *Int J Obes relat Metab Disord* 1996; **20**: 200–205.

118 Xing J, Chen J DZ. Alterations of Gastrointestinal Motility in Obesity. *Obesity Research* 2004; **12**(11): 1723–1732.

119 Jones TF, Lin Z, Sarosiek I, Moncure M, McCallum RW. Assessment of gastric emptying and myoelectric activity in the morbidly obese patients. *Gastroenterology* 2001; **120**: A1500 (abstract)

120 Guyang H, Yin J, Chen JD. Therapeutic potential of gastric electrical stimulation for obesity and its possible mechanism: A preliminary canine study. *Dig Dis Sci* 2003; **48**(4): 698–705.

121 Fraquelli M, Pagliarulo M, Colucci A, Paggi S, Conte D. Gallbladder motility in obesity, diabetes mellitus and celiac disease. *Dig Liv Dis* 2003; **35**: S12–16.

122 Nakeeb A, Comuzzie AG, Al-Azzawi H, Sonnenberg GE, Kissebah AH, Pitt HA. Insulin resistance causes human gallbladder dysmotility. *J Gastrointest Surg* 2006; **10**(7): 948–949.

123 Gielkens HA, Lam WF, Coenraad M *et al.* Effect of insulin on basal and cholecystokinin-stimulated gallbladder motility in humans. *J Hepatol* 1998; **28**: 595–602.

124 Wisen O, Johansson C. Gastrointestinal function in obesity: Motility, secretion and absorption following a liquid test meal. *Metabolism* 1992; **41**: 390–395.

125 Crowell MD, Cheskin LJ, Musial F. Prevalence of gastrointestinal symptoms in obese and normal weight binge eaters. *Am J Gastr* 1994; **8**: 387–391.

126 Delgado-Aros S, Locke R, Camilleri M, Talley N, Fett S, Zinsmeister AR, Melton JM. Obesity is associated with increased risk of gastrointestinal symptoms: A population-based study. *Am J Gastro* 2004; **99**: 1801–1806.

127 Talley NJ, Howell S, Pouton R. Obesity and chronic gastrointestinal tract symptoms in young adults: A birth cohort study. *Am J Gastr* 2004; **99**: 1807–1814.

128 Levy RL, Linde JA, Feld JA, Crowell MD, Jeffrey RW. The association of gastrointestinal symptoms with weight, diet, and exercise in weight-loss program participants. *Clin Gastr Hepatol* 2005; **3**: 992–996.

129 Talley NJ, Quan C, Jones MP, Horowitz M. Association of upper and lower gastrointestinal tract symptoms with body mass index in an Australian cohort. *Neurogastroenterol Motil* 2004; **16**: 413–419.

130 Bulpitt CJ, Palmer AJ, Battersby C, Fletcher AE. Association of symptoms of type 2 diabetic patients with severity of disease, obesity, and blood pressure. *Diabetes Care* 1998; **21**: 111–115.

131 Svelberg P, Johannson S, Wallander MA, Hamelin B, Pedersen NL. Extra-intestinal manifestations associated with irritable bowel syndrome: A twin study. *Aliment Pharmacol Ther* 2002; **16**: 975–983.

132 Clements RH, Gonzalez QH, Foster A, Richards WO, McDowell J, Bondora A, Laws HL. Gastrointestinal symptoms are more intense in morbidly obese individuals and are improved with laparoscopic Roux-en-Y gastric bypass. *Obes Surg* 2003; **13**(4): 610–614.

133 DeMaria EJ. Bariatric surgery for morbid obesity. *N Engl J Med* 2007; **356**: 2176–2183.

134 Sjostrom L, Lindroos AK, Peltonen M *et al.* Lifestyle, diabetes and cardiovascular risk factors 10 years after bariatric surgery. *N Engl J Med* 2004; **351**: 2683–2693.

135 Flum DR, Cheadle A, Chan L *et al.* Early Mortality among Medicare Beneficiaries Undergoing Bariatric Surgical Procedures. *JAMA* 2005; **294**(15): 1903.

136 Livingston EH. Obesity, Mortality, and Bariatric Surgery Death Rates. *JAMA* 2007; **298**(20): 2406–2408.

137 NIH Conference. Consensus development conference. Gastrointestinal surgery for severe obesity. *Ann Intern Med* 1991; **115**, 956–961.

138 Santry HP, Gillen DL, Lauderdale DS. Trends in Bariatric Surgical Procedures. *JAMA* 2005; **294**(15): 1909–1917.

139 Wolfe BM, Morton JM. Weighing in on Bariatric surgery: Procedure use, readmission rates and mortality. *JAMA* 2005; **294**(15): 1960–1963.

140 Huang CS, Farraye FA. Endoscopy in the Bariatric surgery patient. *Gastroenterology Clinics of North America* 2005; **34**(1): 151–166.

141 Lee CW, Kelly J, Wassel WY. Complications of Bariatric surgery. *Current Opinion in Gastroenterology* 2007; **23**: 636–643.

142 Tang S, Rockey DC. The role of endoscopy in Bariatrics. *Gastroentestinal Endoscpy* 2008; **16**(1): 1–4.

143 Liem RK, Niloff PH. Prophylactic cholecystectomy with open gastric bypass operation. *Obes Surg* 2004; **14**: 763–765.

144 Villegas L, Schneider B, Provost D *et al.* Is routine cholecystectomy required during laparascolic gastric bypass? *Obes Surg* 2004; **14**: 60–66.

145 Elton E, Hanson BL, Quaseem T *et al.* Diagnostic and therapeutic ERCP using an enteroscope and pediatric colonoscope in long limb surgical bypass patients. *Gastrointes Endoscopy* 1998; **47**: 62–67.

146 Nutrition Committee, Aills A, Blankenship J, Buffington C, Furtado M, Parrott J. ASBMS Allied Health Nutrition Guidelines for the Surgical Weight Loss Patient. *Surgery for Obes and Related Diseases* 2008. 4(5, Sept–Oct suppl): s73–108.

147 Schweitzer DH, Posthuma EF. Prevention of Vitamin and Mineral Deficiencies after Bariatric surgery: Evidence and Algorithms. *Obes Surg* 2008; **18**: 1028–1034.

148 Villegas T. Sleep Apnea and moderate sedation. *Gastroenterol Nurs* 2004; **27**(3): 121–124.

149 Weaver JM. Increased anaesthetic risk for patients with obesity and obstructive sleep apnea. *Anesth prog* 2004; **51**: 75.

150 Anderson JC, Messina CR, Cohn W *et al.* Factors predictive of difficult colonoscopy. *Gastrointest endosc* 2001; **54**(5): 558–562.

151 Anderson, MA, Gan I, Fanelli RD *et al.* Role of endoscopy in the bariatric surgery Patient. *Gastrointestinal Endoscopy* 2008; **68**: 1–10.

152 Sauerland S, Agrisani L, Belachew M *et al.* Europena Association for Endoscopic Surgery. Obesity Surgery: Evidence based guidelinies of the European Association for Endoscopic Surgery (EAES), *Surg Endosc* 2005; **19**: 200–221.

153 Ceppa DA, Gagne DJ, Papasavas PK *et al.* Laparascopic transgastric endoscopy after RYGB. *Surg Obes Relat Dis* 2007; **3**: 21–24.

154 Martinez J, Guerrero L, Buyers P *et al.* Endoscopi retrograde cholangiopancreatography and gastroduodnoscopy after RYGB. *Surg Endosc* 2006; **20**: 1548–1550.

155 Mason EE, Renquist KE. Gallbladder management in obesity surgery. *Obes Surg* 2002; **12**: 222–229.

156 Miller K, Hell E, Lang B *et al.* Gallstone formation prophylaxis after gastric restrictive procedures for weight loss: A randomized double-blind placebo-controlled trial. *Ann Surg* 2003; **238**: 697–702.

157 Dumonceau JM. Evidence –based review of the Bioenterics intragastric balloon for weight loss. *Obes Surg* 2008; **18**(12): 1611–1617.

158 Swain P. NOTES and anastamosis. *GI Endoscopy clinics of NA* 2008; **8**: 261–277.

II Liver disease

26 Hepatitis C

Keyur Patel, Hans L Tillmann and John G McHutchison

Division of Gastroenterology, Duke Clinical Research Institute *and* Duke University Medical Center, North Carolina, USA

Introduction

Hepatitis C virus (HCV) was identified in 1989 as a major cause of the parenterally transmitted non-A non-B hepatitis. The majority of patients develop chronic hepatitis C infection (CHC) that has a global prevalence of 2.2% and infects over 120 million people worldwide [1]. CHC is characterized by varying degrees of inflammation and hepatic fibrosis, and 20% of patients are likely to develop progressive liver damage with cirrhosis and complications of end-stage liver disease over 20 to 40 years. CHC is now the leading indication for liver transplantation in developed nations and is expected to pose a significant health and economic burden over the next 10 to 20 years.

HCV genome

Hepatitis C virus (HCV) is an enveloped positive-sense virus classified in the *Hepacivirus* genus within the *Flaviviridae* family, and was discovered in 1989 from a cDNA clone derived from blood-borne non-A non-B viral hepatitis genome sequences. The virus consists of a single open reading frame of 9.6 kb flanked by 5′ and 3′ untranslated regions that are required for viral translation and replication. The 5′ UTR contains the internal ribozyme entry site (IRES) that initiates translation of a 3000 aminoacid polyprotein, which is subsequently processed by viral and host cellular proteases into ten mature structural (core, E1, E2 and p7) and non-structural HCV proteins (NS2, NS3, NS4A, NS5A and NS5B). The non-structural proteins encode several key enzymes involved in viral replication such as the NS3 protease and NS5B RNA-dependent RNA polymerase. The lack of small animal model systems for HCV has rather limited our understanding of HCV replication and pathogenesis, but the recent development of *in vitro* and cell culture systems has resulted in significant progress in this regard in recent years [2].

HCV is characterized by a high degree of heterogeneity, resulting from the high replication rate (~10^{12} particles per day) and the lack of a proof-reading repair mechanism in the viral RNA polymerase. The genetic heterogeneity of HCV is complex and may contribute to immune escape and the development of chronic infection in the majority of patients [3].

HCV has evolved into at least six major genetic groups (genotype) and over 50 subtypes, and is recognized by sequence variation in E1 and NS5b regions [4]. Different isolates of the same subtype may vary as much as 5–15%, and differing genotypes by more than 30% in nucleotide sequence. There is significant variation in the geographic distribution of HCV genotypes: genotype 1a is the prototype genotype and found commonly in the USA and Northern Europe; subtype 1b is common in Japan and Southern and Eastern Europe. Genotypes 2a and 2b represent 10–30% of all types and are particularly common in Japan and Northern Italy; genotype 3 is prevalent in the Indian subcontinent and Australasia; genotype 4 is common in Africa and the Middle East; genotypes 5 and 6 are found in South Africa and South East Asia respectively. Clinical studies have been able to identify that viral genotype affects response to antiviral therapy, but it does not have a significant influence on transmission, pathogenesis and the natural history of the disease.

Prevalence and transmission

There are significant differences in the global prevalence of CHC, with seroprevalence rates ranging from 0.6% to 22%. Lower rates are seen in industrialized nations such as Germany (0.6%), France (1.1%), USA (1.8%), Japan (1.5–

Evidence-Based Gastroenterology and Hepatology, 3rd edition.
J. McDonald, A.K. Burroughs, B. Feagan, and M.B. Fennerty. © 2010
Blackwell Publishing Ltd

2.3%), and higher rates in developing nations such as China (3.2%) and Pakistan (2.5–6.5%) [1]. The highest reported seroprevalence rates are in Egypt (22%) due to past exposure through parenteral antischistosomal therapy [5]. HCV infection is transmitted by percutaneous or permucosal exposure to infected blood or body fluids. Although routes of infection may vary by geographic region, injection drug use (IDU) and receipt of a blood transfusion prior to implementation of donor screening in 1992 are the most common factors associated with transmission in developed nations. In these countries, transmission risks have been further reduced following the use of nucleic acid testing for HCV in donor blood, and the American Red Cross estimates that the risk of HCV infection is now 1/2,000,000 blood units [6]. However, most developing countries do not screen blood donations for HCV, and transmission risks from blood product transfusion remain much higher. Injection drug use remains the most significant risk factor for HCV transmission in developed nations, accounting for 68% of newly acquired cases, with high seroprevalence rates of 60–90% amongst those with long-term IDU [7]. In the USA, the incidence of HCV amongst IDU has continued to decline over the last decade, and current prevalence rates among IDU are likely to be lower [8]. Other routes of HCV transmission include sexual exposure to an infected partner, or multiple sex partners that account for 18% of new infections in epidemiological surveys, although transmission is rare between long-term monogamous heterosexual partners. The US Centers for Disease Control does not recommend barrier protection for heterosexual monogamous couples [9]. Nosocomial, iatrogenic and perinatal exposures are responsible for around 1% of cases, but in 9% of cases no definite source is identified. Indeterminate risk factors include household transmission (e.g. sharing razor blades or toothbrushes), tattooing, body piercing, intranasal cocaine use, dental procedures and acupuncture [7]. In general, although screening and testing of blood donors in developed nations has been successful in reducing the risk of HCV transmission, strategies for eliminating transmission from high risk behavior still need to be widely implemented.

Acute hepatitis C infection

Most patients with acute HCV infection are asymptomatic, and only 10–15% may develop symptoms, such as jaundice, febrile illness, abdominal pain and nausea, that may be indicative of acute hepatitis. Marked elevations in serum alanine aminotransferase (ALT) levels of 10–20 times upper limit of normal may be observed at this time. HCV RNA appears in the serum within 1–2 weeks of exposure, and HCV antibodies become detectable over the subsequent 4–6 weeks. Diagnosis of acute infection relies on HCV RNA

detection, as antibody responses such as HCV-IgM antibody remain detectable during both acute and chronic infection [10]. Spontaneous viral clearance and resolution of infection may occur in 10–35% of asymptomatic individuals, but in up to 52% of symptomatic cases [11]. There are no reliable factors in acute hepatitis C that predict progression to chronic infection, but age, gender and mode of transmission may be important [12, 13]. There are no specific guidelines for post-exposure prophylaxis, but HCV RNA and ALT, and HCV antibodies are usually measured at baseline, at 4–8 weeks and at three months after potential exposure, as these tend to fluctuate significantly during the acute phase of illness. Controversies still exist regarding the optimal regimen and timing of antiviral therapy in acute hepatitis C infection. To allow for spontaneous clearance, antiviral therapy may be delayed for three months following exposure. **B4** Depending on viral genotype, HCV RNA levels, and early viral response, sustained virologic response rates of over 80% are possible with a 12–24 week duration of pegylated interferon-alpha (PEG-IFN) therapy, either as monotherapy or in combination with ribavirin [14]. **B4** However, due to inherent difficulties in performing clinical studies in this population, the optimal treatment regimen has yet to be determined [15]. **B4**

Natural history and progression of chronic infection

Persistent or chronic infection, as defined by detectable serum HCV RNA for at least six months, develops in 65–85% of HCV-infected patients, based on data from post-transfusion hepatitis, blood donors and injection drug use cohorts (Figure 26.1). Women and younger patients may have lower rates of chronic infection of 55–71% following exposure to contaminated blood products [12, 13, 16]. Factors such as age at infection, gender, race, severity of acute illness, and immune status likely determine persistence or spontaneous resolution of HCV infection. A broad multispecific CD4+ and CD8+ T-lymphocyte immune response targeting multiple HCV epitopes is associated with viral clearance and resolution of infection, and a weaker cellular immune response is associated with development of chronic infection. Patients with chronic infection are often asymptomatic or may have non-specific complaints of malaise, fatigue and abdominal discomfort. The diagnosis of CHC often follows routine investigations that have noted elevated ALT levels. However, at least one-third of patients may have persistently normal ALT levels and the majority of these patients are likely to have mild and non-progressive disease.

Following a diagnosis of CHC, estimating the duration of infection and an assessment of disease severity may also help guide treatment decisions. The rate of fibrosis pro-

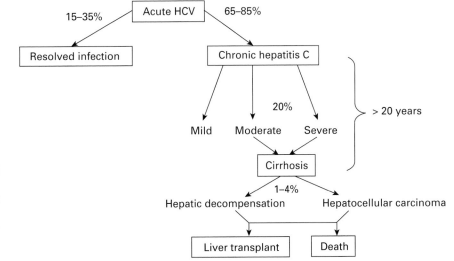

Figure 26.1 Natural history and progression of HCV infection. Following acute infection, 15–35% of patients achieve spontaneous viral clearance. The majority of patients develop chronic infection with variable rates of disease progression. A small proportion of patients with chronic infection will develop progressive disease over >20 years, with subsequent complications of end-stage liver disease.

gression varies amongst CHC infected patients. Host, viral and environmental factors can all influence disease progression in CHC infection (Table 26.1). Some of these co-factors may be potentially modifiable, including alcohol consumption, smoking, metabolic factors (insulin resistance, obesity, steatosis) and HIV co-infection [17, 18]. Studies assessing fibrosis progression have mostly been cross-sectional, and based on a single liver biopsy and estimated duration of infection. Prospective studies have been based on selected cohorts attending tertiary referral centers. These estimates indicate that fibrosis progression is non-linear and may be slow, moderate or rapid. For example, only 0–2% of younger women that acquired HCV from anti-D immune globulin progressed to cirrhosis over a 20-year period, compared to an average of 13 years for older male patients that consumed at least 50 g of alcohol daily [12]. CHC patients with compensated cirrhosis have slowly progressive disease, with an estimated annual hepatic decompensation rate of 4–5%, and 1–4% for incidence of hepatocellular carcinoma (HCC) that remains the most frequent initial complication in these patients [19, 20]. Current estimates of HCC incidence rates are higher in countries such as Japan that have a longer natural history of HCV infection, but these are expected to double in the USA over the next decade.

Diagnosis and evaluation

Diagnostic tests for HCV infection comprise serologic assays for antibodies and molecular techniques for virus particle detection. Anti-HCV is typically identified using second or third generation enzyme immunoassays that detect antibodies directed against various epitopes in the core, NS3, NS4 and NS5 proteins, with a specificity of 99%.

Table 26.1 Host-viral factors associated with disease progression.

Established factors	Possible factors
Age	Genotype 1b
Duration of infection	Quasispecies diversity
Male gender	Race
HIV or HBV co-infection	Smoking, cannabis use
Alcohol abuse	Genetic polymorphisms
Co-morbid disease (NAFLD, iron, schistosomiasis)	Environmental toxins
Increased ALT, necroinflammation or fibrosis	Source of Infection
Metabolic factors (insulin resistance, obesity)	
HLA class II polymorphisms	

NAFLD: non-alcoholic fatty liver disease; ALT: alanine aminotransferase; HLA: human leucocyte antigen.

In low-risk populations, false-positive tests may occur, and recombinant immunoblot assays (RIBA) are used in some centers to confirm positive EIAs. False negative tests may occur in HIV-1 infection, renal failure and HCV-associated cryoglobulinemia. Confirmatory testing involves molecular techniques that are useful in detecting and quantifying viral genomes using target or signal amplification methods. Several reliable qualitative and quantitative assays for detection are now commercially available. The newer real-time PCR and target mediated amplification assays have lower limits of detection for HCV of below 10 IU/ml.

However, these tests are expensive and not recommended for low prevalence population screening. They are used for confirmatory testing in acute infection prior to development of anti-HCV, immunocompromised patients, newborns, and in CHC patients to predict and monitor virologic responses to antiviral therapy.

All patients with confirmed CHC should have genotype testing to determine duration and likelihood of response to currently available antiviral therapy. A liver biopsy in CHC patients also provides useful baseline information in regards to necroinflammatory activity and fibrosis stage that can help determine prognosis, urgency of therapy, prediction of response to treatment, and evaluation of co-morbid states such as steatosis. In the absence of co-morbid issues that preclude treatment, patients with HCV genotype 2 and 3 infection have excellent predicted responses to antiviral therapy, and may not require a biopsy prior to therapy. However, percutaneous liver biopsy is an invasive procedure that is costly, and may be associated with a significant risk of complications that increase with age and the presence of cirrhosis. An additional concern with liver biopsy is that it samples only 1/50000th of the liver, and thus is subject to sampling error, particularly in non-homogenously distributed chronic liver disease. Several studies have highlighted the inaccuracy of liver biopsy even for staging of advanced liver disease [21]. Some countries have adopted non-invasive serum tests of fibrosis, or imaging modalities such as transient elastography, as an alternative to liver biopsy to guide therapeutic decisions in CHC patients [22]. Despite these limitations, most experienced clinicians considering treatment for CHC infection are likely to recommend obtaining a liver biopsy, unless there are obvious contraindications.

Treatment for chronic hepatitis C

The main goal of treatment of patients with CHC infection is the prevention of progressive hepatic fibrosis through long-term eradication of HCV. The benefits of a sustained virologic response (SVR), defined as the absence of serum HCV RNA at 24 weeks after the end of treatment measured by a sensitive molecular assay, include normalization of serum alanine aminotranferase levels, improvement in hepatic necroinflammation and fibrosis, potential health-related quality-of-life benefits, reduced mortality and risk of developing complications of end-stage liver disease, in the majority of patients. Current standard-of-care therapy results in SVR rates that appear to be durable in at least 99% of patients over the subsequent five years, although 1–2% of patients may still harbor intrahepatic virus despite undetectable serum HCV RNA [23, 24]. **A1b** However, the presence of intrahepatic virus alone in these patients is likely to remain clinically insignificant.

Table 26.2 Contraindications to current pegylated IFN and ribavirin therapy.

Definite contraindication	Relative contraindication
Severe cardiovascular disease (e.g. symptomatic coronary artery disease, severe hypertension, severe congestive heart failure)	Poor compliance
Uncontrolled diabetes mellitus	Active substance abuse
Severe pulmonary disease	Chronic renal insufficiency
Recent or active malignancy	Reduced life expectancy from co-morbid illness
Decompensated liver disease	Seizure disorder
Major psychiatric illness	Poorly controlled inflammatory disease (e.g. rheumatoid, connective tissue, inflammatory bowel disease)
Pregnancy or age < 3 yrs	Inability to comply with birth control recommendations
Active autoimmune disease	
Non-liver organ transplant	
Significant anemia (e.g. hemoglobinopathy) or other cytopenia	

Patient selection

All patients with CHC without definite contraindications to currently available IFN-based treatment should be considered as potential candidates for antiviral therapy (Table 26.2) [25]. **A1a** The decision to treat patients must take into account the variable natural history and rate of disease progression, associated co-morbid states, social situation and supports, risk-benefit aspects and cost-effectiveness of therapy in the individual. Patient preferences need to be considered, along with an assessment of behavioral and lifestyle aspects that may influence their ability to adhere to a prolonged duration of therapy associated with significant side effects. Patients also need to be reminded that CHC may be associated with non-specific symptoms such as fatigue, lethargy, asthenia and abdominal discomfort, which may significantly impact upon the quality of life of the individual, but do not correlate with severity of liver disease, and may not remit with successful viral eradication. Patients with significant co-morbid states that pose a relative contraindication to antiviral therapy require assessment and management in a multi-disciplinary setting with experienced health care providers. Several host and virus

Table 26.3 Factors predictive of favorable virologic response to current therapy.

Before therapy
  Treatment naive to IFN
  Genotype 2 or 3
  Low HCV RNA levels (<800,000 IU/mL)
  Absent bridging fibrosis or cirrhosis on liver biopsy
  Age < 40 years
  Female gender
  Absence of steatosis
  Normal BMI
  No insulin resistance
  HCV monoinfection

During therapy
  RVR (week 4)
  EVR (week 12)
  Adherence to therapy
  No dosage reduction

RVR: rapid virologic response; EVR: early virologic response.

factors may determine successful responses to IFN-based therapy, of which the most important appear to be HCV genotype, baseline HCV RNA levels and undetectable virus at week 4 of therapy (rapid virologic response) (Table 26.3).

Treatment options

The current standard-of-care treatment for CHC is a combination of pegylated interferon-alpha (PEG-IFN) and ribavirin [26–28]. **A1a** Interferons (IFN) are a group of naturally occurring cytokines that exhibit a variety of immunomodulatory, antiproliferative and antiviral effects. Pegylation refers to the covalent attachment of an inert, water soluble polymer of polyethylene glycol (PEG) to the IFN molecule in either a linear (Peginterferon alfa-2b (PEGINTRON), Schering-Plough, Kenilworth, NJ) or branch chain configuration (Peginterferon alfa-2a (PEGASYS), Hoffmann-La Roche, Basel, Switzerland) with differing molecular weights. Compared to standard interferon-alpha, the pegylated IFN compounds exhibit improved pharmacokinetic profiles and a prolonged elimination half-life, thus allowing for increased efficacy and a convenient once-weekly subcutaneous dosing schedule (PEGINTRON, 1.5 µg/kg/wk and PEGASYS, 180 µg/wk). Data from a recently completed large randomized multicenter study evaluating individualized dosing efficacy in 3070 HCV genotype 1 infected patients noted similar efficacy (SVR rates 38–41%) and safety and tolerability (discontinuation rate 10–13%) for patients receiving either PEG-IFN-2a or -2b in combination with ribavrin [29]. **A1a**

Ribavirin is a synthetic purine nucleoside analog that likely exhibits antiviral effects through multiple pathogenic mechanisms including immunomodulation, depletion of intracellular guanosine triphosphate, and weak inhibition of HCV RNA-dependent RNA polymerase. Ribavirin acts synergistically with IFN to induce antiviral responses and reduce relapse rates, and is administered orally twice daily at weight-based doses depending on viral genotype (1000–1400 mg/day for HCV genotype 1 (≤75 kg = 1000 mg/d, 75–105 kg = 1200 mg/d and >105 kg = 1400 mg/d) and at a fixed dose of 800 mg/day for HCV genotype 2 and 3) [30, 31]. **A1c**

Combination PEG-IFN and ribavirin therapy can achieve a sustained virologic response in 54–56% of patients, including 42–46% of patients with genotype 1 infection, and around 80% of those with genotype 2 and 3 infection. Most patients with genotype 1 require 48 weeks of combination therapy and those with genotypes 2 and 3 can be treated for only 24 weeks. Many of the large clinical trials have been based in Europe or North America, and there is limited treatment efficacy data available for genotypes 4–6. As a result, these patients should continue to receive treatment as for HCV genotype 1 infection [25, 32]. **A1c**

Early response prediction

Studies of early viral kinetics in response to PEG-IFN and ribavirin indicate a rapid initial first phase decline in HCV RNA, due to virus inhibition, and a slower second phase response due to loss of HCV from infected hepatocytes. This resulted in the development of early virologic predictors in the first 12 weeks of therapy to select patients that would benefit from ongoing therapy, thereby reducing duration of treatment, cost and continued exposure to poorly tolerated drugs for non-responders. Early virologic response (EVR) is defined as a decline in HCV RNA of at least $2\log_{10}$ units or to undetectable levels by the first 12 weeks of treatment. Although 75–85% of patients receiving combination therapy achieve EVR, failure to achieve this early response is associated with a minimal (1.6%) chance of achieving SVR with continued treatment [33]. **B2** Assessment of EVR at week 12 of combination therapy has thus been adopted into clinical practice for HCV genotype 1 patients.

Response predictors at earlier stages during treatment have also been evaluated in relation to shortening the duration of therapy for CHC patients. A study evaluating shorter 24-week duration therapy for HCV genotype 1 patients with low baseline HCV RNA (<600,000 IU/mL) noted SVR rates of 89% in a subgroup of patients that achieve rapid virologic response (RVR, defined as HCV RNA < 29 IU/mL by week 4). This was comparable to SVR rates of 85% observed in historical controls achieving RVR with treatment duration of 48 weeks [34] **A1c** Similar assessments in other study cohorts confirmed that patients with lower baseline HCV RNA and undetectable virus at week 4 of combination therapy achieve SVR rates of over 80% with 24 weeks of treatment [35]. **A1c** In general, 10–15% of HCV genotype 1 infected patients have a low baseline HCV RNA and achieve RVR, and thus may be theoretically considered for reducing treatment duration from 48 weeks to 24 weeks. Until further data is available, HCV genotype 1 infected patients with advanced stage disease, African-Americans, or those requiring early dose adjustments during therapy, should continue to receive the standard-of-care 48 weeks duration treatment. Furthermore, the HCV RNA threshold that defines low baseline viremia has not been clearly delineated and varies from 400,000–800,000 IU/mL. In addition, a sensitive HCV RNA real-time PCR or TMA assay must be utilized to detect minimal residual viremia at week 4 that increases the likelihood of relapse with reduced duration therapy [36]. **B4**

Viral quantitation is not performed routinely during treatment for HCV genotype 2 or 3 infection, as most of these patients become HCV RNA negative early during combination therapy, and achieve excellent SVR rates with 24 weeks of therapy. A number of studies have evaluated shortened treatment duration for HCV genotype 2 or 3 infected patients. Results from a large study of 1469 patients randomized to receive PEG-IFN 2a at 180 μg/wk and ribavirin 800 mg/day for 16 or 24 weeks indicate that SVR rates were higher for the longer duration treatment arm (62% versus 70%) [37]. Based on these results, shortened duration therapy is not recommended for genotype 2 or 3 patients. However, subgroup analysis from this study indicated that two-thirds of patients had RVR, with subsequent SVR rates of 90% with 24 weeks of treatment. Patients with RVR and low baseline HCV RNA (<400,000 IU/mL) had SVR rates of 95% and 90% with 24-week and 16-week treatment regimens respectively. Another study of 283 HCV genotype 2 and 3 infected patients noted overall SVR rates of 85% and 91% for patients that were treated for 12 and 24 weeks respectively, with PEG-IFN-2b and weight-based ribavirin (1000/1200 mg/day), and achieved RVR [38]. **A1c** Thus, an abbreviated treatment regimen may be considered in a proportion of patients that are poorly tolerant to combination therapy.

In contrast to patients that exhibit rapid viral responses, HCV genotype 1 slow responders (patients that have detectable HCV RNA at weeks 4 and 12, but are negative at week 24) may benefit from a longer duration therapy of 72 weeks that reduces relapse rates. One study noted that HCV genotype 1 patients that were still HCV RNA positive at week 12 had higher SVR rates of 29% with 72 weeks of therapy compared to 17% with 48 weeks treatment. However, both discontinuation and relapse rates were around 40% with extended therapy [39]. **A1c** Patient reluctance, cost issues and potential availability of newer anti-

viral therapies in the future, have further limited the implementation of extended therapy for slow responders into routine clinical practice.

Individualized treatment

In recent years, an increased understanding of the host and viral factors that either predict or affect virologic response to current standard-of-care therapy has led to the concept of tailored therapy for CHC patients [36, 40]. The aim of this individualized treatment is to obtain optimal treatment efficacy, reduce risk of side effects, and increase cost-effectiveness of current therapy. For example, as outlined above, prediction of rapid viral responses may reduce duration of therapy for a proportion of CHC patients. Older age, male gender, obesity, insulin resistance, advanced disease, higher HCV RNA levels and race may negatively influence response rates, irrespective of genotype, and some of these patients could potentially benefit from longer duration or higher dose therapy [41]. For example, genotype 3 patients with high HCV RNA (>600,000 IU/mL) may have three-fold higher relapse rates with recommended 24-week combination therapy, compared to those with lower baseline HCV RNA [42]. Retrospective data have also indicated that HCV genotype 2 or 3 infected patients that do not achieve RVR have lower relapse rates with the longer duration 48 weeks of weight-based ribavirin 1000/1200 mg/day combination therapy compared to the standard 24-week fixed dose 800 mg/day ribavirin regimen (4% versus 26% respectively) [43]. Although these studies indicate that a proportion of patients may benefit from intensified dosing and longer duration therapy, it remains important that such treatment decisions are evaluated on an individual basis in clinical practice [44, 45]. **B4**

Management of side effects of therapy

Side effects of current PEG-IFN and ribavirin therapy are relatively common and range from mild, non-specific, flu-like symptoms to major neuropsychiatric disturbance with suicidal ideation. PEG-IFN induced thyroid dysfunction with or without thyroid antibodies may be observed in up to 3–5% of patients [46]. Patients should be screened for thyroid disease at baseline, every three months during treatment, and at least once following completion of antiviral therapy. Other autoantibodies, such as antinuclear and anti-smooth muscle antibodies, are commonly present in low titers in CHC patients, but rarely result in clinical manifestations of autoimmune disease during therapy. One-third of patients with CHC have a history of neuropsychiatric disturbance that may be further exacerbated during PEG-IFN therapy. Symptoms range from mood disturbance and emotional lability to severe depression, suicidal ideation and psychosis. This may lead to premature dose reductions and drug discontinuation, further reducing efficacy of the prescribed antiviral regimen. IFN-induced depression may be a result of changes in cytokine expression and modulation of serotonergic pathways. A multi-disciplinary approach is required to determine risk and management of neuropsychiatric disturbance before and during therapy. Selective serotonin reuptake inhibitors (SSRI) are commonly used before and during therapy, and appear well tolerated in CHC patients [47].

Most side effects abate following the end of treatment. Early recognition and management of symptoms is important in maintaining adherence to therapy. This often requires a multi-disciplinary approach that includes allied health care providers and support groups, along with adjunctive use of simple antipyretics, growth factors, and antidepressants to ensure compliance to the prescribed regimen. Such strategies to improve adherence, particularly in the initial 12 weeks of therapy, may result in improved virologic response rates and associated health-related quality of life (HRQOL) in CHC patients.

PEG-IFN may result in neutropenia that requires dose reduction in 18–20% of patients, although the risk of serious infection remains low even with severe neutropenia (<500/mm^3). Recombinant granulocyte-colony stimulating factor (G-CSF) is often used to stimulate granulopoiesis and maintain PEG-IFN dose, but is associated with significant expense and uncertain benefit. Dose reductions for thrombocytopenia are also relatively frequent in patients with advanced disease receiving PEG-IFN. The ongoing clinical development of thrombopoietin receptor agonists as adjunctive therapy will be important in this regard [48]. Ribavirin results in a risk of dose-dependent hemolytic anemia that is associated with hemoglobin <10 g/dL, requires dose reduction, or drug withdrawal, in 9% of patients, with higher risk estimates observed in Asian cohorts. Recombinant erythropoietin compounds are frequently used to maintain ribavirin dosage and improve HRQOL, but are associated with significant expense, potential for complications such as thrombosis, and at present there is no data indicating benefits in terms of early or sustained virologic response to combination therapy [49]. **B4**

Treatment of specific patient populations

Most of the recommendations for therapy in CHC patients are based on data from selected patients enrolled in tertiary multicenter clinical registration studies. Data from community centers indicate that less than one-third of patients diagnosed with CHC are eligible or actually receive antiviral therapy [50]. These difficult-to-treat CHC patients often have significant co-morbid illness and behavioral factors that reduce eligibility for current combination therapy.

Financial restrictions also limit treatment eligibility for many patients in countries without universal health care, such as the USA. Treatment options in commonly encountered patient cohorts are considered below.

Mild disease

In clinical practice treatment is usually considered for patients with persistent elevations of serum ALT. However, around 30% of CHC patients may have persistently normal ALT levels, and many of these patients will have mild disease, with slow rates of disease progression. Response rates, however, are similar to patients with biochemically active and more advanced histological disease. Treatment decisions again need to be individualized in patients with normal ALT levels, and should consider factors such as genotype, age, liver histology, patient motivation and co-morbid illnesses. Watchful waiting is appropriate for many of these patients, but progression of liver disease may occur in one-third of cases, and a liver biopsy should be repeated at five-yearly intervals [51]. **B4** In the future, patients with mild disease may be considered for newer treatments with improved efficacy and tolerance.

Advanced stage disease

Patients with stable or compensated cirrhosis should also be considered for treatment, but require close monitoring due to the higher risk of complications with PEG-IFN therapy. Subgroup data from the PEG-IFN registration trials that included small numbers of patients with compensated advanced disease (bridging fibrosis or cirrhosis) indicate overall SVR rates of 43–44% [52]. **A1d** Improvement in advanced stage fibrosis may occur in one-half of patients that achieve SVR, but there may also be histological benefits for some patients that fail to respond to therapy [53]. Select patients with decompensated cirrhosis and model for end-stage liver disease (MELD) score <18 may be considered for treatment in experienced transplant centers, given that achievement of SVR prior to transplant reduces recurrence of infection in the allograft [54, 55]. **B4**

Non-responder patients

There are an increasing proportion of patients that have failed PEG-IFN and ribavirin treatment, either as initial therapy or following retreatment of prior standard-IFN alpha based treatment failures. This latter group appear to have incremental SVR rates of 10–15% following re-treatment with current standard-of-care therapies [25]. Patients that relapsed to previous standard IFN based or shorter duration treatment should be retreated with 48 weeks of PEG-IFN and ribavirin. There are limited therapeutic options for true non-responders to PEG-IFN and ribavirin. Re-treatment with higher dose induction PEG-IFN or consensus IFN based combination therapy results in SVR rates of around 10–15%, depending on dose and duration of 48 or 72 weeks [56, 57]. **B4** However, these induction regimens are often poorly tolerated and result in frequent treatment withdrawal. In the absence of factors such as compliance or financial constraints that negatively influenced outcomes to initial therapy, non-responder patients are unlikely to benefit from re-treatment with the same agents. Lifestyle measures such weight loss and reducing alcohol, cannabis use, or smoking tobacco, should be encouraged to reduce progression of disease in all patients.

The rationale for low dose IFN maintenance therapy was based on the antifibrotic and antiproliferative properties of interferon, and the absence of viable therapeutic options for non-responder patients with advanced disease. Maintenance therapy has been evaluated in three large studies utilizing low dose PEG-IFN monotherapy for up to four years. Although there may be possible benefits in terms of reduced portal hypertension with extended duration therapy, data from the large multicenter HALT-C trial, that randomized non-responder patients with advanced disease to receive 90 µg of PEG-IFN 2a or placebo for three and one-half years, indicated no differences in fibrosis progression, development of hepatoma, complications of cirrhosis, need for transplantation, or mortality. **A1d** The COPILOT study indicated no overall differences in clinical endpoints between low dose PEG-IFN 2b and colchicine, although a proportion of patients on PEG-IFN 2b had reduced incidence of variceal bleeding. **A1d** At present, maintenance therapy cannot be recommended for CHC non-responder patients. Such patients with advanced disease should be considered for clinical studies that include the newer specific targeted antiviral therapies (STAT-C) that are currently in phase III evaluation.

Substance abuse
Patients with active or recent injection drug use (IDU) on methadone maintenance treated successfully with combination therapy achieve comparable SVR rates to non-IDU patients [58]. **B4** Interestingly, cannabis use may improve compliance to antiviral therapy in some patients by helping with symptoms such as nausea, reduced appetite and insomnia [59]. These patients need to be evaluated and treated in an experienced multi-disciplinary setting. Alcohol dependence may reduce virologic response rates and increase disease progression. Safe thresholds of alcohol consumption have not been established, and abstinence should be encouraged during therapy and in the long term [9].

HIV co-infection
Around one-third of patients with HIV infection are co-infected with HCV. Liver-related morbidity and mortality has increased significantly among the HIV-HCV co-infected population following the advent of highly active antiretroviral therapy (HAART) for HIV infection, and increased disease progression in this group. Virologic responses to combination therapy are 10–15% lower than HCV mono-infected patients, with SVR rates of 14–38% and 53–73% for HCV genotypes 1–4 and 2–3 respectively [25]. Patients should be treated for 48 weeks regardless of HCV genotype, although shorter duration therapy may be considered for HCV genotype 2 and 3 infected patients with low HCVRNA levels and minimal stage disease. HIV infection should be controlled with HAART, preferably with CD4 cell counts >250/mm^3 prior to initiation of PEG-IFN and ribavirin therapy [60]. **B4** Due to potential drug interactions or adverse event in advanced disease, HAART therapies that include didanosine, stavudine, zidivudine and nevaripine should be avoided in co-infected patients being considered for treatment [61].

End-stage renal disease
Patients with end-stage renal disease requiring hemodialysis have a higher prevalence of HCV infection, increased disease progression, and reduced post-transplant graft and patient survival. There is a substantial risk of ribavirin induced hemolytic anemia as this drug is renally excreted and not removed by dialysis. Treatment needs to be individualized and administered prior to renal transplantation using dose reductions for both PEG-IFN and ribavirin [62]. **B4**

Other patient cohorts
Combination therapy after liver transplantation is poorly tolerated and results in SVR rates <20% [63–65]. However, this has to be balanced against the substantial risk of disease progression in the immunosuppressed patient, resulting in graft loss and reduced patient survival. Treatment also needs to be individualized for other CHC population cohorts with higher likelihood of treatment related toxicity, including elderly patients, or those with co-morbid cardiovascular or respiratory compromise [66]. Patients with thalassemia, inherited coagulation disorders, or other hemoglobinoapthies have a higher incidence of CHC transmitted through repeated transfusion of blood products prior to screening of donors. Small studies have indicated that patients with beta-thalassemia major may achieve SVR rates comparable to non-thalassemic patients, but transfusion requirements and potential iron toxicity require close monitoring [67]. **B4** Children appear to have slower rates of disease progression and response rates are similar to adult cohorts [68]. Treatment is not recommended for those age < 3 years. Patients with extrahepatic manifestation of HCV associated immune complex disease and mixed cryoglobulinemia resulting in cutaneous vasculitis, neuropathy or glomerulonephritis should be offered antiviral therapy, but in practice sustained viral eradication rates and resolution of clinical sequelae are somewhat disappointing [69]. Rituximab (anti-CD 20 monoclonal anti-

body) has been used in combination with PEG-IFN and ribavirin therapy in refractory cases [70]. An increase in HCV RNA may be observed in patients receiving rituximab therapy, but this remains of uncertain clinical significance. Phlebotomy is often performed in select CHC patients with iron overload conditions or porphyria cutanea tarda, but the benefits of iron depletion on virologic response to therapy remain relatively minor and uncertain [71, 72]. **B4**

Future treatment options

Therapeutic approaches in development for CHC include newer IFNs, ribavirin analogues, specific viral inhibitors and immune modulation [73, 74]. Several IFN compounds are in development, including consensus IFN, Omega IFN and albinterferon alfa-2b which is an 85.7-kD protein consisting of recombinant human IFNα-2b genetically fused to recombinant human albumin that allows for two or four-week dosing intervals, and is currently being evaluated in phase III trials for treatment naive CHC patients [75]. Viramidine (taribavirin hydrochloride) is a ribavirin prodrug that does not lead to accumulation in erythrocytes, and results in a lower frequency of anemia. However, recent data indicated that SVR rates were 14% lower for viramidine combined with PEG-IFN compared to ribavirin, although higher doses may result in improved SVR for this compound. Technological advances in high throughput screening have resulted in the preclinical development of many potential compounds that aim at several targets during the HCV lifecycle. Two promising targets are NS5B RNA-dependent RNA polymerase (NS5-RdRP) and NS3 serine proteases. Inhibitors active at these sites are often referred to as STAT-C drugs. Valopicitabine (NM283) is an example of NS5-RdRP inhibitor that demonstrated efficacy in early clinical studies, and did progress to phase III trials in combination with standard-of-care therapy. However, further development of this compound was halted due to poor efficacy and tolerability. Several other NS5-RdRP compounds are currently in clinical development. Recent data indicate that telaprevir (VX-950), an orally bioavailable slow-binding inhibitor of HCV NS3-4A protease, administered for 12 weeks, in combination with PEG-IFN and ribavirin, resulted in significant incremental SVR in both treatment naive and non-responder patients. This compound is currently being evaluated in multicenter phase III clinical trials for both naive and non-responder cohorts. Selection of viral resistant HCV strains is an issue for STAT-C compounds, and future use will require multi-targeted therapy with potent antiviral compounds without cross resistance, most likely in combination with IFN. Other NS3/4A compounds that have shown adequate safety and efficacy during clinical development include Boceprevir (SCH 503034). Immune modulation targets through toll-like receptors, that are present on the cell surface and function to recognize pathogen-associated molecules, are also in early stage clinical development, and may potentially allow for non-IFN based therapy in the future. Several other promising approaches to inhibit viral replication are in development, but at present appear to have limited efficacy without the use of IFN-based therapy. The continued discovery and development of new therapeutic targets that are effective and tolerable will be important for treating the increasing pool of CHC patients that have not responded, have yet to be diagnosed, or are intolerant to, or hesitant to receive currently available therapies.

Summary

HCV infection is a global health problem that leads to significant morbidity and mortality from complications of end-stage liver disease in a proportion of patients. Current standard-of-care therapies can result in long-term eradication of virus, but treatment is not suitable for all patients and is often poorly tolerated. Individualized and tailored therapeutic approaches may be appropriate for some patients to improve efficacy and reduce the potential for side-effects. Implementation of primary prevention methods, providing access to health care, and identification of CHC patients at greatest risk of disease progression remain significant challenges. The recent development of specific targeted antiviral therapies provides optimism for CHC infected patients that have failed to achieve SVR, or remain ineligible to receive current standard-of-care therapy.

References

1 Shepard CW, Finelli L, Alter MJ. Global epidemiology of hepatitis C virus infection. *Lancet Infect Dis* 2005; **5**(9): 558–567.

2 McHutchison JG, Bartenschlager R, Patel K *et al*. The face of future hepatitis C antiviral drug development: recent biological and virologic advances and their translation to drug development and clinical practice. *J Hepatol* 2006; **44**(2): 411–421.

3 Dustin LB, Rice CM. Flying under the radar: the immunobiology of hepatitis C. *Annu Rev Immunol* 2007; **25**: 71–99.

4 Bukh J, Miller RH, Purcell RH. Genetic heterogeneity of hepatitis C virus: quasispecies and genotypes. *Semin Liver Dis* 1995; **15**(1): 41–63.

5 Frank C, Mohamed MK, Strickland GT *et al*. The role of parenteral antischistosomal therapy in the spread of hepatitis C virus in Egypt. *Lancet* 2000; **355**(9207): 887–891.

6 Stramer SL, Glynn SA, Kleinman SH *et al*. Detection of HIV-1 and HCV infections among antibody-negative blood donors by nucleic acid-amplification testing. *N Engl J Med* 2004; **351**(8): 760–768.

7 Alter MJ. Prevention of spread of hepatitis C. *Hepatology* 2002; **36**(5 Suppl. 1): S93–S98.

8 Amon JJ, Garfein RS, Ahdieh-Grant L *et al.* Prevalence of hepatitis C virus infection among injection drug users in the United States, 1994–2004. *Clin Infect Dis* 2008; **46**(12): 1852–1858.

9 Peters MG, Terrault NA. Alcohol use and hepatitis C. *Hepatology* 2002; **36**(5 Suppl. 1): S220–225.

10 Quiroga JA, Campillo ML, Catillo I *et al.* IgM antibody to hepatitis C virus in acute and chronic hepatitis C. *Hepatology* 1991; **14**(1): 38–43.

11 Berg T, Sarrazin C, Hinrichsen H *et al.* Does noninvasive staging of fibrosis challenge liver biopsy as a gold standard in chronic hepatitis C? *Hepatology* 2004; **39**(5): 1456–1457; author reply 1457–1458.

12 Wiese M, Berr F, Lafrenz M *et al.* Low frequency of cirrhosis in a hepatitis C (genotype 1b) single-source outbreak in germany: a 20-year multicenter study. *Hepatology* 2000; **32**(1): 91–96.

13 Kenny-Walsh E. Clinical outcomes after hepatitis C infection from contaminated anti-D immune globulin. Irish Hepatology Research Group. *N Engl J Med* 1999; **340**(16): 1228–1233.

14 Maheshwari A, Ray S, Thuluvath PJ. Acute hepatitis C. *Lancet* 2008; **372**(9635): 321–332.

15 Santantonio T, Wiegand J, Gerlach JT. Acute hepatitis C: current status and remaining challenges. *J Hepatol* 2008; **49**(4): 625–633.

16 Vogt M, Lang T, Frosner G *et al.* Prevalence and clinical outcome of hepatitis C infection in children who underwent cardiac surgery before the implementation of blood-donor screening. *N Engl J Med* 1999; **341**(12): 866–870.

17 Bialek SR, Terrault NA. The changing epidemiology and natural history of hepatitis C virus infection. *Clin Liver Dis* 2006; **10**(4): 697–715.

18 Missiha SB, Ostrowski M, Heathcote EJ. Disease progression in chronic hepatitis C: modifiable and nonmodifiable factors. *Gastroenterology* 2008; **134**(6): 1699–1714.

19 Sangiovanni A, Prati GM, Fasani P *et al.* The natural history of compensated cirrhosis due to hepatitis C virus: a 17-year cohort study of 214 patients. *Hepatology* 2006; **43**(6): 1303–1310.

20 Benvegnu L, Gios M, Boccato S *et al.* Natural history of compensated viral cirrhosis: a prospective study on the incidence and hierarchy of major complications. *Gut* 2004; **53**(5): 744–749.

21 Regev A, Berho M, Jeffers LJ *et al.* Sampling error and intraobserver variation in liver biopsy in patients with chronic HCV infection. *Am J Gastroenterol* 2002; **97**(10): 2614–2618.

22 Rockey DC, Bissell DM. Noninvasive measures of liver fibrosis. *Hepatology* 2006; **43**(2 Suppl. 1): S113–S120.

23 Maylin S, Martinot-Peignoux M, Moucari R *et al.* Eradication of hepatitis C virus in patients successfully treated for chronic hepatitis C. *Gastroenterology* 2008. **135**(3): 821–829.

24 McHutchison JG, Poynard T, Esteban-Mur R *et al.* Hepatic HCV RNA before and after treatment with interferon alone or combined with ribavirin. *Hepatology* 2002; **35**(3): 688–693.

25 Dienstag JL, McHutchison JG. American Gastroenterological Association medical position statement on the management of hepatitis C. *Gastroenterology* 2006; **130**(1): 225–230.

26 Manns MP, McHutchison JG, Gordon SC *et al.* Peginterferon alfa-2b plus ribavirin compared with interferon alfa-2b plus ribavirin for initial treatment of chronic hepatitis C: a randomised trial. *Lancet* 2001; **358**(9286): 958–965.

27 Fried MW, Shiffman ML, Reddy KR *et al.* Peginterferon alfa-2a plus ribavirin for chronic hepatitis C virus infection. *N Engl J Med* 2002; **347**(13): 975–982.

28 Hoofnagle JH, Seeff LB. Peginterferon and ribavirin for chronic hepatitis C. *N Engl J Med* 2006; **355**(23): 2444–2451.

29 McHutchison J, Sulkowski M. Scientific rationale and study design of the individualized dosing efficacy vs flat dosing to assess optimal pegylated interferon therapy (IDEAL) trial: determining optimal dosing in patients with genotype 1 chronic hepatitis C. *J Viral Hepat* 2008; **15**(7): 475–481.

30 Bronowicki JP, Ouzan D, Asselah T *et al.* Effect of ribavirin in genotype 1 patients with hepatitis C responding to pegylated interferon alfa-2a plus ribavirin. *Gastroenterology* 2006; **131**(4): 1040–1048.

31 Jacobson IM, Brown RS, Jr, Freilich B *et al.* Peginterferon alfa-2b and weight-based or flat-dose ribavirin in chronic hepatitis C patients: a randomized trial. *Hepatology* 2007; **46**(4): 971–981.

32 Kamal SM, Nasser IA. Hepatitis C genotype 4: what we know and what we don't yet know. *Hepatology* 2008; **47**(4): 1371–1383.

33 Davis GL, Wong JB, McHutchison JG *et al.* Early virologic response to treatment with peginterferon alfa-2b plus ribavirin in patients with chronic hepatitis C. *Hepatology* 2003; **38**(3): 645–652.

34 Zeuzem S, Buti M, Ferenci P *et al.* Efficacy of 24 weeks' treatment with peginterferon alfa-2b plus ribavirin in patients with chronic hepatitis C infected with genotype 1 and low pretreatment viremia. *J Hepatol* 2006; **44**(1): 97–103.

35 Zeuzem S, Pawlotsky JM, Lukasiewicz E *et al.* International, multicenter, randomized, controlled study comparing dynamically individualized versus standard treatment in patients with chronic hepatitis C. *J Hepatol* 2005; **43**(2): 250–257.

36 Berg T. Tailored treatment for hepatitis C. *Clin Liver Dis* 2008; **12**(3): 507–528, vii–viii.

37 Shiffman ML, Suter F, Bacon R *et al.* Peginterferon alfa-2a and ribavirin for 16 or 24 weeks in HCV genotype 2 or 3. *N Engl J Med* 2007; **357**(2): 124–134.

38 Mangia A, Santoro R, Minerva N *et al.* Peginterferon alfa-2b and ribavirin for 12 vs 24 weeks in HCV genotype 2 or 3. *N Engl J Med* 2005; **352**(25): 2609–2617.

39 Berg T, von Wagner M, Nasser S *et al.* Extended treatment duration for hepatitis C virus type 1: comparing 48 versus 72 weeks of peginterferon-alfa-2a plus ribavirin. *Gastroenterology* 2006; **130**(4): 1086–1097.

40 Pawlotsky JM. Therapy of hepatitis C: from empiricism to eradication. *Hepatology* 2006; **43**(2 Suppl. 1): S207–S220.

41 Fried MW, Jensen D, Rodriguez-Torres M *et al.* Improved outcomes in patients with hepatitis C with difficult-to-treat characteristics: randomized study of higher doses of peginterferon alpha-2a and ribavirin. *Hepatology* 2008; **48**(4): 1033–1043.

42 Zeuzem S, Hultcrantz R, Bourliere M *et al.* Peginterferon alfa-2b plus ribavirin for treatment of chronic hepatitis C in previously untreated patients infected with HCV genotypes 2 or 3. *J Hepatol* 2004; **40**(6): 993–999.

43 Hadziyannis SJ, Sette H, Jr, Morgan TR *et al.* Peginterferon-alpha2a and ribavirin combination therapy in chronic hepatitis C: a randomized study of treatment duration and ribavirin dose. *Ann Intern Med* 2004; **140**(5): 346–355.

44 Lee SS, Ferenci P. Optimizing outcomes in patients with hepatitis C virus genotype 1 or 4. *Antivir Ther* 2008; **13** (Suppl. 1): 9–16.

45 Berg T, Carosi G. Optimizing outcomes in patients with hepatitis C virus genotype 2 or 3. *Antivir Ther* 2008; **13** (Suppl. 1): 17–22.

46 Mandac JC, Chaudhry S, Sherman KE *et al.* The clinical and physiological spectrum of interferon-alpha induced thyroiditis: toward a new classification. *Hepatology* 2006; **43**(4): 661–672.

47 Crone CC, Gabriel GM, Wise TN. Managing the neuropsychiatric side effects of interferon-based therapy for hepatitis C. *Cleve Clin J Med* 2004; **71** (Suppl. 3): S27–32.

48 McHutchison JG, Dusheiko G, Shiffman ML *et al.* Eltrombopag for thrombocytopenia in patients with cirrhosis associated with hepatitis C. *N Engl J Med* 2007; **357**(22): 2227–2236.

49 McHutchison JG, Manns MP, Brown RS, Jr *et al.* Strategies for managing anemia in hepatitis C patients undergoing antiviral therapy. *Am J Gastroenterol* 2007; **102**(4): 880–889.

50 Falck-Ytter Y, Kale H, Mullen KD *et al.* Surprisingly small effect of antiviral treatment in patients with hepatitis C. *Ann Intern Med* 2002; **136**(4): 288–292.

51 Ghany MG, Kleiner DE, Alter H *et al.* Progression of fibrosis in chronic hepatitis C. *Gastroenterology* 2003; **124**(1): 97–104.

52 Wright TL. Treatment of patients with hepatitis C and cirrhosis. *Hepatology* 2002; **36**(5 Suppl. 1): S185–194.

53 Poynard T, McHutchison J, Manns M *et al.* Impact of pegylated interferon alfa-2b and ribavirin on liver fibrosis in patients with chronic hepatitis C. *Gastroenterology* 2002; **122**(5): 1303–1313.

54 Wiesner RH, Sorrell M, Villamil F. Report of the first International Liver Transplantation Society expert panel consensus conference on liver transplantation and hepatitis C. *Liver Transpl* 2003; **9**(11): S1–S9.

55 Everson GT. Treatment of hepatitis C in the patient with decompensated cirrhosis. *Clin Gastroenterol Hepatol* 2005; **3**(10 Suppl. 2): S106–S112.

56 Thomas E, Fried MW. Hepatitis C: current options for nonresponders to peginterferon and ribavirin. *Curr Gastroenterol Rep* 2008; **10**(1): 53–59.

57 Satoskar R, Jensen DM. Retreatment of chronic hepatitis C in previous non-responders and relapsers. *Expert Opin Pharmacother* 2007; **8**(15): 2491–2503.

58 Backmund M, Reimer J, Meyer K *et al.* Hepatitis C virus infection and injection drug users: prevention, risk factors, and treatment. *Clin Infect Dis* 2005; **40**(Suppl. 5): S330–335.

59 Fischer B, Reimer J, Firestone M *et al.* Treatment for hepatitis C virus and cannabis use in illicit drug user patients: implications and questions. *Eur J Gastroenterol Hepatol* 2006; **18**(10): 1039–1042.

60 Andersson K, Chung RT. Hepatitis C virus in the HIV-infected patient. *Clin Liver Dis* 2006; **10**(2): 303–320, viii.

61 Soriano V, Barreiro P, Martin-Carbonero L *et al.* Update on the treatment of chronic hepatitis C in HIV-infected patients. *AIDS Rev* 2007; **9**(2): 99–113.

62 Okoh EJ, Bucci JR, Simon JF *et al.* HCV in patients with end-stage renal disease. *Am J Gastroenterol* 2008; **103**(8): 2123–2134.

63 Chalasani N, Manzarbeitia C, Ferenci P *et al.* Peginterferon alfa-2a for hepatitis C after liver transplantation: two randomized, controlled trials. *Hepatology* 2005; **41**(2): 289–298.

64 Samuel D, Bizollon T, Feray C *et al.* Interferon-alpha 2b plus ribavirin in patients with chronic hepatitis C after liver transplantation: a randomized study. *Gastroenterology* 2003; **124**(3): 642–650.

65 Xirouchakis E, Triantos C, Manousou P *et al.* Pegylated-interferon and ribavirin in liver transplant candidates and recipients with HCV cirrhosis: systematic review and meta-analysis of prospective controlled studies. *J Viral Hepat* 2008; **15**(10): 699–709.

66 Patel K, Muir AJ, McHutchison JG. Diagnosis and treatment of chronic hepatitis C infection. *BMJ* 2006; **332**(7548): 1013–1017.

67 Harmatz P, Jonas MM, Kwiatkowski JL *et al.* Safety and efficacy of pegylated interferon alpha-2a and ribavirin for the treatment of hepatitis C in patients with thalassemia. *Haematologica* 2008; **93**(8): 1247–1251.

68 Gonzalez-Peralta RP, Kelly DA, Haber B *et al.* Interferon alfa-2b in combination with ribavirin for the treatment of chronic hepatitis C in children: efficacy, safety, and pharmacokinetics. *Hepatology* 2005; **42**(5): 1010–1018.

69 Zignego AL, Ferri C, Pileri SA *et al.* Extrahepatic manifestations of hepatitis C virus infection: a general overview and guidelines for a clinical approach. *Dig Liver Dis* 2007; **39**(1): 2–17.

70 Saadoun D, Resche-Rigon M, Sene D *et al.* Rituximab combined with Peg-interferon-ribavirin in refractory hepatitis C virus-associated cryoglobulinaemia vasculitis. *Ann Rheum Dis* 2008; **67**(10): 1431–1436.

71 Teubner A, Richter M, Schuppan D *et al.* Hepatitis C, hemochromatosis and porphyria cutanea tarda. *Dtsch Med Wochenschr* 2006; **131**(13): 691–695.

72 Desai TK, Jamil LH, Balasubramaniam M *et al.* Phlebotomy improves therapeutic response to interferon in patients with chronic hepatitis C: a meta-analysis of six prospective randomized controlled trials. *Dig Dis Sci* 2008; **53**(3): 815–822.

73 Cholongitas E, Papatheodoridis GV. Review article: novel therapeutic options for chronic hepatitis C. *Aliment Pharmacol Ther* 2008; **27**(10): 866–884.

74 Stauber RE, Kessler HK. Drugs in development for hepatitis C. *Drugs* 2008; **68**(10): 1347–1359.

75 Subramanian GM, Fiscella M, Lamouse-Smith A *et al.* Albinterferon alpha-2b: a genetic fusion protein for the treatment of chronic hepatitis C. *Nat Biotechnol* 2007; **25**(12): 1411–1419.

27 Hepatitis B: Prognosis and treatment

Piero Luigi Almasio, Calogero Cammà, Vito Di Marco and Antonio Craxì

Division of Gastroenterology, Academic Department of Internal Medicine, University of Palermo, Palermo, Italy

Background

Hepatitis B virus (HBV) infection, together with hepatitis C and alcohol abuse, is among the leading causes of cirrhosis and hepatocellular carcinoma (HCC) worldwide [1, 2]. It thus represents a major cause of morbidity and mortality [3–5], and induces substantial direct and indirect social costs. Effective treatment of HBV-related conditions in association with extensive mass vaccination for HBV would significantly reduce the global burden of chronic liver disease.

Alpha interferon (IFN) has been the mainstay of therapy for chronic hepatitis B since the early 1980s. Meta-analyses of randomized clinical trials (RCTs) conclusively prove its effectiveness in normalizing alanine aminotransferases (ALT) and clearing HBeAg and HBV-DNA from blood in 25–40% of HBeAg positive treated patients [6–9]. However, no specific data are available from these reviews on improvements of liver histology. Standardized response criteria have been set by the use of these "surrogate" markers of cure on the grounds of clinical and biological plausibility [10, 11]. "True" disease endpoints (i.e. progression to cirrhosis, to HCC and death) cannot usually be assessed in short-term trials of IFN due to the slow natural course of chronic hepatitis B. A major issue of concern is the fact that RCTs of IFN for chronic hepatitis B have been mostly performed in patients without advanced fibrosis or cirrhosis. The transferability of results to the whole spectrum of subjects with chronic liver disease due to HBV is hence questionable. Since IFN is today in widespread use as the first-line therapy for chronic hepatitis B, no addi-

tional prospective cohort studies on the course of untreated disease will be feasible [1, 2, 10, 11]. Long-term retrospective or prospective studies to evaluate the benefits of IFN therapy on true endpoints, that is, prevention of cirrhosis, liver failure, HCC and death, will also be difficult to perform due to the prolonged and slow course of the disease.

In the last few years a new form of IFN, namely pegylated IFN, has become available on the market for treatment of chronic hepatitis B. This drug has been evaluated both alone or in combination with other antiviral molecules, namely nucleoside/nucleotide analogs (see later), in order to increase its efficacy.

A number of molecules which inhibit viral replication by selectively blocking the HBV-DNA polymerase enzyme activity are currently available to treat patients with chronic HBV infection. They include nucleoside analogs, lamivudine (LAM), entecavir (ETV) and telbivudine (LdT), and nucleotide analogs, adefovir dipivoxyl (ADV) and tenofovir (TDF). Some of them, when compared to IFN, are less expensive and better tolerated but their long-term efficacy is limited by inability to obtain sustained viral suppression after withdrawal. As a matter of fact, prolonging the administration of LAM beyond one year of therapy causes the emergence of LAM resistant HBV mutants at a yearly rate of 15–25% [12, 13].

Other drugs, such as Emtricitabine (FTC), are currently undergoing phase II and III evaluation as potential anti-HBV treatments. Initial results would also suggest that other antiviral compounds, current in phase 2 testing, even if endowed with a strong antiviral effect, cannot by themselves eradicate HBV infection. Phase II and III studies of combination therapy using IFN and nucleoside/nucleotide analogs or combinations of analogs are ongoing.

We have appraised the available evidence for drugs which are currently on the market in order to estimate the effectiveness of antiviral therapy on "surrogate markers" of response and its long-term benefit.

Evidence-Based Gastroenterology and Hepatology, 3rd edition.
J. McDonald, A.K. Burroughs, B. Feagan, and B.M. Fennerty. © 2010
Blackwell Publishing Ltd

Evaluation of available evidence

What effect has anti-viral therapy of chronic hepatitis B on "surrogate" markers of response?

IFN in HBeAg positive chronic hepatitis B

Twenty-one RCTs which compared IFN to no treatment in adult patients with chronic hepatitis B due to wild type (HBeAg positive HBV) were recovered by Medline search (1985–2008) (see Table 27.1) [14–34]. These RCTs included a total of 1216 patients, 745 receiving active treatment. Overall, IFN treatment had a favorable, statistically significant effect in comparison to no treatment. Meta-analysis showed the following risk differences, all in favor of IFN:

- Clearance of HBeAg (see Figure 27.1): 0.24 (95% CI: 0.08–0.30, $p < 0.001$); NNT 4.1.
- Loss of HBsAg (see Figure 27.2): 0.05 (95% CI: 0.03–0.08, $p < 0.001$); NNT 18. **A1a**

The amount of IFN used was clearly important. Subjects receiving a total dose of <200 MU had a 1.37 odds ratio (OR, 95% CI: 0.95–1.98) of HBeAg clearance above controls, while those who received >200 MU had an OR of 2.05 (95% CI: 1.5–2.78).

Overall experience suggests that the optimal cost-effectiveness ratio on surrogate endpoints is reached by treating HBeAg positive patients with 9–10 MU IFN tiw for four to six months. Predictive factors of a favourable response are:

- Low serum HBV-DNA or a low amount of HBcAg in the hepatocytes
- High levels of ALT

Table 27.1 Randomized controlled trials of interferon (IFN) treatment of HBeAg positive chronic hepatitis B.

ID	Study	Year	Patients	Schedule	Total dose	Type of IFN
1	Carreno [14]	1987	20	5.5 MU/m² IM daily for 3 weeks then twice weekly for 6 months	380 MU/m²	r-IFNα-2a
2	Mc Donald [15]	1987	41	2.5, 5, 10 MU/m² IM TIW for 6 months	180, 360, 720 MU	r-IFNα-2a
3	Alexander [16]	1987	46	10 MU/m² TIW for 6 months	720 MU	Lymphoblastoid IFN
4	Porres [17]	1988	24	2.5, 5, 10 MU/m² IM TIW for 6 months	180, 360, 720 MU	r-IFNα-2a
5	Pastore [18]	1988	28	0.07 to 0.10 MU/Kg IM daily for 1 month then twice weekly for 2 months	2.52 to 3.6 MU/Kg	Leukocyte IFN
6	Hoofnagle [19]	1988	45	5 MU daily or 10 every other day for 4 months	560 MU	r-IFNα-2b
7	Lok [20]	1988	72	2.5, 5, 10 MU/m² IM TIW for 6 months	180, 360, 720 MU	r-IFNα-2a
8	Saracco [21]	1989	64	5 MU/m² IM TIW for 6 months	360 MU	Lymphoblastoid IFN
9	Brook [22]	1989	71	10 MU/m² TIW IM for 6 months	720 MU	Lymphoblastoid IFN
10	Brook [23]	1989	60	2.5, 5, 10 MU/m² IM TIW for 6 months	180, 360, 720 MU	r-IFNα-2a
11	Williams [24]	1990	30	2.5, 5, 10 MU/m² IM TIW for 6 months	180, 360, 720 MU	r-IFNα-2a
12	Waked [25]	1990	40	5 MU/m² SC 3 or 7 times weekly for 4 months	240 or 560 MU/m²	r-IFNα-2b
13	Realdi [26]	1990	79	4.5 MU IM TIW for 4 months	216 MU	r-IFNα-2a
14	Muller [27]	1990	58	3 MU SC TIW for 4 months	144 MU	r-IFNα-2b
15	Perrillo [28]	1990	125	1 or 5 MU, SC daily for 4 months	112 or 560 MU	r-IFNα-2b
16	Lok [29]	1992	75	10 MU SC TIW for 4 months	480 MU	r-IFNα-2b
17	Di Bisceglie [30]	1993	47	10 MU SC TIW for 4 months	480 MU	r-IFNα-2b
18	Bayraktar [31]	1993	35	5 MU TIW SC for 6 months	360 MU	r-IFNα-2b
19	Wong [32]	1995	50	10 MU/m2 TIW for 3 months	360 MU	r-IFNα-2
20	Sarin [33]	1996	41	3 MU SC TIW for 4 months	144 MU	r-IFNα-2b
21	Janssen [34]	1999	162	10 MU SC TIW for 4 or 8 months	480 or 960 MU	r-IFNα-2b

rIFN: recombinant-interferon.

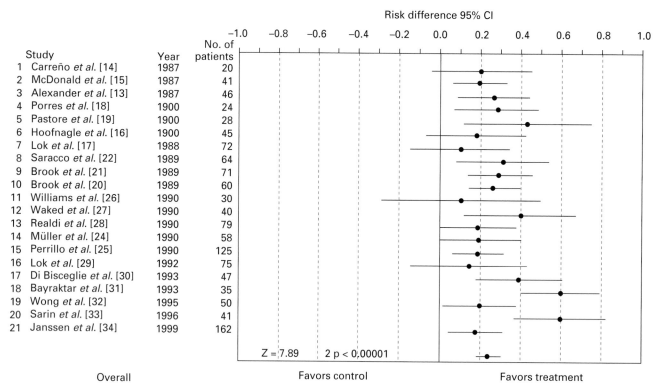

Figure 27.1 Meta-analysis of interferon therapy for HBeAg positive chronic hepatitis B: effect of treatment, measured as risk difference, on HBeAg clearance.

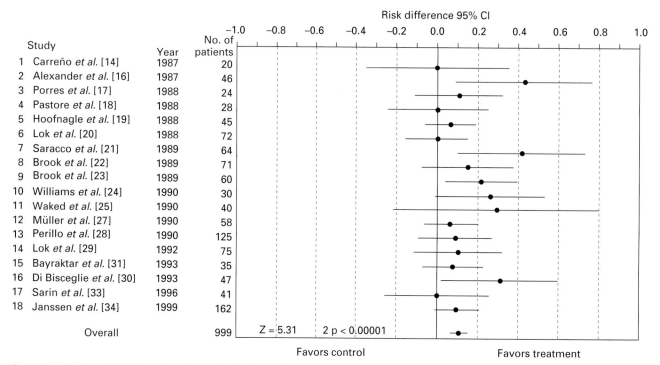

Figure 27.2 Meta-analysis of interferon therapy for HBeAg positive chronic hepatitis B: effect of treatment, measured as risk difference, on loss of HBsAg.

- High value of histological activity index (HAI) at liver biopsy
- Infection acquired in the adult age and/or a history of acute hepatitis
- Non-Asian ethnic origin [8, 9, 25, 28, 29, 35–37]

Pegylated IFN in HBeAg positive chronic hepatitis B

Only two RCTs comparing peginterferons to IFN in patients with HBeAg positive chronic hepatitis B have been published so far [38, 39]. The first study used different doses of pegylated IFN α-2a (90, 180 and 270 μg sc weekly for 24 weeks); in the second one patients received pegylated IFN α-2b at a dose of 1.0 μg/kg weekly for 24 weeks. The rate of combined response at the end of follow-up (HBeAg negative, HBV DNA < $5\log_{10}$ copies/ml, and ALT normalization) was significanlty higher in patients treated with pegylated IFN (21.3% vs 11.2%; OR, 2.16; 95% CI: 1.34–3.51). **A1d**

IFN and corticosteroids in HBeAg positive chronic hepatitis B

An alternative approach to chronic HBV infection is based on the induction of a brief period of immunosuppression by steroids [40, 41], then a withdrawal to provoke an abrupt ALT elevation due to the host immune reconstitution, and a subsequent decline of HBV-DNA. IFN administration is then started 2–4 weeks after stopping steroids. The sequential schedule has been studied in some RCTs and their results have been pooled in a meta-analysis [42]. The overall rate of HBeAg loss in 13 RCTs was significantly higher in the prednisone-IFN group (34.7% vs 29.1%, OR 1.41; 95% CI: 1.03–1.92). Similar results were observed for loss of HBV-DNA (39.7% vs 31.6%; OR, 1.51; 95% CI: 1.12–2.05). However, the loss of HBsAg was similar across the two groups (7.3% vs 5.4%; OR, 1.41; 95% CI: 0.77–2.59). Pre-treatment ALT levels had no impact on evaluated outcomes but only the low dose of prednisone was significantly associated with HBsAg loss (OR, 2.76; 95% CI: 1.18–6.43) as compared to high dose (OR, 0.69; 95% CI: 0.29–1.66).

Even if there could be an advantage in pre-treatment with steroids of this subset of patients, this must be balanced against the risk of flare of liver disease after steroid withdrawal. A severe, sometimes fatal "seroconversion hepatitis" has been reported in subjects with pre-existing cirrhosis [43, 44]. This treatment algorithm is not recommended.

Pegylated IFN and lamivudine in HBeAg positive chronic hepatitis B

Another approach to increase the rate of viral clearance is to add another antiviral drug to the current therapy. Three RCTs have tested this hypothesis and patients were randomized to receive peginterferon plus LAM or peginterferon alone [45–47]. The rate of persistent viral clearance, as evaluated by serum HBV-DNA levels <400 copies/ml at the end of follow-up, was similar across the two groups (11.6% vs 10.9%%; OR, 1.07; 95% CI: 0.73–1.58), and therefore it can be concluded that the association of pegylated IFN with LAM is not superior to peginteferon alone in treating patients with HBeAg positive chronic hepatitis B and this schedule is not recommendable in the clinical practice. **A1c**

IFN in HBeAg negative chronic hepatitis B

Data on the efficacy of IFN therapy in HBeAg negative chronic hepatitis B are few compared to HBeAg positive. The results of published RCTs remain inconsistent and the overall assessment of the treatment effect is difficult to evaluate. The drawing of firm conclusions based on the results of these studies is hampered by the small sample size of the studies and by heterogeneity of baseline severity of patients and the schedule of treatment. An evaluation of treatment efficacy on HBV-DNA clearance and sustained ALT normalization was performed by a meta-analysis on seven RCTs [48–54] enrolling patients infected by the HBe minus mutant. Five RCTs compared IFN regimens with non-active treatment; two trials compared different doses of IFN. We combined the results of IFN arms of these two trials and made a single pair-wise comparison with the overall control rate of the other five RCTs. All the RCTs were performed in centers from the Mediterranean area, indirectly confirming the high geographical prevalence of this mutation. Pooled data totalling 301 subjects, showed a significant effect of IFN therapy on sustained loss of HBV-DNA (Risk difference 0.17; 95% CI: 0.07–0.27; NNT 5.9) (see Figure 27.3). **A1c**

IFN or pegylated IFN and lamivudine in HBeAg negative chronic hepatitis B

No study has properly compared peginterferon to IFN therapy in patients with HBV mutant infection, but, similarly to HBeAg positive patients, the combination therapy of IFN or peginterferon plus LAM in comparison to IFN alone has been tested also in anti-HBeAg positive subjects. One study used IFN-α [55] and three PEG IFN [56–58]. Overall, 225 patients received combination therapy and 219 IFN alone. The rate of HBV-DNA undetectability at the end of follow-up was 18.2% and 21.0% respectively (OR, 0.83; 95% CI: 0.51–1.35), so addiction of LAM does not improve efficacy of IFN.

Nucleoside and nucleotide analogs

Evidence of effectiveness from phase III randomized trials is available in the literature for nucleoside analogs (LAM, LdT and ETV), and nucleotide analogs (ADV and TDF). These drugs are administered by the oral route and display

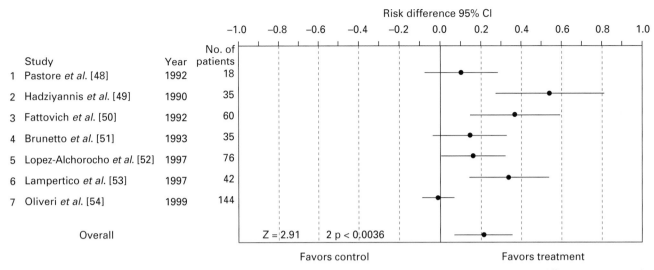

Figure 27.3 Meta-analysis of interferon therapy for HBeAg negative chronic hepatitis B: effect of treatment, measured as risk difference, on sustained loss of HBV-DNA.

a powerful inhibitory effect on HBV-DNA polymerase [59]. The examined "surrogate" endpoints (6–24 months) were ALT normalization, reduction of serum HBV-DNA levels during therapy, the rate of undetectable serum HBV DNA at the end of therapy, the rate of HBeAg loss or anti-HBe seroconversion at the end of therapy for patients with HBeAg positive hepatitis, the rate of HBsAg loss, anti-HBs seroconversion and the histological improvement at the end of treatment. Regarding the values of serum HBV-DNA during treatment and at the end of therapy, the RCTs reported different methods and different units to measure viral load. The serum HBV-DNA load was measured using polymerase chain reaction (PCR) assay or reverse transcription PCR assay or solution hybridization assay. The detection limits to evaluate the response ranged from 1.6 pg/ml (150,000 copies/ml) to 300 copies/ml.

Finally, the majority of studies evaluated the rate of appearance of mutations in specific regions of the polymerase-encoding HBV gene (so-called YMDD mutant and others) which were associated with the loss of efficacy of the drugs [60].

Lamivudine The original observations on the anti-HBV efficacy of LAM came from the treatment of HIV infected subjects who were also HBsAg positive [61–62]. The optimal dosage in immunocompetent patients with HBV chronic hepatitis, found by a dose-ranging study [63] and confirmed by an RCT [64], was 100 mg daily. It is important to consider that only a minority of published full papers are controlled trials with an appropriate control group.

The first two RCTs evaluated the efficacy of LAM therapy in HBeAg positive chronic hepatitis previously untreated and used a control arm treated with placebo. The first RCT performed in China [64], included exclusively Oriental

subjects, and the second trial was performed in USA and included prevalently white patients [65]. Both studies reported that a course of 12 months of LAM had favorable effects on histological, virological, and biochemical features of the disease and was well tolerated. At the end of treatment the rate of HBeAg seroconversion was 16% and 17% respectively in treated groups and 4% and 6% in control groups (OR, 3.06; 95% CI: 1.56–6.01). The histological response, evaluated as a reduction of at least two points of grading Knodell score, was more frequent in treated groups with a rate between 49% and 52%. Finally, the overall incidence of YMDD mutations at the end of treatment was of 14% in the Chinese trial and 32% in the American trial.

RCTs which compared the efficacy of 48–52 weeks LAM therapy versus IFN monotherapy (standard or pegylated IFN) or combination therapy with IFN and LAM [66–70], reported that among patients allocated in the LAM arm the rate of ALT normalization ranged between 23% and 78%, the rate of HBe seroconversion ranged between 19% and 28%, and the incidence of YMDD mutations was 8–40%. The identified predictors of virological relapse were older age, male sex and low levels of aminotransferases at the start of therapy.

The only published RCT including patients with anti-HBe positive chronic hepatitis used a schedule of 52 weeks of therapy with LAM [75]. Patients were randomized to receive 100 mg LAM orally once daily for 52 weeks or placebo for 26 weeks. The primary efficacy endpoint was loss of serum HBV-DNA with a cutoff of 1.6 pg/ml) plus normalization of ALT at week 24. A significantly higher proportion of patients receiving LAM (63%) had a complete response at week 24 compared with patients receiving placebo (6%) (p < 0.001). In a ranked assessment of pretreatment and post-treatment biopsy pairs 11% improved, 86% showed no change, and 2% worsened in fibrosis. At week 52, 27% of patients receiving LAM had YMDD variant HBV.

There are two major problems with LAM treatment: the occurrence of YMDD mutants under therapy and the stability of viral suppression after drug discontinuation. Appearance of the YMDD mutant was associated with an ALT relapse in 30–70% of cases, and usually both the YMDD mutant and the ALT peak subside rapidly upon stopping LAM. The efficacy of LAM to inhibit HBV replication was limited only to the period of drug exposure [72–75].

Telbivudine LdT is a potent and specific inhibitor of HBV-DNA polymerase. A double-blind pre-clinical study evaluated the efficacy and safety of two different doses of LdT (400 or 600 mg/day) alone or plus LAM (100 mg/day) compared with LAM alone in adult patients with HBeAg positive chronic hepatitis [76]. At the end of 52 weeks of therapy, LdT monotherapy showed a significantly greater mean reduction in HBV-DNA levels (6.01 vs 4.57 $\log_{10}$ copies/ml; $p < 0.05$), rate of undetectable HBV-DNA by PCR with a cutoff limit of 10^5 copies/ml (61% vs 32%; $p < 0.05$), and rate of ALT normalization (86% vs 63%; $p < 0.05$) compared with LAM monotherapy. The rate of HBeAg seroconversion (31% vs 22%) was not significantly different. Combination treatment with LdT and LAM was not better than LdT alone. **A1d**

In a phase III RCT [77], 1370 patients (more than 80% Asian) with HBsAg positive chronic hepatitis (921 HBeAg positive and 446 HBeAg negative) were randomly assigned to receive 600 mg of LdT or 100 mg of LAM once daily. At week 52, a significantly higher proportion of HBeAg positive and HBeAg negative patients receiving LdT than of those receiving LAM had a reduction in the serum HBV-DNA levels to fewer than 5 $\log_{10}$ copies/ml (60.0% vs 40.4%, $p = < 0.001$ and 88.3% vs 71.4%, $p < 0.001$ respectively). The histological response was different in HBeAg positive patients (64.7% vs 56.3%, $p = 0.01$), but not in HBeAg negative patients (66.6% vs 66.0%, $p = 0.90$). The rate of HBeAg loss and HBeAg seroconversion was comparable in HBeAg positive patients in both groups of treatment. The incidence of viral resistance during 52 weeks of therapy was lower in patients treated with LdT than in these treated with LAM (5.0% vs 11.0% in HBeAg positive patients, $p < 0.0001$, and 2.2% vs 10.7% in HBeAg negative patients, $p < 0.001$). The frequency of adverse events was similar for patients receiving LdT and LAM, and serious adverse events were reported in 2.6% of patients receiving LdT and 4.8% receiving LAM. **A1c**

In another RCT trial conducted in China, 332 HBeAg positive or HBeAg negative patients were treated with 600 mg of LdT or 100 mg of LAM daily for 104 weeks [78]. The primary efficacy endpoint was reduction in serum HBV-DNA levels at week 52 of treatment. Secondary endpoints included clearance of HBV-DNA to undetectable levels, HBeAg loss, seroconversion and ALT normalization. At week 52, among 290 HBeAg-positive patients, mean reductions of serum HBV-DNA (6.3 $\log_{10}$ versus 5.5 $\log_{10}$, $p < 0.001$) undetectable serum HBV-DNA by PCR (67% vs 38%, $p < 0.001$), ALT normalization (87% vs 75%, $p < 0.007$), and HBeAg loss (31% vs 20%, $p < 0.047$) were significantly more common in the LdT group. Viral resistance in LdT recipients was approximately half that observed with LAM, but this difference was not statistically significant. **A1c**

Finally, a randomized open-label trial compared the antiviral efficacy of LdT and ADV in 135 treatment-naive HBeAg positive patients with chronic hepatitis [79]. Patients were randomly assigned to received 52 weeks of LdT or ADV or 24 weeks of ADV and then LdT for the remaining 28 weeks. The primary efficacy comparison was serum HBV-DNA reduction at week 24 and at week 52. At week 24, mean HBV-DNA reduction was greater in patients with received LdT than in two groups who received ADV (−6.30 vs −4.97 $\log_{10}$ copies/ml; $p < 0.001$), and more patients treated with LdT had undetectable HBV-DNA by PCR, which has a lower limit of detection of 300 copies/ml. (39% vs 12%; $p < 0.001$). At week 52, the rate of undetectable HB-DNA by PCR (60% vs 40%, $p = 0.06$), the rate of HBeAg loss (30% vs 21%, $p = 0.3$), HBeAg seroconversion (18% vs 19%, $p = 0.3$) and the rate of ALT normalization (79% vs 85%, p 0.4) were similar in patients treated with LdT or ADV.

Entecavir ETV is a cyclopentyl guanosine analog that inhibits both the priming and elongation steps of viral replication. In a phase III RCT [80], 715 nucleoside naive patients (60% Asian and 40% white) with HBeAg positive chronic hepatitis were randomized to receive 0.5 mg of ETV or 100 mg of LAM once daily for 52 weeks. The primary efficacy endpoint was histological improvement (a decrease by at least two points in the Knodell necroinflammatory score) at week 48. Secondary endpoints included a reduction in the serum HBV-DNA level, HBeAg loss and seroconversion, and normalization of ALT level.

At 48 weeks, the ETV treated patients had higher rates of histological improvement (72% vs 62%, $p = 0.009$), HBV-DNA reduction (−6.9 vs −5.4 $\log_{10}$), undetectable HBV-DNA (67% vs 36%, $p < 0.001$), and ALT normalization (68% vs 60%, $p = 0.02$). HBeAg seroconversion occurred in 21% of ETV treated patients and 18% of those treated with LAM ($p = 0.33$). Safety was similar in the two groups. **A1c**

Another study showed that the antiviral activity of ETV is greater than that of ADV in patients with HBeAg positive chronic hepatitis who are treatment-naive [81]. In this study 69 patients with high levels of baseline HBV-DNA (>10^8 copies/ml) were treated with ETV 0.5 mg/day or

ADV 10 mg/day for 52 weeks. ETV was superior to ADV for mean change from baseline in serum HBV-DNA levels at week 12 ((−6.23 $\log_{10}$ copies/ml vs −4.42 $\log_{10}$ copies/ml respectively; p < 0.0001). The proportion of patients achieving HBV-DNA less than 300 copies/ml were greater in ETV-treated than ADV-treated patients at weeks 12, 24, and 48. At week 48 only 3% of ETV treated patients versus 47% of ADV treated patients had HBV-DNA of 10^5 copies/ml or more. **A1c**

In HBeAg negative chronic hepatitis only one RCT compared ETV and LAM treatment [82]. A total of 648 patients were randomized to receive either ETV 0.5 mg/day or LAM 100 mg/day for 48 weeks. More patients in the ETV group than in the LAM group had undetectable serum HBV-DNA levels (<300 copies/ml) (90% vs 72 %; p < 0.001) at the end of treatment. ALT normalization was also observed more frequently with ETV than with LAM (78% vs 71%, p = 0.045), but there was no difference in improvement in fibrosis. There was no evidence of resistance to ETV. Safety and adverse-event profiles were similar in the two groups. **A1c**

Adefovir dipivoxyl ADV, a nucleotide analog, has a potent *in vitro* and *in vivo* effect against herpes virus, retroviruses and hepadnaviruses. The drug, when given orally at a dose of 10 mg daily, inhibits both the wild type and LAM-resistant HBV strains with an excellent safety profile [83]. Renal tubular damage has been observed when prolonged treatment with higher doses has been given [84]. Two phase III multicenter RCTs, one in HBeAg positive patients have been published [85, 86]. In the first study, 1515 patients worldwide with HBeAg positive chronic hepatitis B were randomized to receive 10 mg or 30 mg of ADV or placebo for 48 weeks. Most of them were treatment naive, since only 123 had been previously treated with IFN. The observed reduction of HBV-DNA levels was 4.76 with 30 mg vs 3.52 log copies/ml with 10 mg of ADV; in both cases a significantly greater suppression than that observed in the placebo group. The rate of biochemical and histological improvement was comparable between two ADV regimens (59% vs 53% and 55% vs 48% respectively). HBeAg seroconversion, although significantly more common in patients receiving ADV (12% at 30 mg, 14% at 10 mg) than in the control group (6%, p = 0.049 and 0.01 respectively), was relatively uncommon. No ADV-associated resistance mutations were identified in the HBV-DNA polymerase gene. Mild nephrotoxicity was observed with the 30 mg regimen, and thus 10 mg was considered to be the best regimen. In the second RCT 480 Chinese subjects with hepatitis HBeAg positive chronic hepatitis were enrolled in a multicenter, double-blind, randomized, placebo-controlled study of ADV 10 mg once daily [26]. There was a significant difference in reduction of serum HBV-DNA levels after 12 weeks between subjects who received ADV

and those who received the placebo (3.4 and 0.1 $\log_{10}$ copies/ml respectively, p < .001). A higher proportion of subjects with undetectable serum HBV-DNA and with normal ALT was observed in ADV treated subjects at week 52 (median HBV-DNA reduction of 4.5 $\log_{10}$ copies/ml, 67% with HBV-DNA <10^5 copies/ml, 28% with HBV-DNA undetectable, and 79% with ALT normalization). Subjects with YMDD mutant HBV at baseline had virological, biochemical, and serological responses to treatment that were similar to those of subjects with wild-type HBV. The incidence of clinically adverse events was similar in nature and severity between the treatment groups, and there was no evidence of renal toxicity. No ADV related HBV mutations were identified. **A1c**

Patients with chronic HBeAg negative, HBV-DNA positive chronic hepatitis were studied in a multicenter trial [87], comparing the efficacy of 10 mg of ADV daily for 48 weeks to placebo. Viral suppression was obtained in 51% of patients on ADV vs none in the placebo group. The median HBV-DNA level of ADV-treated patients at 48 weeks (3.91 log copies/ml) was lower than observed with placebo (1.35 log copies/ml, p < 0.001). HBsAg seroconversion was never achieved. Histology changed significantly in the ADV group, with 64% of patients improved as compared with 33% of those on placebo, and alanine aminotransferase level normalized in 72% on ADV and 29% on the placebo. In both studies, YMDD or other repetitive mutations in the HBV polymerase region did not occur under either dose of ADV during the 48 weeks of treatment.

Tenofovir TDF is an acyclic nucleotide analog with a molecular structure related to that of ADV. Data from several small studies suggest that TDF might be more potent than ADV in inducing the early and rapid suppression of HBV-DNA in LAM resistant patients [88–90]. In two double-blind, phase III RCTs [91], patients with HBeAg positive or HBeAg negative chronic hepatitis were assigned in a 2:1 ratio to receive 300 mg of TDF or 10 mg ADV once daily for 48 weeks. The primary efficacy endpoint was HBV-DNA level less than 400 copies/ml and histologic improvement (a reduction in the Knodell necroinflammation score of two or more points without worsening of fibrosis) at week 48. The first RCT included 176 HBeAg positive patients which were treated with TDF, and 90 HBeAg positive patients treated with ADV. At 48 weeks, a higher proportion of patients in the TDF arm than in the ADV arm achieved HBV-DNA levels <400 copies/ml (76% vs 13%, p < 0.001). The respective rates for ALT normalization were 69% vs 54% (p = 0.03) and for HBeAg seroconversion were 21% vs 18% (p = 0.02). A higher proportion of patients treated with TDF had HBsAg loss (3% vs 0%, p = 0.02). The incidence of severe adverse events was similar in the TDF and ADV arms. **A1c**

In the second RCT, 375 HBeAg negative patients with chronic hepatitis were randomized to receive TDF 300 mg (250 patients) or ADV 10 mg (125 patients) for 48 weeks. At week 48, a significantly higher proportion of patients treated with TDF achieved the primary endpoint, compared with patients treated with ADV (71% vs 49%, p < 0.001). At the end of treatment, 93% of the patients in the TDF group had HBV-DNA levels greater than 400 copies/ml, compared with 63% of patients in the ADV group (p < 0.001). The rates of ALT normalization were similar in both treatment groups. No patients treated with TDF had a confirmed 0.5 mg increase in serum creatinine level or creatinine clearance of <50 ml/min. **A1c**

What are the long-term benefits of anti-viral therapy for chronic hepatitis B?

IFN therapy and HCC development

We reviewed the available literature to estimate whether IFN reduces the incidence of HCC and liver-related mortality in HBV-related cirrhosis. All potentially relevant papers were initially classified into two subsets (1: controlled trials; 2: cohort studies).

Subset 1: controlled trials The rate of HCC in treated and untreated patients with HBV cirrhosis was reported in 11 studies, including 2560 patients [92–102]. The benefit of IFN on cancer development is shown in Figure 27.4. IFN seemingly decreased the rate of HCC occurrence in all but one trial, and a significant difference was observed in three studies. The pooled estimate of the preventive effect of treatment was significantly in favor of IFN (rate difference: –0.04; 95% CI: –0.01––0.07). A remarkable heterogeneity was detected among studies (heterogeneity: 39.12 with 10 df; p < 0.001).

Since the trials showed a significant inconsistency, subgroup analyses were performed in relation to the ethnic origin of patients (European versus Oriental studies). Consistent results were observed only when assessing data pooled from European reports; in this subgroup no preventive effect of HCC was found. **A1c**

Subset 2: cohort studies It has been suggested from long-term cohort studies that IFN treatment may have a protective effect against HCC development in patients with chronic HBV infection. We reviewed the clinical course and outcome of patients enrolled in long-term, follow-up studies [98, 99, 102, 103–111]. The 12 studies (11 prospective and one retrospective) included a total of 1952 patients, 1187 of them not receiving active treatment. Length of follow-up ranged from 2.1 to 8.9 years. Meta-analysis of longitudinal studies with prolonged follow-up showed no significant differences in the rate of HCC between treated patients (1.9%; 95% CI: 0.8–3.0%) and controls (3.16%; 95% CI: 1.8–4.5%). **A1c**

All data dealing with HCC development coming from studies with prolonged follow-up must be interpreted with caution because possible biases can lead to erroneous estimates:

• Data collected from both prospective and retrospective studies conducted in tertiary care centers with limited generalizability

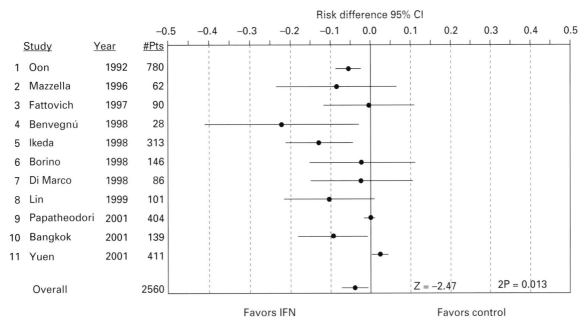

Figure 27.4 Meta-analysis of the 11 controlled trials of IFN for prevention of HCC in patients with HBV-related cirrhosis. Risk difference and 95% CI for each study and the pooled estimate of the treatment effect CI are plotted on the graph. Studies are arranged by publication year.

Loss of HBsAg

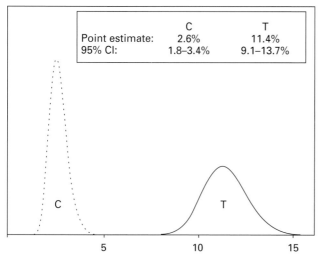

Figure 27.5 Probability distribution of the loss of HBsAg rate in HBeAgpositive chronic hepatitis B from IFN-treated (T) patients and controls (C). Data from cohort studies.

- Lack of randomization reducing the internal and the external validity of the studies
- Heterogeneity of patients enrolled, both in respect of clinical and demographic features and of possible co-factors
- Slow and prolonged course of the disease not allowing an inception cohort
- Few clinically relevant events, relatively small sample size, and duration of follow-up less than eight to ten years
- High mortality from non-hepatic causes
- Selection and increased surveillance for cases with more severe disease and unfavorable course
- Progressive shift over the years of the global spectrum of the disease due to intervening factors (e.g. new diagnostic tests and screening programs; new available treatments)

In conclusion, there is no sound evidence from controlled trials and prospective cohort studies to support a recommendation for widespread use of IFN to prevent HCC in these patients.

IFN therapy and long-term outcome

HBeAg positive chronic hepatitis B   In the setting of HBeAg-positive CHB, the long-term benefits of IFN treatment for chronic HBV infection were assessed by meta-analysis of 12 studies involving 1975 patients in which the length of follow-up ranged from 2.9 to 8.9 years [98, 99, 102, 103–111].

Loss of HBsAg occurred in 11.4% of treated patients, compared to 2.6% of controls, a four-fold benefit (see Figure 27.5). In contrast, a smaller effect was evident for the reduction in the incidence during the observation period of

Disease decompensation

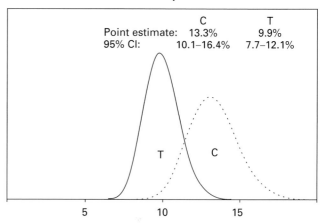

Figure 27.6 Probability distribution of disease decompensation rate in HBeAg-positive chronic hepatitis B from IFN-treated (T) patients and controls (C). Data from cohort studies.

Liver-related mortality

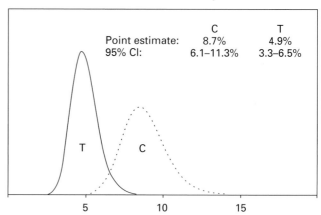

Figure 27.7 Probability distribution of liver-related mortality rate in HBeAg-positive chronic hepatitis B from IFN-treated (T) patients and controls (C). Data from cohort studies.

decompensation (see Figure 27.6) or liver-related deaths (see Figure 27.7), but the differences were not statistically significant. As the authors pointed out, however, all clinically relevant events (such as liver-related deaths) occurred infrequently in these studies to explain the lack of association with the therapy. **A1c**

HBeAg negative chronic hepatitis B   There have been controversies about the long-term benefit of IFN therapy in the HBeAg negative form of chronic hepatitis B. Differences of the baseline severity of illness in the population of the studies, the length of follow-up, type and frequency of post-treatment monitoring, and treatment regimens limit the assessment of the impact of IFN therapy on the course of the disease. Overall, the four cohort studies with a length of follow-up ranging from two to seven years showed that the response appeared to be less durable at long-term follow-up compared to HBeAg positive cases and that relapses can occur even years after therapy [112–115]. The rate of HBsAg loss ranged from 4.5% to 13%.

An RCT performed by Lampertico et al. [116] has demonstrated that long-term suppression of viral replication by 24-month IFN therapy improved the outcome of sustained responders defined as subjects with normal aminotransferase levels and undetectable hepatitis B virus DNA. Liver disease progressed in none of the sustained responders but in 16 with treatment failure (0% vs 22%; p = 0.002) while HCC developed with similar frequency in both groups (7%). Overall, estimated eight-year complication-free survival was longer for the 30 sustained responders than the 71 patients with treatment failure (90% vs 60%, p < 0.001), but eight-year patient survival was similar in the two groups (100% and 90%).

Nucleos(t)ide analogs therapy and HCC development

It has been argued that long-term suppression of HBV replication could reduce hepatocyte turnover and lessen the risk of dysplasia and cancer [117]. In 2004, a large RCT [118] showed a decrease in the incidence of HCC in patients with HBV-related advanced liver disease treated with LAM as compared to untreated controls. In the wake of this study, further controlled trials and retrospective or prospective cohort studies [119–123] were performed, mostly in patients with advanced liver disease. These studies collected cohorts of HBeAg positive and negative patients and showed a marked degree of heterogeneity, making it difficult to assess the actual level of benefit obtained by nucleos(t)ide analogs treatment.

We have pooled the available literature data to evaluate whether nucleos(t)ide treatment reduces the incidence of HCC in patients with HBV-related chronic liver disease. The effect of nucleos(t)ide on cancer incidence was assessed in six studies: two RCTs [118, 122], and four non-randomized or cohort studies [119–121, 123]. The six studies included 2394 patients, 1372 of whom received nucleos(t)ide therapy (1166 as LAM monotherapy and 206 as LAM and ADV combination therapy) and 1022 were untreated controls. Since in the cohort study a control arm of untreated patients was not included, we indirectly compared the rate of HCC development in the treatment arm to the mean control rate pooled from all the other included studies [123].

The percentage of males ranged from 73% to 85%. The sample size of each study varied greatly, ranging from 754 to 105 patients. Mean patient age ranged from 34 to 50 years. The proportion of patients with cirrhosis differed greatly among studies, ranging from 0% [121] to 100% [122]. Similarly, a great variability was observed among trials in the HBeAg status, ranging from 0% [120] to 100%

[121]. A large variability of nucleos(t)ide schedules between trials was found in the length of treatment (ranging between 19 and 96 months) and in the treatment follow-up (ranging between 2.7 and 8.2 years).

Nucleos(t)ide treatment seemingly decreased HCC rate in all the six evaluable studies, a significant difference being observed in three. The pooled estimate of the treatment effect by *random effect model* was significantly in favor of a preventive effectiveness of NA (RR: 0.26, 95% CI: 0.12–0.48). **A1c** We found a remarkable statistical quantitative heterogeneity among the studies, in the difference of the magnitude of the treatment effect on the risk of cancer development. Large differences were observed in the baseline risk of HCC among the different studies: the HCC rate in the untreated group ranged from 2.4% to 32.4%.

The results of this meta-analysis demonstrate that the heterogeneity in the magnitude of the preventive effect of nucleos(t)ide on the risk of cancer is the most impressive feature of these studies. Regarding HBV-related chronic infection, the pooled data suggested a preventive effect of nucleos(t)ide analogs on HCC development in patients without cirrhosis and in subjects with HBeAg positive infection. The benefit on HCC prevention was observed in studies from Asia. As with all meta-analyses, a methodological issue of the meta-analysis described above, is the potential limitation of the generalizability of its results to new populations and settings, particularly in western populations and in real clinical practice outside highly specialized centers.

Nucleos(t)ide analogs therapy and long term outcome

There have been only a few studies assessing the effects of LAM alone or in combination with ADV on hepatic decompensation and mortality. Five previously published long-term studies have shown that continuous treatment with LAM alone or in combination with ADV delays clinical progression in patients with advanced fibrosis or cirrhosis by reducing the incidence of hepatic decompensation [119–123]. In the large RCT by Liaw, 436 LAM-treated patients and 215 controls were followed for a mean time of 32 months. A significant difference was observed in the incidence of the primary endpoint, a composite endpoint combining hepatic decompensation, HCC, spontaneous bacterial peritonitis, bleeding gastresophageal varices or death related to liver disease between treated patients and controls.

Similar results were observed by Di Marco et al. in a large retrospective multicenter observational study [124]. On LAM therapy for four years a virological suppression was obtained in 616 patients (93.9%), and the rate of sustained virological response was 39% after four years. During follow-up, 47 (7.2%) patients underwent liver transplantation, liver disease worsened in 31 (4.7%), HCC developed in 31

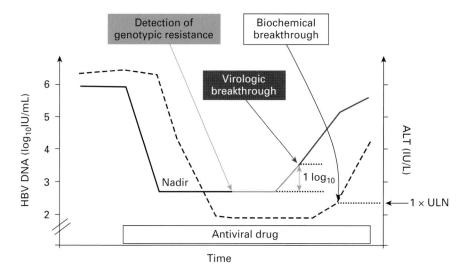

Figure 27.8 Genotypic resistance, virologic rebound and biochemical rebound. From: Ahmed S *et al. Hepatology* 2000; **32**: 1078–1088. Lok ASF, McMahon BJ. *Hepatology* 2007; **45**: 507–539.

(4.7%), and 24 patients (3.6%) died of liver-related causes. Patients who had cirrhosis and who maintained virological response were less likely than those with viral breakthrough to develop disease worsening. Survival was better in Child-Pugh A patients with cirrhosis and sustained virological suppression.

The relationships between HBV suppression, development of viral resistance and disease outcome are clarified in a small single center prospective study enrolling 59 patients mainly with HBeAg negative compensated cirrhosis [125]. Event-free survival was significantly longer in patients who maintained virological suppression than in those who did not have a complete virological response or suffered a breakthrough. Patients with advanced cirrhosis were more likely to develop liver failure after the emergence of YMDD mutants. Profound and maintained HBV-DNA suppression correlates with a better outcome.

Finally, data of the long-term benefit of subjects treated with others nucleos(t)ide analogs are not available as yet.

Resistance rates to nucleos(t)ide analogs associated with therapies for chronic hepatitis B

Antiviral drug resistance reflects reduced susceptibility of a virus to the inhibitory effect of a drug. Resistance results from a process of adaptive mutations under therapy, influenced by:

- High replication rates
- Low fidelity of the viral polymerase
- Selective pressure of the drug
- Genetic barrier of the drug
- Replication space (liver turnover)
- Fitness of mutant

Indications of emergence of drug-resistant HBV is given by:

- Increasing viral load ($\geq 1.0 \log IU/ml$)
- Identification of known genotypic markers of drug resistance within viral polymerase:
    —primary resistance mutations (e.g.: LAM → rtM204I)
    —secondary resistance mutations (e.g.: LAM → rtL180M with rtM204V)
    —compensatory mutations (e.g.: LAM → rtV173L)
- Increasing serum ALT levels
- Clinical deterioration

The following definitions are currently adopted to classify resistance to therapy (see Figure 27.8) [126]:

- Virologic breakthrough: increase in serum HBV DNA by $>1 \log_{10}$ (ten-fold) above nadir after achieving virologic response, during continued treatment
- Viral rebound: increase in serum HBV DNA to $>20,000 IU/ml$ or above pretreatment level after achieving virologic response, during continued treatment
- Biochemical breakthrough: increase in ALT above upper limit of normal after achieving normalization, during continued treatment
- Genotypic resistance: detection of mutations that have been shown in *in vitro* studies to confer resistance to the nucleos(t)ide analog that is being administered
- Phenotypic resistance: *in vitro* confirmation that the mutation detected decreases susceptibility (as demonstrated by increase in inhibitory concentrations) to the nucleos(t)ide analog administered

Long-term use of nucleos(t)ide analogs is associated with an increased risk of developing resistance at varying rates, depending on the drug used. The overall profile of resistance is reported in Table 27.2. The main mutations occurring on treatment with the nucleos(t)ide analogs in current usage are reported in Figure 27.9. Overlap in many of these mutations is remarkable across various analogs. This highlights the importance of careful assessment of virologic response in patients so that drug resistance can be quickly

Table 27.2 Annual prevalent resistance rates for lamivudine, adefovir, entecavir, emtricitabine and telbivudine.

DRUG	Resistance at each year of therapy expressed as percentage of patients				
	1	2	3	4	5
Lamivudine[a]	23	46	55	71	80
Adefovir[b] (naive HBeAg-neg)	0	3	11	18	29
Adefovir (LAM resistant)[c]	0–18	—	—	—	—
Entecavir[d] (naive)	0.1	0.4	1.1	1.1	1.2
Entecavir[d] (LAM resistant)	6	15	35	43	—
Emtricitabine[d]	9–16	19–37	—	—	—
Telbivudine[e] (HBeAg-pos)[f]	4.4[d]	21.6[e]	—	—	—
(HBeAg-neg)[f]	2.7	8.6			

[a] Modified and updated from Lai CL *et al.* 2003 and Leung V *et al.* 2001.
[b] from Locarnini S *et al.* 2005; Hadziyannis S *et al. NEJM* 2005. 352: 2673.
[c] from Lee Y-S *et al. Hepatology* 2006; 43: 1385.
[d] from Perrillo RP *et al.* 2005; and Colonno *et al.* 2006.
[e] In the LAM comparator arm, the percentage was only 8% based on a complex case definition of anti-viral drug resistance/treatment failure. One would thus expect a comparable relative level of
[f] 10–12% based on genotypic resistance compared with lamivudine (25% per annum). Lok A & McMahon B. *Hepatology* 2007; **45**: 507.

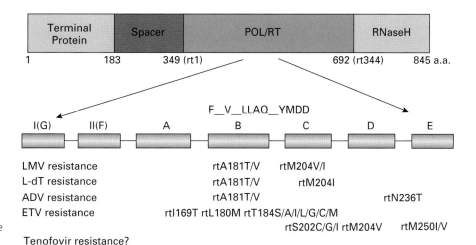

Figure 27.9 Primary resistance mutations occurring on treatment with the nucleos(t)ide analogues.

identified and multidrug resistance can be avoided. If cost and access are not issues because of insurance reimbursement, geographic location, or agent approval, clinicians should choose the most potent nucleoside analog available with the least likelihood of developing resistance. In this regard, the two drugs that would be preferable as monotherapy appear to be ETV and TDF. No head-to-head efficacy or resistance data are available for ETV and TDF in treatment-naive patients. The use of TDF might be warranted over ETV in LAM-resistant patients. **B4**

Management of resistance to one analog must take into account previous exposure to other drugs in this class. Current EASL recommendations are reported in Table 27.3.

Combination vs monotherapy with nucleos(t)ide analogs

A generally accepted concept in virology is that the use of combination therapy may increase the genetic barrier to resistance, resulting in a decrease in the occurrence of viral

Table 27.3 AASLD recommendations for managing virologic breakthrough.

Resistance	Rescue therapy
LAM	• Add ADV (superior to ADV switch) • Switch to ETV (increased risk of ETV resistance development) • Add TDF[a] or switch to FTC/TDF[a]
ADV	• Add LAM (superior to LAM switch) • Switch to or add ETV (only in the absence of LAM resistance) • Switch to FTC/TDF[a]
ETV	• Add or switch to ADV or TDF[a]
LdT	• Add ADV (superior to ADV switch) • Switch to ETV (increased risk of ETV resistance development) • Add TDF[a] or switch to FTC/TDF[a]

[a] Off label.
From Lok A et al. Hepatology 2007; **45**: 507–39.

resistance; this has been well documented in the treatment of HIV. Much discussion has focused on the potential benefits of combination therapy or add-on therapy vs sequential monotherapy. Although many believe that combination therapy may still play a role in improving long-term prevention of resistance, data are currently insufficient regarding the efficacy of combinations of nucleoside analogs or combinations of nucleos(t)ide analogs with peginterferon to determine any significant benefit over monotherapy. Therefore, although a theoretical benefit to combination therapy may exist, it cannot be recommended as a first-line treatment strategy.

The use of a more potent antiviral as de novo monotherapy is the current alternative to the combination of two drugs with low genetic barriers to resistance or suboptimal efficacy. The patient's virologic response should also be monitored, considering the need for a therapy change at 12–24 weeks if a robust virologic suppression is not achieved, depending on the agent with which the patient is treated [127]. In general, choosing the most potent first-line monotherapy, if available, is a reasonable approach.
B4

The ultimate goal is to maintain very low levels of viral replication or undetectable replication for as long as possible; the prevention of viral replication results in preventing development of resistance [128]. To achieve this, potent drugs with a high genetic barrier to resistance should be selected, or, if these drugs are not available de novo combination therapy could be used, while full adherence to the regimen should be strongly encouraged in either circumstance.

Conclusions

Data from studies of natural history and RCTs or non-randomized studies of antiviral treatment give sufficient data to conclude that:

(1) The natural history of chronic hepatitis B is variable, according to phenotypic and ethnic background, and is also influenced by viral co-infections and toxic co-factors. At least 20% of patients develop clinically significant liver disease in the long term.

(2) Presence of significant HBV replication and of continuing liver necroinflammation predict an adverse outcome.

(3) IFN therapy results in stable clearance of HBeAg in 25% of all patients chronically infected by wild type HBV, but only rarely results in HBsAg clearance.

(4) IFN therapy results in stable clearance of HBV-DNA in 25% of all patients chronically infected by HBe minus HBV.

(5) All available oral analogs effectively reduce HBV-DNA and normalize ALT during therapy in at least two-thirds of patients within one year of treatment.

(6) Viral resistance to analogs appear at variable frequency (more with nucleosides, except entecavir, less with nucleotides) and affects their long-term effectiveness.

(7) Effects of anti-viral treatment on survival, although biologically plausible and already evident when treating patients with advanced disease, have yet to be proven in non-cirrhotic chronic hepatitis.

(8) A protective effect of IFN against development of HCC is still unproven.

References

1 Lok AS, McMahon BJ. Chronic hepatitis B. *Hepatology* 2001; **34**: 1225–1241.

2 Lok AS, Heathcote J, Hoofnagle JH. Management of hepatitis B: 2000 – summary of a workshop. *Gastroenterology* 2001; **120**: 1828–1853.

3 Liaw YF, Tai DI, Chu CM, Chen TJ. The development of cirrhosis in patients with chronic type B hepatitis: a prospective study. *Hepatology* 1988; **8**: 493–496.

4 De Jongh FE, Janssen HLA, De Man RA et al. Survival and prognostic indicators in hepatitis B surface antigen-positive cirrhosis of the liver. *Gastroenterology* 1992; **103**: 1630–1635.

5 Fattovich G, Giustina G, Schalm SW et al. Occurrence of hepatocellular carcinoma and decompensation in western European patients with cirrhosis type B. *Hepatology* 1995; **21**: 77–82.

6 Craxì A, Di Bona D, Cammà C. Interferon-alpha for HBeAg-positive chronic hepatitis B. *J Hepatol* 2003; **39**(Suppl. 1): S99–S105.

7 Wong JB, Koff RS, Tiné F, Pauker SG. Cost-effectiveness of interferon-alpha 2b treatment for hepatitis B e antigen-positive chronic hepatitis B. *Ann Intern Med* 1995; **122**: 664–675.

8 Tiné F, Liberati A, Craxì A, Almasio P and Pagliaro L. Interferon treatment in patients with chronic hepatitis B: a meta-

analysis of the published literature. *J Hepatol* 1993; **18**: 154–162.

9 Wong DK, Cheung AM, O'Rourke K, Naylor CD, Detsky AS, Heathcote J. Effect of alpha-interferon treatment in patients with hepatitis B e antigen-positive chronic hepatitis B. A meta-analysis. *Ann Intern Med* 1993; **119**: 312–323.

10 Evans AA, London WT. Interferon for chronic hepatitis B. *Ann Intern Med* 1996; **124**: 276.

11 Carithers RL, Jr. Effect of interferon on hepatitis B. *Lancet* 1998; **351**: 157.

12 Zoulim F, Trépo C. Drug therapy for chronic hepatitis B: antiviral efficacy and influence of hepatitis B virus polymerase mutations on the outcome of therapy. *J Hepatol* 1998; **29**:151–168.

13 Hussain M, Lok AS. Mutations in the hepatitis B virus polymerase gene associated with antiviral treatment for hepatitis B. *J Viral Hepat* 1999; **6**: 183–194.

14 Carreño V, Porres JC, Mora I *et al.* A controlled study of treatment with recombinant interferon alpha in chronic hepatitis B virus infection: induction and maintenance schedules. *Antiviral Res* 1987; **3**: 125–137.

15 McDonald JA, Caruso L, Karayiannis P *et al.* Diminished responsiveness of male homosexual chronic hepatitis B virus carriers with HTLV-III antibodies to recombinant alpha-interferon. *Hepatology* 1987; **7**: 719–723.

16 Alexander GJ, Brahm J, Fagan EA *et al.* Loss of HBsAg with interferon therapy in chronic hepatitis B virus infection. *Lancet* 1987; **2**: 66–69.

17 Porres JC, Carreño V, Mora I *et al.* Different doses of recombinant alpha interferon in the treatment of chronic hepatitis B patients without antibodies against the human immunodeficiency virus. *Hepatogastroenterology* 1988; **35**: 300–303.

18 Pastore G, Santantonio T, Monno L, Milella M, Luchena N, Angarano G. Permanent inhibition of viral replication induced by low dosage of human leukocyte interferon in patients with chronic hepatitis B. *Hepatogastroenterology* 1988; **35**: 57–61.

19 Hoofnagle JH, Peters M, Mullen KD *et al.* Randomized, controlled trial of recombinant human alpha-interferon in patients with chronic hepatitis B. *Gastroenterology* 1988; **95**: 1318–1325.

20 Lok AS, Lai CL, Wu PC, Leung EK. Long-term follow-up in a randomised controlled trial of recombinant alpha 2-interferon in Chinese patients with chronic hepatitis B infection. *Lancet* 1988; **2**: 298–302.

21 Saracco G, Mazzella G, Rosina F *et al.* A controlled trial of human lymphoblastoid interferon in chronic hepatitis B in Italy. *Hepatology* 1989; **10**: 336–341.

22 Brook MG, Chan G, Yap I *et al.* Randomised controlled trial of lymphoblastoid IFN alpha in Europid men with chronic hepatitis B virus infection. *BMJ* 1989; **299**: 652–656.

23 Brook MG, McDonald JA, Karayiannis P *et al.* Randomised controlled trial of interferon alpha 2A (Roferon-A) for the treatment of chronic hepatitis B virus (HBV) infection: factors that influence response. *Gut* 1989; **30**: 1116–1122.

24 Williams SJ, Craig PI, Cooksley WG *et al.* Randomised controlled trial of recombinant human interferon-alpha A for chronic active hepatitis B. *Aust N Z J Med* 1990; **20**: 9–19.

25 Waked I, Amin M, Abd el Fattah S, Osman LM, Sabbour MS. Experience with interferon in chronic hepatitis B in Egypt. *J Chemother* 1990; **2**: 310–318.

26 Realdi G, Fattovich G, Pastore G *et al.* Problems in the management of chronic hepatitis B with interferon: experience in a randomized, multicentre study. *J Hepatol* 1990; **11** (Suppl 1): S129–S132.

27 Müller R, Baumgarten R, Markus R *et al.* Treatment of chronic hepatitis B with interferon alpha-2b. *J Hepatol* 1990; **11** (Suppl 1): S137–S140.

28 Perrillo RP, Schiff ER, Davis GL *et al.* A randomized, controlled trial of interferon alpha-2b alone and after prednisone withdrawal for the treatment of chronic hepatitis B. The Hepatitis Interventional Therapy Group. *N Engl J Med* 1990; **323**: 295–301.

29 Lok AS, Wu PC, Lai CL *et al.* A controlled trial of interferon with or without prednisone priming for chronic hepatitis B. *Gastroenterology* 1992; **102**: 2091–2097.

30 Di Bisceglie AM, Fong TL, Fried MW *et al.* A randomized, controlled trial of recombinant alpha-interferon therapy for chronic hepatitis B. *Am J Gastroenterol* 1993; **88**: 1887–1892.

31 Bayraktar Y, Uzunalimoglu B, Arslan S, Koseoglu T, Kayhan B, Telatar H. Effects of recombinant alpha interferon on chronic active hepatitis B: preliminary results. *Gut* 1993; 34: S101.

32 Wong DK, Yim C, Naylor CD *et al.* Interferon alpha treatment of chronic hepatitis B: randomized trial in a predominantly homosexual male population. *Gastroenterology* 1995; **108**: 165–171.

33 Sarin SK, Guptan RC, Thakur V *et al.* Efficacy of low-dose alpha interferon therapy in HBV-related chronic liver disease in Asian Indians: a randomized controlled trial. *J Hepatol* 1996; **24**: 391–396.

34 Janssen HL, Gerken G, Carreno V *et al.* Interferon alpha for chronic hepatitis B infection: increased efficacy of prolonged treatment. The European Concerted Action on Viral Hepatitis (EUROHEP). *Hepatology* 1999; **30**: 238–243.

35 Thomas HC, Karayiannis P, Brook G. Treatment of hepatitis B virus infection with interferon. Factors predicting response to interferon. *J Hepatol* 1991; **13** (Suppl 1): S4–S7.

36 Carreño V, Castillo I, Molina J, Porres JC and Bartolomé J. Long-term follow-up of hepatitis B chronic carriers who responded to interferon therapy. *J Hepatol* 1992; **15**: 102–106.

37 Krogsgaard K, Christensen E, Bindslev N *et al.* Relation between treatment efficacy and cumulative dose of alpha interferon in chronic hepatitis B. *Journal of Hepatology* 1996; **25**: 795–802.

38 Cooksley WG, Piratvisuth T, Lee SD *et al.* Peginterferon alpha-2a (40 kDa): an advance in the treatment of hepatitis B e antigen-positive chronic hepatitis B. *J Viral Hepat* 2003; **10**: 298–305.

39 Zhao H, Kurbanov F, Wan MB *et al.* Genotype B and younger patient age associated with better response to low-dose therapy: a trial with pegylated/nonpegylated interferon-alpha-2b for hepatitis B e antigen-positive patients with chronic hepatitis B in China. *Clin Infect Dis* 2007; **44**: 541–548.

40 Krogsgaard K. Does corticosteroid pretreatment enhance the effect of alpha interferon treatment in chronic hepatitis B. *J Hepatol* 1994; **20**: 159–162.

41 Krogsgaard K, Marcellin P, Trepo C *et al.* Prednisolone withdrawal therapy enhances the effect of human lymphoblastoid interferon in chronic hepatitis B. *J Hepatol* 1996; **25**: 803–813.

42 Mellerup MT, Krogsgaard K, Mathurin P, Gluud C, Poynard T. Sequential combination of glucocorticosteroids and alfa inter-

feron versus alfa interferon alone for HBeAg-positive chronic hepatitis B. *Cochrane Database Syst Rev.* 2002; (2): CD000345.

43 Perrillo R, Tamburro C, Regenstein F *et al.* Low-dose, titratable interferon alpha in decompensated liver disease caused by chronic infection with hepatitis B virus. *Gastroenterology* 1995; **109**: 908–916.

44 Perrillo RP. Chronic hepatitis B: problem patients (including patients with decompensated disease). *J Hepatol* 1995; **22**: 45–48.

45 Janssen HL, van Zonneveld M, Senturk H *et al.* HBV 99-01 Study Group; Rotterdam Foundation for Liver Research. Pegylated interferon alfa-2b alone or in combination with lamivudine for HBeAg-positive chronic hepatitis B: a randomised trial. *Lancet* 2005; **365**: 123–129.

46 Flink HJ, Hansen BE, Heathcote EJ *et al.* HBV 99-01 Study Group. Successful treatment with peginterferon alfa-2b of HBeAg-positive HBV non-responders to standard interferon or lamivudine. *Am J Gastroenterol* 2006; **101**: 2523–2529.

47 Lau GK, Piratvisuth T, Luo KX *et al.* Peginterferon Alfa-2a HBeAg-Positive Chronic Hepatitis B Study Group. Peginterferon Alfa-2a, lamivudine, and the combination for HBeAg-positive chronic hepatitis B. *N Engl J Med* 2005; **352**: 2682–2695.

48 Pastore G, Santantonio T, Milella M *et al.* Anti-HBe-positive chronic hepatitis B with HBV-DNA in the serum response to a 6-month course of lymphoblastoid interferon. *J Hepatol* 1992; **14**: 221–225.

49 Hadziyannis S, Bramou T, Makris A *et al.* Interferon alfa-2b treatment of HBeAg negative/serum HBV DNA positive chronic active hepatitis type B. *J Hepatol* 1990; **11** (Suppl 1): S133–S136.

50 Fattovich G, Farci P, Rugge M *et al.* A randomized controlled trial of lymphoblastoid interferon-a in patients with chronic hepatitis B lacking HBeAg. *Hepatology* 1992; **15**: 584–589.

51 Brunetto MR, Giarin M, Saracco G *et al.* Hepatitis B virus unable to secrete e antigen and response to interferon in chronic hepatitis B. *Gastroenterology* 1993; **105**: 845–850.

52 Lopez-Alchorocho JM, Bartolome J, Cotonat T, Carreno V. Efficacy of prolonged interferon-alpha treatment in chronic hepatitis B patients with HbeAb: comparison between 6 and 12 months of therapy. *J Viral Hepat* 1997; **4**: 27–32.

53 Lampertico P, Del Ninno E, Manzin A *et al.* A randomized, controlled trial of a 24-month course of interferon alpha 2b in patients with chronic hepatitis B who had hepatitis B virus DNA without hepatitis B e antigen in serum. *Hepatology* 1997; **26**: 1621–1625.

54 Oliveri F, Santantonio T, Bellati G *et al.* Long term response to therapy of chronic anti-HBe-positive hepatitis B is poor independent of type and schedule of interferon. *Am J Gastroenterol* 1999; **94**: 1366–1372.

55 Karabay O, Tamer A, Tahtaci M, Vardi S, Celebi H. Effectiveness of lamivudine and interferon-alpha combination therapy versus interferon-alpha monotherapy for the treatment of HBeAg-negative chronic hepatitis B patients: a randomized clinical trial. *J Microbiol Immunol Infect* 2005; **38**: 262–266.

56 Marcellin P, Lau GK, Bonino F *et al.* Peginterferon Alfa-2a HBeAg-Negative Chronic Hepatitis B Study Group. Peginterferon alfa-2a alone, lamivudine alone, and the two in combination in patients with HBeAg-negative chronic hepatitis B. *N Engl J Med* 2004; **351**: 1206–1217.

57 Kaymakoglu S, Oguz D, Gur G *et al.* Pegylated interferon Alfa-2b monotherapy and pegylated interferon Alfa-2b plus lamivudine combination therapy for patients with hepatitis B virus E antigen-negative chronic hepatitis B. *Antimicrob Agents Chemother.* 2007; **51**: 3020–3022.

58 Gish RG, Lau DT, Schmid P, Perrillo R. A pilot study of extended duration peginterferon alfa-2a for patients with hepatitis B e antigen-negative chronic hepatitis B. *Am J Gastroenterol* 2007; **102**: 2718–2723.

59 Zoulim F. Assessment of treatment efficacy in HBV infection and disease. *J Hepatol* 2006; **44**: S95–S99.

60 Fournier C, Zoulim F. Antiviral therapy of chronic hepatitis B: prevention of drug resistance. *Clin Liver Dis* 2007; **11**: 869–892.

61 Benhamou Y, Dohin E, Lunel-Fabiani F *et al.* Efficacy of lamivudine on replication of hepatitis B virus in HIV-infected patients. *Lancet* 1995; **345**: 396–397.

62 Benhamou Y, Katlama C, Lunel F *et al.* Effects of lamivudine on replication of hepatitis B virus in HIV-infected men. *Ann Intern Med* 1996; **125**: 705–712.

63 Lai CL, Ching CK, Tung AKM *et al.* Lamivudine is effective in suppressing hepatitis B virus DNA in Chinese hepatitis B surface antigen carriers: a placebo-controlled trial. *Hepatology* 1997; **25**: 241–244.

64 Lai CL, Chien RN, Leung NWY *et al.* and Asia Hepatitis Lamivudine Study Group. A one-year trial of lamivudine for chronic hepatitis B. *N Engl J Med* 1998; **339**: 61–68.

65 Dienstag JL, Schiff ER, Wright TL *et al.* Lamivudine as initial treatment for chronic hepatitis B in the United States. *N Engl J Med.* 1999; **341**: 1256–1263.

66 Lau GK, Piratvisuth T, Luo KX *et al.* Peginterferon Alfa-2a, lamivudine, and the combination for HBeAg-positive chronic hepatitis B. *N Engl J Med* 2005; **352**: 2682–2695.

67 han HL, Leung NW, Hui AY *et al.* A randomized, controlled trial of combination therapy for chronic hepatitis B: comparing pegylated interferon-alpha2b and lamivudine with lamivudine alone. *Ann Intern Med* 2005; **142**: 240–250.

68 Schalm SW, Heathcote J, Cianciara J *et al.* Lamivudine and alpha interferon combination treatment of patients withchronic hepatitis B infection: a randomised trial. *Gut* 2000; **46**: 562–568.

69 Sarin SK, Kumar M, Kumar R *et al.* Higher efficacy of sequential therapy with interferon-alpha and lamivudine combination compared to lamivudine monotherapy in HBeAg positive chronic hepatitis B patients. *Am J Gastroenterol* 2005; **100**: 2463–2471.

70 Barbaro G, Zechini F, Pellicelli AM *et al.* Lamivudine Italian Study Group Investigators. Long-term efficacy of interferon alpha-2b and lamivudine in combination compared to lamivudine monotherapy in patients with chronic hepatitis B. An Italian multicenter, randomized trial. *J Hepatol* 2001; **35**: 406–411.

71 Tassopoulos NC, Volpes R, Pastore G *et al.* Efficacy of lamivudine in patients with hepatitis B e antigen-negative/hepatitis B virus DNA-positive (precore mutant) chronic hepatitis B. Lamivudine Precore Mutant Study Group. *Hepatology* 1999; **29**: 889–896.

72 Van Nunen AB, Hansen BE, Suh DJ *et al.* Durability of HBeAg seroconversion following antiviral therapy for chronic hepatitis B: relation to type of therapy and pretreatment serum hepatitis

B virus DNA and alanine aminotransferase. *Gut* 2003; **52**: 420–424.

73 Lee KM, Cho SW, Kim SW, Kim HJ, Hahm KB, Kim JH. Effect of virological response on post-treatment durability of lamivudine-induced HBeAg seroconversion. *J Viral Hepat* 2002; **9**: 208–212.

74 Song BC, Suh DJ, Lee HC, Chung YH, Lee YS. Hepatitis B e antigen seroconversion after lamivudine therapy is not durable in patients with chronic hepatitis B in Korea. *Hepatology* 2000; **32**: 803–806.

75 Dienstag JL, Cianciara J, Karayalcin S *et al*. Durability of serologic response after lamivudine treatment of chronic hepatitis B. *Hepatology* 2003; **37**: 748–755.

76 Lai CL, Leung N, Teo EK *et al*. A 1-year trial of telbivudine, lamivudine, and the combination in patients with hepatitis B e antigen-positive chronic hepatitis B. *Gastroenterology* 2005; **129**: 528–536.

77 Lai CL, Gane E, Liaw YF *et al*. Telbivudine versus lamivudine in patients with chronic hepatitis B. *N Engl J Med* 2007; **357**: 2576–2588.

78 Hou J, Yin YK, Xu D *et al*. Telbivudine versus lamivudine in Chinese patients with chronic hepatitis B:Results at 1 year of a randomized, double-blind trial. *Hepatology* 2008; **47**: 447–454.

79 Chan HL, Heathcote EJ, Marcellin P *et al*. Treatment of hepatitis B e antigen positive chronic hepatitis with telbivudine or adefovir: a randomized trial. *Ann Intern Med* 2007; **147**: 745–754.

80 Chang TT, Gish RG, de Man R *et al*. A comparison of entecavir and lamivudine for HBeAg-positive chronic hepatitis B. *N Engl J Med* 2006; **354**: 100–110.

81 Leung N, Peng CY, Hann HW *et al*. Early hepatitis B virus DNA reduction in hepatitis B e antigen-positive patients with chronic hepatitis B: a randomized international study of entecavir versus adefovir. *Hepatology* 2009; **49**: 72–79.

82 Lai CL, Shouval D, Lok AS *et al*. Entecavir versus lamivudine for patients with HBeAg-negative chronic hepatitis B. *N Engl J Med* 2006; **354**: 1011–1020.

83 Rivkin AM. Adefovir dipivoxil in the treatment of chronic hepatitis B. *Ann Pharmacother* 2004; **38**: 625–633.

84 Izzedine H, Hulot JS, Launay-Vacher V *et al*. Renal safety of adefovir dipivoxil in patients with chronic hepatitis B: two double-blind, randomized, placebo-controlled studies. *Kidney Int* 2004; **66**: 1153–1158.

85 Marcellin P, Chang TT, Lim SG *et al*. Adefovir dipivoxil for the treatment of hepatitis B e antigen-positive chronic hepatitis B. *N Engl J Med* 2003; **348**: 808–816.

86 Zeng M, Mao Y, Yao G *et al*. A double-blind randomized trial of adefovir dipivoxil in Chinese subjects with HBeAg-positive chronic hepatitis B. *Hepatology* 2006; **44**: 108–116.

87 Hadziyannis SJ, Tassopoulos NC, Heathcote EJ *et al*. Adefovir dipivoxyl for the treatment of hepatitis B e antigen-negative chronic hepatitis B. *N Engl J Med* 2003; **348**: 800–807.

88 van Bommel F, Zollner B, Sarrazin C *et al*. Tenofovir for patients with lamivudine-resistant hepatitis B virus (HBV) infection and high HBV DNA level during adefovir therapy. *Hepatology* 2006; **44**: 318–325.

89 van Bommel F, Wunsche T, Mauss S *et al*. Comparison of adefovir and tenofovir in the treatment of lamivudine-resistant hepatitis B virus infection. *Hepatology* 2004; **40**: 1421–1425.

90 van Bommel F, Schernick A, Hopf U *et al*. Tenofovir disoproxil fumarate exhibits strong antiviral effect in a patient with lamivudine-resistant severe hepatitis B reactivation. *Gastroenterology* 2003; **124**: 586–587.

91 Marcellin P, Heathcote EJ, Buti M *et al*. Tenofovir disoproxil fumarate versus adefovir dipivoxil for chronic hepatitis B. *N Engl J Med* 2008; **359**: 2442–2455.

92 Oon CJ. Long-term survival following treatment of hepatocellular carcinoma in Singapore: evaluation of Wellferon in the prophylaxis of high-risk pre-cancerous conditions. *Cancer Chemother Pharmacol* 1992; **31** (Suppl 1): S137–S142.

93 Mazzella G, Accogli E, Sottili S *et al*. Alpha-interferon treatment may prevent hepatocellular carcinoma in HCV-related liver cirrhosis. *J Hepatol* 1996; **24**: 141–147.

94 Fattovich G, Giustina G, Realdi G *et al*. and the European Concerted Action on Viral Hepatitis (EUROHEP). Long-term outcome of hepatitis B e antigen-positive patients with compensated cirrhosis treated with interferon alfa. *Hepatology* 1997; **26**: 1338–1342.

95 Benvegnu` L, Chemello L, Noventa F *et al*. Retrospective analysis of the effect of interferon therapy on the clinical outcome of patients with viral cirrhosis. *Cancer* 1998; **83**: 901–909.

96 Ikeda K, Saitoh S, Suzuki Y *et al*. Interferon decreases hepatocellular carcinogenesis in patients with cirrhosis caused by the hepatitis B virus. *Cancer* 1998; **82**: 827–835.

97 International Interferon-alpha Hepatocellular Carcinoma Study Group. Effect of interferon-alpha on progression of cirrhosis to hepatocellular carcinoma: a retrospective cohort study. *Lancet* 1998; **351**: 1535–1539.

98 Di Marco V, Lo Iacono O, Cammà C *et al*. The long term course of chronic hepatitis B. *Hepatology* 1999; **30**: 257–264.

99 Lin SM, Sheen IS, Chien RN *et al*. Long-term beneficial effect of interferon therapy in patients with chronic hepatitis B virus infection. *Hepatology* 1999; **29**: 971–975.

100 Papatheodoridis GV, Manesis E, Hadziyannis SJ. The long-term outcome of interferon-alpha treated and untreated patients with HBeAg-negative chronic hepatitis B. *J Hepatol* 2001; **34**: 30–13.

101 Tangkijvanich P, Thong-ngam D, Mahachai V, Kladchareon N, Suwangool P, Kullavanijaya P. Long-term effect of interferon therapy on incidence of cirrhosis and hepatocellular carcinoma in Thai patients with chronic hepatitis B. *Southeast Asian J Trop Med Public Health* 2001; **32**: 452–458.

102 Yuen MF, Hui CK, Cheng CC *et al*. Long-term follow-up of interferon alfa treatment in Chinese patients with chronic hepatitis B infection: The effect on hepatitis B e antigen seroconversion and the development of cirrhosis-related complications. *Hepatology* 2001; **34**: 139–145.

103 Niederau C, Heintges T, Lange S *et al*. Long-term follow-up of HBeAg-positive patients treated with interferon alfa for chronic hepatitis B. *N Engl J Med* 1996; **334**: 1422–1427.

104 Chen DK, Yim C, O'Rourke K *et al*. Long-term follow-up of a randomized trial of interferon therapy for chronic hepatitis B in a predominantly homosexual male population. *J Hepatol* 1999; **30**: 557–563.

105 Evans AA, Fine M, London WT. Spontaneous seroconversion in hepatitis B e antigen-positive chronic hepatitis B: implications for interferon therapy. *J Infect Dis* 1997; **176**: 845–850.

106 Korenman J, Baker B, Waggoner J *et al.* Long-term remission of chronic hepatitis B after alpha-interferon therapy. *Ann Intern Med* 1991; **114**: 629–634.

107 Lok AS, Chung HT, Liu VW *et al.* Long-term follow-up of chronic hepatitis B patients treated with interferon alfa. *Gastroenterology* 1993; **105**: 1833–1838.

108 Lau DT, Everhart J, Kleiner DE *et al.* Long-term follow-up of patients with chronic hepatitis B treated with interferon alfa. *Gastroenterology* 1997; **113**: 1660–1667.

109 Fattovich G, Giustina G, Christensen E *et al.* Influence of hepatitis delta virus infection on morbidity and mortality in compensated cirrhosis type B. The European Concerted Action on Viral Hepatitis (Eurohep). *Gut* 2000; **46**: 420–426.

110 Hsu YS, Chien RN, Yeh CT *et al.* Long-term outcome after spontaneous HBeAg seroconversion in patients with chronic hepatitis B. *Hepatology* 2002; **35**: 1522–1527.

111 Lampertico P, Del Ninno E, Viganò M *et al.* Long-term suppression of hepatitis B e antigen-negative chronic hepatitis B by 24-month interferon therapy. *Hepatology* 2003; **37**: 756–763.

112 Benvegnù L, Chemello L, Noventa F, Fattovich G, Pontisso P, Alberti A. Retrospective analysis of the effect of interferon therapy on the clinical outcome of patients with viral cirrhosis. *Cancer* 1998; **83**: 901–909.

113 Papatheodoridis GV, Manesis E, Hadziyannis SJ. Long term outcome of interferon-alpha treated and untreated patients with HBeAg negative chronic hepatitis B. *J Hepatol* 2000; **34**: 306–313.

114 Manesis E, Hadziyannis S. Interferon alpha treatment and retreatment of hepatitis B e antigen-negative chronic hepatitis B. *Gastroenterology* 2001; **121**: 101–109.

115 Brunetto MR, Oliveri F, Coco B *et al.* Outcome of anti-HBe positive chronic hepatitis B in alpha-interferon treated and untreated patients: a long term cohort study. *Hepatology* 2002; **36**: 263–270.

116 Lampertico P, Del Ninno E, Manzin A *et al.* A randomized, controlled trial of a 24-month course of interferon alpha 2b in patients with chronic hepatitis B who had hepatitis B virus DNA without hepatitis B e antigen in serum. *Hepatology* 1997; **26**: 1621–1625.

117 Chien-Jen C, Hwai-I Y, Jun S *et al.* for the REVEAL-HBV Study Group Risk of Hepatocellular Carcinoma Across a biological gradient of serum hepatitis B virus DNA level. *JAMA* 2006; **295**: 65–73.

118 Liaw YF, Sung JJ, Chow WC *et al.* Lamivudine for patients with chronic hepatitis B and advanced liver disease. *New Engl J Med.* 2004; **351**: 1521–1531.

119 Matsumoto A, Tanaka E, Rokuhara A *et al.* Efficacy of lamivudine for preventing hepatocellular carcinoma in chronic hepatitis B: a multicenter retrospective study of 2795 patients. *Hepatol Res* 2005; **32**: 173–184.

120 Patheodoridis GV, Dimou E, Dimakopoulos K *et al.* Outcome of hepatitis B e antigen-negative chronic hepatitis B on long-term nucleos(t)ide analog therapy starting with lamivudine. *Hepatology* 2005; **42**: 121–129.

121 Yuen MF, Seto WK, Chow DH *et al.* Long-term lamivudine therapy reduces the risk of long-term complications of chronic hepatitis B infection even in patients without advanced disease. *Antiviral Therap.* 2007; **12**: 1295–1303.

122 Eun JR, Lee HJ, Lee SH, *et al.* The effect of lamivudine and adefovir dipivoxil on preventing hepatocellular carcinoma in hepatitis B virus-related liver cirrhosis. *Hepatology* 2007; **46** (Suppl 1): 664A–665A.

123 Lampertico P, Viganò M, Manenti E, Lavarone M, Sablon E, Colombo M. Low resistance to adefovir combined with lamivudine: a 3-year study of 145 lamivudine-resistant hepatitis B patients. *Gastroenterology* 2007; **133**: 1718–1721.

124 Di Marco V, Marzano A, Lampertico P *et al.* Clinical outcome of HBeAg-negative chronic hepatitis B in relation to virological response to lamivudine. *Hepatology* 2004; **40**: 883–891.

125 Di Marco V, Di Stefano R, Ferraro D *et al.* HBV-DNA suppression and disease course in HBV cirrhosis patients on long-term lamivudine therapy. *Antivir Ther* 2005; **10**: 431–439.

126 Lok AS, Zoulim F, Locarnini S *et al.* Antiviral drug-resistant HBV: standardization of nomenclature and assays and recommendations for management. *Hepatology* 2007; **45**: 507–539.

127 Keeffe EB, Zeuzem S, Koff RS *et al.* Report of an international workshop: roadmap for management of patients receiving oral therapy for chronic hepatitis B. *Clin Gastroenterol Hepatol* 2007; **5**: 890–897.

128 Hadziyannis SJ, Tassopoulos NC, Heathcote EJ *et al.* Long-term therapy with ADV dipivoxil for HBeAg-negative chronic hepatitis B for up to 5 years. *Gastroenterology* 2006; **131**: 1743–1751.

28 Alcoholic liver disease

Hélène Castel and Philippe Mathurin

Department of Hepatology, Hôpital Claude Huriez, Lille, France

Screening

In heavy drinkers, liver-related mortality is mainly attributed to cirrhosis and hepatocellular carcinoma (HCC). Therefore, the main objectives of the screening are: to identify patients with significant liver injury; to characterize the main risk factors for HCC; and to diagnose HCC early.

We focus on the non-invasive screening of cirrhosis and on screening of HCC.

Non-invasive screening of cirrhosis

Assessment of the stage and severity of liver injury requires liver biopsy, an invasive procedure associated with complications leading to death in 0.02% of patients [1]. Less than 30% of heavy drinkers have significant liver injury such as extensive fibrosis, alcoholic hepatitis or cirrhosis [2]. Routine liver biopsy is not essential in 70% of heavy drinkers. The recent development of non-invasive methods for the screening of extensive fibrosis and/or cirrhosis is an important progress to identify the subgroup with significant alcoholic liver disease (ALD) and will avoid screening with liver biopsy.

Initial development of biomarkers of fibrosis

Serum hyaluronate was identified to be useful for the diagnosis of cirrhosis [3–5], with a good AUROC for the diagnosis of significant fibrosis (Metavir class ≥ F2 versus F0–F1).

Prothrombin time (PT) predicts liver fibrosis and is inversely correlated with the area of fibrosis [4, 6]. A study showed that PT has a high diagnostic accuracy for severe fibrosis or cirrhosis, particularly in those with ALD [7].

Evidence-Based Gastroenterology and Hepatology, 3rd edition. J. McDonald, A.K. Burroughs, B. Feagan, and M.B. Fennerty. © 2010 Blackwell Publishing Ltd

Results of the studies evaluating serum procollagen III propeptide (PIIIP) in assessing fibrosis are controversial [4, 8–11]. A major problem, beside the heterogeneity of the assays, is that even with the same assay the PIIIP screening cutoff is unknown.

Apolipoprotein A-I (ApoA-I) has an independent and discriminative value for the diagnosis of fibrosis [12]. A simple index called PGA, developed by combining PT, γ-glutamyl transpeptidase and ApoA-I was efficient for screening of cirrhosis [6].

Serum α-2 macroglobulin has been evaluated as a marker of cirrhosis. Levels were higher in patients with cirrhosis than in patients without [13, 14]. Based on these results, the hypothesis that serum α-2 macroglobulin could improve the accuracy of PGA index for the diagnostic of cirrhosis was confirmed [15].

These studies constitute the background for the development of the new blood tests for screening of fibrosis. As an example, PT, Apo A-1 and serum α-2 macroglobulin have been incorporated in the formula of non-invasive methods such as Fibrotest® and Fibrometer®.

Non-invasive tests to screen for fibrosis

Several new blood tests combining different biomarkers of fibrosis are now available. These tests have been initially designed for patients with hepatitis C but seem to be as efficient in patients with ALD.

Aspartate aminotransferase (AST) to platelet ratio index (APRI) is an accurate non-invasive marker of fibrosis in chronic hepatitis C, and has been evaluated in heavy drinkers. A total of 1308 subjects from two studies of ALD were evaluated, with a liver biopsy available from 781 non-cirrhotic patients and a history of decompensation in 527 [16]. In the 507 patients with biopsy-confirmed fibrosis, the sensitivity of APRI for significant fibrosis was 13.2% and the specificity 77.6%. Twenty percent were misclassified. Thus, APRI has low sensitivity and specificity for the diagnosis of significant fibrosis in patients with ALD. The use of this test to screen fibrosis is not recommended.

Fibrotest® combines alpha-2-macroglobulin, haptoglobin, GGT, ApoA1 and bilirubin, corrected for age and sex. It was designed to predict advanced fibrosis in chronic hepatitis C, and is also known to have high predictive values for the detection of significant fibrosis in ALD [5, 17]. In a study of 221 consecutive patients with biopsy-proven ALT, the mean Fibrotest® value ranged from 0.29 in those without fibrosis to 0.88 in those with cirrhosis. For the diagnosis of cirrhosis, the AUROC was very high at 0.95 [5]. FibrometerA®, combining PT, alpha-2-macroglobulin, hyaluronic acid and age has similar accuracy in ALD [18]. In the validating step, the Fibrometer® AUROC curve was 0.892 in overall patients and 0.962 in patients with ALD. Hepascore® combines bilirubin, GGT, hyaluronic acid, alpha-2-macroglobulin, age and sex. The diagnostic accuracies of Fibrotest®, Fibrometer® and Hepascore® were compared in patients with ALD [19]. The diagnostic values of FibrometerA® and Hepascore® did not differ from that of FibroTest® for advanced fibrosis (AUROCs around 0.80) and cirrhosis (AUROCs around 0.90), and were significantly greater than those of non-patented biomarkers APRI, Forns, FIB4). The combination of any of these tests was useless to improve diagnostic performance.

In addition to their diagnostic performance in the screening of fibrosis, non-invasive tests may be as useful as biopsy to predict liver-related mortality. A recent study compared the prognostic and diagnostic values of these biomarkers in 218 patients with ALD followed up for a median of 8.2 years. Five-year survival was inversely correlated with baseline Fibrotest® value: 98.7% if baseline Fibotest® between 0–0.31, 92.1% if 0.32–0.58 and 68.3% if 0.59–1 [19]. Among the different tests (FibrometerA®, Hepascore®, APRI, Forns, FIB4) Fibrotest® was the only biomarker strongly associated with overall survival in multivariate analysis.

The estimation of fibrosis by measurement of liver stiffness is another alternative to biopsy. In patients with ALD, liver stiffness was correlated with the amount of fibrosis and ranged from 5.7 kPa in patients with Metavir score F1, 8.3 kPa in F2, 17.5 kPa in F3, to 40.9 kPa in F4. The optimal cutoff (kPa) for the screening of cirrhosis was 22.7 kPa with positive predictive value at 0.85 and negative predictive value at 0.82 [20]. A study comparing the diagnostic performance of transient elastography (TE) to those of biopsy and biomarkers in patients with alcohol abuse demonstrated that TE has a good diagnostic performance [21]. Liver stiffness is correlated with fibrosis. A cutoff at 19.5 kPa identifies cirrhosis with a PPV of 68.6% and a NPV of 87.9%. In this cohort, the diagnostic performance of TE was not significantly different than those of Fibrotest® and Fibrometer® but higher than those of APRI and Hepascore®. Thus, TE is a useful tool for the screening for cirrhosis in populations with chronic alcohol abuse, and could identify patients requiring biopsy.

Screening for hepatocellular carcinoma

Chronic alcohol abuse (>50–80 g/day during at least ten years) increases the risk of hepatocellular carcinoma (HCC) by five [22]. This risk does not decrease with abstinence. In alcoholic cirrhosis, the cumulative risk of developing HCC at five years is approximately 8% [23], with a yearly incidence rate of 1% in decompensated alcoholic cirrhosis [22].

Identification of patients at high risk for HCC, and its early detection are of crucial importance. In heavy drinkers, presence of cirrhosis, age >50 years, male sex, serum alpha fetoprotein (AFP) = 15 ng/ml, HBsAg and antiHCV antibodies were independently associated with the occurrence of HCC [24–26]. A clinicobiological score identifies two groups at low (three-year cumulative incidence, 0%) and high risk of HCC (three-year cumulative incidence, 24%) [27]. The pre-neoplastic role of liver large cell dysplasia (LLCD) has been suggested [28]. A study estimated the cumulative incidence of HCC at three years at 38% in patients with LLCD and 10% in patients without [27]; another study found that LLCD was associated with a five-fold increase in the risk of HCC [29]. Nevertheless, in another study, LLCD was not an independent risk factor for HCC [30]. Taken together, these data do not support LLCD to be a direct precursor for HCC, but support its significance as a marker able to predict HCC development. Patients without the lesions are at low risk of HCC [31]. High grade dysplastic nodules are associated with a high risk of malignant transformation and are clearly classified as pre-neoplastic lesions [32]. Based on these results, biopsy would be useful to identify patients with a higher risk for HCC.

Screening for HCC is usually done with ultrasonography and concentration of AFP. Contrasting data have been reported on the effectiveness of ultrasonography for early detection of HCC: a French center observed that diagnosis of tumour less than 3 cm was made in only 21% of cases [33], but other studies detected small HCC in 76% of cases [34, 35]. A recent Markov model assessed that screening by AFP and ultrasonography was cost-effective [36]. In an RCT evaluating screening in hepatitis B versus no screening, the screening strategy decreased the mortality rate by HCC by 37% [37]. Regardless of these data, screening for HCC by biannual AFP testing and ultrasonography is recommended.

Summary of screening in heavy drinkers

At present, non-invasive methods are available and will be helpful to define the best strategy to identify significant fibrosis in heavy drinkers in routine practice. Patented blood biomarkers (Fibrotest®, Fibrometer® and Hepascore®) and TE are simple, non-invasive, cost-effective and reproducible. As observed in HCV patients, the combination of serum biomarker tests and TE need to be tested in patients with ALD for the screening of fibrosis. This practice can select candidates for liver biopsy and at risk of development of portal hypertension and HCC. HCC screening should be done using biannual AFP dosage and ultrasonography, and the presence of high grade dysplasia at biopsy is a strong predictive marker for high risk of malignant transformation. However, future studies are required to validate these screening strategies.

Treatment

In heavy drinkers, pharmacological treatments and liver transplantation (LT) have been tested to improve survival of heavy drinkers with severe liver injury such as severe alcoholic hepatitis (SAH) or cirrhosis. Except for SAH, the usefulness of pharmacological treatments for controlling the alcohol-induced liver injury is still unsettled.

Pharmacological treatments

Anti-fibrotic therapies

Colchicine Colchicine is an anti-fibrotic therapy which has been widely evaluated in the treatment of alcoholic or non-alcoholic fibrosis. In the first RCT evaluating its effect on long-term survival of patients with alcoholic cirrhosis, five and ten-year survival rates were significantly higher in the colchicine group (75% and 56%, respectively) than in the placebo group (34% and 20%, p < 0.001) [38]. Nevertheless, in patients with AH, two other studies did not observe any effect on short-term survival [39, 40]. A recent RCT did not observe any difference between the colchicine and the placebo groups in terms of liver-related mortality: 32% vs 28% [16]. The ineffectiveness of colchicine was confirmed by a meta-analysis combining all the RCTs evaluating colchicine [41]. **A1a**

Propylthiouracil Two RCTs did not document any effect of propylthiouracil on short-term survival [42, 43]. Meta-analysis of these RCTs confirms the lack of benefit on survival, with a mean difference of 1% (CI: 7–9%) between propylthiouracil-treated and controlled patients.

The effect on long-term survival was analyzed in an RCT with 310 alcoholic patients receiving propylthiouracil (n = 157) or placebo (n = 153) for two years [44], which found that two-year mortality was lower in propylthiouracil group than in placebo group (13% versus 26%, p < 0.05). Nevertheless, this study was limited by two biases: the use

of "per protocol analysis" and the cumulative drop-out rates in both groups were approximately 60%.

A systematic review of six RCTs including 710 patients demonstrated no survival benefit of propylthiouracil compared with placebo (odds ratio 0.99) [45]. Moreover, propylthiouracil was associated with a non-signifiacnt trend towards an increased risk of adverse events and serious adverse events (leukopenia). Taking into account these data, propylthiouracil is not considered as an effective therapy in alcoholic cirrhosis. **A1a**

Other drugs D-penicillamine, vitamin E, (+)-cyanidanol-3, thioctic acid, malotilate and amlodipine have been evaluated in RCTs, but none improved survival [46–51]. **A1d**

Silymarin The first RCT suggested an improvement in long-term survival of patients with cirrhosis [52]. However, another larger RCT involving 200 patients did not confirm any effect on survival [53]. **A1d**

S-adenosyl methionine In an RCT, there was a trend toward greater decrease in overall mortality/liver transplantation in S-adenosyl methionine than in placebo patients (16% vs 30%, p = 0.077) [54]. A sensitivity analysis restricted to patients with Child A or B classes observed a significant lower mortality/liver transplantation in S-adenosyl methionine patients (12 vs 29%, p = 0.025). In summary, because of the absence of statistical difference on overall patients, the benefit of S-adenosyl methionine is still unknown and future studies are needed. **A1d**

Phospatidylcholine This has demonstrated a trend towards a decrease in transaminase and bilirubin levels in heavy drinkers, in a trial on alcoholic cirrhosis. Nevertheless, there was no improvement on survival or histology at 24 months [55].

Therapies for acute severe alcoholic hepatitis

Alcoholic hepatitis (AH) occurs in approximately 20% of heavy drinkers. Several investigators have studied SAH intensively, due to its significant early mortality (50–75% in severe forms) [56]. Despite the impact of abstinence on survival in ALD [57–59], pharmacological treatments are required. The treatment of SAH remains controversial and is one of the main challenges in ALD.

Evaluation of any effect on short-term survival requires identification of patients with significant risk of death at one or two months. Until the Maddrey function became available, no reproducible objective criterion existed to predict the risk of early death. Prior to the era of the Maddrey Discriminant Function (DF), survival in untreated control arms ranged from 0% to 81% [56, 60–71]. Maddrey *et al.* described a DF [56] and later modified it [61]. This modified DF identifies patients at high risk of early mortality: 4.6 (PT-control time in seconds) + bilirubin (in mg/dl). In the absence of treatment, the spontaneous survival of patients with a DF ≥ 32 fluctuated between 50% and 65% [61, 72, 73].

Insulin-glucagon infusion [74–76] and nabolic-androgenic steroids [71, 77–79] are not effective in SAH. A systematic review confirmed that anabolic-androgenic steroids did not have any benefit on mortality and were associated with serious adverse events [80]. **A1a** Furthermore, their use is questionable when considering the potential associated risk of HCC.

Corticosteroids

Thirteen RCTs have evaluated corticosteroids in patients with AH [56, 60–71]. These yielded inconsistent results, attributed to the wide differences between studies, since survival of placebo groups ranged from 0% to 81%. The last two RCTs included only patients with either a DF ≥ 32 or spontaneous encephalopathy [60, 61]. Survival in corticosteroid groups was significantly higher than in placebo groups: 94% vs 65% at 28 days (p = 0.006) [61] and 88% vs 45% at 66 days (p = 0.001) [60]. The response to steroids was lower in case of bleeding [81]. The survival benefit of steroids is restricted to short term [82].

A recent meta-analysis using multivariate statistics to adjust for confounding variables between corticosteroid and control groups concluded that corticosteroids are ineffective [83]. Nevertheless, this was problematic in identifying the effect of steroids because of the limited number of trials (n = 12) and the inclusion of lower-quality trials [84]. Moreover, meta-analysis of published results is not designed to identify the effect of treatment in distinct patients [85]. In the particular setting of AH, this method cannot pool the results restricted to patients with DF ≥ 32, as most of the previous RCTs did not supply the survival data on this subgroup.

To conclude this controversy, individual data of the most recent RCTs were combined [72]. The analysis was restricted to patients with a DF ≥ 32. The findings were: (1) at 28 days, corticosteroid patients had significantly better survival than placebo patients: 84.6 ± 3.4% vs 65.1 ± 4.8%, p = 0.001; (2) steroids, age and creatinine were independently associated with survival at 28 days; (3) steroids induced rapid improvement in liver function by seven days of treatment [72]. The final argument for the benefit of corticosteroids is that all the studies observed that two-month survival of patients treated with corticosteroids was approximately 80% [60, 61, 86–89]. **A1a**

To progress in the management of SAH, a criterion for early identification of non-responders to steroids has been proposed [87]. This criterion, "early change in bilirubin levels (ECBL)" is defined as a bilirubin level at seven days lower than these on the first day of treatment [87]. However, the ECBL was highly specific but not sensitive enough for predicting death. A specific prognostic model, the so-called Lille model, was developed to identify subjects early on who are unlikely to survive and propose new management based on this specific model [90]. Patients above the ideal cutoff of 0.45 showed a marked decrease in six-month survival as compared to others: 25 ± 3.8% vs 85 ± 2.5%, p < 0.0001. Using the 0.45 Lille model cutoff, close to 40% of patients do not benefit from corticosteroids, which is higher than the 25% previously identified by ECBL [90]. In non-responders (i.e. 0.45 ≥ Lille model) corticosteroids should be interrupted at day seven. A recent study evaluating a two-step strategy consisting of early withdrawal of corticosteroids and a switch to pentoxifylline for 28 additional days in non-responders observed that non-responders to corticosteroids do not obtain any benefit from an early switch to pentoxifylline. Thus, the issue of management of non-responders remains unsettled.

In summary, even if steroids improve short-term survival in SAH, new treatments are required to improve the probability of being alive within the year following the onset of the disease.

New therapies

Extracorporeal liver support Liver support devices have been developed to provide additional time for liver regeneration and improvement of liver function. Extracorporeal liver support, consisting of a molecular adsorbent recirculating system (MARS), detoxifies blood of protein-bound toxins having a molecular weight <50 kDa and water-soluble substances. In a recent pilot study, eight patients with SAH were treated with MARS [91]. Improvement in bilirubin, creatinine, DF and International Normalized Ratio (INR), and in circulatory disturbances was observed. The efficacy of MARS is still unsettled and requires future studies.

Enteral nutrition Total enteral tube feeding was compared to corticosteroids in a RCT [92], using a low-fat diet with a lipid content constituted of medium-chain triglycerides and oleic acid, considering the deleterious effects of a high-fat diet on ALD in animal models [93–95]. Mortality occurred earlier in the enteral group: 7 days vs 23 days, p = 0.025. During follow-up after the treatment, deaths were observed more frequently in the corticosteroid group (10/27) than in the enteral group (2/24, p = 0.04). **A1d** The same groups recently suggested that combined treatment (enteral nutrition plus corticosteroids) should be investigated in SAH [96].

Pentoxifylline Pentoxifylline, an inhibitor of TNFα synthesis, was evaluated in a double-blind RCT [97]. In this study 101 patients with SAH randomly received pentoxifylline (n = 49) or a placebo (n = 52). The mean DF in the pentoxifylline and placebo groups was 45.9 and 45.3 respectively. Twenty-four percent of pentoxifylline-treated patients and 46.1% of controls (relative risk: 0.57, p = 0.04) died after a mean of 29 and 33.1 days respectively. The survival benefit of pentoxifylline is related to a significant reduction of hepatorenal syndrome [97]. Contrary to corticosteroids, pentoxifylline did not improve liver function. At the end of the treatment, the two groups had similar values of DF, PT and bilirubin levels. During the treatment, there were no differences between the groups in values or decrease of TNFα. **A1d** The development of a new first-line therapy which is more efficient than corticosteroids or pentoxifylline alone is warranted for improving short and medium-term survival. Amongst available options, a combination of these two drugs remains attractive in light of their potential synergistic action. Indeed, in naive patients, corticosteroids improve liver function, whereas the effect of pentoxifylline was thought to be related to prevention of hepatorenal syndrome, but not to improvement in liver function. This combination warrants comparison with corticosteroids alone or pentoxifylline alone in randomized controlled trials.

Anti-TNFα strategy Production of TNFα by inflammatory cells in response to oxidative stress and endotoxin is a critical mediator of ALD. In animal models, anti-TNFα antibodies attenuated liver injury, and lack of TNFα-receptor-1 avoids the development of ALD [98]. The anti-TNFα strategy was tested in two pilot studies and two RCTs [86, 88, 99, 100], evaluating infliximab (chimeric human/mouse antibody), binding with high affinity to TNFα. The first study randomized 20 patients with SAH, treated by prednisolone 40 mg/day for 28 days, to receive infliximab 5 mg/kg IV (n = 10) or placebo (n = 10) [88]. At day 28, DF and IL-8 decreased significantly, contrary to the placebo group [88]. Infliximab was well tolerated, but the sample size did not allow comparison between two groups. Another study tested a single dose of 5 mg/kg without steroids in 12 patients with SAH [100]. Despite the use of norfloxacine, two patients died from infection within three weeks. The levels of IL-6 and IL-8 decreased the day after infliximab administration. At 28 days, bilirubin, DF and C-reactive protein decreased, whereas PT did not change significantly [100]. Bilirubin levels and DF remained stable during 14 days and began to decrease after 21 days [100], suggesting that the effect of infliximab is delayed compared to steroids [87, 100].

To determine its survival impact, an RCT was conducted [86]. However, the first interim analysis was not performed, because of the unbalanced rate of deaths before the planned enrollment of 38 patients [86]. After 36 patients, 7 deaths in the infliximab group and 3 deaths in the steroid group occurred. Two-month survival was lower in the infliximab group than in placebo (61% vs 82%). The frequency of

severe infections increased in the infliximab group compared to placebo. There were no differences in the course of DF [86]. **A1d** Compared to previous studies, the dosage of infliximab varied drastically: a single dose of 5 mg/kg in other studies, three infusions of 10 mg/kg in the French trial. It was felt that high doses were required to inhibit the higher TNFα levels observed in SAH compared to Crohn's disease. This was controversial, because serum TNFα level was not indicative of treatment response [101]. Second, the discrepancies in disease severity between studies may also explain these different results: in the French study, patients with fatal infection had a DF significantly higher than patients without [86].

A recent RCT evaluated etanercept, a soluble extracellular ligand binding portion of the human p75 TNF receptor which binds and neutralizes unbound serum TNFα, in 48 patients with moderate to severe AH (MELD score ≥ 15) randomized to six injections of either etanercept or placebo. The one-month mortality was similar but the six-month mortality was significantly higher in etanercept than in placebo group (57.7% vs 22.7%). Infectious serious adverse events were significantly more frequent with etanercept group than with placebo (34.6% vs 9.1%). Thus, etanercept is not effective for the treatment of SAH. **A1d**

In summary, the anti-TNF approach is associated with an increased risk of infection and does not seem to be effective with the proposed regimens.

Antioxidants The rationale for the use in SAH is that numerous data suggest that oxidative stress is a key mechanism in ALD. Corticosteroids were compared with antioxidants cocktail in an RCT of 101 patients with SAH. At 30 days there were 16 deaths (30%) in the corticosteroid treated group, compared with 22 deaths (46%) in the antioxidant treated group. The odds of dying by 30 days were 2.4 greater for patients on antioxidants (95%; CI: 1.0–5.6) [102]. **A1d** Another study evaluated N-acetylcysteine plus an antioxidant cocktail in patients with SAH, stratified by gender and corticosteroid use, but did not demonstrate any impact of antioxydants [103]. **A1d**

Liver transplantation

Liver transplantation (LT) is an effective option for end-stage liver disease, leading to survival rates similar in alcoholic and non-alcoholic cirrhosis [104–106]. During the past two decades, the percentage of transplantations performed for ALD patients has increased (20% in the USA and 21% in Europe) [107]. Nevertheless, only 6% of patients at risk of dying from alcoholic cirrhosis receive a LT [108].

Alcohol-related cirrhosis and survival benefit from LT

Timing of LT is crucial to avoid harm due to intervening too early, and ineffectiveness from transplanting too late.

In patients with alcoholic cirrhosis, the efficacy of LT has been estimated by comparison with matched and simulated non-transplanted controls [73, 109]. Among Child class C, transplanted patients had higher one and five-year survival than matched controls, whereas among Child class A or B, there was no survival difference between transplanted patients and controls [73, 109].

At the present time, MELD score is used to prioritize patients on a LT waiting list [110–112], and it is recommended to list only patients with a MELD score ≥ 15 [113]. The MELD score has been validated as a useful prognostic score in patients with a broad spectrum of ALD [114–116].

Abstinence and LT for ALD   Long-term studies showed that moderately heavy drinking did not impact graft or patient survival [117–120]. Conversely, the effect of drinking is controversial. Initial studies focusing on short-term survival did not observe any survival difference between recipients who resumed heavy drinking and others [119–121]. However, the duration of the follow-up period is critical in assessing the effect of alcohol relapse on survival. Recent studies focused on long-term survival [122, 123]. Recipients who resumed drinking consistent with levels within the range of alcohol abuse showed significantly lower long-term survival than those who were abstinent or those with minor relapses. Analysis revealed that recurrent ALD was responsible for 90% of deaths in recipients with heavy levels of drinking. In summary, abusive drinking after LT worsens long-term survival [123].

The main source of concern about LT in alcoholic patients is the risk of relapse into alcohol abuse after transplantation. A documented period of abstinence is generally considered as a good prognostic indicator. Most programs require a six-month period of abstinence prior to evaluation for LT [124]. The six-month period of abstinence is presumed: (1) to permit some patients to recover and obviate the need for LT; and (2) to identify patients likely to maintain abstinence. Nevertheless, this criterion alone cannot predict relapse and its use alone forced numerous candidates with low risk of relapse to wait for listing [118, 125–130]. ROC curve analysis of the value of pre-transplantation abstinence revealed it was a relatively poor indicator [128]. For patients with mild alcoholism, less than six months' abstention does not significantly affect the risk of relapse, but may exclude patients at low relapse risk from prompt listing and transplantation [125].

One important aspect is the absence of consensus concerning the definition of alcohol relapse [131–134]. For some centers, all drinking is considered a relapse, whereas others have defined heavy drinking, which is the only relapse associated with liver injury, as relapse.

In conclusion, patients with alcoholic cirrhosis benefit from LT. Most of the centers recommend six-month absti-nence before listing the patients. However, this sole criterion is insufficient to predict abstinence after transplantation.

References

1 Piccinino F, Sagnelli E, Pasquale G, Giusti G. Complications following percutaneous liver biopsy. A multicentre retrospective study on 68,276 biopsies. *J Hepatol* 1986; **2**: 165–173.

2 Bedossa P, Poynard T, Naveau S, Martin ED, Agostini H, Chaput JC. Observer variation in assessment of liver biopsies of alcoholic patients. *Alcohol Clin Exp Res* 1988; **12**: 173–178.

3 Engstrom-Laurent A, Loof L, Nyberg A, Schroder T. Increased serum levels of hyaluronate in liver disease. *Hepatology* 1985; **5**: 638–642.

4 Oberti F, Valsesia E, Pilette C *et al.* Noninvasive diagnosis of hepatic fibrosis or cirrhosis. *Gastroenterology* 1997; **113**: 1609–1616.

5 Naveau S, Raynard B, Ratziu V *et al.* Biomarkers for the prediction of liver fibrosis in patients with chronic alcoholic liver disease. *Clin Gastroenterol Hepatol* 2005; **3**: 167–174.

6 Poynard T, Aubert A, Bedossa P *et al.* A simple biological index for detection of alcoholic liver disease in drinkers. *Gastroenterology* 1991; **100**: 1397–1402.

7 Croquet V, Vuillemin E, Ternisien C *et al.* Prothrombin index is an indirect marker of severe liver fibrosis. *Eur J Gastroenterol Hepatol* 2002; **14**: 1133–1141.

8 Torres-Salinas M, Pares A, Caballeria J *et al.* Serum procollagen type III peptide as a marker of hepatic fibrogenesis in alcoholic hepatitis. *Gastroenterology* 1986; **90**: 1241–1246.

9 Niemela O, Risteli L, Sotaniemi EA, Risteli J. Aminoterminal propeptide of type III procollagen in serum in alcoholic liver disease. *Gastroenterology* 1983; **85**: 254–259.

10 Annoni G, Colombo M, Cantaluppi MC, Khlat B, Lampertico P, Rojkind M. Serum type III procollagen peptide and laminin (Lam-P1) detect alcoholic hepatitis in chronic alcohol abusers. *Hepatology* 1989; **9**: 693–697.

11 Teare JP, Sherman D, Greenfield SM *et al.* Comparison of serum procollagen III peptide concentrations and PGA index for assessment of hepatic fibrosis. *Lancet* 1993; **342**: 895–898.

12 Poynard T, Abella A, Pignon JP, Naveau S, Leluc R, Chaput JC. Apolipoprotein AI and alcoholic liver disease. *Hepatology* 1986; **6**: 1391–1395.

13 Nalpas B, Boigné JM, Zafrani ES, Zimmermann R, Berthelot P. [Abnormalities of ten plasma proteins in alcoholic liver disease (author's transl)]. *Gastroenterol Clin Biol* 1980; **4**: 646–654.

14 Murray-Lyon IM, Clarke HG, McPherson K, Williams R. Quantitative immunoelectrophoresis of serum proteins in cryptogenic cirrhosis, alcoholic cirrhosis and active chronic hepatitis. *Clin Chim Acta* 1972; **39**: 215–220.

15 Naveau S, Poynard T, Benattar C, Bedossa P, Chaput JC. Alpha-2-macroglobulin and hepatic fibrosis. Diagnostic interest. *Dig Dis Sci* 1994; **39**: 2426–2432.

16 Morgan TR, Weiss DG, Nemchausky B *et al.* Colchicine treatment of alcoholic cirrhosis: a randomized, placebo-controlled clinical trial of patient survival. *Gastroenterology* 2005; **128**: 882–890.

17 Thabut D, Naveau S, Charlotte F *et al.* The diagnostic value of biomarkers (AshTest) for the prediction of alcoholic steatohepatitis in patients with chronic alcoholic liver disease. *J Hepatol* 2006; **44**: 1175–1185.

18 Cales P, Oberti F, Michalak S *et al.* A novel panel of blood markers to assess the degree of liver fibrosis. *Hepatology* 2005; **42**: 1373–1381.

19 Naveau S, Gaude, G, Asnacios A *et al.* Diagnostic and prognostic values of noninvasive biomarkers of fibrosis in patients with alcoholic liver disease. *Hepatology* 2009; **49**: 97.

20 Nahon PKA, Tengher-Barna J, Ziol M *et al.* Assessment of liver fibrosis using transient elastography in patients with alcoholic liver disease. *J Hepatol* 2008; **49**: 1062–1068.

21 Nguyen-Khac E, Chatelain D, Tramier B *et al.* Assessment of asymptomatic liver fibrosis in alcoholic patients using fibroscan: prospective comparison with seven non-invasive laboratory tests. *Aliment Pharmacol Ther* 2008; **28**: 1188–1198.

22 Morgan TR, Mandayam S, Jamal MM. Alcohol and hepatocellular carcinoma. *Gastroenterology* 2004; **127**: S87–96.

23 Fattovich G, Stroffolini T, Zagni I, Donato F. Hepatocellular carcinoma in cirrhosis: incidence and risk factors. *Gastroenterology* 2004; **127**: S35–50.

24 Bruix J, Barrera JM, Calvet X *et al.* Prevalence of antibodies to hepatitis C virus in Spanish patients with hepatocellular carcinoma and hepatic cirrhosis. *Lancet* 1989; **2**: 1004–1006.

25 Di Bisceglie AM, Rustgi VK, Hoofnagle JH, Dusheiko GM, Lotze MT. NIH conference. Hepatocellular carcinoma. *Ann Intern Med* 1988; **108**: 390–401.

26 Poynard T, Aubert A, Lazizi Y *et al.* Independent risk factors for hepatocellular carcinoma in French drinkers. *Hepatology* 1991; **13**: 896–901.

27 Ganne-Carrie N, Chastang C, Chapel F *et al.* Predictive score for the development of hepatocellular carcinoma and additional value of liver large cell dysplasia in Western patients with cirrhosis. *Hepatology* 1996; **23**: 1112–1118.

28 Anthony PP, Vogel CL, Barker LF. Liver cell dysplasia: a premalignant condition. *J Clin Pathol* 1973; **26**: 217–223.

29 Borzio M, Bruno S, Roncalli M *et al.* Liver cell dysplasia is a major risk factor for hepatocellular carcinoma in cirrhosis: a prospective study. *Gastroenterology* 1995; **108**: 812–817.

30 Donato MF, Arosio E, Del Ninno E *et al.* High rates of hepatocellular carcinoma in cirrhotic patients with high liver cell proliferative activity. *Hepatology* 2001; **34**: 523–528.

31 Park YN, Roncalli M. Large liver cell dysplasia: a controversial entity. *J Hepatol* 2006; **45**: 734–743.

32 Libbrecht L, Desmet V, Roskams T. Preneoplastic lesions in human hepatocarcinogenesis. *Liver Int* 2005; **25**: 16–27.

33 Pateron D, Ganne N, Trinchet JC *et al.* Prospective study of screening for hepatocellular carcinoma in Caucasian patients with cirrhosis. *J Hepatol* 1994; **20**: 65–71.

34 Zoli M, Magalotti D, Bianchi G, Gueli C, Marchesini G, Pisi E. Efficacy of a surveillance program for early detection of hepatocellular carcinoma. *Cancer* 1996; **78**: 977–985.

35 Cottone M, Turri M, Caltagirone M *et al.* Screening for hepatocellular carcinoma in patients with Child's A cirrhosis: an 8-year prospective study by ultrasound and alphafetoprotein. *J Hepatol* 1994; **21**: 1029–1034.

36 Patel D, Terrault NA, Yao FY, Bass NM, Ladabaum U. Cost-effectiveness of hepatocellular carcinoma surveillance in patients with hepatitis C virus-related cirrhosis. *Clin Gastroenterol Hepatol* 2005; **3**: 75–84.

37 Zhang BH, Yang BH, Tang ZY. Randomized controlled trial of screening for hepatocellular carcinoma. *J Cancer Res Clin Oncol* 2004; **130**: 417–422.

38 Kershenobich D, Vargas F, Garcia-Tsao G, Perez Tamayo R, Gent M, Rojkind M. Colchicine in the treatment of cirrhosis of the liver. *N Engl J Med* 1988; **318**: 1709–1713.

39 Trinchet JC, Beaugrand M, Callard P *et al.* Treatment of alcoholic hepatitis with colchicine. Results of a randomized double blind trial. *Gastroenterol Clin Biol* 1989; **13**: 551–555.

40 Akriviadis EA, Steindel H, Pinto PC *et al.* Failure of colchicine to improve short-term survival in patients with alcoholic hepatitis. *Gastroenterology* 1990; **99**: 811–818.

41 Rambaldi A, Gluud C. Colchicine for alcoholic and non-alcoholic liver fibrosis and cirrhosis. *Cochrane Database Syst Rev* 2005: CD002148.

42 Halle P, Pare P, Kaptein E, Kanel G, Redeker AG, Reynolds TB. Double-blind, controlled trial of propylthiouracil in patients with severe acute alcoholic hepatitis. *Gastroenterology* 1982; **82**: 925–931.

43 Orrego H, Kalant H, Israel Y *et al.* Effect of short-term therapy with propylthiouracil in patients with alcoholic liver disease. *Gastroenterology* 1979; **76**: 105–115.

44 Orrego H, Blake JE, Blendis LM, Compton KV, Israel Y. Long-term treatment of alcoholic liver disease with propylthiouracil. *N Engl J Med* 1987; **317**: 1421–1427.

45 Rambaldi A, Gluud C. Propylthiouracil for alcoholic liver disease. *Cochrane Database Syst Rev* 2002: CD002800.

46 Bird GL, Prach AT, McMahon AD, Forrest JA, Mills PR, Danesh BJ. Randomised controlled double-blind trial of the calcium channel antagonist amlodipine in the treatment of acute alcoholic hepatitis. *J Hepatol* 1998; **28**: 194–198.

47 Resnick RH, Boitnott J, Iber FL, Makopour H, Cerda JJ. Preliminary observations of d-penicillamine therapy in acute alcoholic liver disease. *Digestion* 1974; **11**: 257–265.

48 de la Maza MP, Petermann M, Bunout D, Hirsch S. Effects of long-term vitamin E supplementation in alcoholic cirrhotics. *J Am Coll Nutr* 1995; **14**: 192–196.

49 Colman JC, Morgan MY, Scheuer PJ, Sherlock S. Treatment of alcohol-related liver disease with (+)-cyanidanol-3: a randomised double-blind trial. *Gut* 1980; **21**: 965–969.

50 Marshall AW, Graul RS, Morgan MY, Sherlock S. Treatment of alcohol-related liver disease with thioctic acid: a six month randomised double-blind trial. *Gut* 1982; **23**: 1088–1093.

51 Keiding S, Badsberg JH, Becker U *et al.* The prognosis of patients with alcoholic liver disease. An international randomized, placebo-controlled trial on the effect of malotilate on survival. *J Hepatol* 1994; **20**: 454–460.

52 Ferenci P, Dragosics B, Dittrich H *et al.* Randomized controlled trial of silymarin treatment in patients with cirrhosis of the liver. *J Hepatol* 1989; **9**: 105–113.

53 Pares A, Planas R, Torres M *et al.* Effects of silymarin in alcoholic patients with cirrhosis of the liver: results of a controlled, double-blind, randomized and multicenter trial. *J Hepatol* 1998; **28**: 615–621.

54 Mato JM, Fernandez de Paz J, Calliera L *et al.* S-adenosylmethionine in alcoholic liver cirrhosis: a randomized,

placebo-controlled, double-blind, multicenter clinical trial. *J Hepatol* 1999; **30**: 1081–1089.

55 Day CP. Treatment of alcoholic liver disease. *Liver Transpl* 2007; **13**: S69–75.

56 Maddrey WC, Boitnott JK, Bedine MS, Weber FL, Jr, Mezey E, White RI, Jr. Corticosteroid therapy of alcoholic hepatitis. *Gastroenterology* 1978; **75**: 193–199.

57 Powell WJ, Jr, Klatskin G. Duration of survival in patients with Laennec's cirrhosis. Influence of alcohol withdrawal, and possible effects of recent changes in general management of the disease. *Am J Med* 1968; **44**: 406–420.

58 Pares A, Caballeria J, Bruguera M, Torres M, Rodes J. Histological course of alcoholic hepatitis. Influence of abstinence, sex and extent of hepatic damage. *J Hepatol* 1986; **2**: 33–42.

59 Pande NV, Resnick RH, Yee W, Eckardt VF, Shurberg JL. Cirrhotic portal hypertension: morbidity of continued alcoholism. *Gastroenterology* 1978; **74**: 64–69.

60 Ramond MJ, Poynard T, Rueff B *et al.* A randomized trial of prednisolone in patients with severe alcoholic hepatitis. *N Engl J Med* 1992; **326**: 507–512.

61 Carithers RL, Jr, Herlong HF, Diehl AM *et al.* Methylprednisolone therapy in patients with severe alcoholic hepatitis. A randomized multicenter trial. *Ann Intern Med* 1989; **110**: 685–690.

62 Helman RA, Temko MH, Nye SW, Fallon HJ. Alcoholic hepatitis. Natural history and evaluation of prednisolone therapy. *Ann Intern Med* 1971; **74**: 311–321.

63 Porter HP, Simon FR, Pope CE, 2nd, Volwiler W, Fenster LF. Corticosteroid therapy in severe alcoholic hepatitis. A double-blind drug trial. *N Engl J Med* 1971; **284**: 1350–1355.

64 Campra JL, Hamlin EM, Jr, Kirshbaum RJ, Olivier M, Redeker AG, Reynolds TB. Prednisone therapy of acute alcoholic hepatitis. Report of a controlled trial. *Ann Intern Med* 1973; **79**: 625–631.

65 Blitzer BL, Mutchnick MG, Joshi PH, Phillips MM, Fessel JM, Conn HO. Adrenocorticosteroid therapy in alcoholic hepatitis. A prospective, double-blind randomized study. *Am J Dig Dis* 1977; **22**: 477–484.

66 Lesesne HR, Bozymski EM, Fallon HJ. Treatment of alcoholic hepatitis with encephalopathy. Comparison of prednisolone with caloric supplements. *Gastroenterology* 1978; **74**: 169–173.

67 Shumaker JB, Resnick RH, Galambos JT, Makopour H, Iber FL. A controlled trial of 6-methylprednisolone in acute alcoholic hepatitis. With a note on published results in encephalopathic patients. *Am J Gastroenterol* 1978; **69**: 443–449.

68 Theodossi A, Eddleston AL, Williams R. Controlled trial of methylprednisolone therapy in severe acute alcoholic hepatitis. *Gut* 1982; **23**: 75–79.

69 Depew W, Boyer T, Omata M, Redeker A, Reynolds T. Double-blind controlled trial of prednisolone therapy in patients with severe acute alcoholic hepatitis and spontaneous encephalopathy. *Gastroenterology* 1980; **78**: 524–529.

70 Bories P, Guedj JY, Mirouze D, Yousfi A, Michel H. Treatment of acute alcoholic hepatitis with prednisolone. 45 patients. *Presse Med* 1987; **16**: 769–772.

71 Mendenhall CL, Anderson S, Garcia-Pont P *et al.* Short-term and long-term survival in patients with alcoholic hepatitis treated with oxandrolone and prednisolone. *N Engl J Med* 1984; **311**: 1464–1470.

72 Mathurin P, Mendenhall CL, Carithers RL, Jr *et al.* Corticosteroids improve short-term survival in patients with severe alcoholic hepatitis (AH): individual data analysis of the last three randomized placebo controlled double blind trials of corticosteroids in severe AH. *J Hepatol* 2002; **36**: 480–487.

73 Poynard T, Barthelemy P, Fratte S *et al.* Evaluation of efficacy of liver transplantation in alcoholic cirrhosis by a case-control study and simulated controls. *Lancet* 1994; **344**: 502–507.

74 Feher J, Cornides A, Romany A, Karteszi M, Szalay L, Gogl A, Picazo J. A prospective multicenter study of insulin and glucagon infusion therapy in acute alcoholic hepatitis. *J Hepatol* 1987; **5**: 224–231.

75 Bird G, Lau JY, Koskinas J, Wicks C, Williams R. Insulin and glucagon infusion in acute alcoholic hepatitis: a prospective randomized controlled trial. *Hepatology* 1991; **14**: 1097–1101.

76 Trinchet JC, Balkau B, Poupon RE *et al.* Treatment of severe alcoholic hepatitis by infusion of insulin and glucagon: a multicenter sequential trial. *Hepatology* 1992; **15**: 76–81.

77 Islam N, Islam A. Testosterone propionate in cirrhosis of the liver. *Br J Clin Pract* 1973; **27**: 125–128.

78 Mendenhall CL, Moritz TE, Roselle GA *et al.* A study of oral nutritional support with oxandrolone in malnourished patients with alcoholic hepatitis: results of a Department of Veterans Affairs cooperative study. *Hepatology* 1993; **17**: 564–576.

79 Wells R. Prednisolone and testosterone propionate in cirrhosis of the liver. A controlled trial. *Lancet* 1960; **2**: 1416–1419.

80 Rambaldi A, Iaquinto G, Gluud C. Anabolic-androgenic steroids for alcoholic liver disease: a Cochrane review. *Am J Gastroenterol* 2002; **97**: 1674–1681.

81 Imperiale TF, McCullough AJ. Do corticosteroids reduce mortality from alcoholic hepatitis? A meta-analysis of the randomized trials. *Ann Intern Med* 1990; **113**: 299–307.

82 Mathurin P, Duchatelle V, Ramond MJ *et al.* Survival and prognostic factors in patients with severe alcoholic hepatitis treated with prednisolone. *Gastroenterology* 1996; **110**: 1847–1853.

83 Christensen E, Gluud C. Glucocorticoids are ineffective in alcoholic hepatitis: a meta-analysis adjusting for confounding variables. *Gut* 1995; **37**: 113–118.

84 Imperiale TF, O'Connor JB, McCullough AJ. Corticosteroids are effective in patients with severe alcoholic hepatitis. *Am J Gastroenterol* 1999; **94**: 3066–3068.

85 Imperiale TF. Meta-analysis: when and how. *Hepatology* 1999; **29**: 26S–31S.

86 Naveau S, Chollet-Martin S, Dharancy S *et al.* A double-blind randomized controlled trial of infliximab associated with prednisolone in acute alcoholic hepatitis. *Hepatology* 2004; **39**: 1390–1397.

87 Mathurin P, Abdelnour M, Ramond MJ *et al.* Early change in bilirubin levels is an important prognostic factor in severe alcoholic hepatitis treated with prednisolone. *Hepatology* 2003; **38**: 1363–1369.

88 Spahr L, Rubbia-Brandt L, Frossard JL *et al.* Combination of steroids with infliximab or placebo in severe alcoholic hepatitis: a randomized controlled pilot study. *J Hepatol* 2002; **37**: 448–455.

89 Duvoux C, Radier C, Roudot-Thoraval F *et al.* Low-grade steatosis and major changes in portal flow as new prognostic factors in steroid-treated alcoholic hepatitis. *Hepatology* 2004; **40**: 1370–1378.

90 Louvet A, Naveau S, Abdelnour M *et al.* The Lille model: a new tool for therapeutic strategy in patients with severe alcoholic hepatitis treated with steroids. *Hepatology* 2007; **45**: 1348–1354.

91 Jalan R, Sen S, Steiner C, Kapoor D, Alisa A, Williams R. Extracorporeal liver support with molecular adsorbents recirculating system in patients with severe acute alcoholic hepatitis. *J Hepatol* 2003; **38**: 24–31.

92 Cabre E, Rodriguez-Iglesias P, Caballeria J *et al.* Short- and long-term outcome of severe alcohol-induced hepatitis treated with steroids or enteral nutrition: a multicenter randomized trial. *Hepatology* 2000; **32**: 36–42.

93 Tsukamoto H, French SW, Benson N *et al.* Severe and progressive steatosis and focal necrosis in rat liver induced by continuous intragastric infusion of ethanol and low fat diet. *Hepatology* 1985; **5**: 224–232.

94 Tsukamoto H, Towner SJ, Ciofalo LM, French SW. Ethanol-induced liver fibrosis in rats fed high fat diet. *Hepatology* 1986; **6**: 814–822.

95 Tsukamoto H, Cheng S, Blaner WS. Effects of dietary polyunsaturated fat on ethanol-induced Ito cell activation. *Am J Physiol* 1996; **270**: G581–586.

96 Alvarez MA, Cabre E, Lorenzo-Zuniga V, Montoliu S, Planas R, Gassull MA. Combining steroids with enteral nutrition: a better therapeutic strategy for severe alcoholic hepatitis? Results of a pilot study. *Eur J Gastroenterol Hepatol* 2004; **16**: 1375–1380.

97 Akriviadis E, Botla R, Briggs W, Han S, Reynolds T, Shakil O. Pentoxifylline improves short-term survival in severe acute alcoholic hepatitis: a double-blind, placebo-controlled trial. *Gastroenterology* 2000; **119**: 1637–1648.

98 Yin M, Wheeler MD, Kono H *et al.* Essential role of tumor necrosis factor alpha in alcohol-induced liver injury in mice. *Gastroenterology* 1999; **117**: 942–952.

99 Mookerjee RP, Sen S, Davies NA, Hodges SJ, Williams R, Jalan R. Tumour necrosis factor alpha is an important mediator of portal and systemic haemodynamic derangements in alcoholic hepatitis. *Gut* 2003; **52**: 1182–1187.

100 Tilg H, Jalan R, Kaser A *et al.* Anti-tumor necrosis factor-alpha monoclonal antibody therapy in severe alcoholic hepatitis. *J Hepatol* 2003; **38**: 419–425.

101 Blendis L, Dotan I. Anti-TNF therapy for severe acute alcoholic hepatitis: what went wrong? *Gastroenterology* 2004; **127**: 1637–1639.

102 Phillips M, Curtis H, Portmann B, Donaldson N, Bomford A, O'Grady J. Antioxidants versus corticosteroids in the treatment of severe alcoholic hepatitis – a randomised clinical trial. *J Hepatol* 2006; **44**: 784–790.

103 Stewart S, Prince M, Bassendine M *et al.* A randomized trial of antioxidant therapy alone or with corticosteroids in acute alcoholic hepatitis. *J Hepatol* 2007; **47**: 277–283.

104 Stefanini GF, Biselli M, Grazi GL *et al.* Orthotopic liver transplantation for alcoholic liver disease: rates of survival, complications and relapse. *Hepatogastroenterology* 1997; **44**: 1356–1359.

105 Starzl TE, Van Thiel D, Tzakis AG *et al.* Orthotopic liver transplantation for alcoholic cirrhosis. *JAMA* 1988; **260**: 2542–2544.

106 Lucey MR, Merion RM, Henley KS *et al.* Selection for and outcome of liver transplantation in alcoholic liver disease. *Gastroenterology* 1992; **102**: 1736–1741.

107 Burroughs AK, Sabin CA, Rolles K *et al.* Three-month and 12-month mortality after first liver transplant in adults in Europe: predictive models for outcome. *Lancet* 2006; **367**: 225–232.

108 Watt KD, McCashland TM. Transplantation in the alcoholic patient. *Semin Liver Dis* 2004; **24**: 249–255.

109 Poynard T, Naveau S, Doffoel M *et al.* Evaluation of efficacy of liver transplantation in alcoholic cirrhosis using matched and simulated controls: 5-year survival. Multi-centre group. *J Hepatol* 1999; **30**: 1130–1137.

110 Kamath PS, Wiesner RH, Malinchoc M *et al.* A model to predict survival in patients with end-stage liver disease. *Hepatology* 2001; **33**: 464–470.

111 Merion RM, Schaubel DE, Dykstra DM, Freeman RB, Port FK, Wolfe RA. The survival benefit of liver transplantation. *Am J Transplant* 2005; **5**: 307–313.

112 Wiesner R, Edwards E, Freeman R *et al.* Model for end-stage liver disease (MELD) and allocation of donor livers. *Gastroenterology* 2003; **124**: 91–96.

113 Olthoff KM, Brown RS, Jr, Delmonico FL *et al.* Summary report of a national conference: Evolving concepts in liver allocation in the MELD and PELD era. 8 December 2003, Washington, DC. *Liver Transpl* 2004; **10**: A6–22.

114 Srikureja W, Kyulo NL, Runyon BA, Hu KQ. MELD score is a better prognostic model than Child-Turcotte-Pugh score or Discriminant Function score in patients with alcoholic hepatitis. *J Hepatol* 2005; **42**: 700–706.

115 Dunn W, Jamil LH, Brown LS *et al.* MELD accurately predicts mortality in patients with alcoholic hepatitis. *Hepatology* 2005; **41**: 353–358.

116 Said A, Williams J, Holden J *et al.* Model for end stage liver disease score predicts mortality across a broad spectrum of liver disease. *J Hepatol* 2004; **40**: 897–903.

117 DiMartini A, Day N, Dew MA *et al.* Alcohol consumption patterns and predictors of use following liver transplantation for alcoholic liver disease. *Liver Transpl* 2006; **12**: 813–820.

118 Bravata DM, Olkin I, Barnato AE, Keeffe EB, Owens DK. Employment and alcohol use after liver transplantation for alcoholic and nonalcoholic liver disease: a systematic review. *Liver Transpl* 2001; **7**: 191–203.

119 Pageaux GP, Bismuth M, Perney P *et al.* Alcohol relapse after liver transplantation for alcoholic liver disease: does it matter? *J Hepatol* 2003; **38**: 629–634.

120 Pageaux GP, Michel J, Coste V *et al.* Alcoholic cirrhosis is a good indication for liver transplantation, even for cases of recidivism. *Gut* 1999; **45**: 421–426.

121 Lucey MR, Carr K, Beresford TP *et al.* Alcohol use after liver transplantation in alcoholics: a clinical cohort follow-up study. *Hepatology* 1997; **25**: 1223–1227.

122 Cuadrado A, Fabrega E, Casafont F, Pons-Romero F. Alcohol recidivism impairs long-term patient survival after orthotopic liver transplantation for alcoholic liver disease. *Liver Transpl* 2005; **11**: 420–426.

123 Pfitzmann R, Schwenzer J, Rayes N, Seehofer D, Neuhaus R, Nussler NC. Long-term survival and predictors of relapse after orthotopic liver transplantation for alcoholic liver disease. *Liver Transpl* 2007; **13**: 197–205.

124 Snyder SL, Drooker M, Strain JJ. A survey estimate of academic liver transplant teams' selection practices for alcohol-dependent applicants. *Psychosomatics* 1996; **37**: 432–437.

125 Yates WR, Martin M, LaBrecque D, Hillebrand D, Voigt M, Pfab D. A model to examine the validity of the 6-month abstinence criterion for liver transplantation. *Alcohol Clin Exp Res* 1998; **22**: 513–517.

126 Miguet M, Monnet E, Vanlemmens C *et al.* Predictive factors of alcohol relapse after orthotopic liver transplantation for alcoholic liver disease. *Gastroenterol Clin Biol* 2004; **28**: 845–851.

127 Bird GL, O'Grady JG, Harvey FA, Calne RY, Williams R. Liver transplantation in patients with alcoholic cirrhosis: selection criteria and rates of survival and relapse. *BMJ* 1990; **301**: 15–17.

128 Foster PF, Fabrega F, Karademir S, Sankary HN, Mital D, Williams JW. Prediction of abstinence from ethanol in alcoholic recipients following liver transplantation. *Hepatology* 1997; **25**: 1469–1477.

129 Kumar S, Stauber RE, Gavaler JS *et al.* Orthotopic liver transplantation for alcoholic liver disease. *Hepatology* 1990; **11**: 159–164.

130 Osorio RW, Ascher NL, Avery M, Bacchetti P, Roberts JP, Lake JR. Predicting recidivism after orthotopic liver transplantation for alcoholic liver disease. *Hepatology* 1994; **20**: 105–110.

131 Lucey MR. How will patients be selected for transplantation in the future? *Liver Transpl* 2004; **10**: S90–92.

132 Lucey MR. Liver transplantation for alcoholic liver disease: past, present, and future. *Liver Transpl* 2007; **13**: 190–192.

133 Tang H, Boulton R, Gunson B, Hubscher S, Neuberger J. Patterns of alcohol consumption after liver transplantation. *Gut* 1998; **43**: 140–145.

134 Tome S, Lucey MR. Timing of liver transplantation in alcoholic cirrhosis. *J Hepatol* 2003; **39**: 302–307.

29 Non-alcoholic fatty liver disease

Christopher P Day

Institute of Cellular Medicine, Newcastle University, Newcastle Upon Tyne, UK

Introduction

Non-alcoholic fatty liver disease (NAFLD) is increasingly diagnosed worldwide and considered to be the commonest liver disorder in Western countries. It comprises a disease spectrum ranging from simple steatosis (fatty liver), through non-alcoholic steatohepatitis (NASH) to fat with fibrosis and ultimately cirrhosis. Simple steatosis is largely benign and non-progressive, whereas NASH, characterized by hepatocyte injury, inflammation and fibrosis can lead to cirrhosis, liver failure and hepatocellular carcinoma (HCC). NAFLD is strongly associated with obesity, insulin resistance, hypertension and dyslipidemia and is now regarded as the liver manifestation of the metabolic syndrome. Rapid spread of the obesity "pandemic" in adults and children, coupled with the realization that the outcomes of obesity-related liver disease are not entirely benign, has led to rapid growth in clinical and basic studies in NAFLD over the past decade.

Epidemiology

NAFLD is often an asymptomatic illness in which the liver blood tests may be completely normal. This has made studies on prevalence extremely difficult, with most relying on ultrasound, which is known to be sensitive only when more than one-third of the liver is affected by steatosis. With this proviso the prevalence of NAFLD appears to be around 20–30% in Western adults [1, 2], and 15% in Asians [3]. Due to the lack of prospective studies, the true inci-dence of NAFLD is not well defined, although from the information available, it appears to be low [4]. Since liver biopsy is the only method of accurately diagnosing steato-hepatitis, incidence/prevalence studies of NASH are rare. According to available data, NASH is much rarer than NAFLD, affecting 2–3% of the general population [5]. NAFLD and NASH are strongly associated with the presence and severity of obesity. Studies in severely obese patients (BMI > 35 kg/m^2) undergoing bariatric surgery have reported prevalences of NAFLD and NASH of 91% and 37% respectively [6], while a large post-mortem study reported NASH to be present in 3% of non-obese, 19% of obese and 50% of a morbidly obese individuals [7]. A recent novel observational study in NAFLD patients has demonstrated that while central obesity correlates with the severity of inflammation, dorsocervical lipohypertrophy correlates with hepatocyte injury, inflammation and fibro-sis [8]. Type 2 diabetes mellitus (T2DM) is the other major association of NAFLD, with a prevalence of 70% recently reported from an ultrasound survey of almost 3000 unse-lected Italian T2DM patients [9, 10]. Even in the absence of obesity and T2DM, NAFLD is closely associated with other features of the metabolic syndrome, with one study of non-diabetics with NAFLD reporting that 18% of normal weight patients and 67% of obese fulfilled criteria for the metabolic syndrome [11].

There are no accurate data regarding temporal changes in the prevalence of NAFLD; however, the rising preva-lence of obesity, diabetes and the metabolic syndrome seems likely to be reflected in an increasing prevalence of NAFLD. This trend is of particular concern in the paediat-ric population where the reported increase in obesity will undoubtedly result in a higher incidence and prevalence of paediatric and adult NAFLD in the future. To date, studies in children have reported a prevalence of NAFLD of 3% in the general paediatric population and 53% in obese chil-dren [12, 13]. Reports of toddlers with NAFLD and primary school children with NAFLD- related cirrhosis are clearly a cause for alarm [14].

Evidence-Based Gastroenterology and Hepatology, 3rd edition.
J. McDonald, A.K. Burroughs, B. Feagan, and M.B. Fennerty. © 2010
Blackwell Publishing Ltd

Natural history of NAFLD

In marked contrast to alcoholic steatohepatitis, the short-term prognosis of NAFLD is good. The largest prospective histological study of the natural history of NAFLD, with a mean follow-up of 13 years, has recently been published [15]. Data from this and other studies suggest that the long-term hepatic prognosis of patients with NAFLD depends on the histological stage of disease at presentation [16]. Among patients with simple steatosis 12–40% will develop NASH with early fibrosis after 8–13 years. For patients presenting with NASH and early fibrosis, around 15% will develop cirrhosis and/or evidence of hepatic decompensation over the same time-period, increasing to 25% of patients with advanced pre-cirrhotic fibrosis at baseline. In the most recent study, weight gain and the presence of portal tract fibrosis on index biopsy were the only significant predictors of fibrosis progression [15]. About 7% of subjects with compensated cirrhosis associated with NAFLD will develop a hepatocellular carcinoma (HCC) within ten years, while 50% will require a transplant or die from a liver-related cause [17]. The risk of HCC in NAFLD-related cirrhosis is comparable to that in cirrhosis associated with alcohol or hepatitis C [18]. This may partly explain the recently reported associations of HCC with high BMI and T2DM [19]. Liver transplantation is increasingly available to those with chronic liver failure and about 10–12% of liver transplants in the USA are for NAFLD cirrhosis [20]. Unfortunately the condition can recur in transplanted organs. The overall and liver-related mortality of patients with NAFLD is higher than in an age and sex-matched population, with adjusted hazard ratios of 1.038 and 9.32 respectively [21, 22].

Susceptibility

While the vast majority of individuals with obesity, insulin resistance and the metabolic syndrome will have steatosis, only a minority will ever develop steatohepatitis, fibrosis and cirrhosis. Potential environmental determinants of NAFLD are dietary factors and small bowel bacterial overgrowth [23, 24]. Recent studies have shown that diets high in saturated fat, fructose-containing soft drinks and meat, and low in antioxidants and omega-3 containing fish are associated with an increased risk of NAFLD/NASH [25, 26, 27]. With respect to alcohol intake, while there is no doubt that obesity increases risk of cirrhosis in heavy drinkers [28], emerging evidence suggests that "sensible" light alcohol intake may be protective versus NAFLD/NASH [29, 30], an effect that appears likely to be due to the beneficial effect of light alcohol intake on insulin sensitiv-

ity. Family studies and inter-ethnic variations in susceptibility suggest that genetic factors may be important in determining disease risk. Thus far, only one genetic association with advanced NAFLD has been replicated in an independent population – an association between a functional polymorphism in the gene encoding the tumor suppressor gene Kruppel-like factor 6 and fibrosis [31]. More recently the first genome-wide association study has been performed in patients with proton magnetic resonance spectroscopy (^{1}H-MRS) diagnosed NAFLD and found an association between hepatic fat content and genetic variation in the *PNPLA3* gene encoding a protein involved in lipid metabolism [32].

Disease associations with NAFLD

Cardiovascular disease

Given the close association between NAFLD and classical cardiovascular risk factors it is perhaps not surprising that, when compared to controls, patients with NAFLD have a higher prevalence of atherosclerosis, as shown by increased carotid wall intimal thickness, increased numbers of atherorosclerotic plaques and increased plasma markers of endothelial dysfunction [9, 33, 34]. This association also extends to children, with the prevalence of coronary and aortic atheroma higher in children with fatty liver compared to controls in an autopsy based report [35]. Consistent with these observations three natural history studies have reported that the increased age-related mortality observed in patients with NAFLD is attributable to cardiovascular as well as liver-related deaths [15, 17, 22]. Although an indirect association between NAFLD and cardiovascular disease is expected, a growing body of evidence supports a direct role for NAFLD in the pathogenesis of atheromatous cardiovascular disease. A recent study of unselected patients with T2DM reported that the prevalence of cardiovascular, cerebrovascular and peripheral vascular disease was significantly greater in those with NAFLD than in those without, independent of the individual components of the metabolic syndrome [10]. A similar finding has been observed for microvascular diseases, nephropathy and retinopathy [36]. The mechanism of any direct effect of NAFLD on cardiovascular risk remains unclear; possibilities include the release of atherogenic inflammatory cytokines and pro-coagulant factors from the steatotic liver [37].

Polycystic ovary syndrome [PCOS]

As with the association between NAFLD and the metabolic syndrome, the now well-established association between

NAFLD and the PCOS seems likely to be indirect as a result of both conditions being characterized by insulin resistance. Up to 30% of females with PCOS have elevated alanine transaminase (ALT) levels [38], and NAFLD prevalence of 42% has been reported in a series of PCOS patients with a mean age of 25 years [39]. More recently, advanced fibrotic liver disease has been reported in patients with PCOS, suggesting that women with this syndrome require careful hepatic evaluation [40].

Obstructive sleep apnoea

Chronic intermittent hypoxia, as seen in obstructive sleep apnoea (OSA), has been associated with cardiovascular disease, the metabolic syndrome and insulin resistance [41]. As might be expected, therefore, a proportion of patients with OSA have elevated liver enzymes and histological features of NASH independent of body weight [42]. The severity of histology and the associated insulin resistance both correlate with the severity of OSA, strongly implicating insulin resistance as the pathogenic mechanism linking OSA to NASH although not entirely excluding a role for hypoxic liver injury. As with PCOS, this and other similar reports suggest that patients with OSA require hepatic evaluation, and that the diagnosis of OSA should be considered in NAFLD patients reporting daytime somnolence, sleep disturbances or any other symptoms suggesting a diagnosis of OSA.

Clinical presentation

NAFLD is a largely asymptomatic condition that may reach an advanced stage before it is suspected or diagnosed. Symptoms such as right upper quadrant discomfort, fatigue and lethargy have been reported in up to 50% of patients, but are uncommon modes of presentation. Fatigue is a significant problem in NAFLD patients and associates with objectively measured inactivity, but not histological disease severity [43]. Most patients with NAFLD are diagnosed after they are found to have hepatomegaly, or, more commonly, unexplained abnormalities of liver blood tests performed as part of routine health checks or during drug monitoring (e.g. statin therapy). NAFLD is the commonest cause of incidental abnormal liver blood tests, accounting for between 60–90% of such cases [44, 45]. Importantly, the vast majority (around 80%) of patients with NAFLD have normal liver blood tests [2], and there is no difference in histological severity between those with and without abnormal tests [46]. Accordingly, NAFLD should be suspected and sought in all patients with established risk factors, including PCOS and OSA, regardless of

liver blood tests. The history should concentrate on determining the presence/absence of conditions commonly associated with "primary" NAFLD – metabolic syndrome components, cardiovascular disease and OSA – and on excluding alternative causes of steatosis, including excessive alcohol intake, previous abdominal surgery (leading to bacterial overgrowth) and drugs causing NAFLD, such as amiodarone and tamoxifen. On examination, most patients are centrally obese and dorsocervical lipohypertrophy (a "buffalo hump") appears to be a particular feature of the fat distribution in patients with advanced NAFLD [8]. Features of PCOS (hyperandrogenism) should be sought in young women with suspected NAFLD [39], and clinical evidence of lipodystrophy should be sought in young, non-obese patients in view of its association with NAFLD [47].

Investigation

In the absence of advanced disease routine liver blood tests are either normal or typically show mild elevations of transaminases, alkaline phosphatase and gamma glutamyl transpeptidase (GGT) 1.5–3 times the upper limit of normal. The ALT/AST ratio is greater than one unless there is advanced fibrotic NAFLD or the patient is a covert heavy drinker. Other blood tests are aimed at detecting associated conditions, such as dyslipidemia, and excluding alternative causes of abnormal liver blood tests. Regarding lipids, it is worth measuring serum levels of apolipoprotein B (apoB) in patients either with no obvious risk factors for NAFLD or with low levels of LDL and HDL cholesterol, looking for evidence of hypobetalipoproteinemia a rare, familial cause of NAFLD [48]. Serum ferritin is often raised in NAFLD patients [49], and has been associated with advanced fibrosis [50]. *HFE* genotyping should be carried out when hyperferritemia is accompanied by raised transferrin saturation. Autoantibodies associated with autoimmune hepatitis (AIH), including ANA SMA, are often present at low titers in patients with NAFLD and have been associated with more advanced disease in some, but not all studies [51, 52]. Around one in ten of these patients have histological features of autoimmune hepatitis on biopsy and fulfil diagnostic criteria for probable/definite AIH [51]. Currently available imaging modalities including ultrasound, CT and routine MR imaging are all excellent at detecting steatosis (once more than around one-third of the liver is affected) but none can reliably detect NASH or fibrosis [53]. Newer imaging techniques, including proton magnetic resonance spectroscopy [54], and transient elastography [55] show promise (particularly in children [56]), but require further study prior to routine use for disease staging.

The role of liver biopsy

Undoubtedly the most important and controversial issue to consider in the investigation of patients with suspected NAFLD is whether or not to perform a liver biopsy. For diagnosis, biopsy is not required in a "typical" patient with abnormal liver blood tests, classical risk factors for NAFLD (obesity, T2DM, dyslipidemia) and an ultrasound showing steatosis; however, a high ferritin with *HFE* mutations, positive autoantibodies (ANA, SMA) or the use of medications associated with drug-induced liver injury all may justify a biopsy to exclude alternative/additional diagnoses. The main indication to perform a biopsy is, however, the accurate staging of the disease since (1) different stages have different prognoses and therefore require different management strategies, and (2) no currently availably imaging techniques can perform this role [53].

Non-invasive markers for staging NAFLD

The current reliance on liver biopsy for disease staging has prompted many studies aimed at defining clinical or laboratory-based variables capable of acting as surrogate markers of disease stage [57]. Various clinical and laboratory markers have been shown to be associated with advanced fibrosis (bridging fibrosis or cirrhosis) in patients with NAFLD, notably advanced age (>45 years), BMI > 30 kg/m², central obesity, T2DM (or raised fasting blood glucose), the severity of OSA [42] an AST:ALT ratio greater than one, hyperferritinemia [50] and positive autoantibodies [45]. In patients with normal ALT increased insulin resistance is the best predictor of advanced fibrotic disease [58]. At present, it would seem reasonable to restrict liver biopsy to patients with at least some, if not all, of these risk factors. Some of these markers (age, BMI, T2DM, AST/ALT ratio) have recently been combined together with platelet count and serum albumin concentration, into a NAFLD fibrosis "score" that accurately predicts the presence or absence of advanced fibrosis in the majority of patients with NAFLD [59]. This score has recently been combined with the European Liver Fibrosis (ELF) panel of serum fibrosis markers [60] and shown to have an accuracy of over 90% in differentiating the fibrosis stages in NAFLD [61]. An even simpler score – the **BARD** score – combining **B**MI, **A**ST/ALT **R**atio and **D**iabetes has recently been developed that reliably identifies patients without advanced disease [62]. With respect to the non-invasive diagnosis of NASH rather than fibrosis stage, serum levels of a caspase cleavage product of the hepatocyte protein cytokeratin-18 (a putative marker of hepatocyte apoptosis) have recently been shown to accurately predict the presence of NASH in a small pilot study [63]. Clearly this and other tests and scoring systems require further validation before they can be used in routine clinical practice but they do appear, at

last, to offer real potential to replace the need for liver biopsy in the majority of patients with NAFLD.

Overall management strategy for NAFLD

Almost no large randomized controlled trials (RCTs) have been published on which to establish evidence-based treatment recommendations for NAFLD. Accordingly, current management strategies are directed at treating, where present, the individual components of the metabolic syndrome since this will reduce risk of cardiovascular disease and may also be beneficial for the liver. Alcohol intake should not exceed "sensible" limits, but there is no need to advise complete abstinence, as an emerging body of data suggest that light to moderate intake may actually reduce the risk of NAFLD [29, 30]. In view of their largely benign prognosis these strategies are all that it is required for patients with simple steatosis who can be managed by general or primary-care physicians with no requirement for formal hepatological follow-up. In contrast, patients with more advanced NAFLD require long-term follow-up by hepatologists in light of their increased propensity for disease progression and the resulting need for surveillance for complications, including esophageal varices and HCC. These patients will also be candidates either for emerging "second-line" therapies currently being evaluated in large RCTs or for entry into these trials. The rationale for NAFLD therapies is based on a growing understanding of disease pathogenesis, with a particular focus on reducing insulin resistance, hepatic free fatty acid (FFA) levels, oxidative, endoplasmic reticulum and cytokine-mediated stress and influencing the balance and effects of profibrotic, pro-inflammatory and antifibrotic, anti-inflammatory adipokines released from adipose tissue [64]. Current and emerging therapies for NAFLD can be divided into those directed at the metabolic syndrome components with potential liver effects and those directed primarily at the liver.

Treatments directed at components of the metabolic syndrome

Obesity

Obesity is a rational target for NAFLD therapy since weight loss should reduce many of the putative mediators of liver injury, including insulin resistance, hepatic FFA supply and pro-inflammatory, profibrotic adipokines.

Diet and exercise

Several small, largely uncontrolled studies have shown an improvement in either ALT or steatosis following diet (with or without exercise) induced weight loss. **B4** There is very little evidence that necroinflammation or fibrosis can be improved by weight loss alone although a few small case series have shown some improvement in these parameters with drastic weight loss [65]. To date, almost all studies of diet-induced weight loss have employed simple calorie restriction, with very few attempting to manipulate specific dietary components. This area seems worthy of study, since intakes of both saturated fat and fiber are known to influence insulin resistance and diets high in saturated fat, soft drinks and meat, and low in omega 3 containing fish appear to be associated with both NAFLD and NASH. Dietary fat intake has also been shown to correlate with liver fat content and insulin resistance in short-term studies of obese, non-diabetic women – independently of changes in total-body, subcutaneous or abdominal fat [66]. The value of exercise in achieving and maintaining weight loss and improving insulin resistance is well established and thus far the only controlled study of weight loss that has reported histological improvement (steatosis) combined calorie restriction with increased exercise [67]. **B2**

Pharmacological anti-obesity agents

Encouraging improvements in liver histology have been reported from pilot studies of the intestinal lipase inhibitor orlistat in patients with NASH [68, 69]. However, there is no evidence as yet that this improvement is over and above what would be expected from the resulting weight loss. Nonetheless, data from currently ongoing large RCTs of orlistat are awaited with interest. The cannabinoid receptor 1 (CB_1) antagonist rimonabant has been shown to be effective in reducing weight and waist circumference, with improvements in several metabolic parameters, including insulin resistance [70]. **A1d** Animal data demonstrating that CB_1 blockade is both anti-steatotic [71] and anti-fibrotic [72] provide strong rationale for drugs directed at the CB_1 receptor in NAFLD. However, their adverse psychological side-effect profile is likely to limit their clinical utility severely.

Bariatric surgery

Various surgical procedures are currently in use for the treatment of obesity. Biliopancreatic diversion appears to carry a significant risk of liver failure and worsening fibrosis, and should therefore be avoided in patients with NAFLD. However, more encouraging results have been reported for gastric bypass and gastric banding surgery [73, 74]. To date all studies have shown improvements in metabolic parameters and steatosis, with some, but not all, reporting improvements in necroinflammation and fibrosis [73]. **B4**

Type 2 diabetes mellitus and insulin resistance

Evidence that insulin resistance may contribute to both inflammation and fibrosis in NAFLD has led to several pilot studies of metformin and other insulin-sensitizing agents in patients with NAFLD with and without diabetes. There is as yet no direct evidence of hyperinsulinemia *per se* adversely affecting the liver; however, evidence from animal studies that insulin is a direct cause of both hepatic steatosis and fibrosis might suggest that insulin or sulphonylureas should be avoided if possible [75]. It is of interest, therefore, that a recent pilot study in patients with T2DM has shown that long-term high dose insulin therapy results in a reduction of transaminases and hepatic steatosis, presumably reflecting the beneficial effects of insulin on blood glucose and adipose tissue lipolysis [76]. Whether or not long-term insulin therapy increases fibrosis in patients with NAFLD is, however, as yet unknown.

Metformin

Pilot studies of metformin in diabetic and non-diabetic patients with NAFLD have shown inconsistent effects on liver blood tests and steatosis (determined by MRI or MR proton spectroscopy). However, the largest RCT to date, in non-diabetic NAFLD patients, has been more encouraging. In this 12-month, randomized open-label trial, metformin treatment (2 g/day) was associated with significantly higher rates of normalized aminotransferase levels and with significant decreases in liver fat, necroinflammation and fibrosis, compared with either vitamin E treatment or weight-reducing diet treated patients [77]. The low number of patients who agreed to a second biopsy does, however, limit the strength of the conclusions that can be drawn from this study. **A1d**

Thiazolidinediones (TZDs)

TZDs act as agonists for the peroxisome proliferator activated receptor-γ (PPARγ). They improve insulin sensitivity, at least in part, via anti-steatotic effects in liver and muscle which may in turn result from an increase in the secretion of the anti-inflammatory, anti-fibrotic adipokine, adiponectin by adipocytes. Moreover, their potential as a therapy for NAFLD is further increased by evidence from animal models that they may also exert direct anti-fibrotic effects in the liver [78]. Pilot studies of the second-generation TZDs, pioglitazone and rosiglitazone, have consistently reported encouraging improvements in insulin sensitivity, liver blood tests and liver histology and several large RCTs are currently in progress. Two placebo-controlled RCTs of pioglitazone in the treatment of patients with NASH have recently reported significant improvements in steatosis, inflammation and ballooning necrosis associated with a non-significant decrease in fibrosis [79, 80]. **A1d** A note of caution over the use of TZDs in the treatment of NASH has arisen recently as a result of several meta-analyses of trials of TZDs in T2DM patients that have consistently shown that rosiglitazone increases the incidence of myocardial infarction and heart failure [81]. **A1a** The risk of heart failure is also increased by pioglitazone but it is associated with a lower risk of myocardial infarction and stroke compared to placebo-treated patients [82]. **A1d** This is reassuring since a recent study suggests that pioglitazone treatment for NASH has to be continued long term since stopping it led to a worsening of steatosis and inflammation [83]. **B4**

Dyslipidemia

Hypertriglyceridemia affects 20–80% of patients with NAFLD. As with anti-obesity and insulin-sensitizing drugs, there are sound scientific reasons to support the use of fibrates – the conventional triglyceride-lowering agents – in patients with NAFLD. Fibrates are agonists for the PPARα receptor, a transcription factor that up-regulates the transcription of genes encoding various proteins that would be expected to reduce hepatic FFA levels and also exerts anti-inflammatory effects. As with many other potential therapies for NAFLD, studies of PPARα agonists in animal models of NASH have been encouraging [84]. However, the only controlled study in patients with histological follow-up reported that one year of clofibrate had no effect on liver biochemistry or histology [85]. **A1d** There is less rationale for using HMG CoA reductase inhibitors (statins) to treat NAFLD; however, they can be safely prescribed for "conventional" indications, including T2DM and high cardiovascular risk. Importantly, there is no evidence that patients with pre-existing NAFLD are at increased risk of statin-induced idiosyncratic hepatotoxicity, or that statins are associated with a higher frequency of hepatic steatosis or serum ALT abnormalities in these subjects [86].

Hypertension

No RCTs have specifically examined the effect of different anti-hypertensive agents on the liver in hypertensive patients with NAFLD. However, a growing body of evidence from animal models of hepatic fibrosis and NASH suggests that therapy directed at the renin-angiotensin system and α-blockers may be beneficial for the liver [87, 88]. As yet, only one pilot study has examined the use of angiotensin II receptor blockade in patients with NASH and showed a reduction in serum markers of fibrosis [89]. Newer angiotensin II receptor blockers with insulin sensitizing effects seem worthy of study in NAFLD [90].

Treatments directed at the liver

An increased understanding of the mechanisms of progressive liver damage in NAFLD has stimulated the search for therapies specifically targeting the liver rather than at the individual components of the metabolic syndrome that may have beneficial effects.

Antioxidants

Several encouraging pilot studies of various agents indicate potential beneficial effects which may be related to their anti-oxidant effects. These include probucol [91], betaine [92], iron depeletion through venesection [93], and vitamin E [94]. However, a recent RCT of vitamin E combined with vitamin C in patients with NASH found no overall improvement in hepatic fibrosis score compared with placebo [95]. **A1d**

Anti-cytokine agents

Beneficial effects of anti-TNFα therapies have been demonstrated in animal models of NASH, and the two pilot studies in patients with NAFLD have reported improvements in aminotransferase levels and histology [96, 97]. Given the emerging importance of pro-inflammatory cytokines in both liver pathology and insulin resistance in obesity, it seems likely that cytokines and their regulatory molecules, including NF-kB, will become major therapeutic targets in both NAFLD and T2DM in the near future.

Ursodeoxycholic acid (UDCA)

Given its long history as a hepatoprotectant and recent evidence that bile acids may act as molecular chaperones capable of reducing ER stress implicated in NASH pathogenesis it is hardly surprising that UDCA has been considered as a potential treatment for NASH [64, 98]. To date, however, the only large, placebo-controlled RCT in patients with NASH showed no benefit of UDCA (13–15 mg/kg/day) on liver histology after two years' treatment [99]. **A1d** More encouraging results have recently been reported from a study combining UCDA with vitamin E [100].

Liver transplantation for patients with NAFLD

Patients with NAFLD who progress to decompensated cirrhosis or who develop HCC are candidates for liver transplantation. A favorable outcome depends on removing the factors that originally caused liver damage. Perhaps unsurprisingly, steatosis recurs in most patients within four years, with 50% developing NASH and fibrosis; cases of recurrent cirrhosis are also reported [101, 102]. Risk factors for recurrence are the presence of insulin resistance or T2DM pre and post-transplantation, weight gain following transplantation and a high cumulative steroid dose. These findings highlight the importance of ensuring weight and metabolic control in reducing the risk of disease recurrence, in a group of patients who will undoubtedly contribute increasing numbers to transplant programmes in the future.

References

1 Bedogni G, Miglioli L, Masutti F *et al.* Prevalence and risk factors for nonalcoholic fatty liver disease: the Dionysos nutrition and liver study. *Hepatology* 2005; **42**: 44–52.

2 Browning JS, Dobbins LS, Nuremberg R *et al.* Prevalence of hepatic steatosis in an urban population in the United States: impact of ethnicity. *Hepatology* 2004; **40**: 1387–1395.

3 Nomura H, Kashiwaqi S, Hayashi J *et al.* Prevalence of fatty liver in a general population of Okinawa Japan. *Jpn J Med* 1988; **27**: 142–149.

4 Bedogni G, Miglioli L, Masutti F *et al.* Incidence and natural course of fatty liver in the general population: the Dionysos Study. *Hepatology* 2007; **46**: 1387–1391.

5 Neuschwander-Tetri B, Caldwell S. Non alcoholic steatohepatitis: summary of an AASLD single topic conference. *Hepatology* 2003; **37**: 1202–1219.

6 Machado M, Marques-Vidal P, Cortez-Pinto H. Hepatic histology in patients undergoing bariatric surgery. *J Hepatol* 2006; **45**: 600–606.

7 Wanless IR, Lentz JS. Fatty liver hepatitis (steatohepatitis) and obesity: an autopsy study with analysis of risk factors. *Hepatology* 1990; **12**: 1106–1110.

8 Cheung P, Kapoor A, Puri P *et al.* The impact of fat distribution on the severity of nonalcoholic fatty liver disease and the metabolic syndrome. *Hepatology* 2007; **46**: 1091–1100.

9 Targher G, Bertolini L, Padovani R *et al.* Relation between carotid artery wall thickness and liver histology in subjects with non-alcoholic fatty liver disease. *Diabetes Care* 2006; **29**: 1325–1330.

10 Targher G, Bertolini L, Padovani R *et al.* Prevalence of nonalcoholic fatty liver disease and its association with cardiovascular disease among type 2 diabetic patients. *Diabetes Care* 2007; **30**: 1212–1218.

11 Marchesini G, Bugianesi E, Forlani G *et al.* Nonalcoholic fatty liver, steatohepatitis and the metabolic syndrome. *Hepatology* 2003; **37**: 917–923.

12 Franzese A, Vajro P, Argenziano A *et al.* Liver involvement in obese children. Ultrasonography and liver enzyme levels at diagnosis and during follow up in an Italian population. *Dig Dis Sci* 1997; **42**: 1428–1432.

13 Tominaga K, Kurata J, Chen Y *et al.* Prevalence of fatty liver in Japanese children and relationship to obesity. An epidemiological ultrasonographic survey. *Dig Dis Sci* 1995; **40**: 2002–2009.

14 Molleston J, White F, Teckman J *et al.* Obese children with steatohepatitis can develop cirrhosis in childhood. *Am J Gastroenterol* 2002; **97**: 2460–2462.

15 Ekstedt M, Franzen LE, Mathiesen UL *et al.* Long-term follow-up of patients with NAFLD and elevated liver enzymes. *Hepatology* 2006; **44**: 865–873.

16 Day CP. Natural history of NAFLD: Remarkably benign in the absence of cirrhosis. *Gastroenterology* 2005; **129**: 375–378.

17 Sanyal AJ, Banas C, Sargeant C *et al.* Similarities and differences in outcomes of cirrhosis due to nonalcoholic steatohepatitis and hepatitis C. *Hepatology* 2006; **43**: 682–689.

18 Nair S, Mason A, Eason J *et al.* Is obesity an independent risk factor for hepatocellular carcinoma in cirrhosis? *Hepatology* 2002; **36**: 150–155.

19 Calle E, Rodriguez C, Walker-Thurmond K *et al.* Overweight, obesity and mortality from cancer in a prospectively studied cohort of US adults. *N Engl J Med* 2003; **348**: 1625–1638.

20 McCullough A. The clinical features, diagnosis and natural history of non alcoholic fatty liver disease. *Clin Liver Dis* 2004; **8**: 521–533.

21 Adams LA, Lymp JF, St Sauver J *et al.* The natural history of nonalcoholic fatty liver disease: a population-based cohort study. *Gastroenterology* 2005; **129**: 113–121.

22 Ong JP, Pitts A, Younossi ZM. Increased overall mortality and liver-related mortality in non-alcoholic fatty liver disease. *J Hepatol* 2008; **49**: 608–612.

23 De Alwis N, Day CP. Genetics of alcoholic liver disease and nonalcoholic fatty liver disease. *Semin Liver Dis* 2007; **27**: 44–54.

24 Siebler J, Galle PR, Weber MM. The gut-liver axis: endotoxemia, inflammation, insulin resistance and NASH. *J Hepatol* 2008; **48**: 1032–1034.

25 Musso G, Gambino R, De Michieli F *et al.* Dietary habits and their relations to insulin resistance and postprandial lipemia in nonalcoholic steatohepatitis. *Hepatology* 2003; **37**: 909–916.

26 Zelber-Sagi S, Nitzan-Kaluski D, Goldsmith R *et al.* Long term nutritional intake and the risk of nonalcoholic fatty liver disease (NAFLD): a Population based study. *J Hepatol* 2007; **47**: 711–717.

27 Ouyang X, Cirillo P, Sautin Y *et al.* Fructose consumption as a risk factor for non-alcoholic fatty liver disease. *J Hepatol* 2008; **48**: 993–999.

28 Naveau S, Giraud V, Borotto E *et al.* Excess weight risk factor for alcoholic liver disease. *Hepatology* 1997; **25**: 108–111.

29 Dixon J, Bhathal P, O'Brian P. Non-alcoholic fatty liver disease: predictors of non-alcoholic steatohepatitis and liver fibrosis in the severely obese. *Gastroenterology* 2001; **121**: 91–100.

30 Dunn W, Xu R, Schwimmer JB. Modest wine drinking and decreased prevalence of suspected nonalcoholic fatty liver disease. *Hepatology* 2008; **47**: 1947–1954.

31 Miele L, Beale G, Patman G *et al.* The Kruppel like factor 6 genotype is associated with fibrosis in nonalcoholic fatty liver disease. *Gastroenterology* 2008; **135**: 282–291.

32 Romeo S, Kozlitina J, Xing C *et al.* Genetic variation in *PNPLA3* confers susceptibility to nonalcoholic fatty liver disease. *Nat Genet* 2008; **40**(12): 1461–1465.

33 Targher G, Bertolini L, Scala L *et al.* Non alcoholic hepatic steatosis and its relation to increased plasma biomarkers of inflammation and endothelial dysfunction in nondiabetic men. Role of visceral adipose tissue. *Diabet Med* 2005; **22**: 1354–1358.

34 Sookoian S, Pirola CJ. Non-alcoholic fatty liver disease is strongly associated with carotid atherosclerosis: A systemic review. *J Hepatol* 2008; **49**: 600–607.

35 Schwimmer J, Deutsch R, Behling C *et al.* Fatty liver as a determinant of atherosclerosis. *Hepatology* 2005; **42**: 610A.

36 Targher G, Bertolini L, Rodella S *et al.* Nonalcoholic fatty liver disease is independently associated with an increased preva-

lence of chronic kidney disease and proliferative/laser treated retinopathy in type 2 diabetic patients. *Diabetologia* 2008; **51**: 444–450.

37 Targher G, Bertolini L, Rodella S *et al.* NASH predicts plasma inflammatory biomarkers independently of visceral fat in men. *Obesity* 2008; **16**: 1394–1399.

38 Schwimmer J, Hhorram O, Chiu V *et al.* Abnormal aminotransferase activity in women with polycystic ovary syndrome. *Fertil Steril* 2005; **83**: 494–497.

39 Cerda C, Perez-Ayuso RM, Riquelme A *et al.* Nonalcoholic fatty liver disease in women with polycystic ovary syndrome. *J Hepatol* 2007; **47**: 412–417.

40 Setji T, Holland N, Sanders L *et al.* Nonalcoholic steatohepatitis and nonalcoholic fatty liver disease in young women with polycystic ovary syndrome. *J Clin Endocrinol Metab* 2006; **91**: 1741–1747.

41 Volk R, Somers V. Obesity related cardiovascular disease: implications of obstructive sleep apnea. *Diabet Obes Met* 2005; **8**: 250–260.

42 Tanne F, Gagnadoux F, Chazouilleres O *et al.* Chronic liver injury during obstructive sleep apnea. *Hepatology* 2005; **41**: 1290–1296.

43 Newton JL, Jones DEJ, Henderson E *et al.* Fatigue in non-alcoholic fatty liver disease (NAFLD) is significant and associates with inactivity and excessive daytime sleepiness but not with liver disease severity or insulin resistance. *Gut* 2008; **57**: 807–813.

44 Skelly M, James P, Ryder S. Findings on liver biopsy to investigate abnormal liver function tests in the absence of diagnostic serology. *J Hepatol* 2001; **35**: 195–199.

45 Pendino G, Mariano A, Surace P *et al.* Prevalence and etiology of altered liver tests: A population based survey in a Mediterranean town. *Hepatology* 2005; **41**: 1151–1159.

46 Mofrad P, Contos MJ, Haque M *et al.* Clinical and histologic spectrum of nonalcoholic fatty liver disease associated with normal ALT values. *Hepatology* 2003; **37**: 1286–1292.

47 Javor E, Ghany M, Cochran E *et al.* Leptin reverses nonalcoholic steatohepatitis in patients with severe lipodystrophy. *Hepatology* 2005; **41**: 753–760.

48 Tanoli T, Tue P, Yablonskiy D *et al.* Fatty liver in familial hypobetalipoproteinaemia: roles of the APOB defects, intra-abdominal adipose tissue, and insulin sensitivity. *J Lipid Res* 2004; **45**: 941–947.

49 Trombini P, Piperno A. Ferritin, metabolic syndrome and NAFLD: elective attractions and dangerous liaisons. *J Hepatol* 2007; **46**: 549–552.

50 Bugianesi E, Manzini P, D'Antico S *et al.* Relative contribution of iron burden, HFE mutations and insulin resistance to fibrosis in nonalcoholic fatty liver. *Hepatology* 2004; **39**: 179–187.

51 Adams LA, Lindor KD, Angulo P. The prevalence of autoantibodies and autoimmune hepatitis in patients with non alcoholic fatty liver disease. *Am J Gastroenterol* 2004; **90**: 1316–1320.

52 Loria P, Carulli N, Lonardo A. The prevalence of autoantibodies and autoimmune hepatitis in patients with nonalcoholic fatty liver disease. *Am J Gastroenterol* 2005; **100**: 1200–1201.

53 Saadeh S, Younossi ZM, Remer ME *et al.* The utility of radiological imaging in nonalcoholic fatty liver disease. *Gastroenterology* 2002; **123**: 745–750.

54 Cox I, Sharif A, Cobbold J *et al.* Current and future applications of in vitro magnetic resonance spectroscopy in hepatobiliary disease. *World J Gastroenterol* 2006; **12**: 4773–4783.

55 Yoneda M, Yoneda M, Mawatari H *et al.* Noninvasive assessment of liver fibrosis by measurement of stiffness in patients with nonalcoholic fatty liver disease (NAFLD). *Gut* 2008; **56**: 1330–1331.

56 Nobili V, Vizzutti F, Arena U *et al.* Accuracy and reproducibility of transient elastography for the diagnosis of fibrosis in pediatric nonalcoholic steatohepatitis. *Hepatology* 2008; **48**: 442–448.

57 Guha IN, Parkes J, Roderick PR *et al.* Non-invasive markers associated with liver fibrosis in non-alcoholic fatty liver disease. *Gut* 2006; **55**: 1650–1660.

58 Francanzani AL, Valenti L, Bugianesi E *et al.* Risk of severe liver disease in nonlcoholic fatty liver disease with normal aminotransferase levels: a role for insulin resistance and diabetes. *Hepatology* 2008; **48**: 792–798.

59 Angulo P, Hui JM, Marchesini G *et al.* The NAFLD fibrosis score: a non-invasive system that accurately identifies liver fibrosis in patients with NAFLD. *Hepatology* 2007; **45**: 846–854.

60 Rosenberg WM, Voelker M, Thiel R *et al.* Serum markers detect the presence of liver fibrosis: a cohort study. *Gastroenterology* 2004; **127**: 1704–1713.

61 Guha I, Parkes J, Roderick P *et al.* Non-invasive markers of fibrosis in non alcoholic fatty liver disease: validating the European Liver Fibrosis panel and exploring simple markers. *Hepatology* 2008; **47**: 455–460.

62 Harrison SA, Oliver D, Arnold HL *et al.* Development and validation of a simple NAFLD scoring system for identifying patients without advanced disease. *Gut* 2008; **57**: 1441–1447.

63 Wieckowska A, Zein NN, Yerian LM *et al.* In vivo assessment of liver cell apoptosis as a novel biomarker of disease severity in nonalcoholic fatty liver disease. *Hepatology* 2006; **44**: 27–33.

64 Day CP. From fat to inflammation. *Gastroenterology* 2006; **130**: 207–210.

65 Harrison SA, Day CP. Benefits of lifestyle modification in NAFLD. *Gut* 2007; **56**: 1760–1769.

66 Westerbacka J, Lammi K, Hakkinen A *et al.* Dietary fat content modifies liver fat in overweight nondiabetic subjects. *J Clin Endocrinol Metab* 2005; **90**: 2804–2809.

67 Ueno T, Sugawara S, Sujaku K *et al.* Therapeutic effects of diet and exercise in obese patients with fatty liver. *J Hepatol* 1997; **27**: 103–110.

68 Harrison SA, Fincke C, Helinski D *et al.* Pilot study of orlistat treatment in obese, nonalcoholic steatohepatitis patients. *Aliment Pharm Ther* 2004; **20**: 623–628.

69 Hussein O, Grosovski M, Schlesinger S *et al.* Orlistat reverses fatty infiltration and improves hepatic fibrosis in obese patients with nonalcoholic steatohepatitis (NASH). *Dig Dis Sci* 2007; **52**: 2512–2519.

70 Van Gaal LF, Rissanen AM, Scheen AJ *et al.* Effects of the cannabinoid-1 receptor blocker rimonabant on weight reduction and cardiovascular risk factors in overweight patients: 1-year experience from the RIO-Europe study. *Lancet* 2005; **365**: 1389–1397.

71 Gary-Bobo M, Elachouri G, Galla J *et al.* Rimonabant reduces obesity associated hepatic steatosis and features of the metabolic syndrome in obese Zucker fa/fa Rats. *Hepatology* 2007; **46**: 122–129.

72 Teixeira-Clerc F, Julien B, Grenard P *et al.* CB1 cannabinoid receptor antagonism: a new strategy for the treatment of liver fibrosis. *Nat Med* 2006; **12**: 671–676.

73 Dixon J, Bhathal P, Hughes N *et al.* Improvement in liver histological analysis with weight loss. *Hepatology* 2004; **39**: 1647–1654.

74 Klein S, Mittendorfer B, Eagon C *et al.* Gastric bypass surgery improves metabolic and hepatic abnormalities associated with nonalcoholic fatty liver disease. *Gastroenterology* 2006; **130**: 1564–1572.

75 Adachi M, Osawa Y, Uchinami H *et al.* The forkhead transcription factor FoxO1 regulates proliferation and transdifferentiation of hepatic stellate cells. *Gastroenterology* 2007; **132**: 1434–1446.

76 Juurinen L, Tiikkainen M, Hakkinen A *et al.* Effects of insulin therapy on liver fat content and hepatic insulin sensitivity in patients with type 2 diabetes. *Am J Physiol Endocrinol Metab* 2006; **292**: E829–835.

77 Bugianesi E, Gentilcore E, Manini R *et al.* A randomized controlled trial of metformin versus vitamin E or prescriptive diet in nonalcoholic fatty liver disease. *Am J Gastroenterology* 2005; **100**: 1082–1090.

78 Galli A, Crabb DW, Ceni E *et al.* Antidiabetic thiazolidinediones inhibit collagen synthesis and hepatic stellate cell activation *in vivo* and *in vitro. Gastroenterology* 2002; **122**: 1924–1940.

79 Belfort R, Harrison SA, Brown K *et al.* A placebo controlled trial of pioglitazone in subjects with non-alcoholic steatohepatitis. *N Engl J Med* 2006; **355**: 2297–2307.

80 Aithal GP, Thomas JA, Kaye PV *et al.* Randomized placebo-controlled trial of pioglitazone in nondiabetic subjects with nonalcoholic steatohepatitis. *Gastroenterology* 2008; **135**: 1176–1184.

81 Singh S, Loke Y, Furberg C. Long-term risk of cardiovascular events with rosiglitazone. A meta-analysis. *J Am Med Ass* 2007; **298**: 1189–1195.

82 Lincoff M, Wolski K, Nicholls S *et al.* Pioglitazone and risk of cardiovascular events in patients with type 2 diabetes mellitus. *J Am Med Ass* 2007; **298**: 1180–1188.

83 Lutchman G, Modi A, Kleiner D *et al.* The effects of discontinuing pioglitazone in patients with nonalcoholic steatohepatitis. *Hepatology* 2007; **46**: 424–429.

84 Ip E, Farrell G, Hall P *et al.* Administration of the potent PPAR alpha agonist, Wy-14,643, reverses nutritional fibrosis and steatohepatitis in mice. *Hepatology* 2004; **39**: 1286–1296.

85 Laurin J, Lindor K, Crippin J *et al.* Ursodeoxycholic acid or clofibrate in the treatment of nonalcoholic induced steatohepatitis: a pilot study. *Hepatology* 1996; **23**: 1464–1467.

86 Browning J. Statins and hepatic steatosis: perspectives from the Dallas Heart Study. *Hepatology* 2006; **44**: 466–471.

87 Hirose A, Ono M, Saibara T *et al.* Angiotensin II type 1 receptor blocker inhibits fibrosis in rat nonalcoholic steatohepatitis. *Hepatology* 2007; **45**: 1375–1381.

88 Yokohama S, Yoneda M, Haneda M *et al.* Therapeutic efficacy of an angiotensinogen II receptor antagonist in patients with nonalcoholic steatohepatitis. *Hepatology* 2004; **40**: 1222–1225.

89 Oben J, Roskams T, Yang S *et al.* Norepinephrine induces hepatic fibrosis in leptin deficient ob/ob mice. *Biochem Biophys Res Commun* 2003; **308**: 284–292.

90 Ichikawa Y. Comparative effects of telmisartan and valsartan on insulin resistance in hypertensive patients with metabolic syndrome. *Intern Med* 2007; **46**: 1331–1336.

91 Merat S, Malekzadeh R, Sohrabi M *et al.* Probucol in the treatment of nonalcoholic steatohepatitis: a double blind randomized controlled study. *J Hepatol* 2003; **38**: 414–418.

92 Abdelmalek M, Angulo P, Jorgensen R *et al.* Betaine, a promising new agent for patients with nonalcoholic steatohepatitis: results of a pilot study. *Am J Gastroenterology* 2001; **96**: 2711–2717.

93 Facchini F, Hua N, Stoohs R. Effect of iron depletion in carbohydrate-intolerant patients with clinical evidence of nonalcoholic fatty liver disease. *Gastroenterology* 2002; **122**: 931–939.

94 Lavine J. Vitamin E treatment of nonalcoholic steatohepatitis in children: a pilot study. *J Pediatr* 2000; **136**: 734–738.

95 Harrison SA, Torgerson S, Hayashi P *et al.* Vitamin E and vitamin C treatment improves fibrosis in patients with nonalcoholic steatohepatitis. *Am J Gastroenterology* 2003; **98**: 2485–2490.

96 Adams LA, Zein C, Angulo P *et al.* A pilot trial of pentoxyfylline in nonalcoholic steatohepatitis. *Am J Gastroenterology* 2004; **99**: 2365–2368.

97 Satapathy S, Sakhuja P, Malhotra V *et al.* Beneficial effects of pentoxifylline on hepatic steatosis, fibrosis and necroinflammation in patients with non alcoholic steatohepatitis. *J Gastroenterol Hepatol* 2007; **22**: 634–638.

98 Ozcan U, Yilmaz E, Ozcan L *et al.* Chemical chaperones reduce ER stress and restore glucose homeostasis in a mouse model of type 2 diabetes. *Science* 2006; **313**: 1137–1140.

99 Lindor K, Kowdley K, Heathcote E *et al.* Ursodeoxycholic acid for treatment of non alcoholic steatohepatitis: results of a randomized trial. *Hepatology* 2004; **39**: 770–778.

100 Dufour J, Oneta C, Gonvers J *et al.* Swiss Association for the Study of the Liver: randomized placebo controlled trial of ursodeoxycholic acid with Vitamin E in nonalcoholic steatohepatitis. *Clin Gastro Hepat* 2006; **4**: 1537–1543.

101 Contos MJ, Cales W, Sterling RK *et al.* Development of nonalcoholic fatty liver disease after orthotopic liver transplantation for cryptogenic cirrhosis. *Liver Transpl* 2001; **7**: 363–373.

102 Ong J, Younossi Z, Reddy V *et al.* Cryptogenic cirrhosis and post-transplantation nonalcoholic fatty liver disease. *Liver Transpl* 2001; **7**: 797–801.

30 Hemochromatosis

Gary P Jeffrey[1] and Paul C Adams[2]
[1] Western Australia Liver Transplantation Service, Sir Charles Gairdner Hospital, Nedlands, Australia
[2] London Health Sciences Centre, London, Ontario, Canada

Introduction

Hemochromatosis is the most common genetic disease in populations of European ancestry. Despite the estimated prevalence in different countries, ranging from 1 in 100 to 1 in 300, hemochromatosis is still considered by many physicians to be a rare disease. The diagnosis can be difficult because of the non-specific nature of the symptoms. The discovery of the major hemochromatosis gene in 1996 has led to new insights into the pathogenesis of the disease and new diagnostic strategies [1, 2].

Pathogenesis of hemochromatosis

The regulation of dietary iron absorption and intracellular iron homeostasis is controlled by hepcidin, a protein synthesized in the liver and rapidly excreted by the kidneys [3, 4]. Hepcidin binds to ferroportin, a membrane bound iron transporter present on the basolateral surface of enterocytes, and regulates the transfer of dietary iron from the enterocyte cytoplasm into the body in response to body iron requirements. Hepcidin also regulates iron export from macrophages via ferroportin. Decreased levels of hepcidin allows for increased dietary iron absorption and vice versa. Inappropriate decreased levels of hepcidin are present in hemochromatosis and this results in increased dietary iron absorption and iron overload [5, 6]. HFE, transferrin receptor 2 and hemojuvelin are three proteins that have been found to regulate the expression of hepcidin [3, 7, 8]. Mutations in any of these five proteins have been associated with hemochromatosis. The C282Y mutation in HFE was the first to be identified and is the most frequent cause of hemochromatosis [1].

Evidence-Based Gastroenterology and Hepatology, 3rd edition.
J. McDonald, A.K. Burroughs, B. Feagan, and M.B. Fennerty. © 2010 Blackwell Publishing Ltd

Diagnosis of hemochromatosis

A paradox of genetic hemochromatosis is the observation that the disease is underdiagnosed in the general population, and overdiagnosed in patients with secondary iron overload.

Underdiagnosis of hemochromatosis

Population studies using genetic testing in patients of northern European ancestry have demonstrated a prevalence of C282Y homozygotes of approximately 1 in 227 [9]. The fact that many physicians consider hemochromatosis to be rare implies either a lack of penetrance of the gene (non-expressing homozygote) or a large number of undiagnosed patients in the community.

Barriers to the diagnosis of hemochromatosis include the lack of symptoms and the non-specific nature of symptoms. An elderly patient who presents with joint pain and diabetes is not often considered to have genetic hemochromatosis. The presenting features vary depending on age and sex but fatigue is the most common complaint. Women are more likely to have fatigue, arthralgia and pigmentation than liver disease [10].

Diagnostic tests for hemochromatosis

Serum iron
An elevated serum iron is found in most but not all cases. Serum iron can vary throughout the day and it has been estimated that approximately 5–10% of C282Y homozygotes have a normal serum iron [11].

Transferrin saturation
The transferrin saturation is the serum iron/total iron binding capacity. The transferrin saturation has a sensitivity of greater than 90% for hemochromatosis in referral studies of iron loaded patients. However, in population studies the sensitivity may be as low as 50% [12, 13]. The

transferrin saturation is often elevated, even in children or young adults with hemochromatosis, before the development of iron overload and a rising ferritin. The threshold to pursue further diagnostic studies has varied from 45% to 62% in previous studies. A lower threshold picks up more patients with hemochromatosis but also leads to more investigations in patients without hemochromatosis. A higher threshold leads to fewer investigations overall, with a greater possibility of missing some patients. These concepts are most relevant when considering population screening. A large population screening study demonstrated wide biological variability in transferrin saturation (see Figure 30.1) and there was no advantage in using fasting blood samples (see Table 30.1) [14].

Serum ferritin

The relationship between serum ferritin and total body iron stores in hemochromatosis has been clearly established by strong correlations with hepatic iron concentra-

tion and amount of iron removed by venesection [15]. However, serum ferritin can be elevated secondary to chronic inflammation and histiocytic neoplasms and not be associated with increased body iron stores. A major diagnostic dilemma in the past was whether the serum ferritin was related to hemochromatosis or another underlying liver disease such as alcoholic liver disease, chronic viral hepatitis or non-alcoholic steatohepatitis. These difficult cases can now be resolved in the majority by HFE genetic testing. The result of the obesity epidemic in developed countries is that the commonest cause of abnormal LFT and mild elevation in ferritin (300–1000 ug/l) is non-alcoholic fatty liver disease. Large population studies have demonstrated that a mild elevation in ferritin (300–1000 micrograms/l) is very common, and may be related to obesity with NAFLD, regular alcohol consumption or inflammation. These observations have limited the use of serum ferritin as a screening test for hemochromatosis because of the lack of specificity for iron overload. **B4**

Iron removed by venesection

Historically hemochromatosis was diagnosed when symptoms developed in the fifth or sixth decade and patients had significant iron overload at the time of diagnosis. The removal of 500 ml of blood weekly (0.25 g iron) was well tolerated, often for years, without the development of significant anemia. If a patient became anemic (hemoglobin < 100 g/l) after only six venesections, this suggested mild iron overload incompatible with the diagnosis of hereditary hemochromatosis. We now know that these guidelines no longer apply as population and pedigree studies uncover patients in their second and third decade

Table 30.1 The use of transferrin saturation as a screening test to detect C282Y homozygotes in a population-based study. There was no advantage to the use of fasting samples (PPV = positive predictive value [14].

Blood test	n	Sensitivity (%)	Specificity (%)	PPV (%)
Fasting TS	31,796	77 (65–86)	93 (92–93)	2.3 (2–3)
Random TS	64,230	75 (67–81)	95 (95–96)	3.5 (3–4)

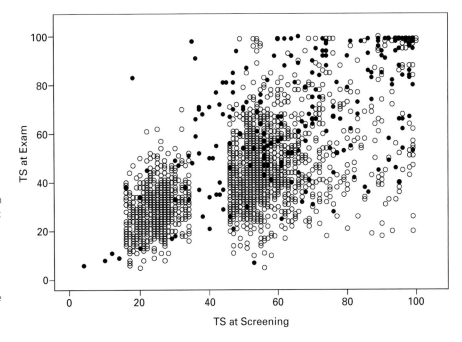

Figure 30.1 A comparison of the transferrin saturation at initial screening (random) and at the clinical examination (fasting) in all participants recalled for a clinical exam (• = C282Y homozygotes, o = non-C282Y homozygote, n = 2285). The apparent gap around 40% is related to the requirement of control participants to have a TS between the 25th and 75th percentile (reprinted with permission from the *Am J Med*).

[16]. At our center only 71% of homozygotes would have met the arbitrary criterion that more than 5 g of iron (20 venesections) were removed without anemia [17]. This historical diagnostic criterion for hemochromatosis is no longer relevant in the era of genetic testing. **B4**

Liver biopsy

Liver biopsy has been the "gold standard" diagnostic test for hemochromatosis, but its use has shifted from a diagnostic tool to staging the degree of fibrosis. The need for liver biopsy seems less apparent in the young asymptomatic patient with a low clinical suspicion of cirrhosis based on history, physical examination and iron studies. Clinical guidelines have been suggested, such as a serum ferritin < 1000 micrograms/l or age < 40 years to reduce the need for liver biopsy [18]. Clinical judgment and assessment of concomitant risk factors (alcohol, viral hepatitis) would be a better guide for the need for liver biopsy than an arbitrary threshold. Most non-cirrhotic patients with hemochromatosis have serum ferritin < 1000 micrograms/l and a normal aspartate transaminase (AST) [19, 20]. Cirrhosis can be predicted non-invasively in C282Y homozygotes if the serum ferritin is >1000 micrograms/l, the platelet count is less than $200 \times 10^6/l$ and the AST is >40 U/l [21]. The presence of fibrosis can also be assessed using hepatic elastography [22].

Patients with cirrhosis have a 5.5-fold relative risk of death compared with non-cirrhotic hemochromatosis patients [23, 24]. Cirrhotic patients are also at risk of hepatocellular carcinoma. The mean age of cirrhotic patients with hepatocellular carcinoma was 68 years in a Canadian series, but was lower in Italian patients with concomitant viral hepatitis [25]. Although early detection of hepatocellular cancer has been clearly demonstrated by serial ultrasound and α-fetoprotein determination, curative treatment options remain limited. An elderly cirrhotic patient may not withstand a major resection and the residual cirrhotic liver remains a fertile ground for new tumor development. Organ shortages often preclude the possibility of immediate liver transplantation, although living related adult liver transplantation may improve this situation in the future.

Hepatic iron concentration and hepatic iron index

The traditional method of assessing iron status by liver biopsy uses the semi-quantitative staining method of Perls. However, when moderate iron overload is present, the degree of iron overload can be difficult to interpret. Iron concentration can be measured using atomic absorption spectrophotometry. This can be done on a piece of paraffin embedded tissue, so special preparation is not required at the time of the biopsy. An advantage of cutting the tissue from the block is that one can be more certain that the tissue assayed is the same as the tissue examined microscopically. The normal reference range for hepatic iron concentration

is 0–35 μmol/g dry weight (<2000 micrograms/g). The hepatic iron index has therefore limited use with the advent of genetic testing. The commentary on liver biopsy reports that a hepatic iron index >1.9 confirms a diagnosis of genetic hemochromatosis should be strongly discouraged.

Imaging studies of the liver

Magnetic resonance imaging (MRI) can demonstrate moderate to severe iron overload of the liver. The technology is advancing and it is possible that eventually it may become as precise as hepatic iron determination [26, 27]. Proponents of MRI have emphasized the non-invasive nature of the test for the diagnosis and alleviated need for liver biopsy. As previously discussed, the role of liver biopsy has now shifted from a diagnostic tool to a prognostic tool. It is likely that the presence of an elevated ferritin with a positive genetic test will satisfy the non-invasive clinician more than an MRI study. MRI can also demonstrate the clinical features of cirrhosis such as nodularity of the liver, ascites, portal hypertension and splenomegaly as well as hepatocellular carcinoma. These features can be more readily assessed by abdominal ultrasound at a lower cost.

Genetic testing for hemochromatosis

A major advance, which stems from the discovery of the HFE gene, is the diagnostic genetic test. The original publication reported that 83% of a group of patients with suspected hemochromatosis had the characteristic C282Y mutation of the HFE gene. In this report, the gene was called HLA-H but this name was later changed to HFE [1]. The C282Y mutation is also reported as 845A in some laboratories, reflecting the base pair change rather than the amino acid change. Subsequent studies in well-defined hemochromatosis pedigrees reported that 90–100% of typical hemochromatosis patients had the C282Y mutation [28]. The presence of a single mutation in most patients was in marked contrast to other genetic diseases in which multiple mutations have been discovered (cystic fibrosis, Wilson's disease, α-1-antitrypsin deficiency). A second minor mutation, H63D, was also described in the original report [1]. This mutation does not cause the same intracellular trafficking defect of the HFE protein and many homozygotes for H63D have been found without iron overload in the general population. Compound heterozygotes (C282Y/H63D) and H63D homozygotes (H63D/H63D) may resemble homozygotes with mild to moderate iron overload, particularly if a co-factor is present, for example NAFLD, HCV, or alcohol. However, these compound heterozygote (C282Y/H63D) patients usually have normal iron studies [9, 29].

The interpretation of the genetic test in several settings is shown in Box 30.1. The test may also be performed on DNA extracted from paraffin embedded tissue such as

BOX 30.1 Interpretation of C282Y, genetic testing for hemochromatosis

C282Y homozygote: This is the classic genetic pattern that is seen in >90% of typical cases. Expression of disease ranges from no evidence of iron overload to massive iron overload with organ dysfunction. Siblings have a one in four chance of being affected and should have genetic testing. For children to be affected the other parent must be at least a heterozygote. If iron studies are normal, false positive genetic testing or a non-expressing homozygote should be considered.

C282Y/H63D (compound heterozygote): This patient carries one copy of the major mutation and one copy of the minor mutation. Most patients with this genetic pattern have normal iron studies. A small percentage of compound heterozygotes have been found to have mild to moderate iron overload. Severe iron overload is usually seen in the setting of another concomitant risk factor (alcoholism, viral hepatitis, NAFLD).

C282Y heterozygote: This patient carries one copy of the major mutation. This pattern is seen in about 10% of the Caucasian population and is usually associated with normal or mildly increased iron studies. In rare cases the iron studies are high in the range expected in a homozygote rather than a heterozygote. These cases may carry an unknown hemochromatosis mutation and measurement of body iron stores is helpful to determine the need for venesection therapy.

H63D homozyote: This patient carries two copies of the minor mutation: Most patients with this genetic pattern have normal iron studies. A small percentage of these cases have been found to have mild to moderate iron overload. Severe iron overload is usually seen in the setting of another concomitant risk factor (alcoholism, or viral hepatitis).

H63D heterozygote: This patient carries one copy of the minor mutation. This pattern is seen in about 20% of the Caucasian population and is usually associated with normal iron studies. This pattern is so common in the general population that the presence of iron overload may be related to another risk factor. Liver biopsy may be required to determine the cause of the iron overload and the need for treatment in these cases.

No HFE mutations: There are currently some newly recognized mutations associated with iron overload that are being studied in research laboratories (ferroportin, transferrin receptor 2, hepcidin, hemojuvelin). There will likely be other hemochromatosis mutations discovered in the future. If iron overload is present without any HFE mutations, a careful history for other risk factors must be reviewed and liver biopsy may be useful to determine the cause of the iron overload and the need for treatment. Many of these cases are isolated, non-familial cases.

Non-expressing C282Y homozygotes: As genetic testing becomes more widespread an increasing number of persons have been found with the hemochromatosis gene without iron overload. Large-scale population studies in North America and northern Europe have demonstrated that approximately 50% of C282Y homozygous women and 86% of homozygous men will have an elevated ferritin. It is apparent that the prevalence of HFE mutations far exceeds the prevalence of biochemical iron overload and clinical symptoms attributable to hemochromatosis. Patients who are homozygous for the C282Y mutation should be considered at risk of developing iron overload, but if there are no abnormalities in transferrin saturation or ferritin in adulthood, it seems more likely that they are non-expressing homozygotes rather than patients who will develop iron overload later in life [36].

Family studies in hemochromatosis: Once the proband case is identified and confirmed with genetic testing for the C282Y mutation, family testing is imperative. Siblings have a one in four chance of carrying the gene and should be screened with the genetic test and serum ferritin. The risk to a child is dependent on the prevalence of heterozygotes in the community and is approximately 1 in 20 and much lower if the spouse is non-Caucasian. A cost-effective strategy now possible with the genetic test is to test the spouse for the C282Y mutation to assess the risk in the children. If the spouse is not a heterozygote or homozygote, the children will be obligate heterozygotes. This assumes paternity and no other gene or mutation causing hemochromatosis. This strategy is particularly advantageous where the children are geographically separated or may be under a different physician or health care system [37]. Genetic testing in general raises many perplexing questions, such as premarital testing, *in utero* testing, and paternity issues, which have not yet been tested in hemochromatosis.

liver explants. Studies of explanted livers have demonstrated that many liver transplant patients classified as hemochromatosis patients are negative for the C282Y mutation [30]. This suggests that those patients may have had iron overload secondary to chronic liver disease rather than hemochromatosis. Therefore any interpretation of iron reaccumulation post liver transplant for hemochromatosis must be done with caution and with the benefit of genetic testing.

Genetic discrimination has been a concern with the widespread use of genetic testing. A positive genetic test even without iron overload could disqualify a patient for health or life insurance. In the case of hemochromatosis, the advantages of early diagnosis of a treatable disease outweigh the disadvantages of genetic discrimination. Recent population studies have demonstrated that genetic discrimination is rare with hemochromatosis genetic testing [31].

Genotypic-phenotypic correlation in hemochromatosis If we define the presence of homozygosity for the C282Y mutation as a predisposition for the development of hemochromatosis, it provides for the first time a benchmark for the assessment of the phenotypic diagnostic tools that have been used for decades. In one study transferrin saturation, ferritin, hepatic iron index and iron removed by venesection were evaluated in *referred* putative homozygotes with a high pre-test probability of hemochromatosis. Ninety-five percent (122/128) patients were homozygous for the C282Y mutation. The hepatic iron index was >1.9 in 91.3% of these cases, transferrin saturation >55% in 90%, serum ferritin >300 micrograms/l in 96% of men and >200 micrograms/l in 97% of women, and iron removed >5 g in 70% of men and 73% of women. Four homozygotes for C282Y had no biochemical evidence of iron overload. The sensitivity of the phenotypic tests in decreasing order was: serum ferritin, hepatic iron index, transferrin saturation and iron removed by venesection. Although the genetic test is useful in the diagnostic algorithm (see Figure 30.3), this study demonstrated both iron loaded patients without the mutation and homozygous patients without iron overload [17].

However, population-based studies have revealed a different clinical profile for C282Y homozygotes. It appears that many C282Y homozygotes will have no obvious symptoms related to iron overload and that 50% of women and 20% of men will have normal serum ferritin [1]. The biochemical clinical expression of hemochromatosis is illustrated in screening studies in Figure 30.2. The prevalence of signs and symptoms of hemochromatosis is more difficult to assess since there are not standardized criteria for their assessment. A recent study by Allen *et al.* suggested that 28% of male and 1% of female C282Y homozygotes from a population screening study had hemochromatosis related symptoms [32, 33]. A screening

study from Norway which utilized 149 liver biopsies, demonstrated cirrhosis in 4% of male and in none of the female C282Y homozygotes [12]. Only the presence of liver disease was significantly different between C282Y homozygotes and a control population in a screening study from San Diego, California [34]. Several studies have demonstrated that there is no increase in diabetes compared to control participants [1, 34, 35].

If an isolated heterozygote is detected by genetic testing, it is recommended to test siblings. Extended family studies are less revealing than a family study with a homozygote but more likely to uncover a homozygote than random population screening.

It is important to remember that there will be patients with a clinical picture indistinguishable from genetic hemochromatosis who will be negative for the C282Y mutation. Most of these patients will be isolated cases, although a few cases of familial iron overload (ferroportin, transferrin receptor 2 and hepcidin mutations) have been reported with negative C282Y testing [38]. A negative C282Y test should alert the physician to question the diagnosis of genetic hemochromatosis and reconsider secondary iron overload related to cirrhosis, alcohol, viral hepatitis, NAFLD or iron loading anemias. If no other risk factors are found, the patient should begin venesection treatment similar to any other hemochromatosis patient.

Population screening

Soon after the development of the genetic test for hemochromatosis, it seemed that hemochromatosis would be an ideal disease for population screening. It seemed to have a high prevalence, could be detected with low-cost iron tests, confirmed by a specific genetic test and could easily be treated. Hemochromatosis meets many of the guidelines

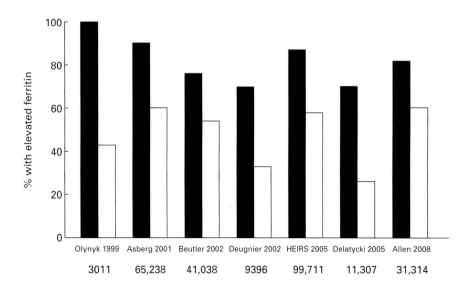

Figure 30.2 The percentage of C282Y homozygotes discovered in population screening studies that have an elevated serum ferritin (>200 ug/l in women, >300 ug/l in men).

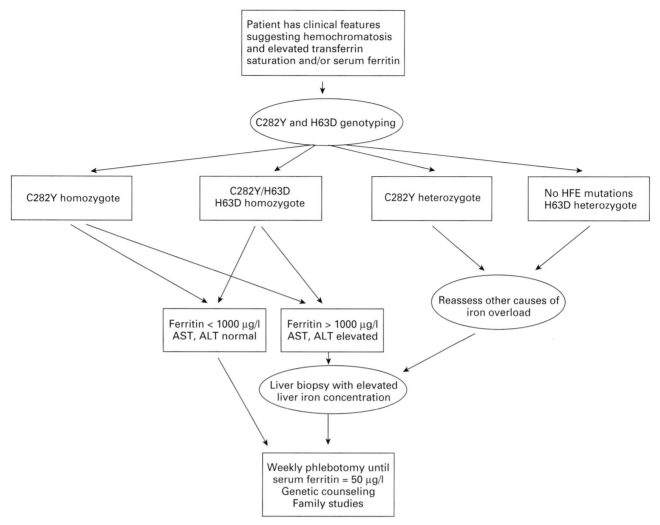

Figure 30.3 Diagnostic algorithm for a patient suspected of having hemochromatosis. AST: aspartate transaminase; ALT: alanine transaminase.

established by the World Health Organization for screening (see Table 30.2). Large population screening studies have been done in North America, Europe and Australia using a variety of approaches and patient populations. A common finding is that there appear to be more genetic mutations than clinical illness. The natural history of untreated disease is the Achilles heel of screening for hemochromatosis. If the survival in untreated patients appears similar to control participants or treated patients, there is little rationale for identifying patients in the general population. Several epidemiological studies performed genetic testing for hemochromatosis many years after the initiation of the study and presented data on the serum ferritin and long-term survival of C282Y homozygotes and other genotypes that were followed for up to 25 years without treatment or awareness of their underlying condition (see Figure 30.4) [33, 39, 40]. A similar longitudinal study in type 2 diabetes found that there was no associa-

tion of HFE mutations or ferritin levels with all cause mortality or cardiovascular complications [41].

Universal screening is unlikely to be widely implemented, but selective screening in high-risk populations, such as men of northern European ancestry may be a preferred strategy. Other strategies include more intense physician and patient education about iron overload and extended pedigree studies. Screening patients with established causes of liver disease (e.g. HCV, HBV, autoimmune liver disease, etc.) for hemochromatosis is important as this will identify another co-factors causing liver damage and potentially fibrosis that is treatable.

Treatment of hemochromatosis

Patients are initially treated by the weekly removal of 500 ml of blood. Patients attend either a blood transfusion

Table 30.2 Population screening for hemochromatosis.

WHO criteria for screening for medical disease	Phenotypic testing (serum iron, transferrin saturation, UIBC, ferritin)	Genotypic testing (C282Y mutation)
Is the disease an important health problem?	Yes (1 in 300)	Yes (1 in 200)
Is there an effective treatment?	Yes	Yes
Are there facilities for diagnosis and treatment?	Yes	Yes
Is there a presymptomatic stage?	Yes	Yes
Is the cost of screening reasonable?	Yes	If limited to few mutations
Is continuous case finding on an ongoing basis feasible?	Yes	Yes
Is there a suitable test?	Yes	Yes
Is the testing acceptable to the population?	Yes	Genetic discrimination?
Is the natural history of disease understood?	Natural history of untreated disease has not been well studied	Uncertain in non-expressing homozygotes
Is there agreement on whom to treat?	Yes, but the impact of treatment is difficult to assess	Yes

WHO; World Health Organization; UIBC: unsaturated iron binding capacity.

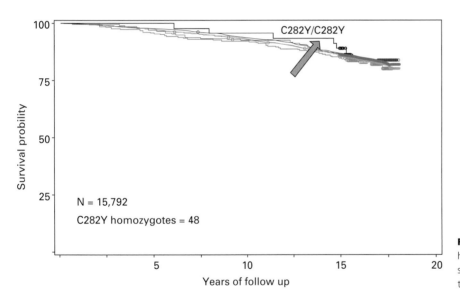

Figure 30.4 The long-term survival in C282Y homozygotes (C282Y/C282Y) was not significantly different from patients with all of the other HFE genotypes in the ARIC study.

service, where red cells and plasma are used for transfusion, or an ambulatory care facility. The venesection is carried out by a nurse using a kit containing a 16-gauge straight needle and collection bag. Blood is removed with the patient lying flat over 15–30 minutes. A haemoglobin test is done at the time of each venesection. If the hemoglobin decreases to less than 100 g/l the venesection schedule is modified to 500 ml every other week. Serum ferritin is measured periodically (every three months in severe iron overload, monthly in mild iron overload) and weekly ven-

esections are continued until the serum ferritin is approximately 50 micrograms/l. Transferrin saturation often remains elevated despite therapy. Patients may then begin maintenance venesections three to four times per year. Iron reaccumulation is an inconsistent observation and many patients will go for years without treatment and without a rise in serum ferritin [41]. Chelation therapy is not commonly used for the treatment of hereditary hemochromatosis. The newest oral iron chelator, deferasirox, has been undergoing a clinical trial in hemochromatosis but its high cost and potential side effects (GI side effects, elevation in serum creatinine) may limit its use to secondary iron overload.

There have been some studies, now, documenting reversal of fibrosis following iron depletion therapy [42, 43].

There are no randomized trials comparing venesection therapy to no treatment. Iron depletion before the development of cirrhosis can prevent cirrhosis and the development of hepatocellular carcinoma. Other disabling diseases such as arthritis, diabetes and impotence will likely be prevented. Therefore the goal is early detection and treatment before the development of cirrhosis.

References

1 Feder JN, Gnirke A, Thomas W *et al.* A novel MHC class I-like gene is mutated in patients with hereditary hemochromatosis. *Nature Genetics* 1996; **13**: 399–408.

2 Adams PC, Barton JC. Haemochromatosis. *Lancet* 2007; **370**: 1855–1860.

3 Andrews NC. Forging a field: the golden age of iron biology. *Blood* 2008; **112**: 219–230.

4 Olynyk J, Trinder D, Ramm GA, Britton R, Bacon BR. Hereditary hemochromatosis in the post-HFE era. *Hepatology* 2008; **48**: 991–1001.

5 Bridle K, Frazer D, Wilkins S *et al.* Disrupted hepcidin regulation in HFE-associated haemochromatosis and the liver as a regulator of body iron homeostasis. *Lancet* 2003; **361**: 661–673.

6 Piperno A, Girelli D, Nemeth E *et al.* Blunted hepcidin response to oral iron challenge in HFE-related hemochromatosis. *Blood* 2007; **110**: 4096–4100.

7 Muckenthaler M, Vujic-Spasic M, Kiss J *et al.* HFE acts in hepatocytes to prevent hemochromatosis. *Cell Metab* 2008; **7**: 173–178.

8 Babitt JL, Huang FW, Wrighting DM *et al.* Bone morphogenetic protein signaling by hemojuvelin regulates hepcidin expression. *Nat Genet* 2006; **38**: 531–539.

9 Adams PC, Reboussin DM, Barton JC *et al.* Hemochromatosis and iron-overload screening in a racially diverse population. *N Eng J Med* 2005; **352**: 1769–1778.

10 Moirand R, Adams PC, Bicheler V, Brissot P, Deugnier Y. Clinical features of genetic hemochromatosis in women compared to men. *Ann Int Med* 1997; **127**: 105–110.

11 Adams PC, Valberg LS. Evolving expression of hereditary hemochromatosis. *Sem Liv Dis* 1996; **16**: 47–54.

12 Asberg A, Hveem K, Thorstensen K *et al.* Screening for hemochromatosis – high prevalence and low morbidity in an unselected population of 65,238 persons. *Scand J Gastroenterol* 2001; **36**: 1108–1115.

13 Beutler E, Felitti V, Gelbart T, Ho N. The effect of HFE genotypes on measurement of iron overload in patients attending a health appraisal clinic. *Ann Int Med* 2000; **133**: 329–337.

14 Adams P, Reboussin D, Press R *et al.* Biological variability of transferrin saturation and unsaturated iron binding capacity. *Am J Med* 2007; **120**: 999.e1–7.

15 Brissot P, Bourel M, Herry D *et al.* Assessment of liver iron content in 271 patients: a re-evaluation of direct and indirect methods. *Gastroenterology* 1981; **80**: 557–565.

16 Adams PC, Kertesz AE, Valberg LS. Clinical presentation of hemochromatosis: a changing scene. *Am J Med* 1991; **90**: 445–449.

17 Adams PC, Chakrabarti S. Genotypic/phenotypic correlations in genetic hemochromatosis: evolution of diagnostic criteria. *Gastroenterology* 1998; **114**: 319–323.

18 Tavill AS. Diagnosis and management of hemochromatosis. *Hepatology* 2001; **33**: 1321–1328.

19 Adams PC. Factors affecting rate of iron mobilization during venesection therapy for hereditary hemochromatosis. *Am J Hematology* 1998; **58**: 16–19.

20 Morrison E, Brandhagen D, Phatak P *et al.* Serum ferritin levels predicts advanced hepatic fibrosis among US patients with phenotypic hemochromatosis. *Ann Int Med* 2003; **138**: 627–633.

21 Beaton M, Guyader D, Deugnier Y, Moirand R, Chakrabarti S, Adams P. Non-invasive prediction of cirrhosis in C282Y-linked hemochromatosis. *Hepatology* 2002; **36**: 673–678.

22 Adhoute X, Foucher J, Laharie D *et al.* Diagnosis of liver fibrosis using FibroScan and other noninvasive methods in patients with hemochromatosis: a prospective study. *Gastroenterol Clin Biol* 2008; **32**: 180–187.

23 Niederau C, Fischer R, Purschel A, Stremmel W, Haussinger D, Strohmeyer G. Long-term survival in patients with hereditary hemochromatosis. *Gastroenterology* 1996; **110**: 1107–1119.

24 Wojcik J, Speechley M, Kertesz A, Chakrabarti S, Adams P. Natural history of C282Y homozygotes for haemochromatosis. *Can J Gastro* 2002; **16**: 297–302.

25 Fargion S, Mandelli C, Piperno A *et al.* Survival and prognostic factors in 212 Italian patients with genetic hemochromatosis. *Hepatology* 1992; **15**: 655–659.

26 Gandon Y, Olivie D, Guyader D *et al.* Non-invasive assessment of hepatic iron stores by MRI. *Lancet* 2004; **363**: 357–360.

27 St Pierre T, Clark P, Chua-anusorn W *et al.* Noninvasive measurement and imaging of liver iron concentrations using proton magnetic resonance. *Blood* 2005; **105**: 855–861.

28 The UK Haemochromatosis Consortium. A simple genetic test identifies 90% of UK patients with haemochromatosis. *Gut* 1997; **41**: 841–845.

29 Rossi E, Olynyk J, Cullen D *et al.* Compound heterozygous hemochromatosis genotype predicts increased iron and erythrocyte indices in women. *Clin Chem* 2000; **46**: 162–166.

30 Minguillan J, Lee R, Britton R *et al.* Genetic markers for hemochromatosis in patients with cirrhosis and iron overload. *Hepatology* 1997; **26**: 158A.

31 Hall M, Barton J, Adams P *et al.* Genetic screening for iron overload: no evidence of discrimination at one year. *J Fam Practice* 2007; **56**: 829–833.

32 Allen KJ, Gurrin LC, Constantine CC *et al.* Iron-overload-related disease in HFE hereditary hemochromatosis. *N Engl J Med* 2008; **358**: 221–230.

33 Gurrin L, Osborne N, Constantine C *et al.* The natural history of serum iron indices for HFE C282Y homozygosity associated with hereditary hemochromatosis. *Gastroenterology* 2008; **135**: 1945–1952.

34 Beutler E, Felitti V, Koziol J, Ho N, Gelbart T. Penetrance of the 845G to A (C282Y) HFE hereditary haemochromatosis mutation in the USA. *Lancet* 2002; **359**: 211–218.

35 McLaren GD, McLaren C, Adams PC *et al.* Clinical manifestations of hemochromatosis in HFE C282Y homozygotes identified by screening. *Can J Gastro* 2008; **11**: 923–930.

36 Yamashita C, Adams PC. Natural history of the C282Y homozygote of the hemochromatosis gene (HFE) with a normal serum ferritin level. *Clinical Gastroenterology and Hepatology* 2003; **1**: 388–391.

37 Adams PC. Implications of genotyping of spouses to limit investigation of children in genetic hemochromatosis. *Clinical Genetics* 1998; **53**: 176–178.

38 Pietrangelo A. Non-HFE hemochromatosis. *Sem Liv Disease* 2005; **25**: 450–460.

39 Andersen R, Tybjaerg-Hansen A, Appleyard M, Birgens H, Nordestgaard B. Hemochromatosis mutations in the general population: iron overload progression rate. *Blood* 2004; **103**: 2914–2919.

40 Pankow J, Boerwinkle E, Adams PC *et al.* HFE C282Y homozygotes have reduced low-density lipoprotein cholesterol: the Atherosclerosis Risk in Communities (ARIC) Study. *Translational Research* 2008; **152**: 3–10.

41 Adams PC, Kertesz AE, Valberg LS. Rate of iron reaccumulation following iron depletion in hereditary hemochromatosis. Implications for venesection therapy. *J Clin Gastroenterol* 1993; **16**: 207–210.

42 Falize L, Guillygomarch A, Perrin M *et al.* Reversibility of hepatic fibrosis in treated genetic hemochromatosis: a study of 36 cases. *Hepatology* 2006; **44**: 472–477.

43 Powell L, Dixon J, Ramm G *et al.* Screening for hemochromatosis in asymptomatic subjects with or without a family history. *Arch Int Med* 2006; **166**: 294–301.

31 Wilson's disease

James S Dooley[1] and Aftab Ala[2]

[1]Centre for Hepatology, University College London Medical School (Royal Free Campus), University College London *and* the Royal Free Sheila Sherlock Liver Centre, Royal Free Hampstead NHS Trust, London, UK
[2]Centre for Gastroenterology, Hepatology and Nutrition, Department of Medicine, Frimley Park Hospital NHS Foundation Trust, Surrey, UK

Introduction

Wilson's disease (WD) is a rare autosomal recessive genetic disorder of copper metabolism. Mutations in the copper transporter ATP7B result in the accumulation of copper in the liver because excretion in bile is defective. Accumulation of copper in the body results in tissue damage which particularly affects the liver and brain so that patients present with either hepatic and/or neurological disease. The prevalence of Wilson's disease is between 1:30,000 and 1:100,000. It was first described as a clinical syndrome in 1912 by Dr Kinnier Wilson. Until the development of oral copper chelators in the 1950s by Dr John Walshe, WD was uniformly fatal. In the majority of patients treatment halts disease progression and allows reversal of organ dysfunction, such that patients, although needing lifelong treatment, usually return to a normal life.

The understanding of the molecular genetics, cellular biology and pathogenesis of WD has advanced over the last twenty years. However, there is still a lack of universal consensus on the optimal treatment regimen, which by implication means that several are effective. There are very few randomized or comparative studies of therapy and current recommendations are based predominantly on observational data published over the last 50 years.

There is no single diagnostic test and evidence-based examination of the diagnostic approach shows that a combination of features is best used. Certain features allow a confident straightforward diagnosis of WD; ruling out WD (particularly in those with liver disease) may be challenging. Clinical issues include delayed diagnosis and deterioration during treatment.

Evidence-Based Gastroenterology and Hepatology, 3rd edition.
J. McDonald, A.K. Burroughs, B. Feagan, and M.B. Fennerty. © 2010 Blackwell Publishing Ltd

Physiological copper metabolism

Around 40% of dietary copper (intake being approximately 2–5 mg/day) is absorbed in the duodenum and upper jejunum. Absorbed copper passes in the portal vein to the liver. The copper is taken up across the sinusoidal aspect of the hepatocyte via the copper transporter 1 (CTR1) (Figure 31.1). This transporter is essential for healthy development and is thought to be the main mammalian process for the uptake of copper into cells [1]. Copper is potentially toxic in the cytoplasm; glutathione and metallothioneins are thought to bind copper, rendering it non-toxic. Another protein (ATOX1) is thought to deliver copper to ATP7B by a copper-dependent protein – protein interaction [2]. ATP7B transports copper into the trans-Golgi where it is incorporated into apoceruloplasmin to produce holoceruloplasmin.

When hepatic copper levels are high, ATP7B is expressed in cytoplasmic vesicles, allowing excretion of copper into bile. This process involves COMMD1 (previously called MURR1), a protein which interacts directly with ATP7B [3]. Copper toxicosis of Bedlington Terriers, where there is deficient biliary copper excretion, is a result of mutations in COMMD1 [3]. Studies in non-Wilsonian copper storage disorders in humans have, to date, shown no abnormality in this protein [4].

The evidence for the normal function of ATP7B is based on studies of the trafficking of this protein between different cellular compartments in response to the concentration of copper [5]. In HepG2 hepatoma cells cultured in medium with a low copper concentration ATP7B localized to the trans-Golgi network. With increased levels of copper there is redistribution of APT7B to vesicles and thence to vacuoles. Immunohistochemical studies on human liver demonstrate punctuate immunoreactivity within the cell and localization also to the apical membrane adjacent to the bile canaliculus [6]. When the intracellular copper concentration is low or normal, ATP7B is found in the trans-Golgi

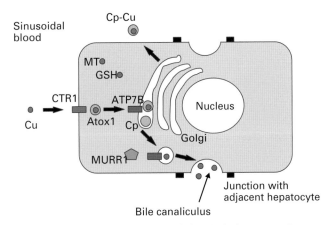

Figure 31.1 Pathways of copper metabolism in the hepatocyte. See text for explanation (Cu=copper, CTR1=copper transporter1. MT=metallothioneins. GSH=glutathione. Cp=ceruloplasmin.)
(reproduced with permission from Ala et al, Lancet 2007; **369**: 397–408)

network described above. With excess intracellular copper the ATP7B moves towards the canalicular pole of the hepatocyte.

Ceruloplasmin (Cp) is a member of the multi copper oxidase family of enzymes. It is also an acute phase protein. Cp itself is not essential for normal copper metabolism; it is for iron metabolism in which it is an important ferroxidase. It seems likely that the reason for the low Cp in WD is not the lack of hepatic expression of apoceruloplasmin (due to a low copper in the secretory pathway) but the change in the proportion of apo- to holoceruloplasmin in the circulation and the lower stability of apoceruloplasmin [7].

Molecular pathogenesis

In WD there are mutations in the ATP7B gene. This gene was identified by three groups in 1993 [8-11].

The ATP7B gene is highly expressed in the liver, kidney and placenta. It encodes a transmembrane ATPase which is a copper-dependent P type ATPase.

Mutations in ATP7B are associated with lack of entry of copper into bile and into the Golgi. This leads to hepatic copper accumulation which, depending on its severity, leads to hepatic and neurological features of WD.

Mutations within the ATP7B gene variously affect the function of the ATP7B protein. The H1069Q mutation (which results in histidine to glutamate substitution at amino acid 1069) is the most common mutation found in patients of European origin. Studies on liver tissue from patients homozygous for this mutation with WD show that the ATP7B resided in the endoplasmic reticulum rather than the trans-Golgi network [12]. This mutation is associ-

ated with defective phosphorylation of ATP7B by adenosine triphosphate (ATP). This finding parallels the fact that the histidine 1069 is in a conserved motif within the ATP binding domain of ATP7B [13].

Techniques are now available for the analysis of various APT7B mutations and show their effect on copper transport activity [14].

Molecular genetics

Phenotype/genotype relationship

Over 400 disease-related mutations in the ATP7B have been reported in WD (www.wilsondisease.med.ualberta.ca/database.aspdatabase). Most patients are compound heterozygotes. This makes phenotype/genotype correlation problematic.

In some populations, particular mutations predominate [15]. Because of this, screening of specific mutations may be fruitful. Thus, around 50–80% of patients with WD from Central, Eastern and Northern Europe carry at least one allele with the H1069Q mutation [15]. There is a wide range of mutations in the Mediterranean region and their frequency varies between different countries. In some countries, for example Sardinia and Spain, other particular mutations are common.

Studies of genotype/phenotype correlations of WD have been more made difficult by the large number of mutations that exist. Because of the prominence of the H1069Q mutation this has received most attention. Homozygosity for this mutation has been reported to correlate with late onset neurological disease in individual studies and in a meta-analysis [16]. There have been studies of genotype/phenotype associations with mutations in other genes but there is as yet no clinically applicable result [17].

Family screening using genetics

Family screening for WD is covered later in this chapter. Clinical and biochemical tests should be done, but molecular genetics with identification of mutations is an invaluable tool. If both mutations are known in the index patient with WD, testing of indeterminate siblings for the same mutations will define whether or not they are either affected, heterozygote carriers or normal.

Clinical manifestations

The clinical spectrum of manifestations of Wilson's disease is wide (Table 31.1). Patients can present acutely with liver failure, hemolysis or both. They may also present with chronic liver disease or neuro-psychiatric problems or a

Table 31.1 Clinical features of Wilson's disease.

Hepatic
Acute liver failure (+/– hemolysis)
Chronic hepatitis (persistent transaminitis)
Cirrhosis (compensated or decompensated)

Neurological
Tremor
Choreiform movements
Parkinsonian or akinetic rigid syndrome – i.e. partial Parkinsonism
Gait disturbances
Dysarthria
Pseudobulbar palsy
Rigid dystonia
Seizures
Migraine headaches
Insomnia

Ophthalmological
Kayser Fleischer rings
Sunflower cataracts

Psychiatric
Depression
Neuroses
Personality changes
Psychosis

Other manifestations
Renal tubular acidosis, aminoaciduria, nephrolithiasis
Skeletal

combination of the two. Patients who present initially with neurological or psychiatric features tend to be older than those who present with clinical manifestations of liver disease or hepatic decompensation.

Classically, WD is recognized as presenting most often in children and young adults, and indeed it had been considered that it did not occur in individuals aged more than 40 years. However, it is now recognized that later presentation does occur, with a recent report of neurological presentation in a group aged 40–52, and hepatic presentation at up to 58 years of age [18]. This emphasizes the need to have WD within the differential diagnosis of patients with unexplained liver disease and particular neurological symptoms presenting anywhere from teenage years to the fifth decade, and beyond.

Most patients with central nervous system involvement are believed to have liver disease at the time of presentation but they may not be symptomatic from their liver disease. However, hepatic histology is not generally available for these patients because the diagnosis is usually established solely on the basis of the presence of Kayser Fleischer rings with a decreased ceruloplasmin concentration.

It is generally the case that those presenting with acute liver disease, even in the younger age group, already have cirrhosis. Deterioration at this stage appears to be based upon the toxic effect of free copper causing decompensation of liver disease [19], or hemolysis [20].

Hepatic disease

Pathology

In the early stages of the disease, diffuse cytoplasmic copper accumulation can only be seen with special immunological stains detecting copper. These are not routinely available. The early accumulation of cytoplasmic copper is associated with macrosteatosis, microsteatosis and glycogenated nuclei.

Ultra structural abnormalities (on electron microscopy) include enlargement and separation of the mitochondrial inner and outer membranes, with widening of the intercrystal spaces, to increases in the density of granularity of the matrix, or presence of larger vacuoles. In the absence of cholestasis, these changes are regarded as pathognomonic of Wilson's disease.

These initial stages of WD progress to an intermediate stage which is characterized by periportal inflammation, mononuclear cellular infiltrates, erosion of the limiting plate, lobular necrosis and bridging fibrosis. These features may be indistinguishable from those of an autoimmune hepatitis [21, 22]. Mallory bodies are seen in up to 50% of liver biopsy specimens [23]. Cirrhosis almost invariably follows with either a micro-nodular or mixed macro-micro nodular pattern.

In patients with fulminant hepatic failure, parenchymal apoptosis, necrosis and collapse may be prominent, often, as already mentioned, on a background of cirrhosis [24]. One series of results of liver biopsy in WD showed cirrhosis in 54% of 83 patients with a hepatic presentation, and 41% in 34 with a neurological presentation [25].

Confirmation of excess copper histologically (rhodanine, rubeanic acid) may be helpful in diagnosis but if absent does not exclude Wilson's disease. The lack of immunoreactivity to copper binding protein (orcein stain) may occur because of the diffuse presence of copper in the cytoplasm and because of the stain's low sensitivity.

Clinical features

Wilson's disease can present as fulminant hepatic failure. There is worsening coagulopathy and encephalopathy. There may be an associated Coombs' negative hemolytic anemia, when there is a substantial increase in serum total and free copper as well as a high urinary copper concentration. This complication is recognized as potentially leading to renal failure. Around 5% of patients present in this manner [26], with most patients being in the second decade of life, when KF rings may not yet be formed. Almost all such patients already have cirrhosis, although some might show evidence of massive necrosis with only bridging fibrosis, which clearly would progress to cirrhosis with time. Concentration of serum alkaline phosphatase is frequently low and this feature has led to the suggestion that a ratio of alkaline phosphatase concentration (in IU/L) to serum bilirubin concentration (mg/dl) is diagnostically useful. A ratio of less than 2 [27, 28] or 4 [29], may be diagnostic or very suggestive of Wilsonian fulminant hepatic disease.

In those with a more chronic hepatic presentation, the clinical picture can be similar to other forms of chronic hepatitis, which, as already noted, emphasizes the need for WD to be in the differential diagnosis of such patients.

Some patients present with an asymptomatic cirrhosis. These would have the usual clinical features, including spider nevi, splenomegaly, portal hypertension and ascites. Cirrhosis may be well compensated.

Hepatocellular carcinoma is very rarely associated with Wilson's disease, but as in other causes of cirrhosis it may occur [30, 31]. In a series of 11 patients reported (from a total cohort of 363) there were cholangiocarcinomas (three cases) and malignancies of uncertain origin (three cases) as well as three hepatocellular carcinomas [30].

If neurological features occur in patients with liver disease, they usually do so 2–5 years later [32].

Eye changes

The classic finding in patients with WD is the Kayser Fleischer (KF) ring. KF rings are caused by the granular deposition of copper on the inner surface of the cornea in Descemet's membrane. They are most apparent at the periphery of the cornea. The upper pole is affected first. Although sometimes visible to the naked eye as a golden-brown ring on the periphery of the cornea, slit lamp examination by an experienced ophthalmologist is necessary to confirm the presence or absence of KF rings. Appearances indistinguishable from KF rings have also been seen in other forms of chronic liver disease, in particular chronic cholestasis, and cryptogenic cirrhosis [33].

Sunflower cataracts, also only visible by slit lamp examination, are brilliantly multi-coloured [34]. Interestingly, they do not impair vision.

Both of these findings disappear with successful medical therapy or after liver transplantation. The re-appearance in "the medically treated" patient suggests non-compliance with therapy [35].

Other less common ophthalmological findings include night blindness, exotropic strabismus, optic neuritis and optic disc pallor.

Neurological and neuro-psychiatric disease

Pathology

Histologically, there is an increase in astrocytes in the grey matter, associated with swollen glia, liquefaction, and appearances of spongiform degeneration. Neuronal loss is often accompanied by gliosis and active glial fibrillary protein. The characteristic astrocytes are Alzheimer type I and type II cells. Opalski cells are distinctive for WD [36]. These cells are thought to be derived from from degenerating astrocytes [37].

Clinical features

Neuropsychiatric signs are present in 40–50% of patients with WD [26].

The neurological changes have been classified as: (1) an akinetic-rigid syndrome similar to Parkinson's disease; (2) pseudosclerosis dominated by a tremor; (3) ataxia; and (4) a dystonic syndrome [38].

Subtle changes can appear before the characteristic neurological features. These include changes in behavior, deterioration of schoolwork or an inability to carry out activities that require good hand-eye coordination. There may be deterioration of hand writing and consequent micrographia – as in Parkinson's disease. Other neurological features include tremor, plasticity, lack of motor coordination, dysarthria, drooling and dystonia. Seizures, migraine, headaches and insomnia have also been reported. As well as behavioral changes already described, depression, anxiety and frank psychosis are seen [39].

Cognitive dysfunction in patients with WD may be present with neurological changes, often in the absence of detectable cortical changes or hepatic encephalopathy. This lends support to pathological changes of basal ganglia as being the primary cause in WD of cognitive deficit [40].

All patients with WD should have a neurological examination. Patients with obvious symptoms or signs need to be seen by a neurologist, preferably with a special interest in movement disorders, before treatment. A specific assessment tool with neurological features (based on that for Huntingdon's disease) has been used in clinical trials to assess patients [41]. However, a new Unified Wilson's Disease Rating Scale (UWDRS) has value in assessing disease severity [42].

Imaging

Structural brain MRI for WD has shown widespread lesions in the putamen, globus pallidus, caudate, thalamus, mid brain, pons and cerebellum as well as cortical atrophy and white matter changes. Broadly, these lesions show high signal intensity on T2 weighted images and low intensity on T1 scanning [43]. These changes tend to be more severe and widespread in patients with neurological WD [44], although MRI changes may be present in those without neurological symptoms or signs.

Other clinical changes

There may be bone and peri-articular abnormalities, including osteomalacia, osteoporosis, spontaneous fractures, adult rickets, osteoarthritis, osteochondritis dissecans, chondrocalcinosis, subchondrial cyst formation and azure lunulae of the fingernails. The most common sites for skeletal and articular abnormalities are the knee joints and spine [45]. Myocardial copper accumulation can cause cardiomyopathy and arrhythmias although these are clinically rare [46].

Other rare extra hepatic/neural manifestations include hypoparathyroidism, infertility, repeated miscarriages [47] and renal abnormalities [48], including renal tubular acidosis with aminoaciduria and nephrocalcinosis.

Diagnostic approach

Certain tests are essential when the possibility of WD has been raised. No single one of these on its own has 100% specificity or sensitivity for WD. A combination of features is necessary for a definitive diagnosis to be made [49].

The important observations or biochemical measurements used in the work-up of patients with suspected WD are: serum ceruloplasmin, serum total and free copper, ophthalmological examination (for KF rings); 24-hour urine excretion of copper, and measurement of liver copper content. One might add to this the presence of two mutations found on molecular analysis of the ATP7B gene, but since some of these may be polymorphisms caution is needed in making a diagnosis based on molecular analysis alone.

Other useful measures include: (1) urinary excretion of copper after penicillamine challenge (this test has been described and validated in the pediatric age group) [50]; (2) the presence of rhodamine staining on liver biopsy histology, if hepatic copper measurement has not been done.

There are potential problems with all the observations and measurements described above. Serum ceruloplasmin concentrations are well recognized to be normal in a proportion of patients presenting particularly with hepatic WD [51]. Urinary copper excretion can be increased in some other types of liver disease. The same is true for liver copper concentration, particularly in cholestatic disease.

However, if an individual with neurological symptoms consistent with Wilson's disease has Kayser Fleischer rings and a low serum ceruloplasmin concentration, the diagnosis is made. Kayser Fleischer rings are usually present in patients presenting with neurological Wilson's disease – 18 of 20 patients in one report [51].

In patients presenting with liver disease, diagnosis can be more difficult [51]. Roberts and Schilsky [49] have provided several valuable algorithms for the diagnostic approach for patients with different initial features suggesting WD. They provide specific recommendations on the basis of previous published work and the authors' experience in caring for pediatric and adult patients with WD.

To provide further help with the diagnostic route, Ferenci *et al.* [52] have proposed a scoring system (Table 31.2). Within this, clinical, biochemical, histological and molecular genetic data are allocated a score. The cumulative total gives an indication of the possibility of a particular individual having WD. This scoring system may be helpful if diagnosis of the disease is being considered [53]. The recent report of a group of pediatric patients as part of the analysis of the Euro Wilson's Group of patients gives some information on this scoring system [54].

Liver function tests

Serum aminotransferase activity is in general abnormal in WD except at a very early stage. The rise in aminotransferase activity is often mild and does not necessarily reflect the severity of liver disease.

The ratio of alkaline phosphatase to serum bilirubin in mg/dl has already been discussed. This may be valuable in raising the possibility of WD in patients with fulminant hepatic failure but again is not 100% specific and may only be valuable in particular patient groups [55].

Ceruloplasmin

A low serum ceruloplasmin concentration (normal range 0.2–0.5 g/l) should raise the question as to whether WD is a possible diagnosis. However, it should be emphasized that many patients presenting to a hepatology clinic can have a low ceruloplasmin, but in only a small fraction is WD diagnosed [56].

On the other hand, a low ceruloplasmin may be found in hypoproteinemic states due, for example, to the nephrotic syndrome, in copper deficient states (due to malabsorption) and in inherited diseases such as aceruloplasminemia [57]. In the latter two situations, the serum ceruloplasmin may be so low as to be undetectable by laboratory methods.

A normal serum ceruloplasmin in WD patients presenting with active liver disease is interpreted as due to an

Table 31.2 Proposed scoring system for diagnosis of Wilson's disease (from Ferenci et al, 2003; ref 52).

		Score
Clinical		
Kayser Fleischer rings (slit lamp exam)		
	present	2
	absent	0
Neuropsychiatric symptoms suggestive of WD (or typical MRI features)		
	present	2
	absent	0
Coombs' negative haemolytic anemia (plus high serum copper)		
	present	1
	absent	0
Laboratory results		
Urinary copper (in absence of acute hepatitis)		
	normal	0
	1–2x upper limit normal	1
	>2x upper limit normal	2
	normal but > 5x normal after D-penicillamine challenge (2x 0.5 gm)	2
Liver copper concentration		
	normal	−1
	up to 5x upper limit normal	1
	>5x upper limit normal	2
Rhodanine positive hepatocytes (only if quantitative Cu measurement not available)		
	absent	0
	present	1
Serum ceruloplasmin (nephelometric assay normal > 20 mg/dl)		
	Normal	0
	10–20	1
	<10	2
Mutation analysis		
Disease causing mutations		
	on both chromosomes	4
	on one chromosome	1
	none detected	0

Suggested likelihead of WD as diagnosis from cumulative score:	
4 or more:	highly likely
2–3:	probable, do more investigations
0–1:	Unlikely

acute phase reaction. The oral contraceptive may also falsely raise the ceruloplasmin.

A further confounding factor in the measurement of serum ceruloplasmin is the technique used. Most laboratories use an immunological reaction which measures both apo as well as holo ceruloplasmin. In WD it is the level in particular of holo ceruloplasmin which is low. This would be measured more accurately by a biological method (oxidase activity), but this method appears only to be used in a small number of laboratories. Thus, the technology used for measuring ceruloplasmin may be responsible for the finding of normal levels in some patients with Wilson's disease, and also the variability between laboratories [58].

Steindl *et al.* found in their group of hepatic patients, that serum ceruloplasmin (measured immunologically) was low in only 65% of patients, but in patients with neurological or neuropsychiatric presentation, low ceruloplasmin was found in 85% [51].

These findings indicate that if the serum ceruloplasmin is low then other investigations are necessary in order to define whether this is related to WD or not. Conversely, in patients in whom WD has been suspected but who have a normal ceruloplasmin, other tests are required to investigate this further.

Kayser Fleischer rings

Examination of the eyes using a slit lamp should be done by an experienced ophthalmologist. Steindl *et al.* found that Kayser Fleischer rings were found in 90% of patients with neurological and/or neuropsychiatric presentation and only 47% in those with hepatic disease [51]. Of ten asymptomatic siblings, only one had Kayser Fleischer rings.

Urinary excretion of copper

Urinary copper is derived from the so-called free "non-ceruloplasmin bound" copper within plasma. In Wilson's disease 24-hour urinary copper excretion is increased; the threshold taken suggestive of disease is greater than 1.6 μmol/24 hour (100 μg/24 hour) [51, 59, 60]. The reference limits for normal 24-hour excretion of copper varies between laboratories, with many taking 0.6 μmol/24 hour (40 μg per 24 hours) as the upper limit of normal.

This limit seems to be a better threshold for diagnosis because sensitivity of detection of WD is increased. Strict precautions during collection to avoid contamination are necessary. The interpretation of 24-hour urinary copper excretion can be difficult because increased copper excretion may be seen in other types of liver disease, especially where there is severe liver injury. In addition, heterozygotes may also have intermediate levels of copper excretion.

Urinary copper output following penicillamine challenge has been found to be a useful diagnostic adjunct, particularly in the pediatric age group. The protocol used has been the administration of 500 mg of d-penicillamine at the start and again twelve hours later during a 24-hour urine collection. A copper excretion greater than 25 μmol/24 hours (1600 μg/24 hours) has been regarded as diagnostic for pediatric Wilson's disease [61]. The penicillamine challenge test for urinary copper excretion has been studied in adults and may been useful but less diagnostically so than in children [62]. **B4**

Hepatic copper concentration

Accurate measurement of the liver copper concentration needs an adequate sample of liver biopsy (at least 1 cm of a 1.6 mm diameter core) [49]. The normal copper content of liver is less than 55 μg per gram dry weight. A hepatic copper concentration greater than 250 μg/gm dry weight is usual in homozygous WD. With some caveats this remains the best biochemical test for WD. Thus, the measurement of copper content in the liver is the most valuable diagnostic test in patients in whom other data are inconclusive. A normal liver copper concentration on an adequate sample of liver rules out Wilson's disease.

Diagnosis is sometimes only considered after liver biopsy has been done and when a sample has not been taken for copper estimations. Under these circumstances quantitative copper measurement can be done from tissue retrieved from paraffin blocks.

There has been discussion about the value of a liver copper measurement between 250 μg/gm dry weight and the upper limit of the normal range of 55 μg/gm dry weight. Values within this range do not exclude or define WD. Therefore results of hepatic copper concentration have to be taken in the context of the histological, clinical and biochemical data [63]. Specimens of liver with extensive fibrosis and few parenchymal cells may provide copper concentrations that are falsely low. Conversely, hepatic copper concentrations can be increased in patients with cholestasis, which may provide further confusion during the diagnostic work up.

Molecular genetic analysis

Mutation analysis of ATP7B in individuals with a suspected diagnosis of Wilson's disease can be done to identify ATP7B mutations. Patients with neurological or hepatic disease sometimes have abnormalities of copper metabolism which do not reach the level of secure diagnosis for WD. For such individuals mutation analysis of ATP7B may be helpful. The finding of two mutations or homozygosity for a single mutation would be highly suggestive of the presence of WD. However, these data should be used in combination with the other clinical data. It is not yet known whether 100% of individuals carrying a mutation in the ATP7B gene on each chromosome 13 will develop WD if left untreated. A recent report suggests that this assumption may be challenged [64].

Family screening using genetics

First degree relatives (siblings) must be screened for Wilson's disease. The probability of a sibling of an index case having WD is 25% and in their children approximately 0.5% (based on an estimated carrier frequency of 1 in 90). Screening should include liver function tests, serum ceruloplasmin and copper concentration, and urinary copper excretion. Depending on the outcome of these investigations, it may be necessary to have ophthalmological examination for KF rings and liver copper estimation.

Previously, haplotype analysis was done to identify siblings at risk. This involved using markers flanking the gene on chromosome 13 to be characterized so that it was then possible to identify siblings who had inherited the same two disease carrying chromosomes.

Molecular genetic analysis for mutations is now becoming more widely available. This will be useful for families in whom both mutations have been detected in the index patient, so that the presence or absence of these can be analysed in siblings. Siblings with a slightly low ceruloplasmin but without KF rings could be affected or carriers. Molecular genetic analysis is an alternative to hepatic copper quantitation to define their clinical status.

Parents of a child with WD have at least to be heterozygote carriers for this condition. Clinicians need to be alert to the rare possibility that one of the two parents is also affected.

Children of patients with WD are obligate heterozygote carriers. However, there is a 1 in 90 chance of the spouse being a carrier, which would result in a 50:50 chance of the child being susceptible. Thus, usually WD patients wish to know whether or not their children are affected. Children may be evaluated using biochemical tests (see below) and also, potentially, genetic screening. There is no evidence base for either approach and recommendations vary between specialists in this condition.

Treatment

The majority of patients with WD are treated with copper chelators which promote copper excretion in the urine. An alternative approach in selected patients is zinc therapy, which results in reduced copper absorption (Table 31.3).

For patients with fulminant liver failure due to WD, or in those with hepatic decompensation unresponsive to medical treatment, liver transplantation is done (see later).

Wilson's disease is rare. It follows that there are very few randomized studies of therapy and therefore the evidence for the use of different therapeutic approaches is based upon publications describing the outcome in series of patients treated with particular regimens.

Table 31.3 Treatment options for Wilson's disease.

Therapy	Mode of action	Pros	Cons	Notes
Penicillamine	Copper chelator • urinary excretion	Long experience Successful in majority of patients	Frequency of side effects • immunological • neutropenia • proteinuria • neurological deterioration	Used by many units despite side effects Need strategy if neurological or hepatic deterioration Efficacy reported in all patient groups
Trientine	Copper chelator • urinary excretion	Less experience than with d-penicillamine Most reported experience in patients intolerant of d-pen transferred to trientine Growing experience as first-line treatment	Some side effects but much fewer than d-penicillamine. Neurological deterioration reported but appears less than d-penicillamine Storage necessary in refrigerator (2–8°C)	Limited data as first-line treatment But increasing use as first-line treatment
Zinc salts	Induces metallothionein • reduces absorption	Few side effects Extent of experience mainly in asymptomatic and neurological patients	Speed of action Gastric intolerance in some patients (change formulation)	Initial treatment reported for asymptomatic/neurological disease; less data for hepatic Has been used post chelator as maintenance therapy
Tetrathiomolybdate	Copper chelator • reduces absorption • biliary excretion	Randomized study suggests low rate of neurological deterioration	Not generally available Some side effects	Investigational Need source for study and use
Albumin dialysis, MARS, plasmapheresis	Removes free copper and other toxins	Bridge to liver transplantation in acute liver failure/hemolysis	Not formally evaluated but case reports of success	Investigational but needs to be considered in acute liver failure/hemolysis
Liver transplantation	Replaces liver	Successful 80–90% Corrects metabolic defect (no WD treatment required) Life-saving	Timing Availability of donor	Only hope in certain patients

Wilson's disease was progressive and uniformly fatal until 1951, when the first chelating agent dimercaprol given intramuscularly was used. The clinical benefit of the orally active chelator penicillamine was reported by Dr John Walshe in 1956 [65]. This revolutionized treatment of the disease. Because some patients could not tolerate penicillamine, Walshe also developed trientine, another copper chelator, which was introduced in 1969 [66]. D penicillamine and trientine have remained the mainstay of chelation therapy. Ammonium tetrathiomolybdate (TTM), a copper chelator used for treating copper poisoning in animals, has been used historically and has been under investigation in the USA, particularly for treatment of patients with neurological disease [67].

Oral zinc therapy was first used in treatment in the early 1960s. It has been further studied particularly in Holland and the USA and as initial therapy has mainly been used for asymptomatic and pre-symptomatic patients. It has also been used as maintenance therapy after an initially period of treatment with a chelator [68].

Historically, the treatment of choice has been penicillamine. This drug does, however, have a range of side effects (see below) and there may be neurological deterioration in some patients after treatment is initiated. These issues have led to the suggestion that trientine may be an effective and safer alternative as initial treatment.

After chelation therapy, usually until clinical improvement has occurred, subsequent maintenance therapy may either be with a reduced dose of chelator or alternatively zinc monotherapy. This choice depends on local experience, expertise and opinion.

Opinions differ as to the rationale and efficacy of treating with both chelator and zinc. These have to be given at separate times; taken together the activity of both would be expected to be compromised. The coordination of combination therapy thus needs very close control, which may be possible as an inpatient, but may suffer from compliance issues with timing at home.

Penicillamine

Penicillamine is cysteine, doubly substituted with methyl groups. Copper is chelated by a free sulphydryl group. After oral administration 40–70% is absorbed and is bioavailable. More than 80% of the penicillamine absorbed is excreted in urine carrying with it chelated copper. Penicillamine may also induce metallothionein, a cysteine rich protein and endogenous chelator of metal.

Food reduces absorption by approximately 50%. Guidelines state that it is important that penicillamine is taken at least one hour before or two hours after eating, that is on an empty stomach [49]. However, Walshe has pointed out that studies with radioactive copper show better mobilization of copper when given before meals not after [69] and that penicillamine should always be given before meals. The target dose of penicillamine is 1000–1500 mg per day taken in 2–4 divided doses. **B4** Because of the concern of side effects, guidelines have recommended starting with a lower dose (250–500 mg per day) increasing by increments over several weeks [49]. This approach may increase tolerance to penicillamine. During the introduction of treatment it is necessary to monitor full blood count and urinary protein (using dipstix) regularly.

Adverse effects to penicillamine occur in 10–20% of patients and may be severe enough to necessitate withdrawal of the drug [37]. Side effects in the first 1–3 weeks include sensitivity reactions, with fever, rash, lymphadenopathy, neutropenia, thrombocytopenia and proteinuria [37]. If there are early immune side effects penicillamine should be discontinued immediately. Historically, reintroduction with steroid coadministration was used. However, with the availability of trientine, it seems more logical to withdraw penicillamine and introduce treatment with trientine, which has fewer side effects.

Later side effects of penicillamine include nephrotoxicity (a lupus-like syndrome) and bone marrow suppression (aplasia, thrombocytopenia).

Long-term use of penicillamine has been associated with skin complications, including progeriatric changes, elastosis perforans serpiginosa, and aphthous stomatitis [37]. Progeriatric changes are reported to occur with long-term

doses greater than 1000 mg a day – a reason for reducing to the maintenance dose as soon as feasible.

Penicillamine may affect pyridoxine metabolism. Supplementation (25–50 mg of vitamin B6 daily) is often prescribed, although the rationale is questionable [49]. Prescription is thought most important for groups at risk, in particular children, pregnant women and patients with malnutrition [70].

Data from Walshe in the UK, and Sternlieb and Scheinberg in the USA have documented the clinical benefit of penicillamine in Wilson's disease [37, 71]. **B4** Hepatic function usually improves in patients with severe liver disease – that is those with high bilirubin, low albumin or prolonged prothrombin time with ascites or high Child Turcott score. If patients deteriorate, the decision is whether to have a trial with a higher dose of penicillamine or consider working the patient up for liver transplantation.

In patients with WD and neurological changes, clinical and cerebral MRI improvement has been well documented [43]. Some studies [71, 72] report initial neurological deterioration in 20–50% of patients with a neurological presentation. In some cases this deterioration does not reverse [72].

Trientine

Trientine has a polyamine structure. The copper is chelated by the formation of stable complexes with four constituent nitrogens in a planar ring. Although widely regarded as a weaker chelator of copper than penicillamine, Walshe has shown that as an initial treatment trientine may result in urinary copper excretion similar to that of penicillamine [73].

The initial dose of trientine is 1200–1800 mg per day in 2–3 divided doses. Again, it is critical for trientine to be taken at least one hour before, or two hours after food. In addition, it is critical to keep trientine refrigerated at around 4°C, since at room temperature over time, or higher temperatures, it becomes inactive. The maintenance dose of trientine is 900–1200 mg per day.

There are few reported side effects of trientine. Pancytopenia occurs rarely, and hypersensitive reactions and renal effects have not been reported. If copper deficiency develops because of excessive treatment with trientine, sideroblastic anemia and hepatic siderosis may occur. Neurological deterioration after treatment with trientine has been reported [74]; data suggest that this is less frequent than with penicillamine, but no direct comparisons have been made.

There are few data on the outcome with initial treatment with trientine in those with liver disease. Askari et al. [75] reported nine adults with severe liver disease identified over a ten-year period treated initially with trientine (1000 mg per day) in combination with zinc (150 mg per day). One of the nine patients had hepatic encephalopathy. During treatment one patient developed mild neurological symptoms and was transferred to TTM and zinc. The remaining eight patients received trientine and zinc for at least four months. This was followed with maintenance zinc therapy. During the first twelve months of treatment prothrombin time, bilirubin and albumin concentrations were reported to return to normal and ascites disappeared. Over a follow-up of between twelve months and fourteen years, the benefit was maintained.

In one of the few randomized trials to have been done in WD, the efficacy of TTM was compared with trientine (both agents combined with zinc) in a series of patients with neurological Wilson's disease [74]. **A1d** In those treated with TTM 1 of 27 patients had neurological deterioration. This compared with 5 of 27 patients in the trientine group. As already pointed out, at present TTM is not available for routine prescription.

Results using trientine, mainly as a substitute for penicillamine after intolerance, have recently been reported in the pediatric age group and efficacy was shown [54]. **B4**

There is evidence now for the effectiveness of trientine in the treatment of patients with WD. Overall there are fewer side effects than with penicillamine and guidelines are now suggesting that trientine can be regarded as an acceptable alternative to penicillamine for initial treatment [49].

Ammonium tetrathiomolybdate (TTM)

This drug forms a complex with copper and protein. When taken with meals these complexes are formed in the food and copper is excreted in stool. Thus, absorption is prevented. If TTM is taken between meals it is absorbed and complexes copper in blood with albumin. These complexes are metabolized by the liver and excreted in the bile [67].

As already noted, TTM is not currently available in England and only in investigational studies in the USA. The randomized trial of TTM against trientine has been referred to in the section on trientine [74]. **A1d** This study suggests that it is associated with less neurological deterioration. Three patients in the TTM group developed anemia or leucopenia; four had increased transaminases. These side effects resolved on dose reduction. More data are required to confirm the benefit of TTM, and it is unfortunate that this agent is not more widely available for study.

Zinc

Oral zinc induces metallothionein in the intestinal cells which will then preferentially bind to intracellular copper in the duodenal enterocytes. Copper absorption is reduced. A small amount of copper is lost normally in the urine and therefore without copper absorption there is negative copper balance.

The therapeutic dose of zinc in adults is 150 mg of elemental zinc. This is given in three divided doses. Since food interferes with absorption, zinc must be taken one hour before meals and more than two hours after meals, otherwise food would interfere with absorption. Untoward effects of zinc include dyspepsia. The timing of administration and different formulations, for example acetate, gluconate or sulphate may help.

Zinc has been reported as being therapeutically successful as a form of treatment in asymptomatic, pre-symptomatic affected family members of index cases with WD [68]. **B4**

In a group of patients with predominantly neurological WD followed up for a mean of twelve years Czlonkowska *et al.* reported that zinc was equally effective as penicillamine in their treatment [76]. **B4**

In patients with severe hepatic disease due to Wilson's disease, maintenance therapy with zinc after initial treatment with trientine was found to be effective [75].

Vitamin E

Copper toxicity in part is due to lipid peroxidation of mitochondrial and other membranes. Experimentally this can be reduced by the administration of vitamin E, the levels of which may be lower in patients with WD [77]. Although currently, however, there is no evidence base to substantiate routine administration of vitamin E in patients with Wilson's disease, it may have a place in those with severe disease.

Diet

Some foods contain a high concentration of copper and the recommendation has been in guidelines that they are generally best avoided [49]. Foods involved include chocolate, liver, nuts, mushrooms and shell fish.

Current choice of medical treatment

Virtually all the data on the treatment options of WD are from clinical series of patients with only one randomized study in those with predominantly neurological disease [74]. Thus, strict recommendations (Table 31.4) are difficult and are predominantly dependent upon reported clinical series from specialist centers.

The choice between treatments depends upon the balance between their efficacy and their side effects. The evidence available shows that treatments available for Wilson's disease are effective for most patients. Clinical deterioration has been reported or alluded to in reviews for all treatments. Thus, none is reliably effective.

Table 31.4 Considerations when choosing treatment for WD.

Initial treatment

General principles
- Take advice if not experienced.
- Monitor closely for therapeutic effects and side effects.
- Have an alternative strategy if side effects/deterioration despite treatment.

Hepatic presentation (compensated)
- Trientine monotherapy appears acceptable and efficacious alternative to penicillamine. Zinc not used because of speed of therapeutic effect.
- Monitor liver function closely.

Acute liver failure
- Refer to liver transplant centre.
- May introduce chelator, vitamin E, nutrition.
- Calculate risk score (see text) on which to determine transplant listing.

Neurological presentation
- Review by movement disorder neurologist.
- Cerebral MRI.
- Chelators usually effective, but deterioration may occur (see text)
- Have strategy if deterioration with treatment.

Pre-symptomatic WD
- Use of chelator or monotherapy with zinc: experience with both.
- If not conversant, liase with WD specialist.

Maintenance therapy (after clinical stabilization with initial treatment)
- Either reduce dose of chelator, or introduce zinc monotherapy.
- With both approaches close monitoring of patient (clinical symptoms and signs, LFTs, free Cu, urinary copper, KF rings).
- Watch for non-compliance (true for all phases of treatment).

Confounding issues evaluating treatments are that patients commence with different phases and patterns of clinical disease. In addition it is not always clear whether there has been treatment failure or lack of compliance.

Although penicillamine in many units remains the first choice of chelator for symptomatic patients, trientine has shown to be effective with fewer side effects. Combined chelation treatment with zinc has been used apparently with success but it is important to emphasize that there must be sufficient separation between taking of chelators and zinc.

For asymptomatic patients, although publications have suggested that zinc therapy is sufficient [68], patients in this group have also been treated with chelators successfully for many years.

There is no evidence or data to show whether for maintenance therapy, reduction of the dose of chelators is any less or more effective than zinc therapy alone.

For patients with hepatic disease who deteriorate despite what appears to be adequate treatment, and who are compliant with treatment, liver transplantation is a successful option. However, in patients with neurological deterioration the choices are more difficult.

Attempts to identify patients with a risk of neurological progression have been made. Studies of brain MRI changes may give hints [78], but evidence for a particular pattern being useful has not been substantiated.

Various approaches have been used to try and reduce the chance of neurological deterioration. Lower initial doses of chelators with gradual step-wise increase over the subsequent weeks have been suggested [49]. However, there is no evidence to suggest that this reduces the risk of neurological deterioration. In another report chelator was withdrawn temporarily, and subsequently reintroduced at a lower dose [78]. In a small number of patients this was thought to contribute to subsequent successful treatment.

As discussed earlier, data suggests that TTM is a useful initial treatment option with a lower risk of neurological deterioration [74, recently reviewed in 79].

In patients who deteriorate neurologically despite treatment with penicillamine, intramuscular use of dimercaprol has been associated with improvement [80].

Monitoring

Clinical review of symptoms, signs and laboratory tests of liver disease are necessary at an interval appropriate to the severity of disease at the start of treatment. Similarly, neurological assessment ideally by a movement disorder neurologist should be done.

Measurements of serum copper and ceruloplasmin as well as 24-hour urinary copper excretion are valuable in showing reduction in free copper levels by treatment. They are also useful in showing whether there is compliance with medication.

The accepted target for non-ceruloplasmin bound copper is 5–15 µg/dl. The accurate calculation of non-ceruloplasmin bound copper (see below) is difficult since ceruloplasmin is almost universally measured immunologically. The problem with this method is discussed earlier. In addition, laboratories may report ceruloplasmin levels as being undetectable (<0.04 g/l, for example). It cannot be assumed however that there is no ceruloplasmin present. Estimation of free copper depends upon calculating the copper contained in the serum ceruloplasmin (3 µg/mg) and subtracting this from the total serum copper, after adjustment of the units (µg to µmol, dl to l, or vica-versa) as necessary (mol wt copper 63) [81].

The non-ceruloplasmin bound copper is an important measure in monitoring patients. It is also useful to see the total serum copper falling with treatment. However, low levels may raise the question of whether there is copper deficiency due to therapy.

A 24-hour urine copper measurements should also be done. During chelation therapy an output of 3–8 μmol/l (200–500 μg) denotes adequate treatment. Whether there is any advantage in measuring urinary copper after temporarily stopping chelating treatment for 48–72 hours is not evidence based. However, proponents of this approach would argue that copper excretion off treatment will give an indication of whether copper deficiency is occurring (when there will be low 24-hour urinary copper).

In some patients after years of treatment the 24-hour urine copper is surprisingly high. One explanation is that the patient restarts chelator after a period of non-compliance.

In patients taking oral zinc, urinary output of zinc as well as copper are measured. Twenty-four hour urinary zinc output of at least 2 mg per 24 hours has been suggested as indicative of a therapeutic level which would control copper metabolism in Wilson's disease [82]. If urinary zinc excretion on 150 mg of oral elemental zinc per day is not in this range, then questions regarding compliance, timing of treatment and formulation have to be raised. The dose of oral zinc can be adjusted in order to bring the urinary output of zinc in 24 hours into this "therapeutic" range.

Prognosis

Long-term studies of survival in WD are difficult to interpret, and indeed the introduction of liver transplantation has improved outcome for those severely affected by liver disease. In a recent report of the cause of death in WD, the importance of early diagnosis is noted; delayed diagnosis was the principal cause of death, and the risk from poor compliance with treatment was emphasized [83].

Pregnancy

A review of treatments used for WD in pregnancy has concluded that penicillamine, trientine and zinc are not associated with increased maternal or foetal risk when used during pregnancy [84]. Cessation of treatment has been associated with development of fulminant liver failure [85], and therefore compliance with treatment is important during pregnancy. It has been recommended that the dose of chelators be reduced during pregnancy, particularly the last trimester [49, 84]. The dose of zinc treatment is recommended to be maintained [49].

Salvage treatment/bridge to transplantation in fulminant liver failure

Patients with WD may present with acute liver failure, often with hemolysis. Although listing for liver transplantation can be done immediately there may be a delay before a donor organ is available. For such patients case reports of plasma exchange, single pass albumin dialysis and MARS therapy have been published and reported in some cases to be beneficial [86–90]. Despite lack of clear evidence base, these approaches need to be considered as a potential life-saving bridge to liver transplantation.

Liver transplantation

Liver transplantation is indicated for patients with acute fulminant hepatic failure (FHF) from WD. It is also indicated for patients with WD in whom medical therapy is ineffectual as defined by a failure to stabilize and prevent progressive hepatic insufficiency. This group includes a subset of who have neurological as well as hepatic disease, but the hepatic symptoms are predominant.

Transplantation of these individuals can be achieved by cadaveric donor [91–93] or living donor liver transplant [94], even if the donor is a heterozygous carrier.

One-year survival rates are 87–90% [91–94], results which compare well with those for other patient groups. The metabolic defect is corrected.

Scoring methods based on clinical features have an important role in the decision to list for transplantation. For children, the King's system uses serum bilirubin, international normalized ratio (INR), aspartate transaminase (AST) and white cell count at presentation [95]. A cutoff score of eleven gave a positive predictive value of 88% for death, and prospective evaluation in 14 patients predicted the need for transplantation. In adults the same scoring system performs well in predicting response to medical therapy in patients with decompensated chronic WD [96].

The clinical dilemmas in patients not responding to medical therapy are how to decide on the duration of an adequate treatment trial, and what is a true failure of medical therapy, so as to aid the decision to transplant. Given the lag between the initiation of treatment and measurable, objective clinical and laboratory response, which may be up to 6–8 weeks, the previous recommended interval for a medical trial was three months. While this three-month period is not an absolute requirement since some will deteriorate before this time has elapsed, careful observation is critical to detect those individuals for whom transplant may be more urgently needed. If the patient can be stabilized over this time period, there is at least hope for the long-term utilization of medical therapy and avoidance of transplantation.

Individuals with long-standing neurological impairment from WD are unlikely to recover after transplantation, although improvement in severe neurological disease has been reported. In this group of patients the indication for transplantation must be considered carefully. The decision of whether to choose transplantation rather than medical treatment is complicated because of the significantly long period of time (up to four years) over which neurologically affected patients may improve whilst on medical therapy. The problem is that the time needed to determine whether medical treatment for neurological disease has failed, is probably longer than the window of opportunity for transplant to have prevented progression.

Summary

(1) WD is rare, but an essential disorder to consider in patients with liver and/or neurological disease, since without treatment the condition is fatal.

(2) Once considered as a potential diagnosis, a group of clinical and laboratory investigations should be done. No investigation is 100% specific on its own. Diagnosis depends upon a combination of findings. A published scoring system has been proposed. Liver copper concentration is a gold standard. Mutation analysis of ATP7B, the gene involved, is more widely available as a clinical tool, and can play an important part in diagnosis.

(3) Screening of siblings of patients with WD is mandatory.

(4) Treatment of WD is based on a copper chelator (penicillamine or treintine), or zinc which inhibits absorption of copper. All may be effective but the clinical features of the patient are relevant to the choice. There is no universal consensus on a standard therapy.

(5) For patients with acute liver failure, liver transplantation is effective. A clinical scoring system aids selection for transplantation particularly in children.

(6) Supportive therapy for patients with acute liver failure/acute hemolysis includes plasmapheresis, albumin dialysis and MARS, as a bridge to transplantation, but there is no definitive evidence base for this.

References

1 Lee J, Prohaska JR, Thiele DJ. Essential role for mammalian copper transporter Ctr1 in copper homeostasis and embryonic development. *Proc Natl Acad Sci USA* 2001; **98**: 6842–6847.

2 van Dongen EM, Klomp LW, Merkx M. Copper-dependent protein-protein interactions studied by yeast two-hybrid analysis. *Biochem Biophys Res Commun* 2004; **323**: 789–795.

3 Tao TY, Liu F, Klomp L, Wijmenga C *et al.* The copper toxicosis gene product Murr1 directly interacts with the Wilson disease protein. *J Biol Chem* 2003; **278**: 41593–41596.

4 Coronado VA, Bonneville JA, Nazer H *et al.* COMMD1 (MURR1) as a candidate in patients with copper storage disease of undefined etiology. *Clin Genet* 2005; **68**: 548–551.

5 Roelofsen H, Wolters H, Van Luyn MJ *et al.* Copper-induced apical trafficking of ATP7B in polarized hepatoma cells provides a mechanism for biliary copper excretion. *Gastroenterology* 2000; **119**: 782–793.

6 Schaefer M, Roelofsen H, Wolters H, *et al.* Localization of the Wilson's disease protein in human liver. *Gastroenterology* 1999; **117**: 1380–1385.

7 Hellman NE, Gitlin JD. Ceruloplasmin metabolism and function. *Annu. Rev. Nutr* 2002; **22**: 439–458.

8 Frydman M, Bonne-Tamir B, Farrer LA *et al.* Assignment of the gene for Wilson disease to chromosome 13: linkage to the esterase D locus. *Proc Natl Acad Sci USA* 1985; **82**: 1819–1821.

9 Bull PC, Thomas GR, Rommens JM *et al.* The Wilson disease gene is a putative copper transporting P-type ATPase similar to the Menkes gene. *Nat Genet* 1993; **5**: 327–337.

10 Tanzi RE, Petrukhin K, Chernov I, *et al.* The Wilson disease gene is a copper transporting ATPase with homology to the Menkes disease gene. *Nat Genet* 1993; **5**: 344–350.

11 Yamaguchi Y, Heiny ME, Gitlin JD. Isolation and characterization of a human liver cDNA as a candidate gene for Wilson disease. *Biochem Biophys Res Commun* 1993; **197**(1): 271–277.

12 Huster D, Hoppert M, Lutsenko S *et al.* Defective cellular localization of mutant ATP7B in Wilson's disease patients and hepatoma cell lines. *Gastroenterology* 2003; **124**: 335–345.

13 Tsivkovskii R, Efremov RG, Lutsenko S. The role of the invariant His-1069 in folding and function of the Wilson's disease protein, the human copper-transporting ATPase ATP7B. *J Biol Chem* 2003; **278**: 13302–13308.

14 His G, Cullen LM, Macintyre G *et al.* Sequence variation in the ATP-transport domain of the Wilson disease transporter, ATP7B, affects copper transport in a yeast model system. *Hum Mutat* 2008; **29**: 491–501.

15 Ferenci P. Regional distribution of mutations of the ATP7B gene in patients with Wilson disease: impact on genetic testing. *Hum Genet* 2006; **120**: 151–159.

16 Stapelbroek JM, Bollen CW, van Amstel JK *et al.* The H1069Q mutation in ATP7B is associated with late and neurologic presentation in Wilson disease: results of a meta-analysis. *J Hepatol* 2004; **41**: 758–763.

17 Schiefermeier M, Kollegger H, Madl C *et al.* The impact of apolipoprotein E genotypes on age at onset of symptoms and phenotypic expression in Wilson's disease. *Brain* 2000; **123**: 585–590.

18 Ferenci P, Czlonkowska A, Merle U *et al.* Late-onset Wilson's disease. *Gastroenterology* 2007; **132**: 1294–1298.

19 Gu M, Cooper JM, Butler P *et al.* Oxidative-phosphorylation defects in liver of patients with Wilson's disease. *Lancet* 2000; **356**: 469–474.

20 McIntyre N, Clink HM, Levi AL *et al.* Hemolytic anemia in Wilson's disease. *N Engl J Med* 1967; **276**: 439–444.

21 Schilsky ML, Scheinberg IH, Sternlieb I. Prognosis of Wilsonian chronic active hepatitis. *Gastroenterology* 1991; **100**: 762–767.

22 Scott J, Gollan JL, Samourian S, Sherlock S. Wilson's disease presenting as chronic active hepatitis. *Gastroenterology* 1978; **74**: 645–651.

23 Muller T, Langner C, Fuchsbichler A *et al.* Immunohistochemical analysis of Mallory bodies in Wilsonian and non-Wilsonian hepatic copper toxicosis. *Hepatology* 2004; **39**(4): 963–969.

24 Strand S, Hofmann WJ, Grambihler A *et al.* Hepatic failure and liver cell damage in acute Wilson's disease involve CD95 (APO-1/Fas) mediated apoptosis. *Nat Med* 1998;**4**:588–93.

25 Ferenci P (2006) Wilson disease. In: Bacon BR, O'Grady JG, Di Bisceglie AM , Lake JR, eds. *Comprehensive Clinical Hepatology*, 2nd edn. St Louis, Mosby, 351–367.

26 Walshe JM. Wilson's disease. The presenting symptoms. *Arch Dis Child* 1962; **37**: 253–256.

27 Tissieres P, Chevret L, Debray D *et al.* Fulminant Wilson's disease in children: appraisal of a critical diagnosis. *Pediatr Crit Care Med* 2003 Jul; **4**(3): 338–343.

28 Sallie R, Katsiyiannakis L, Baldwin D *et al.* Failure of simple biochemical indexes to reliably differentiate fulminant Wilson's disease from other causes of fulminant liver failure. *Hepatology* 1992; **16**: 1206–1211.

29 Korman JD, Volenberg I, Balko J *et al.* Screening for Wilson's disease in acute liver failure: a comparison of currently available diagnostic tests. *Hepatology* 2008; **48**: 1167–1174.

30 Walshe JM, Waldenstrom E, Sams V *et al.* Abdominal malignancies in patients with Wilson's disease. *QJM* 2003; **96**(9): 657–662.

31 Wilkinson ML, Portmann B, Williams R. Wilson's disease and hepatocellular carcinoma: possible protective role of copper. *Gut* 1983; **24**(8): 767–771.

32 Medici V, Mirante VG, Fassati LR *et al.* Monotematica AISF 2000 OLT Study Group. Liver transplantation for Wilson's disease: The burden of neurological and psychiatric disorders. *Liver Transpl* 2005; **11**(9): 1056–1063.

33 Frommer D, Morris J, Sherlock S *et al.* Kayser-Fleischer-like rings in patients without Wilson's disease. *Gastroenterology* 1977; **72**(6): 1331–1335.

34 Cairns JE, Williams HP, Walshe JM. "Sunflower cataract" in Wilson's disease. *Br Med J* 1969; **3**: 95–96.

35 Schilsky ML, Scheinberg IH, Sternlieb I. Liver transplantation for Wilson's disease: indications and outcome. *Hepatology* 1994; **19**: 583–587.

36 Opalski A. Type special de cellules neurologiques dans la degenerescence lenticulaire progressive. *Z Gesamte Neurol Psychiatrie* 1930: **124**: 420.

37 Scheinberg IH, Sternlieb I. *Wilson's Disease*. WB Saunders, Philadelphia, 1984.

38 Svetel M, Kozic D, Stefanova E *et al.* Dystonia in Wilson's disease. *Mov Disord* 2001; **16**: 719–723.

39 Oder W, Grimm G, Kollegger H *et al.* Neurological and neuropsychiatric spectrum of Wilson's disease: a prospective study of 45 cases. *J Neurol* 1991; **238**: 281–287.

40 Medalia A, Galynker I, Scheinberg IH. The interaction of motor, memory, and emotional dysfunction in Wilson's disease. *Biol Psychiatry* 1992; **31**: 823–826.

41 Siesling S, Zwinderman AH, van Vugt JP *et al.* A shortened version of the motor section of the Unified Huntington's Disease Rating Scale. *Mov Disord* 1997; **12**: 229–234.

42 Leinweber B, Möller JC, Scherag A *et al.* Evaluation of the Unified Wilson's Disease Rating Scale (UWDRS) in German patients with treated Wilson's disease. *Mov Disord* 2008; **23**: 54–62.

43 King AD, Walshe JM, Kendall BE *et al.* Cranial MR imaging in Wilson's disease. *Am J Roentgenol* 1996; **167**: 1579–1584.

44 Kozic D, Svetel M, Petrovic B *et al.* MR imaging of the brain in patients with hepatic form of Wilson's disease. *Eur J Neurol* 2003; **10**: 587–592.

45 Golding DN, Walshe JM. Arthropathy of Wilson's disease. Study of clinical and radiological features in 32 patients. *Ann Rheum Dis* 1977; **36**: 99–111.

46 Factor SM, Cho S, Sternlieb I *et al.* The cardiomyopathy of Wilson's disease. Myocardial alterations in nine cases. *Virchows Arch A Pathol Anat Histol* 1982; **397**: 301–311.

47 Sinha S, Taly AB, Prashanth LK *et al.* Successful pregnancies and abortions in symptomatic and asymptomatic Wilson's disease. *J Neurol Sci* 2004; **217**(1): 37–40.

48 Sozeri E, Feist D, Ruder H *et al.* Proteinuria and other renal functions in Wilson's disease. *Pediatr Nephrol* 1997; **11**: 307–311.

49 Roberts EA, Schilsky ML. Diagnosis and treatment of Wilson disease: an update. *Hepatology* 2008; **47**: 2089–2111.

50 Müller T, Koppikar S, Taylor RM *et al.* Re-evaluation of the penicillamine challenge test in the diagnosis of Wilson's disease in children. *J Hepatol* 2007; **47**: 270–276.

51 Steindl P, Ferenci P, Dienes HP *et al.* Wilson's disease in patients presenting with liver disease: a diagnostic challenge. *Gastroenterology* 1997; **113**: 212–218

52 Ferenci P, Caca K, Loudianos G *et al.* Diagnosis and phenotypic classification of Wilson disease. *Liver Int* 2003; **23**: 139–142.

53 Xuan A, Bookman I, Cox DW *et al.* Three atypical cases of Wilson disease: assessment of the Leipzig scoring system in making a diagnosis. *J Hepatol* 2007; **47**: 428–433.

54 Taylor RM, Chen Y, Dhawan A. Triethylene tetramine dihydrochloride (trientine) in children with Wilson disease: experience at King's College Hospital and review of the literature. *Eur J Pediatr* 2009: **168**:1061-1068..

55 O'Brien A, Williams R. Rapid diagnosis of Wilson Disease in acute liver failure: no more waiting for the caeruloplasmin level? *Hepatology* 2008; **48**: 1030–1032.

56 Cauza E, Maier-Dobersberger T, Polli C *et al.* Screening for Wilson's disease in patients with liver diseases by serum ceruloplasmin. *J Hepatol* 1997; **27**: 358–362.

57 Skidmore FM, Drago V, Foster P *et al.* Aceruloplasminaemia with progressive atrophy without brain iron overload: treatment with oral chelation. *J Neurol Neurosurg Psychiatry* 2008; **79**: 467–470.

58 Twomey PJ. Effect of a different caeruloplasmin assay method on the relationship between serum copper and caeruloplasmin. *Postgrad Med J* 2008; **84**: 549–551.

59 Gow PJ, Smallwood RA, Angus PW *et al.* Diagnosis of Wilson's disease: an experience over three decades. *Gut* 2000; **46**: 415–419.

60 Frommer DJ. Urinary copper excretion and hepatic copper concentrations in liver disease. *Digestion* 1981; **21**: 169–178.

61 Martins da Costa C, Baldwin D, Portmann B *et al.* Value of urinary copper excretion after penicillamine challenge in the diagnosis of Wilson's disease. *Hepatology* 1992; **15**: 609–615.

62 Foruny JR, Boixeda D, López-Sanroman A *et al.* Usefulness of penicillamine-stimulated urinary copper excretion in the diagnosis of adult Wilson's disease. *Scan J Gastroenterol* 2008; **43**: 597–603.

63 Ferenci P, Steindl-Munda P, Vogel W *et al.* Diagnostic value of quantitative hepatic copper determination in patients with Wilson's disease. *Clin Gastroenterol Hepatol* 2005; **3**: 811–818.

64 Czlonkowska A, Rodo M, Gromadzka G. Late onset Wilson's disease: therapeutic implications. *Mov Disord* 2008; **23**: 896–898.

65 Walshe JM. Wilson's disease. New oral therapy. *Lancet* 1956; **I**: 25–26.

66 Walshe JM. The management of penicillamine nephropathy in Wilson's disease. A new chelating agent. *Lancet* 1969; **II**: 1401–1402.

67 Brewer GJ, Hedera P, Kluin KJ *et al.* Treatment of Wilson's disease with ammonium tetrathiomolybdate. III. Initial therapy in a total of 55 neurologically affected patients and follow-up with zinc therapy. *Arch Neurol* 2003; **60**: 379–385.

68 Brewer GJ, Dick RD, Johnson *et al.* Treatment of Wilson's disease with zinc: XV. Long-term follow-up studies. *J Lab Clin Med* 1998; **132**: 264–278.

69 Walshe JM. Wilson's disease (letter). *Lancet* 2007; **369**: 902.

70 Gibbs KR, Walshe JM. Penicillamine and pyridoxine requirements in man. *Lancet* 1996; **1**: 175–179.

71 Walshe JM, Yealland M. Chelation treatment of neurological Wilson's disease. *Q J Med* 1993; **86**: 197–204.

72 Brewer GJ, Terry CA, Aisen AM *et al.* Worsening of neurologic syndrome in patients with Wilson's disease with initial penicillamine therapy. *Arch Neurol* 1987; **44**: 490–493.

73 Walshe JM. Copper chelation in patients with Wilson's disease: a comparison of penicillamine and triethylene tetramine dihydrochloride. *Q J Med* 1973; **42**: 441–452.

74 Brewer GJ, Askari F, Lorincz MT *et al.* Treatment of Wilson disease with ammonium tetrathiomolybdate. IV. Comparison of tetrathiomolybdate and trientine in a double-blind study of treatment of the neurologic presentation of Wilson disease. *Arch Neurol* 2006; **63**: 521–527.

75 Askari FK, Greenson J, Dick RD *et al.* Treatment of Wilson's disease with zinc. XVIII. Initial treatment of the hepatic decompensation presentation with trientine and zinc. *J Lab Clin Med* 2003; **142**: 385–390

76 Czlonkowska A, Gajda J, Rodo M. Effects of long-term treatment in Wilson's disease with D-penicillamine and zinc sulphate. *J Neurol* 1996; **243**: 269–273.

77 Sinha S, Christopher R, Arunodaya GR *et al.* Is low serum tocopherol in Wilson's disease a significant symptom? *J Neurol Sci* 2005; **228**: 121–123.

78 Prashanth LK, Taly AB, Sinha S *et al.* Prognostic factors in patients presenting with severe neurological forms of Wilson's disease. *Q J Med* 2005; **98**: 557–563

79 Lorincz MT. Neurologic Wilson's disease. *Ann NY Acad Sci* 2010; **1184**: 173–187.

80 Scheinberg IH, Sternlieb I. Treatment of neurologic manifestations of Wilson's disease. *Arch Neurol* 1995; **52**: 339–340.

81 Twomey PJ, Viljoen A, House IM *et al.* Relationship between serum copper, ceruloplasmin, and non-ceruloplasmin-bound copper in routine clinical practice. *Clin Chem* 2005; **51**: 1558–1559.

82 Brewer GJ, Yuzbasiyan-Gurkan V. Wilson disease. *Medicine* 1992; **71**: 139–164.

83 Walshe JM. Cause of death in Wilson disease. *Mov Disord* 2007; **22**: 2216–2220.

84 Sternlieb I. Wilson's disease and pregnancy. *Hepatology* 2000; **31**: 531–532.

85 Shimono N, Ishibashi H, Ikematsu H *et al.* Fulminant hepatic failure during perinatal period in a pregnant woman with Wilson's disease. *Gastroenterol Jpn* 1991; **26**: 69–73.

86 Sen S, Felidin M, Steiner C *et al.* Albumin dialysis and Molecular Adsorbent Recirculating System (MARS) for acute Wilson's disease. *Liver Transpl* 2002; **8**: 962–967.

87 Jhang JS, Schilsky ML, Lefkowitch JH *et al.* Therapeutic plasma pheresis as a bridge to liver transplantation in fulminant Wilson disease. *J Clin Apher* 2007; **22**: 10–14.

88 Asfaha S, Almansori M, Qarni U *et al.* Plasmapheresis for hemolytic crisis and impending acute liver failure in Wilson's disease. *J Clin Apher* 2007; **22**: 295–298.

89 Collins KL, Roberts EA, Adeli K *et al.* Single pass albumin dialysis (SPAD) in fulminant Wilsonian liver failure: a case report. *Pediatr Nephrol* 2008; **23**: 1013–1016.

90 Chiu A, Tsoi NS, Fan ST. Use of the molecular adsorbent recirculating system as a treatment for acute decompensated Wilson disease. *Liver Transplant* 2008; **14**: 1512–1516.

91 Emre S, Atillasoy EO, Ozdemir S *et al.* Orthotopic liver transplantation for Wilson's disease: a single-centre experience. *Transplantation* 2001; **72**: 1232–1236.

92 Podgaetz E, Chan C, Liver Transplantation team. Liver transplantation for Wilson's disease: our experience with review of the literature. *Ann Hepatol* 2003; **2**: 131–134.

93 Martin AP, Bartels M, Redlich J *et al.* A single-centre experience with liver transplantation for Wilson's disease. *Clin Transplant* 2008; **22**: 216–221.

94 Yoshitoshi EY, Takada Y, Oike F *et al.* Long-term outcomes for 32 cases of Wilson's disease after living-donor liver transplantation. *Transplantation* 2009; **87**: 261–267.

95 Dhawan A, Taylor RM, Cheeseman P *et al.* Wilson's disease in children: 37-year experience and revised King's score for liver transplantation. *Liver Transpl* 2005; **11**: 441–448.

96 Petrasek J, Jirsa M, Sperl J *et al.* Revised King's College Score for liver transplantation in adult patients with Wilson's disease. *Liver Transpl* 2007; **13**: 55–61.

32 Primary biliary cirrhosis

Gideon M Hirschfield and E Jenny Heathcote

Francis Family Liver Centre, Toronto Western Hospital, University Health Network *and* Department of Medicine, University of Toronto, Toronto, Canada

Introduction

Primary biliary cirrhosis (PBC) is the accepted name for a hepato-biliary disease characterized by a chronic non-suppurative granulomatous cholangitis of the interlobular and septal bile ducts [1, 2]. Epidemiological surveys have shown that the disease predominantly, but not exclusively, affects middle-aged women across all racial groups. In some studies the prevalence has been estimated to reach 1 in 1000 of women over 40 years old [3]. It is considered autoimmune in origin because overwhelmingly patients have serological evidence for specific anti-mitochondrial antibodies (AMA). Additionally, other autoimmune disorders are more frequent in those with this disease, and their relatives. The natural history of this chronic cholestatic disease is more variable than traditionally taught, reflecting a wide spectrum of presentation, but untreated progression is often to biliary cirrhosis. This is a result of chronic inflammation (piecemeal necrosis), ductopenia (a consequence of chronic granulomatous bile duct injury) and cholestasis (retention of bile acids).

Diagnosis

The first descriptions of disease were in patients with a profound cholestatic hyperlipidemia and its accompanying pronounced skin xanthoma. With greater use of biochemical testing patients were identified prior to the onset of jaundice, and indeed now most patients are asymptomatic when diagnosed, with no significant fibrosis. The biggest diagnostic advance was made by Doniach and Walker who demonstrated that most individuals had non-organ and non-species specific mitochondrial antibodies, using the

then new technique of immunofluorescence [4, 5]. By the late 1980s, it was clear that the targets of the anti-mitochondrial antibodies were the E2 component of the pyruvate dehydrogenase complex and other members of the family of 2-oxo acid dehydrogenase enzymes located on the inner membrane of mitochondria. Understanding the antigens in greater detail led to better, and more specific assays for AMA using ELISA technology and/or immunoblotting; these confirm that an AMA test is positive in about 95% of patients with PBC [6]. However AMA-M2 is not restricted to PBC alone, with descriptions in the healthy population (~0.5%) [7, 8], in asymptomatic first-degree relatives of patients (as high as 13%) [9], in autoimmune hepatitis [10], hepatitic overlap syndromes [11], and transiently during acute liver injuries [12]. Additionally, of patients who have recurrent urinary tract infections, half test positive for anti–PDC-E2, most likely due to cross-reactivity with *E coli* mitochondrial antigens [13].

Careful assessment of liver pathology codified in greater detail the specific features of this disease, but whilst histological assessment has been very important in studying the progression of disease (and thus identifying risk factors for progression), and as a surrogate for treatment efficacy, its role in routine clinical care has become less prominent [14]. The characteristic lesion of PBC is lymphocytic destruction of the interlobular bile ducts within portal triads. Histological staging systems assess the degree of fibrosis, inflammation and/or bile duct damage. For example, in Ludwig's classification, stage 1 is defined by portal inflammation, and stage 2 is extension of the inflammation beyond the portal tracts into the surrounding parenchyma, with or without associated duct loss. By stage 3, fibrous septa link adjacent portal triads and stage 4 represents cirrhosis. The difficulty for any system is the sampling error inherent in percutaneous liver biopsy (e.g. it being difficult to agree what is an appropriate number of portal tracts that need to be sampled to be sure of adequate representation of cholestatic liver disease). Explant tissue has been used to demonstrate how variable a percutaneous biopsy can

Evidence-Based Gastroenterology and Hepatology, 3rd edition.
J. McDonald, A.K. Burroughs, B. Feagan, and M.B. Fennerty. © 2010
Blackwell Publishing Ltd

actually be if relied upon to stage PBC [15]. Hence, when sections from 50 PBC liver specimens obtained at transplantation were examined only 10 (20%) samples had a consistent degree of fibrosis in all sections scanned. By contrast, the same fibrosis stage was assigned in 30 (60%) specimens examined using a simulated needle biopsy method. When the results obtained by the two methods were compared, there was a discrepancy of one or two stages in 32 samples. This discrepancy was the result of areas with a lesser degree of fibrosis in whole sections compared with a simulated needle biopsy specimen.

In present practice PBC is considered definite in the presence of all three of chronic biochemical cholestasis, antimitochondrial antibodies and typical pathology, but only probable if only two features are present [16]. However, in the correct context cholestasis with AMAs has been confirmed to be virtually diagnostic of PBC without recourse to biopsy [17]. Although asymptomatic individuals with PBC were reported by Sherlock in 1959 the natural history of such patients was more fully described by Long *et al.* in 1977 [18, 19]. Later it became evident that AMA positive subjects with normal liver biochemistry, undergoing serological tests because of the presence of another autoimmune disease, may also have the histological lesions of PBC on biopsy. A longitudinal follow-up study of 29 untreated patients assessed every year from first-detected AMA for a mean of 18 years showed that 24 (83%) developed cholestatic liver tests and 22 (76%) developed fatigue and/or pruritus. The median time to progression from AMA positivity to persistently abnormal liver enzymes was 5.6 years (range, 1–20 years) [20]. Whether all patients who test positive for AMA, particularly those who test positive by the more sensitive ELISA technology, will eventually develop clinical disease is unknown because such studies are yet to be performed. Indeed it seems improbable since the prevalence of AMA in the general population is so much higher than the prevalence of clinical disease, and the male: female ratio of those testing positive does not mirror that of the overwhelmingly female predominant PBC population as a whole [8].

It has also become clear with careful observation that 5% of patients have the clinical, biochemical, and histological features of PBC, as well as the same associated autoimmune diseases, but test repeatedly negative for AMA (by all modalities of testing) [21, 22]. These latter patients tend to be seropositive for antinuclear antibodies (ANA) or smooth muscle antibodies (SMA), often with high titers. The immunologic profile of PBC normally includes ANA and by indirect immunofluorescence is reported as commonly as 50% of the time. The immunofluorescence patterns for PBC-specific ANA are described as a perinuclear/rim-like or multiple nuclear dot pattern. The rim-like pattern results from autoantibodies directed against constituents of the nuclear envelope, including in particular

gp210, a 210-kd transmembrane glycoprotein of the nuclear pore complex. The multiple nuclear dot pattern is caused by autoantibodies against two autoantigens that colocalize: sp100 and promyelocytic leukemia protein. ANA reacting with gp210 occur in 10% to 40% of patients who have AMA positivity and in up to 50% of patients who have AMA-negative PBC and, therefore, are an appropriate second-line investigation in this group of individuals.

Natural history

PBC is a chronic liver disease generally characterized by a slow progression but highly variable clinical course. More than half of patients diagnosed today are asymptomatic at diagnosis and one contemporary series showed how nearly 90% do not have fibrosis when first identified [23]. Some patients will still present jaundiced, or with intractable pruritus, but increasingly patients are generally investigated after the observation of an elevation in serum alkaline phosphatase (ALP) and/or total serum cholesterol, and this often results from a routine health screen. The diagnosis may also be made in patients with an associated autoimmune disease such as scleroderma, hypothyroidism or rheumatoid arthritis, in whom clinicians may routinely screen for PBC (usually with a combination of liver biochemistry and autoantibody screening).

An important question pertains to whether the natural history of the disease is unchanged when compared to prior studies and whether the widespread use of ursodeoxycholic acid (UDCA) explains the apparent change in severity of disease encountered, for example transplant rates for PBC have fallen markedly but this is not the case for PSC [24], and survival similarly appears improved for PBC but not PSC [25]. The Japanese have proposed a natural history model in which so called latent/early PBC (AMA-M2 positive with normal liver tests), passes on through to asymptomatic and then symptomatic PBC [26]. Patients with symptomatic PBC appear to have a more rapid progression to end-stage liver disease and have a worse prognosis than those with asymptomatic disease. Within this latter group, a further division has been suggested into those that develop portal hypertension (anti-centromere positive) and those that develop liver failure (anti-gp210 positive) [27]. How accurate these divisions are remains to be seen, and it perhaps reflects the lack of pathophysiological understanding of autoimmune liver disease that symptoms still play such an important part in classification. In the management of chronic viral hepatitis, the focus is on surrogate viremic endpoints (HBV DNA/HCV RNA) and symptoms do not register in natural history discussions. Conversely, the symptom often thought so "specific" for PBC, fatigue, is in fact also reported by those with other liver diseases [28].

The initial ten-year, follow-up report of asymptomatic disease suggested that 50% of asymptomatic patients became symptomatic over this period of time [19]. More recent studies with longer follow-up indicate that although asymptomatic disease tends to progress at a much slower rate than symptomatic disease, survival of both symptomatic and asymptomatic patients with PBC is significantly less than that of the general population [29, 30]. Mean survival for patients with symptomatic PBC is eight years whereas that for asymptomatic disease is closer to 16 years according to some authors [31]. One UK study suggested absolute survival was the same regardless of symptoms, although notably the cause of death in those who were asymptomatic was more commonly non-hepatic, and those without symptoms had less severe disease at diagnosis [32]. Information from the many randomized controlled trials (RCTs) of therapy in patients with PBC conducted over the past decades also confirms that the course of PBC is not the same for all patients. About one-third of asymptomatic patients develop symptomatic disease within five years. The other two-thirds may not develop symptomatic disease for much longer. A large study from Newcastle reported that 54% of patients with asymptomatic PBC do not die of their liver disease [33]. The age at diagnosis must be noted and may be relevant when trying to compare studies. One study that described asymptomatic patients included predominantly patients who were mostly older than 60 years old [20], and some reports show that the diagnosis of asymptomatic PBC tends to be made in patients who are between and two to ten years older than patients with symptomatic disease [34]. This relationship suggests that asymptomatic disease is not necessarily a precursor of symptomatic disease, but could also be a *form fruste* of symptomatic disease.

Surrogate markers of outcome

As PBC is primarily a disease of the biliary system, when signs of failure of hepatocyte function develop, such as uncorrectable coagulopathy or jaundice, these usually indicate terminal disease, assuming there is no precipitant such as drug injury or a *de novo* autoimmune hepatitis. There are no symptoms present in patients with purely compensated disease which correlate with outcome, for example fatigue does not correlate with the severity of disease as judged by the height of the serum bilirubin or the Mayo risk score [35], and similarly, pruritus is not a marker of disease severity [36], in fact frequently diminishing as the disease progresses. In one report of symptom development in 770 patients who had PBC, ascites was present in 20% and bleeding varices in 10.5% after ten years of follow-up [33]. The outlook for patients who develop these complications is worse and new portal hypertension complicated by

ascites is usually a bad sign. In 143 patients who first developed ascites (n = 111) or peripheral edema (n = 32), the mean time to death was 3.1 years [37]. Occasionally, varices have been reported to develop in PBC before histologic cirrhosis can be documented (nodular regenerative hyperplasia or intense periportal inflammation) and this then carries a better prognosis [38].

Once a patient develops biochemical hyperbilirubinemia, the natural untreated history of this disease is more predictable. The degree of hyperbilirubinemia has been shown to correlate extremely well with survival. This was shown prior to the introduction of liver transplantation and the height of the bilirubin was a valid marker of final outcome, that is, death. The liver insufficiency phase is characterized by worsening jaundice and is a preterminal phase: mean survival once the bilirubin is 34 μmol/l is four years, and when the bilirubin reaches 102 μmol/l mean survival is only two years [39]. This had formed the basis for guidance to refer patients with PBC for transplant once their bilirubin reaches 100 μmol/l. Encephalopathy, when it occurs, is usually (but not always) during this phase. Pruritus, alkaline phosphatase, and cholesterol may all paradoxically improve in the preterminal stage. The introduction of UDCA therapy, which was demonstrated in early studies to reduce serum bilirubin levels [40], has been shown not to invalidate either the absolute serum bilirubin or the Mayo risk score as a prognostic marker [41]. What is less clear is whether the serum bilirubin in patients treated with UDCA remains a valid marker of survival in those with end-stage disease.

The identification of other surrogate markers of outcome remains extremely important in evaluating specific therapies in PBC, particularly as the mean survival time of this disease, in both symptomatic and asymptomatic patients, is long. As more and more asymptomatic patients (whose survival may be influenced by factors external to the liver) are included in drug trials, these trials will need to be very large in size and of long duration to evaluate the effect of therapy on survival effectively. Further, the risk scores discussed below may not necessarily be applicable to asymptomatic patients, since most are derived from cohorts of patients with moderate/severe disease, an exception being the study from Prince and colleagues [33].

More sophisticated risk scores designed to predict prognosis in patients with PBC have been developed. It is not surprising that serum bilirubin features in each of the scores described [42]. The most widely used composite score, the Mayo risk score, is popular because it does not require liver biopsy [43]. The components of the Mayo risk score, age, serum bilirubin and albumin, coagulation time, and the presence of fluid retention and/or use of diuretics, seem to be sufficient to accurately predict outcome in PBC. The Mayo risk score was first developed from a cohort of patients in a randomized trial, and validated for patients who were not treated with a liver transplant for end-stage disease. The original Mayo risk score has been re-evaluated with extended follow-up and inclusion of a number of patients who progressed to receive liver transplantation [44]. In total, progression of primary biliary cirrhosis was studied in 312 patients who were seen at the Mayo Clinic between 1974 and 1984. Follow-up was extended to 1988, by which time 140 of the patients had died and 29 had undergone liver transplantation. These patients generated 1945 patient visits, which enabled the authors to study the change in the prognostic variables of primary biliary cirrhosis from the time of referral. The updated model was superior to the original model for predicting short-term survival (during the two years) after a patient visit. This study also confirmed that updating the model every time a patient is reviewed was statistically acceptable. Although the Mayo score is popular it should be noted that other investigators have also produced similar analyses on their own cohorts [33, 45]. When using risk scores in comparative studies it should also be borne in mind that patients presently may be less severe in their presentation than those included in original studies, and this may lead to an over estimate of mortality; further score validity is usually short (two years) and not long term. The MELD score is of value once the disease is advanced and provides an accurate tool for transplant evaluation since it is a reliable measure of short-term mortality risk [46]; in early stage disease it is clearly not particularly meaningful.

Recent attempts at survival analysis have looked to see if simple assessments of biochemical response to treatment may be useful clinically. Three studies stand out in this regard with particular utility for patients. Pares assessed the course and survival of patients with PBC treated with UDCA and compared this with the survival predicted by the Mayo model and the estimated survival of a standardized population [47]. There were 192 patients with PBC treated with UDCA (15 mg/kg per day) for 1.5–14 years. In this study a response to treatment was defined by an ALP decrease greater than 40% of baseline values or normal levels after one year of treatment. In the timeframe 8.9% of patients met the endpoint (died or fulfilled criteria for liver transplantation) and the observed survival was higher than that predicted by the Mayo model but lower than that of the control Spanish population. Just under two-thirds of patients responded to treatment, according to their definition and the survival of responders was significantly higher than that predicted by the Mayo model and similar to that estimated for the control population (but only if they were treated at an early stage of disease). In a similar vein the biochemical response to UDCA was correlated with long-term prognosis in PBC recently by a French group studying 292 patients [48]. Those showing ALP < 3 ULN, AST < 2 ULN, and bilirubin ≤ 17 μmol/l after one year of UDCA had a ten-year transplant-free survival rate of 90% (95% CI:

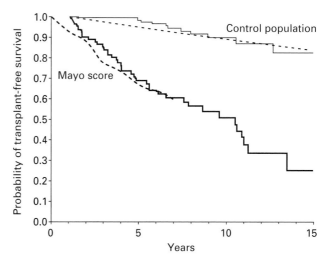

Figure 32.1 Survival without transplantation, according to the one-year biochemical response to UDCA. The thin curve represents survival of responders (n = 179). The thick curve represents survival of non-responders (n = 113). The survival of the control population (thin dotted curve) and the survival predicted for non-responders by the updated Mayo model (thick dotted curve) are indicated. The transplant free survival of responders was significantly higher than that of nonresponders (p < 0.0001; RR, 0.4; 95% CI: 0.3–0.5) and similar to that of the control population (p = 0.8). The transplant-free survival of non-responders was not different from that predicted by the updated Mayo model (p = 0.9). Reproduced with the permission of the American Association for the Study of Liver Diseases [48].

81–95%), compared to 51% (95% CI: 38–64%) for those who did not (see Figure 32.1).

Huet *et al.* [49] have used a different approach, looking at portal hypertension in a study unlikely to be repeated because of its invasive nature. A total of 132 patients had portohepatic gradient and biochemical values measured at inclusion and every two years. After two years of treatment, a decreased or stable portohepatic gradient (hazard ratio, 4.64; 95% CI: 2.01–10.72) and normalization of AST level (hazard ratio, 2.89; 95% CI: 1.03–8.05) were predictive of better survival on multivariate analysis. Responders (defined as either stable or improved portohepatic gradient and normalized AST level at two years) had a 15-year survival similar to that of a matched local Canadian population.

Histology can be a hard endpoint, but only in the context of clinical trials where large numbers of biopsy specimens are available to offset the effect of sampling error. Transition rates between Ludwig histologic stages have been calculated using Markov modelling (namely that, given the present state, the future and past states are independent). In a large randomized trial of D-penicillamine, which was found to have no effect on histologic progression, the mean increase in histologic stage for PBC can be estimated to be one stage every 1.5 years. After four years, 31% of patients whose initial biopsy showed stage 1 had progressed to cirrhosis, and 50% of patients who started in stage 2 had progressed to cirrhosis [50]. An earlier study (on a relatively small number of patients) did indicate that patients who have liver fibrosis or cirrhosis on biopsy had a worse survival than those without fibrosis or cirrhosis [51]. On its own, presence or absence of cirrhosis is not a highly predictive surrogate marker for final outcome, that is, death, presumably because there are other features which factor into progression of disease. A detailed review of liver histology in PBC suggests that the presence of lymphoplasmacytic interface hepatitis is a marker of more rapidly progressive disease [52], and in another report of four cases, rapidly progressive bile duct loss, even in the absence of cirrhosis led to liver failure [53]. Corpechot described the progression toward cirrhosis in 183 UDCA-treated patients with PBC [52]. A total of 254 pairs of liver biopsy specimens collected during 655 patient-years were studied and the incidence of cirrhosis after five years of UDCA treatment was 4%, 12% and 59% among patients followed up from stages I, II and III respectively. At ten years, the incidence was 17%, 27% and 76% respectively. The median time for developing cirrhosis from stages I, II and III was 25 years, 20 years and 4 years respectively. The independent predictive factors of cirrhosis development were serum bilirubin greater than $17\,\mu mol/l$, serum albumin less than $38\,g/l$, and moderate to severe lymphocytic piecemeal necrosis. Validation of the importance of interface hepatitis is important, as are other potential factors (vascular supply to the liver, the presence of various inflammatory mediators and markers of tissue fibrosis). In the latest paper from France already discussed, independent predictive factors of death or transplant were baseline serum bilirubin level $>17\,\mu mol/l$ (RR, 1.7), histologic stage ≥ 3 (RR, 1.5), interface hepatitis (RR, 1.9), and the absence of biochemical response (ALP > 3 ULN or AST > 2 ULN, or bilirubin $> 17\,\mu mol/l$) (RR, 2.3) [48]. There is no good evidence that the AMA titer correlates with the course of PBC [54] (although it can fall with treatment [55]), but some groups have suggested specific anti-nuclear antibodies may delineate subtypes of PBC [27]. This, however, remains to be validated widely [56].

Aside from the increasing rarity of liver deaths from PBC, it has also become very difficult to use death as an endpoint, since most patients with decompensated PBC, if they have no contraindication, are referred for liver transplantation. As liver transplantation has become established for end-stage liver disease in particular, it has been used as a final outcome measure by many. Even transplant has some variability; however, certainly as some patients in the past have been transplanted for symptoms, different centers have longer waiting times, whilst factors such as blood group and body size can alter the duration of waiting. With the advent of scoring systems such as MELD, these issues will be largely addressed. Furthermore, perhaps because of therapy the rates of those patients with PBC

going to transplant continues to fall markedly [24]. Over a 12-year period (1995 to 2006) PBC and PSC transplant data of first-time liver recipients from the United Network for Organ Sharing database were collected. Although the absolute number of liver transplantations in the USA increased by an average of 249 transplants per year the absolute number of transplants performed for PBC decreased by an average of 5.4 cases per year. The absolute number of transplantations for PSC showed no statistical change.

Therapeutic trial design: assessment of credibility

Understanding the limitations of the available evidence is essential for those interested in the evidence base for treatments of PBC. Numerous trials form the basis of the current treatment offered to patients. In evaluating such work a number of concerns arise for a disease such as PBC which is relatively uncommon and has a slow and varied natural history. To establish appropriate study size requires not only a large sample of historical data to chart the natural history of untreated disease but also pilot data, from which an estimate of the expected benefit can be calculated (sample size must also assess the frequency of adverse events). Historical data may not, though, always remain valid, for example the exclusion of chronic hepatitis C was only possible after approximately 1990, and patterns of presentation may change with time. The pivotal patient descriptions in the *New England Journal of Medicine* by Sherlock in 1973 clearly do not reflect those seen now [23, 57]. Recognized improvements in trial management have helped produce more robust data, with much thought given to careful trial design (e.g. double blinded, prior sample size calculation, stopping rules, crossover arms, and intention-to-treat analysis). The intention-to-treat principle is particularly relevant when carrying out statistical analysis of outcome to avoid as much bias as possible when interpreting the data. This means that all patients who are randomized need to be included in the final analysis, even though they may have been censored at a very early point in the trial because of untimely death, need to withdraw from the study, non-compliance, etc. Using the intention to treat principle allows for a very conservative analysis of the effectiveness of therapy, but permits assessment of the "real life" situation, that is, the generalizability of the study.

Meta-analysis can also overcome some concerns, particularly sample size, but many assumptions are made about inclusion and exclusion of studies, and original raw data is not always accessed. Additionally, meta-analysis is a tool to define the gaps in knowledge (and thus to help the design of better studies), rather than a true grading system for an intervention, meaning conclusions drawn may reflect the quality and quantity of the evidence available as much as anything else. Variability in clinical practice, referral biases and varied ethnicity also generate difficulties as clinicians pool their patient resources. Finally, a major challenge relates to early detection of disease such that significant events, for example death or liver transplantation are unlikely to occur during any single trial. The use of surrogate markers (biochemical response, histological change, disease risk scores) as endpoints are by necessity employed, but their own origin and limitations need to be recognized as already discussed [58].

Randomized controlled trials of treatment for primary biliary cirrhosis

Immunosuppression

As the archetypal presumed autoimmune disease, inevitably immunosuppression has been evaluated as a therapy. Because the majority of patients with PBC are women and osteoporosis is prevalent (but not necessarily causally related to PBC [59–61]), corticosteroid therapy has for the most part been avoided. Trials of immunosuppressive therapy in PBC have employed azathioprine, cyclosporin, methotrexate, prednisolone, chlorambucil, thalidomide and, more recently, budesonide and mycophenolate mofetil. Neither of the two trials of azathioprine showed a beneficial effect of this drug on survival [62, 63]. The first trial had an inadequate sample size, lacked a placebo control group and predetermined stopping rules, and the results were not analyzed according to intention to treat. The second trial of azathioprine although much larger (248 patients), did not include a sample size calculation to assure that it had adequate power, and the withdrawal rate was greater than 20% in both the azathioprine and placebo groups. Despite randomization, the two groups were not stratified for factors known to influence survival and were not comparable at baseline. Only after employment of the Cox multiple regression analysis to adjust for these baseline differences was a benefit of treatment on survival observed. This difference in survival between the treatment groups could only be measured in months, which may not be clinically meaningful. Patients were followed for up to ten years, but the number of patients still being followed at that period was only nine in the azathioprine and none in the placebo group. It appears that the intention to treat principle was not used in the analysis, since 32 patients were excluded from the analysis because of incomplete data. Thus, the validity of the small benefit in survival can be further questioned. **A1d** Mycophenolate mofetil similarly has been disappointing, with no important clinical benefits, albeit in data from a single, small pilot study of 25 patients with PBC lasting one year [64].

Several small trials and one large trial (349 patients) of cyclosporin therapy have been published [65–68]. This trial ran into the same problems as had been encountered with the large azathioprine trial, that is, lack of comparability of the two treatment groups at baseline. Even though there were a similar number of deaths, 30 in the cyclosporin group and 31 in the placebo group, the authors concluded that survival was improved in the cyclosporin-treated patients. Renal impairment was observed in 9% and systemic hypertension in 11% of the cyclosporin-treated patients (1.7% and 1% in placebo-treated respectively). These two serious adverse effects in patients whose disease is relatively slowly progressive precludes the use of this drug in the long-term treatment of PBC. **A1d** Tacrolimus, a similar agent, has not been studied to date formally in PBC, neither has the other increasingly popular immunosuppressant, rapamycin.

Methotrexate was suggested to be of value in pilot studies [69, 70]. In one RCT of therapy sixty patients were recruited, 30 randomized to low-dose therapy (2.5 mg three times per week). At the end of six years, the serum bilirubin and Mayo risk score were higher in those receiving methotrexate, suggesting that the drug may be toxic in patients with PBC [71]. In a large NIH effort (placebo-controlled, randomized, multicenter trial comparing the effects of methotrexate plus UDCA to UDCA alone on the course of PBC) methotrexate when added to UDCA for a median period of 7.6 years had no effect on the course of PBC treated with UDCA alone [72]. **A1d** This study illustrates some of the difficulties of trial design: at the time of planning, it was anticipated that the five-year, transplant-free survival would be 83%, whereas the experience in this trial corresponded instead to a 94.5% five-year and 84.3% eight-year transplant free survival probability. The lower event rate meant that patients had to be followed for a longer time period, and this in turn probably contributed to a higher rate of patients discontinuing methotrexate. The authors calculated, using the log rank statistic to compare the distributions of time to an event in a randomized trial, that they needed to observe 88 events in order to have 90% power to detect a two-fold improvement in the risk of an event. With their calculations in a study that followed subjects for an average of eight years (with an expected 7% rate of death and 16% rate of transplant or death), this implied they needed to randomize a total of 1257 subjects when using the endpoint of overall survival, or 550 subjects when using the endpoint of transplant-free survival. If one then appreciates their recruitment reality, the enormous challenges for investigators planning future studies is clear: in this case investigators at 12 centers in the USA screened 535 patients for possible entry into the trial. At screening 393 of the 535 patients were determined to meet the defined inclusion criteria, and 385 patients went on to meet the screening inclusion and exclusion criteria. Three hundred patients progressed to a pre-entry evaluation phase and ultimately 265 patients were randomized with equal probability in a double-blind fashion.

A small, three-year RCT of prednisolone has been done [73]. **A1d** A significant reduction in the serum bilirubin level (a valid surrogate outcome measure) was observed in treated patients, but osteoporosis in those who received corticosteroids worsened. However, a trial with a very small sample size of bisphosphonates in patients with PBC treated with corticosteroids indicates that etidronate significantly stabilizes bone mineral density in vertebrae of patients with PBC receiving corticosteroids [74]. Hence, it may be appropriate that corticosteroids be re-evaluated in the therapy of PBC now that patients can be given preventive therapies to reduce the complication of osteoporosis. Budesonide is an oral corticosteroid which is eliminated on first pass through the liver. Thus it was hoped that this agent could benefit patients with PBC without having a deleterious effect on bone mineral density. In the first small RCT by Leuschner et al., improvement in liver biochemistry, IgM values and liver histology was observed in the few patients studied, most of whom had very early disease [75]. In a second study by Angulo et al., no benefit was observed and the Mayo risk score increased significantly in those randomized to budesonide for a year and bone mineral density measurements deteriorated in the lumbar spine (p < 0.01); it is likely that many of these patients had advanced PBC so that the benefit of the first-pass effect was lost [76]. Subsequent work from Finland has alluded to a histological benefit when combined with UDCA and the observation that interface hepatitis on baseline biopsy is predictive of outcome in PBC (as well as a failure to normalize transaminases with UDCA) does suggest that a subgroup may benefit from immunosuppression [77]. **A1d** Interest therefore remains in using budesonide adjunctively in those with more florid hepatitic features. However, Wolfhagen et al. in another small RCT involving 50 patients with PBC with suboptimal response to UDCA, treated patients with additional prednisone (30 mg/day tapered to 10 mg/day) and azathioprine (50 mg/day) [78]. There was no improvement in bilirubin. The trial was too small and of too short a duration to examine the effect on survival. **A1d**

A small study of 13 patients randomized to 0.5–4 mg daily of chlorambucil (mean 2 mg daily) compared with placebo has been reported [79]. All treated patients developed some degree of bone marrow suppression and discontinuation of therapy was required in four. A 30% withdrawal rate due to drug toxicity indicates that this drug should not undergo further evaluation in patients with PBC. **A1d** A very small and short (six-month) RCT of 18 PBC patients taking thalidomide has been reported, showing little benefit of this treatment [80]. However, this study lacked adequate power to evaluate this form of

therapy in any meaningful way. No benefit on serum bilirubin was observed during the six months of treatment.

An alternative approach has been to use drugs that may not interfere with the primary cause, that is, immune-mediated bile duct destruction, but interfere with the progression of the disease, either by reducing fibrogenesis or by reducing cholestasis. Two potential antifibrotic drugs have been assessed: colchicine in four good studies [81–84] and D-penicillamine in many more [85–92]. The studies of colchicine therapy are interesting, but unfortunately all the size of the populations studied are small. A Cochrane Hepato-Biliary Group systematic review of randomized clinical trials for this agent included ten trials involving 631 patients, only four of which were high-quality [93]. No significant differences were detected between colchicine and placebo/no intervention regarding mortality (relative risk (RR), 1.21; 95% CI: 0.71–2.06), mortality or liver transplantation (RR = 1.00; 95% CI: 0.67–1.49), liver complications, liver biochemical variables, liver histology, or adverse events. **A1c** While the numerous trials of D-penicillamine demonstrated great interest, the results are also disappointing. Unlike patients with Wilson's disease, adverse effects of therapy were particularly common, resulting in a high withdrawal rate, similar to the experience with rheumatoid arthritis. This drug is not recommended for the treatment of PBC and a meta-analysis is consistent with this (including seven trials randomizing 706 patients) [94]. **A1c**

Reduction of cholestasis: ursodeoxycholic acid

The prevailing view remains that UDCA improves the natural history of PBC [95], although the evidence for efficacy has been cumulative, is imperfect, and has been appropriately challenged as dogma [96, 97]. **A1a** Japanese researchers first isolated UDCA from bear bile in 1927; bear bile itself having a track record in traditional medicine as a choleretic [98]. UDCA is the natural intestinal metabolite of chenodeoxycholic acid (7-ß epimer). In the 1960s patients with gallstones were found to have lower biliary levels of cholic acid and chenodeoxycholic acid, which led to trials of oral bile salt supplementation in hepatobiliary disease. UDCA is less hydrophobic and more hydrophilic than other bile acids, with apparently less toxicity towards the hepatobiliary epithelium. Its therapeutic mechanism of action includes expansion of the hydrophilic bile acid pool, a direct choleretic effect (administration results in a bicarbonate-rich choleresis and modulation of biliary transporter proteins), anti-inflammatory effects (UDCA interacts with the glucocorticoid receptor in vitro) and anti-apoptotic effects on hepatic epithelia [99]. Cessation of therapy with UDCA leads to a return of abnormal liver biochemistry in those with PBC who respond, demonstrating that the initiating and perpetuating factors of PBC remain unresolved.

UDCA normally accounts for about 4% of bile acids but with pharmacotherapy UDCA becomes the predominant bile acid. Leuschner showed that when treating gallstones with UDCA in those with histologically confirmed HBsAg-negative chronic active hepatitis a fall in transaminases occurred [100]. In further work to investigate the dose-response relationship for UDCA, three different doses were given to patients with PBC, PSC and chronic hepatitis. This allowed Podda *et al.* to show that significant falls in liver biochemistry occurred at dosages of 4–5 mg/kg daily, but higher doses (8–10 mg/kg and 12–15 mg/kg) induced further improvements, with the changes correlated approximately with the enrichment of bile by UDCA [101]. Subsequent studies confirmed a correlation between the degree of bile enrichment and improvement in liver biochemistries and PBC Mayo risk score, and overall in PBC the data suggest that the optimum dose of UDCA if used should be 13 to 15 mg/kg per day, given as a single daily dose [40, 55, 102, 103]. UDCA at this dose is very safe, with minimal side effects: weight gain (approx. 3 kg in the first 12 months [104]), hair loss and, rarely, diarrhea and flatulence. Additionally, nothing suggests UDCA is teratogenic but it is usually stopped before and during the first trimester, and restarted subsequently, with there being a good safety profile from its use in intrahepatic cholestasis of pregnancy [105].

Justification for the widespread use of UDCA

Many studies have attempted to demonstrate clinical efficacy for UDCA, particularly following initial studies showing a fall in bilirubin levels in patients with PBC, with most trials showing beneficial effects of UDCA on biochemical parameters in particular. With such a slow natural history any individual trial will inevitably lack the power to address endpoints such as death or liver transplantation. Additional criticism can be made for assuming that every patient benefits equally, that is, identifying and treating more patients with mild disease may be self-fulfilling if those patients were never destined to progress. Moreover whilst appealing to assume that the natural history of the disease is unchanged, the absence of a clear cut pathophysiologic understanding means that such an assumption should not necessarily be considered correct.

The cumulative evidence that convinces most to prescribe UDCA, has nevertheless come from individual and pooled analysis. Of note the Mayo Clinic followed up patients with PBC treated with UDCA and have demonstrated a treatment-related prolongation in transplant free survival [106–108]. French cohorts with long-term follow-up similarly demonstrate survival benefit [109], and this was reiterated and furthered by a Spanish cohort including nearly 200 patients treated for a mean of 6.7 years [47]. Pathophysiologically early disease is most likely to respond to intervention before duct loss is established and fibrosis

present. In those with early stage disease, a biochemical response to UDCA (normalization or a 40% reduction from baseline) after one year was associated with a similar survival to the matched control population. In the Netherlands ter Borg and colleagues were able to show a survival benefit without transplant for low-risk patients compared to survival predicted by the Mayo risk model (which, as discussed, may not be a perfect risk score to employ in this case if the comparison group has predominantly early stage disease, as survival may be underestimated); moreover overall survival was nearly the same as for a control population [110]. **B4** A UK study that examined a large cohort not receiving UDCA did not, however, demonstrate differences in outcomes between treated and untreated patients [111]. A recent publication, as discussed, looked at defining the biochemical response a year after treatment, to identify UDCA-treated patients at risk of death or transplant and showed how UDCA responders had a ten-year, transplant-free survival rate of 90%, compared to 51% for those who did not [48]. **B4**

Three larger double-blind randomized trials used the same dose of UDCA (13–15 mg/kg per day), and thus the results have been analyzed according to an intention to treat principle [102, 107, 112, 113]. In two of these a composite "treatment failure" outcome measure was used, and in the third the percentage change in total serum bilirubin over two years was used as the primary outcome measure. Detailed sample size calculations and clear-cut predetermined definition of study duration were only described for this latter study. Few adverse effects of UDCA were reported and the withdrawal rate was less than 20% in all three studies. In two of the three trials, some patients initially randomized to placebo were switched to open label UDCA after the first 24 months, that is, the studies have a crossover design. However, the results were analyzed according to intention to treat (methodologically this can be criticized in studies with large crossover designs), so that those patients initially randomized to receive placebo and subsequently switched to receive UDCA remained in the placebo group for the purposes of analysis. Ultimately, then, this combined analysis of the three trials (548 patients) showed a one-third reduction in the risk of death or transplant, for patients with moderate to severe PBC, that is, UDCA therapy for up to four years led to an increase in time free of liver transplantation. Subgroup analyses did not show any benefit in patients who, at baseline, had a total serum bilirubin of less than 17–68 μmol/l and/or stage I/II liver histology. These subgroup analyses do not prove that UDCA is ineffective in patients with asymptomatic and/or early disease, but they do suggest that clinical trials in such patients would require very large numbers of patients and would be required to be of such long duration to show any benefit of the treatment that they would not be feasible. One other concern raised was the observation that those patients crossed over to UDCA, continued to have a poorer clinical course. A further large trial (151 patients) employed a smaller dose (10–12 mg/kg body-weight daily) and a different preparation of UDCA [114]. After two years of treatment no difference in survival was seen, there being eight deaths in those randomized to UDCA and 12 in those randomized to placebo. Prolonged follow-up also showed no survival benefit [115].

Meta-analysis findings

It should be pointed out that the pooled analysis of the three trials is not a systematic review or meta-analysis, but rather was done by pooling of results from three trials which were of similar design. This procedure differs from a systematic review or formal meta-analysis, which attempts to minimize bias by the consideration and inclusion of all relevant trials, justifies the exclusion of trials from the analysis, and explores heterogeneity between trials and the reasons for variation in results. A formal meta-analysis which demonstrates benefit from an intervention may also include a sensitivity analysis to indicate the number of unpublished or excluded trials of specified size with negative results which would be required to negate the results of the meta-analysis. Meta-analyses may suffer from the opposite weakness cited for the combined analysis of similar trials, that is, they may involve pooled analysis of trials which differ sufficiently in their design that they are not truly comparable. Accordingly, caution should be exercised in interpreting both combined analyses and meta-analyses. For PBC much debate has been generated because the various meta-analyses have been inconsistent. Some conclude no beneficial effect on the incidence of death and/or transplant, despite improvements in serum bilirubin, jaundice and ascites [96, 97]; thus, UDCA treatment offers no benefit. This contrasts with others showing that long-term treatment with the optimal dose of UDCA could improve survival free of transplant [116]. One needs to appreciate the varying, and often inadequate sample size and duration of several studies, as well as inclusion of data from trials using suboptimal doses. Both Goulis *et al.* and the Cochrane group have performed detailed analyses of the heterogeneous studies in which treatment periods ranged from as little as six months up to four years, the daily dose of UDCA ranged from 7.7 mg/kg to 15 mg/kg, and there was a wide range of disease severity. In addition, the Jadad scores for methodological quality were only ≥ 4 in five of the 16 trials. Sensitivity analyses for dose, length of study, and quality did not show differences in the first meta-analysis. The Cochrane group attempted to take these variations into consideration and observed a marginally significant effect of UDCA on liver transplantation only in the later period in which all the patients were treated with open label UDCA, but not in the original period in which patients were treated with

UDCA or placebo/no intervention. However, transplant is not a perfect endpoint, as already alluded to. Survival without transplant was not significantly influenced by UDCA therapy (see Figure 32.2).

Since not all placebo or non-intervention patients were eventually given UDCA (although the majority were), the evaluation of the non-randomized phases of these trials has intrinsic biases and lacks the appropriate basis for an intention-to-treat analysis. Of the 16 randomized clinical trials evaluating UDCA against placebo, nearly half of the trials had high risk of bias [97]. In all studies, the administration of UDCA was associated with an improvement of liver biochemistry. The latest updated Cochrane meta-analysis shows that overt ascites and obvious jaundice are less frequent in patients randomized to UDCA, but there was no difference in the number of patients with bleeding varices or hepatic encephalopathy. These data suggest that prolonged treatment with UDCA, started before onset of severe disease, may be required to exert a beneficial effect on the natural history of PBC; appropriately powered studies have not been performed to date, however, to definitively confirm the concept that patients with early disease benefit most from UDCA.

The meta-analysis that was confined to trials using an appropriate dose of UDCA (>10 mg per kilogram of body weight per day) and with sufficient follow-up (at least two years) included a total of 1038 patients (522 who received UDCA and 516 who received placebo) [116]. Treatment with UDCA resulted in significant improvement in liver biochemical values. Histologic evidence of disease progression was similar for the two treatment groups, but subjects without evidence of fibrosis (stages I and II) who were treated with UDCA had slower disease progression than did subjects in the control group. A total of 160 patients who were treated with UDCA and 186 control subjects died or underwent liver transplantation. This difference was significant in a fixed-effect model (OR, 0.76; 95% CI: 0.57–1.00; p = 0.05) but not in a random-effects model (OR, 0.77; 95% CI: 0.50–1.21; p = 0.30). This particular analysis is open to criticism because of the difference seen between the fixed-effect and random-effects model.

Osteoporosis

There are modest increases in both the absolute and relative fracture risks in people with PBC compared with the general population, with the excess risks similar in those with more severe disease [117, 118]. No effect of UDCA on bone mineral density was, however, demonstrated in the RCT of UDCA in PBC published by Lindor *et al.*, although the study may have lacked power [119]. A small study assessing bone mineral density and vertebral fractures in PBC patients randomized to cyclosporin A or placebo suggested that cyclosporin-treated patients have less bone loss and better biochemical parameters of bone remodelling

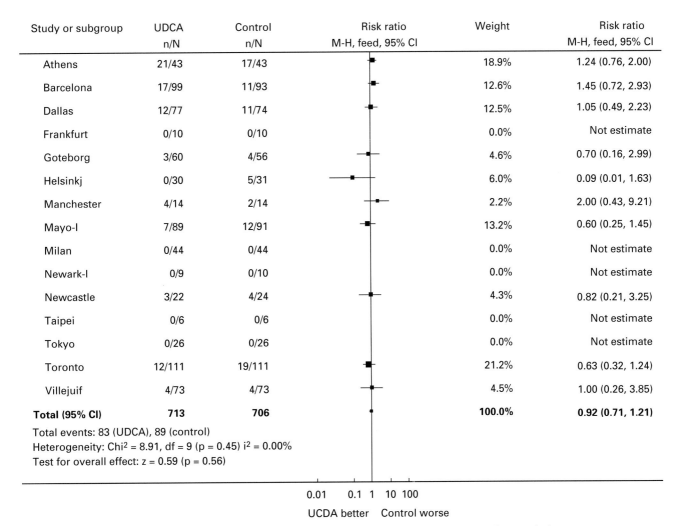

Study or subgroup	UDCA n/N	Control n/N	Risk ratio M-H, feed, 95% CI	Weight	Risk ratio M-H, feed, 95% CI
Athens	21/43	17/43		18.9%	1.24 (0.76, 2.00)
Barcelona	17/99	11/93		12.6%	1.45 (0.72, 2.93)
Dallas	12/77	11/74		12.5%	1.05 (0.49, 2.23)
Frankfurt	0/10	0/10		0.0%	Not estimate
Goteborg	3/60	4/56		4.6%	0.70 (0.16, 2.99)
Helsinkj	0/30	5/31		6.0%	0.09 (0.01, 1.63)
Manchester	4/14	2/14		2.2%	2.00 (0.43, 9.21)
Mayo-I	7/89	12/91		13.2%	0.60 (0.25, 1.45)
Milan	0/44	0/44		0.0%	Not estimate
Newark-I	0/9	0/10		0.0%	Not estimate
Newcastle	3/22	4/24		4.3%	0.82 (0.21, 3.25)
Taipei	0/6	0/6		0.0%	Not estimate
Tokyo	0/26	0/26		0.0%	Not estimate
Toronto	12/111	19/111		21.2%	0.63 (0.32, 1.24)
Villejuif	4/73	4/73		4.5%	1.00 (0.26, 3.85)
Total (95% CI)	**713**	**706**		**100.0%**	**0.92 (0.71, 1.21)**

Total events: 83 (UDCA), 89 (control)
Heterogeneity: Chi^2 = 8.91, df = 9 (p = 0.45) i^2 = 0.00%
Test for overall effect: z = 0.59 (p = 0.56)

0.01 0.1 1 10 100
UCDA better   Control worse

Figure 32.2 Meta-analysis of ursodeoxycholic acid for primary biliary cirrhosis: outcome mortality or liver transplantation [97].

[120]. With regard to specific treatment of osteoporosis in PBC, a number of small trials have been performed. Etidronate was not shown to be beneficial whereas alendronate was well tolerated and did significantly improve bone density in a double-blinded randomized, placebo-controlled trial, including a total of 34 patients followed for one year [121, 122]. Estrogen therapy can be used safely (from the hepatic perspective) and there is limited data on its efficacy [123–125].

Fatigue and pruritus

Although there are now some very sophisticated methods to measure these symptoms [126], none of the RCTs of therapy for PBC employed such instruments to monitor the effect of therapy. There are many anecdotal case reports of marked improvement and marked worsening of both fatigue and pruritus in patients receiving UDCA. Pilot studies of methotrexate have reported dramatic improvement in both fatigue and pruritus, but these uncontrolled studies provide only weak evidence for benefit. The Newcastle group have reported a study of the CNS-acting drug modafinil in patients with PBC suffering from significant daytime somnolence and associated fatigue [127]. Open label modafinil therapy was associated, where tolerated by patients, with improvement in excessive daytime somnolence and associated fatigue in PBC, but clearly placebo-controlled trials are needed. Effective treatments for pruritus, a distressing symptom in PBC are more readily available [128]. Although randomized controlled data is limited [129], treatment approaches include cholestryramine [130, 131], rifampin [132], sertraline [133], opioid antagonists [134, 135] and plasma exchange or albumin dialysis [136–138].

Histology

In the study by Pares *et al.* the apparent benefit of five years of UDCA therapy on liver histology in terms of stage of disease, progression of bile duct destruction and interface hepatitis was significantly greater than that observed in those randomized to placebo [139]. The majority of patients included in this trial had early asymptomatic disease. Assessment of liver histology from the French multicenter study using the Markov model indicated that regression of cirrhosis was never seen, but that the progression to cirrhosis was markedly delayed in those who received UDCA [140]. It must be emphasized that follow-up liver histology was not available in all randomized patients, some refused to have a second biopsy, and more importantly, no second biopsy was obtained from those patients who died or required a liver transplant, that is, those whose liver disease clearly had progressed. Only 44% of patients had second biopsies available for evaluation. This factor introduces the potential for significant bias into observations concerning effect of both UDCA and placebo on histology. However, a further pooled study showed that two years of UDCA treatment reduced periportal necroinflammation and improved ductular proliferation; if UDCA was initiated at the earlier stages disease (I–II) it also delayed the progression of histologic stage [141].

Cost-effectiveness of ursodeoxycholic acid therapy in primary biliary cirrhosis

Cost-efficacy analyses are limited to one paper, which used data from two previously published trials, and determined the effectiveness of UDCA by comparing the annual reduction in the development of ascites, varices, variceal bleeding, encephalopathy, liver transplantation, and death between the treatment groups [142]. Average annual costs for each of these events were estimated based on literature and institutional data. Approximately twice as many major events occurred in the placebo group compared with the UDCA group. Based on the estimated annual cost of managing these events and the then annual costs of UDCA ($2500), there was an annual cost saving per patient of $1372. Compared with the placebo group, patients receiving UDCA had a lower incidence of major complications and lower medical care costs.

Recurrent PBC following liver transplantation

After around five years, perhaps approaching one in five patients transplanted for PBC will have histological evidence of recurrence [143]. Diagnosis needs to be carefully evaluated in view of the broad differential in transplant recipients, but disease progression is slow and retransplantation exceptional. Some data suggests lower recurrence with cyclosporin use as opposed to tacrolimus [144], and whilst UDCA appears to improve liver biochemistry, in the short term it does not alter histological progression [145].

The future for therapy in primary biliary cirrhosis

Although most physicians will prescribe UDCA for patients with PBC, newer and more targeted therapies are needed. Specific targets may arise when there is a better biologic understanding of disease. The group of patients most appropriate for new agents would logically be those who fail to respond adequately to UDCA (around 40% of patients) and a number of agents are worthy of comment. The addition of bezafibrate (which may increase phospholipid translocation into the bile) has been investigated, but the results to date are early and a well-powered study is needed [146, 147]. Atorvastatin, with many anti-inflammatory properties beyond its lipid lowering effects, was recently shown not to be of value for PBC [148]. In view of the cloning of a human retrovirus from a cDNA library derived from PBC biliary epithelia cells, anti-retrovirals have been investigated, but convincing data is still awaited [149, 150]. More selective immunosuppression (e.g. rituximab) is also being studied. More specific approaches focusing on fibrosis modulation may eventually prove efficacious, for example rapamycin, angiotensin blockade, or adhesion molecule modulation. Finally, other ways of targeting the bile acid pathway are being pursued. Modifications to UDCA (e.g. nor-UDCA) may appeal [151], as well as interfering with nuclear hormone receptors [152]. The Farnesoid X receptor (FXR) is a bile acid-activated nuclear receptor highly expressed in both the liver and gastrointestinal tract. It has a role in regulating bile and cholesterol metabolism and FXR agonists (e.g. novel bile acids or small molecule agonists such as INT-747) may have a place in treating cholestatic liver diseases. The first ever genome wide association study in PBC published in 2009 [153] identified the IL-12 signaling axis as highly relevant to disease, and so rational therapy may now truly be on the horizon for patients.

References

1 Kaplan MM, Gershwin ME. Primary biliary cirrhosis. *N Engl J Med* 2005; **353**: 1261–1273.

2 Gershwin ME, Mackay IR. The causes of primary biliary cirrhosis: convenient and inconvenient truths. *Hepatology* 2008; **47**: 737–745.

3 Gross RG, Odin JA. Recent advances in the epidemiology of primary biliary cirrhosis. *Clin Liver Dis* 2008; **12**: 289–303.

4 Reuben A. The serology of the Addison-Gull syndrome. *Hepatology* 2003; **37**: 225–228.

5 Walker JG, Doniach D, Roitt IM, Sherlock S. Serological tests in diagnosis of primary biliary cirrhosis. *Lancet* 1965; **1**: 827–831.

6 Oertelt S, Rieger R, Selmi C *et al*. A sensitive bead assay for antimitochondrial antibodies: Chipping away at AMA-negative primary biliary cirrhosis. *Hepatology* 2007; **45**: 659–665.

7 Turchany JM, Uibo R, Kivik T *et al.* A study of antimitochondrial antibodies in a random population in Estonia. *Am J Gastroenterol* 1997; **92**: 124–126.

8 Mattalia A, Quaranta S, Leung PS *et al.* Characterization of antimitochondrial antibodies in health adults. *Hepatology* 1998; **27**: 656–661.

9 Lazaridis KN, Juran BD, Boe GM *et al.* Increased prevalence of antimitochondrial antibodies in first-degree relatives of patients with primary biliary cirrhosis. *Hepatology* 2007; **46**: 785–792.

10 O'Brien C, Joshi S, Feld JJ *et al.* Long-term follow-up of antimitochondrial antibody-positive autoimmune hepatitis. *Hepatology* 2008; **48**: 550–556.

11 Bhat M, Guindi M, Heathcote EJ, Hirschfield GM. Transient development of anti-mitochondrial antibodies accompanies autoimmune hepatitis-sclerosing cholangitis overlap. *Gut* 2009; **58**(1): 152–153.

12 Leung PS, Rossaro L, Davis PA *et al.* Antimitochondrial antibodies in acute liver failure: implications for primary biliary cirrhosis. *Hepatology* 2007; **46**: 1436–1442.

13 Butler P, Hamilton-Miller J, Baum H, Burroughs AK. Detection of M2 antibodies in patients with recurrent urinary tract infection using an ELISA and purified PBC specific antigens. Evidence for a molecular mimicry mechanism in the pathogenesis of primary biliary cirrhosis? *Biochem Mol Biol Int* 1995; **35**: 473–485.

14 Ludwig J. The pathology of primary biliary cirrhosis and autoimmune cholangitis. *Baillieres Best Pract Res Clin Gastroenterol* 2000; **14**: 601–613.

15 Garrido MC, Hubscher SG. Accuracy of staging in primary biliary cirrhosis. *J Clin Pathol* 1996; **49**: 556–559.

16 Lindor KD, Gershwin ME, Poupon R *et al.* AASLD Practice Guidelines: Primary biliary cirrhosis. *Hepatology* 2009; **50**: 291–308.

17 Zein CO, Angulo P, Lindor KD. When is liver biopsy needed in the diagnosis of primary biliary cirrhosis? *Clin Gastroenterol Hepatol* 2003; **1**: 89–95.

18 Sherlock S. Primary billiary cirrhosis (chronic intrahepatic obstructive jaundice). *Gastroenterology* 1959; **37**: 574–586.

19 Long RG, Scheuer PJ, Sherlock S. Presentation and course of asymptomatic primary biliary cirrhosis. *Gastroenterology* 1977; **72**: 1204–1207.

20 Metcalf JV, Mitchison HC, Palmer JM *et al.* Natural history of early primary biliary cirrhosis. *Lancet* 1996; **348**: 1399–1402.

21 Hirschfield GM, Heathcote EJ. Antimitochondrial antibody-negative primary biliary cirrhosis. *Clin Liver Dis* 2008; **12**: 323–331.

22 Muratori L, Granito A, Muratori P *et al.* Antimitochondrial antibodies and other antibodies in primary biliary cirrhosis: diagnostic and prognostic value. *Clin Liver Dis* 2008; **12**: 261–276, vii.

23 Pla X, Vergara M, Gil M *et al.* Incidence, prevalence and clinical course of primary biliary cirrhosis in a Spanish community. *Eur J Gastroenterol Hepatol* 2007; **19**: 859–864.

24 Lee J, Belanger A, Doucette JT *et al.* Transplantation trends in primary biliary cirrhosis. *Clin Gastroenterol Hepatol* 2007; **5**: 1313–1315.

25 Mendes FD, Kim WR, Pedersen R *et al.* Mortality attributable to cholestatic liver disease in the United States. *Hepatology* 2008; **47**: 1241–1247.

26 Abe M, Onji M. Natural history of primary biliary cirrhosis. *Hepatol Res* 2008; **38**: 639–645.

27 Nakamura M, Kondo H, Mori T *et al.* Anti-gp210 and anti-centromere antibodies are different risk factors for the progression of primary biliary cirrhosis. *Hepatology* 2007; **45**: 118–127.

28 Newton JL, Jones DE, Henderson E *et al.* Fatigue in non-alcoholic fatty liver disease (NAFLD) is significant and associates with inactivity and excessive daytime sleepiness but not with liver disease severity or insulin resistance. *Gut* 2008; **57**: 807–813.

29 Balasubramaniam K, Grambsch PM, Wiesner RH *et al.* Diminished survival in asymptomatic primary biliary cirrhosis. A prospective study. *Gastroenterology* 1990; **98**: 1567–1571.

30 Springer J, Cauch-Dudek K, O'Rourke K *et al.* Asymptomatic primary biliary cirrhosis: a study of its natural history and prognosis. *Am J Gastroenterol* 1999; **94**: 47–53.

31 Mahl TC, Shockcor W, Boyer JL. Primary biliary cirrhosis: survival of a large cohort of symptomatic and asymptomatic patients followed for 24 years. *J Hepatol* 1994; **20**: 707–713.

32 Prince MI, Chetwynd A, Craig WL *et al.* Asymptomatic primary biliary cirrhosis: clinical features, prognosis, and symptom progression in a large population based cohort. *Gut* 2004; **53**: 865–870.

33 Prince M, Chetwynd A, Newman W *et al.* Survival and symptom progression in a geographically based cohort of patients with primary biliary cirrhosis: follow-up for up to 28 years. *Gastroenterology* 2002; **123**: 1044–1051.

34 Newton JL, Jones DE, Metcalf JV *et al.* Presentation and mortality of primary biliary cirrhosis in older patients. *Age Ageing* 2000; **29**: 305–309.

35 Cauch-Dudek K, Abbey S, Stewart DE, Heathcote EJ. Fatigue in primary biliary cirrhosis. *Gut* 1998; **43**: 705–710.

36 Newton JL, Bhala N, Burt J, Jones DE. Characterisation of the associations and impact of symptoms in primary biliary cirrhosis using a disease specific quality of life measure. *J Hepatol* 2006; **44**: 776–783.

37 Chan CW, Carpenter JR, Rigamonti C *et al.* Survival following the development of ascites and/or peripheral oedema in primary biliary cirrhosis: a staged prognostic model. *Scand J Gastroenterol* 2005; **40**: 1081–1089.

38 Colina F, Pinedo F, Solis JA *et al.* Nodular regenerative hyperplasia of the liver in early histological stages of primary biliary cirrhosis. *Gastroenterology* 1992; **102**: 1319–1324.

39 Shapiro JM, Smith H, Schaffner F. Serum bilirubin: a prognostic factor in primary biliary cirrhosis. *Gut* 1979; **20**: 137–140.

40 Poupon R, Chretien Y, Poupon RE *et al.* Is ursodeoxycholic acid an effective treatment for primary biliary cirrhosis? *Lancet* 1987; **1**: 834–836.

41 Kilmurry MR, Heathcote EJ, Cauch-Dudek K *et al.* Is the Mayo model for predicting survival useful after the introduction of ursodeoxycholic acid treatment for primary biliary cirrhosis? *Hepatology* 1996; **23**: 1148–1153.

42 Krzeski P, Zych W, Kraszewska E *et al.* Is serum bilirubin concentration the only valid prognostic marker in primary biliary cirrhosis? *Hepatology* 1999; **30**: 865–869.

43 Dickson ER, Grambsch PM, Fleming TR *et al.* Prognosis in primary biliary cirrhosis: model for decision making. *Hepatology* 1989; **10**: 1–7.

44 Murtaugh PA, Dickson ER, Van Dam GM *et al.* Primary biliary cirrhosis: prediction of short-term survival based on repeated patient visits. *Hepatology* 1994; **20**: 126–134.

45 Hughes MD, Raskino CL, Pocock SJ *et al.* Prediction of short-term survival with an application in primary biliary cirrhosis. *Stat Med* 1992; **11**: 1731–1745.

46 Kamath PS, Wiesner RH, Malinchoc M *et al.* A model to predict survival in patients with end-stage liver disease. *Hepatology* 2001; **33**: 464–470.

47 Pares A, Caballeria L, Rodes J. Excellent long-term survival in patients with primary biliary cirrhosis and biochemical response to ursodeoxycholic Acid. *Gastroenterology* 2006; **130**: 715–720.

48 Corpechot C, Abenavoli L, Rabahi N *et al.* Biochemical response to ursodeoxycholic acid and long-term prognosis in primary biliary cirrhosis. *Hepatology* 2008; **48**: 871–877.

49 Huet PM, Vincent C, Deslaurier J *et al.* Portal hypertension and primary biliary cirrhosis: effect of long-term ursodeoxycholic acid treatment. *Gastroenterology* 2008; **135**: 1552–1560.

50 Locke GRr, Therneau TM, Ludwig J *et al.* Time course of histological progression in primary biliary cirrhosis. *Hepatology* 1996; **23**: 52–56.

51 Roll J, Boyer JL, Barry D, Klatskin G. The prognostic importance of clinical and histologic features in asymptomatic and symptomatic primary biliary cirrhosis. *N Engl J Med* 1983; **308**: 1–7.

52 Corpechot C, Carrat F, Poupon R, Poupon RE. Primary biliary cirrhosis: incidence and predictive factors of cirrhosis development in ursodiol-treated patients. *Gastroenterology* 2002; **122**: 652–658.

53 Vleggaar FP, van Buuren HR, Zondervan PE *et al.* Jaundice in non-cirrhotic primary biliary cirrhosis: the premature ductopenic variant. *Gut* 2001; **49**: 276–281.

54 Van Norstrand MD, Malinchoc M, Lindor KD *et al.* Quantitative measurement of autoantibodies to recombinant mitochondrial antigens in patients with primary biliary cirrhosis: relationship of levels of autoantibodies to disease progression. *Hepatology* 1997; **25**: 6–11.

55 Poupon RE, Balkau B, Eschwege E, Poupon R. A multicenter, controlled trial of ursodiol for the treatment of primary biliary cirrhosis. UDCA-PBC Study Group. *N Engl J Med.* 1991; **324**: 1548–1554.

56 Bogdanos DP, Liaskos C, Pares A *et al.* Anti-gp210 antibody mirrors disease severity in primary biliary cirrhosis. *Hepatology* 2007; **45**: 1583; author reply 1583–1583; author reply 1584.

57 Sherlock S, Scheuer PJ. The presentation and diagnosis of 100 patients with primary biliary cirrhosis. *N Engl J Med* 1973; **289**: 674–678.

58 Gluud C, Brok J, Gong Y, Koretz RL. Hepatology may have problems with putative surrogate outcome measures. *J Hepatol* 2007; **46**: 734–742.

59 Menon KV, Angulo P, Weston S *et al.* Bone disease in primary biliary cirrhosis: independent indicators and rate of progression. *J Hepatol* 2001; **35**: 316–323.

60 Newton J, Francis R, Prince M *et al.* Osteoporosis in primary biliary cirrhosis revisited. *Gut* 2001; **49**: 282–287.

61 Benetti A, Crosignani A, Varenna M *et al.* Primary biliary cirrhosis is not an additional risk factor for bone loss in women receiving regular calcium and vitamin D supplementation: a controlled longitudinal study. *J Clin Gastroenterol* 2008; **42**: 306–311.

62 Heathcote J, Ross A, Sherlock S. A prospective controlled trial of azathioprine in primary biliary cirrhosis. *Gastroenterology* 1976; **70**: 656–660.

63 Christensen E, Neuberger J, Crowe J *et al.* Beneficial effect of azathioprine and prediction of prognosis in primary biliary cirrhosis. Final results of an international trial. *Gastroenterology* 1985; **89**: 1084–1091.

64 Talwalkar JA, Angulo P, Keach JC *et al.* Mycophenolate mofetil for the treatment of primary biliary cirrhosis in patients with an incomplete response to ursodeoxycholic acid. *J Clin Gastroenterol* 2005; **39**: 168–171.

65 Minuk GY, Bohme CE, Burgess E *et al.* Pilot study of cyclosporin A in patients with symptomatic primary biliary cirrhosis. *Gastroenterology* 1988; **95**: 1356–1363.

66 Wiesner RH, Ludwig J, Lindor KD *et al.* A controlled trial of cyclosporine in the treatment of primary biliary cirrhosis. *N Engl J Med* 1990; **322**: 1419–1424.

67 Lombard M, Portmann B, Neuberger J *et al.* Cyclosporin A treatment in primary biliary cirrhosis: results of a long-term placebo controlled trial. *Gastroenterology* 1993; **104**: 519–526.

68 Gong Y, Christensen E, Gluud C. Cyclosporin A for primary biliary cirrhosis. *Cochrane Database of Systematic Reviews* 2007, Issue 3. Art. No.: CD005526. DOI: 10.1002/14651858.CD005526. pub2.

69 Kaplan MM, Knox TA. Treatment of primary biliary cirrhosis with low-dose weekly methotrexate. *Gastroenterology* 1991; **101**: 1332–1338.

70 Kaplan MM, Schmid C, Provenzale D *et al.* A prospective trial of colchicine and methotrexate in the treatment of primary biliary cirrhosis. *Gastroenterology* 1999; **117**: 1173–1180.

71 Hendrickse MT, Rigney E, Giaffer MH. Low-dose methotrexate is ineffective in primary biliary cirrhosis: long-term results of a placebo-controlled trial. *Gastroenterology* 1999; **117**: 400–407.

72 Combes B, Emerson SS, Flye NL *et al.* Methotrexate (MTX) plus ursodeoxycholic acid (UDCA) in the treatment of primary biliary cirrhosis. *Hepatology* 2005; **42**: 1184–1193.

73 Mitchison HC, Palmer JM, Bassendine MF *et al.* A controlled trial of prednisolone treatment in primary biliary cirrhosis. Three-year results. *J Hepatol* 1992; **15**: 336–344.

74 Wolfhagen FH, van Buuren HR, den Ouden JW *et al.* Cyclical etidronate in the prevention of bone loss in corticosteroid-treated primary biliary cirrhosis. a prospective, controlled pilot study. *J Hepatol* 1997; **26**: 325–330.

75 Leuschner M, Maier KP, Schlichting J *et al.* Oral budesonide and ursodeoxycholic acid for treatment of primary biliary cirrhosis: results of a prospective double-blind trial. *Gastroenterology* 1999; **117**: 918–925.

76 Angulo P, Jorgensen RA, Keach JC *et al.* Oral budesonide in the treatment of patients with primary biliary cirrhosis with a suboptimal response to ursodeoxycholic acid. *Hepatology* 2000; **31**: 318–323.

77 Rautiainen H, Karkkainen P, Karvonen AL *et al.* Budesonide combined with UDCA to improve liver histology in primary biliary cirrhosis: a three-year randomized trial. *Hepatology* 2005; **41**: 747–752.

78 Wolfhagen FH, van Hoogstraten HJ, van Buuren HR *et al.* Triple therapy with ursodeoxycholic acid, prednisone and azathioprine in primary biliary cirrhosis: a 1-year randomized, placebo-controlled study. *J Hepatol* 1998; **29**: 736–742.

79 Hoofnagle JH, Davis GL, Schafer DF *et al.* Randomized trial of chlorambucil for primary biliary cirrhosis. *Gastroenterology* 1986; **91**: 1327–1334.

80 McCormick PA, Scott F, Epstein O *et al.* Thalidomide as therapy for primary biliary cirrhosis: a double-blind placebo controlled pilot study. *J Hepatol* 1994; **21**: 496–499.

81 Kaplan MM, Alling DW, Zimmerman HJ *et al.* A prospective trial of colchicine for primary biliary cirrhosis. *N Engl J Med* 1986; **315**: 1448–1454.

82 Warnes TW, Smith A, Lee FI *et al.* A controlled trial of colchicine in primary biliary cirrhosis. Trial design and preliminary report. *J Hepatol* 1987; **5**: 1–7.

83 Bodenheimer HJ, Schaffner F, Pezzullo J. Evaluation of colchicine therapy in primary biliary cirrhosis. *Gastroenterology* 1988; **95**: 124–129.

84 Zifroni A, Schaffner F. Long-term follow-up of patients with primary biliary cirrhosis on colchicine therapy. *Hepatology* 1991; **14**: 990–993.

85 Jain S, Scheuer PJ, Samourian S, McGee JO. A controlled trial of D-penicillamine therapy in primary biliary cirrhosis. *Lancet* 1977; **1**: 831–834.

86 Fleming CR, Ludwig J, Dickson ER. Asymptomatic primary biliary cirrhosis. Presentation, histology, and results with D-penicillamine. *Mayo Clin Proc* 1978; **53**: 587–593.

87 Epstein O, Jain S, Lee RG *et al.* D-penicillamine treatment improves survival in primary biliary cirrhosis. *Lancet* 1981; **1**: 1275–1277.

88 Matloff DS, Alpert E, Resnick RH, Kaplan MM. A prospective trial of D-penicillamine in primary biliary cirrhosis. *N Engl J Med* 1982; **306**: 319–326.

89 Taal BG, Schalm SW, Ten Kate FW *et al.* Low therapeutic value of D-penicillamine in a short-term prospective trial in primary biliary cirrhosis. *Liver* 1983; **3**: 345–352.

90 Bodenheimer HCJ, Schaffner F, Sternlieb I *et al.* A prospective clinical trial of D-penicillamine in the treatment of primary biliary cirrhosis. *Hepatology* 1985; **5**: 1139–1142.

91 Dickson ER, Fleming TR, Wiesner RH *et al.* Trial of penicillamine in advanced primary biliary cirrhosis. *N Engl J Med* 1985; **312**: 1011–1015.

92 Neuberger J, Christensen E, Portmann B *et al.* Double blind controlled trial of d-penicillamine in patients with primary biliary cirrhosis. *Gut* 1985; **26**: 114–119.

93 Gong Y, Gluud C. Colchicine for primary biliary cirrhosis: a Cochrane Hepato-Biliary Group systematic review of randomized clinical trials. *Am J Gastroenterol* 2005; **100**: 1876–1885.

94 Gong Y, Klingenberg SL, Gluud C. D-penicillamine for primary biliary cirrhosis. *Cochrane Database of Systematic Reviews* 2004, Issue 4. Art. No.: CD004789. DOI: 10.1002/14651858.CD004789.pub2.

95 Lindor K. Ursodeoxycholic acid for the treatment of primary biliary cirrhosis. *N Engl J Med* 2007; **357**: 1524–1529.

96 Goulis J, Leandro G, Burroughs AK. Randomised controlled trials of ursodeoxycholic-acid therapy for primary biliary cirrhosis: a meta-analysis. *Lancet* 1999; **354**: 1053–1060.

97 Gong Y, Huang ZB, Christensen E, Gluud C. Ursodeoxycholic acid for primary biliary cirrhosis. *Cochrane Database of Systematic Reviews* 2008, Issue 3. Art. No.: CD000551. DOI: 10.1002/14651858.CD000551.pub2.

98 Makino I, Tanaka H. From a choleretic to an immunomodulator: historical review of ursodeoxycholic acid as a medicament. *J Gastroenterol Hepatol* 1998; **13**: 659–664.

99 Beuers U. Drug insight: Mechanisms and sites of action of ursodeoxycholic acid in cholestasis. *Nat Clin Pract Gastroenterol Hepatol* 2006; **3**: 318–328.

100 Leuschner U, Leuschner M, Sieratzki J *et al.* Gallstone dissolution with ursodeoxycholic acid in patients with chronic active hepatitis and two years follow-up. A pilot study. *Dig Dis Sci* 1985; **30**: 642–649.

101 Podda M, Ghezzi C, Battezzati PM *et al.* Effect of different doses of ursodeoxycholic acid in chronic liver disease. *Dig Dis Sci* 1989; **34**: 59S–65S.

102 Poupon RE, Poupon R, Balkau B. Ursodiol for the long-term treatment of primary biliary cirrhosis. The UDCA-PBC Study Group. *N Engl J Med* 1994; **330**: 1342–1347.

103 Angulo P, Dickson ER, Therneau TM *et al.* Comparison of three doses of ursodeoxycholic acid in the treatment of primary biliary cirrhosis: a randomized trial. *J Hepatol* 1999; **30**: 830–835.

104 Siegel JL, Jorgensen R, Angulo P, Lindor KD. Treatment with ursodeoxycholic acid is associated with weight gain in patients with primary biliary cirrhosis. *J Clin Gastroenterol* 2003; **37**: 183–185.

105 Kondrackiene J, Beuers U, Kupcinskas L. Efficacy and safety of ursodeoxycholic acid versus cholestyramine in intrahepatic cholestasis of pregnancy. *Gastroenterology* 2005; **129**: 894–901.

106 Lindor KD, Dickson ER, Baldus WP *et al.* Ursodeoxycholic acid in the treatment of primary biliary cirrhosis. *Gastroenterology* 1994; **106**: 1284–1290.

107 Lindor KD, Therneau TM, Jorgensen RA *et al.* Effects of ursodeoxycholic acid on survival in patients with primary biliary cirrhosis. *Gastroenterology* 1996; **110**: 1515–1518.

108 Jorgensen R, Angulo P, Dickson ER, Lindor KD. Results of long-term ursodiol treatment for patients with primary biliary cirrhosis. *Am J Gastroenterol* 2002; **97**: 2647–2650.

109 Corpechot C, Carrat F, Bahr A *et al.* The effect of ursodeoxycholic acid therapy on the natural course of primary biliary cirrhosis. *Gastroenterology* 2005; **128**: 297–303.

110 ter Borg PC, Schalm SW, Hansen BE, van Buuren HR. Prognosis of ursodeoxycholic Acid-treated patients with primary biliary cirrhosis. Results of a 10-yr cohort study involving 297 patients. *Am J Gastroenterol* 2006; **101**: 2044–2050.

111 Chan CW, Gunsar F, Feudjo M *et al.* Long-term ursodeoxycholic acid therapy for primary biliary cirrhosis: a follow-up to 12 years. *Aliment Pharmacol Ther* 2005; **21**: 217–226.

112 Heathcote EJ, Cauch-Dudek K, Walker V *et al.* The Canadian Multicenter Double-blind Randomized Controlled Trial of ursodeoxycholic acid in primary biliary cirrhosis. *Hepatology* 1994; **19**: 1149–1156.

113 Poupon RE, Lindor KD, Cauch-Dudek K *et al.* Combined analysis of randomized controlled trials of ursodeoxycholic acid in primary biliary cirrhosis. *Gastroenterology* 1997; **113**: 884–890.

114 Combes B, Carithers RLJ, Maddrey WC *et al.* A randomized, double-blind, placebo-controlled trial of ursodeoxycholic acid in primary biliary cirrhosis. *Hepatology* 1995; **22**: 759–766.

115 Combes B, Luketic VA, Peters MG *et al.* Prolonged follow-up of patients in the US multicenter trial of ursodeoxycholic acid

for primary biliary cirrhosis. *Am J Gastroenterol* 2004; **99**: 264–268.

116 Shi J, Wu C, Lin Y *et al.* Long-term effects of mid-dose ursodeoxycholic acid in primary biliary cirrhosis: a meta-analysis of randomized controlled trials. *Am J Gastroenterology* 2006; **101**: 1529–1538.

117 Solaymani-Dodaran M, Card TR, Aithal GP, West J. Fracture risk in people with primary biliary cirrhosis: a population-based cohort study. *Gastroenterology* 2006; **131**: 1752–1757.

118 Pares A, Guanabens N. Osteoporosis in primary biliary cirrhosis: pathogenesis and treatment. *Clin Liver Dis* 2008; **12**: 407–424.

119 Lindor KD, Janes CH, Crippin JS *et al.* Bone disease in primary biliary cirrhosis: does ursodeoxycholic acid make a difference? *Hepatology* 1995; **21**: 389–392.

120 Guanabens N, Pares A, Navasa M *et al.* Cyclosporin A increases the biochemical markers of bone remodeling in primary biliary cirrhosis. *J Hepatol* 1994; **21**: 24–28.

121 Lindor KD, Jorgensen RA, Tiegs RD *et al.* Etidronate for osteoporosis in primary biliary cirrhosis: a randomized trial. *J Hepatol* 2000; **33**: 878–882.

122 Zein CO, Jorgensen RA, Clarke B *et al.* Alendronate improves bone mineral density in primary biliary cirrhosis: a randomized placebo-controlled trial. *Hepatology* 2005; **42**: 762–771.

123 Menon KV, Angulo P, Boe GM, Lindor KD. Safety and efficacy of estrogen therapy in preventing bone loss in primary biliary cirrhosis. *Am J Gastroenterol* 2003; **98**: 889–892.

124 Pereira SP, O'Donohue J, Moniz C *et al.* Transdermal hormone replacement therapy improves vertebral bone density in primary biliary cirrhosis: results of a 1-year controlled trial. *Aliment Pharmacol Ther* 2004; **19**: 563–570.

125 Boone RH, Cheung AM, Girlan LM, Heathcote EJ. Osteoporosis in primary biliary cirrhosis: a randomized trial of the efficacy and feasibility of estrogen/progestin. *Dig Dis Sci* 2006; **51**: 1103–1112.

126 Jacoby A, Rannard A, Buck D *et al.* Development, validation, and evaluation of the PBC-40, a disease specific health related quality of life measure for primary biliary cirrhosis. *Gut* 2005; **54**: 1622–1629.

127 Jones DE, Newton JL. An open study of modafinil for the treatment of daytime somnolence and fatigue in primary biliary cirrhosis. *Aliment Pharmacol Ther* 2007; **25**: 471–476.

128 Bergasa NV. Pruritus in primary biliary cirrhosis: pathogenesis and therapy. *Clin Liver Dis* 2008; **12**: 385–406.

129 Tandon P, Rowe BH, Vandermeer B, Bain VG. The efficacy and safety of bile Acid binding agents, opioid antagonists, or rifampin in the treatment of cholestasis-associated pruritus. *Am J Gastroenterol* 2007; **102**: 1528–1536.

130 Van Itallie TB, Hashim SA, Crampton RS, Tennent DM. The treatment of pruritus and hypercholesteremia of primary biliary cirrhosis with cholestyramine. *N Engl J Med* 1961; **265**: 469–474.

131 Datta DV, Sherlock S. Cholestyramine for long term relief of the pruritus complicating intrahepatic cholestasis. *Gastroenterology* 1966; **50**: 323–332.

132 Khurana S, Singh P. Rifampin is safe for treatment of pruritus due to chronic cholestasis: a meta-analysis of prospective randomized-controlled trials. *Liver Int* 2006; **26**: 943–948.

133 Mayo MJ, Handem I, Saldana S *et al.* Sertraline as a first-line treatment for cholestatic pruritus. *Hepatology* 2007; **45**: 666–674.

134 Bergasa NV, Talbot TL, Alling DW *et al.* A controlled trial of naloxone infusions for the pruritus of chronic cholestasis. *Gastroenterology* 1992; **102**: 544–549.

135 Wolfhagen FH, Sternieri E, Hop WC *et al.* Oral naltrexone treatment for cholestatic pruritus: a double-blind, placebo-controlled study. *Gastroenterology* 1997; **113**: 1264–1269.

136 Cohen LB, Ambinder EP, Wolke AM *et al.* Role of plasmapheresis in primary biliary cirrhosis. *Gut* 1985; **26**: 291–294.

137 Pusl T, Denk GU, Parhofer KG, Beuers U. Plasma separation and anion adsorption transiently relieve intractable pruritus in primary biliary cirrhosis. *J Hepatol* 2006; **45**: 887–891.

138 Pares A, Cisneros L, Salmeron JM *et al.* Extracorporeal albumin dialysis: a procedure for prolonged relief of intractable pruritus in patients with primary biliary cirrhosis. *Am J Gastroenterol* 2004; **99**: 1105–1110.

139 Pares A, Caballeria L, Rodes J *et al.* Long-term effects of ursodeoxycholic acid in primary biliary cirrhosis: results of a double-blind controlled multicentric trial. UDCA-Cooperative Group from the Spanish Association for the Study of the Liver. *J Hepatol* 2000; **32**: 561–566.

140 Corpechot C, Carrat F, Bonnand AM *et al.* The effect of ursodeoxycholic acid therapy on liver fibrosis progression in primary biliary cirrhosis. *Hepatology* 2000; **32**: 1196–1199.

141 Poupon RE, Lindor KD, Pares A *et al.* Combined analysis of the effect of treatment with ursodeoxycholic acid on histologic progression in primary biliary cirrhosis. *J Hepatol* 2003; **39**: 12–16.

142 Pasha T, Heathcote J, Gabriel S *et al.* Cost-effectiveness of ursodeoxycholic acid therapy in primary biliary cirrhosis. *Hepatology* 1999; **29**: 21–26.

143 Mottershead M, Neuberger J. Transplantation in autoimmune liver diseases. *World J Gastroenterol* 2008; **14**: 3388–3395.

144 Dmitrewski J, Hubscher SG, Mayer AD, Neuberger JM. Recurrence of primary biliary cirrhosis in the liver allograft: the effect of immunosuppression. *J Hepatol* 1996; **24**: 253–257.

145 Charatcharoenwitthaya P, Pimentel S, Talwalkar JA *et al.* Long-term survival and impact of ursodeoxycholic acid treatment for recurrent primary biliary cirrhosis after liver transplantation. *Liver Transpl* 2007; **13**: 1236–1245.

146 Iwasaki S, Ohira H, Nishiguchi S *et al.* The efficacy of ursodeoxycholic acid and bezafibrate combination therapy for primary biliary cirrhosis: A prospective, multicenter study. *Hepatol Res* 2008; **38**: 557–564.

147 Walker LJ, Newton J, Jones DE, Bassendine MF. Comment on biochemical response to ursodeoxycholic acid and long-term prognosis in primary biliary cirrhosis. *Hepatology* 2008; **49**: 337–338.

148 Stojakovic T, Putz-Bankuti C, Fauler G *et al.* Atorvastatin in patients with primary biliary cirrhosis and incomplete biochemical response to ursodeoxycholic acid. *Hepatology* 2007; **46**: 776–784.

149 Mason AL, Farr GH, Xu L *et al.* Pilot studies of single and combination antiretroviral therapy in patients with primary biliary cirrhosis. *Am J Gastroenterol* 2004; **99**: 2348–2355.

150 Mason AL, Lindor KD, Bacon BR *et al.* Clinical trial: randomized controlled trial of zidovudine and lamivudine for patients with primary biliary cirrhosis stabilized on ursodiol. *Aliment Pharmacol Ther* 2008; **28**: 886–894.

151 Fickert P, Wagner M, Marschall HU *et al.* 24-norUrsodeoxycholic acid is superior to ursodeoxycholic acid in the treatment of sclerosing cholangitis in Mdr2 (Abcb4) knockout mice. *Gastroenterology* 2006; **130**: 465–481.

152 Zollner G, Marschall HU, Wagner M, Trauner M. Role of nuclear receptors in the adaptive response to bile acids and cholestasis: pathogenetic and therapeutic considerations. *Mol Pharm* 2006; **3**: 231–251.

153 Hirschfield GM, Liu X, Xu C *et al.* Primary biliary cirrhosis associated with HLA, IL12A, and IL12RB2 variants. *N Engl J Med* 2009; **360**: 2544–2555.

33 Autoimmune hepatitis

Michael MP Manns and Arndt Vogel

Department of Gastroenterology, Hepatology and Endocrinology, Medical School, Hanover, Germany

Introduction

Autoimmune hepatitis is a self-perpetuating necroinflammatory disease of unknown etiology, which is characterized by a loss of tolerance towards the patient's own liver tissue. If left untreated the disease leads to cirrhosis and liver failure. Since the recognition of immunologically based liver disease in the 1950s, efforts have been directed toward the development of tools for diagnosis, classification according to serological markers and clinical course, and distinguishing autoimmune hepatitis from other liver diseases.

In the early years diagnosis of autoimmune hepatitis was hampered by the lack of knowledge about the etiology of most acute and chronic liver diseases. The detection of hepatitis viruses and a better understanding of the etiology of other forms of liver disease allowed for the exclusion of patients with these disorders from studies of autoimmune hepatitis and a more accurate determination of prognosis and effects of immunosuppressive drugs. The characterization of distinctive autoantibodies and the identification of autoantigens led to a more specific diagnosis of the disease and to the ability to characterize distinct subclasses according to prognosis, treatment response and outcome.

Features of autoimmune hepatitis

Autoimmune hepatitis is a syndrome which is characterized by a typical constellation of epidemiological, laboratory and clinical features: female predominance (female: male ratio 4:1), overrepresentation of the human leukocyte antigen (HLA) alleles DR3 and DR4, hypergammaglob-

ulinemia, circulating autoantibodies, response to immunosuppressive therapy and coexistence of extrahepatic autoimmune diseases. The disease is seen in all ethnic groups and at all ages [1–5]. The mean annual incidence of AIH among white Northern Europeans is ~2 per 100,000 inhabitants, and its point prevalence is ~17 per 100,000 [6].

Clinical features

Although autoimmune hepatitis occurs mainly in young women, the disease may develop at any age and in either sex [5]. Patients with AIH frequently complain about non-specific symptoms such as fatigue, jaundice, nausea and abdominal pain at presentation, but the clinical spectrum is wide, ranging from an asymptomatic presentation to fulminant disease. Forty percent of patients present with acute hepatitis [7]. Fulminant liver failure may occur but is rare. Hepatomegaly is common and an enlarged spleen is palpable in 50% of patients. In some patients the disease progresses without major symptoms, and the diagnosis is not made until symptoms of severe liver disease are present. Amenorrhea occurs in women with severe hepatic inflammation.

Coexisting extrahepatic autoimmune diseases are frequently found in patients with autoimmune hepatitis. Whereas arthropathies and periarticular swelling of both large and small joints occurs in 6–36% of patients, arthritis with joint erosions is rarely seen. Additional clinical features are listed in Table 33.1.

The risk of hepatocellular carcinoma in autoimmune liver disease varies considerably between the different diseases PBC, PSC and AIH. Particular PSC can be complicated by cholangiocarcinoma, gallbladder carcinoma and hepatocellular carcinoma [8]. In contrast, the incidence of HCCs in patients with AIH was not well documented for a long time. However, several recent retrospective studies indicate that about 2% of AIH patients eventually develop HCCs [9–11]. Similar to other chronic liver diseases, cirrhosis is the sine qua non for HCC development in AIH.

Evidence-Based Gastroenterology and Hepatology, 3rd edition.
J. McDonald, A.K. Burroughs, B. Feagan, and M.B. Fennerty. © 2010
Blackwell Publishing Ltd

Table 33.1 Extrahepatic autoimmune syndromes in autoimmune hepatitis.

Frequent symptoms	Rare symptoms
Arthritis	Mixed connective tissue disease
Vitiligo	Lichen planus
Autoimmune thyroid	Ulcerative colitis disease
Insulin dependent diabetes	
Hirsutism, cushingoid features	

Serological features

Autoantibodies are an important tool for the diagnosis of AIH [12]. However, autoantibodies are not specific to AIH and their expressions can vary during the course of AIH [13]. Furthermore, a low autoantibody titer does not exclude the diagnosis of AIH and a high titer (in the absence of other supportive findings) does not establish the diagnosis. Importantly, autoantibodies do not cause the disease nor alter in titer in response to treatment (at least in adult populations); as such, they do not need to be serially monitored [12]. ANA, SMA and LKM are pivotal components for the diagnosis of AIH and should be first tested in suspicious patients [14]. ANA were the first autoantibodies to be associated with AIH and led Mackay to create the term "lupoid" hepatitis as early as 1956. ANA are the most nonspecific marker of AIH and can also be found in PBC, PSC, viral hepatitis, drug-related hepatitis, and alcoholic and non-alcoholic, fatty liver disease [15, 16]. Additionally, serum ANAs have been reported to occur in up to 15% of the general healthy populations from different countries, increasing with age. SMA are frequently found in AIH, and are directed against components of the cytoskeleton such as actin and non-actin components, including tubulin, vimentin, desmin and skeletin [15]. They frequently occur in high titers in association with ANA and are, like ANA, present in a variety of liver and non-liver diseases such as rheumatic diseases. Antibodies to LKM were first discovered in 1973 by indirect immunofluorescence and are reactive with the proximal renal tubule and hepatocellular cytoplasm [17, 18]. They form a heterogeneous group and are associated with several immune mediated diseases, including AIH, drug-induced hepatitis, the autoimmune polyendocrinopathy-candidiasis-ectodermal dystrophy (APECED or APS-1), and chronic hepatitis C and D infection [15]. A 50 kilo Dalton antigen of LKM-1 was identified as the cytochrome mono-oxygenase P450 2D6 (CYP2D6). LKM-3 antibodies are directed against family 1 uridine 5′-diphosphate glucuronosyltransferase (UGT1A), which belong to the drug metabolizing enzymes located in the endoplasmatic reticulum.

Patients who present without these antibodies may be tested for other, characterized autoantibodies. Antibodies against LC-1, SLA/LP, pANCA and the asialoglycoprotein receptor may be helpful to extend the diagnosis of AIH in these patients. Anti-LC1 antibodies are visualized by indirect immunofluorescence. However, their characteristic staining may be masked by the more diffuse pattern of LKM-1 antibodies. Therefore, other techniques such as ouchterlony double diffusion, immunoblot and counterimmunoelectrophoresis are also used for their detection. The antigen recognized by anti-LC1 was identified as formiminotransferase cyclodeaminase (FTCD) [19]. Contrary to most other autoantibodies in AIH, anti-LC1 seems to correlate with disease activity and may be useful as a marker of residual hepatocellular inflammation in AIH [20]. Anti-SLA/LP antibodies are detectable by radioimmunoassay and enzyme linked immunosorbent assays (ELISA) but cannot be detected by immunofluorescence [15]. Anti-SLA/LP antibodies are considered to be highly specific for AIH, in which they are detectable in about 10–30% of patients. In some patients, they are the only serological marker of autoimmune hepatitis. Screening of cDNA expression libraries identified a UGA tRNA suppressor as anti-SLA target autoantigen [21]. Several studies suggest that patients with anti-SLA/LP antibodies display a more severe course of the disease [22–25].

Additionally, antibodies against cardiolipin, chromatin and *Saccharomyces cerevisiae* have been described in AIH, which, however, do not define patients with a distinctive clinical phenotype [26–28].

There have been several proposals to classify AIH according to different antibody profiles. According to this approach, AIH type I is characterized by the presence of ANA and/or anti-SMA antibodies. AIH type II is characterized by anti-LKM-1 and with lower frequency against LKM-3 antibodies. AIH type III is characterized by autoantibodies against SLA/LP. AIH-2 displays a regionally variable prevalence, with only 4% in the USA and up to 20% in western Europe [18, 29]. Patients with AIH-II are younger at presentation, show a more severe course at onset and are more likely to progress to cirrhosis [30]. Both entities of AIH are characterized by a high incidence of other organ specific immune mediated diseases, for example autoimmune thyroid disease, which are not only detected in patients with AIH, but also in their first degree relatives.

Histological features

Autoimmune hepatitis cannot be diagnosed by liver histology alone, since there are no pathognomonic histological features. Histology can only support the diagnosis and is used to classify disease activity (grading) and the degree of fibrosis (staging). There is a general agreement that bridging necrosis and multilobular necrosis should be

Table 33.2 HLA alleles and autoimmune hepatitis.

HLA allele	Population	Adults/Children	# Pat.	#Contr.	Risk ratio
DRB1*0301	Argentina	Children	122	208	3.0
DRB1*0301	North America, UK		297	236	3.39
DRB1*0301	India	Adults	20	113	3.79
DRB1*0404	Mexico	Mixed	30	175	7.71
DRB1*0405	Argentina	Adults	84	208	10.4
DRB1*0405	Japan	Adults	77	248	4.97
DRB1*1301	Argentina	Children	122	208	16.3
DRB1*1301	India	Adults	20	113	6.47
DRB1*1302	Argentina	Children	122	208	0.1
DRB1*14	India	Adults	20	113	3.25
DRB1*1501	North America, UK		297	236	0.52
DRB1*0301/ DRB1*0301	North America, UK		297	236	7.61
DRB1*0301/DRB1*04	North America, UK		297	236	5.09

regarded as factors associated with a poor prognosis. Interface hepatitis, also known as piecemeal necrosis or periportal hepatitis, is the histological hallmark and plasma cell infiltration is typical [14, 30–32].

Up to 30% of adult patients have histological features of cirrhosis at diagnosis [5, 33]. Recent data indicate that only a small number of patients develop cirrhosis during therapy and that fibrosis scores are stable or improve in up to 75% patients [34]. However, it is important to note that the presence of cirrhosis at baseline significantly increases the risk of death or liver transplantation [5, 35]. Almost half of children with AIH already have cirrhosis at the time of diagnosis [36, 37]. In elderly patients a more severe histological grade has been reported, but the frequency of cirrhosis does not seem to be different from that in younger patients [38, 39].

Genetic features

It is generally accepted that occurrence and probably the severity of autoimmune hepatitis is influenced by genetic factors. However, the heritable component of AIH is currently regarded as small. The most conclusive genetic association with autoimmune hepatitis is related to the major histocompatibility complex alleles. Among white northern European and Americans there is a well-recognized association between increased susceptibility to AIH and inheritance of HLA DR3 and HLA DR4 (later identified as DRB1*0301 and DRB1*0401 respectively) [40, 41]. HLA DR3 is the main susceptibility factor in white Caucasians, and HLA DR4 is a secondary but independent risk factor for the disease. Eighty-five percent of white patients with type I AIH from the USA and northern Europe have HLA DR3, DR4, or DR3 and DR4. Table 33.2 summarizes confirmed associations of HLA DRB1 alleles in AIH patients

from different populations [42]. Based on these data, different models have been created whereby genetic susceptibility and resistance to AIH is best related to specific amino acid sequence motifs within DRB1 polypeptides. Donaldson has suggested three different models: one, for type I AIH is dependent on histidine or other basic amino acid residues at position 13 of the DRβ polypeptide; the second is based on the amino acid residue LLEQKR at positions 67–72 of the DRβ polypeptide and the third model is based on valine/glycine dimorphism at position 86 [43].

HLA alleles associated with AIH confer not only susceptibility towards AIH but also appear to influence the course of the disease. Most strikingly, patients with the DRB1*0301 were found to be younger at disease onset and have a higher frequency of treatment failure, relapse after treatment withdrawal and liver transplantation. Patients with DRB1*0401 are at greater risk to develop additional autoimmune disorders, but are thought to be associated with milder disease, seen in older patients, which is easier to treat [41, 44, 45].

Diagnosis

Because signs and symptoms of AIH are not specific, an international panel (the International Autoimmune Hepatitis Group (IAIHG)) established a consensus on diagnostic criteria, and its recommendations were published in 1993 [46], and revised in 1999 [14]. These criteria include clinical, laboratory and histological findings at presentation, as well as response to corticosteroid therapy and are in most cases sufficient to make the diagnosis of autoimmune hepatitis and to distinguish it from other forms of chronic hepatitis. Response to corticosteroids may help to clarify the diagnosis even in patients who lack other typical features (see Table 33.3) [14, 30, 42, 47]. Additionally, a scoring system was established assigning points (both negative and positive) to specific findings to allow for the distinction between a definitive diagnosis and a probable diagnosis. Prior to corticosteroid treatment, a definitive diagnosis requires a score greater than 15; after treatment, a definitive diagnosis requires a score greater than 17.

The AIH scoring system was subsequently subjected to validation testing in several studies, which consistently showed that the sensitivity was very high (97–100%) but that the specificity for excluding AIH in patients with biliary disorders was markedly lower (44–65%) (see Table 33.3). The notable weakness of the original system in excluding cholestatic syndromes justified the subsequent revision to further downgrade cholestatic findings [14]. The new scoring system more precisely differentiated between biliary diseases and AIH, and application of the revised system in PBC and PSC patients revealed significantly less patients who scored for definite and probable AIH [48, 49].

However, the above-described criteria were primarily introduced to allow comparison of studies from different centers. Because these criteria are complex and include a variety of parameters of questionable value, the IAIHG decided to devise a simplified scoring system for wider applicability in routine clinical practice. A limited number of routinely available measurements were therefore selected to design the score. Liver histology (demonstration of hepatitis on histology is required), autoantibody titers, gamma-globulin/IgG levels, and the absence of viral hepatitis were found to be independent predictors for the presence of AIH (see Table 33.4) [50]. The score was found to have good sensitivity and specificity in a second validation set. Therefore a simple score based on four measurements may be sufficient to differentiate between patients with or without AIH, with a high degree of accuracy. However, additional studies are required to validate this score in patients with different chronic liver diseases.

Treatment

The indication for treatment of AIH is based on inflammatory activity and not so much on the presence of cirrhosis. In the absence of inflammatory activity immunosuppressive treatment has only limited effects. An indication for treatment is present when aminotransferases are elevated two-fold, gamma globulin levels are elevated two-fold and histology shows moderate to severe periportal hepatitis. Symptoms of severe fatigue are also an indication for treatment. An absolute indication exists in cases with a ten-fold or higher elevation of aminotransferase levels, histological signs of severe inflammation and necrosis, and upon disease progression.

Table 33.3 Scoring system for diagnosis of autoimmune hepatitis.

Parameter	Score
Gender	
Female	+2
Male	0
Serum biochemistry	
Ratio of elevation of serum alkaline phosphatase vs aminotransferase	
>3.0	−2
<3.0	+2
Total serum globulin, γ-globulin or IgG	
Times upper normal limit	
>2.0	+3
1.5–2.0	+2
1.0–1.5	+1
<1.0	0
Autoantibodies (titers by immunfluorescence on rodent tissues)	
Adults	
ANA, SMA or LKM-1	
>1:80	+3
1:80	+2
1:40	+1
<1:40	0
Children	
ANA or LKM-1	
>1:20	+3
1:10 or 1:20	+2
<1:20	0
or SMA	
>1:20	+3
1:20	+2
<1:20	0
Antimitochondrial antibody	
Positive	−2
Negative	0
Viral markers	
IgM anti-HAV, HBsAg orIgM anti-HBc positive	−3
Anti-HCV positive by ELISA and/or RIBA	−2
HCV positive by PCR for HCV RNA	−3
Positive test indicating active infection with any other virus	−3
Seronegative for all of the above	+3
Other etiological factors	
History of recent hepatotoxic drug usage or parenteral exposure to blood products	
Yes	−2
No	+1
Alcohol (average consumption)	
Male < 35 gm/day; female < 25 gm/day	+2
Male 35–50 gm/day; female 25–40 gm/day	0
Male 50–80 gm/day; female 40–60 gm/day	−1
Male > 80 gm/day; female > 60 gm/day	−2
Genetic factors: HLA DR3 or DR4	
Other autoimmune diseases in patient or first degree relatives	+1

Interpretation of aggregate scores: definite AIH, greater than 15 before treatment and greater than 17 after treatment; probable AIH 10 to 15 before treatment and 12 to 17 after treatment. Alvarez F, Berg PA, Bianchi FB *et al.* International Autoimmune Hepatitis Group Report: review of criteria for diagnosis of autoimmune hepatitis. *J Hepatol* 1999; **31**: 929–938.

Conventional corticosteroids and azathioprine

Three controlled trials provided evidence that corticosteroid therapy reduces mortality in autoimmune hepatitis, and this benefit was further substantiated by longer follow-up of the patients in one of these studies (see Table 33.5). The magnitude of the reduction of mortality produced by steroids can be estimated from the original analysis of the study of Cook *et al.* (control 55%, steroid 14%, absolute risk reduction (ARR) 42%, numbers needed to treat (NNT) = 3) and from the analysis conducted after ten-year follow-up of the same patient groups (control 73%, steroid 37%, ARR 36%, NNT = 3) [51, 52]. **A1d**

Treatment with prednisone monotherapy or in combination with azathioprine remains the standard therapy for patients with AIH [53]. Both are equally effective and the decision for either strategy involves the consideration of patient profiles [54]. Data from the randomized trials and from uncontrolled studies suggest that the remission rate is approximately 80% with initial therapy [55]. About 9% percent of patients deteriorate despite compliance to treatment, 13% improve, but not to a degree to reach remission and 13% are intolerant to standard therapy [56, 57]. Long-term remission is maintained by low-dose corticosteroids alone or in combination with azathioprine (1–2 mg/kg body weight) or with azathioprine monotherapy [53]. **B4**

Controlled trials have not been performed in patients with mild asymptomatic autoimmune hepatitis. In these patients, who numerically far outnumber patients with severe liver disease, the role for steroid therapy remains unclear and the decision to treat must be weighed against the risk of medication. A recent study revealed that the overall survival and survival to liver related endpoints of asymptomatic patients who received no therapy was not different to that of the total cohort [5]. **B4** However, asymptomatic patients not receiving therapy require a close follow-up since 25% of this group subsequently developed symptoms [5].

Treatment withdrawal should not be attempted less than 2–3 years from the start of therapy to prevent early relapse. Drug withdrawal should be preceded by liver biopsy if a long-term biochemical remission is not documented. The rate of relapse depends on the degree of continuing inflam-

---

Table 33.4 Simplified criteria for diagnosis of autoimmune hepatitis.

Concentration of serum IgG	
IgG > 16 g/l	1 point
IgG > 18 g/l	2 points
Serum auto antibodies (ANA, SMA, SLA/LP, LKM)	
ANA, SMA or LKM > 1 : 40	1 point
>1 : 80, or SLA/LP positive	2 points
Histology of chronic hepatitis	
Compatible with AIH	1 point
Typical for AIH	2 points
Exclusion of viral hepatitis	2 points

Score > 6 = probable AIH
Score > 7 = definite AIH

Cutoff 6 : 88% sensitivity und 97% specificity
Cutoff 7 : 81% sensitivity und 99% specificity

Table 33.5 Effect of prednisone on mortality in randomized controlled trials of chronic autoimmune hepatitis (CAH).

Study	Patients	Steroid regimen	Control intervention	Mortality		
				Control	Steroid	p
Cook *et al.* (1971)	49 patients with CAH, 35 with cirrhosis; no previous steroids; 5 patients (4 in steroid group) excluded from analysis because of change in diagnosis	Prednisone 15 mg (3–72 months) attempts to withdraw after 1 month	"No specific treatment"	3/22	15/27	<0.01
Soloway *et al.* (1972)	35[a] patients with chronic liver disease biochemically and histologically, 16 with cirrhosis	Prednisone 20 mg after 4 weeks tapering course from 60 mg (3 months to 3.5 years)	Placebo	1/18	7/17	<0.05
Murray-Lyon *et al.* (1973)	47 patients with chronic aggressive hepatitis, 33 with cirrhosis; approximately half had previous steroid or azathioprine	15 mg daily (up to 2 years); discontinued in 1 month if no improvement in liver function	Azathioprine 75 mg	1/22	6/25	N/A[b]

[a] Additional patients were randomized to receive prednisone 10 mg plus azathioprine 50 mg (14 patients), or azathioprine 100 mg (14 patients); see text.
[b] N/A, not available. Estimated probability of survival at two years: steroid 95%, azathioprine 72%.

mation and increases from 20% with complete resolution of hepatic inflammation to 50% with ongoing portal inflammation, and 100% with progression to cirrhosis or persisting periportal hepatitis. The rate of relapse after treatment withdrawal is as high as 80%. Those without relapse have to be regularly assessed by clinical parameters and liver biopsy, as the risk of relapse cannot be predicted reliably. Ongoing inflammation may exist without significantly elevated transaminases. Normal liver histology after two years of steroid therapy does not exclude relapse following treatment withdrawal.

Budesonide

Budesonide, a non-halogenated glucocorticoid, is of particular interest for the treatment of AIH, because it has a 15-fold greater receptor binding capacity than prednisolone, and a high hepatic first-pass clearance, exceeding 90% of the orally administered dose. Several small studies suggested that budesonide might be an interesting alternative for immunosuppression, with fewer side effects than conventional glucosteroids. The potential benefit of budesonide was therefore evaluated in a phase 3 multicenter, multinational clinical study. In this study, patients with newly diagnosed AIH and no signs of cirrhosis were randomized to a six-month treatment period. Randomized patients received either prednisolone (dose: 40 mg for the first four weeks, and then tapered down to 10 mg/day in week nine; upon early biochemical remission start of tapering was allowed already at week three) or 3 mg budesonide tid. Upon biochemical remission budesonide dose was reduced to 3 mg bid. All patients received azathioprine at a dose of 1–2 mg/kg body weight. The primary endpoint was defined as biochemical remission, defined as AST and ALT within normal range without steroid specific side effects throughout the six-month treatment period (complete response). In this largest AIH-trial, ever conducted, 3 mg tid oral budesonide was superior to oral prednisone in inducing biochemical remission in AIH with significantly less steroid specific side effects, suggesting that budesonide is a valid alternative for conventional steroids in selected patients [58]. **A1d**

Other immunosuppressive drugs

If standard treatment fails or drug intolerance occurs, alternative therapies can be considered. Several agents have emerged, especially from the transplantation setting, which might offer greater immunosuppression and which are better tolerated than prednisone and azathioprine. These include cyclosporine A, tacrolimus, cyclophosphamide, mercaptopurine, mycophenolate mofetil or deflazacort, which have been more or less successfully tested in several small studies with AIH patients [59–63]. **B4**

Liver transplantation

Liver transplantation remains the only life-saving option in approximately 10% of AIH patients. The indication for liver transplantation in AIH is similar to that in other chronic liver diseases [64]. The disease accounts for about 4–6% of liver transplantation in the USA and Europe. Candidates for liver transplantation are usually patients who do not show early response at six months of treatment and who do not reach remission within three years of continuous therapy [65. The long-term results of liver transplantation for AIH are excellent and well within the range of other indications for liver transplantation [66]. Studies published during past years indicate that the rate of recurrence of AIH ranges between 10–35%, and that the risk of AIH recurrence is perhaps as high as 68% after five years of follow-up [66, 67]. Prednisone alone or in combination with azathioprine remains the therapy for recurrent autoimmune hepatitis [68, 69]. Addition of rapamycin successfully treats patients with post-transplant hepatitis, not responding to treatment with increasing doses of prednisolone and addition of azathioprine or to calcineurin inhibitors [70]. **B4** Several follow-up studies indicate that patients with recurrent AIH are at risk of developing liver allograft cirrhosis, requiring re-transplantation. Some patients even develop recurrence of AIH within the second graft.

Development of *de novo* autoimmune hepatitis in patients who undergo transplantation for non-autoimmune liver disease is rare (2.5–3.4% of allografts) and predominantly occurs in children. [71–73]. Treatment with prednisolone and azathioprine is effective in these patients.

Prognosis

Data on the natural progression of untreated disease are derived principally from papers published in the 1960s and 1970s, prior to the widespread use of immunosuppressives for AIH. The mortality in untreated autoimmune hepatitis in the placebo control groups of these early clinical trials was greater than 50% within 3–5 years of diagnosis [74, 75]. However, only cases with severe inflammatory activity or fibrosis were included in these early trials. Although the etiology of the chronic hepatitis was not certain, due to the lack of viral markers, the majority of patients in these trials appear to have been suffering from autoimmune hepatitis. However, it was impossible to exclude hepatitis C infection until the early 1990s. Verification of these data on naive patients in whom the diagnosis of hepatitis C has been excluded is not possible, since studies including untreated control groups or cohort studies of untreated patients can no longer be justified ethically.

Several studies have shown that up to 30% of adult patients have histological features of cirrhosis at diagnosis.

In one study on the natural history of AIH from the Mayo clinic, Roberts *et al.* found that the ten-year survival of patients with cirrhosis was similar to that of patients without cirrhosis at baseline (93%) [76]. In contrast, one recent study reported that patients with cirrhosis at baseline had poorer ten-year survival (61.9%; CI: 44.9–78.9%) than those without cirrhosis at presentation (94.0%; CI: 87.4–100%) (p = 0.003) regardless of whether they presented with symptoms or whether they received immunosuppressive therapy [5]. **B4** Furthermore, patients with cirrhosis at presentation were shown to be more likely to die or develop complications of their liver disease during follow-up [35].

Almost half of the children with AIH already have cirrhosis at the time of diagnosis. Long-term follow-up revealed that only a few children can completely stop all treatment and about 70% of children receive long-term treatment [18, 36]. Most of these patients relapse when treatment is discontinued, or if the dose of immunosuppressive drug is reduced. About 15% of patients develop chronic liver failure and are transplanted before the age of 18 years.

In elderly patients, a more severe initial histological grade has been reported, but the frequency of cirrhosis does not differ from that in younger patients. At follow-up, about 30% of patients develop cirrhosis. Response to immunosuppression is similar in older and younger patients and up to 90% of older patients achieve remission. However, in a study from the UK 41% of the elderly patients with AIH received no immunosuppressive therapy and the prognosis was not worse than in younger, usually treated, patients [39, 77, 78]. **B4**

References

1 Fainboim L, Marcos Y, Pando M *et al.* Chronic active autoimmune hepatitis in children: Strong association with a particular HLA-DR6 (DRB1*1301) haplotype. *Hum Immunol* 1994; **41**: 146–150.

2 Seki T, Ota M, Furuta S *et al.* HLA class II molecules and autoimmune hepatitis susceptibility in Japanese patients. *Gastroenterology* 1992; **103**(3): 1041–1047.

3 Bittencourt PL, Palacios SA, Cancado EL *et al.* Autoimmune hepatitis in Brazilian patients is not linked to tumor necrosis factor alpha polymorphisms at position -308. *J Hepatol* 2001; **35**(1): 24–28.

4 Lim KN, Casanova RL, Boyer TD, Bruno CJ. Autoimmune hepatitis in African Americans: presenting features and response to therapy. *Am J Gastroenterol* 2001; **96**(12): 3390–3394.

5 Feld JJ, Dinh H, Arenovich T, Marcus VA, Wanless IR, Heathcote EJ. Autoimmune hepatitis: Effect of symptoms and cirrhosis on natural history and outcome. *Hepatology* 2005; **42**(1): 53–62.

6 Boberg KM, Aadland E, Jahnsen J, Raknerud N, Stiris M, Bell H. Incidence and prevalence of primary biliary cirrhosis, primary sclerosing cholangitis, and autoimmune hepatitis in a Norwegian population. *Scand J Gastroenterol* 1998; **33**: 99–103.

7 Nikias GA, Batts KP, Czaja AJ. The nature and prognostic implications of autoimmune hepatitis with acute presentation. *J Hepatol* 1994; **21**: 866–871.

8 Broome U, Olsson R, Loof L *et al.* Natural history and prognostic factors in 305 Swedish patients with primary sclerosing cholangitis. *Gut* 1996; **38**(4): 610–615.

9 Werner M, Almer S, Prytz H *et al.* Hepatic and extrahepatic malignancies in autoimmune hepatitis. A long-term follow-up in 473 Swedish patients. *J Hepatol* 2009; **50**(2): 388–393.

10 Montano-Loza AJ, Carpenter HA, Czaja AJ. Predictive factors for hepatocellular carcinoma in type 1 autoimmune hepatitis. *Am J Gastroenterol* 2008; **103**(8): 1944–1951.

11 Yeoman AD, Al-Chalabi T, Karani JB *et al.* Evaluation of risk factors in the development of hepatocellular carcinoma in autoimmune hepatitis: Implications for follow-up and screening. *Hepatology* 2008; **48**(3): 863–870.

12 Vergani D, Alvarez F, Bianchi FB *et al.* Liver autoimmune serology: A consensus statement from the committee for autoimmune serology of the International Autoimmune Hepatitis Group. *J Hepatol* 2004; **41**(4): 677–683.

13 Czaja AJ. Current concepts in autoimmune hepatitis. *Ann Hepatol* 2005; **4**(1): 6–24.

14 Alvarez F, Berg PA, Bianchi FB *et al.* International Autoimmune Hepatitis Group Report: Review of criteria for diagnosis of autoimmune hepatitis. *J Hepatology* 1999; **31**: 929–938.

15 Strassburg CP, Manns MP. Autoantibodies and autoantigens in autoimmune hepatitis. *Semin Liver Dis* 2002; **22**(4): 339–352.

16 Adams LA, Lindor KD, Angulo P. The prevalence of autoantibodies and autoimmune hepatitis in patients with nonalcoholic fatty liver disease. *Am J Gastroenterol* 2004; **99**(7): 1316–1320.

17 Rizzetto M, Swana G, Doniach D. Microsomal antibodies in active chronic hepatitis and other disorders. *Clin Exp Immunol* 1973; **15**: 331–344.

18 Homberg JC, Abuaf N, Bernard On *et al.* Chronic active hepatitis associated with anti liver/kidney microsome type 1: A second type of "autoimmune" hepatitis. *Hepatology* 1987; **7**: 1333–1339.

19 Lapierre P, Hajoui O, Homberg J-C, Alvarez F. Fomiminotransferase cyclodeaminase is an organ specific autoantigen recognized by sera of patients with autoimmune hepatitis. *Gastroenterology* 1999; **116**: 643–649.

20 Muratori L, Cataleta M, Muratori P, Lenzi M, Bianchi FB. Liver/kidney microsomal antibody type 1 and liver cytosol antibody type 1 concentrations in type 2 autoimmune hepatitis. *Gut* 1998; **42**(5): 721–726.

21 Wies I, Brunner S, Henninger J *et al.* Identification of target antigen for SLA/LP autoantibodies in autoimmune hepatitis [see comments]. *Lancet* 2000; **355**(9214): 1510–1515.

22 Ma Y, Okamoto M, Thomas MG *et al.* Antibodies to conformational epitopes of soluble liver antigen define a severe form of autoimmune liver disease. *Hepatology* 2002; **35**(3): 658–664.

23 Gelpi CSE, Rodriguez-Sanchez JL. Autoantibodies against a serine tRNA-protein complex implicated in cotranslational selenocysteine insertion. *Proc Natl Acad Sci USA* 1992; **89**(20): 9739–9743.

24 Baeres M, Herkel J, Czaja AJ *et al.* Establishment of standardised SLA/LP immunoassays: Specificity for autoimmune hepatitis,

worldwide occurrence, and clinical characteristics. *Gut* 2002; **51**(2): 259–264.

25 Czaja AJ, Carpenter HA. Progressive fibrosis during corticosteroid therapy of autoimmune hepatitis. *Hepatology* 2004; **39**(6): 1631–1638.

26 Czaja AJ, Shums Z, Donaldson PT, Norman GL. Frequency and significance of antibodies to Saccharomyces cerevisiae in autoimmune hepatitis. *Dig Dis Sci* 2004; **49**(4): 611–618.

27 Czaja AJ, Shums Z, Binder WL, Lewis SJ, Nelson VJ, Norman GL. Frequency and significance of antibodies to chromatin in autoimmune hepatitis. *Dig Dis Sci* 2003; **48**(8): 1658–1664.

28 Liaskos C, Rigopoulou E, Zachou K *et al*. Prevalence and clinical significance of anticardiolipin antibodies in patients with type 1 autoimmune hepatitis. *J Autoimmun* 2005; **24**(3): 251–260.

29 Czaja AJ, Manns MP, Homburger HA. Frequency and significance of antibodies to liver/kidney microsome type 1 in adults with chronic active hepatitis. *Gastroenterology* 1992; **103**(4): 1290–1295.

30 Krawitt EL. Autoimmune hepatis. *N Engl J Med* 1996; **334**: 897–903.

31 Czaja AJ, Carpenter HA, Santrach PJ, Moore B, Taswell HF, Homburger HA. Evidence against hepatitis viruses as important causes of severe autoimmune hepatitis in the United States. *J Hepatol* 1993; **18**: 342–352.

32 Dienes HP, Popper H, Manns M, Baumann W, Thoenes W, Meyer zum Büschenfelde K-H. Histologic features in autoimmune hepatitis. *Z Gastroenterol* 1989; **27**: 327–330.

33 Kogan J, Safadi R, Ashur Y, Shouval D, Ilan Y. Prognosis of symptomatic versus asymptomatic autoimmune hepatitis: A study of 68 patients. *J Clin Gastroenterol* 2002; **35**(1): 75–81.

34 Czaja AJ, Carpenter HA. Decreased fibrosis during corticosteroid therapy of autoimmune hepatitis. *J Hepatol* 2004; **40**(4): 646–652.

35 Verma S, Gunuwan B, Mendler M, Govindrajan S, Redeker A. Factors predicting relapse and poor outcome in type I autoimmune hepatitis: role of cirrhosis development, patterns of transaminases during remission and plasma cell activity in the liver biopsy. *Am J Gastroenterol* 2004; **99**(8): 1510–1516.

36 Gregorio GV, Portman B, Reid F *et al*. Autoimmune hepatitis in childhood: A 20-year experience. *Hepatology* 1997; **25**: 541–547.

37 Oettinger R, Brunnberg A, Gerner P, Wintermeyer P, Jenke A, Wirth S. Clinical features and biochemical data of Caucasian children at diagnosis of autoimmune hepatitis. *J Autoimmun* 2005; **24**(1): 79–84.

38 Schramm C, Bubenheim M, O'Grady JG *et al*. Long term outcome of patients transplanted for autoimmune hepatitis – analysis of the European Liver Transplant Registry. *Journal of Hepatology* 2008; **48**(2): S47.

39 Granito A, Muratori L, Pappas G *et al*. Clinical features of type 1 autoimmune hepatitis in elderly Italian patients. *Aliment Pharmacol Ther* 2005; **21**(10): 1273–1277.

40 Strettel MDJ, Donaldson PT, Thomson LJ *et al*. Allelic basis for HLA-encoded susceptibility to type 1 autoimmune hepatitis. *Gastroenterology* 1997; **112**: 2028–2035.

41 Czaja AJ, Kruger M, Santrach PJ, Breanndan Moore S, Manns MP. Genetic distinctions between types 1 and 2 autoimmune hepatitis. *Am J Gastroenterol* 1997; **92**: 2197–2200.

42 Manns MP, Vogel A. Autoimmune hepatitis, from mechanisms to therapy. *Hepatology* 2006; **43**(2 Suppl. 1): S132–144.

43 Donaldson PT. Genetics in autoimmune hepatitis. *Semin Liver Dis* 2002; **22**(4): 353–364.

44 Czaja AJ, Carpenter HA, Santrach PJ, Moore SB. Significance of HLA DR4 in type 1 autoimmune hepatitis. *Gastroenterology* 1993; **105**: 1502–1507.

45 Donaldson P, Doherty D, Underhill J, Williams R. The molecular genetics of autoimmune liver disease. *Hepatology* 1994; **20**: 225–229.

46 Johnson PJ, McFarlane IG. Meeting report: International autoimmune hepatitis group. *Hepatology* 1993; **18**: 998–1005.

47 Vergani D, Mieli-Vergani G. Mechanisms of autoimmune hepatitis. *Pediatr Transplant* 2004; **8**(6): 589–593.

48 Kaya M, Angulo P, Lindor KD. Overlap of autoimmune hepatitis and primary sclerosing cholangitis: An evaluation of a modified scoring system. *J Hepatol* 2000; **33**(4): 537–542.

49 Talwalkar JA, Keach JC, Angulo P, Lindor KD. Overlap of autoimmune hepatitis and primary biliary cirrhosis: An evaluation of a modified scoring system. *Am J Gastroenterol* 2002; **97**(5): 1191–1197.

50 Hennes EM, Zeniya M, Czaja AJ *et al*. Simplified criteria for the diagnosis of autoimmune hepatitis. *Hepatology* 2008; **48**(1): 169–176.

51 Kirk AP, Jain S, Pocock S, Thomas HC, Sherlock S. Late results of the Royal Free Hospital prospective controlled trial of prednisolone therapy in hepatitis B surface antigen negative chronic active hepatitis. *Gut* 1980; **21**: 7893.

52 Cook GC, Mulligan R, Sherlock S. Controlled prospective trial of corticosteroid therapy in active chronic hepatitis. *Q J Med* 1971; **40**(158): 159–185.

53 Manns MP, Strassburg CP. Autoimmune hepatitis: Clinical challenges. *Gastroenterology* 2001; **120**(6): 1502–1517.

54 Summerskill WHJ, Korman MG, Ammon HV, Baggenstoss AH. Prednisone for chronic active liver disease: Dose titration, standard dose and combination with azathioprine compound. *Gut* 1975; **16**: 876–883.

55 Sanchez-Urdazpal L, Czaja AJ, Van Holk B. Prognostic features and role of liver transplantation in severe corticoid-treated autoimmune chronic active hepatitis. *Hepatology* 1991; **15**: 215–221.

56 Czaja AJ. Treatment of autoimmune hepatitis. *Semin Liver Dis* 2002; **22**(4): 365–378.

57 Czaja AJ, Freese DK. Diagnosis and treatment of autoimmune hepatitis. *Hepatology* 2002; **36**(2): 479–497.

58 Manns MP, Woynarowski M, Kreisel W, Oren R, Rust C, Hultcrantz R, Spengler U, *et al*. Budesonide 3 mg bid in combination with azathioprine as maintenance treatment of autoimmune hepatitis – final results of a large multicenter international trial. *Hepatology* 2008; **48**: 376A–377A.

59 Heneghan MA, McFarlane IG. Current and novel immunosuppressive therapy for autoimmune hepatitis. *Hepatology* 2002; **35**(1): 7–13.

60 Rebollo Bernardez J, Cifuentes Mimoso C, Pinar Moreno A *et al*. Deflazacort for long-term maintenance of remission in type I autoimmune hepatitis. *Rev Esp Enferm Dig* 1999; **91**(9): 630–638.

61 Alvarez F, Ciocca M, Canero-Velasco C *et al*. Short-term cyclosporine induces a remission of autoimmune hepatitis in children. *J Hepatol* 1999; **30**: 222–227.

62 Richardson PD, James PD, Ryder SD. Mycophenolate mofetil for maintenance of remission in autoimmune hepatitis in patients

resistant to or intolerant of azathioprine. *J Hepatol* 2000; **33**(3): 371–375.

63 Kanzler S, Gerken G, Dienes HP, Meyer zum Büschenfelde K-H, Lohse AW. Cyclophosphamide as alternative immunosuppressive therapy for autoimmune hepatitis – report of three cases. *Z Gastroenterol* 1996; **35**: 571–578.

64 Neuberger, J. Transplantation for Autoimmune Hepatitis. *Semin Liver Dis* 2002; **22**(4): 379–386.

65 Tan P, Marotta P, Ghent C, Adams P. Early treatment response predicts the need for liver transplantation in autoimmune hepatitis. *Liver Int* 2005; **25**(4): 728–733.

66 Vogel A, Heinrich E, Bahr MJ *et al.* Long-term outcome of liver transplantation for autoimmune hepatitis. *Clin Transplant* 2004; **18**(1): 62–69.

67 Duclos-Vallee JC, Sebagh M, Rifai K *et al.* A 10 year follow up study of patients transplanted for autoimmune hepatitis: Histological recurrence precedes clinical and biochemical recurrence. *Gut* 2003; **52**(6): 893–897.

68 Andries S, Casamayou L, Sempoux C *et al.* Posttransplant immune hepatitis in pediatric liver transplant recipients: Incidence and maintenance therapy with azathioprine. *Transplantation* 2001; **72**(2): 267–272.

69 Salcedo M, Vaquero J, Banares R *et al.* Response to steroids in de novo autoimmune hepatitis after liver transplantation. *Hepatology* 2002; **35**(2): 349–356.

70 Kerkar N, Dugan C, Rumbo C *et al.* Rapamycin successfully treats post-transplant autoimmune hepatitis. *Am J Transplant* 2005; **5**(5): 1085–1089.

71 Kerkar N, Hadzic N, Davies ET *et al.* De-novo autoimmune hepatitis after liver transplantation. *Lancet* 1998; **351**(9100): 409–413.

72 Miyagawa-Hayashino A, Haga H, Egawa H *et al.* Outcome and risk factors of de novo autoimmune hepatitis in living-donor liver transplantation. *Transplantation* 2004; **78**(1): 128–135.

73 Heneghan MA, Portmann BC, Norris SM *et al.* Graft dysfunction mimicking autoimmune hepatitis following liver transplantation in adults. *Hepatology* 2001; **34**(3): 464–470.

74 Soloway RD, Summerskill WH, Baggenstoss AH *et al.* Clinical, biochemical, and histological remission of severe chronic active liver disease: A controlled study of treatments and early prognosis. *Gastroenterology* 1972; **63**(5): 820–833.

75 Mistilis SP. Natural history of active chronic hepatitis. II. Pathology, pathogenesis and clinico-pathological correlation. *Australas Ann Med* 1968; **17**(4): 277–288.

76 Roberts SK, Therneau TM, Czaja AJ. Prognosis of histological cirrhosis in type 1 autoimmune hepatitis. *Gastroenterology* 1996; **110**: 848–857.

77 Schramm C, Kanzler S, zum Buschenfelde KH, Galle PR, Lohse AW. Autoimmune hepatitis in the elderly. *Am J Gastroenterol* 2001; **96**(5): 1587–1591.

78 Newton JL, Burt AD, Park JB, Mathew J, Bassendine MF, James OF. Autoimmune hepatitis in older patients. *Age Ageing* 1997; **26**(6): 441–444.

79 Murray-Lyon IM, Stern RB, Williams R. Controlled trial of prednisone and azathioprine in active chronic hepatitis. *Lancet* 1973; **I**: 735–737.

34 Primary sclerosing cholangitis

Nishchay Chandra[1], Susan N Cullen[2] and Roger W Chapman[1]
[1]Gastroenterology Unit, John Radcliffe Hospital, Oxford, UK
[2]Buckinghamshire Hospitals NHS Trust, High Wycombe, UK

Introduction

Primary sclerosing cholangitis (PSC) is a chronic cholestatic liver disease in which a progressive obliterating fibrosis of the intrahepatic and extrahepatic bile ducts leads to biliary cirrhosis, portal hypertension and eventually hepatic failure, and in addition 10–30% of patients will develop a cholangiocarcinoma. In comparison with some of the conditions discussed in this book, PSC is a rare disease. But the absence of large randomized clinical trials and meta-analyses in PSC does not prevent gathering the best evidence with which to attempt to answer the many questions posed by patients and clinicians about the etiology, diagnosis, prognosis and management of this disease. Inevitably, where good external evidence is lacking, personal clinical expertise may play a greater role in the decision-making process. This integration of clinical expertise and best available clinical evidence from systematic research constitutes the practice of "evidence-based gastroenterology".

Etiology

A number of causative agents have been implicated in the pathogenesis of PSC but no single hypothesis has provided a unifying explanation for all the clinical and pathological features of this disease. PSC is closely associated with inflammatory bowel disease (IBD), the majority (65–86%) of patients with PSC have coexistent ulcerative colitis and the prevalence of PSC in ulcerative colitis (UC) populations is between 2% and 6% [1–3]. In a patient with ulcerative colitis, abnormal liver function tests, particularly an elevated serum alkaline phosphatase, may be the first indica-

tion of this insidious condition. Magnetic resonance cholangiopancreaticography (MRCP) and endoscopic retrograde cholangiopancreatography (ERCP) are diagnostic, demonstrating the diffuse multifocal strictures and dilatation giving rise to the characteristic "beaded" appearance. The precise etiology and pathogenesis of PSC is still not completely understood. This chapter sets out the evidence that immune mechanisms play a key role in the development of the disease.

Autoimmunity

The 2:1 male to female ratio of patients with PSC and the relatively poor response of the disease to immunosuppression suggest that PSC is not a classic autoimmune disease. PSC patients do have an increased frequency of the HLA B8 DR3 DC2 "autoimmune" haplotype, in common with a number of organ-specific autoimmune diseases such as lupoid chronic active hepatitis, type I diabetes mellitus, myasthenia gravis and thyrotoxicosis [1–3]. PSC is also independently associated with a range of autoimmune diseases, diabetes mellitus and Graves' disease being the most common. Saarinen *et al.* found that 25% of patients with PSC had one or more autoimmune disease, compared with 9% of patients with IBD alone [4].

Autoantibodies

A wide range of autoantibodies can be detected in the serum of patients with PSC, clearly indicating an altered state of immune responsiveness or immune regulation. Although a few studies have demonstrated some correlation between particular clinical parameters and the presence of autoantibodies, there is presently insufficient evidence to make use of any of them in determining prognosis. Most are present at low prevalence rates and at relatively low titers (see Table 34.1).

Anti-neutrophil specific antibodies are commonly found in the sera of PSC patients, occurring in up to 88% of

Evidence-Based Gastroenterology and Hepatology, 3rd edition.
J. McDonald, A.K. Burroughs, B. Feagan, and M.B. Fennerty. © 2010
Blackwell Publishing Ltd

Table 34.1 Serum autoantibodies in primary sclerosing cholangitis.

Antibody[a]	Prevalence
Anti-nuclear antibody	7–77%
Anti-smooth muscle antibody	13–20%
Anti-endothelial cell antibody	35%
Anti-cardiolipin antibody	4–66%
Thyroperoxidase	7–16%
Thyroglobulin	4%
Rheumatoid factor	15%

[a] Antimitochondrial antibody is only rarely detected in PSC (<10%). This is useful in differentiating primary sclerosing cholangitis from primary biliary cirrhosis.

patients. The antineutrophil cytoplasmic antibodies (ANCA) associated with PSC are distinct from cANCA and classic pANCA in that they demonstrate a unique staining pattern on indirect immunofluorescence microscopy. These "atypical pANCA" are non-specific, with a prevalence of 33–88% in PSC, 40–87% in ulcerative colitis, and 50–96% in type I autoimmune hepatitis (AIH) [5]. Work by Terjung and Worman has demonstrated that the target antigen for atypical pANCA is a neutrophil envelope protein termed viz tubulin-beta isotype 5 and appears to be localized to the nuclear periphery [6]. It has been suggested that the anti-neutrophil antibody in PSC therefore be renamed pANNA (anti-neutrophil nuclear antibody).

Over recent years, several autoantibodies have been identified and implicated in the pathogenesis of PSC. The presence of autoantibodies to surface antigens expressed on biliary epithelial cells has been demonstrated in PSC. Preuss et al. evaluated the presence of serum autoantibodies to human recombinant sulphite oxidase (anti-SO) in a variety of chronic liver disorders, and observed the highest incidence in PSC patients [7]. Furthermore, antibody activity decreased significantly during ursodeoxycholic acid (UDCA) treatment. The specificity of glutathione S-transferase theta 1 (GSTT1) as a potential autoantigenic target was evaluated in PSC [8]. Reactivity against GSTT1 was found with PSC and IBD as well as some patients with other autoimmune pathology, indicating that this population of antibodies is neither specific nor a sensitive serologic marker for PSC, but the frequency was clearly higher in autoimmune patients than controls.

The importance of autoantibodies in the development of PSC remains unclear. To date there is no convincing model of the pathogenesis of PSC and it may be that these antibodies are simply a marker for an as yet undetermined immune dysregulation.

Immunogenetics

Studies of genes encoding the key proteins in the immune system have contributed towards our understanding of the influence of the immune system on the development and progression of PSC.

PSC appears to be a "complex" disease in that it is not attributable to a single gene locus. Susceptibility to PSC is probably acquired through inheriting one of a number of patterns of genetic polymorphisms which together cause a predisposition to development of the disease.

MHC genes

The major histocompatibility complex on the short arm of chromosome 6 encodes the HLA molecules which have a central role in T cell response and are highly polymorphic. The major histocompatibility complex (MHC) class I and class II regions encode the classical transplantation antigens of the HLA A, B, CW and DR, DQ and DP families. The class III region encodes a range of immune response genes, including those encoding tumor necrosis factor-α and β (TNF-α and β), the heat shock protein family (HSP-70), complement proteins C2, C4A, C4B, Bf, and the genes encoding the MHC class I chain-related proteins, MICα and β) (MICA and MICB).

An association between the haplotypes HLA A1-B8-DR3, DR6 and DR2 and susceptibility to PSC are well documented, whilst the presence of HLA DR4 is protective [9]. A recent Norwegian study demonstrated that a gene in linkage disequilibrium with the D6S265*122 microsatellite allele contributes to susceptibility to developing PSC in individuals carrying DR6 solely [10]. Furthermore, a possible protective effect of DR11 was observed. MICA*008 homozygosity confers the strongest association with disease susceptibility. However, the MICA*002 allele has been shown to be protective [10]. The technique of molecular genotyping has elucidated six key HLA haplotypes associated with PSC (see Table 34.2).

Karlsen et al. found that HLA associations found in PSC were mostly distinct from those seen in UC [11]. Also, no significant differences were observed between PSC patients with or without concurrent UC, suggesting that UC in PSC may in fact represent a distinct UC/IBD phenotype.

Non-MHC immunoregulatory genes

A range of non-MHC immunoregulatory genes has been studied in relation to PSC. Cytotoxic lymphocyte antigen-4 (CTLA-4) is one of the differentiation antigens exclusively expressed on activated CD4+ and CD8+ T cells. It acts by binding to B7, the same ligand as CD28, thereby disrupting the crucial CD28-B7 interaction, one of the key co-stimula-

Table 34.2 Key HLA haplotypes associated with primary sclerosing cholangitis (PSC).

Haplotype	Significance in PSC
B8-TNF*2-DRB3*0101-DRB1*0301-DQA1*0501-DQB1*0201	Strong association with disease susceptibility
DRB3*0101-DRB1*1301-DQA1*0103-DQB1*0603	Strong association with disease susceptibility
DRB5*0101-DRB1*1501-DQA1*0102-DQB1*0602	Weak association with disease susceptibility
DRB4*0103-DRB1*0401-DQA1*03-DQB1*0302	Strong association with protection against disease
MICA*008	Strong association with disease susceptibility

tory events in the initiation and progression of the T cell immune response. A CTLA-4 gene polymorphism has been associated with susceptibility to several autoimmune diseases, although its role in PSC is controversial, with a recent study failing to demonstrate any association [12].

Recent studies on non-HLA polymorphisms have produced conflicting data. An Australian study demonstrated that a 32 base pair deletion in the chemokine receptor-5 (CCR5-Delta 32) gene resulted in a non-functioning receptor, and that this was strongly associated with PSC [13]. In contrast, a Belgian study concluded that the mutation was in fact protective against PSC [14], whilst a third study failed to demonstrate any association with the deletion and PSC in 363 Scandinavian patients [15]. A subsequent study from the Belgian investigators observed that the −28G promoter polymorphism of the Regulation on Activation Normal T Expressed and Secreted (RANTES, a ligand of the CCR5 receptor) gene was significantly increased in PSC patients compared with IBD patients and healthy controls [16]. The authors hypothesized that the resulting inflammatory response in the gut predisposed to bacterial translocation through the bowel wall.

Intracellular adhesion molecule-1 (ICAM-1) mediates leucocyte adhesion and is found on proliferating bile ductules and interlobular bile ducts in patients with advanced PSC. Yang *et al.* have previously shown that K469E homozygosity for ICAM-1 is associated with protection against PSC in a cohort of British patients [17]. However, no such association was demonstrated in a larger Scandinavian study [18].

The end result of inflammation in PSC is periductal fibrosis. Genes involved in the regulation of the production and destruction of extracellular matrix are therefore also good candidate genes for study. One such family of genes is that

comprising the matrix metalloproteinases (MMPs). A promoter polymorphism of MMP-3 (stromelysin) has been shown to be associated with both susceptibility to PSC and progression to portal hypertension [19]. Wiencke *et al.* could not confirm this association in 165 Norwegian PSC patients [20]. However, the polymorphism was noted to be more prevalent in patients with concurrent PSC and UC in comparison to patients with PSC only.

Karlsen *et al.* found that the genetic polymorphisms conferring susceptibility to IBD (CARD15, TLR-4, CARD4, SLC22A4, SLC22A5, DLG5 and MDR1) did not play a role in the genetic predisposition to PSC in a large cohort of Scandinavian patients [21].

Cellular immune abnormalities

The initiation and maintenance of the immune cascade is determined not only by MHC recognition but also by the presence of accessory cells and molecules to provide co-stimulatory signals and the production of cytokines to amplify or modify the immune response.

The cellular infiltrate at the site of tissue injury is probably more relevant than the circulating population. Although it is clear that there is a T cell predominant portal tract infiltrate in PSC, there is still some uncertainty regarding the relative importance of CD4+ and CD8+ cells in this infiltrate. The hypothesis that these T lymphocytes are involved in the pathogenesis of the disease (rather than simply being markers for its presence) is supported by evidence that these cells are functional. This evidence comes from studies of surface markers expressed on activated and memory T cells.

T cells

Most T cells carry a T cell receptor (TCR) consisting of two disulphide-linked polypeptides, termed α and β. A group of T cells carrying an alternative receptor, termed $\gamma\delta$, has been identified. The significance of $\gamma\delta$ cells in the pathogenesis of PSC is therefore not clear although they might function by modulating $\alpha\beta$ T cell activation or regulating antibody or autoantibody production from B cells.

Although T cell receptor gene rearrangements serve to generate genetic diversity, a particular V$\alpha\beta$ gene segment can play a dominant role in recognition of certain peptide-MHC complexes. Expanded T cell populations using restricted sets of T cell receptor V gene segments have been identified in areas of inflammation in diseases such as rheumatoid arthritis and Sjögren's disease. This suggests the presence of a specific antigen with the capacity of driving the production of T cells with this restricted V$\alpha\beta$ segment product [22, 23]. Studies from Broome *et al.* indicated that the hepatic, but not peripheral, T cells in PSC preferentially have Vβ3 T cell repertoires [24]. An oligo-clonal expansion was not demonstrated in this study, but oligoclonal T cell receptors which proliferate in culture with enterocytes and are cytotoxic to enterocyte cell lines *in vitro* have also been reported in PSC [25].

Biliary epithelial cells

The biliary epithelial cell (BEC) is the target of immune attack in PSC, while at the same time appearing to be an active participant in the immune response. Normal biliary epithelial cells express only HLA class I and not class II antigens. However, the HLA class II antigens HLA-DR, DQ and DP have all been found to be expressed by the biliary epithelial cells of patients with PSC [26, 27]. These antigens have the potential to initiate an immune response by binding autoantigens or exogenous antigens and present-ing the peptides to class II restricted T lymphocytes.

Xu *et al.* identified autoantibodies in 63% of PSC patients, which stimulated BECs to produce increased levels of the pro-inflammatory cytokine IL-6 and induce expression of CD44, the lymphocytic homing receptor [28]. The same group conducted a further study concluding that BECs played an integral role in their own destruction [29]. They demonstrated that stimulation of BECs with PSC IgG, induced the expression of Toll-like receptor (TLR) 4 and TLR9, extracellular signal-related kinase (ERK) 1/2, and transcription factors. Further stimulation of TLR-expressing BECs with lipopolysaccharide and CpG DNA resulted in the production of pro-inflammatory cytokines and chem-okines. Nitric oxide, arising from BECs in response to cytokines, has been shown to cause ductular cholestasis and inhibit cholangiocellular bile formation [30]. Thus, cholangiocytes appear to play a significant role in the pathogenesis of PSC.

Lymphocyte homing

Grant *et al.* have proposed the existence of an enterohepatic circulation of lymphocytes, whereby some mucosal T lym-phocytes produced in the gut during active inflammation persist as memory cells capable of recirculation through the liver [31]. Under certain circumstances these gut-derived lymphocytes might become activated, resulting in bile duct inflammation. The migration of these T cells to the liver is mediated by the aberrant co-expression of endothelial cell adhesion molecules, including vascular adhesion protein-1 (VAP-1) and mucosal addressin cell adhesion molecule-1 (MAdCAM-1), and chemokines in both organs in patients with concomitant PSC and IBD. Eksteen *et al.* demonstrated that the chemokine CCL25, ordinarily confined to the gut, is up-regulated to the liver in PSC, where they recruit CCR9+ T cells by binding to MadCAM-1 [32]. In a second study, the same investigators propose that CXCR3, a chem-okine receptor, promotes the recruitment of regulatory T cells (T regs) to inflamed tissue and CCR10 lymphocytes allow them to respond to the ligand CCL28 secreted by epithelial cells, resulting in the accumulation of CCR10+ T regs at mucosal surfaces [33]. This concept of dual homing lymphocytes helps to explain the observation that PSC runs a course independent of inflammation in the bowel and indeed can develop even after proctocolectomy. Furthermore, the evidence provides a possible explanation as to why patients with IBD develop extra-intestinal manifestations.

Hepatobiliary transporters

Disturbance of the hepatocellular transport processes leads to an alteration of bile composition, impaired biliary secre-tion, and ultimately bile duct injury. Genetic variations of these transport systems may therefore play an important role in the pathogenesis of cholestatic liver diseases such as PSC.

The steroid and xenobiotic receptor (SXR) is a transcrip-tion factor that is involved in endogenous bile acid home-ostasis. A Scandinavian study of 327 PSC patients demonstrated that functional polymorphisms of the SXR gene failed to confer susceptibility to the development of the disease. However, the gene variants did modify disease course [34]. Lithocholic acid (LCA) is a potentially toxic secondary bile acid that once sensed by the SXR, is detoxi-fied via the increased transcription of the enzymes cyto-chrome P450 3A and sulfotransferase. A simultaneous up-regulation of the membrane transporters MDR1 and MRP2 results in the excretion of the LCA metabolites. A recent review suggests that deficiencies in these defence mechanisms are associated with the development of PSC and IBD [35].

The absence of phospholipids in the bile of multidrug resistant gene 2 knockout (Mdr2-/-) mice results in the development of hepatobiliary injury similar to PSC in humans [36]. Variations in Mdr3 gene, the human equiva-lent of the mouse Mdr2 gene, have not been observed in human PSC patients [37]. Studies evaluating the role of the cystic fibrosis transmembrane conductance regulator (CFTR) have reported conflicting results [10].

Role of bacteria in the etiopathogenesis of primary sclerosing cholangitis

The coexistence of inflammatory colitis in around 75% of northern European patients with PSC has led to the hypoth-esis that the initiating step in this disease is the access of intestinal bacteria through an inflamed and leaky bowel wall, to the portal circulation. An abnormal immune response to bacterial antigens (possibly acting as molecular mimics for autoantigens) in an immunogenetically susceptible host might be sufficient to precipitate the cascade of immune reactions detailed above.

Investigation of bacterial growth from human tissue is confounded by the bacterial contamination caused by intubation of the bile duct at ERCP. Several animal models, however, have been used to investigate this proposal. Wistar and Sprague-Dawley rats develop a pattern of hepatic injury somewhat similar to human PSC after artificially induced small bowel bacterial overgrowth, although a subsequent study in humans involving 22 PSC patients failed to confirm this association [38].

Previous studies have implicated *Helicobacter* species in the pathogenesis of PSC. More recently, Krasinskas *et al.* demonstrated an increase in the prevalence of *H.pylori* DNA detected in microdissected hilar hepatic ducts of PSC patients in comparison to controls [39]. However, direct infection of the biliary epithelium with a subsequent inflammatory response could not be confirmed.

Hypotheses for the etiopathogenesis of PSC

A plausible unifying hypothesis for the etiopathogenesis of PSC has been put forward by Vierling [40]. This suggests that the initial insult is the reaction of an immunogenetically susceptible host to bacterial cell wall products entering the portal circulation through a permeable gut wall either due to colitis or possibly during episodes of intestinal infection. The resulting Kupffer cell (hepatic macrophage) activation would result in peribiliary cytokine and chemokine secretion attracting activated neutrophils, monocyte/macrophages, lymphocytes and fibroblasts to the site of infection. The resultant concentric fibrosis around the bile ducts could lead to ischemia and then atrophy of the biliary epithelial cell. The bile duct loss would then lead to progressive cholestasis, fibrosis and secondary biliary cirrhosis. This hypothesis does not explain why there is a relative paucity of patients with PSC and underlying Crohn's colitis, nor the association of PSC with stricturing of the pancreatic duct.

In conclusion, current evidence suggests that PSC is an immune-mediated rather than a classic autoimmune disease. Genetic analysis suggests a pivotal role for certain alleles of the MHC in determining susceptibility to the development of PSC, whilst the importance of non-MHC genes is not so clear-cut. The association with inflammatory colitis suggests that an abnormal immune response may be initiated in an immunogenetically susceptible host by the access of bacterial antigen, through a permeable gut wall, to the portal circulation. This bacterial antigen might then act as a molecular mimic of an autoantigen precipitating an immune reaction leading to PSC initiation. In addition, lymphocytes generated from the inflamed gut may enter the liver via the enterohepatic circulation resulting in bile duct inflammation with the eventual progression to

stricturing and scarring of the intrahepatic and extrahepatic bile ducts, peribiliary fibrosis and ultimately, cirrhosis. There are difficulties in determining which of the wide range of immune abnormalities identified in these patients, are causal and which are the consequence of tissue injury.

Diagnosis

Characteristic cholangiographic features form the mainstay of PSC diagnosis. Over recent years, MRCP has become established over ERCP as the first-line investigation for the diagnosis of PSC. It confers several advantages, including complete visualization of the biliary tree, liver parenchyma and intra-abdominal organs, and planning for potential therapeutic options. Perhaps, most importantly, it negates the significant morbidity and mortality associated with ERCP. Furthermore, over recent years, several studies have demonstrated comparable sensitivities, specificities and diagnostic accuracies between the two modalities [41, 42]. In 2008, Weber *et al.* reported on the results of the largest comparative study to date and found that MRCP had a sensitivity, specificity and diagnostic accuracy of 86%, 77% and 83% respectively [43]. In a recent case-controlled analysis of 36 patients with PSC, interobserver agreement for diagnosing PSC was very good, but very poor in assessing disease severity [44]. Limitations of the investigation due to inferior spatial resolution include detecting PSC in cirrhotics or in the early stages of the disease, and also with the differentiation of cholangiocarcinoma. Two recent clinical decision models have demonstrated that the strategy of initial MRCP, followed by ERCP if required, is the most cost-effective approach to the work-up of patients with suspected PSC [45, 46]. Petrovic and colleagues raised the question as to whether the degree of biliary duct changes on MRCP correlated with patient survival [47]. Using the Mayo risk score as a survival model, they performed a retrospective study including 47 patients and found no such correlation.

There is some evidence that common bile duct wall thickening and layering demonstrated at endoscopic ultrasound (EUS) may be a useful adjunct in the diagnosis of PSC. However, a comparative prospective study with MRCP is required to determine its true value [48].

Epidemiology, natural history and prognosis

Over recent years, emerging evidence suggests a change in both the epidemiology and natural history of PSC. Epidemiological data is scarce and tends to originate from centers with a specialist interest in PSC. The largest population-based cohort epidemiological study to date, comparing 223 PSC patients with 2217 control patients, reported an incidence of 0.41 per 100,000 and a prevalence of 3.85 per 100,000 over a ten-year period in the UK [49]. As with previously published data, PSC was more commonly observed in middle-aged males, although only 50% of cases were associated with IBD. In comparison to the general population, there was a two-fold and three-fold increase in the risk of malignancy and mortality respectively. The authors also found a non-significant rise in incidence of PSC during the study period. Kaplan *et al.* reported an incident rate of 0.92 per 100,000 person years in the largest population-based study of PSC in Canada [50]. In contrast with previous findings, the investigators observed that the risk of developing PSC was similar in patients with UC and Crohn's disease. At least one coexisting autoimmune disorder was observed in 84% of patients, and autoimmune hepatitis overlap was evident in 10% of cases. A Swedish tertiary center observed a change in the clinical presentation amongst 246 PSC patients over a 20-year period, with more recently diagnosed patients, being older at diagnosis, presenting with fewer symptoms, and having a lower frequency of concurrent IBD [51]. Geographic variation also exists, with Japanese studies demonstrating lower incidences of both IBD and cholangiocarcinoma in patients with PSC [52].

The clinical course of PSC is quite variable; the disease is indolent in some patients and more rapidly progressive in others. However, a diagnosis of PSC should be considered in patients presenting with acute liver failure [53]. The natural history of PSC is described in a number of retrospective studies, with the median survival time from diagnosis to death or orthotopic liver transplantation (OLT) reported between 9.6 and 21 years [54, 55]. Differences in survival estimations may reflect the variation in the definition of onset and outcome. As there is no reliable marker of early disease in PSC the onset is difficult to identify clearly. Whether the onset is defined as the occurrence of the first symptoms consistent with PSC, as the time of the first abnormal liver function test, or as the time of diagnosis by ERCP, will result in differences in survival estimates. In retrospective studies details of distant events may be sparse and there is likely to be failure to recognize early signs and symptoms. Patients with late stage disease may predominate, while patients who die from rapidly progressive disease may be missed.

The ideal study of prognosis is prospective and follows patients from a defined point in the disease process, usually diagnosis. There have been no studies using such an inception cohort in PSC because the disease is rare and its slow progression makes a prospective study impractical. A large retrospective study published by Tischendorf *et al.* evaluated the natural history of 273 PSC patients and observed an estimated median survival time from diagnosis to OLT or death of 9.6 years [56]. This is lower in comparison to previously published data, and may be explained by the higher prevalence of cholangiocarcinoma (13.2%), genetic and environmental factors, and the lower threshold for performing OLT as evidence-based practice evolves. Of the cohort, 39.6% proceeded to liver transplantation and 14.3% developed neoplasia affecting the hepatobiliary system. An elevation in serum bilirubin persisting longer than three months following diagnosis was identified as a novel poor prognostic indicator. Using a range of clinical, biochemical and radiological parameters, the authors constructed a prognostic model, which possessed the highest concordance index in comparison to the MELD score, revised Mayo score and Child-Pugh-score. Several prognostic models have been constructed with the aim of predicting survival and determining therapeutic strategies, and whilst they successfully predict the natural history of the disease in a cohort of PSC patients, they are less successful when applied to individual patients. The confounding factor is the development of hepatobiliary or colonic cancer.

Cholangiocarcinoma

Cholangiocarcinoma (CCA) will develop in 10–30% of patients with PSC, with a cumulative lifetime risk of 10–15% [57]. The absence of predictive risk factors and the inability of conventional investigative modalities to differentiate between benign and malignant strictures, contributes to its dismal prognosis. Historically, the use of tumor markers has been limited by their lack of specificity. The benefit of tumor markers, either in combination, or with ERCP, has not been confirmed despite initial promising results. Recently, serum trypsinogen-2 has been found to be superior to several tumor markers, including CA19-9 and CEA, for differentiating patients with PSC and cholangiocarcinoma from patients with PSC alone [58]. Following an initial study describing ^{18}F-fluoro-2-deoxy-D-glucose positron emission tomography (FDG-PET) as a sensitive test for detecting cholangiocarcinomas in PSC patients two prospective studies have reported conflicting results [59]. In 2005, a study from Belgium concluded that FDG-PET was unable to distinguish malignant stenotic hilar lesions from inflammatory abnormalities [60]. Prytz *et al.* performed a blinded study in which 24 PSC patients listed for OLT, and without evidence of cholangiocarcinoma on USS, CT or MRI, underwent FDG-PET scanning [61]. The results were subsequently correlated with explant histology. The modality correctly identified three patients with cholangiocarcinoma but failed to detect one case of high-grade dysplasia.

A prospective study by Tischendorf and colleagues found that transpapillary intraductal ultrasound (IDUS) was superior to ERCP in discriminating between malignant and benign dominant bile duct strictures with a sensitivity, specificity and diagnostic accuracy of 87.5% vs 62.5%, 90.6% vs 53.1%, and 90% vs 55% respectively [62]. Whilst endoscopic ultrasound (EUS) guided fine-needle aspiration is of value in analyzing suspicious biliary strictures, there have been no studies assessing its use in PSC patients. The use of endoscopic cholangioscopy has been investigated in two separate prospective trials as it permits direct visualization of the biliary tree and enables directed tissue sampling of abnormal areas. Tischendorf *et al.* concluded that cholangioscopy with directed biopsies was significantly more sensitive (92% vs 66%) and specific (93% vs 55%) than ERCP and subsequent brush cytology, in diagnosing malignant strictures [63]. In a second study cholangioscopic biopsies detected one out of three cholangiocarcinomas and excluded cancer in 31 patients at a median follow-up of 17 months [64]. Furthermore, approximately 25% of strictures could not be traversed, highlighting the need for more technically advanced miniscopes. Moreno Luna *et al.* demonstrated that advanced analysis of cytological specimens obtained at ERCP using fluorescent in-situ hybridization (FISH) and digital image analysis (DIA), increased the sensitivity for the diagnosis of malignancy over routine cytology in PSC patients with strictures [65].

To date, there is limited data on screening asymptomatic PSC patients for early CCA. Two separate studies have concluded that routine brush cytology at the time of ERCP improves the detection of early neoplastic changes [66, 67]. A study from the Mayo Clinic has proposed combining serum CA19-9 with an abdominal ultrasound scan at 12-monthly intervals as a useful screening/surveillance tool [68].

There is a paucity of data assessing the impact of UDCA on the development of CCA. Rudolph and colleagues evaluated the incidence rate of CCA in 150 PSC patients maintained on UDCA over an 18-year period [69]. Patients developed 0.58 CCA per 100 patient years in years 0–2.5, 0.59 CCA in years 2.5–8.5, and no CCA thereafter. These rates were lower than those of historical controls.

Gallbladder disease

Gallbladder disease, including gallstones and polypoidal lesions, is common in patients with PSC, with two studies reporting a prevalence of 41% [70, 71]. In approximately 60% of cases, gallbladder polyps are malignant, and given the dismal prognosis of such lesions, annual evaluation of the gallbladder using ultrasonography has been recommended. Leung *et al* reported that the size of a polyp could not reliably predict its malignant potential, therefore advocating the use of early cholecystectomy in patients with PSC and polypoidal lesions on imaging [72]. The interval and cost-effectiveness of this strategy has yet to be investigated.

Lewis *et al.* proposed that the metaplastic-dysplastic-carcinoma sequence could be applied to PSC-associated gallbladder cancers. The authors also observed a strong correlation between gallbladder neoplasia and biliary neoplasia, therefore supporting the concept of a "field effect" along the entire biliary tree in patients with PSC [73].

Colonic neoplasia

An increase in the risk or colorectal dysplasia/cancer in patients with concomitant PSC and UC is generally acknowledged. Soetikno *et al.* conducted a meta-analysis that included 11 studies and reported a four-fold increase in the risk of patients with PSC and UC developing colorectal cancer compared to those with UC alone [74]. The predominance for right-sided colonic cancers has suggested a role for carcinogenic secondary bile acids, such as deoxycholic acid (DCA), in the pathogenesis of such tumors. Moreover, it has been demonstrated that UDCA inhibits deoxycholic acid-induced apoptosis by modulating mitochondrial transmembrane potential and reactive oxygen species production [75]. Subsequently, two studies demonstrated the apparent chemoprotective effect of UDCA against the development of colon cancer in patients with PSC and UC [76, 77]. More recently, a third trial failed to reveal a significant reduction in the incidence of dysplasia or cancer in those using UDCA. However, a reduction in cumulative overall mortality was observed [78].

Despite the lack of randomized controlled trials, there is a general consensus that annual surveillance colonoscopy should be performed in patients with coexistant PSC and UC. The same strategy should be adopted in those with concomitant colitis who have undergone OLT, as the risk of colorectal neoplasia remains high, and furthermore increases with time [79]. Although, the colorectal cancer risk in PSC patients with Crohn's colitis is unknown, regular surveillance is advocated.

In the future, it is envisaged that the detection rates of dysplastic lesions will improve with the advent of hi-tech imaging techniques, such as chromoendoscopy. The role of 5-aminosalicylates in chemoprevention remains unclear. Proctocolectomy with ileo-anal pouch formation is the preferred surgical management of PSC-associated colorectal malignancies as it avoids the complication of peristomal varices evident in patients with an ileal stoma [80]. A recent study observed a higher prevalence of mucosal atrophy in the pouches of patients with coexistant PSC and UC compared with UC controls, suggesting a higher risk of neoplastic transformation in the former group [81]. The incidence of pouchitis is also increased in patients with an ileal pouch-anal anastomosis and coexistent PSC [82].

Small duct PSC

The results of three independent studies aimed at determining the natural history and long-term prognosis of small duct PSC (sdPSC) were published in 2002 and although they revealed similar results, they were limited by small patient size and relatively short follow-up periods [83–85]. Björnsson *et al.* extended the follow-up of the sdPSC patients reported in the original three studies and concluded that patients with sdPSC had a significantly better long-term prognosis than appropriately matched patients with large duct PSC over 13-year median follow-up period [86]. Of the 83 patients with sdPSC included in the study, approximately 23% either underwent liver transplantation or died, and this compared favorably to the large duct PSC group in which almost 50% developed similar outcomes. Patients with sdPSC had a significantly longer survival free of liver transplantation than patients with large duct PSC (13 years (IQR, 10–17) vs ten years (IQR, 6–14) respectively; hazard ratio, 3.04; 95% CI: 1.82–5.06; p < 0.0001). In keeping with the findings reported in the original studies, 27.9% of the 68 patients who underwent repeated cholangiography progressed to develop large duct disease, with a median time of progression of 7.4 (IQR, 5.1–14) years. One patient with small duct PSC who proceeded to develop large duct disease was diagnosed with cholangiocarcinoma, although no malignancies were reported in those solely with small duct disease throughout the entire follow-up period. A significantly higher proportion of patients with sdPSC progressing to large duct PSC either died or underwent liver transplantation compared to those who did not progress (47% vs 15.6%, p < 0.004). Importantly, recurrence of small duct disease was evident in the grafts of two patients who had undergone transplantation for end-stage liver disease secondary to sdPSC.

A recent study from the Mayo Clinic evaluated the influence of inflammatory bowel disease (IBD) and UDCA therapy on 42 patients with sdPSC over a median follow-up period of 4.8 years [87]. They observed a relatively low prevalence of IBD in this form of PSC (52%) although not all patients had undergone a colonoscopy in this retrospective cohort study. Interestingly, 27% had Crohn's disease with colonic involvement and this is in keeping with previously published data. Small duct PSC tended to be diagnosed earlier in patients with IBD as evidenced by a lower prevalence of signs of liver disease at presentation. This may be due to earlier detection of abnormal LFTs in patients undergoing active follow-up for their IBD. Concomitant IBD had no influence on long-term prognosis of sdPSC. Treatment with UDCA at a dose of 13–15 mg/kg failed to halt disease progression, although an improvement in liver biochemistry was observed.

Autoimmune pancreatitis (immunoglobulin G4-associated cholangitis)

Autoimmune pancreatitis (AIP) is a recently described clinical entity characterized by stricturing of the pancreatic duct, focal or generalized pancreatic enlargement, a raised serum immunoglobulin G4 (IgG4) level, a lymphoplasmacytic infiltrate on biopsy, and a response to steroid therapy [88]. AIP in association with intra- and extrahepatic bile duct stricturing similar to those evident in PSC is termed autoimmune pancreatitis – sclerosing cholangitis (AIP-SC). Pancreatic abnormalities are not universally found, suggesting that IgG4-associated cholangitis (IAC) may be a more appropriate term to describe the condition [89]. Whether PSC and AIP represent different ends of the same disease spectrum or are separate clinical entities is of debate, although current evidence favors the latter (see Table 34.3).

The association between AIP and IBD is weak, with a small series from Europe finding UC or Crohn's disease in only 30% of patients with AIP [90]. Furthermore, no cases of cholangiocarcinoma in the presence of AIP have been reported to date. Whilst, no randomized trials of therapy in AIP have been conducted, corticosteroids have been shown to improve biliary structuring [91]. Differences in etiopathogenesis have also been observed. Zen *et al.* demonstrated that the over-production of T-helper (Th) 2 and regulatory cytokines resulted in a unique inflammatory disorder in AIP [92]. A recent study reported the almost exclusive detection of CXCR5- and CXCL13- positive cells in patients with AIP when compared to those with PSC [93].

Elevated serum IgG4 in PSC

A study from the Mayo Clinic found an elevated serum IgG4 level (>140 mg/dl) in 9% of their cohort of 127 PSC patients [94]. In comparison to PSC patients with normal IgG4 concentrations, the former group had significantly higher levels of ALP and bilirubin, in addition to higher PSC Mayo risk scores. An association with IBD was less likely in those with elevated IgG4 levels, although biliary and pancreatic involvement were similar in both groups. Although overall survival time was not different, the time to liver transplantation was significantly shorter (1.7 vs 6.5 years) in patients with elevated IgG4 levels, suggesting a more severe disease course. Whether this group of patients respond to corticosteroids in the same way as those with AIP is yet to be determined.

Management of complications

As PSC slowly progresses to biliary cirrhosis and portal hypertension, complications may arise from chronic

Table 34.3 Comparison of PSC and AIP-SC.

	PSC	AIP-SC
Gender	M:F = 2:1	Probably some male predominance
Clinical presentation	Usually insidious. Sometimes with obstructive jaundice secondary to cholangiocarcinoma.	Mild abdo/back pain. Sometimes with short history of obstructive jaundice due to CBD stricture
Associated inflammatory bowel disease	Yes	No
Cholangiographic findings	Diffuse changes throughout intra- and extrahepatic bile ducts. Abnormalities in pancreatic duct common.	Pancreatic duct strictures or narrowing. Often stricture of distal 1/3 of common bile duct. Intrahepatic duct changes less common.
Blood chemistry data	Often cholestatic but bilirubin usually near normal.	May be cholestatic. Bilirubin often high.
Autoantibodies	Atypical pANCA plus range of others.	Antibodies to carbonic anhydrase II plus range of others.
Immunoglobulins	IgG4 levels normal.	IgG4 levels usually elevated.
Histology	Absence of plasma cells positive for IgG4 on immunostaining.	IgG4 positive plasma cells present in bile ducts and portal tracts.
Liver biopsy staging	Range of Ludwig staging including higher stages e.g. III or IV.	Ludwig staging usually only I or II.
Treatment	Ursodeoxycholic acid +/–biliary drainage for dominant strictures	Systemic steroid therapy usually leads to complete resolution of symptoms and signs of disease. Occasionally patients relapse and require longer courses of steroids

cholestasis or chronic liver failure (as in PBC and other liver diseases) or complications specific to PSC such as biliary strictures and the development of cholangiocarcinoma. The general management of the complications of cholestasis is discussed elsewhere in this book. Given the unpredictable course of PSC, several investigators have sought to create simple, non-invasive means of predicting the development of advanced liver disease. In a cohort of 154 patients, an aspartate transaminase to alanine transaminase ratio (AST: ALT) of at least one was observed to be both an indicator of cirrhosis and a predictor for liver-related death/LT and liver-related death [95]. In a prospective study, Corpechot et al. demonstrated that using transient elastography as a measure of liver stiffness provided an accurate and simple means of assessing biliary fibrosis and histological stage in 28 patients with PSC [96].

Management of complications specific to primary sclerosing cholangitis

Dominant biliary strictures may be treated endoscopically, either via balloon dilatation or the placement of a biliary stent. No randomized trials have compared the different endoscopic treatment options. However, balloon dilatation has become the preferred option as biliary stents are prone

to occlusion and therefore predispose to infection [97]. Stenting after dilatation provides no added value. Gluck et al. evaluated the survival of 106 PSC patients who underwent endoscopic therapy over a 20-year period and observed that patient survival at years three and four was significantly higher than that predicted by the Mayo Clinic natural history model for PSC [98]. In a 13-year prospective study Stiehl et al. studied the survival of 106 patients with PSC treated with 750 mg UDCA daily and by endoscopic balloon dilatation of major dominant stenoses whenever necessary [99, 100]. Ten patients had a dominant stricture at entry and over a median follow-up of five years another 43 developed a dominant stenosis. This was not prevented by low dose UDCA treatment, but successfully treated by balloon dilatation in the majority, only five requiring temporary stenting. This combined approach of UDCA and endoscopic intervention significantly improved the survival compared with predicted survival rates. This was an uncontrolled study and provides only relatively weak evidence that UDCA and/or endoscopic therapy prolonged survival, although the results are promising. Where LT is precluded, as in biliary obstruction due to cholangiocarcinoma, endoscopic stenting is undoubtedly the best option for more distal lesions.

Selected non-cirrhotic PSC patients with dominant extrahepatic strictures may benefit from a bilioenteric bypass [101]. Extrahepatic biliary resection (EHBR) is also potentially effective in carefully selected non-cirrhotic patients. In 2008, Pawlik and colleagues published data on the perioperative morbidity and long-term survival of the largest cohort of patients (n = 77) who had undergone EHBR over the longest follow-up period ever reported (median 10.2 years) [102]. Results were promising, with non-cirrhotic patients demonstrating three, five and ten-year survival rates of 89.6%, 83.3% and 60.2% respectively. This compared favorably with PSC patients who had undergone liver transplantation whose corresponding survival rates were 87.4%, 67.3% and 57% respectively. Furthermore, none of the patients treated with EHBR developed cholangiocarcinoma during the follow-up period. There was a striking contrast in short and long-term survival, with approximately 40% of cirrhotic patients dying within one year of surgery, compared to 5% in the non-cirrhotic cohort. A ten-year survival rate of only 12% was observed in cirrhotics. In addition, EHBR was also associated with low perioperative morbidity and mortality, and also a low rate of PSC-related hospital readmissions.

PSC patients with dominant biliary duct strictures are at increased risk of developing secondary bacterial infections necessitating the need for antibiotic therapy. Kulaksiz and colleagues conducted the first study to evaluate the role of fungal infections in patients with PSC [103]. In a prospective, non-randomized trial, 148 bile samples were obtained endoscopically from 67 consecutive patients. *Candida* species were isolated from eight (11.9%) patients and of these, seven had dominant strictures requiring multiple endoscopic dilatations and courses of antibiotics, suggesting these treatment modalities may have predisposed to colonization with the fungus. The efficacy of antifungal agents and the effect of *Candida* infections on the outcome of PSC patients after liver transplantation will need to be evaluated in future trials.

Medical therapy – the prevention of disease progression

In both PBC and PSC the primary site of inflammation and damage is the biliary epithelium. When severely damaged or destroyed the bile ducts do not have the capacity to regenerate like hepatocytes, which are the primary target for injury in various parenchymal liver diseases. Given the finite number of bile ducts in the liver the natural history of PSC, like PBC, is that of progressive loss of functioning intrahepatic bile ducts (ductopenia). This ductopenia leads to a progressive and irreversible failure of hepatic biliary excretion. To delay and reverse this process physicians have tried a variety of agents, but in PSC, in

contrast to PBC, few randomized controlled trials have been done.

Ursodeoxycholic acid

This hydrophilic bile acid has become widely used in the treatment of cholestatic liver of all causes. UDCA appears to exert a number of effects, all of which may be beneficial in chronic cholestasis: a choleretic effect by increasing bile flow; a direct cytoprotective effect; an indirect cytoprotective effect by displacement of the more hepatotoxic endogenous hydrophobic bile acids from the bile acid pool; an immunomodulatory effect; and finally an inhibitory effect on apoptosis.

Using a labeled bile acid analog Jazrawi *et al.* demonstrated a defect in hepatic bile acid excretion, but not in uptake in patients with PBC and PSC, resulting in bile acid retention [104]. They observed an improvement of hepatic excretory function with UDCA in patients with PBC but only a trend towards improvement in the small number of patients with PSC. Not only is hepatic bile acid excretion affected by UDCA but so is ileal reabsorption of endogenous bile acids. The net result is enrichment of the bile acid pool with UDCA. Hydrophobic bile acids are more toxic than UDCA, which can protect and stabilize membranes.

Studies have demonstrated that long-term treatment with UDCA decreases aberrant expression of HLA class I on hepatocytes and reduces levels of soluble cell adhesion molecules (sICAM) in PBC patients. *In vitro* studies have shown that UDCA may alter cytokine production by human peripheral mononuclear cells. In PSC one study has shown that UDCA has been shown to decrease aberrant HLA DR expression on bile ducts [105]. However, a more recent study could not demonstrate any alteration in expression of either HLA class I and II or ICAM-1 on either biliary epithelial cells or hepatocytes [106]. The body of evidence suggests that UDCA does have some modulatory effects on immune function, but how important these are remains unclear.

Numerous studies have attempted to address the clinical efficacy of UDCA treatment in PSC. The majority have been uncontrolled studies in small numbers of patients. In a pilot study O'Brien *et al.* treated 12 patients with UDCA on an open basis over 30 months [107]. They documented improvement in fatigue, pruritus and diarrhea and significant improvement of all liver biochemical tests, particularly alkaline phosphatise, during the two UDCA treatment periods. Symptoms and liver biochemistry relapsed during a six-month withdrawal period between treatment phases. During UDCA treatment the amount of cholic acid declined slightly but the levels of other relatively hydrophobic bile acids did not change significantly.

In the first randomized double-blind controlled trial of UDCA in PSC Beuers *et al.* compared over a 12-month period six patients who received UDCA 13–15 mg/kg bodyweight with eight patients who received placebo [108]. The majority of patients had early disease (Ludwig classification stages I and II). After six months a significant reduction in alkaline phosphatase and aminotransferases was achieved in the treatment group. A significant fall in bilirubin was only noted after 12 months. Using a multiparametric score the UDCA-treated group showed significant improvement in their liver histology, mainly attributed to decreased portal and parenchymal inflammation. Unfortunately treatment did not ameliorate their symptoms.

Similar results were obtained by Stiehl *et al.* who randomized 20 patients to either 750 mg daily of UDCA or placebo [109]. However, in a larger randomized placebo-controlled trial of UDCA in PSC by Lindor *et al.* no benefit was demonstrated [110]. In this trial 105 patients were randomized to treatment with UDCA in conventional doses (13–15 mg/kg bodyweight daily) or placebo and followed up for up to six years (mean 2.9 years). Treatment with UDCA had no effect upon the time until treatment failure, defined as death, liver transplantation, the development of cirrhosis, quadrupling of bilirubin, marked relapse of symptoms or the development of signs of chronic liver disease. Furthermore, the significant improvement in liver biochemical tests seen in the treated group was not reflected by any beneficial changes in liver histology. **A1d**

In the early 2000s, two pilot studies were performed in order to investigate the efficacy of higher than conventional doses of UDCA in the management of patients with PSC. On the basis that the higher dose would provide adequate enrichment of the bile acid pool and enhance immunomodulatory effects, the Oxford group studied the efficacy of UDCA at a daily dose of 20 mg/kg in a double-blinded, placebo-controlled trial involving 26 patients over a two-year period [111]. The investigators reported significant improvements in most outcomes measured, including liver biochemistry, cholangiographic appearances and histological grade of liver fibrosis, in those randomized to the high dose UDCA. Symptomatic improvement was not evident. An open-label study from the Mayo Clinic reported a significant reduction in expected mortality at four years using the Mayo risk score in patients using UDCA at a dose of 25–30 mg/kg/day in comparison to those taking lower doses (13–15 mg/kg/day) or placebo [112]. A significant improvement of liver biochemistry was also noted. However, radiological and histological outcomes were not measured. In 2005, Olsson *et al.* published the findings of the largest placebo-controlled, prospective trial of high-dose UDCA to date [113]. During the five-year study period, 110 PSC patients received UDCA (17–23 mg/kg/day) and their results were compared with 109 patients in the placebo group. Although there was a trend towards increased survival in the UDCA-treated group, this was

statistically insignificant as the study was underpowered. There was no statistical difference between the two groups in symptom profile, quality of life or in the number of patients diagnosed with cholangiocarcinoma. The primary endpoint of the study was liver transplantation or death, and whilst the incidence of this was lower in the UDCA-treated group, it did not reach statistical significance (7.2% vs 10.9%, 95% CI: 12.2– 4.7%, p = 0.368). In all three studies, the higher doses were well tolerated. **A1c**

Cullen and colleagues conducted a double-blinded, randomized dose-ranging trial to determine whether further enrichment of the bile acid pool with UDCA would lead to additional benefits in outcome for PSC patients [114]. Thirty-one patients were randomized to treatment with 10 mg/kg, 20 mg/kg or 30 mg/kg daily of UDCA for two years. **A1d** As expected, higher doses of UDCA led to further improvements in liver biochemistry compared to more conventional lower doses. Greater reductions in the Mayo risk score were noted in patients who had received the higher doses of UDCA. No significant changes in liver histology among the three groups were observed, which was not surprising given the short follow-up period. Biliary enrichment of UDCA increased with increasing dose, and after two years of treatment biliary UDCA represented 65.6% of total bile acids in the 10 mg/kg group, 79.3% in the 20 mg/kg group, and 92.6% in the 30 mg/kg group. This is in contrast to the findings reported by Rost *et al.* who observed a plateau in bile enrichment after daily doses beyond 22–25 mg/kg. High-doses of UDCA were well tolerated, and in particular, exacerbations of diarrhea in those with underlying colitis were not reported [115]. However, a multicenter randomized trial from the USA comparing high dose UDCA (28–30 mg/kg) with placebo in PSC patients has been halted prematurely because of a higher incidence of adverse outcomes in the UDCA group [116] (see Table 34.4). Thus, at present, high dose UCDA cannot be recommended.

By virtue of its different physiological properties to standard UDCA, Fickert *et al.* investigated the therapeutic effects of 24-*nor*ursodeoxycholic acid (*nor*UDCA), a C_{23} homologue of UDCA with one fewer methylene group in its side chain, using mutidrug resistant gene 2 knockout mice (Mdr2-/-) as an animal model for PSC [117]. Mdr2-/- mice that received a diet containing *nor*UDCA demonstrated a significant improvement in their liver biochemistry and histology, in comparison to mice that were fed UDCA. In addition, a marked reduction in hydroxyproline content and the number of infiltrating neutrophils and proliferating hepatocytes and cholangiocytes was observed in the *nor*UDCA group. Proposed mechanisms of action of *nor*UDCA include increased hydrophilicity of biliary bile acids, stimulation of bile flow with flushing of injured bile ducts, and induction of detoxification and elimination routes for bile acids.

Table 34.4 Controlled trials of ursodeoxycholic acid in primary sclerosing cholangitis.

Authors	No of patients	Type of study	Dose	Duration	LFTs improved Alk P	GGT	Bili	AT	Symptoms improved	Liver histology improved	Proportion with early diseases
Beuers et al. (1992) [108]	14	DBPC	13–15 mg/kg daily	12 months	Yes	Yes	Yes	Yes	No	Yes	57%
Lo et al. (1992) [105]	23	DBPC	10 mg/kg	24 months	Trend	Trend	No	Trend	No	No	74% daily
Stiehl et al. (1994) [109]	20	DBPC, Unc	750 mg daily	Controlled for 3 months, uncontrolled up to 4 years	Yes	Yes	No	Yes	No	Yes	35%
Lindor et al. (1997) [110]	105	DBPC	13–15 mg/kg daily	Mean 2.9 years	Yes	Yes	Yes	Yes	No	No	NA
van Hoogstraten et al. (1998) [118]	48	DB	10 mg/kg daily in single (Grp 1) or three (Grp 2) doses	24 months	Yes	Yes	No	Yes	No	NA	NA
Mitchell et al. (2001) [111]	26	DBPC	20–25 mg/kg daily	12 months	Yes	Yes	No	No	No	Yes	30%
Harnois et al. (2001) [112]	30	OL, historical controls	25–30 mg/kg daily	12 months	Yes	NA	Yes	Yes	NA	NA	NA
Okolicsanyi et al. (2003) [119]	86	DBPC	8–13 mg/kg daily	Retrospective (10-year period)	Yes	Yes	Yes	Yes	Yes	NA	NA
Olsson et al. (2005) [113]	219	DBPC	17–23 mg/kg daily	5 years	Trend	NA	Trend	Trend	No	NA	NA
Lindor et al. (2009) [116]	150	DBPC	28–30 mg/kg daily	6 years	yes	NA	Yes	Yes	No	NA	NA

[a] Proportion with early disease, i.e. stages I and II. Unc: uncontrolled; DB: Double blinded trial; PC: Placebo-controlled trial; OL: open label; Alk P: alkaline phosphatase; GGT γ-:glutamyltranspeptidase; Bili: bilirubin; AT: aminotransferase; NA: data not available; LFTs: liver function tests.

Corticosteroids

Systemic and topical corticosteroid therapy has been evaluated in a number of small, often uncontrolled, trials, but there is no direct evidence to suggest that they are beneficial in PSC. Indeed, when PSC patients with coexistent UC are given corticosteroids for treatment of their colitis, this treatment appears to have little influence on the behavior of their liver disease. **B4** A recent finding that a rat model of cholangitis possesses fewer glucocorticoid receptors on hepatic T lymphocytes may explain the ineffectiveness of steroids in human PSC [120].

In one study, ten patients diagnosed by ERCP and liver biopsy with early PSC (elevated serum alkaline phosphatase, but none with biliary cirrhosis) were treated with prednisone without a significant response [121]. In another uncontrolled pilot study ten patients with PSC, selected because they had elevated aminotransferases, were given prednisolone, and the majority responded with improvement in their biochemistry [122]. In a subsequent study Lindor et al. were unable to confirm these optimistic results [123]. They treated 12 patients with a combination of low dose prednisone (10 mg daily) and colchicine (0.6 mg twice daily). The clinical course of the treated patients was compared with a control group, but the study was not randomized. After two years no significant differences in the biochemistry and liver histology were detected between the two groups. In this study treatment did not alter the rate of disease progression or improve survival. The absence of a beneficial response, and the suspicion that corticosteroid therapy enhanced cortical bone loss and hence the risk of developing compression fractures of the spine even in young male patients, led the authors to advise against empirical corticosteroid therapy in these patients. This conclusion was strengthened by the observation that spontaneous fractures in patients who have undergone liver transplantation occur almost exclusively in PSC patients who are already osteopenic at the time of transplantation [124].

Topical corticosteroids are usually administered through a nasobiliary drain left *in situ* following ERCP. The only controlled trial of nasobiliary lavage with corticosteroids from the Royal Free Hospital showed no benefit when compared with a placebo group [125]. Although the numbers were small, the bile of all the treated patients became rapidly colonized with enteric bacteria and a higher incidence of bacterial cholangitis was recorded in the treatment group.

More recent clinical trials have studied the possible benefit of budesonide, a second-generation corticosteroid with a high first-pass metabolism and minimal systemic availability. Unfortunately preliminary results both alone and in combination with UDCA have been disappointing [126, 127]. **A1d**

There is emerging evidence that corticosteroids may be of value in patients who have overlap syndromes between PSC and autoimmune hepatitis, and in the subgroup of PSC patients who have elevated immunoglobulin G4 levels [128].

Other immunosuppressants

Despite the evidence that PSC may be an immune-mediated disease, there have been few randomized controlled trials of immunosuppressive agents containing sufficient numbers of patients with early disease. Immunosuppression is unlikely to be effective in patients with advanced liver disease and irreversible bile duct loss, and this may account for the disappointing results so far seen in PSC with these agents.

No controlled trials of azathioprine in PSC have been reported. In one case report two patients improved clinically on azathioprine but in another the patient deteriorated [129, 130]. The use of cyclosporine in PSC has been evaluated in a randomized controlled trial from the Mayo Clinic involving 34 patients with PSC and, in the majority, coexistent ulcerative colitis [131]. Treatment with cyclosporine reduced the symptoms of ulcerative colitis but had no effect on the course or prognosis of PSC [132]. **A1d** Follow-up liver histology after two years of treatment revealed progression in 9/10 of the placebo group but only 11/20 of the cyclosporine-treated group. This was not reflected by any beneficial effect on the biochemical tests. The prevalence of adverse effects was low; serious renal

complications were not reported. A combination of cyclosporine and prednisolone elicited a beneficial response in a 65-year-old man with PSC accompanied by pancreatic duct abnormalities [133].

Methotrexate

After demonstrating a promising response to low dose oral pulse methotrexate in an open study involving ten PSC patients without evidence of portal hypertension [134], Knox and Kaplan carried out a double-blind, randomized placebo-controlled trial of oral pulse methotrexate at a dose of 15 mg per week [135]. Twelve patients with PSC were entered into each group and followed up for two years. Although, a significant fall in the serum alkaline phosphatase by 31% was observed in those receiving methotrexate, there were no significant improvements in liver histology, treatment failure or mortality rates. **A1d** In a pilot study Lindor *et al.* found that methotrexate given in combination with UDCA to 19 PSC patients was associated with toxicity (alopecia, pulmonary complications), but showed no additional improvement in liver biochemistry compared with a control group of nine patients treated with UDCA alone [136].

Tacrolimus

Preliminary results from a small pilot study evaluating the benefit of tacrolimus were encouraging, with all ten PSC patients displaying a marked improvement in their liver biochemistry, without the development of significant side effects [137]. Talwalker *et al.* conducted an open-label, phase 2 study, during which, 16 patients received tacrolimus at a dose of 0.05 mg/kg twice daily for one year [138]. A considerable proportion (81%) of patients experienced drug-related adverse effects, with 31% developing toxicities necessitating withdrawal from the study. Of the eight patients who completed the year of treatment, significant improvements in median serum ALP and AST levels were observed. It has been suggested that the poor tolerability of the drug may limit its use in the future.

Mycophenolate motefil

Two studies failed to demonstrate a significant benefit of mycophenolate motefil (MMF) in the treatment of patients with PSC. Sterling and colleagues reported results from a randomized-controlled study in which 25 patients received either UDCA (13–15 mg/kg) alone or in combination with MMF at a dose of 1 g twice a day [139]. After two years, no significant differences were demonstrated with respect to liver biochemistry levels, histological and cholangiographic appearances between the two groups. **A1d** An open-label study performed at the Mayo Clinic evaluated the efficacy and safety of MMF as a single agent in 30 patients with established PSC over a one-year period [140]. Although a statistically significant reduction in ALP levels was observed, there was no such improvement in the other liver function tests or Mayo risk score. Furthermore, the drug was not well tolerated, with seven patients withdrawing from the study due to drug-related adverse effects. Both studies included a substantial proportion of patients with advanced fibrosis and therefore immune-mediated inflammation would be minimal, which may account for the lack of efficacy of MMF.

Cladribine, a nucleoside analog with specific antilymphocyte properties, has been used to treat a variety of autoimmune disorders. In a recent pilot study in PSC six patients with early disease were treated for six months and followed for two years. Whilst significant decreases were seen in peripheral and hepatic lymphocyte counts no significant changes were observed in symptom scores, liver function tests or cholangiograms [141].

Anti TNF-α agents

Tumor necrosis factor-α (TNF-α) has been suggested to drive local inflammatory responses in PSC, and on this basis infliximab has been evaluated as a potential therapeutic agent. Hommes *et al.* conducted a double-blind, placebo-controlled study to assess the efficacy and safety of the chimeric monoclonal antibody in PSC patients [142]. Patients were randomized to receive infliximab (5 mg/kg) or placebo for 52 weeks. Patient enrollment was discontinued prematurely after results of an interim analysis failed to identify any clinical or histological benefit. Of ten patients enrolled, only seven patients (four infliximab and three placebo) completed the study through week 52. No apparent differences could be detected in alkaline phosphatase levels, histological parameters, or symptom scores and no serious drug-related adverse events were reported in either group. **A1d** Two other drugs with anti-TNF activity, etanercept and pentoxifylline, have been found to be ineffective in the treatment of PSC in separate pilot studies [143, 144]. **B4**

Miscellaneous treatments

D-penicillamine

Increased hepatic copper levels are detected in all patients with prolonged cholestasis including those with PSC. This observation provided the rationale for the controlled trial of the cupruretic, D-pencillamine, performed by the Mayo Clinic [145]. Seventy patients were randomized to either D-pencillamine or placebo for 36 months. No improvement was observed on disease progression or overall survival in the treatment group. Major adverse effects, including pancytopenia and proteinuria led to the permanent discontinuation of penicillamine in 21% of the treated patients. **A1d**

Silymarin

Silymarin, a flavonolignan extracted from milk thistle (*Silybum marianum*), has shown promise in the treatment of

a variety of chronic liver disorders characterized by degenerative necrosis and functional impairment. It confers hepatoprotection through its antioxidant, immunomodulatory and antifibrotic properties. Angulo *et al.* performed an open-label pilot study in which 30 patients with PSC received silymarin 140 mg three times a day for one year [146]. A statistically significant improvement in ALP and AST levels was observed, and it appeared to be well tolerated, with only one patient developing diarrhea. Overall, 34% of patients demonstrated a ≥50% improvement or normalization of liver biochemistry. No significant change in serum bilirubin, albumin and Mayo risk score was demonstrated. Whilst the results are encouraging, further controlled trials with a larger sample size and extended follow-up period are warranted. **B4**

Colchicine

In the light of initial reports which suggested a positive trend of the antifibrogenic agent colchicine on survival in PBC and other types of cirrhosis, a randomized trial from Sweden compared colchicine in a dose of 1 mg daily by mouth in 44 patients with PSC with a matched placebo group of 40 patients [147]. At three-year follow up there were no differences in clinical symptoms, serum biochemistry, liver histology or survival between the two groups. The evidence, therefore, suggests that colchicine does not appear to have a role in the treatment of PSC. **A1d**

Bezafibrate

Kita *et al.* conducted a study to assess the efficacy of bezafibrate administered at a dose of 400 mg/day for one month in a variety of chronic liver diseases, including six patients with PSC [148]. In addition to a significant reduction in serum ALP and γ-GT, a decline in ALT was observed in the PSC subgroup. Further trials are warranted in order to evaluate the efficacy of bezafibrate in PSC. **B4**

Nicotine

In keeping with ulcerative colitis, there is a strong inverse relationship between PSC and cigarette smoking. This led Angulo *et al.* to test the hypothesis that oral nicotine might have a beneficial effect in PSC [149]. Eight non-smoking patients with PSC were treated with nicotine 6 mg four times daily for up to one year. Adverse effects were frequent, requiring cessation in three patients and no beneficial effects were seen. A transdermal nicotine patch trial in 11 patients also failed to demonstrate any improvement in symptoms or liver biochemistry [150]. **B4**

Probiotics

On the basis that substances originating from the inflamed gut lead to damage of the biliary tree in PSC, Vleggaar *et al.* conducted a double-blinded, placebo-controlled, crossover study to evaluate the efficacy of probiotics in PSC patients with coexistent IBD [151]. Fourteen patients were initially randomized to receive treatment with probiotics or placebo for three months, and following a one-month washout period, a crossover was made. The investigators failed to observe any significant differences in symptoms or liver biochemistry between those treated with probiotics and those receiving placebo. **A1d**

Combined therapy

In an important pilot study, the potential of combination therapy was explored by Schramm *et al.*, who treated fifteen patients with PSC [152]. All patients received low-dose UDCA (500–750 mg daily), prednisolone 1 mg/kg daily and azathioprine 1–1.5 mg/kg daily. After a median follow-up period of 41 months, all patients had a significant improvement in liver function tests. Seven patients had been previously treated with UDCA, but liver enzymes improved only after immunosuppressive therapy was added. More importantly, six out of ten with follow-up biopsies showed histological improvement and significant radiological deterioration was only seen in one of ten patients who had had ERCP. **B4**

Orthotopic liver transplantation

For patients with advanced PSC, OLT is the only therapeutic option. In the absence of prognostic models capable of predicting the course of disease or the onset of complications in individual patients, the timing of OLT continues to be controversial [153]. With improving expertise and technology, five-year survival rates following liver transplantation have exceeded 80% [154]. This has been associated with an increase in the incidence of recurrent PSC (rPSC) within the allograft. Differences in diagnostic criteria and the use and timing of protocols applied to detect biliary strictures at various institutions have resulted in disparities in the reported incidence of rPSC. Furthermore, whilst MRCP provides a simple, non-invasive means of detecting PSC recurrence, the diagnosis of rPSC is challenging, particularly as indistinguishable biliary stricturing can occur due to chronic rejection, graft preservation injury, hepatic artery stenosis, biliary tract infection and the use of an ABO-incompatible allograft. Investigators from the Mayo Clinic have sought to resolve these issues by setting strict diagnostic criteria based on the existence of cholangiographic and/or histological features characteristic of PSC in the absence of any other apparent cause and occurring beyond the third month after transplantation [155].

A meta-analysis conducted by Gautam *et al.* demonstrated a recurrence rate of 17% in over 900 PSC patients [156]. The natural history of rPSC is unpredictable, although in three recent studies evaluating survival outcome and risk factors for recurrence, retransplantation was required in approximately one-third of all patients [157–159]. There was no significant difference in long-term survival between recipients with rPSC and those with non-recurrent disease. In comparison with symptomatic PSC patients pre-liver transplant, those with rPSC had a better prognosis. Predisposing risk factors identified from these studies included the presence of UC post-transplantation (prior colectomy seemed to be protective), male gender, prolonged use of corticosteroid post-transplantation, acute cellular rejection (ACR), steroid-resistant ACR, HLA-DRB1*08, and the presence of cholangiocarcinoma prior to liver transplantation. Recurrent PSC is likely to become more prevalent in the future, hence a better understanding of its pathogenesis and long-term outcome is essential (see Table 34.5).

Approximately one-third of patients will experience a deterioration in their IBD following OLT, despite the use of heavy immunosuppression [160]. Immunosuppressive regimens containing corticosteroids appear to prevent IBD exacerbation, whilst an increase in corticosteroid dose during a flare leads to a response in most patients [161]. Proctocolectomy is required in a minority of patients with medically-refractory colitis. In addition, PSC patients with a long duration of ulcerative colitis and pancolitis are at increased risk of developing colorectal cancer with reduced survival following OLT [162]. Long-term, post-transplant colonic surveillance is therefore recommended. The impact

Table 34.5 Risk factors for PSC recurrence.

Reference	Risk factor
Jeyarajah *et al.* [164]	Recipient age Cytomegalovirus infection Recurrent acute cellular rejection (ACR)
Vera *et al.* [165]	Male gender Presence of intact colon after liver transplantation
Khettry *et al.* [166]	Gender mismatch
Abu-Elmagd *et al.* [167]	Coexistent IBD Recipient age
Brandsaeter *et al.* [168]	Steroid-resistant ACR
Kugelmas *et al.* [169]	Monoclonal CD3 antibody (OKT3) therapy for steroid resistant ACR
Cholongitas *et al.* [158]	Presence of UC post-transplantation Prolonged use of corticosteroid post-transplantation
Alexander *et al.* [159]	HLA-DRB1*08 ACR
Campsen *et al.* [160]	Presence of cholangiocarcinoma prior to OLT

of OLT on the disease course of pouchitis is not clear. However, dysplasia within the pouch has been reported, therefore advocating the need for surveillance pouchoscopies [163]. *De novo* ulcerative colitis may develop post-OLT in those patients not receiving long-term steroids [161].

Conclusion

Over recent years, substantial progress has been made in obtaining a better understanding of this rare yet important condition. The increasing use of MRCP has resulted in fewer patients being exposed to the complications of ERCP. Furthermore, it has enabled clinicians to diagnose PSC at an earlier stage, and consequently this has led to a change in the clinical presentation over the past decade. Advances in endoscopic, radiological and molecular techniques continue to be made, therefore expanding both diagnostic and therapeutic options, and perhaps most importantly, enabling the differentiation between benign and malignant strictures. Unfortunately, there is no established effective medical treatment for PSC. A recent study was suggested that high-dose UDCA may be harmful and should not be used for the treatment of PSC. Larger, prospective, placebo-controlled trials are required in order to determine the true efficacy and safety of previously evaluated and future medical therapies. Greater insight into the pathogenetic mechanisms involved in PSC would enable therapy to be targeted more specifically at the area of initial damage, namely, the biliary epithelium.

References

1 Schrumpf E, Fausa O, Forre O et al. HLA antigens and immunoregulatory T cells in ulcerative colitis associated with hepatobiliary disease. *Scand J Gastroenterol* 1982; **17**: 187–191.

2 Shepherd HA, Selby WS, Chapman RW et al. Ulcerative colitis and persistent liver dysfunction. *QJM* 1983; **52**: 503–513.

3 Chapman RW, Varghese Z, Gaul R et al. Association of primary sclerosing cholangitis with HLA-B8. *Gut* 1983; **24**: 38–41.

4 Saarinen S, Olerup O, Broome U. Increased frequency of autoimmune diseases in patients with primary sclerosing cholangitis. *Am J Gastroenterol* 2000; **95**: 3195–3199.

5 Terjung B, Worman HJ. Anti-neutrophil antibodies in primary sclerosing cholangitis. *Best Pract Res Clin Gastroenterol* 2001; **15**: 629–642.

6 Terjung B, Muennich M, Gottwein J et al. Identification of myeloid-specific tubulin-beta isotype 5 as target antigen of antineutrophil cytoplasmic antibodies in autoimmune liver disease. *Hepatology* 2005; **42**: 411–417.

7 Preuss B, Berg C, Altenberend F et al. Demonstration of autoantibodies to recombinant human sulphite oxidase in patients with chronic liver disorders and analysis of their clinical relevance. *Clin Exp Immunol* 2007; **150**: 312–321.

8 Ardesjo B, Hansson CM, Bruder CE et al. Autoantibodies to glutathione S-transferase theta 1 in patients with primary sclerosing cholangitis and other autoimmune diseases. *J Autoimmun* 2008; **30**: 273–282.

9 Maggs JR, Chapman RW. Sclerosing cholangitis. *Curr Opin Gastroenterol* 2007; **23**: 310–316.

10 Weismuller T, Wedemeyer J, Kubicka S. The challenges in primary sclerosing cholangitis–aetiopathogenesis, autoimmunity, management and malignancy. *J Hepatol* 2008; **48**(Suppl 1): S38–57.

11 Karlsen TH, Boberg KM, Vatn M et al. Different HLA class II associations in ulcerative colitis patients with and without primary sclerosing cholangitis. *Genes Immun* 2007; **8**: 275–278.

12 Wiencke K, Boberg KM, Donaldson P et al. No major effect of the CD28/CTLA4/ICOS gene region on susceptibility to primary sclerosing cholangitis. *Scand J Gastroenterol* 2006; **41**: 586–591.

13 Eri R, Jonnson JR, Pandeya N et al. CCR5-Delta32 mutation is strongly associated with primary sclerosing cholangitis. *Genes Immun* 2004; **5**: 444–450.

14 Henckaerts L, Fevery J, Van Steenbergen W et al. CC-type chemokine receptor 5-Delta32 mutation protects against primary sclerosing cholangitis. *Inflamm Bowel Dis* 2006; **12**: 272–277.

15 Melum E, Karlsen TH, Broome U et al. The 32-base pair deletion of the chemokine receptor 5 gene (CCR5-Delta32) is not associated with primary sclerosing cholangitis in 363 Scandinavian patients. *Tissue Antigens* 2006; **68**: 78–81.

16 Henckaerts L, Fevery J, Van Steenbergen et al. The RANTES -28 g polymorphism is associated with primary sclerosing cholangitis. *Gut* 2007; **56**: 891–892.

17 Yang X, Cullen SN, Li Jh et al. Susceptibility to primary sclerosing cholangitis is associated with polymorphisms of intercellular adhesion molecule-1. *J Hepatol* 2004; **40**: 375–379.

18 Bowlus CL, Karlsen TH, Broome U et al. Analysis of MAdCAM-1 and ICAM-1 polymorphisms in 365 Scandinavian patients with primary sclerosing cholangitis. *J Hepatol* 2006; **45**: 704–710.

19 Satsangi J, Chapman RW, Haldar N et al. A functional polymorphism of the stromelysin gene (MMP-3) influences susceptibility to primary sclerosing cholangitis. *Gastroenterology* 2001; **121**: 124–130.

20 Wiencke K, Louka AS, Spurkland A et al. Association of matrix metalloproteinase-1 and -3 promoter polymorphisms with clinical subsets of Norwegian primary sclerosing cholangitis patients. *J Hepatol* 2004; **41**: 209–214.

21 Karlsen TH, Hampe J, Wiencke K et al. Genetic polymorphisms associated with inflammatory bowel disease do not confer risk for primary sclerosing cholangitis. *Am J Gastroenterol* 2007; **102**: 115–121.

22 Sumida T, Yonaha F, Maeda T et al. T cell receptor repertoire of infiltrating T cells in lips of Sjogren's syndrome patients. *J Clin Invest* 1992; **89**: 681–685.

23 Imberti L, Sottini A, Primi D. T cell repertoire and autoimmune diseases. *Immunol Res* 1993; **12**: 149–167.

24 Broome U, Grunewald J, Scheynius A et al. Preferential V beta3 usage by hepatic T lymphocytes in patients with primary sclerosing cholangitis. *J Hepatol* 1997; **26**: 527–534.

25 Probert CS, Christ AD, Saubermann LJ et al. Analysis of human common bile duct-associated T cells: Evidence for oligoclonal-

ity, T cell clonal persistence, and epithelial cell recognition. *J Immunol* 1997; **158**: 1941–1948.

26 Chapman RW, Kelly PM, Heryet A *et al.* Expression of HLA-DR antigens on bile duct epithelium in primary sclerosing cholangitis. *Gut* 1988; **29**: 422–427.

27 Broome U, Glaumann H, Hultcrantz R, Forsum U. Distribution of HLA-DR, HLA-DP, HLA-DQ antigens in liver tissue from patients with primary sclerosing cholangitis. *Scand J Gastroenterol* 1990; **25**: 54–58.

28 Xu B, Broome U, Ericzon BG *et al.* High frequency of autoantibodies in patients with primary sclerosing cholangitis that bind biliary epithelial cells and induce expression of CD44 and production of interleukin 6. *Gut* 2002; **51**: 120–127.

29 Karrar A, Broome U, Sodergen T *et al.* Biliary epithelial cell antibodies link adaptive and innate immune responses in primary sclerosing cholangitis. *Gastroenterology* 2007; **132**: 1504–1514.

30 Spirli C, Fabris L, Duner E *et al.* Cytokine-stimulated nitric oxide production inhibits adenylyl cyclase and cAMP-dependent secretion in cholangiocytes. *Gastroenterology* 2003; **124**: 737–753.

31 Grant AJ, Lalor PF, Salmi M *et al.* Homing of mucosal lymphocytes to the liver in the pathogenesis of hepatic complications of inflammatory bowel disease. *Lancet* 2002; **359**: 150–157.

32 Eksteen B, Miles AE, Grant AJ *et al.* Lymphocyte homing in the pathogenesis of extra-intestinal manifestations of inflammatory bowel disease. *Clin Med* 2004; **4**: 173–180.

33 Eksteen B, Miles A, Curbishley SM *et al.* Epithelial inflammation is associated with CCL28 production and the recruitment of regulatory T cells expressing CCR10. *J Immunol* 2006; **177**: 593–603.

34 Karlsen TH, Lie BA, Frey Froslie K *et al.* Polymorphisms in the steroid and xenobiotic receptor gene influence survival in primary sclerosing cholangitis. *Gastroenterology* 2006; **131**: 781–787.

35 Elias E, Mills CO. Coordinated defence and the liver. *Clin Med* 2007; **7**: 180–184.

36 Fickert P, Fuchsbichler A, Wagner M *et al.* Regurgitation of bile acids from leaky bile ducts causes sclerosing cholangitis in Mdr2 (Abcb4) knockout mice. *Gastroenterology* 2004; **127**: 261–274.

37 Pauli-Magnus C, Kerb R, Fattinger K *et al.* BSEP and MDR3 haplotype structure in healthy Caucasians, primary biliary cirrhosis and primary sclerosing cholangitis. *Hepatology* 2004; **39**: 779–791.

38 Bjornsson E, Cederborg A, Akvist A *et al.* Intestinal permeability and bacterial growth of the small bowel in patients with primary sclerosing cholangitis. *Scand J Gastroenterol* 2005; **40**: 1090–1094.

39 Krasinskas AM, Yoa Y, Randhawa P *et al.* *Helicobacter pylori* may play a contributory role in the pathogenesis of primary sclerosing cholangitis. *Dig Dis Sci* 2007; **52**: 2265–2270.

40 Vierling J. Aetiopathogenesis of primary sclerosing cholangitis. In: Manns PCR, Stieihl A, Wiesner R (eds). *Primary Sclerosing Cholangitis.* London: Kluwer Academic Publishers, 1998.

41 Moff SL, Kamel IR, Eustace J *et al.* Diagnosis of primary sclerosing cholangitis: A blinded comparative study using magnetic resonance cholangiography and endoscopic retrograde cholangiography. *Gastrointest Endosc* 2006; **64**: 219–223.

42 Berstad AE, Aabakken L, Smith HJ *et al.* Diagnostic accuracy of magnetic resonance and endoscopic retrograde cholangiography in primary sclerosing cholangitis. *Clin Gastroenterol Hepatol* 2006; **4**, 514–520.

43 Weber C, Kuhlencordt R, Grotelueschen R *et al.* Magnetic resonance cholangiopancreatography in the diagnosis of primary sclerosing cholangitis. *Endoscopy* 2008; **40**: 739–745.

44 Fulcher AS, Turner MA, Franklin KJ *et al.* Primary sclerosing cholangitis: Evaluation with MR cholangiography – a case-control study. *Radiology* 2000; **215**: 71–80.

45 Talwalkar JA, Angulo P, Johnson C *et al.* Cost-minimisation analysis of MRC versus ERCP for the diagnosis of primary sclerosing cholangitis. *Hepatology* 2004; **40**, 39–45.

46 Meagher S, Yusoff I, Kennedy W *et al.* The roles of magnetic resonance and endoscopic retrograde cholangiopancreatography (MRCP and ERCP) in the diagnosis of patients with suspected sclerosing cholangitis: A cost-effectiveness analysis. *Endoscopy* 2007; **39**: 222–228.

47 Petrovic BD, Nikolaidis P, Hamond NA *et al.* Correlation between findings on MRCP and Gadolinium-enhanced MR of the liver and a survival model for primary sclerosing cholangitis. *Dig Dis Sci* 2007; **52**: 3499–3506.

48 Mesenas S, Vu C, Doig L, Meenan J. Duodenal EUS to identify thickening of the extrahepatic biliary tree wall in primary sclerosing cholangitis. *Gastrointestinal Endoscopy* 2006; **63**: 403–408.

49 Card T, Solaymani-Dodaran M, West J. Incidence and mortality of primary sclerosing cholangitis in the UK: A population-based cohort study. *J Hepatol* 2008; **48**: 939–944.

50 Kaplan GG, Laupland KB, Butzner D *et al.* The burden of large and small duct primary sclerosing cholangitis in adults and children: A population-based analysis. *Am J Gastroenterol* 2007; **102**: 1042–1049.

51 Bergquist A, Said K, Broomé U. Changes over a 20-year period in the clinical presentation of primary sclerosing cholangitis in Sweden. *Scand J Gastroenterol* 2007; **42**: 88–93.

52 Tanaka A, Takamori Y, Toda G *et al.* Outcome and prognostic factors of 391 Japanese patients with primary sclerosing cholangitis. *Liver Int* 2008; **28**: 983–989.

53 Bergquist A, Glaumann H, Lindberg B, Broomé U. Primary sclerosing cholangitis can present with acute liver failure: Report of two cases. *Journal of Hepatology* 2006; **44**: 1005–1008.

54 Broome U, Olsson R, Loof L *et al.* Natural history of prognostic factors in 305 Swedish patients with primary sclerosing cholangitis. *Gut* 1996; **38**: 610–615.

55 Farrant JM, Hayllar KM, Wilkinson ML *et al.* Natural history and prognostic variables in primary sclerosing cholangitis. *Gastroenterology* 1991; **100**: 1710–1717.

56 Tischendorf JJ, Meier PN, Strassburg CP *et al.* Characterization and clinical course of hepatobiliary carcinoma in patients with primary sclerosing cholangitis. *Scand J Gastroenterol* 2006; **41**: 1227–1234.

57 Kitiyakara T, Chapman RW. Chemoprevention and screening in primary sclerosing cholangitis. *Postgrad Med J* 2008; **84**: 228–237.

58 Lempinem M, Isoniemi H, Mäkisalo H *et al.* Enhanced detection of cholangiocarcinoma with serum trypsinogen-2 in patients with severe bile duct strictures. *J Hepatol* 2007; **47**: 677–683.

59 Keiding S, Hansen SB, Rasmussen HH *et al*. Detection of cholangiocarcinoma in primary sclerosing cholangitis by positron emission tomography. *Hepatology* 1998; **28**: 700–706.

60 Fevery J, Buchel O, Nevens F *et al*. Positron emission tomography is not a reliable method for the early diagnosis of cholangiocarcinoma in patients with primary sclerosing cholangitis. *J Hepatol* 2005; **43**: 358–360.

61 Prytz H, Keiding S, Bjornsson E *et al*. Dynamic FDG-PET is useful for detection of cholangiocarcinoma in patients with PSC listed for liver transplantation. *Hepatology* 2006; **44**: 1572–1580.

62 Tischendorf JJ, Meier PN, Schneider A *et al*. Transpapillary intraductal ultrasound in the evaluation of dominant bile duct stenoses in patients with primary sclerosing cholangitis. *Scand J Gastroenterol* 2007; **42**: 1011–1017.

63 Tischendorf JJ, Krüger M, Trautwein C *et al*. Cholangioscopic characterization of dominant bile duct stenoses in patients with primary sclerosing cholangitis. *Endoscopy* 2006; **38**: 665–669.

64 Awadallah NS, Chen YK, Piraka C *et al*. Is there a role for cholangioscopy in patients with primary sclerosing cholangitis? *Am J Gastroenterol* 2006; **101**: 284–291.

65 Moreno Luna LE, Kipp B, Halling KC *et al*. Advanced cytologic techniques for the detection of malignant pancreatobiliary strictures. *Gastroenterology* 2006; **131**: 1064–1072.

66 Boberg KM, Jebsen P, Clausen OP *et al*. Diagnostic benefit of biliary brush cytology in cholangiocarcinoma in primary sclerosing cholangitis. *J Hepatol* 2006; **45**: 568–574.

67 Moff SL, Clark DP, Maitra A *et al*. Utility of bile duct brushings for the early detection of cholangiocarcinoma in patients with primary sclerosing cholangitis. *J Clin Gastroenterol* 2006; **40**: 336–341.

68 Charatcharoenwitthaya P, Enders FB, Halling KC, Lindor KD. Utility of serum tumor markers, imaging, and biliary cytology for detecting cholangiocarcinoma in primary sclerosing cholangitis. *Hepatology* 2008; **48**: 1106–1117.

69 Rudolph G, Kloeters-Plachky P, Rost D, Stiehl A. The incidence of cholangiocarcinoma in primary sclerosing cholangitis after long-time treatment with ursodeoxycholic acid. *Eur J Gastroenterol Hepatol* 2007; **19**: 487–491.

70 Brandt DJ, MacCarty RL, Charboneau JW *et al*. Gallbladder disease in patients with primary sclerosing cholangitis. *AJR Am J Roentgenol* 1988; **150**: 571–574.

71 Said K, Glaumann H, Bergquist A. Gallbladder disease in patients with primary sclerosing cholangitis. *J Hepatol* 2008; **48**: 598–605.

72 Leung UC, Wong PY, Roberts R, Koea J. Gall bladder polyps in sclerosing cholangitis: Does the 1-cm rule apply? *ANZ J Surg* 2007; **77**: 355–357.

73 Lewis JT, Talwalkar JA, Rosen CB *et al*. Prevalence and risk factors for gallbladder neoplasia in patients with primary sclerosing cholangitis: Evidence for a metaplasia-dysplasia-carcinoma sequence. *Am J Surg Pathol* 2007; **31**: 907–913.

74 Soetikno RM, Lin OS, Heidenreich PA *et al*. Increased risk of colorectal neoplasia in patients with primary sclerosing cholangitis and ulcerative colitis: A meta-analysis. *Gastrointest Endosc* 2002; **56**: 48–54.

75 Rodrigues CM, Fan G, Wong PY, Kren BT, Steer CJ. Ursodeoxycholic acid may inhibit deoxycholic acid-induced aopotosis by modulating mitochondrial trans membrane potential and reactive species production. *Mol Med* 1998; **4**: 165–178.

76 Tung BY, Edmond MJ, Haggitt RC *et al*. Ursodiol use is associated with lower prevalence of colonic neoplasia in patients with ulcerative colitis and primary sclerosing cholangitis. *Ann Intern Med* 2001; **134**: 89–95.

77 Pardi DS, Loftus EV, Kremers WK *et al*. Ursodeoxycholic acid as a chemoprotective agent in patients with ulcerative colitis and primary sclerosing cholangitis. *Gastroenterology* 2003; **124**: 889–893.

78 Wolf JM, Rybicki LA, Lashner BA. The impact of ursodeoxycholic acid on cancer, dysplasia and mortality in ulcerative colitis patients with primary sclerosing cholangitis. *Aliment Pharmacol Ther* 2005; **22**: 783–788.

79 Vera A, Gunson BK, Ussatoff V *et al*. Colorectal cancer in patients with inflammatory bowel disease after liver transplantation for primary sclerosing cholangitis. *Transplantation* 2003; **75**: 1983–1988.

80 Broome U, Bergquist A. Primary sclerosing cholangitis, inflammatory bowel disease, and colon cancer. *Semin Liver Dis* 2006; **26**: 31–41.

81 Stahlberg D, Veress B, Tribukait B, Broome U. Atrophy and neoplastic transformation of the ileal pouch mucosa in patients with ulcerative colitis and primary sclerosing cholangitis: A case control study. *Dis Colon Rectum* 2003; **46**: 770–778.

82 Penna C, Dozois R, Tremaine WJ *et al*. Pouchitis after pouchanal anastomosis for ulcerative colitis occurs with increased frequency in patients with associated primary sclerosing cholangitis. *Gut* 1996; **38**: 234–239.

83 Bjornsson E, Boberg KM, Cullen S *et al*. Patients with small duct primary sclerosing cholangitis have a favourable long term prognosis. *Gut* 2002; **51**: 731–735.

84 Broome U, Glaumann H, Lindstom E *et al*. Natural history and outcome in 32 Swedish patients with small duct primary sclerosing cholangitis (PSC). *J Hepatol* 2002; **36**: 586–589.

85 Angulo P, Maor-Kendler Y, Lindor KD. Small-duct primary sclerosing cholangitis: A long-term follow-up study. *Hepatology* 2002; **35**: 1494–1500.

86 Björnsson E, Olsson R, Bergquist A *et al*. The natural history of small-duct primary sclerosing cholangitis. *Gastroenterology* 2008; **134**: 975–980.

87 Charatcharoenwitthaya P, Angulo P, Enders FB, Lindor KD. Impact of inflammatory bowel disease and ursodeoxycholic acid therapy on small-duct primary sclerosing cholangitis. *Hepatology* 2008; **47**: 133–142.

88 Kim KP, Kim MH, Lee SS *et al*. Autoimmune pancreatitis: It may be a worldwide entity. *Gastroenterology* 2004; **126**: 1214.

89 Bjornsson E, Chari ST, Smyrk TC *et al*. Immunoglobulin associated cholangitis: Description of a developing clinical entity based on review of the literature. *Hepatology* 2007; **45**: 1547–1554.

90 Church NI, Pereira SP, Hatfield ARW *et al*. Autoimmune pancreatitis: Response to therapy in a UK series. *Gastroenterology* 2006; **1300**: A–326.

91 Kamisawa T, Yoshiike M, Egawa N *et al*. Treating patients with autoimmune pancreatitis: results from a long-term follow-up study. *Pancreatology* 2005; **5**: 234–238.

92 Zen Y, Fujii T, Harada K *et al*. Th2 and regulatory immune reactions are increased in immunoglobulin G-4 related sclerosing pancreatitis and cholangitis. *Hepatology* 2007; **45**: 1538–1546.

93 Esposito I, Born D, Bergmann F *et al.* Autoimmune pancreato-cholangitis, non-autoimmune pancreatitis and primary sclerosing cholangitis: A comparative morphological and immunological analysis. *PLoS ONE* 2008; **3**: e2539.

94 Mendes FD, Levy C, Enders FB *et al.* Elevated serum IgG4 concentration in patients with primary sclerosing cholangitis. *Am J Gastroenterol* 2006; **101**: 2070–2075.

95 Nyblom H, Nordlinder H, Olsson R. High aspartate to alanine amintransferase ratio is an indicator of cirrhosis and poor outcome in patients with primary sclerosing cholangitis. *Liver International* 2007; **27**: 694–699.

96 Corpechot C, Naggar AE, Poujol-Robert A *et al.* Assessment of biliary fibrosis by transient elastography in patients with PBC and PSC. *Hepatol* 2006; **43**: 1118–1124.

97 Stiehl A. Primary sclerosing cholangitis: The role of endoscopic therapy. *Semin Liver Dis* 2006; **26**: 62–68.

98 Gluck M, Cantone NR, Brandabur JJ *et al.* A twenty-year experience with endoscopic therapy for symptomatic primary sclerosing cholangitis. *J Clin Gastroenterol* 2008; **42**: 1032–1039.

99 Stiehl A, Rudolph G, Sauer P *et al.* Efficacy of ursodeoxycholic acid treatment and endoscopic dilatation of major duct stenoses in primary sclerosing cholangitis. A 8 years prospective study. *J Hepatol* 1997; **26**: 56–61.

100 Stiehl A, Rudolph G, Kloteis-Plodsky P *et al.* Development of dominant bile duct stenoses in patients treated with ursodeoxycholic acid, outcome after endoscopic treatment. *J Hepatol* 2002; **36**: 151–156.

101 Hepburgh JA. Surgical biliary drainage in primary sclerosing cholangitis. The role of the Hepp-Couinaud approach. *Arch Surg* 1994; **129**: 1057–1062.

102 Pawlick TM, Olbrecht VA, Pitt HA *et al.* Primary sclerosing cholangitis: Role of extrahepatic biliary resection. *J Am Coll Surg* 2008; **206**: 822–830.

103 Kulaksiz H, Rudolph G, Kloeters-Plachky P *et al.* Biliary candida infections in primary sclerosing cholangitis. *Journal of Hepatology* 2006; **45**: 711–716.

104 Jazrawi RP, de-Caestecker JS, Goggin PM *et al.* Kinetics of hepatic bile acid handling in cholestatic liver disease: effect of ursodeoxycholic acid. *Gastroenterology* 1994; **106**: 134–142.

105 Lo SK, Hermann R, Chapman RW *et al.* Ursodeoxycholic acid in primary sclerosing cholangitis; A double blind controlled trial. *Hepatology* 1992; **16**: 54–59.

106 van Milligen, de Wit AW, Kuiper H *et al.* Does ursodeoxycholic acid mediate immunomodulatory and anti-inflammatory effects in patients with primary sclerosing cholangitis? *Eur J Gastroenterol Hepatol* 1999; **11**: 129–136.

107 O'Brien CB, Senior JR, Arora-Mirchandani R *et al.* Ursodeoxycholic acid for the treatment of primary sclerosing cholangitis: A 30-month pilot study. *Hepatology* 1991; **14**: 838.

108 Beuers U, Spengler U, Kruis W *et al.* Ursodeoxycholic acid for treatment of primary sclerosing cholangitis: A placebo-controlled trial. *Hepatology* 1992; **16**: 707–714.

109 Stiehl A, Walker S, Stiehl L *et al.* Effect of ursodeoxycholic acid on liver and bile duct disease in primary sclerosing cholangitis. A 3-year pilot study with a placebo-controlled study period. *J Hepatol* 1994; **20**: 57–64.

110 Lindor KD. The Mayo PSC/UDCA Study Group. Ursodiol for primary sclerosing cholangitis. *N Engl J Med* 1997; **336**: 691–695.

111 Mitchell SA, Bansi DS, Hunt N *et al.* A preliminary trial of high-dose ursodeoxycholic acid in primary sclerosing cholangitis. *Gastroenterology* 2001; **121**: 900–907.

112 Harnois DM, Angulo P, Jorgensen RA *et al.* High-dose ursodeoxycholic acid as a therapy for patients with primary sclerosing cholangitis. *Am J Gastroenterol* 2001; **96**: 1558–1562.

113 Olsson R, Boberg KM, de Muckadell OS *et al.* High-dose ursodeoxycholic acid in primary sclerosing cholangitis: a 5-year multicenter, randomized, controlled study. *Gastroenterology* 2005; **129**: 1464–1472.

114 Cullen SN, Rust C, Fleming K *et al.* High dose ursodeoxycholic acid for the treatment of primary sclerosing cholangitis is safe and effective. *J Hepatol* 2008; **48**: 792–800.

115 Rost D, Rudolph G, Kloeters-Plachky P, Stiehl A. Effect of high-dose ursodeoxycholic acid on its biliary enrichment in primary sclerosing cholangitis. *Hepatology* 2004; **40**: 693–698.

116 Lindor KD, Enders FB, Schmoll JA *et al.* Randomized, double-blind controlled trial of high-dose ursodeoxycholic acid for primary sclerosing cholangitis. *Hepatology* 2009; **50**: 808–814.

117 Fickert P, Wagner M, Marschall HU *et al.* 24-norUrsodeoxycholic acid is superior to ursodeoxycholic acid in the treatment of sclerosing cholangitis in Mdr2 (Abcb4) knockout mice. *Gastroenterology* 2006; **130**: 465–481.

118 van Hoogstraten HJ, Wolfhagen FH, van de Meeberg PC *et al.* Ursodeoxycholic acid therapy for primary sclerosing cholangitis: Results of a 2-year randomized controlled trial to evaluate single versus multiple daily doses. *J Hepatol* 1998; **29**: 417–423.

119 Okolicsanyi L, Groppo M, Floreani A *et al.* Treatment of primary sclerosing cholangitis with low-dose ursodeoxycholic acid: Results of a retrospective Italian multicentre survey. *Dig Liver Dis* 2003; **35**: 325–331.

120 Tjandra K, Le T, Swain MG. Glucocorticoid receptors are down-regulated in hepatic T lymphocytes in rats with experimental cholangitis. *Gut* 2003; **52**: 1363–1370.

121 Sivak M Jr, Farmer RG, Lalli AF. Sclerosing cholangitis: Its increasing frequency of recognition and association with inflammatory bowel disease. *J Clin Gastroenterol* 1981; **3**: 261–266.

122 Burgert SL, Brown BP, Kirkpatrick RB, LaBrecque DR. Positive corticosteroid response in early primary sclerosing cholangitis (Abstract). *Gastroenterology* 1984; **86**: 1037.

123 Lindor KD, Wiesner RH, Colwell LJ *et al.* The combination of prednisone and colchicine in patients with primary sclerosing cholangitis. *Am J Gastroenterol* 1994; **86**: 57–61.

124 Porayko MK, Wiesner RH, Hay JE *et al.* Bone disease in liver transplant recipients: incidence, timing and risk factors. *Transplant Proc* 1991; **23**: 1462–1465.

125 Allison MC, Burroughs AK, Noone P, Summerfield JA. Biliary lavage with corticosteroids in primary sclerosing cholangitis. A clinical, cholangiographic and bacteriological study. *J Hepatol* 1986; **3**: 118–122.

126 Angulo P, Batts KP, Jorgensen A, Lindor KD. Oral budesonide in the treatment of primary sclerosing cholangitis. *Am J Gastroenterol* 2000; **95**: 2333–2227.

127 van Hoogstraten HJF, Vieggar FP, Boland GI *et al.* Budesonide or prednisone in combination with ursodeoxycholic acid in primary sclerosing cholangitis. A randomized double-blind pilot study. *Am J Gastroenterol* 2000; **95**: 2015–2022.

128 Cullen SN, Chapman RWC. The medical management of primary sclerosing cholangitis. *Semin Liver Dis* 2006; **26**: 52–61.

129 Javett SL. Azathioprine in primary sclerosing cholangitis. *Lancet* 1971; **1**: 810–811.

130 Wagner A. Azathioprine treatment in primary sclerosing cholangitis. *Lancet* 1971; **ii**: 663–664.

131 Wiesner RH, Steiner B, LaRusso NF *et al.* A controlled clinical trial evaluating cyclosporine in the treatment of primary sclerosing cholangitis (Abstract). *Hepatology* 1991; **14**: 63A.

132 Sandborn WJ, Wiesner RH, Tremaine WJ, Larusso NE. Ulcerative colitis disease activity following treatment of associated primary sclerosing cholangitis with cyclosporin. *Gut* 1993; **34**: 242–246.

133 Kyokane K, Ichihara T, Horisawa M *et al.* Successful treatment of primary sclerosing cholangitis with cyclosporine and corticosteroid. *Hepatogastroenterology* 1994; **41**: 449–452.

134 Sterling RK, Salvatori JJ, Luketic VA *et al.* A prospective, randomized-controlled pilot study of ursodeoxycholic acid combined with mycophenolate mofetil in the treatment of primary sclerosing cholangitis. *Aliment Pharmacol Ther* 2004; **20**: 943–949.

135 Talwalkar JA, Angulo P, Keach JC *et al.* Mycophenolate mofetil for the treatment of primary sclerosing cholangitis. *Am J Gastroenterol* 2005; **100**: 308–312.

136 Lindor KD, Jorgensen RA, Anderson ML *et al.* Ursdeoxycholic acid and methotrexate for primary sclerosing cholangitis: A pilot study. *Am J Gastroenterol* 1996; **91**: 511–515.

137 Van Thiel DH, Carroll P, Abu-Elmagd K *et al.* Tacrolimus (FK506), a treatment for primary sclerosing cholangitis: results of an open-label preliminary trial. *Am J Gastroenterol* 1995; **90**: 455–459.

138 Talwalkar JA, Gossard AA, Keach JC *et al.* Tacrolimus for the treatment of primary sclerosing cholangitis. *Liver Int* 2007; **27**: 451–453.

139 Sterling RK, Salvatori JJ, Luketic VA *et al.* A prospective, randomized-controlled pilot study of ursodeoxycholic acid combined with mycophenolate mofetil in the treatment of primary sclerosing cholangitis. *Aliment Pharmacol Ther* 2004; **20**: 943–949.

140 Talwalkar JA, Angulo P, Keach JC *et al.* Mycophenolate mofetil for the treatment of primary sclerosing cholangitis. *Am J Gastroenterol* 2005; **100**: 308–312.

141 Duchini A, Younossi ZM, Saven A *et al.* An open-label pilot trial of cladibrine (2-cloolordeoxyadenosine) in patients with primary sclerosing cholangitis. *J Clin Gastroenterol* 2000; **31**: 271–273.

142 Hommes DW, Erkelens W, Ponsioen C *et al.* A double-blind, placebo-controlled, randomized study of infliximab in primary sclerosing cholangitis. *J Clin Gastroenterol* 2008; **42**: 522–526.

143 Epstein MP, Kaplan MM. A pilot study of etanercept in the treatment of primary sclerosing cholangitis. *Dig Dis Sci* 2004; **49**: 1–4.

144 Bharucha AE, Jorgensen R, Lichtman SN *et al.* (2000) A pilot study of pentoxifylline for the treatment of primary sclerosing cholangitis. *Am J Gastroenterol* **95**, 2338–2342.

145 LaRusso NF, Wiesner RH, Ludwig J *et al.* Prospective trial of penicillamine in primary sclerosing cholangitis. *Gastroenterology* 1998; **95**: 1036–1042.

146 Angulo P, Jorgensen RA, Kowdley KV, Lindor KD. Silymarin in the treatment of patients with primary sclerosing cholangitis: An open-label pilot study. *Dig Dis Sci* 2008; **53**: 1716–1720.

147 Olsson R, Broome U, Danielsson A *et al.* Colchicine treatment of primary sclerosing cholangitis. *Gastroenterology* 1995; **108**: 1199–1203.

148 Kita R, Takamatsu S, Kimura T *et al.* Bezafibrate may attenuate biliary damage associated with chronic liver diseases accompanied by high serum biliary enzyme levels. *J Gastroenterol* 2006; **41**: 686–692.

149 Angulo P, Bharucha AE, Jorgensen RA *et al.* Oral nicotine in treatment of primary sclerosing cholangitis: A pilot study. *Dig Dis Sci* 1999; **44**: 602–607.

150 Vleggaar FP, van Buuren HR, van Berge Henegouwen GP *et al.* No beneficial effects of transdermal nicotine in patients with primary sclerosing cholangitis: Results of a randomized double-blind placebo-controlled cross-over study. *Eur J Gastroenterol Hepatol* 2001; **13**: 171–175.

151 Vleggaar FP, Monkelbaan JF, van Erpecum KJ. Probiotics in primary sclerosing cholangitis: a randomized placebo-controlled crossover pilot study. *Eur J Gastroenterol Hepatol* 2008; **20**: 688–692.

152 Schramm C, Schirmacher P, Helmreich-Becker I *et al.* Combined therapy with azathioprine prednisolone and ursodiol in patients with primary sclerosing cholangitis. A case series. *Ann Intern Med* 1999; **131**: 943–946.

153 Gow PJ, Chapman RW. Liver transplantation for primary sclerosing cholangitis. *Liver* 2000; **20**: 97–103.

154 LaRusso NF, Shneider BL, Black D *et al.* Primary sclerosing cholangitis: Summary of a workshop. *Hepatology* 2006; **44**: 746–764.

155 Graziadei IW, Wiesner RH, Batts KP *et al.* Recurrence of primary sclerosing cholangitis following liver transplantation. *Hepatology* 1999; **29**: 1050–1056.

156 Gautam M, Cheruvattath R, Balan V. Recurrence of autoimmune liver disease after liver transplantation: a systematic review. *Liver Transpl* 2006; **12**: 1813–1824.

157 Cholangitas E, Shusang V, Papatheodoridis GV *et al.* Risk factors for recurrence of primary sclerosing cholangitis after liver transplantation. *Liver Transpl* 2008; **14**: 138–143.

158 Charatcharoenwitthaya P, Lindor KD. Recurrence of primary sclerosing cholangitis: What do we learn from several transplant centers? *Liver Transpl* 2008; **14**: 130–132.

159 Alexander J, Lord JD, Yeh MM *et al.* Risk factors for recurrence of primary sclerosing cholangitis after liver transplantation. *Liver Transpl* 2008; **14**: 245–251.

160 Bjøro K, Brandsaeter B, Foss A, Schrumpf E. Liver transplantation in primary sclerosing cholangitis. *Semin Liver Dis* 2006; **26**: 69–79.

161 Papatheodoridis GV, Hamilton M, Mistry PK *et al.* Ulcerative colitis has an aggressive course after orthotopic liver transplantation for primary sclerosing cholangitis. *Gut* 1998; **43**: 639–644.

162 Vera A, Gunson BK, Ussatoff V *et al.* Colorectal cancer in patients with inflammatory bowel disease after liver transplantation for primary sclerosing cholangitis. *Transplantation* 2003; **75**: 1983–1988.

163 Mathis KL, Dozios EJ, Larson DW *et al.* Ileal pouch-anal anastomosis and livertransplantation for ulcerative colitis complicated by primary sclerosing cholangitis. *Br J Surg* 2008; **95**: 882–886.

164 Jeyarajah DR, Netto GJ, Lee SP *et al*. Recurrent primary sclerosing cholangitis after orthotopic liver transplantation: Is chronic rejection part of the disease process? *Transplantation* 1998; **27**: 1300–1306.

165 Abu-Elmagd KD, Rakela J, Kang Y *et al*. Recurrence of primary sclerosing cholangitis after hepatic transplantation: single centre experience with 380 grafts. *Hepatology* 1998; **28**: 739A.

166 Vera A, Moledina S, Gunson B *et al*. Risk factors for recurrence of primary sclerosing cholangitis of liver allograft. *Lancet* 2002; **360**: 1943–1944.

167 Khettry U, Keaveny A, Goldar-Najafi A *et al*. Liver transplantation for primary sclerosing cholangitis; a long-term clinico-pathologic study. *Hum Pathol* 2003; **34**: 1127–1136

168 Brandsaeter B, Schrumpf E, Bentdal O *et al*. Recurrent primary sclerosing cholangitis after liver transplantation: A magnetic resonance cholangiography study with analyses of predictive factors. *Liver Transpl* 2005; **11**: 1361–1369.

169 Kugelmas M, Spiegelman P, Osgood MJ *et al*. Different immunosuppressive regimens and recurrence of primary sclerosing cholangitis after liver transplantation. *Liver Transpl* 2003; **9**: 727–732.

35 Non-histological assessment of liver fibrosis

Dominique Thabut and Marika Simon-Rudler

UPMC Service d'Hépato-Gastroentérologie, Assistance Publique-Hôpitaux de Paris, Groupe Hospitalier Pitié-Salpêtrière, Université Pierre et Marie Curie, Paris, France

Management and prognosis of chronic liver diseases depend mainly on the amount of liver fibrosis. Therefore, assessment of liver fibrosis is crucial, not only to evaluate the severity of the disease, but also to monitor disease progression and treatment efficacy. Recent reviews recommend liver biopsy as the gold standard for the evaluation of fibrosis [1]. However, liver biopsy has several well-known limitations, that is, sampling error and intra/inter-observer variability [2–8], and risks, with a morbidity ranging from 0.3 to 0.6%, and a mortality of 0.05% [9]. Moreover, liver biopsy is costly. All these pitfalls have stimulated the search for new, non-invasive techniques for the assessment of liver fibrosis. There is a consensus that ideally, non-invasive methods should be easily repeatable, with minimal sampling error or observer variability, and be less expensive than liver biopsy. Assessment of liver fibrosis has been extensively evaluated during the past five years, with over 400 original articles. There are two categories of non-invasive tests: serum markers and methodologies related to liver imaging techniques, the most innovative of which being the measurement of liver stiffness by transient elastography. In this chapter we describe the main methods available for the detection of liver fibrosis, discuss their performance as a diagnostic test, their advantages and limits, and try to determine when and how to use them. We will focus on the most validated techniques that are available for clinical practice.

Serum markers of liver fibrosis

Description of the different serum markers and indices

Serum markers can be direct or indirect. Several direct markers have been evaluated, measuring components of

Evidence-Based Gastroenterology and Hepatology, 3rd edition.
J. McDonald, A.K. Burroughs, B. Feagan, and M.B. Fennerty. © 2010 Blackwell Publishing Ltd

extracellular matrix in the serum (e.g. hyaluronic acid, collagen IV, procollagen III, laminin, YKL-40) as well as enzymes and cytokines involved in the fibrogenetic and fibrolytic process (metalloproteases (MMPs) and tissue inhibitors of metalloproteases (TIMPs)). Indirect markers include markers of liver function and liver inflammation, and are generally routinely available tests, like prothrombin time, serum bilirubin, platelet count, transaminases, but also include apolipoprotein A1, and alpha2-macroglobulin. Taken separately, none of these markers are sufficiently discriminative to consider avoiding liver biopsy. However, combination of different serum markers considerably improves their performance. Therefore, algorithms combining the results of panels of markers have been developed in order to assess liver fibrosis. Before evaluating the performance of the different tests, one must know which stage of development the tests have reached. Indeed, some tests are still at the exploratory stage, which is the first phase of development of the test. Following this comes the very important validation step, either internal validation, or, even better, an external and independent validation. Before use of any test in clinical practice, an external and prospective validation of the test is mandatory. Also important is the formulation of pre-analytical and analytical recommendations, precautions required for use, and algorithms for false positive and false negatives. Lastly, there are steps concerning patents and commercialization.

To date, and since the publication of the first index, which was the PGA index, in alcoholic patients in 1991 [10], more than 30 indexes have been published. As well as PGA, 17 have been validated at least twice [11–26], and five are patented and on the market: FibroTest-FibroSure, ELF index, Fibrometer, FibroSpect II and HepaScore [11, 13, 16, 23, 26]. Table 35.1 describes the components of the 17 tests that were validated twice; 14 were derived and validated for chronic hepatitis C liver disease (HCV). The first commercialized test, and also the most validated, is the FibroTest-FibroSure [16]. The results of this test range from 0 to 1. FibroTest has now been validated in hepatitis C by

Table 35.1 Summary of the 18 tests that have been validated at least twice for the diagnosis of liver fibrosis.

Test	Year 1st publication	Key leader	Components	Liver disease
PGA	1991	Poynard	PT, GGT, ApoA1	ALD
AP	1997	Poynard	Age, Plt	HCV
Bonacini	1997	Lindsay	Plt, AST, ALT	HCV
Pohl	2001	Pohl	Plt, AST	HCV
Forns	2002	Forns	Plt, cholesterol, age	HCV
APRI	2003	Lok	Plt, AST	HCV
FibroTest/Fibrosure	2001	Poynard	A2M, haptoglobin, ApoA1, Bili, GGT, age, gender	HCV
MP3	2004	Leroy	PIIINP, MMP1	HCV
FibroSpectII	2004	Oh	A2M, HA, TIMP1	HCV
ELF	2004	Rosenberg	HA, PIIINP, TIMP	HCV
FibroMeter	2005	Cales	Plt, AST, A2M, HA, PT, age, gender	Mixed
HepaScore	2005	Adams	A2M, HA, GGT, age, gender	HCV
Hui	2005	Hui	BMI, Plt, albumin, Bili	HBV
SHASTA	2005	Kelleher	HA, AST, albumin	HCV/HIV
AST/ALT	2005	Park	AST, ALT	HCV
FIB-4	2006	Sterling	Plt, AST, ALT, age	HCV/HIV
Fibroindex	2007	Koda	Plt, AST, gammaGlobulins	HCV

the original authors [27] and independent teams [13, 28–32], and also in other settings: HBV [33–35], NAFLD [36], HCV-HIV co-infection [37], alcoholic liver disease [38, 39], and in renal transplants and hemodialysed patients [40].

Diagnostic performance of the different serum markers of fibrosis

The performance of a test can be studied with the Area Under the Receiving Operating Curve (AUROC), which reflects the specificity and sensitivity of the test, that is, its discriminatory power. However, one pitfall is that the liver biopsy, which is considered to be the gold standard, is not a perfect standard as it suffers inherent problems of sampling [2]. Another problem is the dichotomous categorization of liver biopsy, that is, mild versus significant fibrosis in the METAVIR scoring system (F0F1 vs F2F3F4), or if the test is aimed to detect severe fibrosis (F0F1F2 vs F3F4) or cirrhosis (F0F1F2F3 vs F4). However, grouping different stages may not be relevant [2]. These categories are descriptive and do not reflect an arithmetical progression of fibrosis in numerical terms, that is, F4 is not twice the amount of fibrosis as F2, and those categories which happen to have numbers and not names cannot be used as a continuous variable in a statistical analysis. Moreover, the AUROC will depend on the prevalence of each fibrosis stage in the population under study. For example, the AUROC for the detection of significant fibrosis will be higher if the population sampled is mainly composed of F0 and F4 patients, than of F1 and F2 patients [41]. Therefore, comparison of

different tests must be performed on the same population, and if this is not the case, comparison of AUROC provided by different studies makes no sense. Use of standardized AUROCs is a better way to assess comparisons [41] but has seldom been used.

A recent overview reported standardized AUROCs for the diagnosis of significant fibrosis (F2F3F4) of 0.84 (95% CI: 0.83–0.86) for FibroTest, without any differences amongst the different causes of liver disease [42]. This meta-analysis also compared FibroTest to the other patented biomarkers, and did not show any significant differences between the AUROCs of these markers for advanced fibrosis. **A1c** However, because of the limited number of patients included in the direct comparisons a clinically significant difference cannot be excluded, particularly between Hepascore with a smaller AUROC (0.04 difference) versus FibroTest and Fibrometer [42]. To date, in hepatitis C, two independent studies compared three of the five patented tests [30, 43], that is, FibroTest, Fibrometer and Hepascore. There was no difference between these tests, when considering the AUROC for the detection of significant fibrosis (F2F3F4), severe fibrosis (F3F4) or cirrhosis (F4). **A1d** For other etiologies of liver disease, there are no published comparisons of the diagnostic performance of the different tests.

Another way to compare these tests could be to compare their accuracy, or its opposite, the proportion of misclassified patients, for each stage of fibrosis. Then a Profile Performance Test can be established. Halfon et al. did this for FibroTest and Fibrometer [30]. In this study, with similar accuracy between the two tests (71% and 72% all stages together, p = ns), the FibroTest classified more F1 patients correctly, whereas the Fibrometer classified more F2 and F3 patients correctly [30]. These results have to be confirmed by other studies.

The study of discordant cases is of major importance when interpreting the results of a test. To date, FibroTest is the test for which discordant results have been the best studied. With Fibrotest there are well-described causes of false positives (hemolysis, Gilbert's syndrome and sepsis) and false negatives (inflammation). In an independent study, discordant results were attributed to FibroTest in 29% of cases (5% of entire population), 21% to liver biopsy, and in the remainder attribution was undetermined. Not surprisingly, the main reason for discordant results were patients with an intermediate stage of fibrosis [31]. However, the performance of liver biopsy in discriminating between two intermediate stages, can also be poor [2]. Although performing an entire liver biopsy is certainly the gold standard, a liver biopsy 15 mm long (the median biopsy length in tertiary centers) is not. It has an AUROC of 0.82 between F1 and F2, That is, there are around 20% false positives or false negatives [2]. Therefore, a test with an AUROC of 0.66 (usually described as a "weak" value when using a true gold standard) between F1 and F2 has a relative AUROC versus the best AUROC possible of 0.66/0.82 = 0.80, which can be considered acceptable for a non-invasive test. The size of liver biopsy is not solely responsible for discordance [44], but few studies have made evaluations with cohorts with optimal size biopsies.

The number of liver biopsies that could be avoided could also represent a target for comparing tests. However, one must be aware that the number of biopsies avoided depends on the specificity and sensitivity required of a test. For example, in the first publication of FibroTest by Imbert-Bismuth, which suggested a requirement of 95% specificity and 100% sensitivity for the diagnosis of significant liver fibrosis, only 46% of biopsies could be avoided [16]. Similarly, Parkes *et al.* arbitrarily defined the "inaccurate" zone of a marker when one "cannot reliably attribute test results" in comparison to tests with lower sensitivities/specificities at thresholds with positive predictive values < 90%, and negative predictive values > 95% [45]. Choosing these thresholds could be acceptable if a true gold standard existed. However, if this definition was applied to 15 mm liver biopsies, the biopsy would be inaccurate in 40% of cases for a diagnosis between F1 and F2.

In summary, non-invasive tests for fibrosis are difficult to compare, and independent validations have not identified one as being better than any other. **B4** Tests have different profiles, and the overall proportion of discordant results between tests and liver biopsy is in the range of 20%, considering all fibrosis stages together.

Limitations of serum markers

One of the main limitations of serum markers is their availability. The tests on the market are available, but not often reimbursed by health authorities or insurance companies. The reproducibility of some indirect components is not good, for example for platelet count. For FibroTest, as mentioned before, the interpretation should take into account the well-described causes of discordances: false positives because of hemolysis (decrease in haptoglobin and bilirubin), false negatives because of inflammation.

Transient elastography

Principles

Transient elastography measures the liver stiffness, using a device including an ultrasound transducer probe that is mounted on the axis of a vibrator [46]. Vibrations transmitted by the transducer induce an elastic shear wave propagating through the underlying tissues. Pulse-echo ultrasound acquisitions are used to follow the propagation of the wave and to measure its velocity, which is directly related to tissue stiffness: the stiffer the tissue, the faster the shear wave propagates. This procedure is non-invasive, painless, fast and easy to perform. Results are immediately available, are expressed as kilopascals, correspond to median values of ten validated measurements and range between 2,5 to 75 kPa [47]. The results of a transient elastography examination can be considered valid only when several conditions are fulfilled: the interquartile range (IQR), reflecting the variability between the different measurements, should not exceed 30% of the median value, and the success rate must reach 60%. An expert in the field should always perform the clinical interpretation of transient elastography [48].

Diagnostic performance of transient elastography

As for serum markers, elastography was first validated in patients with chronic hepatitis C [49]. The diagnostic performance of transient elastography was fairly good, with AUROCs ranging from 0.79 to 0.83 for the diagnosis of clinically significant fibrosis, and 0.95 to 0.97 for cirrhosis [29, 49]. Cutoffs with optimal accuracy were proposed for each METAVIR fibrosis stage, which, however, differ between etiologies of liver diseases so that the diagnosis must be known for the correct interpretation. As for serum markers, a substantial overlap of stiffness values was observed between adjacent stages of fibrosis. However, as already mentioned, the diagnostic performance of liver biopsy when compared to the whole liver, is also far from satisfactory. Transient elastography has also been validated in diseases other than chronic hepatitis C: chronic hepatitis B [50, 51], HIV-HCV coinfection [52, 53], NASH [54], alcoholic liver disease [55], cholestatic diseases [56] and liver transplant patients (57, 58].

In a recent meta-analysis, the sensitivity and specificity for the diagnosis of cirrhosis with transient elastography was very good (87% and 91% respectively) [59]. **A1c** However, there was significant heterogeneity that could be explained by a "cutoff effect". Indeed, optimal cutoffs for cirrhosis remain variable, ranging from 10,3 kPa for hepatitis B to 17,3 kPa for cholestatic diseases with no consensus. Similar to serum markers, the AUROCs for transient elastography depend on the prevalence of cirrhosis in the different populations [41].

Transient elastography was compared to FibroTest in one study: the diagnostic performance measured by AUROCs was similar [29]. Looking at the discordant results between transient elastography and FibroTest, more false negatives were observed with elastography than with FibroTest [60]. However, FibroTest more frequently overestimated the fibrosis found in the liver biopsy. In another study, elastography had the best diagnostic performance for early detection of cirrhosis in patients with chronic hepatitis C [61].

Limitations of transient elastography

Liver stiffness measurements can be difficult in overweight patients or in those with narrow intercostal space, and impossible in patients with ascites [48]. Recent studies suggest that liver stiffness is influenced by ALT flares, with a risk of overestimation of fibrosis. Reproducibility of liver stiffness is excellent with good inter- and intra-observer agreement [62], but this is less good in patients with low degree of fibrosis, or steatosis or with an increased BMI.

Is there a way to optimize the performance of the tests?

The combination of different serum markers together with transient elastography result in much better estimation of the degree of fibrosis. Sebastiani proposed stepwise algorithms in patients with compensated chronic hepatitis C, by performing sequentially APRI, FibroTest and in the remaining patients liver biopsy. With this approach, liver biopsy could be avoided in 71% of cases with an accuracy of 93% [63]. The same approach was also suggested for chronic hepatitis B [35]. Castera proposed the combination of FibroTest and transient elastography, and significantly improved the performance compared to each non-invasive test alone, with an accuracy of 84% when combining the tests [29]. This is probably a very promising approach. The

most important point, when analysing results of non-invasive tests for the screening of liver fibrosis, is to consider their results according to the clinical setting, and to establish if there are clinical situations that may lead to discordant results. If there are such situations then repeat the tests after a few months in order to see if the discordant result remains or not.

Can we expect more from non-invasive tests?

Non-expert physicians and patients aspire to having an almost perfect test, that is, more than 99% applicability and with less than 10% of false positive or false negative results. This is not possible, even with a liver biopsy [34]. A 25 mm non-fragmented biopsy is obtained in less than 50% of all large reported series [44], and the rate of false positives or negatives of such a 25 mm non-fragmented biopsy in one study was about 20%, for the diagnosis of advanced fibrosis, in comparison with the whole liver, which is a virtual gold standard [2]. Among the discordant results observed between biopsy and biomarker estimates of fibrosis, the cause of failure is frequently due to an inadequate biopsy size or interpretation [44, 64]. Therefore, it is far-fetched to expect to obtain an almost perfect biomarker with an AUROC greater than 90% for the diagnosis of advanced fibrosis. Hence, in France, clinical practice is evolving rapidly and a nationwide survey recently found that among 546 hepatologists, 81% used non-invasive biomarkers (FibroTest-ActiTest) and 32% used elastography (Fibroscan), with a dramatic decrease in the use of liver biopsy in more than 50% of patients with chronic hepatitis C, but with an increase in the number of patients treated [65]. A recent overview by French health authorities officially approved non-invasive biomarkers FT and FS as first-line estimates of fibrosis in patients with chronic hepatitis C, and recommended reimbursement by the social security system. Liver biopsy was only approved as second-line test in case of discordant results or non-interpretability of non-invasive markers [66].

Correlation with clinical events and survival

As liver biopsy is not a perfect gold standard, and as the non-invasive tests of fibrosis were constructed taking liver biopsy as the reference, the diagnostic performance of different non-invasive markers is difficult to interpret. Therefore, survival and clinical events related to liver disease could be considered as better endpoints to establish the clinical usefulness of these tests. One group of authors found serum markers to be correlated with survival and survival without liver-related complications [64, 67], and others to response to antiviral therapy [68–70]. FibroTest and transient elastography results have also been found to correlate with the presence and degree of portal hypertension [71–75], although the relationship between elastography and esophageal varices is not good [61, 75, 76]. The ELF score was predictive of liver-related morbidity and mortality, with better sensitivity than liver biopsy [23]. However studies evaluating the prognostic value of non-invasive markers of fibrosis will need to compare these with established prognostic markers, such as hepatic venous pressure gradient, and Child-Pugh and MELD scores. Prognostic scores that are currently used in chronic liver disease rarely include histology in their formulae.

Proposed algorithm for the prediction of liver fibrosis in HCV patients

As liver biopsy is an imperfect gold standard, an algorithm can be proposed which contains few indications for liver biopsy (see Figure 35.1). One starts with two non-invasive tests, and in case of discordant results, clinical causes of this must be evaluated. If none are found, then the tests should be repeated after a few months in order to see if the discordant result persists. If this persists and if the clinical findings do not help to resolve the issue, then liver biopsy or another test could be performed, particularly if a therapeutic decision depends on this. If this is the case, liver biopsy should be considered as complementary to the non-invasive markers, providing histological information at baseline that can help integrate the results of the non-invasive tests.

Conclusion

During the last five years, there has been a major improvement in the non-invasive diagnosis of liver fibrosis, especially for patients with chronic hepatitis C. Independent validations, assessment of preanalytical and analytical recommendations, and study of discordances are of major importance before considering using these tests in clinical practice. All the patented tests seem comparable to one another, and have good performance characteristics, which is also true of transient elastography. The most important issue is to consider the results of non-invasive tests in the correct clinical setting. Because liver biopsy, has its own inherent false positive and false negative results in terms of staging fibrosis (due to sample size and interpretation) any comparison with it cannot lead to establishing a perfect non-invasive marker. In France, where most of these markers have been developed, liver biopsy is no longer mandatory as a first-line test to stage fibrosis in HCV patients and indeed many current guidelines in other countries do not require a liver biopsy before starting therapy at least for genotype 2 and 3 infections. For other etiologies of liver disease, non-invasive staging of fibrosis still requires more validation. Further studies are needed on the prognostic value of these non-invasive tests, with appropriate validation of prognostic models. This involves not only good discrimination (AUROC), but good calibration, that is, the proportion of times the expected result is observed as being correct.

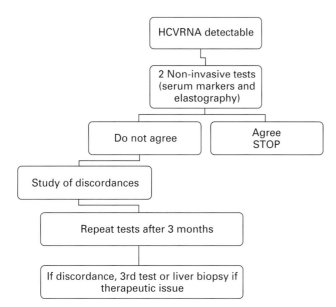

Figure 35.1 Proposed algorithm for detection of liver fibrosis in HCV patients.

References

1 Bravo AA, Sheth SG, Chopra S. Liver biopsy. *N Engl J Med* 2001; **344**: 495–500.

2 Bedossa P, Dargere D, Paradis V. Sampling variability of liver fibrosis in chronic hepatitis C. *Hepatology* 2003; **38**: 1449–1457.

3 Bedossa P, Poynard T, Naveau S, Martin ED, Agostini H, Chaput JC. Observer variation in assessment of liver biopsies of alcoholic patients. *Alcohol Clin Exp Res* 1988; **12**: 173–178.

4 Colloredo G, Guido M, Sonzogni A, Leandro G. Impact of liver biopsy size on histological evaluation of chronic viral hepatitis: the smaller the sample, the milder the disease. *J Hepatol* 2003; **39**: 239–244.

5 Labayle D, Chaput JC, Albuisson F, Buffet C, Martin E, Etienne JP. Comparison of the histological lesions in tissue specimens taken from the right and left lobe of the liver in alcoholic liver disease (author's transl). *Gastroenterol Clin Biol* 1979; **3**: 235–240.

6 McHutchison J, Poynard T, Afdhal N. Fibrosis as an end point for clinical trials in liver disease: a report of the international fibrosis group. *Clin Gastroenterol Hepatol* 2006; **4**: 1214–1220.

7 Ratziu V, Charlotte F, Heurtier A *et al.* Sampling variability of liver biopsy in nonalcoholic fatty liver disease. *Gastroenterology* 2005; **128**: 1898–1906.

8 Regev A, Berho M, Jeffers LJ *et al.* Sampling error and intraobserver variation in liver biopsy in patients with chronic HCV infection. *Am J Gastroenterol* 2002; **97**: 2614–2618.

9 Poynard T, Ratziu V, Bedossa P. Appropriateness of liver biopsy. *Can J Gastroenterol* 2000; **14**: 543–548.

10 Poynard T, Aubert A, Bedossa P *et al.* A simple biological index for detection of alcoholic liver disease in drinkers. *Gastroenterology* 1991; **100**: 1397–1402.

11 Adams LA, Bulsara M, Rossi E *et al.* Hepascore: an accurate validated predictor of liver fibrosis in chronic hepatitis C infection. *Clin Chem* 2005; **51**: 1867–1873.

12 Bonacini M, Hadi G, Govindarajan S, Lindsay KL. Utility of a discriminant score for diagnosing advanced fibrosis or cirrhosis in patients with chronic hepatitis C virus infection. *Am J Gastroenterol* 1997; **92**: 1302–1304.

13 Cales P, Oberti F, Michalak S *et al.* A novel panel of blood markers to assess the degree of liver fibrosis. *Hepatology* 2005; **42**: 1373–1381.

14 Forns X, Ampurdanes S, Llovet JM *et al.* Identification of chronic hepatitis C patients without hepatic fibrosis by a simple predictive model. *Hepatology* 2002; **36**: 986–992.

15 Hui AY, Chan HL, Wong VW *et al.* Identification of chronic hepatitis B patients without significant liver fibrosis by a simple noninvasive predictive model. *Am J Gastroenterol* 2005; **100**: 616–623.

16 Imbert-Bismut F, Ratziu V, Pieroni L, Charlotte F, Benhamou Y, Poynard T. Biochemical markers of liver fibrosis in patients with hepatitis C virus infection: a prospective study. *Lancet* 2001; **357**: 1069–1075.

17 Kelleher TB, Mehta SH, Bhaskar R *et al.* Prediction of hepatic fibrosis in HIV/HCV co-infected patients using serum fibrosis markers: the SHASTA index. *J Hepatol* 2005; **43**: 78–84.

18 Koda M, Matunaga Y, Kawakami M, Kishimoto Y, Suou T, Murawaki Y. FibroIndex, a practical index for predicting significant fibrosis in patients with chronic hepatitis C. *Hepatology* 2007; **45**: 297–306.

19 Leroy V, Monier F, Bottari S *et al.* Circulating matrix metalloproteinases 1, 2, 9 and their inhibitors TIMP-1 and TIMP-2 as serum markers of liver fibrosis in patients with chronic hepatitis C: comparison with PIIINP and hyaluronic acid. *Am J Gastroenterol* 2004; **99**: 271–279.

20 Park G, Jones DB, Katelaris P. Value of AST/ALT ratio as fibrotic predictor in chronic hepatitis C. *Am J Gastroenterol* 2005; **100**: 1623–1624; author reply 1624.

21 Pohl A, Behling C, Oliver D, Kilani M, Monson P, Hassanein T. Serum aminotransferase levels and platelet counts as predictors of degree of fibrosis in chronic hepatitis C virus infection. *Am J Gastroenterol* 2001; **96**: 3142–3146.

22 Poynard T, Bedossa P. Age and platelet count: a simple index for predicting the presence of histological lesions in patients with antibodies to hepatitis C virus. METAVIR and CLINIVIR Cooperative Study Groups. *J Viral Hepat* 1997; **4**: 199–208.

23 Rosenberg WM, Voelker M, Thiel R *et al.* Serum markers detect the presence of liver fibrosis: a cohort study. *Gastroenterology* 2004; **127**: 1704–1713.

24 Sterling RK, Lissen E, Clumeck N *et al.* Development of a simple noninvasive index to predict significant fibrosis in patients with HIV/HCV coinfection. *Hepatology* 2006; **43**: 1317–1325.

25 Wai CT, Greenson JK, Fontana RJ, Kalbfleisch JD, Marrero JA, Conjeevaram HS, Lok AS. A simple noninvasive index can predict both significant fibrosis and cirrhosis in patients with chronic hepatitis C. *Hepatology* 2003; **38**: 518–526.

26 Zaman A, Rosen HR, Ingram K, Corless CL, Oh E, Smith K. Assessment of FIBROSpect II to detect hepatic fibrosis in chronic hepatitis C patients. *Am J Med* 2007; **120**: 280, e289–214.

27 Poynard T, Imbert-Bismut F, Munteanu M *et al.* Overview of the diagnostic value of biochemical markers of liver fibrosis (FibroTest, HCV FibroSure) and necrosis (ActiTest) in patients with chronic hepatitis C. *Comp Hepatol* 2004; **3**: 8.

28 Callewaert N, Van Vlierberghe H, Van Hecke A *et al.* Noninvasive diagnosis of liver cirrhosis using DNA sequencer-based total serum protein glycomics: overview of the diagnostic value of biochemical markers of liver fibrosis (FibroTest, HCV FibroSure) and necrosis (ActiTest) in patients with chronic hepatitis C. *Nat Med* 2004; **10**: 429–434.

29 Castera L, Vergniol J, Foucher J *et al.* Prospective comparison of transient elastography, Fibrotest, APRI, and liver biopsy for the assessment of fibrosis in chronic hepatitis C. *Gastroenterology* 2005; **128**: 343–350.

30 Halfon P, Bacq Y, De Muret A *et al.* Comparison of test performance profile for blood tests of liver fibrosis in chronic hepatitis C. *J Hepatol* 2007; **46**: 395–402.

31 Halfon P, Bourliere M, Deydier R *et al.* Independent prospective multicenter validation of biochemical markers (fibrotest-actitest) for the prediction of liver fibrosis and activity in patients with chronic hepatitis C: the fibropaca study. *Am J Gastroenterol* 2006; **101**: 547–555.

32 Rossi E, Adams L, Prins A *et al.* Validation of the FibroTest biochemical markers score in assessing liver fibrosis in hepatitis C patients. *Clin Chem* 2003; **49**: 450–454.

33 Myers RP, Tainturier MH, Ratziu V *et al.* Prediction of liver histological lesions with biochemical markers in patients with chronic hepatitis B: diagnostic and prognostic values of noninvasive biomarkers of fibrosis in patients with alcoholic liver disease. Biomarkers for the prediction of liver fibrosis in patients with chronic alcoholic liver disease. *J Hepatol* 2003; **39**: 222–230.

34 Poynard T, Ratziu V, Benhamou Y, Thabut D, Moussalli J. Biomarkers as a first-line estimate of injury in chronic liver diseases: time for a moratorium on liver biopsy? *Gastroenterology* 2005; **128**: 1146–1148; author reply 1148.

35 Sebastiani G, Vario A, Guido M, Alberti A. Sequential algorithms combining non-invasive markers and biopsy for the assessment of liver fibrosis in chronic hepatitis B. *World J Gastroenterol* 2007; **13**: 525–531.

36 Ratziu V, Massard J, Charlotte F *et al.* Diagnostic value of biochemical markers (FibroTest-FibroSURE) for the prediction of liver fibrosis in patients with non-alcoholic fatty liver disease. Prediction of liver histological lesions with biochemical markers in patients with chronic hepatitis B. Diagnostic and prognostic values of noninvasive biomarkers of fibrosis in patients with alcoholic liver disease. Biomarkers for the prediction of liver fibrosis in patients with chronic alcoholic liver disease. *BMC Gastroenterol* 2006; **6**: 6.

37 Myers RP, Benhamou Y, Imbert-Bismut F *et al.* Serum biochemical markers accurately predict liver fibrosis in HIV and hepatitis C virus co-infected patients. Sequential algorithms combining non-invasive markers and biopsy for the assessment of liver fibrosis in chronic hepatitis B. Longitudinal assessment of histology surrogate markers (FibroTest-ActiTest) during lamivudine therapy in patients with chronic hepatitis B infection. *Aids* 2003; **17**: 721–725.

38 Naveau S, Gaude G, Asnacios A *et al.* Diagnostic and prognostic values of noninvasive biomarkers of fibrosis in patients with alcoholic liver disease. Biomarkers for the prediction of liver fibrosis in patients with chronic alcoholic liver disease. *Hepatology* 2009; **49**: 97–105.

39 Naveau S, Raynard B, Ratziu V *et al.* Biomarkers for the prediction of liver fibrosis in patients with chronic alcoholic liver disease. *Clin Gastroenterol Hepatol* 2005; **3**: 167–174.

40 Varaut A, Fontaine H, Serpaggi J *et al.* Diagnostic accuracy of the fibrotest in hemodialysis and renal transplant patients with chronic hepatitis C virus. *Transplantation* 2005; **80**: 1550–1555.

41 Poynard T, Halfon P, Castera L *et al.* Standardization of ROC curve areas for diagnostic evaluation of liver fibrosis markers based on prevalences of fibrosis stages. *Clin Chem* 2007; **53**: 1615–1622.

42 Poynard T, Morra R, Halfon P *et al.* Meta-analyses of Fibrotest diagnostic value in chronic liver disease. *BMC Gastroenterol* 2007; **7**: 40.

43 Leroy V, Hilleret MN, Sturm N *et al.* Prospective comparison of six non-invasive scores for the diagnosis of liver fibrosis in chronic hepatitis C. *J Hepatol* 2007; **46**: 775–782.

44 Poynard T, Munteanu M, Imbert-Bismut F *et al.* Prospective analysis of discordant results between biochemical markers and biopsy in patients with chronic hepatitis C. *Clin Chem* 2004; **50**: 1344–1355.

45 Parkes J, Guha IN, Roderick P, Rosenberg W. Performance of serum marker panels for liver fibrosis in chronic hepatitis C. *J Hepatol* 2006; **44**: 462–474.

46 Sandrin L, Fourquet B, Hasquenoph JM *et al.* Transient elastography: a new noninvasive method for assessment of hepatic fibrosis. *Ultrasound Med Biol* 2003; **29**: 1705–1713.

47 Roulot D, Czernichow S, Le Clesiau H, Costes JL, Vergnaud AC, Beaugrand M. Liver stiffness values in apparently healthy subjects: influence of gender and metabolic syndrome. *J Hepatol* 2008; **48**: 606–613.

48 Castera L, Forns X, Alberti A. Non-invasive evaluation of liver fibrosis using transient elastography. *J Hepatol* 2008; **48**: 835–847.

49 Ziol M, Handra-Luca A, Kettaneh A *et al.* Noninvasive assessment of liver fibrosis by measurement of stiffness in patients with chronic hepatitis C. *Hepatology* 2005; **41**: 48–54.

50 Coco B, Oliveri F, Maina AM *et al.* Transient elastography: a new surrogate marker of liver fibrosis influenced by major changes of transaminases. *J Viral Hepat* 2007; **14**: 360–369.

51 Marcellin P, Ziol M, Bedossa P *et al.* Non-invasive assessment of liver fibrosis by stiffness measurement in patients with chronic hepatitis B. *Liver Int* 2008; **4**: 471–477.

52 de Ledinghen V, Douvin C, Kettaneh A *et al.* Diagnosis of hepatic fibrosis and cirrhosis by transient elastography in HIV/hepatitis C virus-coinfected patients. *J Acquir Immune Defic Syndr* 2006; **41**: 175–179.

53 Vergara S, Macias J, Rivero A *et al.* The use of transient elastometry for assessing liver fibrosis in patients with HIV and hepatitis C virus coinfection. *Clin Infect Dis* 2007; **45**: 969–974.

54 Yoneda M, Mawatari H, Fujita K *et al.* Noninvasive assessment of liver fibrosis by measurement of stiffness in patients with nonalcoholic fatty liver disease (NAFLD). *Dig Liver Dis* 2008; **40**: 371–378.

55 Nahon P, Kettaneh A, Tengher-Barna I *et al.* Assessment of liver fibrosis using transient elastography in patients with alcoholic liver disease. *J Hepatol* 2008; **49**: 1062–1068.

56 Corpechot C, El Naggar A, Poujol-Robert A *et al.* Assessment of biliary fibrosis by transient elastography in patients with PBC and PSC. *Hepatology* 2006; **43**: 1118–1124.

57 Carrion JA, Navasa M, Bosch J, Bruguera M, Gilabert R, Forns X. Transient elastography for diagnosis of advanced fibrosis and portal hypertension in patients with hepatitis C recurrence after liver transplantation. *Liver Transpl* 2006; **12**: 1791–1798.

58 Rigamonti C, Donato MF, Fraquelli M *et al.* Transient elastography predicts fibrosis progression in patients with recurrent hepatitis C after liver transplantation. *Gut* 2008; **57**: 821–827.

59 Talwalkar JA, Kurtz DM, Schoenleber SJ, West CP, Montori VM. Ultrasound-based transient elastography for the detection of hepatic fibrosis: systematic review and meta-analysis. *Clin Gastroenterol Hepatol* 2007; **5**: 1214–1220.

60 Poynard T, Ingiliz P, Elkrief L *et al.* Concordance in a world without a gold standard: a new non-invasive methodology for improving accuracy of fibrosis markers. *PLoS ONE* 2008; **3**: e3857.

61 Castera L, Bail BL, Roudot-Thoraval F *et al.* Early detection in routine clinical practice of cirrhosis and oesophageal varices in chronic hepatitis C: comparison of transient elastography (FibroScan) with standard laboratory tests and non-invasive scores. *J Hepatol* 2009; **50**: 59–68.

62 Fraquelli M, Rigamonti C, Casazza G *et al.* Reproducibility of transient elastography in the evaluation of liver fibrosis in patients with chronic liver disease. *Gut* 2007; **56**: 968–973.

63 Sebastiani G, Vario A, Guido M *et al.* Stepwise combination algorithms of non-invasive markers to diagnose significant fibrosis in chronic hepatitis C. *J Hepatol* 2006; **44**: 686–693.

64 Ngo Y, Munteanu M, Messous D *et al.* A prospective analysis of the prognostic value of biomarkers (FibroTest) in patients with chronic hepatitis C. *Clin Chem* 2006; **52**: 1887–1896.

65 Castera L, Denis J, Babany G, Roudot-Thoraval F. Evolving practices of non-invasive markers of liver fibrosis in patients with chronic hepatitis C in France: time for new guidelines? *J Hepatol* 2007; **46**: 528–529; author reply 529–530.

66 La Haute Autorité de Santé (HAS) in France – The HAS recommendations for the management of the chronic hepatitis C using non-invasive biomarkers. http://www.has-sante.fr/portail/display.jsp?id=c_476486 (accessed August 2007).

67 Ngo Y, Benhamou Y, Thibault V *et al.* An accurate definition of the status of inactive hepatitis B virus carrier by a combination of biomarkers (FibroTest-ActiTest) and viral load. *PLoS ONE* 2008; **3**: e2573.

68 d'Arondel C, Munteanu M, Moussalli J *et al.* A prospective assessment of an "a la carte" regimen of PEG-interferon alpha2b and ribavirin combination in patients with chronic hepatitis C using biochemical markers. *J Viral Hepat* 2006; **13**: 182–189.

69 Poynard T, Ngo Y, Marcellin P, Hadziyannis S, Ratziu V, Benhamou Y, for the Adefovir Dipivoxil 437 and 438 Study Groups. Impact of adefovir dipivoxil on liver fibrosis and activity assessed with biochemical markers (FibroTest-ActiTest) in patients infected by hepatitis B virus. *J Viral Hepat* 2008; **16**: 203–213.

70 Poynard T, Zoulim F, Ratziu V *et al*. Longitudinal assessment of histology surrogate markers (FibroTest-ActiTest) during lamivudine therapy in patients with chronic hepatitis B infection. *Am J Gastroenterol* 2005; **100**: 1970–1980.

71 Bureau C, Metivier S, Peron JM *et al*. Transient elastography accurately predicts presence of significant portal hypertension in patients with chronic liver disease. *Aliment Pharmacol Ther* 2008; **27**: 1261–1268.

72 Lemoine M, Katsahian S, Ziol M *et al*. Liver stiffness measurement as a predictive tool of clinically significant portal hypertension in patients with compensated hepatitis C virus or alcohol-related cirrhosis. *Aliment Pharmacol Ther* 2008; **28**: 1102–1110.

73 Thabut D, Imbert-Bismut F, Cazals-Hatem D *et al*. Relationship between the Fibrotest and portal hypertension in patients with liver disease. *Aliment Pharmacol Ther* 2007; **26**: 359–368.

74 Thabut D, Trabut JB, Massard J *et al*. Non-invasive diagnosis of large oesophageal varices with FibroTest in patients with cirrhosis: a preliminary retrospective study. *Liver Int* 2006; **26**: 271–278.

75 Vizzutti F, Arena U, Romanelli RG *et al*. Liver stiffness measurement predicts severe portal hypertension in patients with HCV-related cirrhosis. *Hepatology* 2007; **45**: 1290–1297.

76 Kazemi F, Kettaneh A, N'Kontchou G *et al*. Liver stiffness measurement selects patients with cirrhosis at risk of bearing large oesophageal varices. *J Hepatol* 2006; **45**: 230–235.

36

Portal hypertensive bleeding

Christos Triantos[1,3]*, John Goulis*[2] *and Andrew K Burroughs*[3]

[1] Division of Gastroenterology, Department of Internal Medicine, University Hospital, Patras, Greece
[2] Fourth Department of Medicine, Aristotelian University of Thessaloniki, Hippokration General Hospital of Thessaloniki, Thessaloniki, Greece
[3] The Royal Free Sheila Sherlock Liver Centre, Royal Free Hospital, *and* University College London, London, UK

Introduction

Portal hypertension is a major complication of chronic liver disease, most frequently cirrhosis, leading to the development of portosystemic collaterals, of which the most clinically significant are those that form gastroesophageal varices. Variceal hemorrhage is the most serious complication of portal hypertension and is still associated with a high mortality rate, although it has diminished over the past three decades, probably because of several new therapeutic approaches for the prevention and treatment of variceal bleeding. The therapeutic armamentarium for portal hypertensive bleeding has been considerably expanded by the introduction of pharmacological therapy with various vasoactive agents, the endoscopic ligation of esophageal varices and the covered transjugular intrahepatic portosystemic shunt (TIPS).

As a result, the number of randomized clinical trials dealing with the treatment of portal hypertension is ever increasing. However, most of the new treatments are inadequately or poorly evaluated in trials using heterogeneous criteria for the definition of their main endpoints and usually lacking adequate statistical power.

We evaluated randomized controlled trials for prevention of first bleeding, treatment of acute bleeding and prevention of recurrent bleeding from esophageal varices, using meta-analysis where applicable. The main endpoints selected for analysis were the following: (1) first bleeding episode (for primary prevention trials), or failure to control bleeding including very early re-bleeding (for trials of acute bleeding) or re-bleeding (for trials for prevention of re-bleeding); (2) mortality (short term or long term); and (3) incidence of complications. Pooled estimates of efficacy are presented as pooled odds ratios (POR), obtained by the Mantel-Haenszel method (fixed effect model). We used a statistical evaluation of heterogeneity by χ^2 test to assess whether the variation in treatment effect within trials of the same group was greater than might be expected. We considered heterogeneity to be present if $p < 0.05$; if so the calculation of POR was carried out by the DerSimonian and Laird method [1], which is recommended for meta-analysis of studies with significant heterogeneity.

Prediction of the presence and development of esophageal varices

At the time of diagnosis, esophageal varices are present in 30% of patients with well compensated cirrhosis and 60% of patients with decompensated cirrhosis. Their size is reported to increase by 10–20% in the 1–2 years following their first endoscopic observation [2]. The presence of esophageal varices has been correlated to platelet count, the size of the spleen, the presence of ascites, albumin level, Child Pugh score, and the presence of spider nevi. Esophageal varices are formed if portal pressure exceeds 10–12 mmHg. However, not all patients in this group have varices at endoscopic examination. There have been efforts towards diagnosing varices without endoscopy using various indirect indices such as platelet count, albumin, spleen size, Child Pugh score, but without a final consensus as to whether these can substitute endoscopy [3–7]. Currently, there are no satisfactory non-endoscopic indicators for the presence of varices and consequently endoscopic screening is still the best practice to detect varices. The hepatic vein pressure gradient (HVPG) is presently the most reliable predictor of variceal development [8–11]. The recently developed PillCam ESO esophageal capsule has been shown to be an accurate diagnostic tool for the detection of esophageal varices and portal hypertensive gastropathy [12–15], but cannot substitute endoscopy unless this cannot be done. **A1c**

Evidence-Based Gastroenterology and Hepatology, 3rd edition.
J. McDonald, A.K. Burroughs, B. Feagan, and M.B. Fennerty. © 2010
Blackwell Publishing Ltd

Prevention of the development and growth of varices

Pre-primary prophylaxis is the term used for the prevention of varices. Beta-blockers reduce portal pressure by an average of 15–20%. The decrease of portal pressure is neither dependent on liver function nor the degree of initial portal hypertension or other systemic hemodynamic parameters. However, propranolol does not seem to affect the size of varices, although it reduces variceal pressure [16].

Two studies have addressed the role of beta-blockers in the progression of esophageal varices. In the first study Cales et al. [17] studied 206 cirrhotics with small varices or without varices; 102 patients received propranolol and 104 patients received placebo. After two years of follow-up the proportion of patients with large varices was 31% in the propranolol group compared with 14% in the placebo group (p < 0.05). More recently, Merkel et al. compared nadolol (83 patients) with placebo (78 patients) with a mean follow-up of 60 months [18]. A significantly lower rate of esophageal varices enlargement in patients randomized to nadolol was observed and a significantly lower probability of variceal bleeding. Survival was not improved.

However, in a third study that randomized 213 patients without esophageal varices (minimal HVPG of 6 mm Hg) to receive either timolol (108 patients) or placebo (105 patients), beta-blockers did not prevent varices formation (39% and 40% respectively; p = 0.89) [9]. **A1d** The majority of patients (88%) were Child A liver status and 12% Child B. Median follow-up was 54.9 months, while mean daily dose of timolol was 10.8 mg. Serious adverse events were more common among patients in the timolol group (p = 0.006). Varices developed less frequently among patients with a baseline HVPG < 10 mmHg and among those in whom the HVPG decreased by more than 10% at one year. To date there is only one study with evidence that beta-blockers can reduce the progression of small to large varices in patients with cirrhosis [18]. However, taking into consideration the available data regarding the risk of bleeding in patients with small varices we consider that these drugs are a reasonable therapeutic option, particularly for patients with advanced liver disease, or living far from endoscopic units. **A1d**

Risk of first variceal bleeding

Mortality of the first bleeding episode can be high, depending on severity of liver disease (10–30%). Hence the identification of patients with varices who will bleed, before they do so, is clearly important in order to offer effective prophylactic therapy to those who need it, and avoid it in those who do not, particularly if the therapy is invasive or costly. The risk factors for the first episode of variceal bleeding in patients with cirrhosis are the severity of liver dysfunction, large size of varices (increased tension of the variceal wall), and the presence of endoscopic red color signs. The combination of these three factors is the basis of the North Italian Endoscopic Club (NIEC) index for the prediction of the first variceal bleeding [19]. It is important to realize that patients with small varices and grade C severity cirrhosis have comparable risk of first bleeding compared to patients with large varices and grade A severity cirrhosis, emphasizing the importance of liver dysfunction [20]. However, only a third of patients who present with variceal hemorrhage have the above risk factors [21]. Hence there is a need to define new predictive factors that could be combined in the NIEC index to improve its validity. The main interest has been the identification of hemodynamic factors that could more readily reflect the pathophysiological changes that lead to variceal bleeding. It is now well accepted that bleeding is extremely rare if HVPG falls below 12 mmHg [8]. The severity of HVPG has been shown to be an independent risk factor for bleeding.

Randomized controlled trials for prevention of first variceal bleeding

Shunt surgery versus non-active treatment

There have been four prophylactic shunt trials [22–25], which were the first randomized controlled trials in portal hypertension, including 302 patients. A meta-analysis of these trials has been published [26]. Variceal bleeding was significantly reduced (odds ratio (OR) 0.31; 95% CI: 0.17–0.56) in the treated group, but survival was significantly worse (OR 1.6; 95% CI: 1.02–2.57). In addition, the risk of chronic or recurrent encephalopathy was significantly increased (OR 2.0; 95% CI: 1.2–3.1) in shunted patients. In view of the mortality data and the serious adverse effects, prophylactic shunt surgery has been abandoned worldwide. Moreover the advent of liver transplantation removes any rationale for prophylactic surgery of any kind in cirrhotic patients. **A1a**

Thus, the results of Inokuchi et al. from Japan, who compared devascularization procedures or selective shunts with non-active treatment [27], showing a significant reduction in bleeding risk and mortality with prophylactic surgery, are not clinically relevant today, over and above the issue of the method of randomization, which complicates the validity of the data.

Sclerotherapy versus non-active treatment

The success of endoscopic sclerotherapy in the treatment of acute variceal bleeding led to extensive evaluation of sclerotherapy for the prevention of the first variceal bleed.

There are 21 trials [28–48], of which four are published in abstract form [42–45], including a total of 1922 patients. The main characteristic of these trials was the statistically significant heterogeneity (p < 0.001) in the direction and size of the treatment effect on bleeding and death, so that meta-analysis cannot be interpreted correctly. The first trials reported promising results, with a reduction in bleeding rate, and in some a reduction in overall mortality [29, 35, 36]. However, they were of poor quality [49]. Subsequent larger trials did not confirm benefit and indeed some trials have suggested that prophylactic sclerotherapy is deleterious [40, 48]. In evaluating endoscopic sclerotherapy it must be remembered that it is an expensive and invasive treatment, which is associated with potentially serious complications. Hence prophylactic sclerotherapy would have to be clearly superior to no prophylactic treatment by a considerable margin before it could be recommended for widespread use. **Ala**

Variceal ligation versus non active treatment

In recent years, endoscopic variceal ligation has replaced endoscopic sclerotherapy as the method of choice for the prevention of re-bleeding. In randomized trials and a meta-analysis, ligation was more effective than sclerotherapy in preventing re-bleeding, in part because it resulted in faster eradication of varices and had fewer complications [50]. For primary prophylaxis, ligation has been compared to no treatment in seven trials [51–57], four full papers [53, 54, 56, 57] (see Table 36.1). Meta-analysis of randomized trials shows that EVL reduced both the risk of first portal hypertensive bleeding (OR 0.25; 95% CI: 0.17–0.37) and mortality (OR 0.42; 95% CI: 0.29–0.60) compared to no treatment [57]. Some adverse effects of variceal ligation (retrosternal pain, dysphagia, etc.) were transient, but two patients died, one because of esophageal perforation related to the insertion of the overtube (although this is no longer necessary in current practice)[53], and others after postligation ulcer

bleeding [54, 58], raising concerns about iatrogenic bleeding [59].

B-blockers versus non-active treatment

The optimal prophylactic treatment should be easy to administer, have relatively few adverse effects, and be reasonably effective. Drug therapy potentially fulfils these criteria best. In addition, drug therapy has the potential to protect against gastric mucosal bleeding, which accounts for a sizeable proportion of first bleeding episodes [67]. There are nine prophylactic trials using β-receptor blockade in cirrhotic patients with large varices comprising 996 patients; seven trials of propranolol [38, 44, 48, 61, 64–66], and two of nadolol [62, 63]; two of these as abstracts [44, 66] (see Table 36.2). One of the latter trials was an outlier, reporting a very low bleeding rate in non-treated patients [66]. This study causes statistically significant heterogeneity in the evaluation of first bleeding in a comprehensive analysis evaluating the effect of B-blockade therapy in the prevention of variceal bleeding. The heterogeneity disappears when this trial is excluded from the analysis [66]. There was a statistically significant bleeding risk reduction with β-blocker treatment when the outlier trial was included (OR 0.54; 95% CI: 0.39–0.74) or excluded (OR 0.48; 95% CI: 0.35–0.66). The number of patients needed to be treated (NNT) with β-blockers to prevent one bleeding episode was estimated to be 11. There was no heterogeneity in the evaluation of mortality (p = 0.19). Mortality was reduced with β-blockers but not significantly so (OR 0.75; 95% CI: 0.57–1.06).

β-blockers have been shown to be effective independently of cause and severity of cirrhosis, presence of ascites and variceal size in an analysis of individual patient data from four of the above trials [68]. However, bleeding may occur after stopping β-blocker therapy, suggesting that therapy should be maintained lifelong [69]. Finally, propranolol has been shown to prevent both acute and chronic

Table 36.1 Randomized controlled trials of variceal ligation versus non-treatment for the primary prophylaxis of variceal bleeding.

Study	Child C (%)	No. of patients	Event rate			
			Ligation Bleeding	Controls Bleeding	Ligation Mortality	Controls Mortality
Gameel et al. [52]	N R	33	0/16	3/17	1/16	0/17
Sarin et al. [56]	31	68	3/35	13/33	4/35	8/33
Chen and Chang [51]	NR	156	7/80	28/76	15/80	31/76
Lay et al. [53]	38	126	12/62	38/64	17/62	37/64
Lo et al. [54]	28	127	8/64	14/63	16/64	23/63
Svoboda et al. [60]	N R	102	15/52	27/50	12/52	19/50
Triantos et al. [57]	42	52	5/25	2/27	7/25	11/27

Table 36.2 Randomized controlled trials of β-blockers versus non-active treatment for the prevention of first variceal bleeding.

Study	No. of patients C/T	Child C (%)	Bleeding C/T	Mortality C/T
Pascal and Cales [61]	111/116	46	30/20	40/25
Ideo [62]	49/30	—	11/1	9/3
Lebrec [63]	53/53	—	10/7	10/10
The Italian Multicenter Project for Propranolol in Prevention of Bleeding [64]	89/85	7	31/18	28/37
Andreani et al. [38]	41/43	28	13/2	18/13
Conn et al. [65]	51/51	8	11/2	11/8
PROVA [48]	51/51	8	13/12	14/7
Strauss et al. [44]	16/20	NR	4/4	7/7
Colman et al. [66]	25/23	NR	2/8	7/6

C: control; T: β-blockers; NR: not reported.

bleeding from portal hypertensive gastropathy in a single blind randomized study [67]. Adverse effects of β-blockers are usually reversible after discontinuation of the drug, and no fatal complications have been reported. **A1a**

β-Blockers versus nitrates and beta blockers

A randomized trial first published in 1996 [84] and further evaluated in 2000 [85] showed that nadolol and isosorbide dinitrate combined were more effective than nadolol alone for prevention of first variceal bleeding.

In this study [85] 146 patients with cirrhosis and known esophageal varices, but no bleeding, were treated for seven years. Sixteen in the nadolol group and eight in the combination group bled (logrank test, p = 0.02). The cumulative bleeding risk was 29% and 12% respectively (95% CI for the difference 1–23%). Addition of isosorbide 5-mononitrate did not increase the incidence of liver failure, development of ascites or renal insufficiency; five patients requested discontinuation of nitrates due to adverse effects. However, the results of the most recent multicenter and larger randomized controlled trial are conflicting. In this study 349 cirrhotic patients with gastroesophageal varices were randomized to receive propranolol + placebo (n = 174) or propranolol + isosorbide mononitrate (ISMN) (n = 175) [86]. There were no significant differences in the one and two-year actuarial probability of variceal bleeding between the two groups (propranolol + placebo 8.3% and 10.6% respectively; propranolol + ISMN, 5% and 12.5% respectively). Survival was also similar. Adverse effects were signifi-

cantly more frequent in the propranolol + ISMN group, mainly due to a greater incidence of headache. The combination was otherwise safe and did not produce any deleterious effects on renal function.

β-blockers effectively prevent variceal bleeding. Adding nitrates does not further decrease the low residual risk of bleeding in patients receiving propranolol. Current data do not support a recommendation for additive medication to non-selective β-blockers for primary prophylaxis of variceal bleeding. **A1d**

Variceal ligation versus β-blockers

There are 15 randomized trials comparing endoscopic band ligation of high risk esophageal varices to propranolol [58, 70–83] (see Table 36.3). In the first trial, Sarin et al. found that ligation was more effective than propranolol for prevention of bleeding (actuarial survival, propranolol 43%, ligation 15%, p < 0.05) [71]. However, the rate of bleeding in the propranolol group was higher than has been observed in some other studies. This may be because of the lower mean dose of propranolol used (70 mg/day compared with 123 mg/day in previous studies). Alternatively, the difference in bleeding rates between groups may have occurred because of the relatively small number of patients studied and the resultant rather wide confidence intervals. The rate of bleeding in the propranolol group was the same as that in the non-treated group in a previous trial by the same authors in which the same selection criteria were used [53]. In the meta-analysis of the 15

Table 36.3 Randomized controlled trials of variceal ligation versus β-blockers for the primary prophylaxis of variceal bleeding.

Study	No. of patients	Variceal bleeding Ligation	Variceal bleeding Controls	Mortality Ligation	Mortality Controls
Chen et al. [70]	54	1/26	2/28	3/26	3/28
Sarin et al. [71]	99	4/45	12/44	5/45	5/44
De et al. [72]	30	2/15	1/15	NR	NR
De la Mora et al. [73]	24	1/12	2/12	0/12	1/12
Song et al. [74]	61	6/31	7/30	5/31	8/30
Lui et al. [75]	100	3/44	9/66	11/44	18/66
Gheorge et al. [76]	53	3/25	13/28	1/25	5/28
Drastich et al. [77]	77	4/40	7/33	2/40	3/33
Schepke et al. [58]	152	19/75	22/77	34/75	33/75
Lo et al. [78]	100	8/50	13/50	12/50	11/50
Jutabha et al. [79]	62	0/31	6/31	0/31	4/31
Thuluvath et al. [80]	31	2/16	1/15	6/16	3/15
Psilopoulos et al. [81]	60	2/30	9/30	12/30	10/30
Lay et al. [82]	100	11/50	12/50	14/50	12/50
Norberto et al. [83]	62	2/31	3/31	3/31	3/31

NR: not reported.

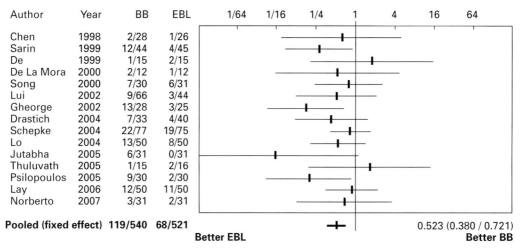

Figure 36.1 Primary prevention: Forrest plot of randomized trials of banding ligation of esophageal varices versus beta-blockers in primary prevention of variceal bleeding. Portal hypertensive bleeding. BB: beta-blockers; EBL: Endoscopic band ligation. Data are expressed as OR (95% CI) in a log scale.

studies variceal ligation significantly reduced the risk of first variceal bleeding compared with propranolol (POR 0.52; 95% CI: 0.38–0.72). However, the same meta-analysis did not find any difference in terms of mortality, with a trend in a favor of drug treatment (POR 0.94; 95% CI: 0.69–1.28), and iatrogenic bleeding due to ligation causing death [57, 59]. Recently Wang et al. reported similar efficacy of ligation to the combination of nadolol plus ISMN (see Figures 36.1 and 36.2) [87]. **Ala**

The conflicting results of these studies and the small number of patients randomized and events observed, as

well as the cost of endoscopic variceal ligation, do not provide sufficient evidence for recommending any change in the current practice of prescribing propranolol as the treatment of first choice for the primary prevention of variceal bleeding and using band ligation if there are contraindications or intolerance to beta-blockers. **Ala**

Variceal ligation versus sclerotherapy

Variceal ligation was compared with sclerotherapy for the primary prevention of variceal bleeding in three small

Author	Year	BB	EBL								
Chen	1998	3/28	3/26								
Sarin	1999	5/44	5/45								
De La Mora	2000	1/12	0/12								
Song	2000	8/30	5/31								
Lui	2002	18/66	11/44								
Gheorge	2002	5/28	1/25								
Drastich	2004	3/33	2/40								
Schepke	2004	33/77	34/75								
Lo	2004	11/50	12/50								
Jutabha	2005	4/31	0/31								
Thuluvath	2005	3/15	6/16								
Psilopoulos	2005	10/30	12/30								
Lay	2006	12/50	14/50								
Norberto	2007	3/31	3/31								

Pooled (fixed effect) 119/525 108/506 0.942 (0.692 / 1.282)

Better EBL   Better BB

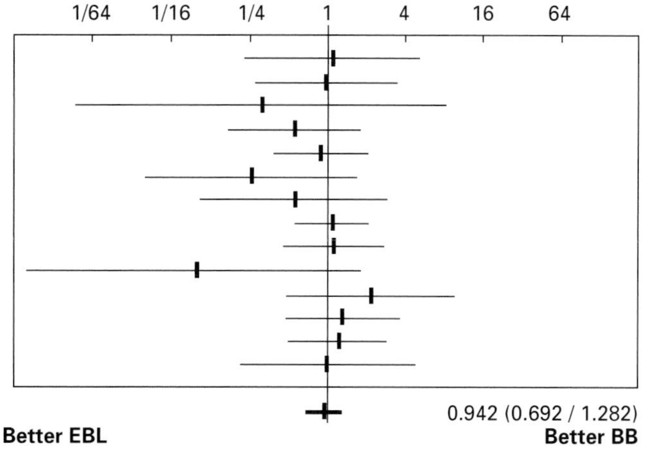

Figure 36.2 Primary prevention: Forrest plot of randomized trials of banding ligation of esophageal varices versus beta-blockers in primary prevention of variceal bleeding. Mortality. BB: beta-blockers; EBL: Endoscopic band ligation. Data are expressed as OR (95% CI) in a log scale.

studies [52, 60, 88] of which one was published only in abstract form [52]. The results were conflicting. One study indicated that sclerotherapy was more effective [88], the second that ligation was more effective [60], and the third that the two interventions are of similar efficacy [52]. Thus, it is not surprising that there is significant heterogeneity in the meta-analysis (p = 0.045) for bleeding, and combining the data in a meta-analysis may not be justified. There was no significant difference for mortality (POR 0.84; 95% CI: 0.35–2.05).

Conclusion

The data from prophylactic trials suggest that screening for varices in cirrhotic patients should be part of routine clinical practice, and if these are found, prophylactic treatment to prevent first variceal bleeding should be offered [89, 90]. Shunt surgery prevents bleeding but the increase in mortality and the long-term risk of encephalopathy make this treatment unacceptable. Prophylactic sclerotherapy should not be used as it is relatively ineffective, costly and potentially dangerous. The treatment of first choice is prophylactic β-blocker therapy; it is inexpensive, easy to administer, and effective for prevention of the first variceal hemorrhage and of bleeding from gastric mucosa. Primary prophylaxis with variceal ligation appears to be safe and may be a reasonable alternative for: (1) patients with contraindications to β-blockers; (2) patients who cannot tolerate or have no hemodynamic response to the drug therapy. However, it is unlikely to be a routine prophylactic treatment as it is much more expensive and less available than β-blockers and it will not prevent gastric mucosal bleeding [57]. The trend towards increased mortality with banding needs further observation, as increased mortality was seen with prophylactic sclerotherapy.

Outcome of acute variceal bleeding

Acute variceal bleeding is a life-threatening complication in patients with cirrhosis and portal hypertension, with mortality that ranges from 10% to 40% [91]. Although overall survival is improving [1], because of new therapeutic approaches, mortality is still closely related to failure to control hemorrhage or early re-bleeding, which is a distinct characteristic of portal hypertensive bleeding and occurs in between 15% and 50% of patients in the first days to six weeks after admission [92].

HVPG has been shown to be prognostic for both survival and the course of acute bleeding. In 1986 Vinel et al. documented that short term prognosis in alcoholic cirrhotics with variceal bleeding was independently associated with portohepatic gradient measured within 48 hr of admission [93]. This was confirmed in a small study of 22 patients, in which the best cutoff for continued bleeding or early re-bleeding was HVPG > 16 mmHg [94]. Villanueva et al. showed that HVPG > 20 mmHg and a decrease ≤10 mmHg under vaso-active therapy were independent predictors of further bleeding [95]. An HVPG > 20 mmHg has been shown to correlate with important clinical outcomes, such as more difficulty in controlling acute variceal bleeding, more early re-bleeding, more blood transfusion need, more days in intensive care and increased hospital mortality [96]. Avgerinos et al. showed that HVPG > 16 mmHg was independently associated with death and/or early re-bleeding, evaluating HVPG measurements before and immediately after endoscopic treatment and every 24 hours for a five-day period [97]. Interestingly, there was sustained rise of portal pressure after sclerotherapy, but not band ligation. In addition, Vlachogiannakos et al. showed that somatostatin but not octreotide effectively prevents the post-endoscopic increase of HVPG [98]. With the prognostic association of high HVPG with the course of bleeding (using vasoactive drugs and endoscopic therapy) and mortality, a randomized study showed that urgent TIPS in patients with HVPG > 20 mmHg, protected against continued or repeated bleeding and reduced mortality [96]. This study clearly demonstrated the therapeutic benefit of intervention based on HVPG measurement and validated the value of 20 mmHg HVPG as a cutoff. The question then arises about the applicability of measuring HVPG in this setting, which although accurate and reproducible, with little co-efficient of variation in measurement, and with few complications is not currently feasible outside a research setting [99].

Several studies have evaluated factors associated with failure to control bleeding and mortality. A consensus has determined that control of variceal bleeding spans the first five days and mortality is death within six weeks of onset of bleeding [89]. Ben-Ari et al. showed that in 385 cirrhotics treated initially with vasoactive drugs and then endosopic therapy if bleeding continued or recurred (within five days) active bleeding at endoscopy (independent of the interval from onset of melena and/or haematemesis or the interval to admission to hospital), the severity of liver disease (mainly Child-Pugh grade C) as well as encephalopathy, platelet count and history of alcoholism were all independently associated with failure to control bleeding (internal validation of the model was performed) [100]. There were some interactions between variables in that active bleeding was associated with transfusion need and transfusion need was associated with Child-Pugh class, and shorter interval to admission. Interestingly a higher Child-Pugh score and increased mortality was independent of transfusion requirement. Independent factors associated with mortality within 30 days were failure to control bleeding within five days, raised bilirubin, encephalopathy, shorter interval to admission to hospital and plasma urea. Lecleire et al. evaluated prospectively 468 consecutive patients with cirrhosis and upper gastrointestinal bleeding (23.5% died during hospitalization) [101]. The independent factors associated with in hospital mortality were: presentation with hematemesis, bleeding starting in hospital, prothrombin time <40% (the strongest association, reflecting severity of liver disease), recent use of steroid drugs within seven days of bleeding, age >60 years and a concomitant hepatocellular cancer. Thomopoulos et al. retrospectively evaluated 141 patients with acute variceal bleeding (18.6% 6 week mortality) treated with somatostatin started before endoscopy and endoscopic ligation [102]. Early re-bleeding, Child-Pugh grade C and shock at admission were independent predictors of mortality at six weeks, whilst active bleeding and presence of infection (prophylactic antibiotics were not routinely used) were not adverse factors.

Lo et al. also found active bleeding to be independently associated with recurrent bleeding, but not mortality, although this was higher in the group with active bleeding at endoscopy [103]. In addition, the presence of hepatocellular carcinoma may alter the immediate prognosis [101, 104, 105] so that early imaging (large tumors will be detected by a bedside ultrasound) to detect HCC may alter the therapeutic algorithm, for example TIPS rescue therapy may not be indicated and only vasoactive and endoscopic methods applied. A concomitant portal vein thrombosis, whether due to tumor or not may also worsen prognosis as often bleeding is more difficult to control.

The use of prophylactic antibiotics should be standard therapy for patients with cirrhosis who have variceal bleeding [106]. The association with failure to control was shown prospectively [107], following a hypothesis that proposed infection as a trigger for bleeding [108], and the causal association was shown in two randomized trials [109, 110]. Antibiotics result in better control of bleeding and less early re-bleeding. **A1c** The prognostic models that assess control of bleeding should now be based in cohorts of patients who have had prophylactic antibiotics.

In a prospectively evaluated cohort of 117 patients with cirrhosis [111], HVPG was measured within 48 hours. As in a previous study HVPG > 20 mmHg was independently predictive of failure to control bleeding at five days, together with shock (systolic blood pressure at admission <100 mmHg) and non-alcoholic etiology of cirrhosis, giving an optimal discrimination using an AUROC curve with a c statistic of 0.79 [96]. However, removing HVPG, the model contained Child-Pugh class, shock at admission and non-alcoholic cirrhosis as independent associations with a c statistic of 0.8, that is, the same discriminatory capacity. The authors devised a simple point score which will be useful in clinical practice as it identifies a subgroup with 40% or more chance of failure to control variceal bleeding. Indeed the authors confirm what is already known clinically about these patients with difficult bleeding with the added data; this is associated with a higher HVPG [89]. This should intensify clinical research into more effective vasoactive regimens to lower portal pressure and treatment algorithms which will result in more effective therapy to control bleeding *ab initio*, for example early TIPS after diagnostic endoscopy, or first-line injection with glues at diagnostic endoscopy, or indeed the recently described self-expanding covered esophageal stent [112]. A randomized trial of early TIPS, reproposing a management scheme used by Orloff et al. with emergency porto-caval shunt [113].

Although survival following variceal bleeding has progressively improved [91, 114], it remains to be proven that "complete" or better control of bleeding with early TIPS or other measures over and above what is current practice after failed vasoactive drugs and endoscopy will result in improved survival. In the large study by Ben-Ari *et al.* mortality in Child-Pugh grade C was independent of transfusion need, that is, of severity of bleeding [100]. Thus there may be an inexorable train of events which is initiated by bleeding in this group of patients, leading to death, independent of good control of bleeding. This concept of "going past the point of no return" is seen in the development of renal failure, despite the prompt resolution of sepsis (not associated with spontaneous bacterial peritonitis) in cirrhosis, where just over 20% of such patients have the complication of renal failure despite optimal treatment and resolution of the precipitating septic event [115].

Intravenous third-generation cephalosporines, compared to oral quinolones are a good option for prophylaxis in upper GI bleeding in cirrhosis being active against Gram-negative bacteria and non-enterococcal streptococci [116]. In addition, many cirrhotics receive quinolones already as prophylaxis for spontaneous bacterial peritonitis, and quinolone resistant bacteria are currently sensitive to cephalosporins. Current trials have started antibiotics after endoscopic diagnosis. Possibly the administration should be started at admission before endoscopy with the potential to increase therapeutic benefit.

The clinician should be aware that most clinical trials have focused on esophageal varices, with very few designed to evaluate therapy for gastric varices. Gastric varices may lead to more severe bleeding initially, and tend to re-bleed frequently [117]. The following sections refer to esophageal varices unless specified.

Randomized controlled trials for the treatment of acute variceal bleeding

Pharmacologic treatment

Vasoactive drug treatment is the only treatment that does not require sophisticated equipment or the skills of a specialist and is immediately available, even before the patient is admitted to hospital [118]. Furthermore, as evidence suggests that those patients with high variceal or portal pressure are likely to continue to bleed or re-bleed early, prolonged drug therapy that lowers portal pressure over days may be the optimal treatment [8, 119]. The vasoactive drugs that are currently used in the management of acute variceal bleeding are vasopressin, glypressin, somatostatin, octreotide and vapreotide. Vasopressin, which is a powerful vasoconstrictor, lowers portal pressure through the induction of smooth muscle contraction, particularly in splanchnic arterioles. However, the drug also causes systemic vasoconstriction which leads to serious side effects, such as cardiac arrhythmias, myocardial ischemia, mesenteric ischemia and cerebrovascular episodes, resulting in cessation of therapy in up to 25% of cases [120, 121].

Terlipressin is a synthetic analogue of vasopressin (triglycyl lysine vasopressin). It has an intrinsic effect as well as being converted *in vivo* into vasopressin by enzymatic cleavage of the triglycyl residues. This prolongs its biological half-life, so that a continuous intravenous infusion is unnecessary. Somatostatin has been used in the pharmacological treatment of variceal bleeding because it reduces splanchnic blood flow [122], portal pressure and azygous blood flow in patients with cirrhosis [123], although only the findings regarding the reduction in azygous flow are consistent. Bolus injections of somatostatin appear to have greater hemodynamic effects as compared with continuous infusion. Finally, octreotide has been reported to cause a reduction in portal pressure [124], and a transient decrease in azygous blood flow [125], but there are some studies that do not confirm these data, using similar or even greater doses of the drug [126].

Randomized controlled trials of vasoactive drug treatment of acute variceal bleeding

Drugs versus placebo

See Table 36.4.

Vasopressin versus placebo

Vasopressin was compared with non-active treatment or placebo in four randomized controlled trials [121, 127–129], including only 157 patients. In two trials the intra-arterial route of administration was used [121, 129]. There was a significant heterogeneity in the evaluation of failure to control bleeding. There was a clear trend in favor of vasopressin but the result was not statistically significant by the Der Simonian and Laird method (POR 0.23; 95% CI: 0.05–1.02). Moreover there was no difference in mortality (POR 0.98; 95% CI: 0.47–2.1). Complications were reported in up to 64% of patients, which led to discontinuation of treatment in 25% of cases. In order to minimize the systemic complications of vasopressin, nitroglycerin has been added to the regimen. This drug is a powerful venous dilator, reduces the portal vascular resistance and improves myocardial performance. Three randomized controlled trials have compared vasopressin alone with vasopressin plus nitroglycerin (transdermally [120], sublingually [130], and intravenously [131]), including 176 patients. Failure to control bleeding was significantly less common with vasopressin plus nitroglycerin (POR 0.39; 95% CI: 0.21–0.72) but there was no difference in mortality (POR 0.94; 95% CI: 0.49–1.79). In two of the trials [130, 131], adverse effects were significantly reduced with the combination treatment. However, nitroglycerin, because of portocollateral shunting, bypasses the liver, and can cause significant sys-

Table 36.4 Randomized controlled trials of drugs versus placebo for the treatment of the acute bleeding episode.

Study	No. of patients C/T	Child C (%)	Failure to control bleeding (n) C/T	Death (n) C/T
Vasopressin vs placebo				
Merigan et al. (1962) [129]	24/29	NR	24/13	23/28
Conn et al. (1975) [121]	16/17	NR	12/5	10/9
Mallory et al. (1980) [128]	20/18	NR	17/10	9/8
Fogel et al. (1982) [127]	19/14	NR	12/10	8/7
Terlipressin vs placebo				
Walker et al. (1986) [136]	25/25	50	12/5	8/3
Freeman et al. (1989) [132]	16/15	29	10/6	4/3
Soderlund et al. (1990) [135]	29/31	33	13/5	11/3
Pauwels et al. (1994) [134]	14/17	NR	6/7	5/6
Levacher et al. (1995) [118]	43/41	81	23/12	20/12
Patch et al. (1999) [133]	66/66	62	40/37	28/22
Somatostatin vs placebo or inactive treatment				
Flati et al. (1986) [140]	16/19	40	9/2	7/4
Testoni et al. (1986) [142]	14/15	17	1/1	0/1
Loperfido et al. (1987) [141]	25/22	19	21/17	7/6
Valenzuela et al. (1989) [139]	36/48	32	9/21	10/15
Burroughs et al. (1990) [137]	59/61	41	35/22	7/9
Gotzsce (2003) [138]	44/42	NR	NR	16/16
Octreotide vs placebo				
Burroughs et al. (1996) [146]	139/123	40	85/71	37/35
Variceal bleeding only	109/88	40	75/56	32/24
Octreotide vs placebo for early re-bleeding				
Primignani et al. (1995) [147]	32/26		10/9	
D'Amico et al. (1998) [148]	131/131	31	37/31	20/26

C: placebo; T: drug; NR: not reported.

temic effects. Hence, this combination therapy must be monitored very closely and is less applicable as an immediate therapy.

Terlipressin versus placebo

The clinical efficacy of terlipressin has been evaluated in six randomized placebo-controlled studies [118, 132–136] including 388 patients. In two studies endoscopic sclerotherapy was employed at the initial diagnostic endoscopy [118, 133]. In one trial the drug was given while the patient was transferred to hospital. There was a statistically significant reduction in failure to control bleeding with terlipressin compared with placebo (POR 0.49; 95% CI: 0.33–0.75) and more importantly the same meta-analysis showed that terlipressin is the only vasoconstrictor that significantly reduces mortality (POR 0.51; 95% CI: 0.33–0.79). However, there is some criticism of these studies. The sample sizes were small, allowing a large type 2 error in the first three trials [132, 135, 136], and the evidence in the early administration trial [118] of the effect of terlipressin, given only

as three doses up to eight hours, does not readily explain the apparent benefit on mortality (only in group C patients) via an effect on the control of bleeding. **A1c**

Somatostatin versus placebo

Three placebo-controlled trials of somatostatin exhibit divergent results [137–139]. The trials by Valenzuela et al. [139] and Gotzse et al. [138] suggested that somatostatin was no more effective than placebo. Unfortunately both studies had a very long recruitment period, suggesting marked patient selection. Moreover, Gotzse et al. did not evaluate the endpoint of failure to control bleeding [138], while Valenzuela et al. reported an extremely high response rate (83%) in the placebo group (the highest ever reported) [139]. In contrast, the study by Burroughs et al. reported a statistically significant benefit for somatostatin in controlling variceal bleeding over a five-day treatment period [137]. These differences in the reported results caused statistically significant heterogeneity (p = 0.006) in the meta-analysis of the six studies which compare somatostatin with placebo or inactive treatment [140–142].There was a trend in favor of somatostatin but the result was not statistically significant by the Der Simonian and Laird method (POR 0.6; 95% CI: 0.21–1.65). There was no difference in mortality between the two treatment groups (POR 1.02; 95% CI: 0.64–1.61). **A1c**

Moitinho *et al.* evaluated a total of 174 patients with acute variceal bleeding who were randomized to receive somatostatin for 48 h: (A) one 250 µg bolus +250 µg/h infusion; (B) three 250 µg boluses +250 µg/h infusion; (C) three 250 µg boluses +500 µg/h infusion [143]. The 500 µg/h infusion dose achieved a higher rate of control of bleeding (82 vs 60%, p < 0.05), less transfusions (3.7 +/− 2.7 vs 2.5 +/− 2.3 units, p = 0.07) and better survival (93 vs 70%, p < 0.05) than schedules A and B. Others have confirmed the above results using somatostatin 500 µg/h [144, 145]. **A1d**

Octreotide versus placebo

There is only one double blind randomized trial of octreotide versus placebo (n = 262) in the management of acute variceal bleeding, currently available only in abstract form [146]. In this study a continuous five-day infusion of 50 µg/ hour octreotide, started as soon as possible after admission was not more effective than placebo, whether or not injection sclerotherapy was needed for active bleeding or drug failure. Infections were treated if suspected on clinical grounds and were similar in the two trial groups. Moreover, two other studies using octreotide (100 µg eight-hourly, subcutaneously) or placebo after the control of the initial bleeding episode failed to show any difference in early rebleeding or mortality between the two treatment groups [147, 148].

Drugs versus balloon tamponade

Six trials compared vasoactive drugs with balloon tamponade. The drugs were terlipressin in three studies [149–151], somatostatin in two studies [152, 153] and octreotide in one study [154]. Meta-analysis of these six trials showed that the drugs were as effective as balloon tamponade for prevention of failure to control bleeding (POR 1.04; 95% CI: 0.63–1.72) or death (POR 0.65; 95% CI: 0.36–1.16). **A1c** Sensitivity analysis showed that there was no difference according to the type of drug. However, the sample sizes were small and the endpoints not very clear, indicating that these results should be interpreted with caution. Tamponade, if used properly, provides good control of bleeding. However, the balloons should not be inflated for more than 12 hours and preferably less, and bleeding frequently recurs when the balloons are deflated. From the trial reports it is not always clear when efficacy is being assessed, for example during therapy or at the end of an interval of 24 hours after termination of drug therapy or tamponade.Whether the new expanding oesophageal stent will replace tamponade will be known from RCTs [112].

Drugs versus drugs

See Table 36.5.

Terlipressin versus vasopressin

Terlipressin was compared with vasopressin in five small, unblinded studies involving only 247 patients [155–158, 170]. In two studies, vasopressin was associated with nitroglycerin [157, 158]. Failure to control bleeding was less frequent with terlipressin, but the result was not statistically significant (POR 0.74; 95% CI: 0.36–1.14). There was no difference in mortality between the two treatment arms (POR 1.48; 95% CI: 0.85–2.57). More importantly, the complication rate was significantly lower with terlipressin even when vasopressin was combined with nitroglycerin. **A1c**

Somatostatin versus vasopressin

Somatostatin was compared with vasopressin in eight trials including 343 patients [159–165, 171]. Although these trials showed a trend in favor of somatostatin, the difference was not statistically significant (POR 0.74; 95% CI: 0.48–1.13). There was no difference in mortality between the two vasoactive agents (POR 0.97; 95% CI: 0.6–1.5). However, a statistically significant reduction in complications was observed in the group receiving somatostatin (POR 0.11; 95% CI: 0.07–0.19) as the mean complication rate was 51% with vasopressin and only 10% with somatostatin. **A1c**

Somatostatin versus terlipressin

Three studies have compared somatostatin with terlipressin involving 326 patients [166, 167, 172]. These studies showed that the two drugs were similarly effective in preventing failure to control variceal bleeding and death. Moreover, in one of these studies a significantly lower incidence of complications in the somatostatin group was reported [166]. **[A1c]**

Octreotide versus other drugs

The efficacy of octreotide treatment in comparison to other vasoactive drugs, for acute variceal bleeding, has not been adequately evaluated. Octreotide was found to be comparable to vasopressin in two low quality studies (n = 89 in total) [168, 173], and to terlipressin plus nitroglycerin in another (n = 87 patients) [169]. However, the sample sizes were small and the trials may have lacked power to show differences, and the endpoints are not very clear, indicating that these results should be interpreted with caution.

Somatostatin versus other drugs

In a single center randomized trial 62 cirrhotics with variceal bleeding were randomized to receive somatostatin

Table 36.5 Randomized controlled trials of comparisons between drugs for the treatment of the acute bleeding episode.

Study	No. of patients C/T	Child C (%)	Failure to control bleeding (n) C/T	Death (n) C/T	Complications C/T
Vasopressin vs vasopressin plus nitroglycerin					
Tsai et al. (1986) [130]	20/19	34	11/15	11/11	NR
Gimson et al. (1986) [131]	38/34	61	12/19	9/9	NR
Bosch et al. (1989) [120]	30/35	51	8/16	9/10	NR
Terlipressin vs vasopressin					
Freeman et al. (1989) [132]	11/10	15	10/3	3/2	NR
Desaint et al. (1987) [155]	6/10	43	1/2	2/3	NR
Lee et al. (1988) [156]	24/21	27	16/17	8/10	NR
Chiu et al. (1990) [157]	28/26	60	13/13	10/12	NR
D'Amico et al. (1994) [158]	55/56	9	13/5	9/14	NR
Somatostatin vs vasopressin					
Kravetz et al. (1984) [159]	31/30	41	13/14	17/16	22/3
Jenkins et al. (1985) [160]	12/10	54	8/3	4/2	2/0
Bagarani et al. (1987) [161]	25/24	69	17/8	10/6	3/1
Cardona et al. (1989) [162]	18/20	26	8/12	3/6	15/6
Hsia et al. (1990) [163]	24/22	65	15/10	15/14	11/4
Saari et al. (1990) [164]	22/32	46	10/11	15/22	11/1
Rodriguez-Moreno (1991) [165]	16/15	30	6/9	3/3	11/0
Somatostatin vs terlipressin					
Feu et al. (1996) [166]	80/81	29	16/13	13/13	31/19
Walker et al. (1996) [167]	53/53	12	5/10	11/11	0/3
Octreotide vs vasopressin					
Hwang et al. (1992) [168]	24/24	44	13/9	12/11	11/3
Octreotide vs terlipressin					
Silvain et al. (1993) [169]	41/46	47	17/10	11/10	31/19

C: control; T: treatment; NR: not reported.

(n = 35) versus somatostatin plus nitroglycerine (n = 26) [174]. Similar proportions of patients achieved control of bleeding in the two groups (88.6% vs 92.3% respectively). The authors concluded that the addition of nitrates does not improve the control of bleeding or prevent early re-bleeding. **A1d**

Recombinant activated factor VIIa

In a placebo-controlled double blind randomized trial, recombinant factor VIIa was safe but no clear-cut benefit in control of bleeding or mortality was seen [175]. More recently a randomized controlled trial assessed the efficacy and safety of rFVIIa in patients with advanced cirrhosis and active variceal bleeding [176]. At 31 hospitals in an emergency setting, 256 patients (Child-Pugh > 8; Child-Pugh B = 26%, C = 74%) were randomized equally to: placebo; 600 μg/kg rFVIIa (200 + 4x 100 μg/kg); or 300 μg/kg rFVIIa (200 + 100 μg/kg). The primary composite endpoint consisted of failure to control bleeding within 24 hours, or failure to prevent re-bleeding or death by day five. Administration of rFVIIa had no significant effect on the composite endpoint compared with placebo (p = 0.37). There was no significant difference in five-day mortality between groups; however, 42-day mortality was significantly lower, with 600 μg/kg rFVIIa compared with placebo (odds ratio 0.31; 95% CI: 0.13–0.74), and bleeding-related deaths were reduced from 12% (placebo) to 2% (600 μg/kg), but this was not associated with differences in control of bleeding. There is no evidence that recombinant activated factor VIIa improves outcome in acute variceal bleeding. **A1b**

Randomized controlled trials of emergency sclerotherapy in the management of acute variceal bleeding

Injection sclerotherapy, first introduced in 1939 and "redis-covered" in the late 1970s, has been used for the control of acute variceal bleeding over the past two decades. Paradoxically the best evidence for the value of sclerotherapy in the management of acute variceal bleeding has come from a more recently published study by the Veterans Affairs Cooperative Variceal Sclerotherapy Group [177]. In this study sclerotherapy, compared with sham sclerotherapy, stopped hemorrhage from actively bleeding esophageal varices (91% in sclerotherapy arm compared with 60% in sham sclerotherapy, p < 0.001, ARR = 29%, NNT = 3) and significantly increased hospital survival (75% vs 51%, p = 0.04 ARR = 24%, NNT = 3). **A1d**

Today it is generally accepted that sclerotherapy should be carried out at the diagnostic endoscopy, which should take place as soon as possible, because there is evidence that this is beneficial compared with delayed injection [178, 179]. No more than two injection sessions should be used to arrest variceal bleeding within a five-day period [92]. Several sclerosing agents have been used for injection, polidocanol 1–3%, ethanolamine oleate 5%, sodium tetradecyl sulfate 1–2% and sodium morrhuate 5%. There is no evidence that any one sclerosant can be considered the optimal sclerosant for acute injection, as it has been shown that a substantial proportion of intravariceal sclerosant ends up in the paravariceal tissue and vice versa. **B4** There is no evidence that one technique is better than the other. One of the main shortcomings of sclerotherapy is the risk of local and systemic complications, although this varies greatly between trials and may be related to the experience of the operator [180].

Sclerotherapy plus drugs/balloon tamponade versus drugs/balloon tamponade

The five trials, three papers [181–183] and two abstracts [184, 185] comprised 400 patients (413 episodes): three used

vasopressin [181, 182, 184], one somatostatin [183] and one octreotide [185]. Treatment effect was evaluated within 24 hours up to 120 hours, except in one study at two weeks [181]. Specific definitions of failure to control bleeding are given in four [181–183, 185]; only three [181, 182, 186] report complications; blood transfusion was reported in four [181–183, 185]; three report less transfusion with sclerotherapy [181–183]; and one no difference [185]. Median quality score was 58 (49–68.5). Failure to control bleeding was reported: 214 episodes of variceal bleeding in the sclerotherapy and vasoactive drugs/balloon tamponade group and 199 in the vasoactive drugs/balloon tamponade alone. Failure to control bleeding was significantly more frequent without sclerotherapy, with pooled difference being 16.3% (95% CI: 8.7–23.9%; p = 0.0001)). **A1c** The NNT was 6 (95% CI: 4–11). The publication bias assessment was 15 null or negative studies. The sensitivity analyses differed from the main metanalysis as follows: abstracts alone showed no differences between trial groups. In only one study, octreotide added to sclerotherapy did not improve control of bleeding. Fewer deaths occurred with sclerotherapy combined with drugs than with drugs/balloon tamponade alone (Q, p = 1.0), with a 5.5% difference (95% CI: –1.8–12.7%; p = 0.138) with no significant changes in the sensitivity analyses. Complications: reported in three studies [181–183] and two [181, 183] did not report per patient. A systematic evaluation was not possible (see Table 36.6).

Sclerotherapy versus drugs

There are 15 studies comprising 1296 patients (1324 episodes), 11 papers [187–197] and four abstracts [198–201]; one used vasopressin [196], one used terlipressin [188], four used somatostatin [191–193, 198] and nine used octreotide [187, 189, 190, 194, 195, 197, 199–201]. Treatment effect

Table 36.6 Randomized controlled trials of sclerotherapy plus drugs/balloon tamponade versus drugs/balloon tamponade alone for the treatment of the acute bleeding episode.

Study	Compared treatment	No. of patients S + D/D	Child C n (%)	Failure to control bleeding n (S + D/D)	Death n (S + D/D)	Complications n (S + D/D)
Soderlund and Ihre (1985) [182]	Vasopressin ± tamponade	57/50	70 (65)	3/8	16/18	10/8
Larson et al. (1986) [181]	Vasopressin ± tamponade	44/38	47 (57)	5/14	2/5	25/42
Alexandrino et al. (1990) [184]	Vasopressin/ nitroglycerin ± tamponade	41/42	41 (49)	12/12	16/17	NR
Novella et al. (1996) [185]	Octreotide	22/19	NR	3/7	3/2	NR
Villanueva et al. (1999) [183]	Somatostatin	50/50	25 (26)	7/21	7/10	11/4

S + D/D: sclerotherapy + drugs/drugs; NR: not reported.

Table 36.7 Randomized controlled trials of sclerotherapy versus drugs for the treatment of the acute bleeding episode.

Study	Compared treatment	No. of pts S/D	Child C (%)	Failure to control bleeding (S/D)	Death n (S/D)	Complications (S/D)
Westaby et al. (1989) [196]	Vasopressin	33/31	22 (34)	4/11	9/12	NR
Di Febo et al. (1990) [198]	Somatostatin	24/23	19 (40)	2/5	5/6	2/1
Shields et al. (1992) [193]	Somatostatin	41/39	42 (52–5)	7/9	8/12	12/5
Sung et al. (1993) [195]	Octreotide	49/49	43 (43)	13/15	20/14	18/5
Planas et al. (1994) [191]	Somatostatin	35/35	24 (34)	6/7	8/10	10/5
Poo et al. (1996) [201]	Octreotide	21/22	20 (47)	2/1	5/3	1/1
Jenkins et al. (1997) [190]	Octreotide	77/73	80 (53)	14/11	13/22	15/19
El-Jackie et al. (1998) [199]	Octreotide	50/50	NR	3/21	NR	NR
Lopez et al. (1999) [200]	Octreotide	33/31	NR	4/5	7/6	NR
Escorsell et al. (2000) [188]	Terlipressin	114/105	69 (31)	36/35	19/26	34/21
Bildozola et al., (2000) [187]	Octreotide	25/25	5 (10)	7/10	2/5	8/9
Freitas et al. (2000) [189]	Octreotide	53/58	39 (35)	12/12	8/13	NR
Sivri et al. (2000) [194]	Octreotide	36/30	35 (53)	9/8	1/1	5/1
Yousuf et al. (2000) [197]	Octreotide	48/48	20 (21)	2/4	5/5	6/8
Ramires et al. (2000) [192]	Somatostatin	19/21	12 (30)	5/5	6/6	NR

S: sclerotherapy; D: drugs; NR: not reported.

was evaluated at the end of drug infusion (12–168 hours). The efficacy of sclerotherapy was 83% (57–94%) in studies of 12–48-hour drug infusion [189–192, 194–196, 198–201] and 73% (68–83%) when 120–168 hours [187, 188, 193]. All except three trials [189, 199, 200] report complications. One study had less transfusion with sclerotherapy (units, 2.1 ± 0.41 vs 2.9 ± 0.79; p < 0.05) [199], ten found no difference [187–195, 197], one study did not state [201], and three had no report [196, 198, 200]. Median quality score was 60 [51–73]. Considering failure to control bleeding, there was significant heterogeneity (p = 0.01), but only in the magnitude and not in the direction of treatment effect; in only two were drugs better than sclerotherapy, but without reaching statistical significance [190, 201]. Excluding abstracts there was no heterogeneity (p = 0.4). Failure to control bleeding was less frequent with sclerotherapy with a difference of 3.4% (95% CI: −1.8–8.5%; p = 0.2) with no change following sensitivity analyses. If all papers are considered then sclerotherapy was more effective, with a 5.9% difference (95% CI: 1.5–10.3%) (p = 0.008). The other sensitivity analyses showed that octreotide in nine studies (p = 0.04) and vasopressin (one study) as well as the combined group of somatostatin and octreotide were significantly worse than sclerotherapy. In the trials there were no differences between treatment groups considering only patients with cirrhosis, or abstracts, or somatostatin, or drug infusion more or less than 120 hours, or combined group of vasopressin and terlipressin or terlipressin alone. There were fewer deaths with sclerotherapy – 4.3% (95% CI: 0.6–8.1%) (p = 0.02). **Ala** The NNT was 23 (95% CI: 12–157). The effect is not robust, as publication bias assessment was four null or negative studies. Sensitivity analyses did not change the main meta-analysis. Complications in 12 studies [187, 188, 190–198, 201] had significant heterogeneity (p = 0.0001) and were less frequent with any drug 8.8% (95% CI: 0.2–15.6%; p = 0.01) (see Table 36.7).

Sclerotherapy plus drugs versus sclerotherapy alone

The eight trials, six papers [189, 202, 205–208] and two abstracts [203, 204] (the first with two treatment arms) comprised 1026 patients; four studies were placebo controlled [202, 203, 205, 206, 208]. Vasoactive drug was administered for 120 hours in six trials [202–206, 208] and 48 hours in two [189, 207]. The efficacy of sclerotherapy was 82.5% (81–84%) with 48 hour drug administration and 61.5% (36–77%) with 120 hours (p = ns). In all studies but one the average units transfused were significantly less with combination therapy [189]. Median quality score was 60 (49.5–75). Failure to control bleeding was less frequent with sclerotherapy combined with drugs: 13.2% (95% CI: 8.4–18.1%; p < 0.0001). **Ala** The NNT was 8 (95% CI: 5–15). The publication bias assessment was 47 null or negative studies, that is, the result is very robust. In the sensitivity analyses, terlipressin did not have an advantage: there was no advantage of any drug added to sclerotherapy for 48 hours administration and no advantage of combined therapy when no placebo drug was used. The difference in mortality was 3.4% (95% CI: −0.4–7.1%) in favor of combined therapy (p = 0.08). Sensitivity

Table 36.8 Randomized controlled trials of sclerotherapy plus drugs versus sclerotherapy alone for the treatment of the acute bleeding episode.

Study	Compared treatment	No. of patients S/S + D	Child C (%)	Failure to control bleeding (S/S + D)	Death *n* (S/S + D)	Complications (S/S + D)
Besson *et al.* (1995) [202]	Sclerotherapy + octreotide	101/98	73(37)	25/11	12/12	33/34
Signorelli *et al.* (1996) [203]	Sclerotherapy + somatostatin	30/33	NR	11/6	5/4	NR
Signorelli *et al.* (1996) [203]	Sclerotherapy + octeotide	30/31	NR	11/8	5/5	NR
Signorelli *et al.* (1999) [204]	Sclerotherapy + octreotide	45/43	NR	18/8	NR	NR
ABOVE (1997) [205]	Sclerotherapy + somatostatin	75/77	NR	48/31	24/27	37/37
Zuberi and Balock (2000) [206]	Sclerotherapy + octreotide	35/35	0(0)	13/4	1/1	NR
Freitas *et al.* (2000) [189]	Sclerotherapy + octreotide	42/44	29(37)	18/9	13/12	NR
Farooqi 2000 [207]	Sclerotherapy + octreotide	69/72	38(27)	11/3	6/1	27/31
Cales *et al.* (2001) [208]	Sclerotherapy + vapreotide	98/98	73(37)	49/33	7/5	8/6

S: sclerotherapy; S + D: sclerotherapy plus drugs; NR: not reported.

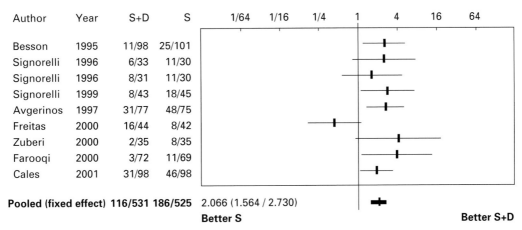

Figure 36.3 Acute bleeding: Forrest plot of risk difference for control of bleeding in trials of sclerotherapy (S) vs sclerotherapy combined with vasoactive agents (S + D).

analysis showed that in placebo controlled trials in which drug was given for 120 hours the difference was 1.3% (95% CI: −3.3–5.8%), strongly suggesting no benefit in mortality despite benefit for control of bleeding. For complications, five studies had data but only two reported per patient [202, 205], with no statistical differences (see Table 36.8 and Figures 36.3 and 36.4).

Sclerotherapy versus variceal ligation

The twelve trials, eight papers [209–216] and four abstracts [217–220], comprised 1309 patients. In seven trials only patients with cirrhosis were included [209–213, 216, 219]. The same ligating device (Bard Interventional Products, Tewksbury, Massachusetts) with an overtube was used in eight [209–212, 214–216]; in three this was not mentioned [217–219] and one used a six-shooter [220]. A definition of failure to control bleeding is stated in five [209, 210, 212,

213, 216]. The efficacy of sclerotherapy for initial hemostasis at the end of endoscopy was 95% (76–100%) compared with 97% (86–100%) with ligation EBL group (p = 0.4). In only one [213] of documenting transfusion requirements [211–213, 215, 216, 218], was this less in the ligation group (units, 4.5 ± 1.8 (0–12) versus 3.2 ± 1.2 (0–6) p < 0.01); in others there was no difference. Median quality score was 68.5 (50.5–79). Failure to control of bleeding: there was a difference favoring ligation −2.5% (95% CI: 0.4–4.6%) (p = 0.018). **Ala** Sensitivity analyses did not show differences from the main metanalysis, including an evaluation defining failure versus those in which there was no failure.

Regarding mortality, the percentage difference was 1.3% favoring ligation (95% CI: −2.3–4.9%, p = 0.46). Sensitivity analyses did not show differences from the main metanalysis.

In another recent trial [221] patients admitted with acute gastrointestinal bleeding and with suspected cirrhosis

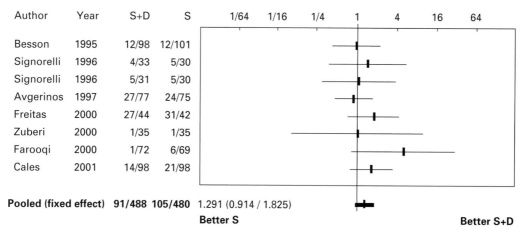

Pooled (fixed effect) 91/488 105/480 1.291 (0.914 / 1.825)

Figure 36.4 Acute bleeding: Forrest plot of risk difference for mortality in trials of sclerotherapy (S) vs sclerotherapy combined with vasoactive agents (S + D).

Table 36.9 Randomized controlled trials of sclerotherapy versus variceal ligation for the prevention of re-bleeding.

Study	No. of pts (S/L)	Child C (%)	Failure of initial hemostasis	Re-bleeding S/L	Death S/L	Variceal obliteration S/L	Variceal recurrence S/L
Stiegmann et al. (1992) [216]	65/64	19	3:13/2:14	31/23	29/18	22/27	11:22/9:27
Laine et al. (1993) [211]	39/38	23	1:9/1:9	17/10	6/4	27/22	—
Gimson et al. (1993) [209]	23/21	26	3/3	26/16	17/21	27/32	—
Jensen et al. (1993) [242]	18/14	NR	0/3	9/6	3/2	NR	—
Mundo et al. (1993) [243]	11/8	37	NR	3/2	4/2	4/4	—
Young et al. (1993) [244]	13/10	78	NR	5/2	4/2	11/9	—
Lo et al. (1995) [212]	59/61	48	3:15/1:18	30/20	19/10	37/45	—
Hou et al. (1995) [210]	67/67	39	2:16/0:20	28/13	11/14	53/58	—
Jensen et al. (1993) [242]	26/24	NR	NR	9/7	9/4	NR	—
Jain et al. (1996) [218]	24/22	46[a]	2/3	5/9	NR	24/20	2:24/5:20
Mostafa et al. (1996) [245]	89/69	NR	1:21/1:18	9/6	2/3	82/63	7:82/12:63
Baroncini et al. (1997) [246]	54/57	27	NR	10/9	12/12	50/53	7:50/17:53
Lo et al. (1997) [213]	34/37	60	8/1	10/6	12/7	NR	—
Sarin et al. (1997) [214]	48/47	14	1:7/1:5	10/3	3/3	45/44	3:45/10:44
Masci et al. (1997) [247]	50/50	NR	NR	26/16	10/12	41/43	6:37/11:37
Avgerinos et al. (1997) [248]	40/37	8	NR	19//0	8/8	39/35	17:39/11:35
Shiha and Farag (1997) [249]	43/42	NR	4:19/2:17	10/6	2/2	37/37	6:37/11:37
Fakhry et al. (1997) [217]	41/43	NR	1:17/1:18	6/7	NR	40/42	8:41/9:42
De la Pena et al. (1998) [250]	46/42	NR	NR	23/13	10/8	29/31	13:29/19:31
Shafqat et al. (1998) [215]	28/24	NR	6/1	NR	6/3	NR	NR
Salem et al. (1999) [220]	180/180	NR	32/16	NR	NR	NR	—

S: sclerotherapy; L: variceal ligation; NR: not reported.

received somatostatin infusion for five days. Endoscopy was performed within six hours and those with esophageal variceal bleeding were randomized to receive either sclerotherapy (n = 89) or ligation (n = 90). Therapeutic failure occurred in 21 patients treated with sclerotherapy (24%) and in nine treated with ligation (10%) (RR = 2.4, 95% CI: 1.1–4.9). However, in those with active bleeding there was no difference between ligation and sclerotherapy. Failure

to control bleeding occurred in 15% vs 4%, respectively (p = 0.02). Treatment group, shock and HVPG > 16 mmHg were independent predictors of failure. Side effects occurred in 28% of patients receiving sclerotherapy vs 14% with ligation (RR = 1.9; 95% CI: 1.1–3.5), being serious in 13% vs 4% (p = 0.04). Six-week survival probability without therapeutic failure was better with ligation (p = 0.01) (see Table 36.9 and Figures 36.5 and 36.6).

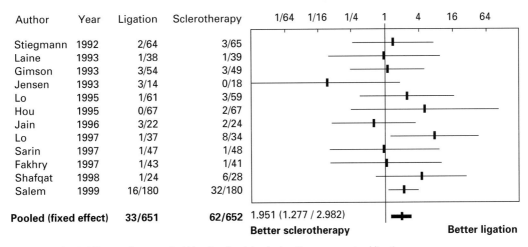

Figure 36.5 Forrest plot of risk difference for control of bleeding in trials of sclerotherapy vs variceal ligation.

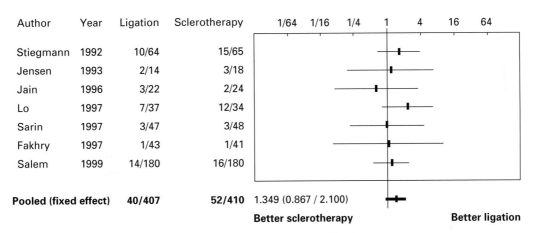

Figure 36.6 Forrest plot of risk difference for mortality in trials of sclerotherapy vs variceal ligation.

Ligation plus sclerotherapy vs ligation

There were 113 patients with either active bleeding or stigmata of recent bleeding from esophageal varices who were randomly assigned to receive ligation plus sclerotherapy, or ligation alone. Hemostasis of active bleeding was achieved at the time of the index treatment in eight of ten of the patients in the combined group (80%) and in ten of twelve of the patients in the ligation group (83%, p > 0.05) [222].

Ligation + terlipressin vs ligation + octreotide

In a recent randomized trial [223] 88 patients with cirrhosis with variceal bleeding allocated to terlipressin (n = 43) or octreotide (n = 45) succesfull hemostasis was achieved in 98% of patients. Early re-bleeding, which included re-bleeding within six weeks of therapy was seen in 28% of terlipressin group and 24% of octreotide group. The two treatments were equally effective for acute esophageal

variceal bleeding with regard to hemostatic effect and prevention of re-bleeding.

Randomized controlled trials of emergency surgery in the management of acute variceal bleeding

Four randomized trials, carried out in the 1980s, compared sclerotherapy to emergency staple transaction [224–226]. Failure to control bleeding was reported only in two of these studies, with divergent results. Teres *et al.* reported that efficacy of transection in their study was only 71%, the lowest in the literature, compared with 83% in the sclerotherapy arm [226]. In contrast, in the largest study by Burroughs *et al.*, a five-day bleeding-free interval was achieved in 90% of the patients who underwent transection (none re-bled from varices) compared with 80% in those who had two emergency injection sessions [227]. There was no difference in mortality between the two treatment modalities. Cello *et al.* showed that emergency portacaval shunt was more effective than emergency sclerotherapy (followed by elective sclerotherapy) in preventing early re-bleeding (19% vs 50%) [228]. Hospital and 30-day mortality were not significantly different. **A1c** Finally, Orloff *et al.* in a small study, reported that portacaval shunt, carried out in less than eight hours from admission, was significantly better than medical treatment (vasopressin/ balloon tamponade) in the control of acute variceal bleeding [229]. Survival was also better in the patients who had shunts, but the difference was not statistically significant.

Randomized controlled trials of other endoscopic therapies in the management of acute variceal bleeding

Two types of tissue adhesives (n-butyl-2-cyanoacrylate, Histoacryl and isobutyl-2-cyanoacrylate, Bucrylate) have been used for the control of variceal bleeding [230]. The adhesives potentially result in better immediate control of bleeding because they harden within seconds upon contact with blood. However, extra care must be taken to ensure that the adhesive does not come into contact with the endoscope and block suction and operator channels. This can be prevented if the adhesive is mixed with lipiodol to delay hardening. Moreover, the sclerotherapy needle must be carefully placed within the varix prior to injection, to avoid leak. A small randomized trial showed that cyanoacrylate was superior to conventional sclerotherapy with 3% ethanolamine oleate solution for control of bleeding and reduction of hospital mortality in Child-Pugh class C patients [231]. Two randomized controlled trials compared sclerotherapy alone with the combination of sclerotherapy and n-butyl-2-cyanoacrylate [232, 233]. The combined treatment was more effective than sclerotherapy alone in both studies. **A1c** Moreover, in two studies n-butyl-2-cyanoacrylate was compared with variceal ligation for the control of bleeding from esophageal [234] or esophagogastric varices [235]. The overall success rate for initial hemostasis of both treatment modalities was similar in these studies. **A1c** However, n-butyl-2-cyanoacrylate was superior to variceal ligation for the control of fundal variceal bleeding, but it was less effective for the prevention of re-bleeding (67% vs 28%). In a small randomized study [236], a biological fibrin glue (Tissucol) was more effective than sclerotherapy with polidocanol in the prevention of early re-bleeding and had a significantly lower incidence of complications. Finally, another study found that fibrin glue was as effective and safe as ligation for acute bleeding and for prevention of re-bleeding from esophageal varices, but had superior tissue compatibility [237]. More studies are necessary to confirm these data and examine the potential risks

of activating coagulation, systemic embolism and particularly transmission of infections with the human plasma-derived fibrin glue. The literature available on thrombin is limited. Bovine thrombin was effective in small series, but has been withdrawn due to its infection risk [238].

In addition, in a prospective randomized controlled trial [239], cirrhotic patients with acute or recent esophageal variceal bleeding were assigned randomly to percutaneous transhepatic varices embolization, PTVE (52 patients) or EVL (50 patients). During the follow-up period (median 24 and 25 months in the PTVE and EVL groups respectively) UGI re-bleeding developed in eight patients in the PTVE group and 21 patients in EVL group (p = 0.004). Recurrent bleeding from esophageal varices occurred in three patients in the PTVE group and 12 in the EVL group (p = 0.012, relative risk 0.24, 95% CI: 10.05–0.74). Survival in these two groups was not significantly different.

An endoscopic detachable snare is another ligation device which has the advantage of allowing an unlimited number of ligations by reloading the nylon minisnare while the endoscope remains in the esophagus. The first prospective randomized trial showed that the mini snare performed equally well when compared with a multiple variceal ligator [240]. **A1d** In another study 50 patients with acute esophageal variceal bleeding were recruited: 25 were treated by elastic band ligation and 25 by endoloop ligation: re-bleeding 12% endoloop group and 28% ligation was not significantly different [241].

Gastric varices

The incidence of bleeding from gastric varices varies between 3% and 30%, but in most series it is less than 10% [251]. Patients with gastric variceal hemorrhage bleed more profusely and require more transfusions than patients with esophageal variceal bleeding [252]. **B4** Moreover, these patients have a higher risk of re-bleeding and a decreased survival rate compared with patients bleeding from esophageal varices. The optimal treatment of gastric variceal bleeding is not known. Limited information is available on the role of vasoactive drugs in the control of gastric fundal bleeding and balloon tamponade has been used with little success. Use of standard sclerosants is associated with unacceptable re-bleeding, particularly from necrotic ulceration, as the gastric mucosa appears much more sensitive to this than the esophagus.

Because of this, alternative sclerosant agents have been evaluated. The tissue adhesives n-butyl-2-cyanoacrylate and isobutyl-2-cyanoacrylate, mixed with lipiodol to delay premature hardening, have been evaluated, and found to be efficacious in observational, studies [253]. Isobutyl-2-cyanoacrylate has been shown to be superior to ethanolamine, in a non-randomized study, achieving hemostasis in 90% of 23 patients, as opposed to 67% of 24 patients (p < 0.005) [254].

In a randomized controlled trial of 37 patients with isolated fundic varices (acute and recent bleeding) with follow-up of 15 months, cyanoacrylate glue was shown to be more effective than sclerotherapy with alcohol for variceal obliteration (100% vs 44%, p < 0.005) [255]. There was a trend in favor of cyanoacrylate glue for the control of acute bleeding (89% vs 62%) and the need of surgical intervention (10% vs 35%), although both were statistically non-significant. Mortality was similar in the two groups. **Ald**

In another randomized trial [256] 48 patients received endoscopic band ligation (GVL) and another 49 patients received endoscopic n-butyl-2-cyanoacrylate injection (GVO). Both treatments were equally successful in controlling active bleeding (14/15 vs 14/15, p = 1.000). More of the patients who underwent GVL had GV re-bleeding (GVL vs GVO, 21/48 vs 11/49; p = 0.044). The two-year and three-year cumulative rate of GV re-bleeding were 63.1% and 72.3% for GVL, and 26.8% for both periods with GVO; p = .0143, log-rank test. Multivariate Cox regression indicated that concomitance with HCC (relative hazard: 2.453, 95% CI: 1.036–5.806, p = 0.041) and the treatment method (GVL vs GVO, relative hazard: 2.660, 95% CI: 1.167–6.061, p = 0.020) were independent factors predictive of GV re-bleeding. There was no difference in survival between the two groups.

In the study by Lo *et al.* cirrhotic patients with a history of gastric variceal bleeding were randomized to two groups [257]. The group receiving endoscopic obturation (group A) comprised 31 patients and the group receiving band ligation (group B) comprised 29 patients. Butyl cyanoacrylate and pneumatic-driven ligator were applied, respectively. Active bleeding occurred in 15 patients in group A and 11 patients in group B. Initial hemostatic rate was 87% in group A and 45% in group B (p = 0.03). The sessions required to achieve variceal obliteration and obliteration rates were similar in both the groups. However, re-bleeding rates were significantly higher in group B (54%) than group A (31%) (p = 0.0005). Nine patients of group A and 14 patients of group B died (p = 0.05). Authors concluded that endoscopic obturation using cyanoacrylate proved more effective and safer than band ligation in the management of bleeding gastric varices.

However, reports of cerebral embolism, with tissue adhesives identified at postmortem as well splenic embolization and development of retrogastric abscesses, cause concern. Interest has therefore focused on thrombin. This is much easier to administer, and has been shown to provide good early hemostasis [258]. However, in all of these studies, re-bleeding rates have remained high. Hence, in patients with re-bleeding or uncontrolled bleeding from gastric varices, devascularization surgery or portosystemic shunting has been proposed. "Salvage" TIPS is very effec-

tive in this situation, with more than 95% success rate for initial hemostasis and an early re-bleeding rate of less than 20% [251]. TIPS appears to be as effective for gastric varices as for esophageal varices.

Non-actively bleeding patients with fundal varices constitute a discrete population. The efficacy of cyanoacrylate in these patients is controversial and bleeding rates in this group can be relatively high. The Japanese experience with balloon-occluded transvenous obliteration as a prophylactic procedure in this patient population appears promising [259, 260]. TIPS, shunt surgery and, of course, liver transplantation are the only other therapeutic options for recurrent bleeding from gastric varices. The consensus at Baveno IV was to use endoscopic therapy with tissue adhesive (e.g. N-butyl-cyanoacrylate) [89]. Lastly, in a recent trial TIPS proved more effective than glue injection in preventing re-bleeding from gastric varices, with similar survival and frequency of complications [261].

Uncontrolled variceal bleeding

The definition of uncontrolled variceal bleeding includes the continued/early variceal re-bleeding (within five days) despite two sessions of therapeutic endoscopy, continued variceal bleeding despite balloon tamponade and continued/early gastric or ectopic variceal bleeding despite vasoconstrictor therapy.

Predictive models indicate grade C patients with signs of significant bleeding are the patients at risk of failure. Balloon tamponade has most often been used to arrest life-threatening hemorrhage or if other measures fail. It has also been used in the absence of a definite diagnosis if bleeding from varices is strongly suspected. The usual tube is a modified four-lumen Sengstaken-Blakemore tube (SBT). The airway should be protected by an endotracheal tube under a short general anesthetic, as the risk of aspiration is very high, particularly in unskilled hands [262]. If blood is still coming up the gastric aspiration lumen, then varices are less likely to be the cause of blood loss, although gastric fundal varices are not always controlled by tamponade. In fact, whenever this occurs, if the position of the SBT has been checked and adequate traction applied, the diagnosis of variceal bleeding should be questioned, and emergency angiography performed.

In a recent report the use of self-expandable metallic stents was evaluated to arrest uncontrollable acute variceal bleeding (20 patients mean age 52, 8 Child pugh C) [112]. The patients had not been successfully managed with prior pharmacologic or endoscopic therapy. The stents were successfully placed in all of the patients and were left in place for 2–14 days. Bleeding from the esophageal varices ceased immediately after implantation of the stent in all cases. No recurrent bleeding, morbidity, or mortality occurred during treatment with the esophageal stent. All of the stents were extracted without any complications after definitive treatment had been started.

Randomized trials of TIPS

TIPS stops bleeding in a significant percentage of patients [263]. In uncontrolled studies TIPS is effective in stopping variceal hemorrhage [251, 264, 265], but there is still a high mortality [266]. Monescillo *et al.* evaluated variceal bleeders with HVPG ≥ 20 mmHg randomly allocated to receiving transjugular intrahepatic portosystemic shunt (TIPS; HR-TIPS group, n = 26) within the first 24 hours after admission or not (HR-non-TIPS group) [96]. The HR-non-TIPS group had more treatment failures (p = 0.0001). Early TIPS placement reduced treatment failure (p = 0.003), in-hospital and one-year mortality (p < 0.05). Overall TIPS remains a good choice as a rescue therapy although when it is not available staple transection of the esophagus could be considered [267]. **Ald** In another multicentre trial an early decision for PTFE-TIPS improved survival in high risk cirrhotic patients admitted with acute variceal bleeding [268].

New diagnostic and treatment algorithms of acute variceal bleeding are needed using known predictive factors of failure to control bleeding and mortality in order to identify the group of bleeders with poor outcome. In this group more effective vasoactive regimens, early TIPS after diagnostic endoscopy, and the use of self-expanding covered esophageal stents could be considered [269].

Conclusion

The available data suggest that emergency endoscopic treatment with banding ligation or sclerotherapy, at the time of the initial diagnostic endoscopy, should be the gold standard for the management of the acute variceal bleeding episode. Sclerotherapy may be more applicable in some acute situations compared with ligation. A diagnostic endoscopy, with visualization unhindered by the ligation device, should be done first as varices may not be the source of bleeding. If ligation is to be used then this entails a double intubation and does lengthen the procedure.

Sclerotherapy is also significantly better than drug treatment alone and there is no need for further studies directly comparing sclerotherapy or ligation with one of the currently available drugs. However, the combination of sclerotherapy with a drug, given as soon as possible after admission is currently the best option. The drugs of choice for this combination are terlipressin (as mortality is reduced albeit in small placebo-controlled studies) and somatostatin (which has less side effects and has been successfully tested over five days). Further studies are needed to assess the role of tissue adhesives or fibrin glues in patients' unresponsive to vasoactive drugs or sclerotherapy.

The role of emergency TIPS as "salvage therapy" for uncontrolled bleeding from esophageal or gastric varices is now common practice but only certain centres can offer an emergency service. Randomized trials with other therapies such as esophageal stent should be performed.

Prevention of recurrent variceal bleeding

Patients surviving the first episode of variceal bleeding are at very high risk of recurrent bleeding (70% or more) and death (30–50%). All patients who have previously bled from varices should have secondary therapy to prevent further variceal bleeding [89]. There is no role for an observational policy, as all randomized studies have shown active therapy to be better than observation alone. **Ala** Hence, in clinical practice the risk indicators of long-term re-bleeding are of less clinical value, than those for first variceal bleeding. However, severity of liver disease, continued alcohol abuse and variceal size have been associated with variceal re-bleeding.

A recent development has been the proposed use of hemodynamic indices to identify patients who are more likely to re-bleed. Two such indices have been reported, using the technique of hepatic venous pressure measurement as an indicator of portal pressure. From the analysis of the Barcelona-Boston-New Haven Primary Prophylaxis trial, it was concluded that variceal bleeding did not occur with an HVPG < 12 mmHg, in patients with predominantly sinusoidal portal hypertension. However, with an HVPG > 12 mmHg, the correlation between portal pressure and bleeding risk is inconsistent.

An hemodynamic index was proposed by Feu *et al.* [270]. Patients who had a percentage reduction of HVPG of 20% or more from baseline had a re-bleeding rate of 15% compared with 50% in those who did not achieve this hemodynamic target. Unfortunately, these HVPG targets are achieved in only about one-third of patients on β-blockers, hence the introduction of combined pharmacologic therapy. Several studies on secondary prevention have used hemodynamic monitoring during combination pharmacotherapy in their design. In these studies the target values are reached only in 45–60% of patients subjected to therapy with β-blockers and nitrates. Moreover, because most re-bleeding episodes occur within one month of the index bleed, early repeat HVPG measurements are needed in order to identify the nonresponders. However, the above approach has not been confirmed in one study [271]. A randomized study has shown greater likelihood of HVPG reduction with sequential monitoring of portal pressure but no reduction in rebleeding compared to combined ligation and nadolol without monitoring of HVPG [272].

There are several options including pharmacologic, endoscopic and surgical/radiological therapies.

Randomized controlled trials for the prevention of variceal re-bleeding

β-blockers versus no treatment

A comprehensive meta-analysis of 12 trials comprising 769 patients [273–284] has been published [285]. The mean follow-up was 21 ± 5 months. There was significant heterogeneity in the evaluation of re-bleeding (p < 0.01). Treatment with β-blockers significantly decreased the risk of re-bleeding (Der Simonian and Laird method: POR 21%; 95% CI: 10–32%). The NNT with β-blockers to prevent one re-bleeding episode was 5. Survival was also significantly improved in patients treated with β-blockers. (Der Simonian and Laird method: POR 5.4%, 95% CI: 0–11%) although there was significant heterogeneity in this analysis (p < 0.01). **A1a** The NNT to prevent one death is 14. Adverse events occurred in 17% of patients and were generally mild. No fatal complication has been reported with β-blockers.

The use of hemodynamic targets (20% reduction of HVPG and/or fall <12 mmHg) to identify patients who are "non-responders" to pharmacological therapy could be a useful tool in the planning of treatment for secondary prevention of variceal bleeding. These patients could then be offered alternative therapy such as variceal ligation, or combination drug therapies, before they have further bleeding. The applicability of hemodynamic monitoring has been questioned [286], and non-responders have a 60% of re-bleeding [287]. β-blockers in association with oral nitrates have been shown to induce a greater drop in portal pressure than β-blockers alone [288] Other drugs that may work in combination with β-blockers include angiotensin-converting enzyme (ACE) inhibitors and angiotensin-II receptor antagonists [289], α-adrenoreceptor antagonists like prazosin [290] and spironolactone [291], but problems with their adverse effects, particularly hypotension and lack of efficacy, preclude their use.

β-blockers plus nitrates versus β-blockers alone

The rationale behind the use of combination therapy is that agents acting through different mechanisms may be additive or synergestic in terms of their benefit. In a recent randomized trial the addition of ISMN significantly improved the efficacy of propranolol alone in the prevention of variceal re-bleeding, but only after stratification according to age (i.e. <50 years of age vs >50 years of age; p = 0.03), or after evaluation of prolonged follow-up (3 years; p = 0.05) [292]. However, no significant difference was found in the overall rate of re-bleeding and survival. Moreover, more patients in the combination treatment group had to discontinue therapy due to adverse effects [293]. Similarly, no additional benefit from the combination

of β-blockers and ISMN was reported in an abstract [293]. **A1d** Of note is that in this study, a higher mortality was observed in the combination-therapy group. Recently, combination therapy and its effectiveness in preventing re-bleeding was assessed by hemodynamic monitoring. Although the number of patients studied was small (n = 34) and the β-blocker dose was fixed (160 mg of long-acting propranolol) the investigators reported that the addition of ISMN increased the number of responders (HVPG < 12 mmHg or >20% from baseline value) from 38% to 59%, and these patients experienced less bleeding (10% vs 64% for non-responders; p < 0.05)[294].

Sclerotherapy versus no treatment

There are seven trials, including 1111 patients [182, 281, 295–299]. The re-bleeding rate was reduced in all studies except one [295]. Meta-analysis showed that the pooled odds ratio was significantly reduced (POR 0.63; 95% CI: 0.49–0.79). Mortality was also reduced significantly in the sclerotherapy arm (POR 0.77; 95% CI: 0.61–0.98). **A1a** However, complications were frequent and did not differ from those of prophylactic or emergency sclerotherapy.

Sclerotherapy versus drugs

Eleven trials, involving 971 patients compared sclerotherapy with drugs (propranolol in ten studies [281, 300–307, 309] and nadolol plus ISMN in one study [308] for the prevention of recurrent bleeding (from any source, for example varices, portal hypertensive bleeding, or sclerotherapy ulcers) (see Table 36.10). There was a striking heterogeneity in the evaluation of re-bleeding (p = 0004): in five studies [281, 301, 305, 306, 308] re-bleeding was less frequent in patients randomized to drugs and in six studies in patients randomized to sclerotherapy [300, 302–304, 307, 309] the POR showed that there was no significant difference between the two treatment modalities (Der Simonian and Laird method: POR 0.88; 95% CI: 0.72–1.25). **A1a** There was no significant heterogeneity in the evaluation of survival (p = 0.15). More patients randomized to sclerotherapy survived, but the result was not statistically significant (POR 0.95; 95% CI: 0.58–1.32). Moreover, the number of patients free of adverse events was significantly higher in the drug group compared with sclerotherapy group (POR 0.85; 95% CI: 0.65–1.11).

Sclerotherapy plus drugs versus sclerotherapy

Twelve trials of sclerotherapy and drugs (eight propranolol [310–317], three nadolol [318–320] and one isosorbide-5-mononitrate [321] versus sclerotherapy alone, comprising 853 patients are summarized in Table 36.11). Theoretically the administration of drugs might prevent re-bleeding

Table 36.10 Randomized controlled trials of sclerotherapy versus β-blockers for the prevention of re-bleeding.

Study	No. of patients D/S	Child C (%)	Bleeding D/S	Death D/S	Adverse events D/S
Alexandrino et al. [300]	34/31	—	25/17	11/9	24/28
Dollet et al. [301]	27/28	27	11/18	12/15	0/10
Fleig et al. [302]	57/58	NR	26/26	16/20	NR
Westaby et al. [303]	52/56	—	29/28	22/21	4/0
Liu et al. [304]	58/60	NR	33/20	27/17	NR
Martin et al. [305]	34/42	24	18/23	8/13	0/19
Rossi et al. [281]	27/26	38	13/13	7/6	3/8
Andreani et al. [306]	35/40	35	12/17	9/17	ND
Dasarathy et al. [307]	53/51	34	31/19	19/10	5/9
Teres et al. [226]	58/58	14	37/26	23/21	10/23
Villanueva et al. [308]	43/43	—	11/23	4/9	—

D; drug; S: sclerotherapy; NR: not reported.

Table 36.11 Randomized controlled trials of sclerotherapy plus drugs versus sclerotherapy for the prevention of re-bleeding.

Study	No. of patients S/S + D	Bleeding S/S + D	Death S/S + D
Westaby et al. [317]	27/26	8/7	7/9
Jensen and Krarup [313]	26/25	12/3	1/1
Lundell et al. [314]	22/19	11/12	NR
Bertoni et al. [318]	14/14	4/1	3/1
Gerunda et al. [319]	30/30	7/6	3/1
Vinel et al. [316]	36/39	10/4	5/5
Avgerinos et al. [311]	40/45	21/14	9/8
Villanueva et al. [320]	18/22	7/12	0/2
Acharya et al. [310]	56/58	12/10	7/5
Vickers et al. [315]	34/39	14/17	9/9
Bertoni et al. [321]	37/39	15/4	9/2
Elsayed et al. [312]	87/91	34/13	10/11

S: sclerotherapy; S + D: sclerotherapy plus drugs; NR: not reported.

before variceal obliteration. One problem with this group of studies is that only one study evaluated β-blockers after obliteration [313]. In the others, the drug was stopped at eradication. There was statistically significant heterogeneity caused by differences between studies both in the direction and in the size of the effect of treatment: three studies were in favor of sclerotherapy alone [314, 315, 320], while nine were in favor of sclerotherapy plus β-blockers [310, 313, 316–319, 321], statistically significant difference reported in three [312, 313, 321] POR showed that there was statistically significantly less re-bleeding in the combined treatment arm (Der Simonian and Laird method: POR 0.55; 95% CI: 0.35–0.86). There was no statistically significant heterogeneity in the evaluation of survival, with no signifi-

cant difference between the treatments treatments (POR 0.77; 95% CI: 0.5–1.1) (see Figures 36.7 and 36.8). **Ala**

Combination sclerotherapy plus subcutaneous octreotide was also compared with sclerotherapy alone for the prevention of early re-bleeding, as well as for long-term management of patients after variceal hemorrhage [322]. This last study showed significantly less re-bleeding and mortality rates in the combined treatment group. However, the possibility of a severe selection bias was raised due to the exceedingly high re-bleeding rates in the sclerotherapy group. Therefore the clinical efficacy of subcutaneous octreotide in reducing re-bleeding rates remain uncertain, despite the post-prandial increase in portal pressure being blunted by octreotide but not by propranolol.

Sclerotherapy plus drugs vs drugs

In a single randomized trial 131 patients were randomly assigned to sclerotherapy plus propranolol with propranolol alone. Twenty-eight patients from the propranolol group but only 12 patients from the propranolol-plus-sclerotherapy group had recurrent bleeding from esophageal variceal rupture (p less than 0.01). The total number of blood units per patient with recurrent bleeding was slightly but not significantly more important in the propranolol group (8 +/− 7) than in thepropranolol-plus-sclerotherapy group (5 +/− 5; p = 0.09) [323]. **Ald**

Sclerotherapy versus variceal ligation

Sclerotherapy does significantly decrease re-bleeding rates and mortality, but it has been associated with serious complications, the most common of which are esophageal stricture and bleeding from treatment-induced ulcers. Variceal ligation was developed with the aim to provide an endo-

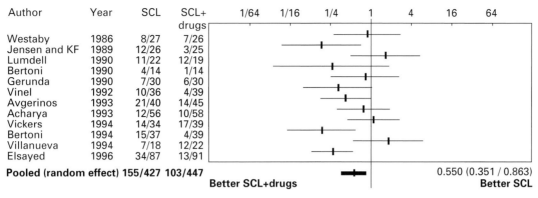

Author	Year	SCL	SCL+drugs		
Westaby	1986	8/27	7/26		
Jensen and KF	1989	12/26	3/25		
Lumdell	1990	11/22	12/19		
Bertoni	1990	4/14	1/14		
Gerunda	1990	7/30	6/30		
Vinel	1992	10/36	4/39		
Avgerinos	1993	21/40	14/45		
Acharya	1993	12/56	10/58		
Vickers	1994	14/34	17/39		
Bertoni	1994	15/37	4/39		
Villanueva	1994	7/18	12/22		
Elsayed	1996	34/87	13/91		
Pooled (random effect)		**155/427**	**103/447**		0.550 (0.351 / 0.863)

Figure 36.7 Secondary prevention: Forrest plot of randomized trials of sclerotherapy plus drugs versus sclerotherapy in secondary prevention of variceal bleeding. Variceal bleeding. SCL: sclerotherapy. Data are expressed as OR (95% CI) in a log scale.

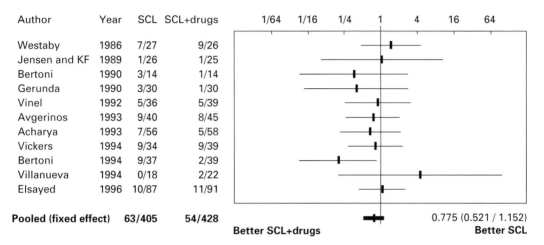

Author	Year	SCL	SCL+drugs		
Westaby	1986	7/27	9/26		
Jensen and KF	1989	1/26	1/25		
Bertoni	1990	3/14	1/14		
Gerunda	1990	3/30	1/30		
Vinel	1992	5/36	5/39		
Avgerinos	1993	9/40	8/45		
Acharya	1993	7/56	5/58		
Vickers	1994	9/34	9/39		
Bertoni	1994	9/37	2/39		
Villanueva	1994	0/18	2/22		
Elsayed	1996	10/87	11/91		
Pooled (fixed effect)		**63/405**	**54/428**		0.775 (0.521 / 1.152)

Figure 36.8 Secondary prevention: Forrest plot of randomized trials of sclerotherapy plus drugs versus sclerotherapy in secondary prevention of variceal bleeding. Mortality. SCL: sclerotherapy. Data are expressed as OR (95% CI) in a log scale.

scopic therapy at least as effective as sclerotherapy, but with fewer complications. There are 20 studies [209, 210, 212–218, 220, 242–249, 324, 325] (n = 1634) comparing sclerotherapy to variceal ligation for the prevention of recurrent bleeding.

Thirteen studies included only patients with cirrhosis [209–213, 216, 242–244, 246–248, 324], six studies involved patients with cirrhosis or non-cirrhotic portal hypertension [214, 215, 218, 220, 245, 249], and one study included only patients with hepatic fibrosis due to schistosomiasis [217]. The sclerosing agent used was sodium tetradecyl sulfate (eight trials [210–213, 216, 242, 244, 324]), ethanolamine oleate (four trials [209, 217, 245, 248]) polidocanol (two trials [243, 246]) absolute alcohol (one trial [214]) and was not reported in five studies [215, 218, 220, 247, 249]. The same ligation equipment (Bard Interventional Products, Tewksbury, Massachusetts, USA) was used in all trials. All treatment sessions were done at intervals of 1–3 weeks. Meta-analysis showed that re-bleeding was significantly less common with variceal ligation than with sclerotherapy

(POR 0.53; 95% CI: 0.42–0.67), without significant heterogeneity amongst trials. **Ala** The NNT with variceal ligation rather than with sclerotherapy to prevent one re-bleeding episode is 10 (95% CI: 7–17). Publication bias assessment showed that 121 null or negative studies would be needed to render the results of the meta-analysis statistically nonsignificant. Variceal ligation was also associated with significantly lower mortality when compared with sclerotherapy as the result just reached statistical significance (POR 0.77; 95% CI: 0.59–0.99, p = 0.048). Complications were also less common in patients treated with variceal ligation in all studies except one [209], although the size of the difference varied between studies, causing significant heterogeneity (p = 0.004). Meta-analysis showed that the difference was statistically significant in favor of variceal ligation (Der Simonian and Laird method: POR 0.29; 95% CI: 0.19–0.44). In addition, the number of treatment sessions needed to achieve variceal obliteration was less with variceal ligation in all studies (2.7–4.1 sessions with variceal ligation compared with 4–6.5 sessions with sclerotherapy).

Table 36.12 Randomized controlled trials of variceal ligation versus variceal ligation plus sclerotherapy for the prevention of re-bleeding.

Study	No. of patients L/L + S	Child C (%)	Re-bleeding L/L + S	Death L/L + S	Variceal eradication L/L + S	Complications L/L + S
Combined						
Laine et al. (1996) [325]	20/21	44	6/6	3/3	12/15	2/3
Djurdjevic et al. (1999) [222]	51/52	21%	5/7	6/7	47/46	1/3
Argonz et al. (2000) [327]	29/30	NR	11/5	9/4	16/24	1/8
Saeed et al. (1997) [328]	25/22	28	6/8	4/8	16/12	5/13
Traif et al. (1999) [329]	31/29	25	7/5	7/3	NR	7/6
El-Khayat et al. (1997) [330]	30/34	NR	2/2	¾	NR	4/6
Hou et al. (2001) [331]	47/47	20	11/13	6/7	40/41	23/31
Bobadilla-Diaz et al. (2002) [332]	15/18	NR	1/0	NR	NR	NR
Sequential						
Bhargava and Pokharna (1997) [333]	25/25	18	4/5	NR	5/20	8/14
Lo et al. (1998) [334]	35/37	21	11/3	10/7		

L, variceal ligation; L + S, variceal ligation plus sclerotherapy; NR, not reported.

There was no difference between the endoscopic modalities in the number of patients with varices obliterated (POR 1.23; 95% CI: 0.93–1.61), while the recurrence of varices was more frequent in patients treated with variceal ligation (POR 1.36; 95% CI: 0.96–1.92). **A1a** However, re-bleeding after initial eradication seems unusual especially if patients are in a regular endoscopic follow-up, and varices that recur are re-obliterated (see Table 36.12) [326].

Variceal ligation versus variceal ligation plus sclerotherapy

To further improve the results achieved with variceal ligation, which requires between three and four therapeutic sessions for variceal eradication (and 25% of patients would have an episode of recurrent bleeding before completion of therapy), variceal ligation combined with low-volume sclerotherapy has been assessed. This could lead to more rapid eradication of varices than the use of variceal ligation alone. Sclerotherapy obliterates deeper paraesophageal varices that serve as feeder vessels for the submucosal vessels, whereas ligation can only be applied to submucosal varices.

Eight studies, involving 501 patients have tested this hypothesis: six were published as peer-reviewed articles [222, 325, 327–329, 331] and two as abstracts [330, 332] (see Table 36.12). Meta-analysis showed no significant differences between the two endoscopic treatments in the number of patients with varices eradicated (POR 1.32; 95% CI: 0.77–2.25), in re-bleeding (POR 0.93; 95% CI: 0.58–1.4) or deaths (POR 0.94; 95% CI: 0.57–1.55). However, complications were significantly higher from the combined therapy compared with variceal ligation alone (POR 2.71;

95% CI: 1.48–4.96). **A1c** Moreover, the number of sessions required to achieve eradication was greater in the combined therapy arm in all studies and significantly in one [325]. A detailed meta-analysis has been published [335].

Two other randomized studies investigated whether there was an additive effect of sclerotherapy for small varices (not amenable to variceal ligation) after the completion of repeated variceal ligation treatment. Bhargava and Pokharna reported that the combined treatment eradicated the varices in a significantly greater number of patients than variceal ligation alone, but they did not find any difference in re-bleeding [333]. In contrast Lo et al. reported that the combined treatment resulted in significantly less recurrence of esophageal varices and re-bleeding [334].

Finally, three studies of comparison between combined variceal ligation and sclerotherapy with sclerotherapy alone have been reported [330, 336, 337]. There was no difference in re-bleeding and mortality between the two treatment modalities in any of these studies. Moreover, this comparison is now redundant since sclerotherapy has been replaced by variceal ligation for the secondary prevention of variceal bleeding.

Variceal ligation versus drug combination (β-blockers plus nitrates)

Six randomized controlled trials [186, 338–342] (two published as abstracts [338, 339], two using propranolol [339, 340] and the others nadolol), involving 719 patients, assessed the efficacy of variceal ligation versus drug combination of β-blockers (propranolol or nadolol) and nitrates (ISMN). We performed a meta-analysis including the updated results [342] of a previous trial [343]. There is no

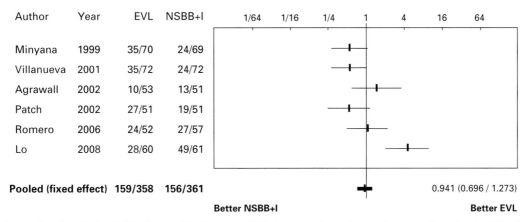

Figure 36.9 Forrest plot of randomized trials of variceal ligation versus β-blockers plus nitrates in secondary prevention of variceal bleeding. Variceal bleeding. EVL: variceal ligation; NSBB + I: β-blockers plus nitrates. Data are expressed as OR (95% CI) in a log scale.

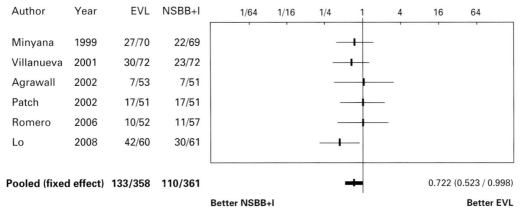

Figure 36.10 Forrest plot of randomized trials of variceal ligation versus β-blockers plus nitrates in secondary prevention of variceal bleeding. Mortality (EVL: variceal ligation, NSBB + I: β-blockers plus nitrates). Data are expressed as OR (95% CI) in a log scale.

difference in re-bleeding rate (REM, OR 0.98; 95% CI: 0.5–1.9). Importantly, regarding survival combined medical therapy is better than ligation (FEM, OR 0.72; 95% CI: 0.5–0.9). **Ala** One randomized trial has compared obliteration of n-butyl-2-cyanoacrylate versus propranolol, with no difference in re-bleeding rates nor survival, but with more complications with the adhesive injection (see Table 36.13 and Figures 36.9 and 36.10) [344].

Variceal ligation plus drugs vs ligation

In a prospective randomized trial, a total of 122 patients with a history of esophageal variceal bleeding were randomized to receive EVL only (group A, 62 patients) or triple therapy (group B, 60 patients, ligation plus nadolol and sucralfate) [345].

After a median follow-up of 21 months, recurrent upper gastrointestinal bleeding developed in 29 patients (47%) in group A and 14 patients (23%) in group B (p = 0.005). Recurrent bleeding from esophagogastric varices occurred

in 18 patients in group A and 7 patients in group B (p = 0.001). Twenty-one patients in group A (50%) and 12 patients (26%) in group B experienced variceal recurrence after variceal obliteration (p < 0.05). Treatment failure occurred in 11 patients (18%) in group A and in 4 patients (7%) in group B (p = 0.05). Twenty patients from group A and 10 patients from group B died (p = 0.08); 9 and 4 of these deaths, respectively, were attributed to variceal hemorrhage (p = 0.26). The combination of ligation, nadolol and sucralfate (triple therapy) proved more effective than banding ligation alone in terms of prevention of variceal recurrence and upper gastrointestinal re-bleeding as well as variceal re-bleeding. **Ald** In another multicentre trial 80 patients randomized to receive EVL plus nadolol or EVL alone [250]. The variceal bleeding recurrence rate was 14% in the EVL plus nadolol group and 38% in the EVL group (p = 0.006). Mortality was similar in both groups. The actuarial probability of variceal recurrence at one year was lower in the EVL plus nadolol group (54%) than in the EVL group (77%; p = 0.06). **Ald**

TIPS versus drug therapy

Escorsell *et al.* compared TIPS with drug therapy and found that the two-year re-bleeding rate was significantly lower in the TIPS group [346]. A total of 91 Child-Pugh class B/C cirrhotic patients surviving their first episode of variceal bleeding were randomized to receive TIPS (n = 47) or drug therapy (propranolol + isosorbide-5-mononitrate) (n = 44) to prevent variceal re-bleeding. Re-bleeding occurred in six (13%) TIPS-treated patients versus 17 (39%) drug-treated

patients (p = 0.007). The two-year re-bleeding probability was 13% versus 49% (p = .01). Encephalopathy was more frequent in TIPS than in drug-treated patients (38% vs 14%, p = 0.007). Child-Pugh class improved more frequently in drug-treated than in TIPS-treated patients (72% vs 45%; p = 0.04). The two-year survival probability was identical (72%). Medical therapy was less effective than TIPS in preventing re-bleeding. However, it caused less encephalopathy, identical survival, and more frequent improvement in Child-Pugh class with lower costs than TIPS in high-risk cirrhotic patients.

Table 36.13 Randomized controlled trials of variceal ligation versus β-blockers plus nitrates.

Study	No. of patients Lig/D	Re-bleeding Lig/D	Death Lig/D
Minyana *et al.* (1999) [338]	70/69	35/24	27/22
Villanueva *et al.* (2001) [186]	72/72	35/24	30/23
Agrawall *et al.* (2002) [339]	53/51	10/13	7/7
Romero *et al.* (2006) [341]	52/57	24/27	10/11
Patch *et al.* (2002) [340]	51/51	27/19	17/17
Lo *et al.* (2008) [342]	60/61	28/49	42/30

Lig: variceal ligation; D: β-blockers + nitrates; NR: not reported.

TIPS versus sclerotherapy or variceal ligation and covered stents

Thirteen trials, involving 948 patients, compared TIPS with endoscopic treatment (with or without the addition of propranolol): nine with sclerotherapy [347–355] and four with variceal ligation [356–359] (one in abstract form [350]) (see Table 36.14). The median range of follow up was from 10 to 32 months. Re-bleeding was significantly less common in patients randomized to TIPS (POR 3.28; 95% CI: 2.28–4.72). However, there was a trend toward fewer deaths in the endoscopic treatment arm, although the difference was not statistically significant (POR 0.87; 95% CI: 0.65–1.17). **Ald** In addition, hepatic encephalopathy was statistically significantly more common in patients randomized to TIPS (POR 0.48; 95% CI: 0.34–0.67). These results are a mirror image of the surgical trials for the secondary prevention of variceal bleeding. However, an important difference is that the mean follow up was less than two years in all but two of these trials [354, 359], whereas the surgical shunt trials had a much greater average follow-up (3–4 years). As TIPS

Table 36.14 Randomized controlled trials of TIPS versus sclerotherapy/variceal ligation for the prevention of re-bleeding.

Study	No. of patients TIPS/Scl	Child C (%)	Re-bleeding TIPS/Scl	Death TIPS/Scl	PSE TIPS/Scl
GEAIH (1995) [350]	32/33	100	13/20	16/14	—
Cabrera *et al.* (1996) [347]	31/32	10	7/16	6/5	10/4
Sanyal *et al.* (1997) [354]	41/39	49	10/9	12/7	12/5
Cello *et al.* (1997) [348]	24/25	NR	3/12	8/8	12/11
Rossle *et al.* (1997) [353]	61/65	18	9/29	8/8	18/9
Sauer *et al.* (1997) [355]	42/41	24	6/21	12/11	14/3
Merli *et al.* (1998) [351]	38/43	12	7/17	9/8	21/10
Garcia-Villarreal *et al.* (1999) [349]	22/24	32	2/12	1/8	5/6
Jalan *et al.* (1997) [356]	31/27	47	3/15	13/10	5/3
Pomier-Layrargues *et al.* (1997) [357]	41/39	NR	10/22	17/12	13/10
Narahara *et al.* (2001) [352]	38/40	NR	7/13	11/7	13/6
Gulberg *et al.* (2002) [358]	28/26	11	7/7	4/4	2/1
Sauer *et al.* (2002) [359]	43/42	29	7/10	8/7	17/9

Scl: sclerotherapy; NR: not reported; POR: pooled odds ratio; TIPS: transjugular intrahepatic portosystemic shunt; PSE: porto-systemic encephalopathy.

stenosis occured in 50–70% of patients within the first year, this approach involves regular monitoring with Doppler/ultrasound, and repeat procedures for recanalization [359]. A similar conclusion was reached in a trial comparing TIPS to propranolol and ISMN in 91 patients with cirrhosis and a Child-Pugh score >7 [346]. TIPS, although effective in reducing re-bleeding did not improve survival, caused hepatic encephalopathy and had a worse cost-benefit profile than pharmacological treatment. However, current TIPS shunts are covered stents with a much reduced chance of dysfunction. Finally, in a recent trial patients who required TIPS for the prevention of esophageal variceal re-bleeding were randomized to either TIPS alone (n = 39, group 1) or TIPSS plus VBL (n = 40, group 2) [361]. In group 1, patients underwent long-term TIPS angiographic surveillance. In group 2, patients entered a banding programme with TIPS surveillance only continued for up to one year. There was a tendency to higher variceal re-bleeding in group 2, although this did not reach statistical significance (8% vs 15%; relative hazard 0.58; 95% CI: 0.15–2.33, p = 0.440). Mortality (47% vs 40%; relative hazard 1.31; 95% CI: 0.66–2.61, p = 0.434) was similar in the two groups. Hepatic encephalopathy was significantly less in group 2 (20% vs 39%; relative hazard 2.63; 95% CI: 1.11–6.25; p = 0.023). Hepatic encephalopathy was not statistically different after correcting for sex and portal pressure gradient (p = 0.136). Therefore, VBL with short-term TIPS surveillance is an alternative to long-term TIPS surveillance in the prevention of esophageal variceal bleeding. A covered stent was evaluated in a randomized trial of 80 patients with cirrhosis with uncontrolled bleeding (n = 23) or recurrent bleeding (n = 25), or refractory ascites (n = 32) who received either a polytetrafluoroethylene-covered stent (group 1: 39 patients) or the usual uncovered prosthesis (group 2: 41 patients) [361]. After a median follow-up of 300 days, five patients (13%) in group 1 and 18 (44%) in group 2 experienced shunt dysfunction (p < 0.001). Clinical relapse occurred in three patients (8%) in group 1 and 12 (29%) in group 2 (p < 0.05). Actuarial rates of encephalopathy were 21% in group 1 and 41% in group 2 at one year (not significant). Estimated probabilities of survival were 71% and 60% at one year and 65% and 41% at two years in groups 1 and 2 respectively (not significant). Thus, the use of polytetrafluoroethylene-covered prostheses improves transjugular intrahepatic portosystemic shunt patency and decreases the number of clinical relapses and reinterventions without increasing the risk of encephalopathy, and is the standard stent to be used.

Endoscopic histoacryl obliteration vs propranolol and other studies

In a randomized study 41 patients with a first bleeding from esophageal (n = 31) or gastric (n = 10) varices were after primary hemostasis with obliteration using Histoacryl® were randomly allocated either to undergo complete Histoacryl® obliteration of the remaining varices (group A, n = 21) or to long-term propranolol administration (group B, n = 20), for the prevention of re-bleeding [344]. No significant difference was observed between groups A and B with regard to the incidence of early re-bleeding (during the first 6 weeks; 5/21 and 3/20), bleeding-related deaths by six weeks (3/21 and 6/20), long-term re-bleeding (11/21 and 5/20), or overall number of deaths (9/21 and 9/20). The incidence of complications was higher in group A (10/21) than group B (2/20) (p < 0.03). **Ald** In two trials treatment with ligation followed by argon plasma coagulation (APC) was superior compared with ligation alone [363, 364]. In another randomized trial 50 cirrhotic patients with esophageal varices randomized into two groups: endoscopic sclerotherapy (ES) (n = 25) vs EUS-guided sclerotherapy (EUS-ES) (n = 25)[365]. EUS-ES was as safe and effective as ES in variceal eradication. Recurrence tended to be less frequent and occured later.

Surgical shunts

The ideal patients for a decompressive surgical shunt, should be well compensated patients with cirrhosis, who have had troublesome bleeding, either failing at least one other modality of therapy (drugs or sclerotherapy), or had bleeding from gastric varices despite medical or endoscopic therapy, or who live far from suitable medical services. These shunts achieve an overall re-bleeding rate of 14.3% and a survival rate of 86%, but they may cause encephalopathy in 20.6% of patients (severe encephalopathy in 3%). The advent of TIPS has had a major impact on the need for these operations. Today, a common indication for a surgical shunt is in patients who have had TIPS, without major encephalopathy, but have had recurrent symptomatic TIPS dysfunction. In essence, they have had a non-surgical trial of shunting, and have selected themselves as good candidates. Small diameter portacaval H-graft or distal splenorenal shunts are probably the favored surgical option, as the portal vein is then still available should liver transplantation be required.

Randomized controlled trials of surgical therapy

Total portacaval shunt versus selective distal splenorenal shunt

Selective distal splenorenal shunt (DSRS) was designed to reduce the incidence of hepatic encephalopathy and liver failure following total portacaval shunt (PCS) by partially maintaining portal liver perfusion while decreasing portal blood flow to varices. Six trials, including 336 patients, compared PCS with DSRS [366–371]. A meta-analysis of these trials has been published [26]. There was no statistical significance in re-bleeding between the two surgical treatments (POR 0.88; 95% CI: 0.54–1.45). Patients with DSRS showed a trend toward less hepatic encephalopathy (POR 1.29; 95% CI: 0.76–2.17) and better long-term survival (POR 1.28; 95% CI: 0.82–2.01), but the differences were not statistically significant. **Ala** The calibrated small-diameter portacaval H-graft shunt (PCHGS) is effective in the control of variceal hemorrhage and has been associated with reduced hepatic encephalopathy when compared with total PCS [372]. **Ald**

Surgery versus drugs

A randomized controlled trial including 119 patients compared the effectiveness of portal blood flow preserving procedures (selective shunts and the Sugiura-Futagawa operation), β-blockers and sclerotherapy for secondary prevention of variceal hemorrhage [373]. The re-bleeding rate was significantly lower in the surgical group compared with patients receiving drugs (16.6% vs 77.5%, p < 0.0001) and survival was better for Child's A cirrhosis in all groups, but there was no significant difference between treatment groups considered as a whole. **Ald**

Surgery versus sclerotherapy

DSRS was compared with sclerotherapy in four trials, involving 292 patients (see Table 36.15) [374–377]. A comprehensive meta-analysis of these studies, using individual patient data provided by the principal authors, has been previously published [378]. **Ala** Re-bleeding was statistically significantly reduced by DSRS (pooled relative risk (PRR) 0.16; 95% CI: 0.10–0.27). There was statistically significant heterogeneity in the evaluation of mortality, as the risk of death was increased in one study [376] and decreased in the other three [374, 375, 377]. The pooled relative risk was not statistically significant between the treatment modalities (PRR 0.78; 95% CI: 0.47–1.29). Chronic hepatic

encephalopathy was increased after DSRS but the difference was not statistically significant (PRR 1.86; 95% CI: 0.90–3.86). **Ala** The results of this meta-analysis are in accordance with the trial discussed above in which significantly lower re-bleeding rates were documented in the surgical compared with sclerotherapy group (16.7% vs 63%, p < 0.0001), but no difference in mortality was observed [309]. However, this study was heavily criticized for the different exclusion criteria that were used in different treatment arms, the lack of information regarding cause of portal hypertension and differences in the surveillance endoscopy program. Finally, two trials [379, 380] (one an abstract [379]) have compared PCS with sclerotherapy in the elective treatment of variceal hemorrhage. Re-bleeding was significantly less in the portacaval shunt group. However, the incidence of hepatic encephalopathy was significantly increased with the surgical treatment and there was no difference in survival.

Surgery versus TIPS

Recently Rosemurgy *et al.* extended the follow-up (median four years) of a previously published randomized trial comparing 8 mm prosthetic H-graft portacaval shunts (HGPCS) with TIPS as definitive therapy for bleeding varices who failed non-operative management [381]. **Ald** The trial included 132 patients and shunting was carried out as an elective, urgent or emergency procedure. Placement of TIPS (non-covered stents) resulted in more re-bleeding (16% vs 3%), liver transplantations (7.5% vs 0%) and late deaths (34% vs 13.2%). According to a cost-benefit analysis carried out by the same group of investigators, TIPS was associated with much higher costs than HGPCS, due to subsequent occlusion and re-bleeding [382]. DSRS has also been shown to be superior to TIPS in terms of recurrent bleeding (6.25% vs 25.7%), encephalopathy (18.75% vs 42.86%) and shunt occlusion (6.25% vs 68.57%) in a comparative study with 67 patients with Child's A and B cirrhosis [383]. Finally Zachs *et al.* recently showed that in a population of Child's A cirrhosis, DSRS is a more cost-effective treatment than TIPS [384]. Given

Table 36.15 Randomized controlled trials of DSRS versus sclerotherapy for the prevention of re-bleeding.

Study	No. of patients DSRS/Scl	Child C (%)	Re-bleeding DSRS/Scl	Death DSRS/Scl	PSE DSRS/Scl
Henderson *et al.* (1990) [376]	35/37	43	1/22	20/12	5/3
Teres *et al.* (1987) [375]	57/55	7.3a	6/18	9/15	8/3
Rikkers *et al.* (1987) [374]	30/30	42	5/18	12/20	6/4
Spina *et al.* (1990) [377]	34/32	0	1/10	4/8	2/2

aChild score. DSRS: distal splenorenal shunt; Scl: sclerotherapy; NR: not reported; PSE: porto-systemic encephalopathy.

the better results with covered stents it is likely that if TIPS is available, surgical shunts will be reserved for patients in whom TIPS cannot be placed for technical reasons.

Conclusion

Pharmacological treatment with β-blockers is a safe and effective long-term treatment for the prevention of recurrence of variceal bleeding. The combination of β-blockers with isosorbide-5-mononitrate needs further testing in randomized controlled trials. The use of hemodynamic targets of HVPG response should be further evaluated for their applicability in clinical practice during pharmacologic therapy for the prevention of re-bleeding. If endoscopic treatment is chosen, variceal ligation is the modality of choice. The combination of simultaneous variceal ligation and sclerotherapy does not offer any benefit. However, the use of additional sclerotherapy for the complete eradication of small varices after variceal ligation should be further addressed in future trials. The results of randomized controlled trials comparing variceal ligation with pharmacologic treatment showed that combination treatment with non-selective β-blockers and nitrates and variceal ligation are equally effective. Combined endoscopic and pharmacological therapy gives the lowest re-bleeding rates but survival is no different. However non-selective beta-blockers also prevent other complications of cirrhosis [385–389] and so will be a fixed component of combination therapy. Finally, the use of TIPS for the secondary prevention of variceal bleeding is not supported by the current data, mainly because of its worse cost-benefit profile compared with other treatments. However, this conclusion is based on uncovered stents. Covered stents may be more effective, and are the stent of choice. There is a limited role for the selective surgical shunts (DSRS or HGPCS) in the modern management of portal hypertension. The ideal patient should have well compensated cirrhosis, have had troublesome bleeding, have failed at least one other modality of therapy (drugs or ligation), or have bled from gastric varices despite medical or endoscopic therapy or live far from suitable medical services, or for whom TIPS is not available.

Summary

In conclusion, this critical review of the studies of treatment in portal hypertension has highlighted several issues with regard to the design of clinical trials and the analysis of the data that should be addressed in future trials. The quality of future trials will also be significantly improved if standardized definitions of critical endpoints (for example bleeding or re-bleeding episodes, treatment failure, etc.), agreed upon in consensus conferences are applied. This will aid the reduction of the heterogeneity

that is present in randomized controlled trials in portal hypertension and lead to better evidence for the optimal treatment options.

References

1 DerSimonian R, Laird N. Meta-analysis in clinical trials. *Control Clin Trials* 1986; **7**(3): 177–188.

2 D'Amico G, Luca A. Natural history. Clinical-haemodynamic correlations. Prediction of the risk of bleeding. *Baillière's Clin Gastroenterol* 1997; **11**(2): 243–256.

3 Fleig WE. To scope or not to scope: still a question. *Hepatology* 2001; **33**(2): 471–472.

4 Ong J. Clinical predictors of large esophageal varices: how accurate are they? *Am J Gastroenterol* 1999; **94**(11): 3103–3105.

5 Pilette C, Oberti F, Aube C, Rousselet MC *et al.* Non-invasive diagnosis of esophageal varices in chronic liver diseases. *J Hepatol* 1999; **31**(5): 867–873.

6 Schepis F, Camma C, Niceforo D *et al.* Which patients with cirrhosis should undergo endoscopic screening for esophageal varices detection? *Hepatology* 2001; **33**(2): 333–338.

7 Burton JR, Jr, Liangpunsakul S, Lapidus J, Giannini E, Chalasani N, Zaman A. Validation of a multivariate model predicting presence and size of varices. *J Clin Gastroenterol* 2007; **41**(6): 609–615.

8 Armonis A, Patch D, Burroughs A. Hepatic venous pressure measurement: an old test as a new prognostic marker in cirrhosis? *Hepatology* 1997; **25**(1): 245–248.

9 Groszmann RJ, Garcia-Tsao G, Bosch J *et al.* Beta-blockers to prevent gastroesophageal varices in patients with cirrhosis. *N Engl J Med* 2005; **353**(21): 2254–2261.

10 Nevens F, Bustami R, Scheys I, Lesaffre E, Fevery J. Variceal pressure is a factor predicting the risk of a first variceal bleeding: a prospective cohort study in cirrhotic patients. *Hepatology* 1998; **27**(1): 15–19.

11 Ripoll C, Groszmann R, Garcia-Tsao G *et al.* Hepatic venous pressure gradient predicts clinical decompensation in patients with compensated cirrhosis. *Gastroenterology* 2007; **133**(2): 481–488.

12 Eisen GM, Eliakim R, Zaman A *et al.* The accuracy of PillCam ESO capsule endoscopy versus conventional upper endoscopy for the diagnosis of esophageal varices: a prospective three-center pilot study. *Endoscopy* 2006; **38**(1): 31–35.

13 Gralnek IM, Adler SN, Yassin K, Koslowsky B, Metzger Y, Eliakim R. Detecting esophageal disease with second-generation capsule endoscopy: initial evaluation of the PillCam ESO 2. *Endoscopy* 2008; **40**(4): 275–279.

14 de Franchis R, Eisen GM, Laine L *et al.* Esophageal capsule endoscopy for screening and surveillance of esophageal varices in patients with portal hypertension. *Hepatology* 2008; **47**(5): 1595–1603.

15 Lapalus MG, Dumortier J, Fumex F *et al.* Esophageal capsule endoscopy versus esophagogastroduodenoscopy for evaluating portal hypertension: a prospective comparative study of performance and tolerance. *Endoscopy* 2006; **38**(1): 36–41.

16 Feu F, Bordas JM, Garcia-Pagan JC, Bosch J, Rodes J. Double-blind investigation of the effects of propranolol and placebo on

the pressure of esophageal varices in patients with portal hypertension. *Hepatology* 1991; **13**(5): 917–922.

17 Cales P, Oberti F, Payen JL *et al.* Lack of effect of propranolol in the prevention of large oesophageal varices in patients with cirrhosis: a randomized trial. French-Speaking Club for the Study of Portal Hypertension. *Eur J Gastroenterol Hepatol* 1999; **11**(7): 741–745.

18 Merkel C, Marin R, Angeli P *et al.* A placebo-controlled clinical trial of nadolol in the prophylaxis of growth of small esophageal varices in cirrhosis. *Gastroenterology* 2004; **127**(2): 476–484.

19 Prediction of the first variceal hemorrhage in patients with cirrhosis of the liver and esophageal varices. A prospective multicenter study. The North Italian Endoscopic Club for the Study and Treatment of Esophageal Varices. *N Engl J Med* 1988; **319**(15): 983–989.

20 Merli M, Nicolini G, Angeloni S *et al.* Incidence and natural history of small esophageal varices in cirrhotic patients. *J Hepatol* 2003; **38**(3): 266–272.

21 Grace ND, Groszmann RJ, Garcia-Tsao G *et al.* Portal hypertension and variceal bleeding: an AASLD single topic symposium. *Hepatology* 1998; **28**(3): 868–880.

22 Conn HO, Lindenmuth WW. Prophylactic portacaval anastomosis in cirrhotic patients with esophageal varices: a progress report of a continuing study. *N Engl J Med* 1965; **272**: 1255–1263.

23 Jackson FC, Perrin EB, Smith AG, Dagradi AE, Nadal HM. A clinical investigation of the portacaval shunt. II. Survival analysis of the prophylactic operation. *Am J Surg* 1968; **115**(1): 22–42.

24 Resnick RH, Chalmers TC, Ishihara AM *et al.* A controlled study of the prophylactic portacaval shunt. A final report. *Ann Intern Med* 1969; **70**(4): 675–688.

25 Conn HO, Lindenmuth WW, May CJ, Ramsby GR. Prophylactic portacaval anastomosis. *Medicine (Baltimore)* 1972; **51**(1): 27–40.

26 D'Amico G, Pagliaro L, Bosch J. The treatment of portal hypertension: a meta-analytic review. *Hepatology* 1995; **22**(1): 332–354.

27 Inokuchi K. Improved survival after prophylactic portal nondecompression surgery for esophageal varices: a randomized clinical trial. Cooperative Study Group of Portal Hypertension of Japan. *Hepatology* 1990; **12**(1): 1–6.

28 Paquet KJ. Prophylactic endoscopic sclerosing treatment of the esophageal wall in varices – a prospective controlled randomized trial. *Endoscopy* 1982; **14**(1): 4–5.

29 Witzel L, Wolbergs E, Merki H. Prophylactic endoscopic sclerotherapy of oesophageal varices. A prospective controlled study. *Lancet* 1985; **1**(8432): 773–775.

30 Koch H, Henning H, Grimm H, Soehendra N. Prophylactic sclerosing of esophageal varices – results of a prospective controlled study. *Endoscopy* 1986; **18**(2): 40–43.

31 Kobe E, Zipprich B, Schentke KU, Nilius R. Prophylactic endoscopic sclerotherapy of esophageal varices – a prospective randomized trial. *Endoscopy* 1990; **22**(6): 245–248.

32 Wordehoff D, Spech HJ. Prophylactic sclerosing of esophageal varices. Results of a prospective randomized 7-year longitudinal study. *Dtsch Med Wochenschr* 1987; **112**(24): 947–951.

33 Santangelo WC, Dueno MI, Estes BL, Krejs GJ. Prophylactic sclerotherapy of large esophageal varices. *N Engl J Med* 1988; **318**(13): 814–818.

34 Sauerbruch T, Wotzka R, Kopcke W *et al.* Prophylactic sclerotherapy before the first episode of variceal hemorrhage in patients with cirrhosis. *N Engl J Med* 1988; **319**(1): 8–15.

35 Piai G, Cipolletta L, Claar M *et al.* Prophylactic sclerotherapy of high-risk esophageal varices: results of a multicentric prospective controlled trial. *Hepatology* 1988; **8**(6): 1495–1500.

36 Potzi R, Bauer P, Reichel W, Kerstan E, Renner F, Gangl A. Prophylactic endoscopic sclerotherapy of oesophageal varices in liver cirrhosis. A multicentre prospective controlled randomised trial in Vienna. *Gut* 1989; **30**(6): 873–879.

37 Russo A, Giannone G, Magnano A, Passanisi G, Longo C. Prophylactic sclerotherapy in nonalcoholic liver cirrhosis: preliminary results of a prospective controlled randomized trial. *World J Surg* 1989; **13**(2): 149–153.

38 Andreani T, Poupon RE, Balkau BJ *et al.* Preventive therapy of first gastrointestinal bleeding in patients with cirrhosis: results of a controlled trial comparing propranolol, endoscopic sclerotherapy and placebo. *Hepatology* 1990; **12**(6): 1413–1419.

39 Triger DR, Smart HL, Hosking SW, Johnson AG. Prophylactic sclerotherapy for esophageal varices: long-term results of a single-center trial. *Hepatology* 1991; **13**(1): 117–123.

40 Prophylactic sclerotherapy for esophageal varices in men with alcoholic liver disease. A randomized, single-blind, multicenter clinical trial. The Veterans Affairs Cooperative Variceal Sclerotherapy Group. *N Engl J Med* 1991; **324**(25): 1779–1784.

41 de Franchis R, Primignani M, Arcidiacono PG *et al.* Prophylactic sclerotherapy in high-risk cirrhotics selected by endoscopic criteria. A multicenter randomized controlled trial. *Gastroenterology* 1991; **101**(4): 1087–1093.

42 Saggioro A, Pallini P, Chiozzini G, Nardin M, Ancilotto F. Prophylactic sclerotherapy – a controlled-study (Abstract). *Dig Dis Sci* 1986; **31**: S504.

43 Fleig WE, Stange EF, Wordehoff D *et al.* Prophylactic (Ps) Vs therapeutic sclerotherapy (Ts) In cirrhotic patients with large esophageal varices and no previous hemorrhage – a randomized clinical trial (Abstract). *Hepatology* 1988; **8**: 1242.

44 Strauss E, Desa MG, Albano A, Lacet CC, Leite MO, Maffei RA. A randomized controlled trial for the prevention of the 1st upper gastrointestinal bleeding due to portal hypertension in cirrhosis – sclerotherapy or propranolol versus cintrol groups (Abstract). *Hepatology* 1988; **8**: 1395.

45 Planas R, Boix J, Dominguez M *et al.* Prophylactic sclerosis of esophageal varices (EV). Prospective trial (Abstract). *J Hepatol* 1989; **9**: S73.

46 Paquet KJ, Kalk JF, Klein CP, Gad HA. Prophylactic sclerotherapy for esophageal varices in high-risk cirrhotic patients selected by endoscopic and hemodynamic criteria: a randomized, single-center controlled trial. *Endoscopy* 1994; **26**(9): 734–740.

47 Van Buuren HR, Rasch MC, Batenburg PL *et al.* Endoscopic sclerotherapy compared with no specific treatment for the primary prevention of bleeding from esophageal varices. A randomized controlled multicentre trial (ISRCTN03215899). *BMC Gastroenterol* 2003; **3**(1): 22.

48 PROVA. Prophylaxis of first hemorrhage from esophageal varices by sclerotherapy, propranolol or both in cirrhotic patients: a randomized multicenter trial. The PROVA Study Group. *Hepatology* 1991; **14**(6): 1016–1024.

49 Pagliaro L, D'Amico G, Sorensen TI et al. Prevention of first bleeding in cirrhosis. A meta-analysis of randomized trials of nonsurgical treatment. *Ann Intern Med* 1992; **117**(1): 59–70.

50 Laine L, Cook D. Endoscopic ligation compared with sclerotherapy for treatment of esophageal variceal bleeding. A meta-analysis. *Ann Intern Med* 1995; **123**(4): 280–287.

51 Chen C, Chang TT. Prophylactic endoscopic variceal ligation (EVL) for esophageal varices. *Gastroenterology* 1997; **112**: A1240.

52 Gameel K, Waked I, Saleh S, Sallam M, Abdel-Fatah S. Prophylactic endoscopic variceal band ligation (EVL) versus sclerotherapy (ES) for the prevention of variceal bleeding: an interim report of a prospective randomized controlled trial in schistosomal portal hypertension. *Hepatology* 1995; **22**: 251A.

53 Lay CS, Tsai YT, Teg CY et al. Endoscopic variceal ligation in prophylaxis of first variceal bleeding in cirrhotic patients with high-risk esophageal varices. *Hepatology* 1997; **25**(6): 1346–1350.

54 Lo GH, Lai KH, Cheng JS, Lin CK, Hsu PI, Chiang HT. Prophylactic banding ligation of high-risk esophageal varices in patients with cirrhosis: a prospective, randomized trial. *J Hepatol* 1999; **31**(3): 451–456.

55 Omar MM, Attia MH, Mostafa IM. Prophylactic band ligation to prevent first bleeding from large esophageal varices. *Gastrointest Endosc* 2000; **51**: AB122.

56 Sarin SK, Guptan RK, Jain AK, Sundaram KR. A randomized controlled trial of endoscopic variceal band ligation for primary prophylaxis of variceal bleeding. *Eur J Gastroenterol Hepatol* 1996; **8**(4): 337–342.

57 Triantos C, Vlachogiannakos J, Armonis A et al. Primary prophylaxis of variceal bleeding in cirrhotics unable to take blockers: a randomized trial of ligation. *Alimentary Pharmacology and Therapeutics* 2005; **21**(12): 1435–1443.

58 Schepke M, Kleber G, Nurnberg D et al. Ligation versus propranolol for the primary prophylaxis of variceal bleeding in cirrhosis. *Hepatology* 2004; **40**(1): 65–72.

59 Triantos C, Vlachogiannakos J, Manolakopoulos S, Burroughs A, Avgerinos A. Is banding ligation for primary prevention of variceal bleeding as effective as beta-blockers, and is it safe? *Hepatology* 2006; **43**(1): 196–197.

60 Svoboda P, Kantorova I, Ochmann J, Kozumplik L, Marsova J. A prospective randomized controlled trial of sclerotherapy vs ligation in the prophylactic treatment of high-risk esophageal varices. *Surg Endosc* 1999; **13**(6): 580–584.

61 Pascal JP, Cales P. Propranolol in the prevention of first upper gastrointestinal tract hemorrhage in patients with cirrhosis of the liver and esophageal varices. *N Engl J Med* 1987; **317**(14): 856–861.

62 Ideo G, Bellati G, Fesce E, Grimoldi D. Nadolol can prevent the first gastrointestinal bleeding in cirrhotics: a prospective, randomized study. *Hepatology* 1988; **8**(1): 6–9.

63 Lebrec D, Poynard T, Capron JP et al. Nadolol for prophylaxis of gastrointestinal bleeding in patients with cirrhosis. A randomized trial. *J Hepatol* 1988; **7**(1): 118–125.

64 Propranolol prevents first gastrointestinal bleeding in non-ascitic cirrhotic patients. Final report of a multicenter randomized trial. The Italian Multicenter Project for Propranolol in Prevention of Bleeding. *J Hepatol* 1989; **9**(1): 75–83.

65 Conn HO, Grace ND, Bosch J et al. Propranolol in the prevention of the first hemorrhage from esophagogastric varices: a multi-center, randomized clinical trial. The Boston-New Haven-Barcelona Portal Hypertension Study Group. *Hepatology* 1991; **13**(5): 902–912.

66 Colman J, Jones P, Finch C, Dudley F. Propranolol in the prevention of variceal hemorrhage in alcoholic cirrhotic patients (Abstract). *Hepatology* 1990; **8**: 1395A.

67 Perez-Ayuso RM, Pique JM, Bosch J et al. Propranolol in prevention of recurrent bleeding from severe portal hypertensive gastropathy in cirrhosis. *Lancet* 1991; **337**(8755): 1431–1434.

68 Poynard T, Cales P, Pasta L et al. Beta-adrenergic-antagonist drugs in the prevention of gastrointestinal bleeding in patients with cirrhosis and esophageal varices. An analysis of data and prognostic factors in 589 patients from four randomized clinical trials. Franco-Italian Multicenter Study Group. *N Engl J Med* 1991; **324**(22): 1532–1538.

69 Abraczinskas DR, Ookubo R, Grace ND et al. Propranolol for the prevention of first esophageal variceal hemorrhage: a lifetime commitment? *Hepatology* 2001; **34**(6): 1096–1102.

70 Chen C, Sheu M, Su S. Prophylactic endoscopic variceal ligation (EVL) with multiple band ligator for esophageal varices (Abstract). *Gastroenterology* 1998; **144**(4): A1224.

71 Sarin SK, Lamba GS, Kumar M, Misra A, Murthy NS. Comparison of endoscopic ligation and propranolol for the primary prevention of variceal bleeding. *N Engl J Med* 1999; **340**(13): 988–993.

72 De BK, Ghoshal UC, Das T, Santra A, Biswas PK. Endoscopic variceal ligation for primary prophylaxis of oesophageal variceal bleed: preliminary report of a randomized controlled trial. *J Gastroenterol Hepatol* 1999; **14**(3): 220–224.

73 De la Mora J, Farca-Belsaguy A, Uribe M, De Hoyos-Garza A. Ligation vs propranolol for primary prophylaxis of variceal bleeding using a multiple band ligator and objective measurements of treatment adequacy: preliminary results. *Gastroenterology* 2000; **1118**(4): 6512.

74 Song I, Shin J, Kim I et al. A prospective randomized trial between the prophylactic endoscopic variceal ligation and propranolol administration for prevention of first bleeding in cirrhotic patients with high risk esophageal varices (Abstract). *J Hepatol* 2000; **32**(suppl. 2): 41.

75 Lui HF, Stanley AJ, Forrest EH et al. Primary prophylaxis of variceal hemorrhage: a randomized controlled trial comparing band ligation, propranolol, and isosorbide mononitrate. *Gastroenterology* 2002; **123**(3): 735–744.

76 Gheorge C, Gheorge L, Vadan R, Hrehoret D, Popescu I. Prophylactic banding ligation of high risk esophageal varices in patients on the waiting list for liver transplantation: an interim report (Abstact). *J Hepatol* 2002; **36**(suppl. 1): 38.

77 Drastich P, Lata J, Petryl J et al. Endoscopic variceal band ligation in comparison with propranolol in prophylaxis of first variceal bleeding in patients with liver cirrhosis (Abstract). *J Hepatol* 2005; **42**(suppl. 2): 79.

78 Lo GH, Chen WC, Chen MH et al. Endoscopic ligation vs nadolol in the prevention of first variceal bleeding in patients with cirrhosis. *Gastrointest Endosc* 2004; **59**(3): 333–338.

79 Jutabha R, Jensen DM, Martin P, Savides T, Han SH, Gornbein J. Randomized study comparing banding and propranolol to prevent initial variceal hemorrhage in cirrhotics with high-risk esophageal varices. *Gastroenterology* 2005; **128**(4): 870–881.

80 Thuluvath PJ, Maheshwari A, Jagannath S, Arepally A. A randomized controlled trial of beta-blockers versus endoscopic band ligation for primary prophylaxis: a large sample size is required to show a difference in bleeding rates. *Dig Dis Sci* 2005; **50**(2): 407–10.

81 Psilopoulos D, Galanis P, Goulas S *et al.* Endoscopic variceal ligation vs propranolol for prevention of first variceal bleeding: a randomized controlled trial. *Eur J Gastroenterol Hepatol* 2005; **17**(10): 1111–1117.

82 Lay CS, Tsai YT, Lee FY *et al.* Endoscopic variceal ligation versus propranolol in prophylaxis of first variceal bleeding in patients with cirrhosis. *J Gastroenterol Hepatol* 2006; **21**(2): 413–419.

83 Norberto L, Polese L, Cillo U *et al.* A randomized study comparing ligation with propranolol for primary prophylaxis of variceal bleeding in candidates for liver transplantation. *Liver Transpl* 2007; **13**(9): 1272–1278.

84 Merkel C, Marin R, Enzo E *et al.* Randomised trial of nadolol alone or with isosorbide mononitrate for primary prophylaxis of variceal bleeding in cirrhosis. Gruppo-Triveneto per L'ipertensione portale (GTIP). *Lancet* 1996; **348**(9043): 1677–1681.

85 Merkel C, Marin R, Sacerdoti D *et al.* Long-term results of a clinical trial of nadolol with or without isosorbide mononitrate for primary prophylaxis of variceal bleeding in cirrhosis. *Hepatology* 2000; **31**(2): 324–329.

86 Garcia-Pagan JC, Morillas R, Banares R *et al.* Propranolol plus placebo versus propranolol plus isosorbide-5-mononitrate in the prevention of a first variceal bleed: a double-blind RCT. *Hepatology* 2003; **37**(6): 1260–1266.

87 Wang HM, Lo GH, Chen WC *et al.* Comparison of endoscopic variceal ligation and nadolol plus isosorbide-5-mononitrate in the prevention of first variceal bleeding in cirrhotic patients. *J Chin Med Assoc* 2006; **69**(10): 453–460.

88 Gotoh Y, Iwakiri R, Sakata Y *et al.* Evaluation of endoscopic variceal ligation in prophylactic therapy for bleeding of oesophageal varices: a prospective, controlled trial compared with endoscopic injection sclerotherapy. *J Gastroenterol Hepatol* 1999; **14**(3): 241–244.

89 de Franchis R. Evolving consensus in portal hypertension. Report of the Baveno IV consensus workshop on methodology of diagnosis and therapy in portal hypertension. *J Hepatol* 2005; **43**(1): 167–176.

90 Garcia-Tsao G, Sanyal AJ, Grace ND, Carey W. Prevention and management of gastroesophageal varices and variceal hemorrhage in cirrhosis. *Hepatology* 2007; **46**(3): 922–938.

91 McCormick PA, O'Keefe C. Improving prognosis following a first variceal haemorrhage over four decades. *Gut* 2001; **49**(5): 682–685.

92 Burroughs AK, Mezzanotte G, Phillips A, McCormick PA, McIntyre N. Cirrhotics with variceal hemorrhage: the importance of the time interval between admission and the start of analysis for survival and re-bleeding rates. *Hepatology* 1989; **9**(6): 801–807.

93 Vinel JP, Cassigneul J, Levade M, Voigt JJ, Pascal JP. Assessment of short-term prognosis after variceal bleeding in patients with alcoholic cirrhosis by early measurement of portohepatic gradient. *Hepatology* 1986; **6**(1): 116–117.

94 Ready JB, Robertson AD, Goff JS, Rector WG, Jr. Assessment of the risk of bleeding from esophageal varices by continuous monitoring of portal pressure. *Gastroenterology* 1991; **100**(5 Pt 1): 1403–1410.

95 Villanueva C, Ortiz J, Minana J *et al.* Somatostatin treatment and risk stratification by continuous portal pressure monitoring during acute variceal bleeding. *Gastroenterology* 2001; **121**(1): 110–117.

96 Monescillo A, Martinez-Lagares F, Ruiz-Del-Arbol L *et al.* Influence of portal hypertension and its early decompression by TIPS placement on the outcome of variceal bleeding. *Hepatology* 2004; **40**(4): 793.

97 Avgerinos A, Armonis A, Stefanidis G *et al.* Sustained rise of portal pressure after sclerotherapy, but not band ligation, in acute variceal bleeding in cirrhosis. *Hepatology* 2004; **39**(6): 1623–1630.

98 Vlachogiannakos J, Kougioumtzian A, Triantos C *et al.* Clinical trial: the effect of somatostatin vs octreotide in preventing post-endoscopic increase in hepatic venous pressure gradient in cirrhotics with bleeding varices. *Aliment Pharmacol Ther* 2007; **26**(11–12): 1479–1487.

99 Groszmann RJ, Wongcharatrawee S. The hepatic venous pressure gradient: anything worth doing should be done right. *Hepatology* 2004; **39**(2): 280–282.

100 Ben Ari Z, Cardin F, McCormick AP, Wannamethee G, Burroughs AK. A predictive model for failure to control bleeding during acute variceal haemorrhage. *J Hepatol* 1999; **31**(3): 443–450.

101 Lecleire S, Di Fiore F, Merle V *et al.* Acute upper gastrointestinal bleeding in patients with liver cirrhosis and in noncirrhotic patients: epidemiology and predictive factors of mortality in a prospective multicenter population-based study. *J Clin Gastroenterol* 2005; **39**(4): 321–327.

102 Thomopoulos K, Theocharis G, Mimidis K, Lampropoulou-Karatza C, Alexandridis E, Nikolopoulou V. Improved survival of patients presenting with acute variceal bleeding. Prognostic indicators of short- and long-term mortality. *Dig Liver Dis* 2006; **38**(12): 899–904.

103 Lo GH, Chen WC, Chen MH *et al.* The characteristics and the prognosis for patients presenting with actively bleeding esophageal varices at endoscopy. *Gastrointest Endosc* 2004; **60**(5): 714–720.

104 Amitrano L, Guardascione MA, Bennato R, Manguso F, Balzano A. MELD score and hepatocellular carcinoma identify patients at different risk of short-term mortality among cirrhotics bleeding from esophageal varices. *J Hepatol* 2005; **42**(6): 820–825.

105 Lang BH, Poon RT, Fan ST, Wong J. Outcomes of patients with hepatocellular carcinoma presenting with variceal bleeding. *Am J Gastroenterol* 2004; **99**(11): 2158–2165.

106 Bernard B, Grange JD, Khac EN, Amiot X, Opolon P, Poynard T. Antibiotic prophylaxis for the prevention of bacterial infections in cirrhotic patients with gastrointestinal bleeding: a meta-analysis. *Hepatology* 1999; **29**(6): 1655–1661.

107 Goulis J, Armonis A, Patch D, Sabin C, Greenslade L, Burroughs AK. Bacterial infection is independently associated with failure to control bleeding in cirrhotic patients with gastrointestinal hemorrhage. *Hepatology* 1998; **27**(5): 1207–1212.

108 Goulis J, Patch D, Burroughs AK. Bacterial infection in the pathogenesis of variceal bleeding. *Lancet* 1999; **353**(9147): 139–142.

109 Hou MC, Lin HC, Liu TT, Kuo BI, Lee FY, Chang FY *et al.* Antibiotic prophylaxis after endoscopic therapy prevents re-bleeding in acute variceal hemorrhage: a randomized trial. *Hepatology* 2004; **39**(3): 746–753.

110 Jun CH, Park CH, Lee WS *et al.* Antibiotic prophylaxis using third generation cephalosporins can reduce the risk of early re-bleeding in the first acute gastroesophageal variceal hemorrhage: a prospective randomized study. *J Korean Med Sci* 2006; **21**(5): 883–890.

111 Abraldes JG, Tarantino I, Turnes J, Garcia-Pagan JC, Rodes J, Bosch J. Hemodynamic response to pharmacological treatment of portal hypertension and long-term prognosis of cirrhosis. *Hepatology* 2003; **37**(4): 902–908.

112 Hubmann R, Bodlaj G, Czompo M *et al.* The use of self-expanding metal stents to treat acute esophageal variceal bleeding. *Endoscopy* 2006; **38**(9): 896–901.

113 Orloff MJ, Bell RH, Jr., Hyde PV, Skivolocki WP. Long-term results of emergency portacaval shunt for bleeding esophageal varices in unselected patients with alcoholic cirrhosis. *Ann Surg* 1980; **192**(3): 325–340.

114 Carbonell N, Pauwels A, Serfaty L, Fourdan O, Levy VG, Poupon R. Improved survival after variceal bleeding in patients with cirrhosis over the past two decades. *Hepatology* 2004; **40**(3): 652–659.

115 Terra C, Guevara M, Torre A *et al.* Renal failure in patients with cirrhosis and sepsis unrelated to spontaneous bacterial peritonitis: value of MELD score. *Gastroenterology* 2005; **129**(6): 1944–1953.

116 Fernandez J, Escorsell A, Zabalza M *et al.* Adrenal insufficiency in patients with cirrhosis and septic shock: effect of treatment with hydrocortisone on survival. *Hepatology* 2006; **44**(5): 1288–1295.

117 Sarin SK. Long-term follow-up of gastric variceal sclerotherapy: an eleven-year experience. *Gastrointest Endosc* 1997; **46**(1): 8–14.

118 Levacher S, Letoumelin P, Pateron D, Blaise M, Lapandry C, Pourriat JL. Early administration of terlipressin plus glyceryl trinitrate to control active upper gastrointestinal bleeding in cirrhotic patients. *Lancet* 1995; **346**(8979): 865–868.

119 Moitinho E, Escorsell A, Bandi JC *et al.* Prognostic value of early measurements of portal pressure in acute variceal bleeding. *Gastroenterology* 1999; **117**(3): 626–631.

120 Bosch J, Groszmann RJ, Garcia-Pagan JC *et al.* Association of transdermal nitroglycerin to vasopressin infusion in the treatment of variceal hemorrhage: a placebo-controlled clinical trial. *Hepatology* 1989; **10**(6): 962–968.

121 Conn HO, Ramsby GR, Storer EH *et al.* Intraarterial vasopressin in the treatment of upper gastrointestinal hemorrhage: a prospective, controlled clinical trial. *Gastroenterology* 1975; **68**(2): 211–221.

122 Sonnenberg GE, Keller U, Perruchoud A, Burckhardt D, Gyr K. Effect of somatostatin on splanchnic hemodynamics in patients with cirrhosis of the liver and in normal subjects. *Gastroenterology* 1981; **80**(3): 526–532.

123 Bosch J, Kravetz D, Rodes J. Effects of somatostatin on hepatic and systemic hemodynamics in patients with cirrhosis of the liver: comparison with vasopressin. *Gastroenterology* 1981; **80**(3): 518–525.

124 Jenkins SA, Baxter JN, Corbett WA, Shields R. Effects of a somatostatin analogue SMS 201–995 on hepatic haemodynamics in the pig and on intravariceal pressure in man. *Br J Surg* 1985; **72**(12): 1009–1012.

125 McCormick PA, Biagini MR, Dick R *et al.* Octreotide inhibits the meal-induced increases in the portal venous pressure of cirrhotic patients with portal hypertension: a double-blind, placebo-controlled study. *Hepatology* 1992; **16**(5): 1180–1186.

126 Escorsell A, Bandi JC, Andreu V *et al.* Desensitization to the effects of intravenous octreotide in cirrhotic patients with portal hypertension. *Gastroenterology* 2001; **120**(1): 161–169.

127 Fogel MR, Knauer CM, Andres LL *et al.* Continuous intravenous vasopressin in active upper gastrointestinal bleeding. *Ann Intern Med* 1982; **96**(5): 565–569.

128 Mallory A, Schaefer JW, Cohen JR, Holt SA, Norton LW. Selective intra-arterial vasopression in fusion for upper gastrointestinal tract hemorrhage: a controlled trial. *Arch Surg* 1980; **115**(1): 30–32.

129 Merigan TC, Jr., Plotkin GR, Davidson CS. Effect of intravenously administered posterior pituitary extract on hemorrhage from bleeding esophageal varices. A controlled evaluation. *N Engl J Med* 1962; **266**: 134–135.

130 Tsai YT, Lay CS, Lai KH *et al.* Controlled trial of vasopressin plus nitroglycerin vs vasopressin alone in the treatment of bleeding esophageal varices. *Hepatology* 1986; **6**(3): 406–409.

131 Gimson AE, Westaby D, Hegarty J, Watson A, Williams R. A randomized trial of vasopressin and vasopressin plus nitroglycerin in the control of acute variceal hemorrhage. *Hepatology* 1986; **6**(3): 410–413.

132 Freeman JG, Cobden I, Record CO. Placebo-controlled trial of terlipressin (glypressin) in the management of acute variceal bleeding. *J Clin Gastroenterol* 1989; **11**(1): 58–60.

133 Patch D, Caplin M, Greenslade L, Burroughs A. Randomized double blind controlled trial of 5 day terlipressin vs placebo in acute variceal hemorrhage (Abstract). *J Hepatol* 1999; **30**: 55.

134 Pauwels A, Florent C, Desaint B, Guivarch P, Van H, Levy VG. Terlipressin and somatostatin in the treatment of hemorrhages from rupture of esophageal varices. *Gastroenterol Clin Biol* 1994; **18**(4): 388–389.

135 Soderlund C, Magnusson I, Torngren S, Lundell L. Terlipressin (triglycyl-lysine vasopressin) controls acute bleeding oesophageal varices. A double-blind, randomized, placebo-controlled trial. *Scand J Gastroenterol* 1990; **25**(6): 622–630.

136 Walker S, Stiehl A, Raedsch R, Kommerell B. Terlipressin in bleeding esophageal varices: a placebo-controlled, double-blind study. *Hepatology* 1986; **6**(1): 112–115.

137 Burroughs AK, McCormick PA, Hughes MD, Sprengers D, D'Heygere F, McIntyre N. Randomized, double-blind, placebo-controlled trial of somatostatin for variceal bleeding. Emergency control and prevention of early variceal re-bleeding. *Gastroenterology* 1990; **99**(5): 1388–1395.

138 Gøtzsche PC, Hróbjartsson A. Somatostatin analogues for acute bleeding oesophageal varices. *Cochrane Database of Systematic Reviews* 2008, Issue 3. Art. No.: CD000193. DOI: 10.1002/14651858. CD000193.pub3.

139 Valenzuela JE, Schubert T, Fogel MR *et al.* A multicenter, randomized, double-blind trial of somatostatin in the management of acute hemorrhage from esophageal varices. *Hepatology* 1989; **10**(6): 958–961.

140 Flati G, Negro P, Flati D *et al.* Somatostatin. Massive upper digestive hemorrhage in portal hypertension. Results of a controlled study. *Rev Esp Enferm Apar Dig* 1986; **70**(5): 411–414.

141 Loperfido S, Godena F, Tosolini G *et al.* Somatostatin in the treatment of hemorrhaging esophago-gastric varices. Controlled clinical trial in comparison with ranitidine. *Recenti Prog Med* 1987; **78**(2): 82–86.

142 Testoni PA, Masci E, Passaretti S *et al.* Comparison of somatostatin and cimetidine in the treatment of acute esophageal variceal bleeding. *Curr Ther Res* 1986; **39**: 759–766.

143 Moitinho E, Planas R, Banares R *et al.* Multicenter randomized controlled trial comparing different schedules of somatostatin in the treatment of acute variceal bleeding. *J Hepatol* 2001; **35**(6): 712–718.

144 Palazon JM, Such J, Sanchez-Paya J *et al.* A comparison of two different dosages of somatostatin combined with sclerotherapy for the treatment of acute esophageal variceal bleeding: a prospective randomized trial. *Rev Esp Enferm Dig* 2006; **98**(4): 249–254.

145 Villanueva C, Planella M, Aracil C *et al.* Hemodynamic effects of terlipressin and high somatostatin dose during acute variceal bleeding in nonresponders to the usual somatostatin dose. *Am J Gastroenterol* 2005; **100**(3): 624–630.

146 Burroughs A, International Octreotide Varices Study Group. Double blind RCT of 5 day octreotide versus placebo, associated with sclerotherapy for trial failures (Abstract). *Hepatology* 1996; **24**: 352A.

147 Primignani M, Andreoni B, Carpinelli L *et al.* Sclerotherapy plus octreotide versus sclerotherapy alone in the prevention of early re-bleeding from esophageal varices: a randomized, double-blind, placebo-controlled, multicenter trial. New Italian Endoscopic Club. *Hepatology* 1995; **21**(5): 1322–1327.

148 D'Amico G, Politi F, Morabito A *et al.* Octreotide compared with placebo in a treatment strategy for early re-bleeding in cirrhosis. A double blind, randomized pragmatic trial. *Hepatology* 1998; **28**(5): 1206–1214.

149 Colin R, Giuli N, Czernichow P, Ducrotte P, Lerebours E. Prospective comparison of glypressin, tamponade and their association in the treatment of bleeding esophageal varices. In: Lebrec D, Blei AT, eds. *Vasopressin Analogs and Portal Hypertension*. John Libbey Eurotext, Paris, 1987.

150 Fort E, Sautereau D, Silvain C, Ingrand P, Pillegand B, Beauchant M. A randomized trial of terlipressin plus nitroglycerin vs balloon tamponade in the control of acute variceal hemorrhage. *Hepatology* 1990; **11**(4): 678–681.

151 Blanc P, Bories J, Desprez D *et al.* Balloon tamponade with Linton-Michel tube versus terlipressin in the treatment of acute oesophageal and gastric variceal bleeding (Abstract). *J Hepatol* 1994; **21**: S133.

152 Jaramillo JL, de la MM, Mino G, Costan G, Gomez-Camacho F. Somatostatin versus Sengstaken balloon tamponade for primary haemostasia of bleeding esophageal varices. A randomized pilot study. *J Hepatol* 1991; **12**(1): 100–105.

153 Avgerinos A, Klonis C, Rekoumis G, Gouma P, Papadimitriou N, Raptis S. A prospective randomized trial comparing somatostatin, balloon tamponade and the combination of both methods in the management of acute variceal haemorrhage. *J Hepatol* 1991; **13**(1): 78–83.

154 McKee R. A study of octreotide in oesophageal varices. *Digestion* 1990; **45**(Suppl. 1): 60–64.

155 Desaint B, Florent C, Levy VG. A randomized trial of triglycyl-lysine vasopressin versus lysine vasopressin in active cirrhotic variceal hemorrhage. In: Lebrec D, Blei AT, eds. John Libbey Eurotext, Paris, 1987.

156 Lee FY, Tsai YT, Lai KH *et al.* A randomized controlled study of triglycyl-vasopressin and vasopressin plus nitroglycerin in the control of acute esophageal variceal hemorrhage. *Chin J Gastroenterol* 1988; **5**: 131–138.

157 Chiu KW, Sheen IS, Liaw YF. A controlled study of glypressin versus vasopressin in the control of bleeding from oesophageal varices. *J Gastroenterol Hepatol* 1990; **5**(5): 549–553.

158 D'Amico G, Traina M, Vizzini G *et al.* Terlipressin or vasopressin plus transdermal nitroglycerin in a treatment strategy for digestive bleeding in cirrhosis. A randomized clinical trial. Liver Study Group of V. Cervello Hospital. *J Hepatol* 1994; **20**(2): 206–212.

159 Kravetz D, Bosch J, Teres J, Bruix J, Rimola A, Rodes J. Comparison of intravenous somatostatin and vasopressin infusions in treatment of acute variceal hemorrhage. *Hepatology* 1984; **4**(3): 442–446.

160 Jenkins SA, Baxter JN, Corbett W, Devitt P, Ware J, Shields R. A prospective randomised controlled clinical trial comparing somatostatin and vasopressin in controlling acute variceal haemorrhage. *Br Med J* (Clin Res Ed) 1985; **290**(6464): 275–278.

161 Bagarani M, Albertini V, Anza M *et al.* Effect of somatostatin in controlling bleeding from esophageal varices. *Ital J Surg Sci* 1987; **17**(1): 21–26.

162 Cardona C, Vida F, Balanzo J, Cusso X, Farre A, Guarner C. Therapeutic efficiency of somatostatin versus vasopressin in nitroglycerin in more active bleeding esophagogastric varices. *Gastroenterol Hepatol* 1989; **12**: 30–34.

163 Hsia HC, Lee FY, Tsai YT *et al.* Comparison of somatostatin and vasopressin in the control of acute esophageal variceal hemorrhage. A randomized, controlled study. *Chin J Gastroenterol* 1990; **7**: 71–78.

164 Saari A, Klvilaakso E, Inberg M *et al.* Comparison of somatostatin and vasopressin in bleeding esophageal varices. *Am J Gastroenterol* 1990; **85**(7): 804–807.

165 Rodriguez-Moreno F, Santolaria F, Gles-Reimers E *et al.* A randomized trial of somatostatin vs vasopressin plus nitroglycerin in the treatment of acute variceal bleeding (Abstract). *J Hepatol* 1991; **13**: S162.

166 Feu F, Ruiz del Arbol L, Banares R, Planas R, Bosch J. Double-blind randomized controlled trial comparing terlipressin and somatostatin for acute variceal hemorrhage. Variceal Bleeding Study Group. *Gastroenterology* 1996; **111**(5): 1291–1299.

167 Walker S, Kreichgauer HP, Bode JC. Terlipressin (glypressin) versus somatostatin in the treatment of bleeding esophageal varices – final report of a placebo-controlled, double-blind study. *Z Gastroenterol* 1996; **34**(10): 692–698.

168 Hwang SJ, Lin HC, Chang CF, Lee FY, Lu CW, Hsia HC *et al.* A randomized controlled trial comparing octreotide and vasopressin in the control of acute esophageal variceal bleeding. *J Hepatol* 1992; **16**(3): 320–325.

169 Silvain C, Carpentier S, Sautereau D *et al.* Terlipressin plus transdermal nitroglycerin vs octreotide in the control of acute

bleeding from esophageal varices: a multicenter randomized trial. *Hepatology* 1993; **18**(1): 61–65.

170 Freeman JG, Cobden I, Lishman AH, Record CO. Controlled trial of terlipressin ("Glypressin") versus vasopressin in the early treatment of oesophageal varices. *Lancet* 1982; **2**(8289): 66–68.

171 Lee HY, Lee HJ, Lee SM *et al.* A prospective randomized controlled clinical trial comparing the effects of somatostatin and vasopressin for control of acute variceal bleeding in the patients with liver cirrhosis. *Korean J Intern Med* 2003; **18**(3): 161–166.

172 Chelarescu D, Gabor O, Lunca C. Terlipressin vs somatostatin in acute variceal bleeding: a prospective, randomized trial. *J Hepatol* 2001; **34**(Suppl. 1): 78.

173 Huang CC, Sheen IS, Chu CM *et al.* A prospective randomized controlled trial of sandostatin and vasopressin in the management of acute bleeding esophageal varices. *Changing Yi Xue Za Zhi* 1992; **15**(2): 78–83.

174 Rallabandi SM, Batra Y, Gulati G, Madan K, Sharma S, Acharya SK. Somatostatin versus somatostatin plus nitroglycerine infusion in the control of acute variceal bleeding and prevention of re-bleeding in cirrhotics (Abstract). *Journal of Gastroenterology and Hepatology* 2006; **21**(suppl. 6): A458.

175 Bosch J, Thabut D, Albillos A *et al.* recombinant factor VIIa (RFVIIa) for active variceal bleeding in patients with advanced cirrhosis: a multi-centre randomized double-blind placebo-controlled trial . *J Hepatol* 2007; **46**(suppl. 1): 295.

176 Bosch J, Thabut D, Albillos A *et al.* Recombinant factor VIIa for variceal bleeding in patients with advanced cirrhosis: A randomized, controlled trial. *Hepatology* 2008; **47**(5): 1604–1614.

177 Hartigan PM, Gebhard RL, Gregory PB. Sclerotherapy for actively bleeding esophageal varices in male alcoholics with cirrhosis. Veterans Affairs Cooperative Variceal Sclerotherapy Group. *Gastrointest Endosc* 1997; **46**(1): 1–7.

178 Prindiville T, Trudeau W. A comparison of immediate versus delayed endoscopic injection sclerosis of bleeding esophageal varices. *Gastrointest Endosc* 1986; **32**(6): 385–388.

179 Shemesh E, Czerniak A, Klein E, Pines A, Bat L. A comparison between emergency and delayed endoscopic injection sclerotherapy of bleeding esophageal varices in nonalcoholic portal hypertension. *J Clin Gastroenterol* 1990; **12**(1): 5–9.

180 De Franchis R, Banares R, Silvain C. Emergency endoscopy strategies for improved outcomes. *Scand J Gastroenterol Suppl* 1998; **226**: 25–36.

181 Larson AW, Cohen H, Zweiban B *et al.* Acute esophageal variceal sclerotherapy. Results of a prospective randomized controlled trial. *JAMA* 1986; **255**(4): 497–500.

182 Soderlund C, Ihre T. Endoscopic sclerotherapy v. conservative management of bleeding oesophageal varices. A 5-year prospective controlled trial of emergency and long-term treatment. *Acta Chir Scand* 1985; **151**(5): 449–456.

183 Villanueva C, Ortiz J, Sabat M *et al.* Somatostatin alone or combined with emergency sclerotherapy in the treatment of acute esophageal variceal bleeding: a prospective randomized trial. *Hepatology* 1999; **30**(2): 384–389.

184 Alexandrino P, Alves P, Fidalgo M *et al.* Is sclerotherapy the first choice treatment for active oesophageal variceal bleeding in cirrhotic patients? Final report of a randomized controlled trial (Abstract). *J.Hepatol* 1990; **11**: S1.

185 Novella M, Villanueva C, Ortiz J *et al.* Octreotide vs sclerotherapy and octreotide for acute variceal bleeding. A pilot study (Abstract). *Hepatology* 1996; **24**: 207A.

186 Villanueva C, Minana J, Ortiz J *et al.* Endoscopic ligation compared with combined treatment with nadolol and isosorbide mononitrate to prevent recurrent variceal bleeding. *N Engl J Med* 2001; **345**(9): 647–655.

187 Bildozola M, Kravetz D, Argonz J *et al.* Efficacy of octreotide and sclerotherapy in the treatment of acute variceal bleeding in cirrhotic patients. A prospective, multicentric, and randomized clinical trial. *Scand J Gastroenterol* 2000; **35**(4): 419–425.

188 Escorsell A, Ruiz DA, Planas R *et al.* Multicenter randomized controlled trial of terlipressin versus sclerotherapy in the treatment of acute variceal bleeding: the TEST study. *Hepatology* 2000; **32**(3): 471–476.

189 Freitas DS, Sofia C, Pontes JM *et al.* Octreotide in acute bleeding esophageal varices: a prospective randomized study. *Hepatogastroenterology* 2000; **47**(35): 1310–1314.

190 Jenkins SA, Shields R, Davies M *et al.* A multicentre randomised trial comparing octreotide and injection sclerotherapy in the management and outcome of acute variceal haemorrhage. *Gut* 1997; **41**(4): 526–533.

191 Planas R, Quer JC, Boix J *et al.* A prospective randomized trial comparing somatostatin and sclerotherapy in the treatment of acute variceal bleeding. *Hepatology* 1994; **20**(2): 370–375.

192 Ramires RP, Zils CK, Mattos AA. Sclerotherapy versus somatostatin in the treatment of upper digestive hemorrhage caused by rupture of esophageal varices. *Arq Gastroenterol* 2000; **37**(3): 148–154.

193 Shields R, Jenkins SA, Baxter JN *et al.* A prospective randomised controlled trial comparing the efficacy of somatostatin with injection sclerotherapy in the control of bleeding oesophageal varices. *J Hepatol* 1992; **16**(1–2): 128–137.

194 Sivri B, Oksuzoglu G, Bayraktar Y, Kayhan B. A prospective randomized trial from Turkey comparing octreotide versus injection sclerotherapy in acute variceal bleeding. *Hepatogastroenterology* 2000; **47**(31): 168–173.

195 Sung JJ, Chung SC, Lai CW *et al.* Octreotide infusion or emergency sclerotherapy for variceal haemorrhage. *Lancet* 1993; **342**(8872): 637–641.

196 Westaby D, Hayes PC, Gimson AE, Polson RJ, Williams R. Controlled clinical trial of injection sclerotherapy for active variceal bleeding. *Hepatology* 1989; **9**(2): 274–277.

197 Yousuf M, Rauf A, Baig I, Akram M, Rizwan Z. Initial management of acute variceal haemorrhage.Comparison of octreotide and sclerotherapy. *J Coll Phys Surg Pak* 2000; **10**: 95–97.

198 Di Fedo G, Siringo S, Vacirca M *et al.* Somatostatin (SMS) and urgent sclerotherapy (US) in active oesophageal variceal bleeding (Abstract). *Gastroenterology* 1990; **98**: 583A.

199 El-Jackie A, Rowaisha I, Waked I, Saleh S, Abdel Ghaffar Y. Octreotide vs Sclerotherapy in the control of acute variceal bleeding in schistosomal portal hypertension: a randomized trial (Abstract). *Hepatology* 1998; **28**(4): 553.

200 Lopez F, Vargas R, Margarita G, Rizo T, Arguelles D. Octreotide vs sclerotherapy in the treatment of acute variceal bleeding (Abstract). *Hepatology* 1999; **30**: 574A.

201 Poo J, Bosques S, Guarduno R *et al.* Octreotide versus emergency sclerotherapy in acute variceal hemorrhage in liver

cirrhosis. A randomized multicenter study (Abstract). *Gastroenterology* 1996; **110**: A1297.

202 Besson I, Ingrand P, Person B *et al.* Sclerotherapy with or without octreotide for acute variceal bleeding. *N Engl J Med* 1995; **333**(9): 555–560.

203 Signorelli S, Negrini F, Paris B, Bonelli M, Girola M. Sclerotherapy with or without somatostatin or octreotide in the treatment of acute variceal haemorrhage: our experience. *Gastroenterology* 1996; **110**: 1326A.

204 Signorelli S, Paris B, Negrini F, Cesareni P, Minola E, Auriemma L. Octreotide and endoscopic variceal sclerotherapy in the management of acute variceal haemorrhage (Abstract). *Endoscopy* 1999; **31**: E66.

205 Avgerinos A, Nevens F, Raptis S, Fevery J. Early administration of somatostatin and efficacy of sclerotherapy in acute oesophageal variceal bleeds: the European Acute Bleeding Oesophageal Variceal Episodes (ABOVE) randomised trial. *Lancet* 1997; **350**(9090): 1495–1499.

206 Zuberi BF, Baloch Q. Comparison of endoscopic variceal sclerotherapy alone and in combination with octreotide in controlling acute variceal hemorrhage and early re-bleeding in patients with low-risk cirrhosis. *Am J Gastroenterol* 2000; **95**(3): 768–771.

207 Farooqi J, Farooqi R, Haq N, Siddiq-u-Rehman, Mahmood S. Treatment and outcome of variceal bleeding – a comparison of two methods. *JCPSP* 2000; **10**(4): 131–133.

208 Cales P, Masliah C, Bernard B *et al.* Early administration of vapreotide for variceal bleeding in patients with cirrhosis. French Club for the Study of Portal Hypertension. *N Engl J Med* 2001; **344**(1): 23–28.

209 Gimson AE, Ramage JK, Panos MZ *et al.* Randomised trial of variceal banding ligation versus injection sclerotherapy for bleeding oesophageal varices. *Lancet* 1993; **342**(8868): 391–394.

210 Hou MC, Lin HC, Kuo BI, Chen CH, Lee FY, Lee SD. Comparison of endoscopic variceal injection sclerotherapy and ligation for the treatment of esophageal variceal hemorrhage: a prospective randomized trial. *Hepatology* 1995; **21**(6):1517–1522.

211 Laine L, el Newihi HM, Migikovsky B, Sloane R, Garcia F. Endoscopic ligation compared with sclerotherapy for the treatment of bleeding esophageal varices. *Ann Intern Med* 1993; **119**(1): 1–7.

212 Lo GH, Lai KH, Cheng JS *et al.* A prospective, randomized trial of sclerotherapy versus ligation in the management of bleeding esophageal varices. *Hepatology* 1995; **22**(2): 466–471.

213 Lo GH, Lai KH, Cheng JS *et al.* Emergency banding ligation versus sclerotherapy for the control of active bleeding from esophageal varices. *Hepatology* 1997; **25**(5): 1101–1104.

214 Sarin SK, Govil A, Jain AK *et al.* Prospective randomized trial of endoscopic sclerotherapy versus variceal band ligation for esophageal varices: influence on gastropathy, gastric varices and variceal recurrence. *J Hepatol* 1997; **26**(4): 826–832.

215 Shafqat F, Khan AA, Alam A *et al.* Band ligation vs endoscopic sclerotherapy in esophageal varices: a prospective randomized comparison. *J Pak Med Assoc* 1998; **48**(7): 192–196.

216 Stiegmann GV, Goff JS, Michaletz-Onody PA *et al.* Endoscopic sclerotherapy as compared with endoscopic ligation for bleeding esophageal varices. *N Engl J Med* 1992; **326**(23): 1527–1532.

217 Fakhry S, Omar M, Mustafa A, El-Behairy N, Hunter S, Bilharz T. Endoscopic sclerotherapy versus endoscopic variceal ligation in the management of bleeding esophageal varices: a final report of a prospective randomized study in schistosomal heaptic fibrosis (Abstract). *Hepatology* 1997; **26**(4 (Pt 2)): 137A.

218 Jain AK, Ray RP, Gupta J. Management of acute variceal bleed: randomized trial of variceal ligation and sclerotherapy (Abstract). *Hepatology* 1996; **23**(1): I–51.

219 Jensen D, Kovacs T, Jutabha R *et al.* Randomized, blinded prospective study of banding vs. sclerotherapy for preventing recurrent variceal hemorrhage for patients without active bleeding at endoscopy (Abstract). *Gastrointest Endosc* 1993; **41**: 315A.

220 Salem S, Shiha G. A prospective randomized trial of sclerotherapy versus saeed six-shooter multiband ligation in the control of acute bleeding from oesophageal varices (Abstract). *Gut* 1999; **44**(Suppl. 1): A19.

221 Villanueva C, Piqueras M, Aracil C *et al.* A randomized controlled trial comparing ligation and sclerotherapy as emergency endoscopic treatment added to somatostatin in acute variceal bleeding. *J Hepatol* 2006; **45**(4): 560–567.

222 Djurdjevic D, Janosevic S, Dapcevic B *et al.* Combined ligation and sclerotherapy versus ligation alone for eradication of bleeding esophageal varices: a randomized and prospective trial. *Endoscopy* 1999; **31**(4): 286–290.

223 Cho SB, Lee CH, Park CH *et al.* Comparison of terlipressin and octreotide as a combination therapy with endoscopic variceal ligation in the control of acute esophageal variceal bleeding: a randomized controlled trial (Abstract) *J Hepatol* 2006; **44**(Suppl. 2): S91.

224 Cello JP, Crass R, Trunkey DD. Endoscopic sclerotherapy versus esophageal transection of Child's class C patients with variceal hemorrhage. Comparison with results of portacaval shunt: preliminary report. *Surgery* 1982; **91**(3): 333–338.

225 Huizinga WK, Angorn IB, Baker LW. Esophageal transection versus injection sclerotherapy in the management of bleeding esophageal varices in patients at high risk. *Surg Gynecol Obstet* 1985; **160**(6): 539–546.

226 Teres J, Baroni R, Bordas JM, Visa J, Pera C, Rodes J. Randomized trial of portacaval shunt, stapling transection and endoscopic sclerotherapy in uncontrolled variceal bleeding. *J Hepatol* 1987; **4**(2): 159–167.

227 Burroughs AK, Hamilton G, Phillips A, Mezzanotte G, McIntyre N, Hobbs KE. A comparison of sclerotherapy with staple transection of the esophagus for the emergency control of bleeding from esophageal varices. *N Engl J Med* 1989; **321**(13): 857–862.

228 Cello JP, Grendell JH, Crass RA, Weber TE, Trunkey DD. Endoscopic sclerotherapy versus portacaval shunt in patient with severe cirrhosis and acute variceal hemorrhage. Long-term follow-up. *N Engl J Med* 1987; **316**(1): 11–15.

229 Orloff MJ, Bell RH, Jr., Orloff MS, Hardison WG, Greenburg AG. Prospective randomized trial of emergency portacaval shunt and emergency medical therapy in unselected cirrhotic patients with bleeding varices. *Hepatology* 1994; **20**(4 Pt 1): 863–872.

230 Soehendra N, Grimm H, Nam VC, Berger B. N-butyl-2-cyanoacrylate: a supplement to endoscopic sclerotherapy. *Endoscopy* 1987; **19**(6): 221–224.

231 Maluf-Filho F, Sakai P, Ishioka S, Matuguma SE. Endoscopic sclerosis versus cyanoacrylate endoscopic injection for the first

episode of variceal bleeding: a prospective, controlled, and randomized study in Child-Pugh class C patients. *Endoscopy* 2001; **33**(5): 421–427.

232 Feretis C, Dimopoulos C, Benakis P, Kalliakmanis B, Apostolidis N. N-butyl-2-cyanoacrylate (Histoacryl) plus sclerotherapy versus sclerotherapy alone in the treatment of bleeding esophageal varices: a randomized prospective study. *Endoscopy* 1995; **27**(5): 355–357.

233 Thakeb F, Salama Z, Salama H, Abdel RT, Abdel KS, Abdel HH. The value of combined use of N-butyl-2-cyanoacrylate and ethanolamine oleate in the management of bleeding esophagogastric varices. *Endoscopy* 1995; **27**(5): 358–364.

234 Sung JY, Lee YT, Suen R, Chung SC. Banding is superior to cyanoacrylate for the treatment of esophageal variceal bleeding: a prospective randomized study (Abstract). *Gastrointest Endosc* 1998; **47**: 210.

235 Duvall GA, Haber G, Kortan P et al. A prospective randomized trial of cyanoacrylate (CYA) vs endoscopic variceal ligation (EVL) for acute esophagogastric variceal hemorrhage (Abstract). *Gastrointest Endosc* 1997; **45**: 172.

236 Zimmer T, Rucktaschel F, Stolzel U et al. Endoscopic sclerotherapy with fibrin glue as compared with polidocanol to prevent early esophageal variceal re-bleeding. *J Hepatol* 1998; **28**(2): 292–297.

237 Zimmer T, Faiss T, Liehr RM et al. Fibrin glue versus variceal ligation for acute hemostasis and prevention of re-bleeding from esophageal varices. Results of a German multi-centre trial. *Gastroenterology* 2005; **128**(4 suppl. 2): A681.

238 Ferguson JW, Tripathi D, Hayes PC. Review article: the management of acute variceal bleeding. *Aliment Pharmacol Ther* 2003; **18**(3): 253–262.

239 Zhang CQ, Liu FL, Liang B et al. A modified percutaneous transhepatic variceal embolization with 2-octyl cyanoacrylate versus endoscopic ligation in esophageal variceal bleeding management: randomized controlled trial. *Dig Dis Sci* 2008; **53**(8): 2258–2267.

240 Shim CS, Cho JY, Park YJ et al. Mini-detachable snare ligation for the treatment of esophageal varices. *Gastrointest Endosc* 1999; **50**(5): 673–676.

241 Naga MI, Okasha HH, Foda AR et al. Detachable endoloop vs elastic band ligation for bleeding esophageal varices. *Gastrointest Endosc* 2004; **59**(7): 804–809.

242 Jensen DM, Kovacs T, Randall GM et al. Initial results of a randomized prospective study of emergency banding vs sclerotherapy for bleeding gastric or esophageal varices (Abstract). *Gastrointest Endosc* 1993; **39**: 128A.

243 Mundo F, Mitrani C, Rodriguez G, Farca A. Endoscopic variceal treatment, is band ligation taking over sclerotherapy? (Abstract). *Am J Gastroenterol* 1993; **88**: 1493A.

244 Young MF, Sanowski RA, Rasche R. Comparison and characterization of ulcerations induced by endoscopic ligation of esophageal varices versus endoscopic sclerotherapy. *Gastrointest Endosc* 1993; **39**(2): 119–122.

245 Mostafa I, Omar M, Fakhry S et al. Prospective randomized comparative study of injection sclerotherapy and band ligation for bleeding esophageal varices (Abstact). *Hepatology* 1996; **23**(1): I–63.

246 Baroncini D, Milandri GL, Borioni D et al. A prospective randomized trial of sclerotherapy versus ligation in the elective treatment of bleeding esophageal varices. *Endoscopy* 1997; **29**(4): 235–240.

247 Masci E, Norberto L, D'Imperio N et al. Prospective multicentric randomized trial comparing banding ligation with sclerotherapy of esophageal varices (Abstract). *Gastrointest.Endosc* 1997; **45**: 847A.

248 Avgerinos A, Armonis A, Manolakopoulos S et al. Endoscopic sclerotherapy versus variceal ligation in the long-term management of patients with cirrhosis after variceal bleeding. A prospective randomized study. *J Hepatol* 1997; **26**(5): 1034–1041.

249 Shiha GE, Farag FM. Endoscopic variceal ligation versus endoscopic sclerotherapy for the management of bleeding varices (Abstract). *Hepatology* 1997; **26**: 136A.

250 de la Pena J, Brullet E, Sanchez-Hernandez E et al. Variceal ligation plus nadolol compared with ligation for prophylaxis of variceal re-bleeding: a multicenter trial. *Hepatology* 2005; **41**(3): 572–578.

251 Chau TN, Patch D, Chan YW, Nagral A, Dick R, Burroughs AK. "Salvage" transjugular intrahepatic portosystemic shunts: gastric fundal compared with esophageal variceal bleeding. *Gastroenterology* 1998; **114**(5): 981–987.

252 Sarin SK, Lahoti D, Saxena SP, Murthy NS, Makwana UK. Prevalence, classification and natural history of gastric varices: a long-term follow-up study in 568 portal hypertension patients. *Hepatology* 1992; **16**(6): 1343–1349.

253 Ramond MJ, Valla D, Mosnier JF et al. Successful endoscopic obturation of gastric varices with butyl cyanoacrylate. *Hepatology* 1989; **10**(4): 488–493.

254 Oho K, Iwao T, Sumino M, Toyonaga A, Tanikawa K. Ethanolamine oleate versus butyl cyanoacrylate for bleeding gastric varices: a nonrandomized study. *Endoscopy* 1995; **27**(5): 349–354.

255 Sarin SK, Jain AK, Jain M, Gupta R. A randomized controlled trial of cyanoacrylate versus alcohol injection in patients with isolated fundic varices. *Am J Gastroenterol* 2002; **97**(4): 1010–1015.

256 Tan PC, Hou MC, Lin HC et al. A randomized trial of endoscopic treatment of acute gastric variceal hemorrhage: N-butyl-2-cyanoacrylate injection versus band ligation. *Hepatology* 2006; **43**(4): 690–697.

257 Lo GH, Lai KH, Cheng JS, Chen MH, Chiang HT. A prospective, randomized trial of butyl cyanoacrylate injection versus band ligation in the management of bleeding gastric varices. *Hepatology* 2001; **33**(5): 1060–1064.

258 Williams SG, Peters RA, Westaby D. Thrombin – an effective treatment for gastric variceal haemorrhage. *Gut* 1994; **35**(9): 1287–1289.

259 Ninoi T, Nishida N, Kaminou T et al. Balloon-occluded retrograde transvenous obliteration of gastric varices with gastrorenal shunt: long-term follow-up in 78 patients. *AJR Am J Roentgenol* 2005; **184**(4): 1340–1346.

260 Cho SK, Shin SW, Lee IH et al. Balloon-occluded retrograde transvenous obliteration of gastric varices: outcomes and complications in 49 patients. *AJR Am J Roentgenol* 2007; **189**(6): W365–W372.

261 Lo GH, Liang HL, Chen WC et al. A prospective, randomized controlled trial of transjugular intrahepatic portosystemic shunt versus cyanoacrylate injection in the prevention of gastric variceal re-bleeding. *Endoscopy* 2007; **39**(8): 679–685.

262 Vlavianos P, Gimson AE, Westaby D, Williams R. Balloon tamponade in variceal bleeding: use and misuse. *BMJ* 1989; **298**(6681): 1158.

263 Vangeli M, Patch D, Burroughs AK. Salvage tips for uncontrolled variceal bleeding. *J Hepatol* 2002; **37**(5): 703–704.

264 Azoulay D, Castaing D, Majno P *et al.* Salvage transjugular intrahepatic portosystemic shunt for uncontrolled variceal bleeding in patients with decompensated cirrhosis. *J Hepatol* 2001; **35**(5): 590–597.

265 Sanyal AJ, Freedman AM, Luketic VA *et al.* Transjugular intrahepatic portosystemic shunts for patients with active variceal hemorrhage unresponsive to sclerotherapy. *Gastroenterology* 1996; **111**(1): 138–146.

266 Patch D, Nikolopoulou V, McCormick A *et al.* Factors related to early mortality after transjugular intrahepatic portosystemic shunt for failed endoscopic therapy in acute variceal bleeding. *J Hepatol* 1998; **28**(3): 454–460.

267 Samonakis DN, Triantos CK, Thalheimer U, Patch DW, Burroughs AK. Management of portal hypertension. *Postgrad Med J* 2004; **80**(949): 634–641.

268 Garcia-Pagan JC, Caca K, Bureau C *et al.* An early decision for PTFE-TIPS improves survival in high risk cirrhotic patients admitted with an acute variceal bleeding. a multicenter RCT (Abstract). *J Hepatol* 2008; **48**: S371.

269 Burroughs AK, Triantos CK. Predicting failure to control bleeding and mortality in acute variceal bleeding. *J Hepatol* 2008; **48**(2): 185–188.

270 Feu F, Garcia-Pagan JC, Bosch J *et al.* Relation between portal pressure response to pharmacotherapy and risk of recurrent variceal haemorrhage in patients with cirrhosis. *Lancet* 1995; **346**(8982): 1056–1059.

271 McCormick PA, Patch D, Greenslade L, Chin J, McIntyre N, Burroughs AK. Clinical vs haemodynamic response to drugs in portal hypertension. *J Hepatol* 1998; **28**(6): 1015–1019.

272 Villanueva C, Aracil C, Colomo A, *et al.* Clinical trial: a randomized controlled study on prevention of variceal rebleeding comparing nadolol and ligation vs hepatic vanous pressure gradient guided pharmacological therapy. *Aliment Pharmacol Ther* 2009; **29**(4): 397–408.

273 Burroughs AK, Jenkins WJ, Sherlock S *et al.* Controlled trial of propranolol for the prevention of recurrent variceal hemorrhage in patients with cirrhosis. *N Engl J Med* 1983; **309**(25): 1539–1542.

274 Cerbelaud P, Lavignolle A, Perrin D *et al.* Propranolol et prevention des recidives de rupture de varice oesophagienne du cirrhotique (Abstract). *Gastroenterol Clin Biol* 1986; **18**: A10.

275 Colombo M, de Franchis R, Tommasini M, Sangiovanni A, Dioguardi N. Beta-blockade prevents recurrent gastrointestinal bleeding in well-compensated patients with alcoholic cirrhosis: a multicenter randomized controlled trial. *Hepatology* 1989; **9**(3): 433–438.

276 Garden OJ, Mills PR, Birnie GG, Murray GD, Carter DC. Propranolol in the prevention of recurrent variceal hemorrhage in cirrhotic patients. A controlled trial. *Gastroenterology* 1990; **98**(1): 185–190.

277 Gatta A, Merkel C, Sacerdoti D *et al.* Nadolol for prevention of variceal re-bleeding in cirrhosis: a controlled clinical trial. *Digestion* 1987; **37**(1): 22–28.

278 Kobe E, Schentke KU. Unsichere rezidivprophylaxe von osophagusvarizenblutungen durch Propranolol bei Leberzirrhotikern: eine prospektive kontrolliertr studie. Zeitschrift Fur Klinische Medizin-Zkm. *Zeitschrift Fur Klinische Medizin-Zkm* 1987; **42**: 507–510.

279 Lebrec D, Poynard T, Hillon P, Benhamou JP. Propranolol for prevention of recurrent gastrointestinal bleeding in patients with cirrhosis: a controlled study. *N Engl J Med* 1981; **305**(23): 1371–1374.

280 Queuniet AM, Czernichow P, Lerebours E, Ducrotte P, Tranvouez JL, Colin R. Controlled study of propranolol in the prevention of recurrent hemorrhage in cirrhotic patients. *Gastroenterol Clin Biol* 1987; **11**(1): 41–47.

281 Rossi V, Cales P, Burtin P *et al.* Prevention of recurrent variceal bleeding in alcoholic cirrhotic patients: prospective controlled trial of propranolol and sclerotherapy. *J Hepatol* 1991; **12**(3): 283–289.

282 Sheen IS, Chen TY, Liaw YF. Randomized controlled study of propranolol for prevention of recurrent esophageal varices bleeding in patients with cirrhosis. *Liver* 1989; **9**(1): 1–5.

283 Villeneuve JP, Pomier-Layrargues G, Infante-Rivard C *et al.* Propranolol for the prevention of recurrent variceal hemorrhage: a controlled trial. *Hepatology* 1986; **6**(6): 1239–1243.

284 Colman J, Jones P, Finch C, Dudley F. Propranolol in the prevention of variceal hemorrhage in alcoholic cirrhotic patients (Abstract). *Hepatology* 1990; **12**: 851.

285 Bernard B, Lebrec D, Mathurin P, Opolon P, Poynard T. Beta-adrenergic antagonists in the prevention of gastrointestinal rebleeding in patients with cirrhosis: a meta-analysis. *Hepatology* 1997; **25**(1): 63–70.

286 Lebrec D, Poynard T, Bernuau J *et al.* A randomized controlled study of propranolol for prevention of recurrent gastrointestinal bleeding in patients with cirrhosis: a final report. *Hepatology* 1984; **4**(3): 355–358.

287 Thalheimer U, Bosch J, Burroughs AK. How to prevent varices from bleeding: shades of grey – the case for nonselective beta blockers. *Gastroenterology* 2007; **133**(6): 2029–2036.

288 Garcia-Pagan JC, Feu F, Bosch J, Rodes J. Propranolol compared with propranolol plus isosorbide-5-mononitrate for portal hypertension in cirrhosis. A randomized controlled study. *Ann Intern Med* 1991; **114**(10): 869–873.

289 Gonzalez-Abraldes J, Albillos A, Banares R *et al.* Randomized comparison of long-term losartan versus propranolol in lowering portal pressure in cirrhosis. *Gastroenterology* 2001; **121**(2): 382–388.

290 Albillos A, Garcia-Pagan JC, Iborra J *et al.* Propranolol plus prazosin compared with propranolol plus isosorbide-5-mononitrate in the treatment of portal hypertension. *Gastroenterology* 1998; **115**(1): 116–123.

291 Abecasis R, Kravetz D, Fassio E *et al.* Nadolol plus spironolactone in the prophylaxis of first variceal bleed in nonascitic cirrhotic patients: a preliminary study. *Hepatology* 2003; **37**(2): 359–365.

292 Gournay J, Masliah C, Martin T, Perrin D, Galmiche JP. Isosorbide mononitrate and propranolol compared with propranolol alone for the prevention of variceal re-bleeding. *Hepatology* 2000; **31**(6): 1239–1245.

293 Patti R, D'Amico G, Pasta H *et al.* Isosorbite mononitrate with nadolol compared to nadolol alone for prevention of recurrent

bleeding in cirrhosis. Double-blind placebo controlled randomized trial (Abstract). *J Hepatol* 1999; **30**: 81.

294 Bureau C, Peron JM, Alric L *et al.* "A La Carte" treatment of portal hypertension: Adapting medical therapy to hemodynamic response for the prevention of bleeding. *Hepatology* 2002; **36**(6): 1361–1366.

295 Terblanche J, Bornman PC, Kahn D *et al.* Failure of repeated injection sclerotherapy to improve long-term survival after oesophageal variceal bleeding. A five-year prospective controlled clinical trial. *Lancet* 1983; **2**(8363): 1328–1332.

296 Sclerotherapy after first variceal hemorrhage in cirrhosis. A randomized multicenter trial. The Copenhagen Esophageal Varices Sclerotherapy Project. *N Engl J Med* 1984; **311**(25): 1594–1600.

297 Westaby D, Macdougall BR, Williams R. Improved survival following injection sclerotherapy for esophageal varices: final analysis of a controlled trial. *Hepatology* 1985; **5**(5): 827–830.

298 Korula J, Balart LA, Radvan G *et al.* A prospective, randomized controlled trial of chronic esophageal variceal sclerotherapy. *Hepatology* 1985; **5**(4): 584–589.

299 Burroughs AK, McCormick PA, Siringo S, Phillips A, McIntyre N. Prospective randomized trial of long term sclerotherapy for variceal re-bleeding, using the same protocol to treat re-bleeding in all patients . Final report (Abstract). *J Hepatol* 1989; **9**: S12.

300 Alexandrino PT, Alves MM, Pinto CJ. Propranolol or endoscopic sclerotherapy in the prevention of recurrence of variceal bleeding. A prospective, randomized controlled trial. *J Hepatol* 1988; **7**(2): 175–185.

301 Dollet JM, Champigneulle B, Patris A, Bigard MA, Gaucher P. Endoscopic sclerotherapy versus propranolol after hemorrhage caused by rupture of esophageal varices in patients with cirrhosis. Results of a 4-year randomized study. *Gastroenterol Clin Biol* 1988; **12**(3): 234–239.

302 Fleig WE, Stange EF, Schonborn W *et al.* Final analysis of a randomized trial of propranolol (P) Vs sclerotherapy (Eps) For the prevention of recurrent variceal hemorrhage (Abstract). *Hepatology* 1988; **8**: 1220.

303 Westaby D, Polson RJ, Gimson AE, Hayes PC, Hayllar K, Williams R. A controlled trial of oral propranolol compared with injection sclerotherapy for the long-term management of variceal bleeding. *Hepatology* 1990; **11**(3): 353–359.

304 Liu JD, Jeng YS, Chen PH, Siauw CP, Lin KY. Endoscopic injection sclerotherapy and propranolol in the prevention of recurrent variceal bleeding (Abstract). *Gastroenterology World Congress Abstract Book* 1990; FP: 1181.

305 Martin T, Taupignon A, Lavignolle A, Perrin D, Le Bodic L. Prevention of recurrent hemorrhage in patients with cirrhosis. Results of a controlled trial of propranolol versus endoscopic sclerotherapy. *Gastroenterol Clin Biol* 1991; **15**(11): 833–837.

306 Andreani T, Poupon RE, Balkau BJ *et al.* Efficacite comparée du propranolol et des scleroses endoscopiques du varices oesophagiennes dans la prevention des recidives d'hemorragies digestives au cours des cirrhoces (Abstract). *Etude controlee Gastroenterol Clin Biol* 1991; **15**: A215.

307 Dasarathy S, Dwivedi M, Bhargava DK, Sundaram KR, Ramachandran K. A prospective randomized trial comparing repeated endoscopic sclerotherapy and propranolol in decompensated (Child class B and C) cirrhotic patients. *Hepatology* 1992; **16**(1): 89–94.

308 Villanueva C, Balanzo J, Novella MT *et al.* Nadolol plus isosorbide mononitrate compared with sclerotherapy for the prevention of variceal re-bleeding. *N Engl J Med* 1996; **334**(25): 1624–1629.

309 Teres J, Bosch J, Bordas JM *et al.* Endoscopic sclerotherapy (ES) vs propranolol (Pr) In the elective treatment of variceal bleeding – preliminary results of a randomized controlled clinical-trial (Abstract). *J Hepatol* 1987; **5**: S210.

310 Acharya SK, Dasarathy S, Saksena S, Pande JN. A prospective randomized study to evaluate propranolol in patients undergoing long-term endoscopic sclerotherapy. *J Hepatol* 1993; **19**(2): 291–300.

311 Avgerinos A, Rekoumis G, Klonis C *et al.* Propranolol in the prevention of recurrent upper gastrointestinal bleeding in patients with cirrhosis undergoing endoscopic sclerotherapy. A randomized controlled trial. *J Hepatol* 1993; **19**(2): 301–311.

312 Elsayed SS, Shiha G, Hamid M, Farag FM, Azzam F, Awad M. Sclerotherapy versus sclerotherapy and propranolol in the prevention of re-bleeding from oesophageal varices: a randomised study. *Gut* 1996; **38**(5): 770–774.

313 Jensen LS, Krarup N. Propranolol in prevention of re-bleeding from oesophageal varices during the course of endoscopic sclerotherapy. *Scand J Gastroenterol* 1989; **24**(3): 339–345.

314 Lundell L, Leth R, Lind T, Lonroth H, Sjovall M, Olbe L. Evaluation of propranolol for prevention of recurrent bleeding from esophageal varices between sclerotherapy sessions. *Acta Chir Scand* 1990; **156**(10): 711–715.

315 Vickers C, Rhodes J, Chesner I *et al.* Prevention of re-bleeding from oesophageal varices: two-year follow up of a prospective controlled trial of propranolol in addition to sclerotherapy. *J Hepatol* 1994; **21**(1): 81–87.

316 Vinel JP, Lamouliatte H, Cales P *et al.* Propranolol reduces the re-bleeding rate during endoscopic sclerotherapy before variceal obliteration. *Gastroenterology* 1992; **102**(5): 1760–1763.

317 Westaby D, Melia W, Hegarty J, Gimson AE, Stellon AJ, Williams R. Use of propranolol to reduce the re-bleeding rate during injection sclerotherapy prior to variceal obliteration. *Hepatology* 1986; **6**(4): 673–675.

318 Bertoni G, Fornaciari G, Beltrami M *et al.* Nadolol for prevention of variceal re-bleeding during the course of endoscopic injection sclerotherapy: a randomized pilot study. *J Clin Gastroenterol* 1990; **12**(3): 364–365.

319 Gerunda GE, Neri D, Zangrandi F *et al.* Nadolol does not reduce early re-bleeding in cirrhotics undergoing endoscopic variceal sclerotherapy (Evs) – a multicenter randomized controlled trial (Abstract). *Hepatology* 1990; **12**: 988.

320 Villanueva C, Martinez FJ, Torras X *et al.* Nadolol as an adjuvant to sclerotherapy of esophageal varices for prevention of recurrent hemorrhaging. *Rev Esp Enferm Dig* 1994; **86**(1): 499–504.

321 Bertoni G, Sassatelli R, Fornaciari G *et al.* Oral isosorbide-5-mononitrate reduces the re-bleeding rate during the course of injection sclerotherapy for esophageal varices. *Scand J Gastroenterol* 1994; **29**(4): 363–370.

322 Vorobioff JD, Gamen M, Kravetz D *et al.* Effects of long-term propranolol and octreotide on postprandial hemodynamics in cirrhosis: a randomized, controlled trial. *Gastroenterology* 2002; **122**(4): 916–922.

323 Ink O, Martin T, Poynard T, Reville M *et al.* Does elective sclerotherapy improve the efficacy of long-term propranolol for

prevention of recurrent bleeding in patients with severe cirrhosis? A prospective multicenter, randomized trial. *Hepatology* 1992; **16**(4): 912–919.

324 Jensen DM, Kovacs T, Jutabha R, Randall G, Cheng S, Freeman M. Randomized, blinded prospective study of banding vs sclerotherapy for preventing recurrent variceal hemorrhage for patients without active bleeding at endoscopy (Abstract). *Gastrointest Endosc* 1995; **41**: 315A.

325 Laine L, Stein C, Sharma V. Randomized comparison of ligation versus ligation plus sclerotherapy in patients with bleeding esophageal varices. *Gastroenterology* 1996; **110**(2): 529–533.

326 de la Pena J, Rivero M, Hernandez ES *et al.* Variceal recurrence after ligation and endoscopic sclerotherapy (Abstract). *Hepatology* 1998; **28**: 1173.

327 Argonz J, Kravetz D, Suarez A *et al.* Variceal band ligation and variceal band ligation plus sclerotherapy in the prevention of recurrent variceal bleeding in cirrhotic patients: a randomized, prospective and controlled trial. *Gastrointest Endosc* 2000; **51**(2): 157–163.

328 Saeed ZA, Stiegmann GV, Ramirez FC *et al.* Endoscopic variceal ligation is superior to combined ligation and sclerotherapy for esophageal varices: a multicenter prospective randomized trial. *Hepatology* 1997; **25**(1): 71–74.

329 Al Triaf, I, Fachartz FS, Al Jumah A *et al.* Randomized trial of ligation versus combined ligation and sclerotherapy for bleeding esophageal varices. *Gastrointest Endosc* 1999; **50**(1): 1–6.

330 El Khayat HR, Omar MM, Moustafa I. Comparative evaluation of combined endoscopic variceal ligation together with low volume sclerotherapy versus ligation alone for bleeding esophageal varices (Abstract). *Hepatology* 1997; **26**: 38.

331 Hou MC, Chen WC, Lin HC, Lee FY, Chang FY, Lee SD. A new "sandwich" method of combined endoscopic variceal ligation and sclerotherapy versus ligation alone in the treatment of esophageal variceal bleeding: a randomized trial. *Gastrointest Endosc* 2001; **53**(6): 572–578.

332 Bobadilla-Diaz J, Castro-Narro G, Chavez El *et al.* Prospective study of endoscopic variceal ligation (EVL) plus endoscopic sclerotherapy vs EVL alone for the treatment of esophageal varices (Abstract). *J Hepatol* 2002; **36**: 702A.

333 Bhargava DK, Pokharna R. Endoscopic variceal ligation versus endoscopic variceal ligation and endoscopic sclerotherapy: a prospective randomized study. *Am J Gastroenterol* 1997; **92**(6): 950–953.

334 Lo GH, Lai KH, Cheng JS *et al.* The additive effect of sclerotherapy to patients receiving repeated endoscopic variceal ligation: a prospective, randomized trial. *Hepatology* 1998; **28**(2): 391–395.

335 Singh P, Pooran N, Indaram A, Bank S. Combined ligation and sclerotherapy versus ligation alone for secondary prophylaxis of esophageal variceal bleeding: a meta-analysis. *Am J Gastroenterol* 2002; **97**(3): 623–629.

336 Jensen DM, Jutabha R, Kovacs TOG *et al.* Final results of a randomized prospective study of combination banding and sclerotherapy versus sclerotherapy alone for hemostasis of bleeding esophageal varices (Abstract). *Gastrointest Endosc* 1998; **47**: 184A.

337 Koutsomanis D. Endoscopic variceal ligation combined with sclerotherapy versus sclerotherapy alone: 5-years follow-up (Abstract). *Gastroenterology* 1997; **112**: 1308A.

338 Minyana J, Gallego A, Sola V *et al.* Endoscopic ligation versus nadolol plus isosorbide-5-monouitrate for the prevention of variceal re-bleeding. A prospective and randomized trial. *Hepatology* 1999; **30**: 214A.

339 Agrawall SR, Gupta R, Marthy NS *et al.* Comparable efficacy of propranolol plus isosorbide monitrate and endoscopic variceal ligation in prevention of variceal re-bleed (Abstract). *J Hepatol* 2002; **36**: 631A.

340 Patch D, Sabin CA, Goulis J *et al.* A randomized, controlled trial of medical therapy versus endoscopic ligation for the prevention of variceal re-bleeding in patients with cirrhosis. *Gastroenterology* 2002; **123**(4): 1013–1019.

341 Romero G, Kravetz D, Argonz J *et al.* Comparative study between nadolol and 5-isosorbide mononitrate vs. endoscopic band ligation plus sclerotherapy in the prevention of variceal re-bleeding in cirrhotic patients: a randomized controlled trial. *Aliment Pharmacol Ther* 2006; **24**(4): 601–611.

342 Lo GH, Chen WC, Lin CK *et al.* Improved survival in patients receiving medical therapy as compared with banding ligation for the prevention of esophageal variceal re-bleeding. *Hepatology* 2008; **48**(2): 580–587.

343 Lo GH, Chen WC, Chen MH *et al.* Banding ligation versus nadolol and isosorbide mononitrate for the prevention of esophageal variceal re-bleeding. *Gastroenterology* 2002; **123**(3): 728–734.

344 Evrard S, Dumonceau JM, Delhaye M, Golstein P, Deviere J, Le Moine O. Endoscopic histoacryl obliteration vs propranolol in the prevention of esophagogastric variceal re-bleeding: a randomized trial. *Endoscopy* 2003; **35**(9): 729–735.

345 Lo GH, Lai KH, Cheng JS *et al.* Endoscopic variceal ligation plus nadolol and sucralfate compared with ligation alone for the prevention of variceal re-bleeding: a prospective, randomized trial. *Hepatology* 2000; **32**(3): 461–465.

346 Escorsell A, Banares R, Garcia-Pagan JC *et al.* TIPS versus drug therapy in preventing variceal re-bleeding in advanced cirrhosis: a randomized controlled trial. *Hepatology* 2002; **35**(2): 385–392.

347 Cabrera J, Maynar M, Granados R *et al.* Transjugular intrahepatic portosystemic shunt versus sclerotherapy in the elective treatment of variceal hemorrhage. *Gastroenterology* 1996; **110**(3): 832–839.

348 Cello JP, Ring EJ, Olcott EW *et al.* Endoscopic sclerotherapy compared with percutaneous transjugular intrahepatic portosystemic shunt after initial sclerotherapy in patients with acute variceal hemorrhage. A randomized, controlled trial. *Ann Intern Med* 1997; **126**(11): 858–865.

349 Garcia-Villarreal L, Martinez-Lagares F, Sierra A *et al.* Transjugular intrahepatic portosystemic shunt versus endoscopic sclerotherapy for the prevention of variceal re-bleeding after recent variceal hemorrhage. *Hepatology* 1999; **29**(1): 27–32.

350 Groupe d Etude des Anastomoses Intrahepatiques. TIPS vs sclerotherapy plus propranolol in the prevention of variceal re-bleeding – preliminary results of a multicenter randomized trial (Abstract). *Hepatology* 1995; **22**: 761.

351 Merli M, Salerno F, Riggio O *et al.* Transjugular intrahepatic portosystemic shunt versus endoscopic sclerotherapy for the prevention of variceal bleeding in cirrhosis: a randomized multicenter trial. Gruppo Italiano Studio TIPS (GIST). *Hepatology* 1998; **27**(1): 48–53.

352 Narahara Y, Kanazawa H, Kawamata H *et al.* A randomized clinical trial comparing transjugular intrahepatic portosystemic shunt with endoscopic sclerotherapy in the long-term management of patients with cirrhosis after recent variceal hemorrhage. *Hepatol Res* 2001; **21**(3): 189–198.

353 Rossle M, Deibert P, Haag K *et al.* Randomised trial of transjugular-intrahepatic-portosystemic shunt versus endoscopy plus propranolol for prevention of variceal re-bleeding. *Lancet* 1997; **349**(9058): 1043–1049.

354 Sanyal AJ, Freedman AM, Luketic VA *et al.* Transjugular intrahepatic portosystemic shunts compared with endoscopic sclerotherapy for the prevention of recurrent variceal hemorrhage. A randomized, controlled trial. *Ann Intern Med* 1997; **126**(11): 849–857.

355 Sauer P, Theilmann L, Stremmel W, Benz C, Richter GM, Stiehl A. Transjugular intrahepatic portosystemic stent shunt versus sclerotherapy plus propranolol for variceal re-bleeding. *Gastroenterology* 1997; **113**(5): 1623–1631.

356 Jalan R, Forrest EH, Stanley AJ *et al.* A randomized trial comparing transjugular intrahepatic portosystemic stent-shunt with variceal band ligation in the prevention of re-bleeding from esophageal varices. *Hepatology* 1997; **26**(5): 1115–1122.

357 Pomier-Layrargues G, Dufresne MP, Bui B *et al.* TIPS versus endoscopic variceal ligation in the prevention of variceal re-bleeding in cirrhotic patients: a comparative randomized clinical trial (interim analysis) (Abstract). *Hepatology* 1997; **26**: 35.

358 Gulberg V, Schepke M, Geigenberger G *et al.* Transjugular intrahepatic portosystemic shunting is not superior to endoscopic variceal band ligation for prevention of variceal re-bleeding in cirrhotic patients: a randomized, controlled trial. *Scand J Gastroenterol* 2002; **37**(3): 338–343.

359 Sauer P, Hansmann J, Richter GM, Stremmel W, Stiehl A. Endoscopic variceal ligation plus propranolol vs. transjugular intrahepatic portosystemic stent shunt: a long-term randomized trial. *Endoscopy* 2002; **34**(9): 690–697.

360 Casado M, Bosch J, Garcia-Pagan JC *et al.* Clinical events after transjugular intrahepatic portosystemic shunt: correlation with hemodynamic findings. *Gastroenterology* 1998; **114**(6): 1296–1303.

361 Tripathi D, Lui HF, Helmy A *et al.* Randomised controlled trial of long term portographic follow up versus variceal band ligation following transjugular intrahepatic portosystemic stent shunt for preventing oesophageal variceal re-bleeding. *Gut* 2004; **53**(3): 431–437.

362 Bureau C, Garcia-Pagan JC, Otal P *et al.* Improved clinical outcome using polytetrafluoroethylene-coated stents for TIPS: results of a randomized study. *Gastroenterology* 2004; **126**(2): 469–475.

363 Nakamura S, Mitsunaga A, Murata Y, Suzuki S, Hayashi N. Endoscopic induction of mucosal fibrosis by argon plasma coagulation (APC) for esophageal varices: a prospective randomized trial of ligation plus APC vs ligation alone. *Endoscopy* 2001; **33**(3): 210–215.

364 Cipolletta L, Bianco MA, Rotondano G, Marmo R, Meucci C, Piscopo R. Argon plasma coagulation prevents variceal recurrence after band ligation of esophageal varices: preliminary results of a prospective randomized trial. *Gastrointest Endosc* 2002; **56**(4): 467–471.

365 de Paulo GA, Ardengh JC, Nakao FS, Ferrari AP. Treatment of esophageal varices: a randomized controlled trial comparing endoscopic sclerotherapy and EUS-guided sclerotherapy of esophageal collateral veins. *Gastrointest Endosc* 2006; **63**(3): 396–402.

366 Reichle FA, Fahmy WF, Golsorkhi M. Prospective comparative clinical trial with distal splenorenal and mesocaval shunts. *Am J Surg* 1979; **137**(1): 13–21.

367 Fischer JE, Bower RH, Atamian S, Welling R. Comparison of distal and proximal splenorenal shunts: a randomized prospective trial. *Ann Surg* 1981; **194**(4): 531–544.

368 Langer B, Taylor BR, Mackenzie DR, Gilas T, Stone RM, Blendis L. Further report of a prospective randomized trial comparing distal splenorenal shunt with end-to-side portacaval shunt. An analysis of encephalopathy, survival, and quality of life. *Gastroenterology* 1985; **88**(2): 424–429.

369 Millikan WJ, Jr., Warren WD, Henderson JM *et al.* The Emory prospective randomized trial: selective versus nonselective shunt to control variceal bleeding. Ten year follow-up. *Ann Surg* 1985; **201**(6): 712–722.

370 Harley HA, Morgan T, Redeker AG *et al.* Results of a randomized trial of end-to-side portacaval shunt and distal splenorenal shunt in alcoholic liver disease and variceal bleeding. *Gastroenterology* 1986; **91**(4): 802–809.

371 Grace ND, Conn HO, Resnick RH *et al.* Distal splenorenal vs portal-systemic shunts after hemorrhage from varices: a randomized controlled trial. *Hepatology* 1988; **8**(6): 1475–1481.

372 Fernandez-Aguilar JL, Bondia Navarro JA, Santoyo SJ *et al.* Calibrated portacaval H-graft shunt in variceal hemorrhage. Long-term results. *Hepatogastroenterology* 2003; **50**(54): 2000–2004.

373 Orozco H, Mercado MA, Chan C, Guillen-Navarro E, Lopez-Martinez LM. A comparative study of the elective treatment of variceal hemorrhage with beta-blockers, transendoscopic sclerotherapy, and surgery: a prospective, controlled, and randomized trial during 10 years. *Ann Surg* 2000; **232**(2): 216–219.

374 Rikkers LF, Burnett DA, Volentine GD, Buchi KN, Cormier RA. Shunt surgery versus endoscopic sclerotherapy for long-term treatment of variceal bleeding. Early results of a randomized trial. *Ann Surg* 1987; **206**(3): 261–271.

375 Teres J, Bordas JM, Bravo D *et al.* Sclerotherapy vs. distal splenorenal shunt in the elective treatment of variceal hemorrhage: a randomized controlled trial. *Hepatology* 1987; **7**(3): 430–436.

376 Henderson JM, Kutner MH, Millikan WJ, Jr *et al.* Endoscopic variceal sclerosis compared with distal splenorenal shunt to prevent recurrent variceal bleeding in cirrhosis. A prospective, randomized trial. *Ann Intern Med* 1990; **112**(4): 262–269.

377 Spina GP, Santambrogio R, Opocher E *et al.* Distal splenorenal shunt versus endoscopic sclerotherapy in the prevention of variceal re-bleeding. First stage of a randomized, controlled trial. *Ann Surg* 1990; **211**(2): 178–186.

378 Spina GP, Henderson JM, Rikkers LF *et al.* Distal spleno-renal shunt versus endoscopic sclerotherapy in the prevention of variceal re-bleeding. A meta-analysis of 4 randomized clinical trials. *J Hepatol* 1992; **16**(3): 338–345.

379 Korula J, Yellin A, Yamada S, Weiner J, Cohen H, Reynolds TB. A prospective randomized controlled comparison of chronic endoscopic variceal sclerotherapy and portalsystemic shunt for

variceal hemorrhage in Child's class a cirrhotics (Abstract). *Hepatology* 1988; **8**: 1242.

380 Planas R, Boix J, Broggi M, Cabre E, Gomes-Vieira MC, Morillas R *et al.* Portacaval shunt versus endoscopic sclerotherapy in the elective treatment of variceal hemorrhage. *Gastroenterology* 1991; **100**(4): 1078–1086.

381 Rosemurgy AS, Goode SE, Zwiebel BR, Black TJ, Brady PG. A prospective trial of transjugular intrahepatic portasystemic stent shunts versus small-diameter prosthetic H-graft portacaval shunts in the treatment of bleeding varices. *Ann Surg* 1996; **224**(3): 378–384.

382 Rosemurgy AS, Bloomston M, Zervos EE *et al.* Transjugular intrahepatic portosystemic shunt versus H-graft portacaval shunt in the management of bleeding varices: a cost-benefit analysis. *Surgery* 1997; **122**(4): 794–799.

383 Khaitiyar JS, Luthra SK, Prasad N, Ratnakar N, Daruwala DK. Transjugular intrahepatic portosystemic shunt versus distal splenorenal shunt – a comparative study. *Hepatogastroenterology* 2000; **47**(32): 492–497.

384 Zacks SL, Sandler RS, Biddle AK, Mauro MA, Brown RS, Jr. Decision-analysis of transjugular intrahepatic portosystemic

shunt versus distal splenorenal shunt for portal hypertension. *Hepatology* 1999; **29**(5): 1399–1405.

385 Thalheimer U, Bosch J, Burroughs AK. How to prevent varices from bleeding: shades of grey–the case for nonselective beta blockers. *Gastroenterology* 2007; **133**(6): 2029–2036.

386 Senzolo M, Cholongitas E, Burra P, Leandro G, Thalheimer U, Patch D, *et al.* beta-Blockers protect against spontaneous bacterial peritonitis in cirrhotic patients: a meta-analysis. *Liver Int* 2009; **29**(8): 1189–1193.

387 Abraldes JG, Tarantino I, Turnes J, Garcia-Pagan JC, Rodes J, Bosch J. Hemodynamic response to pharmacological treatment of portal hypertension and long-term prognosis of cirrhosis. *Hepatology* 2003; **37**(4): 902–908.

388 Villanueva C, Lopez-Balaguer JM, Aracil C, Kolle L, Gonzalez B, Minana J, *et al.* Maintenance of hemodynamic response to treatment for portal hypertension and influence on complications of cirrhosis. *J Hepatol* 2004; **40**(5): 757–765.

389 Triantos C, Samonakis D, Thalheimer U, Patch D, Burroughs A. The relationship between liver function and portal pressure: what comes first, the chicken or the egg? *J Hepatol* 2005; **42**(1): 146–147.

37

Hepatic outflow syndromes and splanchnic venous thrombosis

Marco Senzolo[1], *Neeral Shah*[2], *David Patch*[3] *and Stephen Caldwell*[2]

[1]Department of Surgical and Gastroenterological Sciences, University-Hospital of Padua, Padua, Italy
[2]Department of Hepatology, University of Virginia, Charlottesville, Virginia, USA
[3]The Royal Free Sheila Sherlock Liver Centre, Royal Free Hospital, *and* University College London, London, UK

Budd-Chiari syndrome

Introduction

Budd-Chiari syndrome (BCS) is caused by obstruction of hepatic venous outflow at any level from the small hepatic veins to the junction of the inferior vena cava (IVC) with the right atrium in the absence of right heart failure or constrictive pericarditis [1]. It occurs in 0.2 per million inhabitants per year with a prevalence ranging from 1/1,000,000 of the general population in Eastern countries to 1/100,000 in Nepal [2–4]. The most common presentation is with ascites, but the range is from fulminant liver failure to asymptomatic forms. Obstruction of hepatic venous outflow is mainly caused by primary intravascular thrombosis, which may occur suddenly or repeatedly over time, accompanied by some revascularization accounting for the variable parenchymal hepatic damage and presentation. An important differential diagnosis is constrictive pericarditis or other obstructive cardiac causes. The prognosis of BCS is dictated by the rapidity of disease onset, the severity of liver dysfunction, anatomical sites of thrombosis and etiology.

Staging the venous obstruction

Budd-Chiari syndrome is classified into four disease types according to the site of the venous obstruction and in addition to the presence or absence of portal vein thrombosis: hepatic vein obstruction/thrombosis without IVC obstruction/compression; hepatic vein obstruction/thrombosis with IVC obstruction (as a result of compensatory caudate lobe hypertrophy, or IVC thrombosis) [5]; isolated hepatic webs; isolated IVC webs. Concomitant portal vein thrombosis occurs about 15% of patients with BCS, and when extensive, may preclude shunting. Coexisting PVT is associated with a mean survival of one month compared with 6.3 years without PVT [6]. Moreover, five-year survival was reported to be 85% in non-PVT BCS patients versus 58% when PVT was present [7]. Medical or mechanical thrombectomy combined with TIPS is, however, changing this poor prognosis [8, 9]. Primary membranous obstruction of the IVC is a sequela of thrombosis, occurring without hepatic vein thrombosis and accounting for 60% of BCS patients in Asia [2, 10]. However this pattern has changed over time and IVC obstruction now accounts for a lesser proportion of cases in India [11].

Diagnosis is based on the demonstration of an obstructed hepatic venous outflow tract. Color and pulsed Doppler ultrasound has a diagnostic sensitivity of almost 80% and is the recommended first-line investigation [12]. CT scan or MRI, in addition, shows the typical diagnostic feature of patchy enhancement of hepatic parenchyma which is typical of all diseases involving perfusion defects of the liver. Three-dimensional contrast-enhanced magnetic resonance angiography has been shown to have similar sensitivity to hepatic venography which was considered the most accurate diagnostic imaging [13].

Although non-invasive imaging is sufficient for the diagnosis, hepatic venography is still useful to determine the extent of the thrombosis, as well as to measure caval pressures. In addition, the portal vein can be outlined by CO_2 portography. A transjugular liver biopsy and dilatation and/or stenting of hepatic venous and IVC webs can also be performed, as well as disruption of portal vein thrombus and placement of a TIPS [14]. If a TIPS procedure is planned and hepatic veins cannot be cannulated, the portal vein can sometimes be reached via a transcaval puncture [15].

Liver histology is of potential importance when thrombosis is limited to the small intrahepatic veins as well as to estimate liver reserve and potential reversibility of the liver injury when deciding whether shunting procedures will be

Evidence-Based Gastroenterology and Hepatology, 3rd edition.
J. McDonald, A.K. Burroughs, B. Feagan, and M.B. Fennerty. © 2010
Blackwell Publishing Ltd

safe. However, sampling error is an under-studied but potentially important consideration in this setting.

Functional staging and clinical presentation

A typical patient with BCS is female, about 35 years old, with underlying thrombophilia, and often taking oral contraception [3, 4]. BCS should be suspected in patients with acute abdominal pain; an enlarged liver, particularly with known thrombophilic disorders; or when fulminant liver failure is associated with ascites [16]. Chronic BCS should be excluded when there is refractory ascites, particularly if liver function tests are relatively normal [17]. Leg edema and venous collaterals on the trunk indicate IVC compression/thrombosis [10]. Ascitic fluid typically reveals a high serum-ascites albumin gradient and total protein above 25 g/l, that is, non-cirrhotic ascites.

The severity of presentation has led to a traditional classification of fulminant (5%) [18], acute (20%) [7], subacute or chronic BCS (60%) [17], with these proportions seen in reported series. However, the prognostic value of this classification has not been prospectively validated and several authors no longer recommend it to predict mortality [19–21]. Asymptomatic BCS accounts for about 15% of cases (no ascites or abdominal pain) and is usually diagnosed fortuitously, following investigation of slightly abnormal results of liver function tests [17]. The absence of ascites is attributed to long-standing, venous collaterals. In acute BCS, 58% of patients have histological evidence of chronic disease as recent thromboses compound previous subclinical thromboses [22].

Hepatocellular carcinoma appears to complicate BCS with an incidence similar to other chronic liver diseases. HCC developed in 11 of 97 patients in a recent cohort followed up for a mean of five years [23]. However, the incidence of HCC in patients with membranous IVC obstruction is reported to range from 25% to 47.5% [24].

Etiology

A recent advance in the diagnosis of myeloproliferative disorders as aetiological factors in both Budd Chiari and splanchnic venous thrombosis is the identification of a mutation in the auto-inhibitory domain of a growth factor receptor kinase-the Janus tyrosine kinase-2 (JAK2) gene in myeloid cells, resulting in disinhibited kinase activity. This is a routine investigation in patients with Budd Chiari syndrome and splanchnic venous thrombosis, and the JAK2 mutation has been detected in 50–80% of patients with MPD, 37–45% of BCS patients, and 80% of BCS patients with MPD [28]. In the remaining patients bone marrow biopsy should be performed to exclude the diagnosis.

Amongst other acquired thrombophylic conditions, Behcet's disease is the leading cause of BCS in endemic areas. Paroxysmal nocturnal hemoglobinuria is an extremely rare disease with a severe prognosis and a close association with BCS. The incidence of BCS during the course of the disease is about 35%. Flow cytometry on peripheral blood for detection of the CD55 and CD59 deficient clone is the current standard for diagnosis. Treatment therapies include monoclonal antibodies and bone marrow transplant.

The diagnosis of antiphospholipid syndrome is difficult due to the high prevalence of anticardiolipin antibodies in chronic liver disease. Using lupus anticoagulant as diagnostic criteria, a prevalence of antiphospholipid syndrome is seen in about 15% of BCS patients [4]. Other thrombophilic disorders are seen as a cause of BCS in 20%; the factor V Leiden mutation is commonly found [26]. However, the G20210A prothrombin gene mutation appears to be less over represented among BCS patients. Diagnosing protein C and S deficiency is not straightforward as reduced concentrations can be caused by impaired hepatic synthesis. However, a normal factor II concentration together with a 20% or more reduction of protein C or S can confirm the presence of true deficiency [29].

Oral contraceptive use is a risk factor for BCS, (particularly high estrogen content pills), related to heterozygosity or homozygosity for thrombophilic defects, including ones as yet unknown [30]. BCS in pregnancy (usually postpartum) is associated with estrogen changes, IVC compression and physiologic hyperfibrinogenemia. A summary of prevalence of BCS prothrombotic defects with suggested diagnostic panel is represented in Table 37.1.

Prognosis and survival

The natural history of BCS is not well known, as most publications report on treated patients. Mortality rates have decreased over time [17, 31]. In 120 patients, five-year survival before 1985 was 50%, compared with 75% thereafter. Mortality is highest within two years of diagnosis and independent of treatment in one study, with 77%, 65% and 57% of patients surviving one, six and ten years respectively [31].

Clinicopathological factors, including treatment variables, derived from multivariable prognostic models are shown in Table 37.2 [7, 19–21, 31, 32]. In the largest cohort of 237 patients the severity of encephalopathy, ascites, serum prothrombin time and bilirubin resulted in defining three groups with statistically different five-year survival rates of 89%, 74% and 42% [7].

Histopathological features do not help to determine prognosis [7, 21, 31, 33]; in only one study of surgical shunts (n = 24) was advanced fibrosis associated with increased mortality [32]. Chronic histological changes accompanying an acute presentation of BCS resulted in lower survival compared to acute or chronic BCS [19].

IVC obstruction has a good short-term prognosis, but there is a lack of long-term data [2]. In Japan, patients with

Table 37.1 Prevalence of thrombophilic conditions and suggested screening in Budd Chiari Syndrome.

	Prevalence (%)	
Inherited conditions		
Antithrombin deficiency	5	Plasma level ATIII if no marked liver dysfunction
Protein C deficiency	20	Plasma level protein C if no marked liver dysfunction
Protein S deficiency	7	Plasma level protein S if no marked liver dysfunction
Heterozygous factor V Leiden	20	Activated protein C resistance if molecular test reveals Factor V Leiden mutation
Heterozygous G20210A prothrombin	7	Molecular test for G20210A prothrombin gene mutation
Hyperhomocysteinaemia	(?)	B12 folate, homocysteine level and MTHFR polyporphism
Acquired conditions		
V617F JAK2 positive MPD	40	V617F JAK2 mutation in peripheral blood granulocytes
V617F JAK2 negative MPD	10	Bone marrow biopsy looking for clusters of dystrophic megakaryocytes
Antiphosholipid syndrome	10	Lupus anticoagulant, anti beta2-glycoprotein-1 antibodies, anticardiolipin antibodies
Behcet's disease	5	Specific diagnostic criteria
PNH	2	Flow cytometry for CD55 and CD59 deficient blood cells
Other conditions	5	Detailed medical history
External factors		
Oral contraceptives in women	50	Medical history
Multiple factors including local factors	35	Search always for all possible causes
No factor	5	Screening for familiar prothrombotic conditions

MPD: Myeloproliferative disorders.

PHN: Parosysmal nocturnal hemoglobinuria.

Table 37.2 Clinicopathological factors associated with prognosis of Budd-Chiari syndrome.

	Henderson *et al.* [30]	Tang *et al.* [18]	Langlet *et al.* [17]	Zeitoun *et al.* [29]	Murad *et al.* [16]
Number of patients	24[a]	45	73	120	237
Histological features	yes	no	yes	no	no
Higher serum transaminases	ND	yes	ND	no	no
Higher Child-Pugh score	no	yes	yes	yes	yes
Ascites	ND	no	no	yes	yes
Hepatic encephalopathy	ND	no	ND	ND	yes
Worse prothrombin time	ND	no	yes	no	yes
Higher serum bilirubin	ND	no	yes	no	yes
Older age at diagnosis	ND	yes	ND	yes	no
Higher serum creatinine	yes	no	no	yes	no

[a] Patients who had shunt.

ND: not determined.

obliterative cavopathy have a 25% mortality rate over 15 years; most die from variceal bleeding, liver failure and hepatocellular carcinoma [10].

Treatment

Medical therapy and management of complications

All patients should receive anticoagulation, unless contraindicated, starting with intravenous heparin, then warfarin, to maintain the international normalized ratio of at least 2.5, if not higher. This treatment will control the disease in 10% of cases when the thrombosis is mild and prevent progression, although there are no randomized trials [17, 31, 34].

Fulminant BCS is usually associated with abundant necrosis that ideally requires liver transplantation. Even in the setting of immediate shunting (surgical or TIPS), hepatic regeneration will rarely take place and liver transplantation must be available as the liver failure may worsen [35]. In patients with acute BCS, early thrombolytic therapy used within 72 hours from diagnosis and infused directly into the thrombosed hepatic vein for 24 hours, has had variable success [36]. Adjunctive angioplasty or stent placement may not be of further therapeutic benefit [37].

Angioplasty

Short-segment obstruction or webs in hepatic veins or the IVC are treated successfully by balloon dilatation or intravascular stents. Membranous vena caval obstruction can be relieved initially in 90% of patients, but 20–30% will need additional angioplasty [38, 39]. Eapen *et al.* reported 94% and 87% survival at one and five years in BCS patients with mild disease, according to the Murad classification, who were treated only by radiological intervention at a single center [40].

Approximately half of all cases of rethrombosis are due to suboptimal anticoagulation therapy. When there is diffuse thrombosis of hepatic veins, angioplasty alone is only successful in 56% of patients, even with additional thrombolytic therapy. On the other hand, stents result in long-term patency rates of 80–90%, requiring further angioplasty in 50% [41]. Failure of thrombolysis or angioplasty and the presence of a diffuse hepatic vein thrombosis are indications for shunting.

Portosystemic shunting

The therapeutic principle of portosystemic shunting is the conversion of the portal vein into an outflow tract (reversed portal flow), thus decompressing the sinusoids. Thrombosis or compression of the IVC maintains a high pressure in the infrahepatic IVC. Therefore a portacaval or mesocaval shunt will not provide decompression, whereas a shunt from the portal or mesenteric vein to the suprahepatic IVC or right atrium will be effective.

Surgical shunts Patients with a non-fulminant presentation of BCS and those without significant hepatic fibrosis who have a chronic presentation, can be considered for surgical shunting, providing the portal vein is patent. A side-to-side portal caval shunt (or meso-caval shunt) not only decompresses the liver, but also relieves ascites and eliminates the risk of variceal bleeding. A differential of 10 mmHg or more between the portal and intrahepatic IVC is considered essential [32]. A hypertrophied caudate lobe often makes the side-to-side portal caval shunt difficult to construct. Orloff *et al.* reported no technical failures, one operative death, 95% survival, a complete resolution of ascites and no encephalopathy in 60 patients, followed for a range of 3.5 to 27 years. Normal liver histology was found in 48% of patients, and stable fibrosis in the other patients, but cirrhosis did not regress. All shunts, with the exception of two patients who experienced late thrombosis, remained hemodynamically effective, despite some patients not receiving anticoagulation [42]. Contrary to this study,

another series reported a survival rate between 57–75% [35, 43] suggesting Orloff *et al.* either possessed greater experience or used more favorable selection criteria.

If the IVC is patent but severely compressed, a self-expanding stent can be placed in the intrahepatic IVC, followed by a surgical infrahepatic shunt [44]. Retrospective series have questioned the benefits of surgical shunts due to the lack of a survival advantage, independent of liver disease severity, the type of shunt (including TIPS), and the interval between diagnosis and procedure; an exception was patients with mild hepatic impairment (82% vs 68% survival at five years) [19, 21]. This lack of effect on survival could be explained by the average 25% hospital/perioperative mortality (range 0–30%) [35], and late shunt dysfunction/thrombosis [45]. Increased fibrosis at surgery was associated with higher mortality [32]. Some perioperative mortality can be attributed to acute hepatic decompensation, which is remedied only by emergency salvage liver transplantation.

Thus, shunting should be performed in a liver transplantation center where rescue therapy is possible. Moreover a TIPS procedure should be attempted before a surgical one, allowing a trial of shunting; if this fails, a liver transplantation is indicated. **B4**

Transjugular intrahepatic portosystemic shunts (TIPS) The use of TIPS has improved the management of BCS. TIPS avoids laparotomy, overcomes caudate lobe compression and occlusion of the IVC, with less periprocedure mortality than surgical shunting, particularly in patients with poor liver function. Using TIPS does not preclude subsequent surgical shunting or liver transplantation [14, 46–48]. With TIPS, the porto-caval pressure gradient should be normalized (≤6 mmHg). In three series, mortality rates ranged from 9–30% during a mean follow-up of four years. Among 65 patients, seven died: one with fulminant liver failure (transplantation contraindicated), four with severe liver disease (acute on chronic presentation) and three with underlying hematological disorders.

Long-term patency, despite routine anticoagulation therapy, only averaged 50%, with 36–72% of patients needing reintervention. TIPS can be placed even if there is portal vein thrombosis [11]. Polytetrafluoroethylene-covered stents result in patency rates of 67% at one year compared with 19% with uncovered stents, a very low rate compared with other series [46]. A recent cohort study on 124 patients with BCS who underwent TIPS in six centers in Europe showed that TIPS was able to improve survival according to Rotterdam score prediction with five years survival of 71% in high risk patients [49].

TIPS should be considered as first-line therapy, if variceal bleeding occurs, for acute and chronic BCS and also in patients with fulminant BCS if a liver donor is not available within 2–3 days. **B4** A recent report demonstrated that

Table 37.3 Liver transplantation for Budd-Chiari syndrome.

	Halff et al. [52]	Jamieson et al. [53]	Ringe et al. [35]	Srinivastan et al. [54]	Ulrich et al. [55]	Metha et al. [58]	Segev et al. [57]
Patients	17	12	43	19	27	248	510
Mean interval from diagnosis to OLT (months)	13	ND	ND	8	ND	55.8	NA
Follow-up (years)	3	5	10	10	5	10	3
Survival	88%	50%	69%	95%	87%	68%	80%
Recurrence of disease/thrombosis	17%	13%	9%	21%	15%	11%	NA

Legend: ND: not determined.

among five patients with FHF, TIPS allowed resolution of the disease in one, and acted as a bridge to liver transplantation within one month in three patients [50]. TIPS intervention should be managed carefully if the patient's liver reserve is sub-optimal and rescue liver transplantation should be available. **B4**

Liver transplantation

In the remaining 10% of patients, when percutaneous angioplasty or TIPS fail, liver transplantation should be considered. Emergency liver transplantation is indicated for fulminant BCS, and has been used as a salvage procedure for fulminant liver failure induced by surgical shunting [35, 43, 51].

There are seven major transplant series, with more than ten patients each, totaling 162 patients (see Table 37.3), with survival rates between 50% and 95% with a mean follow-up of 4.5 years [35, 52–55]. Twenty patients (12%) had acute portal vein or hepatic arterial thrombosis, or late thrombosis, which was fatal in eight and resulted in retransplantation in eight. Despite anticoagulation recurrent BCS occurred in two of seven transplanted patients [56].

Recently a retrospective analysis of series from USA and Europe has shown a five-year survival rate of 80% [57, 58]. However, a TIPS was placed in only 4% of patients before transplant in the European series and anticoagulation was used in less than 60%. Recurrence of venous thrombosis or BCS occurred in about 10% of patients, confirming the need of anticoagulation.

Although almost all genetic thrombophilic disorders are cured by transplantation [43, 59], thrombosis still occurs and routine anticoagulation therapy is necessary. Careful monitoring is necessary as complications of anticoagulation were seen in 40% and in 17/197 (11%) after liver transplantation who had bleeding complications due to anticoagulation leading to two deaths in the European series [56].

In patients with myeloproliferative disorders, use of hydroxyurea and aspirin is safe and effective [60]. So far

malignant transformation is anecdotal [54, 58]. A suggested algorithm of treatment for BCS is shown in Figure 37.1.

Portal and splanchnic vein thrombosis

Splanchnic thrombotic disease has a wide spectrum of presentation and a wide range of severity. The disorders can be challenging and sometimes overlapping; appropriate management hinges on accurate diagnosis and especially on the broad distinction between cirrhosis-associated thrombotic disease and non-cirrhotic splanchnic venous thrombosis. The complexity of these cases, especially with non-cirrhotic acute PVT or cavernoma, usually warrants a multidisciplinary approach with involvement of both hematology and GI/hepatology, as well as other support services. Below, we have focused on portal vein thrombosis (PVT) and isolated splenic vein thrombosis (SVT), with emphasis on adult disease from a practical clinical perspective. Several recent reviews also offer excellent and comprehensive examination of the disorder [61–63].

Portal vein thrombosis (PVT): epidemiology

The exact annual incidence of PVT is not known although it is a common condition in most tertiary care centers. The difficulty in determining clear epidemiology of PVT results in part from its highly variable associations. In an autopsy series, PVT was discovered in 254 of 23,796 autopsies (1%) performed over a 12-year period from Uppsala Sweden [64]. Among those with PVT, 28% had cirrhosis (one-third with and two-thirds without hepatocellular cancer), 23% had primary hepatobiliary cancer (two-thirds hepatocellular cancer and one-third biliary), 44% had metastatic cancer, 10% had intra-abdominal infection or inflammatory conditions, 3% had myeloproliferative disease and 14% were without an apparent association. As discussed below, up to 20% of patients with cirrhosis develop portal thrombosis, which probably constitutes the single most common association encountered in liver centers. However, PVT in

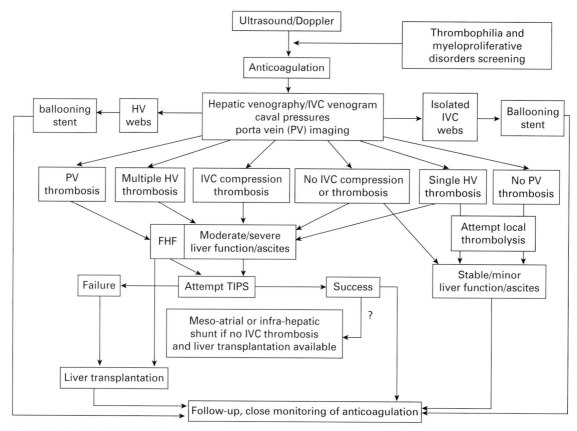

Figure 37.1 Flow chart in and management of Budd-Chiari syndrome.

cirrhosis is frequently discovered incidentally and, while it may result in liver atrophy and warrants a close examination for an associated hepatocellular cancer, it is a less urgent clinical situation than acute PVT in the non-cirrhotic patient in whom the presentation can be dramatic.

In all cases, additional diagnostic investigation is warranted and the risk-benefit of anticoagulation therapy needs to be carefully considered. However, as a result of the broad array of presentations and relatively low prevalence, controlled data treatment is limited and much of the literature, including two efforts at consensus or summary statements, are reflections more of experience and expert opinion than evidence-based on randomized trials [65, 66].

Portal vein thrombosis: overview of clinical presentation and evaluation

The typical clinical presentation ranges from sudden onset of abdominal pain and ascites with acute PVT, to acute variceal hemorrhage in the setting of chronic PVT, to incidentally discovered cavernoma (cavernous transformation of the portal vein) found, for example, during an evaluation of low platelets due to hypersplenism and splenomegaly. These clinical situations can present the clinician with diagnostic and therapeutic problems which need to be systematically worked through. For example, the presence of splenomegaly may be both part of PVT secondary to the thrombus and localized portal hypertension and also part of an underlying myeloproliferative disorder. Ascites can be seen even in patients without cirrhosis and its evaluation can be confusing (see below).

These studies, especially CT and MR, may also help to establish whether the thrombus is recent (absence of collateralisation) or chronic (presence of cavernous transformation.) Long standing portal vein thrombosis may result in irregularity of the liver outline, probably due to asymmetry of blood flow, resulting in the radiological appearance of cirrhosis-in these instances a biopsy is required, as the prognosis will be significantly altered by the histology.

The clinician then needs to exclude the presence of varices by endoscopy which then helps to weigh the risk-benefit of anticoagulation therapy. Laboratory tests should be performed to evaluate for hypercoagulable conditions and the history must be carefully explored to evaluate for any evidence of prior liver abnormalities, use of prothrombotic agents such as estrogen preparations, and prior thrombotic disease, including family history and prior intra-abdominal inflammation. Detailed questioning is needed regarding any history of neonatal illness which would suggest possible umbilical vein cannulation, and any distant episodes of intra-abdominal illnesses which might suggest prior appendicitis or diverticulitis.

Acute non-cirrhotic PVT

Acute, non-cirrhotic PVT is the least common cause of PVT but perhaps the most dramatic. Among 3655 liver disease patients recorded in a University of Virginia liver disease registry kept between approximately 1995 and 2004, 19 patients (0.5%) presented with this condition (unpublished observations). Although these patients have not yet been thoroughly evaluated about one-third of these had an underlying myeloproliferative disorder and another third had an identifiable pro-thrombotic condition. The most common presentation in our patients was abdominal pain and ascites, with intractable variceal bleeding in a minority. Similarly, Condat *et al.* observed significantly less gastrointestinal bleeding in acute PVT compared to cavernoma (see below) [67]. Bloody diarrhea may also be evident, especially if the thrombosis extends into the superior mesenteric vein distribution. Ascites can also be seen in one-third of patients with non-cirrhotic acute PVT [61]. Opening of portosystemic collaterals dissipates the portal hypertension and thus the ascites, although a transition to chylous ascites indicates rupture of the pressurized lymphatic vessels [68]. The ascites fluid characteristics may be difficult to interpret as the fluid (in non-chylous situations) derives from bowel edema rather than the typical liver-derived transudate as in cirrhosis [69].

Although 20–40% of patients have no identifiable underlying thrombophilic risk factors and there is a degree of regional variation, myeloproliferative disorders (polycythemia vera, essential thrombocythemia or myelofibrosis) are the most common identifiable causes of acute PVT, while specific factor abnormalities such as protein C, S or anti-thrombin III deficiency, factor V Leiden or prothrombin mutation, and anti-phospholipid abnormalities are associated risk-factor in the remaining cases [67, 70].

Myeloproliferative disorders underlie PVT more often than previously thought, and it is here that the test for the JAK2 mutation has been particularly eye-opening, as it has provided a non-invasive screening test for bone marrow disorders allowing one to select patients for the more invasive bone marrow biopsy [71]. This test probably should become a part of the routine laboratory evaluation of these patients but this remains to be determined. It should be considered if available.

Morbidity in acute PVT can be substantial, but prolonged survival in acute non-cirrhotic PVT is common. Consistent with our own experience, Janssen *et al.* reported ten-year survival of 81% in this group provided that cirrhosis and underlying malignancy were excluded [72]. As discussed further below, long-term morbidity related to recurrent thrombi and/or transformation to cavernoma can be influenced by early anticoagulation, although controlled data is lacking, and the benefits must be weighed against the risk of severe portal hypertensive bleeding and other complications of anticoagulation.

Portal cavernoma

This entity was first reported in 1869 by Balfour and Stewart to describe the post-thrombotic dilatation of the portal vein, which we now know to be commonly associated with prior and often unrecognized PVT. The term "cavernoma" was subsequently used by Köbrich in 1928 to describe the spongy appearance of the network of blood vessels in the portal vein location related to re-canalization of the thrombosis. Local infections (portal phlebitis, omphalitis), abdominal trauma and a history of prothrombotic disorders are implicated in the development of the PVT, but many cases remain unexplained. Cavernoma develops as the portal vein thrombus undergoes reorganization and remodeling into a network of collateral vessels which overcome the occlusion and restore, to a variable degree, hepatopedal blood flow. Cavernous transformation can occur rapidly even within 6–20 days and thus the presence of cavernoma, while usually suggesting chronicity, does not necessarily indicate a very distant event [73]. Hematemesis and splenomegaly are the most common presenting symptoms occurring in about 50% of these patients [74].

Portal biliopathy (biliary obstruction and stricturing) due to ischemia, duct compression by collateral vessels or possible local infection causes symptomatic disease in 4 to 24%, although abnormal cholestatic liver chemistries and cholangiographic abnormalities are much more common [75]. Treatment options include medical therapy with ursodeoxycholic acid, endoscopic therapy including biliary stenting, and in severe cases surgical or radiological shunting. In chronic cases, pre-operative decompression of the portal cavernoma is being explored to avoid life-threatening hemorrhage and other complications following surgical intervention [76]; decompression can be feasible by the placement of TIPS [77].

Strategies to avoid the complications of portal cavernomas have involved early anticoagulation, in cases with early diagnosis, to promote recanalization [67]. Long-term therapy is essential in those with an identified pre-thrombotic condition such as underlying protein C or S deficiency. However, intervention with anticoagulation requires careful exclusion and management of varices if present. It is also important to recall that portal cavernoma may be stable over many years, even without aggressive intervention, especially among patients presenting with more indolent symptoms, which is also our experience. In such cases, we have typically used low-dose forms of anti-coagulation provided varices have been excluded endoscopically.

PVT in cirrhosis

Portal vein thrombosis (PVT) occurs in 10–20% of all cirrhotic patients, and conversely cirrhosis is responsible for about 20% of all cases of PVT [78]. Symptoms of acute abdominal pain, variceal bleeding, and ascites develop in 57% of cirrhotic patients with PVT [79]. Portal vein thrombosis in this setting can develop due to hepatic fibrosis and the resistance to blood flow (stasis), but there can also be many other factors, including a genetic predisposition to prothrombotic disorders, or abdominal infections, or local factors, for example pancreatitis [80]. Thrombosis can extend distally into right and left portal vein branches or proximally into the superior mesenteric vein (see Table 37.4). More often the thrombosis in the portal vein is incomplete and does not result in complete occlusion [81].

Complications of PVT in cirrhosis include splenomegaly, esophageal varices, gastric varices, and portal hypertensive gastropathy. PVT has traditionally been a contraindication to liver transplantation due to technical difficulties in intra-operative anastomases. This situation has led to evaluation of a trial of anticoagulation in patients with cirrhosis and PVT [82]. However, monitoring anticoagulation in cirrhosis with an underlying coagulopathy is a challenge. Traditional measures such as INR (international normalized ratio) are of limited use because it is not only affected by oral anticoagulation medication, such as coumadin, but also factor deficiencies from hepatic dysfunction.

Low weight molecular heparins may be safer than oral anticoagulation in cirrhosis. Recently, repermeation was obtained in 50% of 38 patients with cirrhosis and portal vein thrombosis with only one episode of non-severe variceal bleeding [83].

Further study is clearly essential to determine the relative utility and the risk-benefit of this type of intervention. Surgical techniques involving thrombectomy and bypass

grafts also remain to be fully evaluated but should be used cautiously as these may be associated with high morbidity and mortality [84].

The use of transjugular intrahepatic portosystemic shunt is feasible in patients with portal vein thrombosis given the patency of intrahepatic portal branches, even in the presence of cavernous transformation and allows treatment of portal hypertensive complications when anticoagulation fails to prevent progression of thrombosis. Moreover TIPS allows the undertaking of thrombectomy in 50% of cases [85]. An integrated algorithm of treatment of portal vein thrombosis including easy anticoagulation and radiological treatments when progression of thrombosis or portal hypertensive complications occur could be the best option, but this needs to be prospectively explored. **B4**

Portal vein thrombosis and hepatocellular cancer (HCC)

The incidence of PVT in patients with cirrhosis and hepatocellular carcinoma (HCC) has been found to be as high as 35% [86]. Indeed, the development of PVT in previously stable cirrhosis warrants a close evaluation for neoplasia. Hypercoagulability due to the underlying malignancy can explain the higher rate of PVT, but tumor invasion into the portal vein can also cause mechanical obstruction. Clinically, it can be difficult to discern between thrombosis or tumor invasion using current imaging modalities.

The concurrence of PVT and HCC imparts a severe prognosis. HCC without PVT has a median prognosis of 24 months, but when associated with PVT and possible portal vein tumor invasion, this drops to a dismal 2.7 months [87]. This striking difference may relate to tumor aggressiveness or possibly to limitations of therapeutic intervention. Several different techniques for HCC treatment are currently being used: percutaneous ethanol injection, radiofrequency ablation, transcatheter arterial chemoembolization, and glass radioactive microspheres. In the setting of PVT and compromised portal flow, extensive or multiple arterial embolization techniques can increase the risk of liver failure, but radioactive microspheres may offer the best risk-benefit ratio.

In experienced centers, super-selective, segmental drug delivery can avoid these complications but still has clinical limitations [88]. In addition, the diagnostic dilemma of thrombus versus tumor invasion, limited by current imaging techniques, usually precludes the possibility of liver transplantation. With tumor invasion into the portal vein, transplantation has limited success and is associated with rapid recurrence [89]. Together, these complex associations are indicative of the need for careful clinical investigation in patients suffering the triad of cirrhosis, HCC and PVT.

Table 37.4 Grades of portal vein thrombosis (PVT).

Grade	Description
Grade 1 PVT	Thrombosis of intrahepatic portal vein branches
Grade 2 PVT	Thrombosis of right or left portal branches
Grade 3 PVT	Partial obstruction of portal vein trunk
Grade 4 PVT	Complete obstruction of portal vein trunk

Adapted from Nonami *et al.* [86].

Isolated splenic vein thrombosis

Isolated splenic vein thrombosis presents most commonly with abdominal pain and UGI bleeding, frequently due to gastric varices, although there is regional variation in the major clinical manifestations and associated symptoms [70, 90]. Underlying malignancy (50%) and pancreatitis (15%) are the two most common predisposing factors although identifiable hypercoagulable states and myeloproliferative disorders can be present in a small minority (7%) in some series [70]. While intractable gastric variceal bleeding is the most serious complication, a natural history study from North Carolina indicates, surprisingly, that this occurs in only about 4% of SVT patients, in the setting of pancreatitis over a mean follow-up of 40 months [91].

From the perspective of gastric variceal bleeding, SVT is the cause in only about 10% of new onset GVB, with the majority being related to cirrhosis and portal hypertension without associated thrombotic disease [92]. Nonetheless, GV bleeding in the setting of SVT is challenging and associated with a high rate of recurrent bleeding following local therapy such as with cyanoacrylate injection. This may be due to the origin of GV in SVT from the short gastric veins rather than gastro-spleno-renal anastomases as seen in cirrhosis. In our experience, most cases of such non-cirrhotic SVT complicate either local pancreatic or gastric cancer (50%), or chronic pancreatitis (50%) [92]. In the latter case, splenectomy, although lacking controlled data, is the optimal intervention [93]. **B4** In the former, palliative measures are more often appropriate.

Several unique circumstances can also be seen in this clinical scenario, such as pregnancy-related SVT [96]. Notably, bleeding due to pregnancy related splenic vein thrombosis can be treated with local injection of cyanoacrylate polymers as occurred in one case we have described [92]. Delivery was successful and post-partum endoscopic evaluation revealed no recurrence of the gastric varices.

Anti-coagulation in portal vein thrombosis

Patients with a procoagulant disorder should be anticoagulated to prevent thrombus extension, or the development of de-novo thromboses. The concern is that patients with varices may bleed if anticoagulated. Yet the evidence suggests that the lethality of subsequent thrombosis is higher than that of bleeding [94]. Thus pragmatically, the approach should be: if pro-coagulant, and never bled, then anticoagulate. If pro-coagulant and previous variceal bleeding- then balance of risk may favour (brief) variceal obliteration and/or betablockers followed by anticoagulation.

The data on thrombolytic therapy in patients with acute portal vein thrombosis is peppered with anecdote and case reports. Whilst outstanding results have been documented, catastrophic complications are also recognised (though usually less reported). A recent review suggested this should only be considered in those who are least likely to re-canalise with anticoagulant therapy-patients with ascites, acute splenic and portal vein thrombosis [95].

Current evidence favours early institution of heparin anticoagulation followed by warfarinisation whilst a search for precipitant factors occurs. Patients with an identified prothrombotic tendency, even in the presence of varices, should be anti-coagulated [97].

Veno occlusive disease/sinusoidal obstruction syndrome

Introduction

Hepatic veno-occlusive/sinusoidal obstruction syndrome (VOD/SOS) disease is a clinical syndrome characterized by hepatomegaly, ascites, weight gain and jaundice [98, 99]. It was first described in a patient who drank an infusion made with pyrrolizidine alkaloids.

Early histological abnormalities include sinusoidal congestion associated with centrilobular necrosis, and later fibrous obliterative lesions in the hepatic venules occur with histologic damage located to zone 3 of the acinus.

VOD is also associated with other toxins such as alcohol, oral contraceptives, toxic oil, terbinafine, or radiation injury. The first case associated with hematopoietic stem cell transplantation (STC) was reported in 1979 [100]. Since then SCT has become the most important and frequent cause of VOD. In this setting diagnosis is made using the same clinical signs as for other etiologies. Other causes are infrequent but require exclusion. VOD after SCT is a part of the spectrum of multi organ syndromes which include idiopathic pneumonitis, diffuse alveolar hemorrhage, thrombotic microangiopathy and capillary leak syndrome.

The incidence of VOD after STC ranges from 0 to 70%, dependent on the particular application of specific diagnostic criteria, the sample size and risk factors which are heterogenous amongst different cohorts [101]. Currently, the incidence and severity of VOD after SCT is decreasing due to earlier timing of SCT in patients with leukemia, the use of non-myeloablative regimens and the decrease of HCV infection amongst transplant candidates [102]. However, the incidence of VOD remains high in patients undergoing aggressive chemotherapy regimens to eradicate cancer. New chemotherapeutic agents, in particular gemtuzumab and ozogamicin have been associated with a frequent occurrence of sinusoidal toxicity.

Veno-occlusive disease is also reported after other solid organ transplantation, particularly, kidney transplantation.

The largest series report an incidence of 2–5% (5/200 kidney transplants), mainly related to azathioprine toxicity. In liver transplant recipients the largest series reported an incidence of 1.9% (19/1023 liver transplants) clinical VOD, related to the number and severity of rejection episodes and azathioprine use. In contrast, reversible hepatic venule stenosis, including cases diagnosed histologically, is reported in 43% after liver transplantation and is mainly related to azathioprine [103].

Pathophysiology and histology

After SCT the high dose cytoreductive therapy used in patients who have a particular susceptibility, produces endothelial injury of both sinusoids and small hepatic venules (the latter only if the damage is more severe). Due to the inconspicuous presence of venular damage in patients with less severe VOD/SOS, and evidence from experimental models of the primary target being sinusoidal endothelial cells, the denomination of sinusoidal obstruction syndrome has been proposed to replace the term VOD.

The sinusoidal damage leads to activation of the coagulation cascade and clot formation. Fibrin-related plugs, intracellular fluid entrapment and cellular debris progressively occlude sinusoids, causing intrahepatic post-sinusoidal portal hypertension, responsible for the clinical signs of fluid retention (weight increase), hepatomegaly, ascites and jaundice. Usually fibrosis occurs several weeks after the onset of the disease. An early deposition of matrix metalloproteinases-2 has also been reported in the sinusoids. Several factors other than cytoreductive therapy contribute to the damage in VOD. Release of cytokines such as TNF-alfa, IL1 and 2 released due to the endothelial injury, but also due to cyclosporine given to patients with GVHD, have procoagulant activity. Immunological mechanisms have been implicated based on the observation of a lower incidence of VOD following T cell depleted and autologous SCT, and a higher incidence amongst mismatched transplants.

All these injuries cause depletion of glutathione from hepatocytes, resulting in increased sensitivity to zone 3 damage due to other compounds, which can further deplete this antioxidant compound, such as cyclophosphamide, busulfan and BCNU. In parallel with the decline in hepatic venous flow, nitric oxide (NO) levels in the hepatic vein decreases [104]. This change suggests that vasoconstriction related to NO depletion occurs, further incrementing the damage.

Clinical presentation and diagnosis

The classic presentation of VOD is characterized by the triad of weight gain caused by fluid retention, tender hepatomegaly and hyperbilirubinemia without any known cause [104, 105]. Usually this occurs within 10–20 days after

SCT when regimens containing cyclophosphamide have been used. With other regimens it occurs later on [106]. After liver transplantation VOD occurs over a wide interval, with a mean of nine weeks after transplant. Diagnosis is usually based on signs and symptoms, having ruled out other conditions which can mimic the disease, particularly after STC, such as viral infections and graft versus host disease, cholestatic secondary sepsis, heart failure and tumoral infiltration of the liver [107].

Nowadays, clinical criteria have been formalized in the Baltimore and Seattle criteria (see Table 37.5). The Baltimore criteria are more restrictive, and usually patients fulfilling these are diagnosed at a more severe stage of the disease [108].

Endothelial injury can be suspected even before the appearance of the clinical or other laboratory signs by finding elevated serum levels of PAI-1, procollagen III, and its precursor propeptide (P-III-P) [109]. Serum hyaluronic acid, vWF-cleaving protease ADAMTS13 and Ca-125 have also been evaluated as early markers of VOD.

Ultrasound of the liver and abdomen with Doppler examination is the first-line imaging investigation. Findings include the presence of ascites, hepatomegaly, attenuated hepatic veins and/or biliary dilatation. However, none of these signs are specific for the diagnosis and must be interpreted within the clinical context [110].

Pulsed Doppler ultrasound can suggest VOD on the basis of a decreased or reversed portal venous flow [111]. Significant elevation of the hepatic artery resistive index in duplex sonography may be a sensitive index of liver

Table 37.5 Diagnostic criteria of veno occlusive disease after SCT.

Seattle criteria
At least two of the three following criteria: within the first month after stem cell transplantation (SCT):
(1) Jaundice
(2) Hepatomegaly and right upper quadrant pain
(3) Ascites and/or unexplained weight gain

Baltimore criteria
Elevated total serum bilirubin (≥2 mg/dl) before day 21 after SCT and two of the following three criteria:
(1) Tender hepatomegaly
(2) Weight gain > 5% from baseline
(3) Ascites

Modified Seattle criteria
Occurrence of two of the following events within 20 days of SCT:
(1) Hyperbilirubinaemia (≥2 mg/dl)
(2) Hepatomegaly or right upper quadrant pain of liver origin
(3) Unexplained weight gain (> 2% of baseline bodyweight) because of fluid accumulation

damage related to VOD. In infants, a segmental portal flow reversal has also been shown to be strongly associated with early VOD [112].

Hemodynamics and hepatic vein catetherization

The transjugular access is a safe route to perform measurement of the hepatic venous pressure gradient (HVPG) and liver biopsy [113]. The absence of a significant gradient (<6 mmHg) along the hepatic veins and in the IVC can exclude anatomical causes of outflow obstruction. In one study 82% of patients with VOD had HVPG greater than 9 mmHg, but this was not found in those with GVHD. In another study an HVPG greater than 10 mmHg was significantly correlated with VOD (91% specificity and 86% positive predictive value) [114].

HVPG can be also helpful to determine prognosis, as patients who will survive with VOD have less severe portal hypertension. An HVPG greater than 20 mmHg is correlated with poor prognosis [98]. The transjugular access allows liver biopsy to be performed safely even if coagulation is impaired (without the need of blood product transfusion), which is often the case. Another advantage of TJLB is the possibility of performing multiple passes in different sites of the liver, which offers a theoretical advantage in diagnosing diseases with patchy distribution like VOD or hepatic venous obstruction syndromes [113].

Prognosis and outcome

Bearman *et al.* have developed a model to estimate survival in patients with VOD based on a large cohort of SCT patients. Percentage of weight gained, bilirubin, ascites and peripheral edema were associated with worse survival. Severe VOD was associated with 98% mortality at day 100 after SCT (see Table 37.3). Moreover HVPG greater than 20 mmHg was confirmed as an independent prognostic marker of mortality [98].

Outcome of VOD after liver transplantation is reported by Sebagh *et al.* with 63% mortality (12 of 19 patients) in the largest series published. Because of the low incidence of this complication after LT, no specific prognostic factors have been evaluated, but clinical features derived from SCT groups could be used to assess severity of VOD after LT as well. Mortality after liver transplantation is related mainly to liver failure and development of renal insufficiency due to portal hypertensive complications [103].

Therapy

Prevention

Treatment of VOD is primary supportive and spontaneous recovery is reported in 70–85% of mild forms after stem cell transplantation. However, as severe forms do not resolve

and given the paucity of effective therapies, prevention is a priority. The use of non-myeloablative regimens in patients with risk factors for VOD is now possible. Busulfan has been shown to be less hepatotoxic when administered intravenously rather than orally. The study of genetic polymorphisms of glutathione S transferase and TNF-alfa have been evaluated and allow identification of the patients at risk, but further studies are needed.

Prophylactic administration of ursodeoxycholic acid, being an antioxidant and antiapoptotic agent, has been evaluated in four randomized trials [115–118]. Two trials have shown a significant benefit of UDCA 600 mg daily in preventing VOD after SCT (VOD incidence 15% vs 40% and 3% vs 18.5%) [115, 117], but in the most recent two (one in combination with heparin) no benefit of UDCA administration per se or when added to heparin was seen. In the trial in which UDCA was given alone at the dose of 12 mg/kg daily, there was a decrease in overall mortality, with a decreased incidence of GVHD [116, 118].

Prostaglandin E1 is a vasodilator with protective properties for the endothelium and has antithrombotic activity. One non-randomized trial in which PGE1 was given in combination with heparin or heparin and tPA showed a lower incidence of VOD in the PGE1 group (12.2% vs 25.5%). However, the most recent prospective study, enrolling 24 patients using PGE1 alone, failed to show any advantage and was associated with severe toxicity in all [119].

Treatment

Treatment of the classical syndrome also includes supportive measure. Ascites is treated with sodium restriction, diuretics and paracentesis. Mechanical organ support may be needed when renal or respiratory failure develops. Correction of coagulopathy and prevention of infections in severe forms are often used to avoid bacterial translocation from the gut by intestinal disinfection.

Based on the histological presence of microthrombosis and fibrin deposition in the hepatic venules of patients with VOD, the principal specific therapy has been to promote fibrinolysis with or without anticoagulation [102]. To date, about 130 patients have been treated with tPA; the response rate is about 30% in the largest series, with the addition of concomitant heparin [120]. However, no response was seen amongst patients with MOF, renal or respiratory failure. Moreover, 24% developed severe bleeding. Thus, administration of antifibrinolytics and anticoagulants should be avoided in these patients, but conversely should be given early in the course of VOD. **B4**

Administration of ATIII and protein C or PGE1 have not been shown to be effective [121]. However, there is some evidence for the use of defibrotide. **B4** This is a polydeoxyribonucleic acid derived from porcine and bovine mucosa that has antifibrinolytic and antithrombotic properties; it also decreases leucocyte rolling and adherence to the

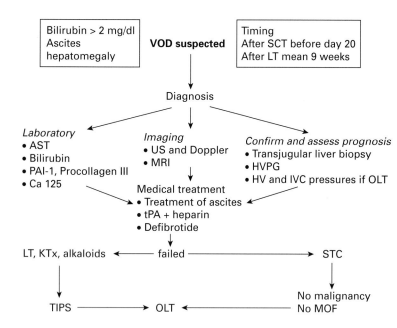

Figure 37.2 Flow chart in diagnosis and management of veno-occlusive disease.
VOD: veno occlusive disease; SCT: stem cell transplantation; OLT: ortothopic liver transplantation; HVPG: hepatic venous pressure gradient; HV: hepatic vein; IVC: inferior vena cava; KT: kidney transplantation; MOF: multi organ failure; TIPS: transjugula, intrahepatic, portosystemic shunt.

endothelium as well as decreasing thrombin generation and lowering circulating levels of PAI-1.

In the largest series published, treatment with 10–60 mg/kg/day infusion of defibrotide every six hours achieved a response rate of 36% and overall survival rate of 35% at 100 days after SCT, without adverse events [122].

The high mortality rate of VOD after liver transplantation leads to the need of specific therapy. In the only two patients treated with defibrotide for VOD after LT, only one survived [123]. No effective medical therapy has been reported.

Decompression of the engorged sinusoids by a transjugular, intrahepatic, portosystemic shunt can relieve portal hypertension and prevent renal failure in patients with VOD. The recent review on clinical practice guidelines for transjugular intrahepatic portosystemic shunt (TIPS) did not recommend TIPS for veno-occlusive disease (VOD). **B4** However, it was implied that VOD is only seen after SCT, whereas it can be seen in other settings, in which TIPS may offer a potentially useful treatment.

To date, 27 VOD patients treated with TIPS, have survived, 20% of the total. All but three (two with previous liver and one with previous kidney transplantation) had bone marrow transplantation [124, 125]. The most common causes of death usually occurring within one to three weeks following diagnosis were multi-organ failure (MOF), sepsis and hemorrhage, due to underlying hematological disease. The interval could influence the success of TIPS. If MOF is already present, patients are probably being treated too late. Earlier intervention may be worthwhile, but it needs formal assessment. Indeed, the causes of death in patients with VOD are usually renal and cardiopulmonary failure and sepsis, rather than liver

failure per se. In liver transplantation six patients with VOD have been treated with TIPS, one died, one was retransplanted, but information in these two patients about the course or the cause of liver failure or death were not reported. Thus, although TIPS is not recommended for patients with severe VOD, this may apply only to SCT patients in whom MOF conditions the prognosis. If a severe VOD is diagnosed in a liver transplanted patient and if medical therapy fails, a transjugular portosystemic shunt should be considered.

Liver transplantation has been reported anedoctically as a rescue therapy in patients with VOD after SCT not responding to medical therapy. Currently, 18 patients have been reported in the literature for transplantation due to VOD/SOS, with 13 deaths (72%), primarily due to infective complications [126]. The presence of malignancies and multiple organ failure (if VOD is advanced) contraindicates OLT. When VOD develops after liver transplantation itself, retransplantation can be performed as a rescue therapy as the liver is the only organ damaged. Previous placement of TIPS allows more time for the clinician to re-list the patients for OLT and it does not jeopardize subsequent OLT.

A flow-chart for the suggested diagnosis and management of VOD is shown in Figure 37.2.

References

1 Okuda K, Kage M, Shrestha SM. Proposal of a new nomenclature for Budd-Chiari syndrome: hepatic vein thrombosis versus thrombosis of the inferior vena cava at its hepatic portion. *Hepatology* 1998; **28**(5): 1191–1198.

2 Okuda H, Yamagata H, Obata H *et al.* Epidemiological and clinical features of Budd-Chiari syndrome in Japan. *J Hepatol* 1995; **22**(1): 1–9.

3 Valla DC. The diagnosis and management of the Budd-Chiari syndrome: consensus and controversies. *Hepatology* 2003; **38**(4): 793–803.

4 Valla DC. Primary Budd-Chiari syndrome. *J Hepatol* 2009; **50**(1): 195–203.

5 Gupta S, Barter S, Phillips GW, Gibson RN, Hodgson HJ. Comparison of ultrasonography, computed tomography and 99mTc liver scan in diagnosis of Budd-Chiari syndrome. *Gut* 1987; **28**(3): 242–247.

6 Mahmoud AE, Helmy AS, Billingham L, Elias E. Poor prognosis and limited therapeutic options in patients with Budd-Chiari syndrome and portal venous system thrombosis. *Eur J Gastroenterol Hepatol* 1997; **9**(5): 485–489.

7 Murad SD, Valla DC, de Groen PC *et al.* Determinants of survival and the effect of portosystemic shunting in patients with Budd-Chiari syndrome. *Hepatology* 2004; **39**(2): 500–508.

8 Mancuso A, Watkinson A, Tibballs J, Patch D, Burroughs AK. Budd-Chiari syndrome with portal, splenic, and superior mesenteric vein thrombosis treated with TIPS: who dares wins. *Gut* 2003; **52**(3): 438.

9 Senzolo M, Patch D, Miotto D, Ferronato C, Cholongitas E, Burroughs AK. Interventional treatment should be incorporated in the algorithm for the management of patients with portal vein thrombosis. *Hepatology* 2008; **48**(4): 1352–1353.

10 Okuda K. Inferior vena cava thrombosis at its hepatic portion (obliterative hepatocavopathy). *Semin Liver Dis* 2002; **22**(1): 15–26.

11 Amarapurkar DN, Punamiya SJ, Patel ND. Changing spectrum of Budd-Chiari syndrome in India with special reference to non-surgical treatment. *World J Gastroenterol* 2008; **14**(2): 278–285.

12 Ohta M, Hashizume M, Tomikawa M, Ueno K, Tanoue K, Sugimachi K. Analysis of hepatic vein waveform by Doppler ultrasonography in 100 patients with portal hypertension. *Am J Gastroenterol* 1994; **89**(2): 170–175.

13 Erden A, Erden I, Karayalcin S, Yurdaydin C. Budd-Chiari syndrome: evaluation with multiphase contrast-enhanced three-dimensional MR angiography. *AJR Am J Roentgenol* 2002; **179**(5): 1287–1292.

14 Mancuso A, Fung K, Mela M *et al.* TIPS for acute and chronic Budd-Chiari syndrome: a single-centre experience. *J Hepatol* 2003; **38**(6): 751–754.

15 Vlachogiannakos J, Patch D, Watkinson A, Tibballs J, Burroughs AK. Carbon-dioxide portography: an expanding role? *Lancet* 2000; **355**(9208): 987–988.

16 Janssen HL, Garcia-Pagan JC, Elias E, Mentha G, Hadengue A, Valla DC. Budd-Chiari syndrome: a review by an expert panel. *J Hepatol* 2003; **38**(3): 364–371.

17 Hadengue A, Poliquin M, Vilgrain V *et al.* The changing scene of hepatic vein thrombosis: recognition of asymptomatic cases. *Gastroenterology* 1994; **106**(4): 1042–1047.

18 Valla DC. Hepatic vein thrombosis (Budd-Chiari syndrome). *Semin Liver Dis* 2002; **22**(1): 5–14.

19 Langlet P, Escolano S, Valla D *et al.* Clinicopathological forms and prognostic index in Budd-Chiari syndrome. *J Hepatol* 2003; **39**(4): 496–501.

20 Singh V, Sinha SK, Nain CK *et al.* Budd-Chiari syndrome: our experience of 71 patients. *J Gastroenterol Hepatol* 2000; **15**(5): 550–554.

21 Tang TJ, Batts KP, de Groen PC *et al.* The prognostic value of histology in the assessment of patients with Budd-Chiari syndrome. *J Hepatol* 2001; **35**(3): 338–343.

22 Ibarrola C, Castellano VM, Colina F. Focal hyperplastic hepatocellular nodules in hepatic venous outflow obstruction: a clinicopathological study of four patients and 24 nodules. *Histopathology* 2004; **44**(2): 172–179.

23 Moucari R, Rautou PE, Cazals-Hatem D *et al.* Hepatocellular carcinoma in Budd-Chiari syndrome: characteristics and risk factors. *Gut* 2008; **57**(6): 828–835.

24 Shrestha SM, Okuda K, Uchida T *et al.* Endemicity and clinical picture of liver disease due to obstruction of the hepatic portion of the inferior vena cava in Nepal. *J Gastroenterol Hepatol* 1996; **11**(2): 170–179.

25 Denninger MH, Beldjord K, Durand F, Denie C, Valla D, Guillin MC. Budd-Chiari syndrome and factor V Leiden mutation. *Lancet* 1995; **345**(8948): 525–526.

26 Janssen HL, Meinardi JR, Vleggaar FP *et al.* Factor V Leiden mutation, prothrombin gene mutation, and deficiencies in coagulation inhibitors associated with Budd-Chiari syndrome and portal vein thrombosis: results of a case-control study. *Blood* 2000; **96**(7): 2364–2368.

27 Hirshberg B, Shouval D, Fibach E, Friedman G, Ben Yehuda D. Flow cytometric analysis of autonomous growth of erythroid precursors in liquid culture detects occult polycythemia vera in the Budd-Chiari syndrome. *J Hepatol* 2000; **32**(4): 574–578.

28 James C, Ugo V, Le Couedic JP *et al.* A unique clonal JAK2 mutation leading to constitutive signalling causes polycythaemia vera. *Nature* 2005; **434**(7037): 1144–1148.

29 Mohanty S, Saxena R, Acharya SK. Activated protein C resistance in Budd-Chiari syndrome. *Int J Hematol* 2000; **72**(2): 255.

30 Minnema MC, Janssen HL, Niermeijer P, de Man RA. Budd-Chiari syndrome: combination of genetic defects and the use of oral contraceptives leading to hypercoagulability. *J Hepatol* 2000; **33**(3): 509–512.

31 Zeitoun G, Escolano S, Hadengue A *et al.* Outcome of Budd-Chiari syndrome: a multivariate analysis of factors related to survival including surgical portosystemic shunting. *Hepatology* 1999; **30**(1): 84–89.

32 Henderson JM, Warren WD, Millikan WJ, Jr. *et al.* Surgical options, hematologic evaluation, and pathologic changes in Budd-Chiari syndrome. *Am J Surg* 1990; **159**(1): 41–48.

33 Dilawari JB, Bambery P, Chawla Y *et al.* Hepatic outflow obstruction (Budd-Chiari syndrome). Experience with 177 patients and a review of the literature. *Medicine (Baltimore)* 1994; **73**(1): 21–36.

34 Plessier A, Sibert A, Consigny Y *et al.* Aiming at minimal invasiveness as a therapeutic strategy for Budd-Chiari syndrome. *Hepatology* 2006; **44**(5): 1308–1316.

35 Ringe B, Lang H, Oldhafer KJ *et al.* Which is the best surgery for Budd-Chiari syndrome: venous decompression or liver transplantation? A single-center experience with 50 patients. *Hepatology* 1995; **21**(5): 1337–1344.

36 Frank JW, Kamath PS, Stanson AW. Budd-Chiari syndrome: early intervention with angioplasty and thrombolytic therapy. *Mayo Clin Proc* 1994; **69**(9): 877–881.

37 Sharma S, Texeira A, Texeira P, Elias E, Wilde J, Olliff SP. Pharmacological thrombolysis in Budd-Chiari syndrome: a single centre experience and review of the literature. *J Hepatol* 2004; **40**(1): 172–180.

38 Bilbao JI, Pueyo JC, Longo JM *et al*. Interventional therapeutic techniques in Budd-Chiari syndrome. *Cardiovasc Intervent Radiol* 1997; **20**(2): 112–119.

39 Fisher NC, McCafferty I, Dolapci M *et al*. Managing Budd-Chiari syndrome: a retrospective review of percutaneous hepatic vein angioplasty and surgical shunting. *Gut* 1999; **44**(4): 568–574.

40 Eapen CE, Velissaris D, Heydtmann M, Gunson B, Olliff S, Elias E. Favourable medium term outcome following hepatic vein recanalisation and/or transjugular intrahepatic portosystemic shunt for Budd-Chiari syndrome. *Gut* 2006; **55**(6): 878–884.

41 Zhang CQ, Fu LN, Xu L *et al*. Long-term effect of stent placement in 115 patients with Budd-Chiari syndrome. *World J Gastroenterol* 2003; **9**(11): 2587–2591.

42 Orloff MJ, Daily PO, Orloff SL, Girard B, Orloff MS. A 27-year experience with surgical treatment of Budd-Chiari syndrome. *Ann Surg* 2000; **232**(3): 340–352.

43 Slakey DP, Klein AS, Venbrux AC, Cameron JL. Budd-Chiari syndrome: current management options. *Ann Surg* 2001; **233**(4): 522–527.

44 Gillams A, Dick R, Platts A, Irving D, Hobbs K. Dilatation of the inferior vena cava using an expandable metal stent in Budd-Chiari syndrome. *J Hepatol* 1991; **13**(2): 149–151.

45 Bachet JB, Condat B. Long term survival after portosystemic shunting for Budd-Chiari syndrome, shunt patency is determinant. *Hepatology* 2002; **36**(4): 416A.

46 Hernandez-Guerra M, Turnes J, Rubinstein P *et al*. PTFE-covered stents improve TIPS patency in Budd-Chiari syndrome. *Hepatology* 2004; **40**(5): 1197–1202.

47 Perello A, Garcia-Pagan JC, Gilabert R *et al*. TIPS is a useful long-term derivative therapy for patients with Budd-Chiari syndrome uncontrolled by medical therapy. *Hepatology* 2002; **35**(1): 132–139.

48 Rossle M, Olschewski M, Siegerstetter V, Berger E, Kurz K, Grandt D. The Budd-Chiari syndrome: outcome after treatment with the transjugular intrahepatic portosystemic shunt. *Surgery* 2004; **135**(4): 394–403.

49 Garcia-Pagan JC, Heydtmann M, Raffa S *et al*. TIPS for Budd-Chiari syndrome: long-term results and prognostics factors in 124 patients. *Gastroenterology* 2008; **135**(3): 808–815.

50 Attwell A, Ludkowski M, Nash R, Kugelmas M. Treatment of Budd-Chiari syndrome in a liver transplant unit, the role of transjugular intrahepatic porto-systemic shunt and liver transplantation. *Aliment Pharmacol Ther* 2004; **20**(8): 867–873.

51 Thompson NP, Miller AD, Hamilton G, Alexander G, Friend PJ, Burroughs AK. Emergency rescue hepatic transplantation following shunt surgery for Budd-Chiari syndrome. *Eur J Gastroenterol Hepatol* 2004; **6**(9): 835–837.

52 Halff G, Todo S, Tzakis AG, Gordon RD, Starzl TE. Liver transplantation for the Budd-Chiari syndrome. *Ann Surg* 1990; **211**(1): 43–49.

53 Jamieson NV, Williams R, Calne RY. Liver transplantation for Budd-Chiari syndrome, 1976–1990. *Ann Chir* 1991; **45**(4): 362–365.

54 Srinivasan P, Rela M, Prachalias A *et al*. Liver transplantation for Budd-Chiari syndrome. *Transplantation* 2002; **73**(6): 973–977.

55 Ulrich F, Steinmuller T, Lang M *et al*. Liver transplantation in patients with advanced Budd-Chiari syndrome. *Transplant Proc* 2002; **34**(6): 2278.

56 Knoop M, Lemmens HP, Langrehr JM *et al*. Liver transplantation for Budd-Chiari syndrome. *Transplant Proc* 1994; **26**(6): 3577–358.

57 Segev DL, Nguyen GC, Locke JE *et al*. Twenty years of liver transplantation for Budd-Chiari syndrome: a national registry analysis. *Liver Transpl* 2007; **13**(9): 1285–1294.

58 Mentha G, Giostra E, Majno PE *et al*. Liver transplantation for Budd-Chiari syndrome: A European study on 248 patients from 51 centres. *J Hepatol* 2006; **44**(3): 520–528.

59 Klein AS, Molmenti EP. Surgical treatment of Budd-Chiari syndrome. *Liver Transpl* 2003; **9**(9): 891–896.

60 Melear JM, Goldstein RM, Levy MF *et al*. Hematologic aspects of liver transplantation for Budd-Chiari syndrome with special reference to myeloproliferative disorders. *Transplantation* 2002; **74**(8): 1090–1095.

61 Bittencourt PL, Couto CA, Ribeiro DD. Portal vein thrombosis and budd-Chiari syndrome. *Clin Liver Dis* 2009; **13**(1): 127–144.

62 Garcia-Pagan JC, Hernandez-Guerra M, Bosch J. Extrahepatic portal vein thrombosis. *Semin Liver Dis* 2008; **28**(3): 282–292.

63 Webster GJ, Burroughs AK, Riordan SM. Review article: portal vein thrombosis – new insights into aetiology and management. *Aliment Pharmacol Ther* 2005; **21**(1): 1–9.

64 Ogren M, Bergqvist D, Bjorck M, Acosta S, Eriksson H, Sternby NH. Portal vein thrombosis: prevalence, patient characteristics and lifetime risk: a population study based on 23,796 consecutive autopsies. *World J Gastroenterol* 2006; **12**(13): 2115–2119.

65 de Franchis R. Evolving consensus in portal hypertension. Report of the Baveno IV consensus workshop on methodology of diagnosis and therapy in portal hypertension. *J Hepatol* 2005; **43**(1): 167–176.

66 Sarin SK, Kumar A. Noncirrhotic portal hypertension. *Clin Liver Dis* 2006; **10**(3): 627–651, x.

67 Condat B, Pessione F, Helene DM, Hillaire S, Valla D. Recent portal or mesenteric venous thrombosis: increased recognition and frequent recanalization on anticoagulant therapy. *Hepatology* 2000; **32**(3): 466–470.

68 Cohen J, Edelman RR, Chopra S. Portal vein thrombosis: a review. *Am J Med* 1992; **92**(2): 173–182.

69 Baggenstoss AH, Wollaeger EE. Portal hypertension due to chronic occlusion of the extrahepatic portion of the portal vein: its relation to ascites. *Am J Med* 1956; **21**(1): 16–25.

70 Ertugrul I, Koklu S, Basar O *et al*. Thrombosis of the portal venous system: a prospective study. *J Clin Gastroenterol* 2008; **42**(7): 835–838.

71 McMahon C, bu-Elmagd K, Bontempo FA, Kant JA, Swerdlow SH. JAK2 V617F mutation in patients with catastrophic intra-abdominal thromboses. *Am J Clin Pathol* 2007; **127**(5): 736–743.

72 Janssen HL, Wijnhoud A, Haagsma EB *et al*. Extrahepatic portal vein thrombosis: aetiology and determinants of survival. *Gut* 2001; **49**(5): 720–724.

73 De Gaetano AM, Lafortune M, Patriquin H, De FA, Aubin B, Paradis K. Cavernous transformation of the portal vein: pat-

terns of intrahepatic and splanchnic collateral circulation detected with Doppler sonography. *AJR Am J Roentgenol* 1995; **165**(5): 1151–1155.

74 Webb LJ, Sherlock S. The aetiology, presentation and natural history of extra-hepatic portal venous obstruction. *Q J Med* 1979; **48**(192): 627–639.

75 Condat B, Vilgrain V, Asselah T *et al*. Portal cavernoma-associated cholangiopathy: a clinical and MR cholangiography coupled with MR portography imaging study. *Hepatology* 2003; **37**(6): 1302–1308.

76 Vibert E, Azoulay D, Aloia T *et al*. Therapeutic strategies in symptomatic portal biliopathy. *Ann Surg* 2007; **246**(1): 97–104.

77 Senzolo M, Cholongitas E, Tibballs J *et al*. Relief of biliary obstruction due to portal vein cavernoma using a transjugular intrahepatic portosystemic shunt (TIPS) without the need for long-term stenting. *Endoscopy* 2006; **38**(7): 760.

78 Fimognari FL, Violi F. Portal vein thrombosis in liver cirrhosis. *Intern Emerg Med* 2008; **3**(3): 213–218.

79 Amitrano L, Guardascione MA, Brancaccio V *et al*. Risk factors and clinical presentation of portal vein thrombosis in patients with liver cirrhosis. *J Hepatol* 2004; **40**(5): 736–741.

80 Mangia A, Villani MR, Cappucci G *et al*. Causes of portal venous thrombosis in cirrhotic patients: the role of genetic and acquired factors. *Eur J Gastroenterol Hepatol* 2005; **17**(7): 745–751.

81 Gaiani S, Bolondi L, Li BS, Zironi G, Siringo S, Barbara L. Prevalence of spontaneous hepatofugal portal flow in liver cirrhosis. Clinical and endoscopic correlation in 228 patients. *Gastroenterology* 1991; **100**(1): 160–167.

82 Francoz C, Belghiti J, Vilgrain V *et al*. Splanchnic vein thrombosis in candidates for liver transplantation: usefulness of screening and anticoagulation. *Gut* 2005; **54**(5): 691–697.

83 Senzolo M, Ferronato C, Burra P, Sartori MT. Anticoagulation for portal vein thrombosis in cirrhotic patients should be always considered. *Intern Emerg Med* 2009; **4**(2): 161–162.

84 Shelat VG, Diddapur RK. An early experience of liver transplantation in portal vein thrombosis. *Singapore Med J* 2008; **49**(2): e37–41.

85 Senzolo M, Tibbals J, Cholongitas E, Triantos CK, Burroughs AK, Patch D. Transjugular intrahepatic portosystemic shunt for portal vein thrombosis with and without cavernous transformation. *Aliment Pharmacol Ther* 2006; **23**(6): 767–775.

86 Nonami T, Yokoyama I, Iwatsuki S, Starzl TE. The incidence of portal vein thrombosis at liver transplantation. *Hepatology* 1992; **16**(5): 1195–1198.

87 Llovet JM, Bustamante J, Castells A *et al*. Natural history of untreated nonsurgical hepatocellular carcinoma: rationale for the design and evaluation of therapeutic trials. *Hepatology* 1999; **29**(1): 62–67.

88 Salem R, Lewandowski R, Roberts C *et al*. Use of Yttrium-90 glass microspheres (TheraSphere) for the treatment of unresectable hepatocellular carcinoma in patients with portal vein thrombosis. *J Vasc Interv Radiol* 2004; **15**(4): 335–345.

89 Sato K, Lewandowski RJ, Bui JT *et al*. Treatment of unresectable primary and metastatic liver cancer with yttrium-90 microspheres (TheraSphere): assessment of hepatic arterial embolization. *Cardiovasc Intervent Radiol* 2006; **29**(4): 522–529.

90 Keck T, Marjanovic G, Fernandez-del CC *et al*. The inflammatory pancreatic head mass: significant differences in the ana-

tomic pathology of German and American patients with chronic pancreatitis determine very different surgical strategies. *Ann Surg* 2009; **249**(1): 105–110.

91 Heider TR, Azeem S, Galanko JA, Behrns KE. The natural history of pancreatitis-induced splenic vein thrombosis. *Ann Surg* 2004; **239**(6): 876–880.

92 Caldwell SH, Hespenheide EE, Greenwald BD, Northup PG, Patrie JT. Enbucrilate for gastric varices: extended experience in 92 patients. *Aliment Pharmacol Ther* 2007; **26**(1): 49–59.

93 Rousso D, Mamopoulos A, Goulis J, Mandala E, Mavromatidis G. Postpartum mesenteric, splenic and portal vein thrombosis. *J Obstet Gynaecol* 2008; **28**(4): 441–443.

94 Condat B, Pessione F, Hillaire S *et al*. Current Outcome of Portal Vein Thrombosis in Adults: Risk and Benefits of Anticoagulant Therapy. *Gastro* 2001; **120**: 490–497.

95 Plessier A, Darwish-Murad S, Hernandez-Guerra M *et al*. Acute Portal Vein Thrombosis Unrelated to Cirrhosis: A Prospective Multicenter Follow-up Study. *Hepatology* 2010; **51**: 210–218.

96 Turnes J, Garcia-Pagan JC, Gonzalez M *et al*. Portal hypertension-related complications after acute portal vein thrombosis: impact of early anticoagulation. *Clin Gastroenterol Hepatol* 2008; **6**(12): 1412–1417.

97 Smalberg JH, Spaander MV, Jie KS *et al*. Risks and benefits of transcatheter thrombolytic therapy in patients with splanchnic venous thrombosis. *Thromb Haemost* 2008; **100**(6): 1084–1088.

98 Bearman SI, Anderson GL, Mori M, Hinds MS, Shulman HM, McDonald GB. Venoocclusive disease of the liver: development of a model for predicting fatal outcome after marrow transplantation. *J Clin Oncol* 1993; **11**(9): 1729–1736.

99 McDonald GB, Hinds MS, Fisher LD *et al*. Veno-occlusive disease of the liver and multiorgan failure after bone marrow transplantation: a cohort study of 355 patients. *Ann Intern Med* 1993; **118**(4): 255–267.

100 Kumar S, DeLeve LD, Kamath PS, Tefferi A. Hepatic veno-occlusive disease (sinusoidal obstruction syndrome) after hematopoietic stem cell transplantation. *Mayo Clin Proc* 2003; **78**(5): 589–598.

101 Carreras E, Bertz H, Arcese W *et al*. Incidence and outcome of hepatic veno-occlusive disease after blood or marrow transplantation: a prospective cohort study of the European Group for Blood and Marrow Transplantation. European Group for Blood and Marrow Transplantation Chronic Leukemia Working Party. *Blood* 1998; **92**(10): 3599–3604.

102 Lee JH, Choi SJ, Lee JH *et al*. Decreased incidence of hepatic veno-occlusive disease and fewer hemostatic derangements associated with intravenous busulfan vs oral busulfan in adults conditioned with busulfan + cyclophosphamide for allogeneic bone marrow transplantation. *Ann Hematol* 2005; **84**(5): 321–330.

103 Sebagh M, Debette M, Samuel D *et al*. "Silent" presentation of veno-occlusive disease after liver transplantation as part of the process of cellular rejection with endothelial predilection. *Hepatology* 1999; **30**(5): 1144–1150.

104 DeLeve LD, Shulman HM, McDonald GB. Toxic injury to hepatic sinusoids: sinusoidal obstruction syndrome (veno-occlusive disease). *Semin Liver Dis* 2002; **22**(1): 27–42.

105 Jones RJ, Lee KS, Beschorner WE *et al*. Venoocclusive disease of the liver following bone marrow transplantation. *Transplantation* 1987; **44**(6): 778–783.

106 Toh HC, McAfee SL, Sackstein R, Cox BF, Colby C, Spitzer TR. Late onset veno-occlusive disease following high-dose chemotherapy and stem cell transplantation. *Bone Marrow Transplant* 1999; **24**(8): 891–895.

107 Costa F, Choy CG, Seiter K, Hann L, Thung SN, Michaeli J. Hepatic outflow obstruction and liver failure due to leukemic cell infiltration in chronic lymphocytic leukemia. *Leuk Lymphoma* 1998; **30**(3–4): 403–410.

108 Blostein MD, Paltiel OB, Thibault A, Rybka WB. A comparison of clinical criteria for the diagnosis of veno-occlusive disease of the liver after bone marrow transplantation. *Bone Marrow Transplant* 1992; **10**(5): 439–443.

109 Eltumi M, Trivedi P, Hobbs JR et al. Monitoring of veno-occlusive disease after bone marrow transplantation by serum aminopropeptide of type III procollagen. *Lancet* 1993; **342**(8870): 518–521.

110 Helmy A. Review article: updates in the pathogenesis and therapy of hepatic sinusoidal obstruction syndrome. *Aliment Pharmacol Ther* 2006; **23**(1): 11–25.

111 Lassau N, Auperin A, Leclere J, Bennaceur A, Valteau-Couanet D, Hartmann O. Prognostic value of doppler-ultrasonography in hepatic veno-occlusive disease. *Transplantation* 2002; **74**(1): 60–66.

112 Ghersin E, Brook OR, Gaitini D, Engel A. Color Doppler demonstration of segmental portal flow reversal: an early sign of hepatic veno-occlusive disease in an infant. *J Ultrasound Med* 2003; **22**(10): 1103–1106.

113 Kalambokis G, Manousou P, Vibhakorn S et al. Transjugular liver biopsy–indications, adequacy, quality of specimens, and complications – a systematic review. *J Hepatol* 2007; **47**(2): 284–294.

114 Shulman HM, McDonald GB, Matthews D et al. An analysis of hepatic venocclusive disease and centrilobular hepatic degeneration following bone marrow transplantation. *Gastroenterology* 1980; **79**(6): 1178–1191.

115 Essell JH, Schroeder MT, Harman GS et al. Ursodiol prophylaxis against hepatic complications of allogeneic bone marrow transplantation. A randomized, double-blind, placebo-controlled trial. *Ann Intern Med* 1998; **128**(12 Pt 1): 975–981.

116 Giles F, Garcia-Manero G, Cortes J, Thomas D, Kantarjian H, Estey E. Ursodiol does not prevent hepatic venoocclusive disease associated with Mylotarg therapy. *Haematologica* 2002; **87**(10): 1114–1116.

117 Ohashi K, Tanabe J, Watanabe R et al. The Japanese multicenter open randomized trial of ursodeoxycholic acid prophylaxis for hepatic veno-occlusive disease after stem cell transplantation. *Am J Hematol* 2000; **64**(1): 32–38.

118 Park SH, Lee MH, Lee H, Kim HS et al. A randomized trial of heparin plus ursodiol vs. heparin alone to prevent hepatic veno-occlusive disease after hematopoietic stem cell transplantation. *Bone Marrow Transplant* 2002; **29**(2): 137–143.

119 Bearman SI, Shen DD, Hinds MS, Hill HA, McDonald GB. A phase I/II study of prostaglandin E1 for the prevention of hepatic venocclusive disease after bone marrow transplantation. *Br J Haematol* 1993; **84**(4): 724–730.

120 Bearman SI, Shuhart MC, Hinds MS, McDonald GB. Recombinant human tissue plasminogen activator for the treatment of established severe venocclusive disease of the liver after bone marrow transplantation. *Blood* 1992; **80**(10): 2458–2462.

121 Morris JD, Harris RE, Hashmi R et al. Antithrombin-III for the treatment of chemotherapy-induced organ dysfunction following bone marrow transplantation. *Bone Marrow Transplant* 1997; **20**(10): 871–878.

122 Richardson P, Guinan E. The pathology, diagnosis, and treatment of hepatic veno-occlusive disease: current status and novel approaches. *Br J Haematol* 1999; **107**(3): 485–493.

123 Mor E, Pappo O, Bar-Nathan N et al. Defibrotide for the treatment of veno-occlusive disease after liver transplantation. *Transplantation* 2001; **72**(7): 1237–1240.

124 Senzolo M, Cholongitas E, Patch D, Burroughs AK. TIPS for veno-occlusive disease: Is the contraindication real? *Hepatology* 2005; **42**(1): 240–241.

125 Senzolo M, Patch D, Cholongitas E et al. Severe venoocclusive disease after liver transplantation treated with transjugular intrahepatic portosystemic shunt. *Transplantation* 2006; **82**(1): 132–135.

126 Senzolo M, Germani G, Cholongitas E, Burra P, Burroughs AK. Veno occlusive disease: update on clinical management. *World J Gastroenterol* 2007; **13**(29): 3918–3924.

38 Ascites, hepatorenal syndrome and spontaneous bacterial peritonitis

Pere Ginès, Andrés Cárdenas, Vicente Arroyo and Juan Rodés

Liver Unit and GI Unit, Hospital Clínic and University of Barcelona, Institut d'Investigacions Biomèdiques August Pi-Sunyer (IDIBAPS), Ciber de Enfermedades Hepáticas y Digestivas (CIBERHED), Barcelona, Spain

Introduction

Patients with cirrhosis frequently develop disturbances in body fluid regulation that result in an increase in the volume of extracellular fluid, which accumulates in the peritoneal cavity as ascites and in the interstitial tissue as edema [1]. Although the pathogenesis of ascites is incompletely understood, most available evidence indicates that fluid retention is the consequence of the homeostatic activation of vasoconstrictor and sodium-retaining systems triggered by marked arterial vasodilation mainly in the splanchnic vascular bed [2]. Marked abnormalities in the splanchnic microcirculation due to portal hypertension facilitate the accumulation of the retained fluid in the peritoneal cavity. Ascites is frequently complicated by abnormalities of renal function such as impaired ability to eliminate solute-free water and vasoconstriction of the renal circulation, which may lead to development of dilutional hyponatremia and hepatorenal syndrome respectively [1, 3]. Finally, coexistence of ascites and abnormalities in the host defense mechanisms against bacterial infection, which occur frequently in patients with advanced cirrhosis, accounts for the spontaneous infection of ascitic fluid, a condition known as spontaneous bacterial peritonitis [4, 5].

The aim of this chapter is to review, on the basis of available evidence, the efficacy of various therapeutic methods in the management of ascites, hepatorenal syndrome and spontaneous bacterial peritonitis in cirrhosis. The pathogenesis of these complications is briefly discussed to provide the reader with an understanding of the pathophysiological basis of the different therapeutic approaches. A comprehensive review of the pathophysiology of these disorders may be found elsewhere [1, 6].

Evidence-Based Gastroenterology and Hepatology, 3rd edition. J. McDonald, A.K. Burroughs, B. Feagan, and M.B. Fennerty. © 2010 Blackwell Publishing Ltd

Ascites

A large body of evidence indicates that in cirrhosis, sodium retention with subsequent ascites and edema formation, results from the action of neurohumoral factors on the kidney, which are activated during the homeostatic response to a disturbed systemic circulation (see Figure 38.1) [1, 2, 6, 7]. The initial abnormality is sinusoidal portal hypertension causing marked arterial vasodilation mainly in the splanchnic circulation. The mechanism of this vasodilation is not known, but may involve the increased synthesis/release of vasodilating substances, including nitric oxide and/or vasodilator peptides [2, 8]. Arterial vasodilation results in an abnormal distribution of blood volume, with reduced effective arterial blood volume (the blood volume in the heart, lungs and central arterial tree), sensed by the arterial receptors with subsequent renal sodium retention due to the activation of vasoconstrictor and sodium-retaining factors.

Sodium restriction

In all diseases associated with generalized edema (cirrhosis, heart failure, renal failure), the amount of exogenous fluid retained depends on the balance between sodium intake and the renal excretion of sodium. Because sodium is retained iso-osmotically in the kidney, 1 liter of extracellular fluid is gained for every 130–140 mmol of sodium that is retained. If sodium excretion remains constant, the gain in extracellular fluid volume (and the consequent increase in weight) depends exclusively on sodium intake and increases proportionally to the amount of sodium in the diet. Nevertheless, because sodium excretion may be increased pharmacologically by the administration of diuretics, the sodium balance depends not only on sodium intake but also on the natriuretic response to the diuretics.

With this background, it seems reasonable that a reduction in sodium intake (low salt diet) will favor a negative

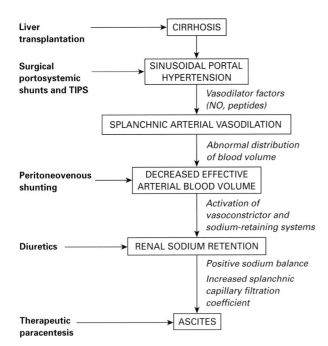

Figure 38.1 Proposed pathogenesis of ascites formation in cirrhosis according to the arterial vasodilatation hypothesis and available therapeutic interventions (in bold).
TIPS: transjugular intrahepatic portosystemic shunt; NO: nitric oxide.

sodium balance and the elimination of ascites and edema. This was demonstrated in earlier studies and is supported by the common clinical observation that the management of ascites is more difficult in patients who do not comply with a low sodium diet [9, 10]. **C5 B4** Non-compliant patients usually require higher doses of diuretics to achieve resolution of ascites and are readmitted more frequently to hospital for recurrence of ascites. Surprisingly, however, an advantage of low sodium diet as compared with an unrestricted sodium diet in the management of ascites has not been demonstrated in randomized controlled trials [11–13]. **A1d** Nevertheless, it should be pointed out that in these studies most patients had mild sodium retention (urine sodium in the absence of diuretic therapy was close to sodium intake) and showed an excellent response to diuretic therapy (less than 5% of patients did not respond to diuretics).

Therefore, on the basis of available evidence, it can be concluded that in patients with mild sodium retention, restriction of dietary sodium is probably not necessary; the hypothetical benefit of low salt diet in the achievement of a negative sodium balance is overridden by the marked natriuretic effect of diuretics. In contrast, in patients with marked sodium retention, who usually have a less intense natriuretic response to diuretics compared with patients with moderate sodium retention, dietary sodium restriction (80 mmol of sodium per day) may facilitate the elimination of ascites and delay the reaccumulation of fluid. A

more severe restriction of sodium is not recommended because it is poorly accepted by patients and may impair their nutritional status. **C5**

Therapeutic paracentesis

Therapeutic paracentesis has progressively replaced diuretics as the treatment of choice in the management of patients with cirrhosis and large volume ascites [14, 15]. This change in treatment strategy is based on the results of several randomized controlled trials comparing paracentesis (either removal of all ascitic fluid in a single tap or repeated taps of 4–6 liters/day) associated with plasma volume expansion versus diuretics [16–20]. **A1d** Because paracentesis does not affect renal sodium retention, patients should be given diuretics after paracentesis to avoid reaccumulation of fluid [21]. **A1d**

Two aspects concerning the use of therapeutic paracentesis in patients with cirrhosis and ascites deserve to be specifically discussed: (1) the population of patients with cirrhosis in whom therapeutic paracentesis should be used; and (2) the use of plasma expanders to prevent disturbances in circulatory function after paracentesis. While most physicians consider that therapeutic paracentesis is the treatment of choice for all patients with large volume ascites [14, 15], others believe that therapeutic paracentesis should be used only in those patients who show a poor or no response to diuretics [22]. Results of randomized trials indicate that therapeutic paracentesis is faster and in several trials was associated with lower incidence of adverse effects compared with diuretics (see Table 38.1) [16–20]. **A1d** Moreover, therapeutic paracentesis may have a better cost-effectiveness profile compared with diuretic treatment that can result in prolonged hospitalization. Therefore, on the basis of the available evidence, it seems clear that the use of therapeutic paracentesis should not be restricted to patients failing to respond to diuretics but should be considered the treatment of choice for all patients with large volume ascites (see Box 38.1).

The removal of large volumes of ascitic fluid is associated with circulatory dysfunction characterized by a reduction of effective blood volume [23–29]. Several lines of evidence indicate that this circulatory dysfunction and/or the mechanisms activated to maintain circulatory homeostasis have detrimental effects in cirrhotic patients. First, circulatory dysfunction is associated with rapid reaccumulation of ascites [29]. Second, approximately 20% of these patients develop hepatorenal syndrome and/or water retention leading to dilutional hyponatremia [23]. Third, portal pressure increases in patients developing circulatory dysfunction after paracentesis, probably owing to an increased intrahepatic resistance due to the action of vasoconstrictor systems on the hepatic vascular bed [27]. Finally,

Table 38.1 Adverse effects in randomized trials comparing the efficacy and safety of diuretics versus therapeutic paracentesis and plasma volume expansion in patients with cirrhosis and large volume ascites[a].

Adverse effect	No. of patients with adverse effects			P
	Type of plasma expander	Diuretics (%)	Paracentesis and plasma volume expansion (%)	
Renal impairment				
Ginès et al. [16]	Albumin	16/59[b] (27)	3/58 (5)	0.003
Salerno et al. [17]	Albumin	1/21 (5)	1/20 (5)	NS
Hagège et al. [18]	Albumin	1/27 (4)	1/26 (4)	NS
Acharya et al. [19]	Dextran-40	1/20 (5)	0/20 (0)	NS
Solà et al. [20]	Dextran-40	5/40 (12)	1/40 (2)	NS
Hyponatremia				
Ginès et al. [16]	Albumin	18/59 (30)	3/58 (5)	0.0009
Salerno et al. [17]	Albumin	—	—	—
Hagège et al. [18]	Albumin	8/27 (30)	2/26 (8)	0.07
Acharya et al. [19]	Dextran-40	1/20 (5)	3/20 (15)	NS
Solà et al. [20]	Dextran-40	8/40 (20)	5/40 (12)	NS
Encephalopathy				
Ginès et al. [16]	Albumin	17/59 (29)	6/58 (10)	0.02
Salerno et al. [17]	Albumin	3/21 (14)	2/20 (10)	NS
Hagège et al. [18]	Albumin	4/27 (15)	1/26 (4)	NS
Acharya et al. [19]	Dextran-40	1/20 (5)	0/20 (0)	NS
Solà et al. [20]	Dextran-40	12/40 (30)	1/40 (2)	0.0015

[a] Differences in the rate of adverse effects among the studies may be due, at least in part, to differences in the populations of patients included.
[b] Figures represent the number of patients developing the adverse effects compared with the total number of patients in each treatment group.

BOX 38.1 Recommendations for the management of patients with cirrhosis and large volume ascites [1]

(1) Total paracentesis plus intravenous albumin[a] (8 g/l of ascites removed). Patients can be treated as outpatients. Hospitalization is recommended for patients with associated complications (i.e. encephalopathy, bacterial infection, gastrointestinal bleeding).
(2) After removal of ascitic fluid, start with moderate sodium restriction (80 mmol/day) and diuretics, either aldosterone antagonists alone (i.e. spironolactone 50–400 mg/day) or in combination with loop diuretics (i.e. furosemide 20–100 mg/day). If patients were on diuretics before the development of large volume ascites, check compliance with sodium diet and diuretic therapy. Compliant patients should be given doses of diuretics higher than those given before paracentesis in order to prevent the recurrence of ascites. Non-compliant patients should be instructed to comply with therapy.
(3) Consider liver transplantation.

[a] Although a survival benefit of albumin over other plasma expanders has not been demonstrated, albumin is more effective than other plasma expanders in the prevention of paracentesis-induced circulatory dysfunction when more than 5 l of ascitic fluid are removed.

the development of circulatory dysfunction is associated with shortened survival [29].

The most studied effective method to prevent circulatory dysfunction is the administration of plasma expanders. A randomized trial has shown that albumin is more effective than other plasma expanders (dextran-70, polygeline) for the prevention of circulatory dysfunction as estimated by changes in plasma renin activity, probably owing to its persisting longer in the intravascular compartment [29]. **A1c** When less than five liters of ascites are removed, dextran-70, polygeline or saline show efficacy similar to that of albumin. However, albumin is more effective than these other plasma expanders when more than five liters of ascites are removed [29]. **A1c** Despite this greater efficacy, randomized trials have not shown differences in survival of patients treated with albumin compared with those treated with other plasma expanders [29–33]. Larger trials would be required to demonstrate a benefit of albumin on survival as well as on renal function. Table 38.2 shows the incidence of adverse effects observed in randomized trials comparing therapeutic paracentesis without plasma volume expansion or with three different plasma expanders in patients with cirrhosis and large ascites.

In summary, conclusive results from a randomized trial with adequate power to demonstrate a benefit of albumin

Table 38.2 Adverse effects reported in randomized trials assessing the efficacy and safety of therapeutic paracentesis without plasma volume expansion or with different plasma volume expanders in patients with cirrhosis and large ascites.

Adverse effect	No. of patients with adverse effects					p
	No plasma expander (%)	Polygeline (%)	Dextran-70 (%)	Saline (%)	Albumin (%)	
Renal impairment						
Ginès et al. [23]	6/531 (11)	—	—		0/52 (0)	0.03
Ginès et al. [29]	—	10/100 (10)	8/93 (9)		7/97 (7)	N S
Planas et al. [30]	—	—	1/42 (2)		1/43 (2)	NS
Salerno et al. [31]	—	1/27 (4)	—		1/27 (4)	NS
Fassio et al. [32]	—	—	1/20 (5)		1/21 (5)	NS
Sola-Vera et al. [33]	—	—		3/21 (14)	1/21 (5)	0.02
Hyponatremia						
Ginès et al. [23]	9/53 (17)	—	—		1/52 (2)	0.02
Ginès et al. [29]	—	19/100 (19)	23/93 (25)		14/97 (14)	NS
Planas et al. [30]	—	—	4/45 (9)		3/43 (7)	NS
Salerno et al. [31]	—	5/27 (18)	—		4/27 (15)	NS
Fassio et al. [32]	—	—	3/20 (15)		4/21 (19)	NS
Sola-Vera et al. [33]	—	—		4/21 (19)	0/21 (0)	0.02

Figures represent the number of patients developing the adverse effect compared with the total number of patients in each treatment group.

administration after therapeutic paracentesis on mortality are not available. However, the currently available data indicate that circulatory dysfunction after removal of large amounts of ascitic fluid is potentially harmful to patients with cirrhosis. Albumin appears to be the plasma expander of choice when more than five liters of ascites are removed.

Diuretics

Diuretics eliminate the excess extracellular fluid presenting as ascites and edema by increasing renal sodium excretion, thus achieving a negative sodium balance. The diuretics most frequently used in patients with cirrhosis and ascites are aldosterone antagonists, mainly spironolactone and potassium canrenoate, drugs that selectively antagonize the sodium-retaining effects of aldosterone in the renal collecting tubules, and loop diuretics, especially furosemide, that inhibit the Na^+-K^+-$2Cl^-$ co-transporter in the loop of Henle [34].

Despite the use of diuretics in clinical practice for more than 30 years, few randomized trials have been reported comparing the efficacy of different diuretic agents in the treatment of ascites [34–36]. In patients without renal failure, the aldosterone antagonist spironolactone at a dose of 150 mg/day (increased to 300 mg/day if there was no response) was shown in one randomized trial to be more effective than the loop diuretic furosemide at a dose of 80 mg/day (increased to 160 mg/day if there was no response) [35]. **A1d** This increased efficacy of aldosterone

antagonists has also been suggested in several studies [13, 37–40]. Based on these findings, aldosterone antagonists are considered the diuretics of choice in the management of cirrhotic ascites.

In clinical practice, aldosterone antagonists are frequently given in combination with loop diuretics. Theoretical advantages of this combination include greater natriuretic potency, earlier onset of diuresis, and reduced tendency to induce hyperkalemia. Two different regimens of diuretic administration have been proposed. In the first, the dose of aldosterone antagonists is increased progressively (usually up to 400 mg/day of spironolactone) and loop diuretics (furosemide up to 160 mg/day) are added only if no response is achieved with the highest dose of spironolactone. In the second, the two drugs are given in combination from the start of therapy. Both regimens are similar with respect to efficacy and incidence of complications. The only difference is that when the combination of spironolactone and furosemide is used from the beginning of therapy there is a more frequent need to reduce the dose of the drugs in responsive patients compared with the other stepwise regimen [41]. **Ald** Diuretic therapy is effective in the elimination of ascites in 80–90% of all patients, a percentage that may increase to 95% when only patients without renal failure are considered [13, 16–20, 35–40]. **Ald B4** The remaining patients either do not respond to diuretic therapy or develop diuretic-induced adverse effects that prevent the use of high doses of these drugs. This condition is known as refractory ascites [42]. These adverse effects include hepatic encephalopathy, hyponatremia, renal impairment, potassium disturbances, gynecomastia and muscle cramps [34, 40–43]. The incidence of renal and electrolyte disorders and encephalopathy vary depending on the population of patients studied, and is higher in patients with marked sodium retention and renal failure (who require higher doses of diuretics) and lower in patients with moderate sodium retention and without renal failure. Although some of these complications may be unrelated to diuretic therapy and due to the existence of advanced liver disease [44], there is no doubt that diuretics are a major cause of these complications because their frequency is markedly lower if ascites is removed by therapeutic paracentesis (see Table 38.1). Spironolactone-induced gynecomastia is common and may be important enough to lead to the discontinuation of the drug in some patients. An alternative treatment for these patients is amiloride, although its potency is much lower than that of spironolactone [36]. **Ald** Eplerenone, a new aldosterone antagonist has fewer endocrine adverse effects compared with spironolactone and could be a good alternative to spironolactone in patients with spironolactone-induced gynecomastia [45]. However, its effectiveness in patients with cirrhosis and ascites has not been assessed. Finally, muscle cramps of variable intensity, sometimes severe, may also occur as an adverse effect of diuretics. Effective therapies for muscle cramps include quinidine (300 mg/day) [46], or albumin (25 g/week) [43]. Zinc sulfate (440 mg/day) also appeared effective in an uncontrolled study including a small number of patients [47]. **B4**

Because therapeutic paracentesis has replaced diuretics as the treatment of choice for hospitalized cirrhotic patients with large volume ascites in most centers, at present the main indications for use of diuretics in cirrhosis are as follows [15]:
• Treatment of patients with mild or moderate ascites or those with large volume ascites in whom paracentesis is not effective because of compartmentalization of ascitic fluid due to peritoneal adhesions.
• Treatment of patients with edema without ascites.
• Prevention of recurrence of ascites after therapeutic paracentesis.

Peritoneovenous shunt

A peritoneovenous shunt is a device designed to transfer ascitic fluid from the abdominal cavity to the systemic circulation via an abdominal tube and a thoracic tube ending in the superior vena cava connected through a one-way valve. This device was used extensively in the 1970s and 1980s for the treatment of refractory ascites in cirrhosis. Although the system was pathophysiologically sound, its use declined progressively during the 1990s due to a high incidence of severe adverse effects, a high rate of obstruc-

tion, lack of demonstration of a significant survival benefit, and development of new procedures, such as the transjugular intrahepatic portosystemic shunt (TIPS) [48–54]. For all these reasons, this procedure is rarely used nowadays.

Transjugular intrahepatic portosystemic shunt

TIPS was introduced in clinical practice in the 1990s for the management of refractory variceal bleeding, with the objective of creating a portosystemic shunt, without the need of surgery. The procedure consists of the placement of an intrahepatic stent between one hepatic vein and the portal vein using a transjugular approach [55]. It soon became evident that in patients with variceal bleeding and ascites treated with TIPS there was an increased natriuretic effect of diuretics, leading to the reduction or elimination of ascites in most patients. These beneficial effects of TIPS on ascites are similar to those reported in earlier studies in patients treated with surgical portosystemic shunts, especially side-to-side portacaval shunts.

A large number of uncontrolled studies have shown that TIPS is effective in preventing recurrence of ascites in patients with refractory ascites. This effect is due to reduction in the activity of sodium-retaining mechanisms and amelioration of renal function, which lead to an improvement of the renal response to diuretics [56–61]. **B4** The main disadvantages of TIPS include shunt stenosis or obstruction (up to 75% of patients develop stenosis within 6–12 months, leading to reaccumulation of ascites in most cases), but this has been reduced with covered stents. In addition, there is a high rate of encephalopathy due to the shunting of blood from the splanchnic to the systemic circulation [62, 63]. Other adverse effects include impairment in liver function, which is usually transient, hemolytic anemia and heart failure [55, 64]. Because of its efficacy and the paucity of good alternative therapies (except for that of repeated large-volume paracentesis with concomitant administration of intravenous albumin), TIPS became a widely used treatment for patients with refractory ascites during the 1990s despite the initial lack of randomized controlled trials comparing it with medical therapy.

Five randomized trials comparing uncovered TIPS versus repeated large volume paracentesis with concomitant intravenous albumin in patients with cirrhosis and refractory ascites have been published [65–69]. **Alc** The trials demonstrate that TIPS controls ascites effectively and is associated with a lower rate of ascites recurrence. The main results of these trials are summarized in Table 38.3. Although there are some discrepancies between the results of the trials these studies demonstrate the following:
• TIPS is clearly more effective than large volume paracentesis in the prevention of recurrence of ascites [65–69]. However, normalization of renal sodium homeostasis is

Table 38.3 Complications and survival in randomized trials comparing transjugular intrahepatic portosystemic shunt (TIPS) and large volume paracentesis in patients with cirrhosis and refractory ascites.

Study	TIPS	Paracentesis[a]	p
Recurrent ascites			
Lebrec et al. [65]	5/10 (50)[b]	12/12 (100)	< 0.05
Rössle et al. [66]	3/23 (13)	15/22 (68)	< 0.04
Ginès et al. [67]	17/35 (49)	29/35 (82)	< 0.01
Sanyal et al. [68]	22/52 (42)	48/57 (84)	< 0.001
Salerno et al. [69]	13/33 (39)	32/33 (97)	< 0.005
Severe hepatic encephalopathy			
Lebrec et al. [65]	2/10 (20)	0/12 (0)	NS
Rössle et al. [66]	NR	NR	—
Ginès et al. [67]	21/35 (60)	12/34 (35)	0.03
Sanyal et al. [68]	20/52 (38)	12/57 (21)	0.058
Salerno et al. [69]	20 (61)	13 (39)	NS
TIPS stenosis/obstruction			
Lebrec et al. [65]	3/10 (30)	—	—
Rössle et al. [66]	13/29 (45)	—	—
Ginès et al. [67]	13/35 (37)	—	—
Sanyal et al. [68]	NR	—	—
Salerno et al. [69]	12/33 (36)	—	—
Hepatorenal syndrome type 1			
Lebrec et al. [65]	NR	NR	—
Rössle et al. [66]	NR	NR	—
Ginès et al. [67]	3/35 (9)	11/35 (31)	0.03
Sanyal et al. [68]	NR	NR	—
Salerno et al. [69]	3/33(9)	5/15(15)	0.05
Mortality during follow-up			
Lebrec et al. [65	9/10 (90)	4/12 (33)	<0.05
Rössle et al. [66]	15/29 (51)	23/31 (74)	NS
Ginès et al. [67]	20/35 (57)	18/35 (51)	NS
Sanyal et al. [68]	18/52 (34)	19/57 (33)	NS
Salerno et al. [69]	13/33 (39)	20 (61)	0.02

[a] In all studies, except that of Rössle et al. [66] IV albumin (6–8 g/l ascites removed) was given routinely to all patients treated with paracentesis.
[b] Patients/total number of patients included.
NR: not reported; IV: intravenous.

not completely achieved and most patients treated with TIPS still require sodium restriction and diuretics during follow-up [67–68].
• TIPS reduces the risk of developing hepatorenal syndrome type 1 [67].
• TIPS is associated with an increased risk of severe hepatic encephalopathy and does not reduce significantly the risk of other complications of cirrhosis, such as gastrointestinal bleeding or spontaneous bacterial peritonitis [67, 68].

• There is a high rate of TIPS stenosis or obstruction that requires frequent intervention to maintain shunt patency [65–69].
• Hepatic encephalopathy after TIPS occurs in approximately 30–50% of patients [65–69].
• Despite better control of ascites and a reduction in the number of hospitalizations for ascites, TIPS does not appear to improve the quality of life compared with repeated large volume paracentesis with concomitant intravenous albumin [67, 68].
• The cost of TIPS is higher than that of conventional therapy with repeated large volume paracentesis and concomitant intravenous albumin [67].
• TIPS does not improve either overall or transplant-free survival compared with therapy with repeated large volume paracentesis with intravenous albumin [67, 68, 70].

A high quality meta-analyses of these randomized controlled studies concluded that TIPS is better at controlling ascites but does not improve survival compared with paracentesis [70]. **A1c** However, another recent meta-analysis that reviewed individual patient data of three trials indicates that TIPS significantly improves transplant-free survival of cirrhotic patients with refractory ascites [66, 68, 69, 71]. **A1c** Although meta-analysis using individual data seems a more reliable tool compared with standard meta-analysis, it cannot overcome deficiencies of individual studies, such as inclusion of patients who did not have refractory ascites in two of the studies [66, 69], use of large-volume paracentesis without albumin in one study [66], and use of TIPS as rescue therapy in a large proportion of patients treated with large-volume paracentesis in another study [69]. Until more information becomes available, the higher frequency of hepatic encephalopathy as well as the higher cost of TIPS compared with large-volume paracentesis plus albumin, in the context of a lack of survival benefit, leaves TIPS as a second-line therapy in the management of refractory ascites. The first line of treatment for refractory ascites is repeated large-volume paracentesis associated with albumin [14, 15]. TIPS placement may be an option for patients with preserved liver function (bilirubin < 3 mg/dl, serum sodium level > 130 mEq/l, Child-Pugh score < 12, model for end-stage liver disease (MELD) score < 18), aged < 70, without hepatic encephalopathy, central hepatocellular carcinoma, or cardiopulmonary disease.

The recommendations for the treatment of refractory ascites based on these conclusions are summarized in Box 38.2.

Liver transplantation

Liver transplantation has become a frequent intervention for patients with advanced cirrhosis. Although randomized trials comparing liver transplantation with conventional

BOX 38.2 Recommendations for the management of patients with cirrhosis and refractory ascites

(1) Total paracentesis plus intravenous albumin (8 g/l of ascites removed). Repeat paracentesis during follow-up whenever needed. Patients can be treated as outpatients. Consider liver transplantation.

(2) Patients should be on sodium restriction (80 mmol/day) and maximum tolerated closes of diuretics (up to spironolactone 400 mg/day and furosemide 160 mg/day). Check urine sodium under diuretic therapy. If urine sodium is greater than 30 mmol/day, diuretic therapy may be maintained because it may help to delay the recurrence of ascites. If urine sodium is lower than 30 mmol/day or diuretic treatment induces complications, diuretics should be withdrawn.

(3) Consider the use, of transjugular intrahepatic portosystemic shunt (TIPS) in patients with preserved liver function and with low acceptance of repeated total paracentesis or in those in whom paracentesis is not effective because of the presence of peritoneal adhesions.

medical therapy in patients with ascites are not available for obvious reasons, the 80% five-year probability of survival obtained in adult cirrhotic patients treated with liver transplantation in most centers is markedly greater than the expected 20% in non-transplanted patients with cirrhosis and ascites [72]. **B2**

Earlier recommendations suggested that ascites per se was not an indication for liver transplantation, and patients had to be considered for transplantation only when ascites was refractory to diuretic therapy or was associated with severe complications, such as spontaneous bacterial peritonitis or hepatorenal syndrome. However, with these guidelines a large proportion of these patients die while registered on the transplantation waiting list. This is because of the short survival associated with these conditions. The median survival time is less than one year for patients with refractory ascites and those recovering from spontaneous bacterial peritonitis, and is even shorter in patients with hepatorenal syndrome, particularly in those with the progressive form of this syndrome – type 1 – who have a median survival time of less than one month [50, 51, 73].

With the growing understanding of the natural history of ascites in cirrhosis, it is now known that a number of factors predictive of survival can be used to identify candidates for liver transplantation [74]. The most useful predictive factors are related to abnormalities in renal function and systemic hemodynamics and include:

• An impaired ability to excrete a water load (urine volume < 8 ml/min after a water load of 5% dextrose 20 ml/kg intravenous (IV)).

• Spontaneous dilutional hyponatremia (serum sodium < 130 mmol/l).

• Arterial hypotension (mean arterial pressure < 80 mmHg in the absence of diuretic therapy).

• Reduced glomerular filtration rate (even moderate reductions, as indicated by serum creatinine levels between 1.2 (106 µmol/l and 1.5 mg/dl (133 µmol/l) in the absence of diuretic therapy).

• Marked sodium retention (urine sodium < 10 mmol/day under a moderate sodium-restricted diet and in the absence of diuretic therapy).

Interestingly, in patients with ascites these parameters are better than liver function tests as predictors of prognosis [74]. Therefore, patients with one or more of these predictive factors have a poor survival expectancy and should be referred to transplant centers for evaluation. **B4**

The MELD score (Model for End-stage Liver Disease score, which includes serum bilirubin, international normalized ratio (INR) and serum creatinine) may be suitable for the evaluation of prognosis of patients with cirrhosis and ascites, as it includes a variable that estimates the degree of impairment of renal function [75]. In addition, many patients with advanced cirrhosis and refractory ascites may have low serum sodium (levels less than 130 mEql/l), which is an independent poor prognostic factor for outcome and survival. In fact both the MELD score and the serum sodium concentration are independent predictors of mortality. Thus, a new score incorporating MELD and serum sodium (MELD-NA) has been proposed, since serum sodium improves the prognostic accuracy of the MELD score in the prediction of survival in these patients [76, 77]. Nevertheless, the inclusion of serum sodium in a new score for survival prediction in cirrhosis has some limitations given that serum sodium is a very labile parameter. In addition, this new score needs to be validated in prospective studies.

Hepatorenal syndrome

Hepatorenal syndrome is at the most severe end of the clinical spectrum of abnormalities of renal function in patients with cirrhosis and ascites [3, 6, 42, 78]. It may occur in two different clinical patterns [42, 78]. Type 1 hepatorenal syndrome is characterized by rapid and progressive impairment of renal function as defined by a 100% increase of the initial serum creatinine to a level greater than 2.5 mg/dl (221 µmol/l) or a 50% reduction of the initial 24-hour creatinine clearance to a level lower than 20 ml/min in less than two weeks; in some patients, this type of hepatorenal syndrome develops spontaneously without any identifiable precipitating factor, while in others it occurs in close chronological relationship with some complicating event, particularly in relation to bacte-

---

BOX 38.3 Diagnostic criteria of hepatorenal syndrome

(1) Cirrhosis with ascites.
(2) Serum creatinine > 1.5 mg/dl (133 μmol/l).
(3) No improvement of serum creatinine (decrease to a level lower than 1.5 mg/dl–133 μmol/l– after at least two days off diuretics and volume expansion with albumin (1 g/kg body weight up to a maximum of 100 g/day).
(4) Absence of shock.
(5) No current or recent treatment with nephrotoxic drugs.
(6) Absence of signs of parenchymal renal disease, as suggested by proteinuria (>500 mg/day) or hematuria (<50 red blood cells per high power field), and/or abnormal renal ultrasound.

Adapted from Salerno *et al. Gut* 2007; **56**: 1310–1318.

---

rial infections such as spontaneous bacterial peritonitis [79].

Type 2 hepatorenal syndrome is characterized by a less severe and non-progressive reduction of glomerular filtration rate (at least in the short term); the main clinical consequence of this type of hepatorenal syndrome is refractory ascites.

Because of the lack of specific diagnostic tests, the diagnosis of hepatorenal syndrome is currently made according to several criteria, as proposed by the International Ascites Club, which are based on demonstration of a marked reduction in glomerular filtration rate (serum creatinine > 1.5 mg/dl in the absence of diuretic therapy) and the exclusion of other causes of renal failure that may occur in patients with cirrhosis (see Box 38.3) [42, 78].

For many years, no effective therapy existed for patients with hepatorenal syndrome, except for liver transplantation. Recently, several effective, new interventions have been introduced.

Vasoconstrictors

A number of observational studies published in the 1990s showed that the administration of vasoconstrictor drugs to patients with cirrhosis and hepatorenal syndrome causes a marked improvement of renal function in a large proportion of patients [80–92]. **B4**, **C5** The rationale for the use of vasoconstrictors in patients with hepatorenal syndrome is to improve effective arterial blood volume by causing a vasoconstriction of the extremely dilated splanchnic vascular bed. The improvement in the arterial circulatory function leads to a suppression in the activity of vasoconstrictor systems and a subsequent increase in renal perfusion and glomerular filtration rate.

Two types of vasoconstrictor drugs have been used in patients with hepatorenal syndrome: vasopressin ana-

logues (terlipressin and ornipressin) andα-adrenergic agonists (norepinephrine, noradrenaline and midodrine), which act on V1 vasopressin receptors and α1-adrenergic receptors, respectively, present in the smooth muscle cells of the vessel wall. The drug most frequently used in published studies is terlipressin, which is marketed in many countries for the indication of acute variceal bleeding in cirrhosis. In most studies terlipressin has been combined with intravenous albumin to further improve the arterial underfilling. Ornipressin is no longer available and there is limited information on the efficacy of α-adrenergic agonists [89–92]. There are four randomized placebo controlled trials investigating the efficacy and safety of terlipressin and albumin in patients with hepatorenal syndrome [93–96]. **A1c** The information currently available on terlipressin can be summarized as follows:

(1) In uncontrolled trials, the administration of terlipressin improves renal function in 50–75% of patients [82–88]. Although there are no dose-efficacy studies, treatment is usually started with 1 mg/4–6 h IV, and the dose is increased up to a maximum of 2 mg/4–6 h after two days if there is no response to therapy as defined by a reduction of serum creatinine > 25% of pre-treatment values.

(2) Results from two large randomized placebo controlled studies indicate that treatment with terlipressin together with albumin is associated with marked improvement of renal function in approximately 40% of patients [93, 94]. **A1c** The overall population of patients treated with terlipressin and albumin in these two studies did not have an improved survival compared to that of patients treated with albumin alone. However, both studies showed that responders in terms of improvement of renal function after therapy had a significant (but moderate) increase in survival compared to non-responders [93, 94]. **A1c** A summary of the results of the four randomized studies are shown in Table 38.4 [93–96].

(3) In most studies, treatment with terlipressin is usually maintained until serum creatinine decreases below 1.5 mg/dl or for a maximum of 15 days. It is unknown whether the continued administration of the drug after the endpoint of 1.5 mg/dl of serum creatinine has been reached may cause a further improvement of renal function.

(4) The incidence of ischemic side effects requiring the discontinuation of treatment is approximately 10%. Some patients may develop myocardial ischemia, arrhythmia, intestinal ischemia or transient pulmonary edema during the first few days of therapy [82–88, 93–96]. Therefore, patients with HRS treated with terlipressin should be closely followed with cardiac monitoring, ideally in semi-intensive or intensive care unit, and if signs of cardiovascular disturbances develop, terlipressin should be discontinued promptly.

(5) A consistent finding in all studies is that the recurrence of hepatorenal syndrome after treatment withdrawal is

Table 38.4 Response rate, survival, recurrence, and adverse effects in patients with cirrhosis and hepatorenal syndrome treated with terlipressin and albumin in randomized controlled trials.

Response (ref)	Terlipressin/ Albumin (%)	Placebo/ Albumin (%)	p
Response			
Sanyal et al. [93]	19/56(34)	7/56 (12.5)	0.08
Martin-Llahi et al. [94]	10/23 (44)	2/23(9)	0.01
Solanki et al. [95]	5/12 (42)	0/12	0.001
Neri et al. [96]	21/26(80)	5/26(19)	0.001
Survival			
Sanyal et al. [93][a]	24/56 (43)	21/56 (37.5)	0.84
Martin-Llahi et al. [94][b]	6/23 (27)	4/23 (19)	0.7
Solanki et al. [95][c]	5/12 (41)	0/15	NR
Neri et al. [96][b]	14/26 (54)	4/26 (18)	NR
Recurrence			
Sanyal et al. [93]	1/19 (5)	1/5(14)	NR
Martin-Llahi et al. [94]	1/10 (10)	NR	—
Solanki et al. [95][c]	NR	NR	—
Neri et al. [96][b]	NR	NR	—
Adverse effects			
Sanyal et al. [93]	18/56 (32)	12/56 (22)	NR
Martin-Llahi et al. [94][d]	10/23 (43)	4/23 (17)	0.10
Solanki et al. [95]	2/12 (16)	0/12	NR
Neri et al. [96]	9/26	0/26	NR

[a] Survival at 180 days.
[b] Survival at 90 days.
[c] Survival at 15 days.
[d] Myocardial ischemia, arrhythmia, intestinal ischemia, circulatory overload.
NR: not reported.

uncommon (approximately 5–15% of patients) (Table 38.4). The explanation for this low recurrence rate is unknown. Treatment of recurrence is usually effective.

(6) The above observations refer mainly to type 1 hepatorenal syndrome, as the majority of patients included in the published studies were in this category. Although some reports suggest that vasoconstrictors also improve renal function in patients with type 2 hepatorenal syndrome, their efficacy in this setting remains to be confirmed [94].

Transjugular intrahepatic portosystemic shunt

There is limited information on the effects of TIPS in patients with type 1 hepatorenal syndrome. Two uncontrolled studies reported that TIPS improves renal function in patients with this syndrome [97, 98]. **B4** Improvement in renal function after TIPS placement alone is slow and successful in approximately 60% of patients. Median survival after TIPS in patients with type 1 HRS ranges between two and four months. Studies assessing TIPS for type 1 HRS have included patients with preserved liver function and excluded those with a history of hepatic encephalopathy, Child-Pugh scores ≥ 12 or serum bilirubin > 5 mg/dl. The applicability of TIPS in patients with type 1 HRS is low because TIPS is considered contraindicated in patients with severe liver failure (high serum bilirubin levels and/or Child-Pugh score greater than 12) and hepatic encephalopathy, which are common findings in the setting of type 1 HRS. No studies have been reported that compared TIPS with vasoconstrictor drugs in patients with type 1 hepatorenal syndrome.

There have been no specific studies assessing the efficacy of TIPS in type 2 hepatorenal syndrome. However, in a subgroup analysis of patients with refractory ascites and type 2 hepatorenal syndrome included in one randomized trial, TIPS reduced the recurrence rate of ascites and the risk of progression from type 2 to type 1 hepatorenal syndrome, but did not improve survival compared to control patients treated with repeated therapeutic paracentesis with intravenous albumin [67]. **A1d**

Other therapeutic methods

Hemodialysis or continuous hemodiafiltration are frequently used in the management of type 1 hepatorenal syndrome in many centers, particularly in patients who are candidates for liver transplantation, with the aim of preventing the complications associated with acute renal failure and maintaining patients alive until transplantation is done [99]. Complications during hemodialysis in these patients are common and include arterial hypotension, bleeding and infections. On the other hand, clinical or biochemical features indicating the need for renal replacement therapy, such as heart or respiratory failure, severe acidosis or severe hyperkalemia are uncommon, at least in early stages of type 1 hepatorenal syndrome. In contrast, these features are usually seen in patients with cirrhosis and acute renal failure caused by conditions other than hepatorenal syndrome, especially acute tubular necrosis due to septic or hemorrhagic shock and acute glomerulonephritis. Considering all these facts and the efficacy of measures aimed at improving circulatory function (especially vasoconstrictors), the use of hemodialysis or continuous hemodiafiltration in the management of patients with hepatorenal syndrome needs to be re-evaluated and perhaps used as a second-line therapy for those patients not responding to vasoconstrictors. Recently, a new method of dialysis, the extracorporeal albumin dialysis or molecular adsorbent recirculating system (MARS), a system that uses an albumin-containing dialysate that is used to remove albumin-bound and water-soluble toxic metabolites, has been reported to improve renal function and survival in a small uncontrolled study in patients with hepatorenal syndrome

[100]. **B4** These promising results, however, require confirmation.

Liver transplantation

Liver transplantation is the only definitive treatment for patients with hepatorenal syndrome without contraindications to the procedure [101]. Even patients showing a complete response to vasoconstrictors or TIPS with normalization of serum creatinine have a poor prognosis if not transplanted [85, 86, 93, 94]. **B4 A1c** Main causes of death in these patients include liver failure and/or bacterial infections [85, 86]. Ideally, patients with hepatorenal syndrome should be prioritized for liver transplantation due to the high mortality rate; otherwise, most patients may die while awaiting liver transplantation. The implemented system of organ allocation in the USA based on the MELD score may be useful in this respect, because it includes serum creatinine in addition to parameters of liver function (bilirubin and INR) [75, 102]. Therefore, patients with hepatorenal syndrome usually achieve high values in the MELD score and may receive transplants within a short period of time. In addition to prioritization, these patients should probably be treated with vasoconstrictors, whenever possible, while awaiting transplantation in order to improve renal function and maintain life while they are on the waiting list. The reversal of HRS before transplantation may help patients not only reach transplantation, but also reduce the relatively high morbidity and mortality after liver transplantation characteristic of HRS [103, 104]. A small study indicates that patients with hepatorenal syndrome treated with vasopressin analogues before transplantation have a complication rate and short-term and long-term survival which are not different from those observed in transplant patients without hepatorenal syndrome [105].

Dilutional hyponatremia

Patients with advanced cirrhosis often develop spontaneous dilutional hyponatremia due to impairment of the renal excretion of free water. This disorder always occurs in the setting of ascites with severe sodium retention, and most patients have poor or no response to diuretics [106]. In this condition, renal retention of solute-free water is disproportionate to that of sodium retained and serum sodium levels decrease despite the existence of increased total body sodium. Dilutional hyponatremia in cirrhosis is defined as a reduction in serum sodium concentration below 130 mEq/l in the setting of ascites and/or edema [106]. **C5** The impaired solute-free water excretion is due to high circulating levels of vasopressin (antidiuretic hormone) secondary to a hypersecretion of the hormone from the neurohypophysis triggered by a non-osmotic (vasoactive) stimulus [107, 108]. The clinical consequences of dilutional hyponatremia are incompletely understood,

but it has been linked to some neurological and non-neurological symptoms seen frequently in patients with advanced cirrhosis. Dilutional hyponatremia impairs the quality of life of patients with cirrhosis because it requires the restriction of fluid intake to a level similar to that of urine output in order to prevent a positive fluid balance that would lead to a further increase in total body water and impairment of hyponatremia.

There is no effective therapy currently available in clinical practice to treat spontaneous dilutional hyponatremia. Fluid restriction is effective in preventing further reduction of serum sodium concentration but usually is not followed by an increase in serum sodium. The administration of hypertonic saline solutions does not make much sense from a pathophysiological perspective, because total body sodium and extracellular fluid volume are increased in patients with dilutional hyponatremia. It invariably leads to marked increase in ascites and edema and has only modest effects on serum sodium concentration and therefore is not recommended. There are anecdotal reports of the efficacy of albumin infusions, but this remains to be proved in larger series [109]. **B4** In recent years, several orally active drugs, the so-called vaptans, that selectively antagonize the vasopressin V2 receptor (the receptor present in collecting duct cells in the kidney responsible for water reabsorption in the distal parts of the nephron), have been developed [108, 110]. **C5** The rationale behind the use of these drugs in patients with cirrhosis and dilutional hyponatremia is to selectively antagonize the effects of vasopressin in the kidney so that solute-free water excretion is increased, the abnormal water balance restored, the increased body water reduced, and serum sodium concentration normalized [108]. **C5** So far, the results of a few phase II and III studies in patients with cirrhosis have confirmed the beneficial effects of these drugs. Two multicenter, randomized, placebo-controlled trials evaluated the use of lixivaptan in cirrhotic patients with dilutional hyponatremia [111, 112] **A1c** In these two studies this agent caused a dose-related increase in serum sodium levels and solute-free water clearance. Unfortunately, the drug caused significant dehydration in some patients at the effective doses in one study [111]. In the other study, which evaluated two doses of the drug versus placebo, a small amount of patients in each group was included and the effects of lixivaptan were only evaluated until serum sodium normalized, without information on long-term response [112]. A large multicenter randomized controlled study evaluating the use of tolvaptan in patients with euvolemic or hypervolemic hyponatremia (SIADH, congestive heart failure and cirrhosis) indicates that this agent is effective in raising serum sodium concentration when used for 30 days [113]. **A1c** In this study, a subgroup of patients with cirrhosis and dilutional hyponatremia were assigned tolvaptan or placebo in ascending doses according to response [113].

A1c There were no significant side effects compared to placebo. Tolvaptan rapidly improved serum sodium, fluid balance and caused significant weight loss in patients with cirrhosis and hyponatremia compared to placebo and markedly increased solute-free water clearance without adversely affecting renal function. In patients with cirrhosis and dilutional hyponatremia, normalization of sodium levels (>135 mEq/l) occurred in 30% and 22% of subjects at days 4 and 30 respectively [113]. This agent therefore seems to be safe, effective and is likely to be promising in the treatment of dilutional hyponatremia. Another multicenter randomized study evaluated short- term use (14 days) of satavaptan at doses of 5 mg, 12.5 mg, 25 mg once daily in 110 patients with cirrhosis and hyponatremia receiving 100 mg of spironolactone [114]. **A1c** Satavaptan treatment was associated with improved control of ascites (measured by a reduction in body weight) and a reduction in abdominal girth. This beneficial effect on ascites was associated with improvements in serum sodium in all patients. A major side effect was thirst in the satavaptan group, and in a few patients a large volume diuresis of 5 liters or more in less than 24 hours. V2 receptor antagonists seem to not only improve ascites control, but also increase serum sodium in patients with cirrhosis, ascites and hyponatremia on diuretics.

Although a number of issues remain to be answered about the efficacy, clinical usefulness, tolerability, drug interactions and adverse effects of vaptans, they represent a powerful pharmacological tool for the management of patients with advanced cirrhosis and dilutional hyponatremia.

Spontaneous bacterial peritonitis

Spontaneous bacterial peritonitis is a common and severe complication in cirrhotic patients with ascites characterized by infection of ascitic fluid with no apparent intra-abdominal source of infection [4, 5]. Spontaneous bacterial peritonitis is generally caused by Gram-negative bacteria from the intestinal flora, especially *Escherichia coli*. However, Gram-positive cocci, particularly *Staphylococcus aureus*, are being isolated with increasing frequency, mainly in hospitalized patients [115–117]. The diagnosis of spontaneous bacterial peritonitis is based on the demonstration of an absolute number of polymorphonuclear cells in ascitic fluid greater than 250/mm^3 [5]. **C5** The clinical spectrum is very variable and ranges from complete absence of symptoms to a classic clinical picture of peritonitis [4, 5, 118]. For this reason and because of its high prevalence, spontaneous bacterial peritonitis should be ruled out in patients with cirrhosis admitted to hospital with ascites, outpatients undergoing large volume paracentesis, and hospitalized patients who develop signs and/or symptoms suggestive of peritoneal or systemic infection (i.e. abdominal pain, rebound tenderness, ileus, fever, leukocytosis, shock), hepatic encephalopathy or impairment in renal function [5, 118]. Cirrhotic patients with hydrothorax may also develop a spontaneous infection of pleural fluid that is pathogenically similar to spontaneous bacterial peritonitis and should be managed in a similar fashion [119].

Therapy

Antibiotic therapy should be started whenever the polymorphonuclear count in ascitic fluid is greater than 250/mm^3 and before obtaining microbiological culture results [5]. **C5** Third-generation cephalosporins are the antibiotics of choice as initial empiric treatment for spontaneous bacterial peritonitis, because of their broad antibacterial spectrum, high efficacy and safety [5, 120–123]. **A1c** Resolution of infection occurs in up to 90% of patients. Cefotaxime (2 g/8–12 hours) has been the drug most commonly used in randomized trials, but other third-generation cephalosporins have similar efficacy [124]. **A1c** Cefotaxime has been shown to be more effective than other antibiotics, such as aztreonam or the combination of aminoglycosides plus ampicillin [120–125]. Amoxicillin-clavulinic acid is as effective as third-generation cephalosporins [126]. Quinolones (ofloxacin, ciprofloxacin) administered orally are also effective and may be an alternative to third-generation cephalosporins or amoxicillinclavulanic acid except in patients who are severely ill (i.e. septic shock, severe renal failure) or with complications that may impair the absorption of the drug (gastrointestinal hemorrhage or ileus) [127]. **A1c** Given the increased frequency of Gram-positive cocci isolates in nosocomial spontaneous bacterial peritonitis, the empiric antibiotic treatment for this condition should probably include an antibiotic active against these bacteria, particularly *S. aureus*, until the results of ascitic fluid or blood cultures are available [115–117]. **C5** Antibiotic therapy is maintained until the complete disappearance of all signs of infection and decrease of polymorphonuclear count in ascitic fluid below the threshold value of 250/mm^3. In most patients, resolution is achieved in a short period of time, usually less than six days.

The development of hepatorenal syndrome, which is one of the most common and severe complications of spontaneous bacterial peritonitis can be effectively prevented by the administration of albumin together with the antibiotic therapy [79, 128]. **B4** The incidence of hepatorenal syndrome is markedly lower in patients receiving albumin plus antibiotics compared with patients receiving antibiotics alone. The prevention of hepatorenal syndrome achieved by administration of albumin improves survival of these patients [128]. **B4** This may be particularly important for liver transplant candidates. The beneficial effect of albumin is probably related to its capacity to prevent the

(1) After diagnosis of peritonitis has been made (>250
polymorphonuclear cells/mm^3 in ascitic fluid), start
with third-generation cephalosporins (i.e. cefotaxime
2 g/8–12 hourly intravenously or ceftriaxone 1 g/24
hours intravenously) or amoxicillin-clavulinic acid
(500 mg/125 mg/8 hourly intravenously). In patients on
antibiotic prophylaxis, third-generation cephalosporins
are the treatment of choice. In nosocomial spontaneous
bacterial peritonitis, consider the addition of an
antibiotic active against Gram-positive cocci.
(2) Give albumin 1.5 g/kg intravenously at the time of
diagnosis of the infection and 1 g/kg 48 hours later.
(3) Maintain antibiotic therapy until disappearance of signs
of infection and reduction of polymorphonuclear cells
in ascitic fluid below 250/mm^3.
(4) After resolution of infection, start long-term norfloxacin
400 mg/day per os (orally).

reduction in the effective arterial blood volume and subsequent activation of vasoconstrictor systems that occurs during the infection.

Recommendations for the management of spontaneous bacterial peritonitis are summarized in Box 38.4.

Hospital mortality in patients with spontaneous bacterial peritonitis was around 30% in most series published during the 1980s and 1990s. In the series that included patients treated with intravenous albumin, hospital mortality has decreased to 10–15% [128]. Advanced liver failure and associated complications (i.e. gastrointestinal hemorrhage, hepatorenal syndrome) are the main causes of death in these patients. As previously discussed, the most important predictor of survival in patients with spontaneous bacterial peritonitis is the development of hepatorenal syndrome during the infection [79, 128]. Long-term prognosis of patients who have recovered from an episode of spontaneous bacterial peritonitis is poor, and patients should be evaluated for liver transplantation. Recurrent spontaneous bacterial peritonitis is very common in these patients and constitutes a major cause of death [4].

Prophylaxis

The identification of subsets of patients with an increased risk of developing spontaneous bacterial peritonitis has stimulated the search for interventions to prevent the development of this complication. Conditions associated with an increased risk of spontaneous bacterial peritonitis include: gastrointestinal bleeding, low protein concentration in ascitic fluid, advanced liver failure (high serum bilirubin and/or markedly prolonged prothrombin time), and past history of spontaneous bacterial peritonitis [4, 5]. Because

most episodes are caused by Gram-negative bacteria present in the normal intestinal flora, the rationale for the prophylaxis of spontaneous bacterial peritonitis has been based mainly on the administration of antibiotics that produce a selective decontamination of the gastrointestinal tract, with elimination of aerobic Gram-negative bacteria without affecting aerobic Gram-positive bacteria and anaerobes.

The efficacy of this approach has been demonstrated in patients with gastrointestinal hemorrhage and in patients who have recovered from the first spontaneous bacterial peritonitis episode (see Table 38.5) [129–136]. **A1c** In patients with gastrointestinal hemorrhage, the short-term administration of norfloxacin markedly reduces the incidence of spontaneous bacterial peritonitis or bacteremia as compared with patients not receiving prophylactic antibiotics [130]. In patients with advanced liver disease who are actively bleeding, intravenous ceftriaxone (1 g/day for seven days) is the preferred dose due to problems with oral absorption in this setting [133]. **A1c** Other effective approaches consist of the administration of parenteral antibiotics, such as ofloxacin or the combination of ciprofloxacin and amoxicillin-clavulinic acid [131, 132]. **B4** The absolute risk reduction in four trials of antibiotic prophylaxis in patients with gastrointestinal hemorrhage ranges from 9% to 23%. The results of a meta-analysis indicate that antibiotic prophylaxis in patients with gastrointestinal bleeding not only prevents infection but also improves survival [134, 135] **A1c**

Long-term norfloxacin administration is very effective in the prevention of spontaneous bacterial peritonitis recurrence (Table 38.5) [136]. This approach is effective and is recommended to prevent recurrence in patients who have recovered from an initial episode [5, 136]. **A1d** Antibiotic prophylaxis (norfloxacin, ciprofloxacin, or trimethoprim-sulfamethoxazole) also appears to be effective in the prevention of the first episode of spontaneous bacterial peritonitis (primary prophylaxis) in patients with low ascitic fluid protein (<10–15 g/l), who have a high risk of developing spontaneous bacterial peritonitis (Table 38.5) [137–144]. **A1d** A recent randomized placebo controlled study showed that long-term treatment with norfloxacin (400 mg/day) in patients with advanced cirrhosis and ascites with low protein level (< 15 g/l) in the ascitic fluid was associated with a lower risk of development of hepatorenal syndrome compared to a control group of patients receiving placebo [144]. **A1c** Norfloxacin reduced the one-year probability of developing spontaneous bacterial peritonitis and hepatorenal syndrome, and significantly improved the three-month and the one-year survival compared with placebo [144]. **A1c** Additional randomized controlled trials involving larger numbers of patients with longer periods of follow-up are needed in order to determine the potential problems such as bacterial resistance and duration of therapy.

Table 38.5 Incidence of spontaneous bacterial peritonitis in randomized trials of antibiotic prophylaxis in cirrhosisa.

	Spontaneous bacterial peritonitis			p
	Antibiotic regimen	Control	Antibiotic	
Primary prophylaxisb				
Gastrointestinal hemorrhage				
Rimola et al. [129]	Non-absorbable antibiotics po	15/72 (21)	6/68 (9)	0.05
Soriano et al. [130]	Norfloxacin 400 twice daily po	10/59 (17)	2/60 (3)	0.02
Blaise et al. [131]	Ofloxacin 400 mg/day IV	7/45 (16)	3/46 (7)	NS
Pauwels et al. [132]	Ciprofloxacin 200 mg IV+ amoxicillin and clavulanic acid 1 g/200 mg po thrice daily	7/34 (21)	1/30 (3)	0.05
Fernandez et al. [133]	Ceftriaxone 1g/day IV	7/57 (12%)c	1/54 (2%)	0.06
Ascites				
Soriano et al. [138]	Norfloxacin 400 mg/day po	7/31 (23)	0/32 (0)	0.005
Rolanchon et al. [139]	Ciprofloxacin 750 mg weekly po	7/32 (22)	1/28 (4)	0.05
Singh et al. [140]	Trimethoprim-sulfamethoxazole 160 mg/800 mg 5 days a week po	8/30 (27)	1/30 (3)	0.03
Novella et al. [141]	Norfloxacin 400 mg/day po	9/53 (17)d	1/56 (2)	0.007
Grange et al. [142]	Norfloxacin 400 mg/day po	4/54 (7)	0/53 (0)	NS
Terg et al. [143]	Ciprofloxacin 500 mg/day po	7/50 (14)	2/50 (4)	NS
Fernandez et al. [144]	Norfloxacin 400 mg/day po	10/33 (30)	2/35 (6)	0.02
Secondary prophylaxis				
Ginès et al. [136]	Norfloxacin 400 mg/day po	14/40 (35)	5/40 (12)	0.03

a Figures represent the number of patients developing spontaneous bacterial peritonitis during follow up compared with the total number of patients in each treatment group.
b Refers to antibiotic prophylaxis given to prevent the first episode of spontaneous bacterial peritonitis.
c Control group received norfloxacion 400 mg/day po.
d The control group received norfloxacin only during hospitalizations, po, per os (orally).

Acknowledgement

Some of studies reported in this chapter have been performed with the support of grants from the Fondo de Investigación Sanitaria- Ministerio de Ciencia e Innovación: Fondo de Instituto de Salud Carlos III, FIS08; PI080126.

References

1 Arroyo V, Ginès P, Planas R, Rodés J. Pathogenesis, diagnosis and treatment of ascites in cirrhosis. In: McIntyre N, Benhamou JP, Bircher J, Rizetto M, Rodés J, eds. *Oxford Textbook of Clinical Hepatology*, 2nd edn. Oxford University Press, Oxford, 1999: 697–732.

2 Cárdenas A, Ginès P. Mechanisms of ascites formation. In: Sanyal A, Shah V, eds. *Portal Hypertension*. Humana Press, New Jersey, 2005: 65–84.

3 Ginès P, Cárdenas A, Schrier R. Liver disease and the kidney. In: Schrier R, ed. *Diseases of the Kidney and Urinary Tract*, 8th edn. Lippincott Williams & Wilkins, Philadelphia, 2007: 2179–2205.

4 Tandon P, Garcia-Tsao G. Bacterial infections, sepsis, and multiorgan failure in cirrhosis. *Semin Liver Dis* 2008; **28**(1): 26–42.

5 Rimola A, García-Tsao G, Navasa M *et al*. Diagnosis, treatment and prophylaxis of spontaneous bacterial peritonitis: a consensus document. International Ascites Club. *J Hepatol* 2000; **32**(1): 142–153.

6 Cárdenas A, Ginès P, Arroyo V, Rodes J. Complications of cirrhosis: ascites, hyponatremia, hepatorenal syndrome, and spontaneous bacterial peritonitis. In: O'Grady J, Bacon B, eds. *Comprehensive Clinical Hepatology*, 2nd edn. Elsevier, Philadelphia, 2006: 153–168.

7 Schrier RW, Arroyo V, Bernardi M *et al*. Peripheral arterial vasodilation hypothesis: a proposal for the initiation of renal sodium and water retention in cirrhosis. *Hepatology* 1988; **8**: 1151–1157.

8 Iwakiri Y, Groszmann R. The hyperdynamic circulation of chronic liver diseases: from the patient to the molecule. *Hepatology* 2006; **43**: S121–131.

9 Farnsworth EB, Krakusin JS. Electrolyte partition in patients with edema of various origins. *J Lab Clin Med* 1948; **33**: 1545–1554.

10 Eisenmenger WJ, Blondheim SH, Bongiovanni AM, Kunkel HG. Electrolyte studies on patients with cirrhosis of the liver. *J Clin Invest* 1950; **29**: 1491–1499.

11 Reynolds TB, Lieberman FL, Goodman AR. Advantages of treatment of ascites without sodium restriction and without complete removal of excess fluid. *Gut* 1978; **19**: 549–553.

12 Gauthier A, Levy VG, Quinton A *et al*. Salt or no salt in the treatment of cirrhotic ascites: a randomized study. *Gut* 1986; **27**: 705–709.

13 Bernardi M, Laffi G, Salvagnini M *et al*. Efficacy and safety of the stepped care medical treatment of ascites in liver cirrhosis: a randomized controlled clinical trial comparing two diets with different sodium content. *Liver* 1993; **13**: 156–162.

14 Moore KP, Wong F, Gines P *et al*. The management of ascites in cirrhosis: report on the consensus conference of the International Ascites Club. *Hepatology* 2003; **1**(38): 258–266.

15 Moore KP, Aithal GP. Guidelines on the management of ascites in cirrhosis. *Gut* 2006; **55**(Suppl. 6): vi1–12.

16 Ginès P, Arroyo V, Quintero E *et al*. Comparison of paracentesis and diuretics in the treatment of cirrhotics with tense ascites. Results of a randomized study. *Gastroenterology* 1987; **93**: 234–241.

17 Salerno F, Badalamenti S, Incerti P *et al*. Repeated paracentesis and IV albumin infusion to treat "tense" ascites in cirrhotic patients: a safe alternative therapy. *J Hepatol* 1987; **5**: 102–108.

18 Hagège H, Ink O, Ducreux M *et al*. Traitement de l'ascite chez les malades atteints de cirrhose sans hyponatrémie ni insuffisance rénale. Résultats d'une étude randomisée comparant les diurétiques et les ponctions compensées par l'albumine. *Gastroenterol Clin Biol* 1992; **16**: 751–755.

19 Acharya SK, Balwinder S, Padhee AK *et al*. Large-volume paracentesis and intravenous dextran to treat tense ascites. *J Clin Gastroenterol* 1992; **14**: 31–35.

20 Solà R, Vila MC, Andreu M *et al*. Total paracentesis with dextran 40 vs diuretics in the treatment of ascites in cirrhosis: a randomized controlled study. *J Hepatol* 1994; **20**: 282–288.

21 Fernández-Esparrach G, Guevara M, Sort P *et al*. Diuretic requirements after therapeutic paracentesis in nonazotemic patients with cirrhosis. A randomized double-blind trial of spironolactone versus placebo. *J Hepatol* 1997; **26**: 614–620.

22 Runyon BA. Mangagement of patients with cirrhosis and ascites. *Hepatology* 2004; **39**(3): 841–856.

23 Ginès P, Titó Ll, Arroyo V *et al*. Randomized comparative study of therapeutic paracentesis with and without intravenous albumin in cirrhosis. *Gastroenterology* 1988; **94**: 1493–1502.

24 Pozzi M, Osculati G, Boari G *et al*. Time course of circulatory and humoral effects of rapid total paracentesis in cirrhotic patients with tense, refractory ascites. *Gastroenterology* 1994; **106**: 709–719.

25 Luca A, Garcia-Pagan JC, Bosch J *et al*. Beneficial effects of intravenous albumin infusion on the hemodynamic and humoral changes after total paracentesis. *Hepatology* 1995; **22**: 753–758.

26 Saló J, Ginès A, Ginès P *et al*. Effect of therapeutic paracentesis on plasma volume and transvascular escape rate of albumin in patients with cirrhosis. *J Hepatol* 1997; **27**: 645–653.

27 Ruiz del Arbol L, Monescillo A, Jiménez W *et al*. Paracentesis-induced circulatory dysfunction: mechanism and effect on hepatic hemodynamics in cirrhosis. *Gastroenterology* 1997; **113**: 579–586.

28 Vila MC, Solà R, Molina L *et al*. Hemodynamic changes in patients developing effective hypovolemia after total paracentesis. *J Hepatol* 1998; **28**: 639–645.

29 Ginès A, Fernández-Esparrach G, Monescillo A *et al*. Randomized trial comparing albumin, dextran-70 and polygelin in cirrhotic patients with ascites treated by paracentesis. *Gastroenterology* 1996; **111**: 1002–1010.

30 Planas R, Ginès P, Arroyo V *et al*. Dextran 70 vs albumin as plasma expanders in cirrhotic patients with tense ascites treated with total paracentesis. Results of a randomized study. *Gastroenterology* 1990; **99**: 1736–1744.

31 Salerno F, Badalamenti S, Lorenzano E *et al*. Randomized comparative study of Hemaccel vs albumin infusion after total paracentesis in cirrhotic patients with refractory ascites. *Hepatology* 1991; **13**: 707–713.

32 Fassio E, Terg R, Landeira G *et al*. Paracentesis with dextran 70 vs paracentesis with albumin in cirrhosis with tense ascites: results of a randomized study. *J Hepatol* 1992; **14**: 310–316.

33 Sola-Vera J, Miñana J, Ricart E *et al*. Randomized trial comparing albumin and saline in the prevention of paracentesis-induced circulatory dysfunction in cirrhotic patients with ascites. *Hepatology* 2003; **37**(5): 1147–1153.

34 Angeli P, Gatta A. Medical treatment of ascites in cirrhosis. In: Ginès P, Arroyo V, Rodes J, Schrier R, eds. *Ascites and Renal Dysfunction in Liver Disease*, 2nd edn. Blackwell Publishing, Oxford, 2005: 227–240.

35 Pérez-Ayuso RM, Arroyo V, Planas R *et al*. Randomized comparative study of efficacy of furosemide versus spironolactone in nonazotemic cirrhosis with ascites. Relationship between the diuretic response and the activity of the renin-aldosterone system. *Gastroenterology* 1983; **84**: 961–968.

36 Angeli P, Pria MD, De Bei E *et al*. Randomized clinical study of the efficacy of amiloride and potassium canreonate in nonazotemic cirrhotic patients with ascites. *Hepatology* 1994; **19**: 72–79.

37 Campra JL, Reynolds TB. Effectiveness of high-dose spironolactone therapy in patients with chronic liver disease and relatively refractory ascites. *Dig Dis Sci* 1978; **23**: 1025–1030.

38 Eggert RC. Spironolactone diuresis in patients with cirrhosis and ascites. *Br Med J* 1970; **4**: 401–403.

39 Strauss E, De SaMF, Lacet CM *et al*. Standardization of a therapeutic approach for ascites due to chronic liver disease. A prospective study of 100 patients. *Gastrointest Endosc Digest* 1985; **4**: 79–86.

40 Gatta A, Angeli P, Caregaro L *et al*. A pathophysiological interpretation of unresponsiveness to spironolactone in a stepped-care approach to the diuretic treatment of ascites in nonazotemic cirrhotic patients. *Hepatology* 1991; **14**: 231–236.

41 Santos J, Planas R, Pardo A *et al*. Spironolactone alone or in combination with furosemide in the treatment of moderate ascites in nonazotemic cirrhosis. A randomized comparative study of efficacy and safety. *J Hepatol* 2003; **39**: 187–192.

42 Arroyo V, Ginès P, Gerbes A *et al*. Definition and diagnostic criteria of refractory ascites and hepatorenal syndrome in cirrhosis. *Hepatology* 1996; **23**: 164–167.

43 Angeli P, Albino G, Carraro P *et al*. Cirrhosis and muscle cramps: evidence of a causal relationship. *Hepatology* 1996; **23**: 264–273.

44 Gregory PB, Broekelschen PH, Hill MD *et al.* Complications of diuresis in the alcoholic patient with ascites: a controlled trial. *Gastroenterology* 1977; **73**: 534–538.

45 Mimidis K, Papadopoulos V, Kartalis G. Eplerenone relieves spironolactone-induced painful gynaecomastia in patients with decompensated hepatitis B-related cirrhosis. *Scand J Gastroenterol* 2007; **42**(12): 1516–1517.

46 Lee FY, Lee SD, Tsai YT *et al.* A randomized controlled trial of quinidine in the treatment of cirrhotic patients with muscle cramps. *J Hepatol* 1991; **12**: 236–240.

47 Kugelmas M. Preliminary observation: oral zinc sulfate replacement is effective in treating muscle cramps in cirrhotic patients. *J Am Coll Nutr* 2000; **19**: 13–15.

48 Blendis LM, Greig PD, Langer B *et al.* Renal and hemodynamic effect of the peritoneovenous shunt for intractable hepatic ascites. *Gastroenterology* 1979; **77**: 250–257.

49 Greig PD, Blendis LM, Langer B *et al.* Renal and hemodynamic effect of the peritoneovenous shunt. II. Long-term effect. *Gastroenterology* 1981; **80**: 119–125.

50 Ginès P, Arroyo V, Vargas V *et al.* Paracentesis with intravenous infusion of albumin as compared with peritoneovenous shunting in cirrhosis with refractory ascites. *N Engl J Med* 1991; **325**: 829–835.

51 Ginès A, Planas R, Angeli P *et al.* Treatment of patients with cirrhosis and refractory ascites by LeVeen shunt with titanium tip. Comparison with therapeutic paracentesis. *Hepatology* 1995; **22**: 124–131.

52 Epstein M. Peritoneovenous shunt in the management of ascites and hepatorenal syndrome. In: Epstein M, ed. *The Kidney in Liver Disease*, 4th edn. Hanley and Belfus, Philadelphia, 1996.

53 Ring-Larsen H. Treatment of refractory ascites. In: Arroyo V, Ginès P, Rodés J, Schrier RW, eds. *Ascites and Renal Dysfunction in Liver Disease. Pathogenesis, Diagnosis and Treatment*. Blackwell Science, Malden, 1999.

54 LeVeen HH, Vujic I, D'Ovidio N *et al.* Peritoneovenous shunt occlusion. Etiology, diagnosis, therapy. *Ann Surg* 1984; **200**: 212–223.

55 Boyer TD. Transjugular intrahepatic portosystemic shunt in the management of complications of portal hypertension. *Curr Gastroenterol Rep* 2008; **10**(1): 30–35.

56 Ferral H, Bjarnason H, Wegryn SA *et al.* Refractory ascites: early experience in treatment with transjugular intrahepatic portosystemic shunt. *Radiology* 1993; **189**: 7905–7801.

57 Somberg KA, Lake JR, Tomlanovich SJ *et al.* Transjugular intrahepatic portosystemic shunt for refractory ascites: assessment of clinical and humoral response and renal function. *Hepatology* 1995; **21**: 709–716.

58 Quiroga J, Sangro B, Nunez M *et al.* Transjugular intrahepatic portal-systemic shunt in the management of refractory ascites: effect on clinical, renal, humoral and hemodynamic parameters. *Hepatology* 1995; **21**: 986–994.

59 Wong F, Sniderman K, Liu P *et al.* Transjugular intrahepatic portosystemic stent shunt: effects on hemodynamics and sodium homeostasis in cirrhosis and refractory ascites. *Ann Intern Med* 1995; **122**: 816–822.

60 Ochs A, Rossle M, Haag K *et al.* The transjugular intrahepatic portosystemic stent shunt procedure for refractory ascites. *N Engl J Med* 1995; **332**: 1192–1197.

61 Bureau C, García-Pagan JC, Otal P *et al.* Improved clinical outcome using polytetrafluoroethylene-coated stents for TIPS: results of a randomized study. *Gastroenterology* 2004; **126**: 469–475.

62 Sanyal AJ, Freedman AM, Shiffman ML *et al.* Porto systemic encephalopathy after transjugular intrahepatic portosystemic shunt: results of a prospective controlled study. *Hepatology* 1994; **20**: 46–55.

63 Casado M, Bosch J, Garcia-Pagan JC *et al.* Clinical events after transjugular, intrahepatic portosystemic shunt: correlation with hemodynamic findings. *Gastroenterology* 1998; **114**: 1296–1303.

64 Braverman AC, Steiner MA, Picus D *et al.* High-output congestive heart failure following transjugular intrahepatic portalsystemic shunting. *Chest* 1995; **107**: 1467–149.

65 Lebrec D, Giuily N, Hadengue A *et al.* Transjugular intrahepatic portosystemic shunts: comparison with paracentesis in patients with cirrhosis and refractory ascites: a randomized trial. *J Hepatol* 1996; **25**: 135–144.

66 Rössle M, Ochs A, Gulberg V *et al.* A comparison of paracentesis and transjugular intrahepatic portosystemic shunting in patients with ascites. *N Engl J Med* 2000; **342**: 1701–1707.

67 Ginès P, Uriz J, Calahorra B *et al.* Transjugular intrahepatic portosystemic shunting versus paracentesis plus albumin for refractory ascites in cirrhosis. *Gastroenterology* 2002; **123**: 1839–1847.

68 Sanyal AJ, Genning C, Reddy KR *et al.* The North American Study for the Treatment of Refractory Ascites. *Gastroenterology* 2003; **124**: 634–641.

69 Salerno F, Merli M, Riggio O *et al.* Randomized controlled study of TIPS versus paracentesis plus albumin in cirrhosis with severe ascites. *Hepatology* 2004; **40**: 629–635.

70 Saab S, Nieto JM, Lewis SK, Runyon BA. TIPS versus paracentesis for cirrhotic patients with refractory ascites. *Cochrane Database of Systematic Reviews* 2006, Issue 4. Art. No.: CD004889. DOI: 10.1002/14651858.CD004889.pub2.

71 Salerno F, Camma C, Enea M *et al.* Transjugular intrahepatic portosystemic shunt for refractory ascites: a meta-analysis of individual patient data. *Gastroenterology* 2007; **133**: 825–834.

72 Rimola A, Navasa M, Grande L, Garcia-Valdecaseas JC. Liver transplantation in cirrhotic patients with ascites. In: Ginès P, Arroyo V, Rodes J, Schrier R, eds. *Ascites and Renal Dysfunction in Liver Disease*, 2nd edn. Blackwell Publishing, Oxford, 2005: 271–285.

73 Ginès A, Escorsell A, Ginès P *et al.* Incidence, predictive factors, and prognosis of the hepatorenal syndrome in cirrhosis with ascites. *Gastroenterology* 1993; **105**: 229–236.

74 Guevara M, Cárdenas A, Uriz J, Ginès P. Prognosis of patients with ascites and cirrhosis. In: Ginès P, Arroyo V, Rodes J, Schrier R, eds. *Ascites and Renal Dysfunction in Liver Disease*, 2nd edn. Blackwell Publishing, Oxford, 2005: 260–270.

75 Kamath P, Wiesner R, Malinchoc M *et al.* A model to predict survival in patients with end-stage liver disease. *Hepatology* 2001; **33**: 464–470.

76 Biggins SW, Kim WR, Terrault NA *et al.* Evidence-based incorporation of serum sodium concentration into MELD. *Gastroenterology* 2006; **130**: 1652–1660.

77 Kim WR, Biggins SW, Kremers WK *et al.* Hyponatremia and mortality among patients on the liver-transplant waiting list. *N Engl J Med* 2008; **359**(10): 1018–1026.

78 Salerno F, Gerbes A, Wong F *et al.* Diagnosis, prevention and treatment of the hepatorenal syndrome in cirrhosis. A consensus workshop of the international ascites club. *Gut* 2007; **56**: 1310–1318.

79 Fasolato S, Angeli P, Dallagnese L *et al.* Renal failure and bacterial infections in patients with cirrhosis: epidemiology and clinical features. *Hepatology* 2007; **45**: 223–229.

80 Guevara M, Ginès P, Fernández-Esparrach G *et al.* Reversibility of hepatorenal syndrome by prolonged administration of ornipressin and plasma volume expansion. *Hepatology* 1998; **27**: 35–41.

81 Gullberg V, Bilzer M, Gerbes AL. Long-term therapy and retreatment of hepatorenal syndrome type 1 with ornipressin and dopamine. *Hepatology* 1999; **30**: 870–875.

82 Hadengue A, Gadano A, Moreau R *et al.* Beneficial effects of the 2-day administration of terlipressin in patients with cirrhosis and hepatorenal syndrome. *J Hepatol* 1998; **29**: 565–570.

83 Ganne-Carrié N, Hadengue A, Mathurin P *et al.* Hepatorenal syndrome. Long-term treatment with terlipressin as a bridge to liver transplantation. *Dig Dis Sci* 1996; **41**: 1054–1056.

84 Uriz J, Ginès P, Cardenas A *et al.* Terlipressin plus albumin infusion is an effective and safe therapy of hepatorenal syndrome. *J Hepatol* 2000; **33**: 43–48.

85 Moreau R, Durand F, Poynard T *et al.* Terlipressin in patients with cirrhosis and type 1 hepatorenal syndrome: a restrospective multicenter study. *Gastroenterology* 2002; **122**: 923–930.

86 Ortega R, Ginès P, Uriz J *et al.* Terlipressin therapy with and without albumin for patients with hepatorenal syndrome. Results of a prospective, non-randomized study. *Hepatology* 2002; **36**: 941–948.

87 Halimi C, Bonnard P, Bernard B *et al.* Effect of terlipressin (Glypressin) on hepatorenal syndrome in cirrhotic patients: results of a multicentre pilot study. *Eur J Gastroenterol Hepatol* 2002; **14**: 153–158.

88 Colle I, Durand F, Pessione F *et al.* Clinical course, predictive factors and prognosis in patients with cirrosis and type 1 hepatorenal syndrome treated with terlipressin: a retrospective analysis. *J Gastroenterol Hepatol* 2002; **17**: 882–888.

89 Duvoux C, Zanditenas D, Hezode C *et al.* Effects of noradrenalin and albumin in patients with type I hepatorenal syndrome: a pilot study. *Hepatology* 2002; **36**: 374–380.

90 Angeli P, Volpin R, Gerunda G *et al.* Reversal of type 1 hepatorenal syndrome with the administration of midodrine and octreotide. *Hepatology* 1999; **29**: 1690–1697.

91 Wong F, Pantea L, Sniderman K. Midodrine, octreotide, albumin, and TIPS in selected patients with cirrhosis and type 1 hepatorenal syndrome. *Hepatology* 2004; **40**: 55–64.

92 Alessandria C, Ottobrelli A, Debernardi-Venon W *et al.* Noradrenalin vs terlipressin in patients with hepatorenal syndrome: a prospective, randomized, unblinded, pilot study. *J Hepatol* 2007; **47**: 499–505.

93 Sanyal A, Boyer T, Garcia-Tsao G *et al.* A prospective, randomized, double-blind, placebo-controlled trial of terlipressin for type 1 hepatorenal syndrome (HRS). *Gastroenterology* 2008; **134**: 1360–1368.

94 Martín-Llahí M, Pépin MN, Guevara M *et al.* Randomized comparative study of terlipressin and albumin vs albumin alone in patients with cirrhosis and hepatorenal syndrome. *Gastroenterology* 2008; **134**: 1352–1359.

95 Solanki P, Chawla A, Garg R *et al.* Beneficial effects of terlipressin in hepatorenal syndrome: a prospective, randomized placebo-controlled clinical trial. *J Gastroenterol Hepatol* 2003; **18**: 152–156.

96 Neri S, Pulvirenti D, Malaguarnera M *et al.* Terlipressin and albumin in patients with cirrhosis and type I hepatorenal syndrome. *Dig Dis Sci* 2008; **53**: 830–835.

97 Guevara M, Ginès P, Bandi JC *et al.* Transjugular intrahepatic portosystemic shunt in hepatorenal syndrome: effects on renal function and vasoactive systems. *Hepatology* 1998; **28**: 416–422.

98 Brensing KA, Textor J, Perz J *et al.* Long-term outcome after transjugular intrahepatic portosystemic stent-shunt in non-transplant patients with hepatorenal syndrome: a phase II study. *Gut* 2000; **47**: 288–295.

99 Wong LP, Blackley MP, Andreoni KA *et al.* Survival of liver transplant candidates with acute renal failure receiving renal replacement therapy. *Kidney Intern* 2005; **68**: 362–370.

100 Mitzner SR, Stange J, Klammt S *et al.* Improvement of hepatorenal syndrome with extracorporeal albumin dialysis MARS: results of a prospective, randomized controlled clinical trial. *Liver Transpl* 2000; **6**: 277–286.

101 Wadei HM, Mai ML, Ahsan N, Gonwa TA. Hepatorenal syndrome: pathophysiology and management. *Clin J Am Soc Nephrol* 2006; **1**(5): 1066–1079.

102 Wiesner R, Edwards E, Freeman R *et al.* Model for end-stage liver disease (MELD) and allocation of donor livers. *Gastroenterology* 2003; **124**: 91–96.

103 Gonwa TA, Morris CA, Goldstein RM *et al.* Long-term survival and renal function following liver transplantation in patients with and without hepatorenal syndrome – experience in 300 patients. *Transplantation* 1991; **51**: 428–430.

104 Nair S, Verma S, Thuluvath PJ. Pretransplant renal function predicts survival in patients undergoing orthotopic liver transplantation. *Hepatology* 2002; **35**: 1179–1185.

105 Restuccia T, Guevara M, Ginès P *et al.* Impact of pretransplant treatment of hepatorenal syndrome (hrs) with vasopressin analogues on outcome after liver transplantation (ltx). A case-control study. *J Hepatol* 2004; **40**: 140–146.

106 Ginès P, Berl T, Bernardi M *et al.* Hyponatremia in cirrhosis: from pathogenesis to treatment. *Hepatology* 1998; **28**: 851–864.

107 Schrier RW. Water and sodium retention in edematous disorders: role of vasopressin and aldosterone. *Am J Med* 2006; **119**(7 Suppl. 1): S47–53.

108 Gines P, Guevara M. Hyponatremia in cirrhosis: pathogenesis, clinical significance, and management. *Hepatology* 2008; **48**(3): 1002–1010.

109 McCormick PA, Mistry P, Kaye G *et al.* Intravenous albumin infusion is an effective therapy for hyponatraemia in cirrhotic patients with ascites. *Gut* 1990; **31**: 204–207.

110 Decaux G, Soupart A, Vassart G. Non-peptide arginine-vasopressin antagonists: the vaptans. *Lancet* 2008; **371**(9624): 1624–1632.

111 Wong F, Blei AT, Blendis LM, Thuluvath PJ. A vasopressin receptor antagonist (VPA-985) improves serum sodium concentration in patients with hyponatremia: a multicenter, randomized, placebo-controlled trial. *Hepatology* 2003; **37**: 182–191.

112 Gerbes A, Gülberg V, Ginès P *et al.* The VPA Study Group. Therapy of hyponatremia in cirrhosis with a vasopressin recep-

tor antagonist: a randomized double-blind multicenter trial. *Gastroenterology* 2003; **124**: 933–939.

113 Schrier RW, Gross P, Gheorghiade M *et al.* Tolvaptan, a selective oral vasopressin V2-receptor antagonist, for hyponatremia. *N Engl J Med* 2006; **355**: 2099–2112.

114 Ginès P, Wong F, Watson H *et al.* Effects of satavaptan, a selective vasopressin V(2) receptor antagonist, on ascites and serum sodium in cirrhosis with hyponatremia: a randomized trial. *Hepatology* 2008; **48**(1): 204–213.

115 Fernández J, Navasa M, Gómez J *et al.* Bacterial infections in cirrhosis: epidemiological changes with invasive procedures and norfloxacin prophylaxis. *Hepatology* 2002; **35**: 140–148.

116 Campillo B, Richardet JP, Kheo T, Dupeyron C. Nosocomial spontaneous bacterial peritonitis and bacteremia in cirrhotic patients: impact of isolate type on prognosis and characteristics of infection. *Clin Infect Dis* 2002; **35**: 1–10.

117 Bert F, Andreu M, Durand F *et al.* Nosocomial and community-acquired spontaneous bacterial peritonitis: comparative microbiology and therapeutic implications. *Eur J Clin Microbiol Infect Dis* 2003; **22**: 10–15.

118 Evans LT, Kim WR, Poterucha JJ, Kamath PS. Spontaneous bacterial peritonitis in asymptomatic outpatients with cirrhotic ascites. *Hepatology* 2003; **37**: 745–747.

119 Castellvi JM, Guardiola J, Sesé E *et al.* Spontaneous bacterial empyema of cirrhotic patients: a prospective study. *Hepatology* 1996; **23**: 719–724.

120 Felisart J, Rimola A, Arroyo V *et al.* Cefotaxime is more effective than is ampicillin-tobramycin in cirrhotics with severe infections. *Hepatology* 1985; **5**: 457–462.

121 Toledo C, Salmerón JM, Rimola A *et al.* Spontaneous bacterial peritonitis in cirrhosis: predictive factors of infection resolution and survival in patients treated with cefotaxime. *Hepatology* 1993; **17**: 251–257.

122 Rimola A, Salmerón JM, Clemente G *et al.* Two different dosages of cefotaxime in the treatment of spontaneous bacterial peritonitis in cirrhosis: results of a prospective, randomized, multicenter study. *Hepatology* 1995; **21**: 674–679.

123 Runyon BA, McHutchinson JG, Antillon MR. Short-course versus long-course antibiotic treatment of spontaneous bacterial peritonitis: a randomized, controlled study of 100 patients. *Gastroenterology* 1991; **100**: 1737–1742.

124 Gómez-Jimènez J, Ribera E, Gasser I *et al.* Randomized trial comparing ceftriaxone with cefonicid for treatment of spontaneous bacterial peritonitis in cirrhotic patients. *Antimicrob Agents Chemother* 1993; **37**: 1587–1592.

125 Ariza J, Xiol X, Esteve M *et al.* Aztreonam vs Cefotaxime in the treatment of Gram-negative spontaneous peritonitis in cirrhotic patients. *Hepatology* 1991; **14**: 91–98.

126 Ricart E, Soriano G, Novella MT *et al.* Amoxicillinclavulanic acid versus cefotaxime in the therapy of bacterial infections in cirrhotic patients. *J Hepatol* 2000; **32**: 596–602.

127 Navasa M, Follo A, Llovet JM *et al.* Randomized, comparative study of oral ofloxacin versus intravenous cefotaxime in spontaneous bacterial peritonitis. *Gastroenterology* 1996; **111**: 1011–1017.

128 Sort P, Navasa M, Arroyo V *et al.* Effect of intravenous albumin on renal impairment and mortality in patients with cirrhosis and spontaneous bacterial peritonitis. *N Engl J Med* 1999; **341**: 403–409.

129 Rimola A, Bory F, Terés J *et al.* Oral non-absorbable antibiotics prevent infection in cirrhosis with gastrointestinal hemorrhage. *Hepatology* 1985; **5**: 463–467.

130 Soriano G, Guarner C, Tomás A *et al.* Norfloxacin prevents bacterial infection in cirrhotics with gastrointestinal hemorrhage. *Gastroenterology* 1992; **103**: 1267–1272.

131 Blaise M, Pateron D, Trinchet JC *et al.* Systemic antibiotic therapy prevents bacterial infections in cirrhotic patients with gastrointestinal hemorrhage. *Hepatology* 1994; **20**: 34–38.

132 Pauwels A, Mostefa-Kara N, Debenes B *et al.* Systemic antibiotic prophylaxis after gastrointestinal hemorrhage in cirrhotic patients with a high risk of infection. *Hepatology* 1996; **24**: 802–806.

133 Fernández J, Ruiz del Arbol L, Gomez C *et al.* Norfloxacin versus ceftriaxone in the prophylaxis of infections in patients with advanced cirrhosis and hemorrhage. *Gastroenterology* 2006; **131**: 1049–1056

134 Bernard B, Grangé JD, Khac NE *et al.* Antibiotic prophylaxis for the prevention of bacterial infections in cirrhotic patients with gastrointestinal bleeding: a meta-analysis. *Hepatology* 1999; **29**: 1655–1661.

135 Soares-Weiser K, Brezis M, Tur-Kaspa R, Leibovici L. Antibiotic prophylaxis for cirrhotic patients with gastrointestinal bleeding. *Cochrane Database of Systematic Reviews* 2002, Issue 2. Art. No.: CD002907. DOI: 10.1002/14651858.CD002907.

136 Ginès P, Rimola A, Planas R *et al.* Norfloxacin prevents spontaneous bacterial peritonitis recurrence in cirrhosis: results of a double blind, placebo-controlled trial. *Hepatology* 1990; **12**: 716–724.

137 Bauer TM, Follo A, Navasa M *et al.* Daily norfloxacin is more effective than weekly rufloxacin in prevention of spontaneous bacterial peritonitis recurrence. *Dig Dis Sci* 2002; **47**: 1356–1361.

138 Soriano G, Guarner C, Teixidó M *et al.* Selective intestinal decontamination prevents spontaneous bacterial peritonitis. *Gastroenterology* 1991; **100**: 77–81.

139 Rolanchon A, Cordier L, Bacq Y *et al.* Ciprofloxacin and long-term prevention of spontaneous bacterial peritonitis: results of a prospective controlled trial. *Hepatology* 1995; **22**: 1171–1174.

140 Singh N, Gayowski T, Yu VL *et al.* Trimethoprimsulfamethoxazole for the prevention of spontaneous bacterial peritonitis in cirrhosis: a randomized trial. *Ann Intern Med* 1995; **122**: 595–598.

141 Novella M, Sold R, Soriano G *et al.* Continuous versus inpatient prophylaxis of the first spontaneous bacterial peritonitis with norfloxacin. *Hepatology* 1997; **25**: 532–536.

142 Grange JD, Roulot D, Pelletier G *et al.* Norfloxacin primary prophylaxis of bacterial infections in cirrhotic patients with ascites: a double-blind randomized trial. *J Hepatol* 1998; **29**: 430–436.

143 Terg R, Fassio E, Guevara M. Ciprofloxacin in primary prophylaxis of spontaneous bacterial peritonitis: a randomized, placebo-controlled study. *J Hepatol* 2008; **48**: 774–779.

144 Fernández J, Navasa M, Planas R *et al.* Primary prophylaxis of spontaneous bacterial peritonitis delays hepatorenal syndrome and improves survival in cirrhosis. *Gastroenterology* 2007; **133**: 818–824.

39 Hepatic encephalopathy: Treatment

Peter Ferenci and Christian Müller

Division of Gastroenterology and Hepatology, Medical University Vienna, Vienna, Austria

Because the pathogenesis of hepatic encephalopathy (HE) is unknown, no truly "specific" treatment exists [1]. Nevertheless, a variety of compounds have been introduced for treatment of HE (see Table 39.1). Some of these treatments are based on clinical observations, some on extrapolation of experimental data obtained in animal models of HE. Research on hepatic encephalopathy is hampered by the imprecise definition of this disabling complication of liver disease. In view of this, the Organisation Mondiale de Gastroentérologie (OMGE) commissioned a working party to reach a consensus in this area and to present it at the Eleventh World Congress of Gastroenterology in Vienna (1998). The working party continued its work thereafter and published their final report.

In summary, the working party has suggested a modification of current nomenclature for clinical diagnosis of hepatic encephalopathy (see Table 39.2), proposed guidelines for the performance of future clinical trials in hepatic encephalopathy, and felt the need for a large study to redefine neuropsychiatric abnormalities in liver disease, which would allow the diagnosis of minimal (= subclinical) encephalopathy to be made on firm statistical grounds [2]. These new definitions will be the basis to improve the design of clinical studies but cannot be applied to already published trials. Nevertheless, the new nomenclature was used in this analysis.

Design of clinical trials in hepatic encephalopathy

A large spectrum of clinical conditions is summarized under the term "HE" and includes a variety of neuropsychiatric symptoms, ranging from minor, not readily discernible signs of altered brain function, overt psychiatric and/or neurological symptoms, to deep coma. Accordingly, the methods to quantify treatment effects and treatment endpoints are highly variable. Another variable is the treatment of control groups. Most studies compare a new drug to "standard treatment" (which by itself may be highly effective) such as oral lactulose, for which efficacy has not been demonstrated in a randomized placebo controlled trial for ethical reasons. However, in view of the natural history of HE, the inclusion of a placebo group in trials of new agents is highly desirable. In studies comparing a new drug with effective "standard treatment" demonstration of effectiveness of the new drug will require a very large sample size. Table 39.3 summarizes the appropriate study endpoints in various patient groups.

Natural history of HE

The natural history of HE is not well studied. However, examination of the outcomes in the placebo treatment groups in nine randomized controlled trials (see Table 39.4) reveals that patients with grade III and IV HE may have recovery rates from 22% to greater than 90%. Therefore, in studies of new agents which lack controls, high response rates may be anticipated, and trials of new agents may require quite large numbers of patients to demonstrate benefits. In the short term mortality of patients with HE appears to be low if unstable patients are excluded. The course of patients with subclinical HE is unknown, and it is by definition impossible to detect clinical improvement in such cases. Studies of new agents with subclinical illness should focus on progression to more severe levels of HE. The grade of encephalopathy of patients selected for clinical trials may be expected to have a substantial influence on results.

Evidence-Based Gastroenterology and Hepatology, 3rd edition.
J. McDonald, A.K. Burroughs, B. Feagan, and M.B. Fennerty. © 2010
Blackwell Publishing Ltd

Table 39.1 Treatments for hepatic encephalopathy.

	Controlled studies	
	vs lactulose	vs placebo
Decrease of ammoniagenic substrates		
Enemas with lactulose		+
Reduction of dietary protein		?
Inhibition of ammonia production		
Antibiotics		
Neomycin	=	=
Rifaximin	+	nd
Vancomycin	= / +	nd
Disaccharides		
Lactulose		? =
Lactitol	=	nd
Lactose in lactase deficiency		+
Modification of colonic flora		
Lactobacillus SF 68	=	nd
Metabolic ammonia removal		
Ornithine aspartate iv		+
Benzoate	=	nd
L-Carnitin		+
BCAA supplementation		
Modified AA solutions ("FO80" type)	=	±
Dietary BCAA supplementation		+
Neuroactive drugs		
Flumazenil iv		+
L-Dopa, bromocriptine		=

+ Superior to control treatment; = equal to control treatment; ± conflicting results; nd: not done.

Table 39.2 Proposed nomenclature of hepatic encephalopathy [2].

HE type	Nomenclature	subcategory	subdivisions
A	Encephalopathy associated with **a**cute liver failure		
B	Encephalopathy associated with portal-systemic **b**ypass and no intrinsic hepatocellular disease.		
C	Encephalopathy associated with **c**irrhosis and portal hypertension/or portal-systemic shunts	Episodic hepatic encephalopathy	precipitated
			spontaneous[a]
		Persistent hepatic encephalopathy	recurrent mild
			severe treatment-dependent
		Minimal hepatic encephalopathy	

[a] Without recognized precipitating factors.

Methods to quantify

Clinical assessment

The simplest assessment of HE is a description of the mental state, according to Conn [12], which grades HE in stages I–IV based on changes in consciousness, intellectual function and behavior. It does not include neurological changes or asterixis. The Glasgow Coma scale is useful in stages III and IV.

The PSE (portal–systemic encephalopathy) index

In 1977 the "PSE index" was introduced in a trial comparing neomycin with lactulose and has been subsequently used by other investigators [13]. The main problem with this index is the inclusion of arterial ammonia estimations. Hyperammonemia is possibly a cause, but not a symptom or effect of HE. Measurements of arterial ammonia concentrations require serial arterial punctures. The scoring of actual arterial ammonia concentrations is arbitrary and not based on a sound statistical analysis. Furthermore, the other parameters of the PSE index – mental state, EEG and number connection tests (NCT) – are also graded by arbitrary units. No age-dependent normal values are used for NCT [14]. Finally, the PSE index does not discriminate between overt, mild or subclinical HE and has not been validated prospectively. In clinically overt HE the PSE index does not appear to be superior to simple clinical grading.

Psychometric tests

Grading of HE does not allow the documentation of subtle changes. To quantify the impairment of mental function in mild stages of HE several psychometric tests have been evaluated [15, 16, 17]. Detailed psychometric testing is more sensitive in the detection of minor deficits of mental

Table 39.3 Methods to assess treatment in various groups of patients with hepatic encephalopathy.

Study group	Treatment endpoint	Assessment of treatment effects	Natural history	Problems
Episodic HE, type C	Clinical improvement	Clinical grading, EEG, SEP	Well documented	High mortality, precipitating factors
Persistent HE, type C	Clinical improvement	Clinical grading, PSE index[a]	Well documented	
Episodic HE, type C, recurrent	Recurrence	PSE index, MDF	Variable	Compliance
TIPS or portocaval shunts (surgical)	Prevention of HE	Psychometry, MDF, PSE index[a]	Well documented	
minimal HE	Psychometry EEG	Psychometry, MDF, P300	Unknown	Clinical meaning of certain tests

[a] PSE index according to Conn *et al.* [2] (the use of this index was not recommended by the WCOG-Working party 1a).
SEP: somatosensory evoked potentials; MDF: mean dominant frequency; P300: event related acoustic evoked responses.

Table 39.4 Survival rates and improvement of hepatic encephalopathy in placebo treated patients in randomized controlled trials.

Study	Test drug	HE grade	No. of patients	Observation time	Exclusion criteria	Survival % (on placebo)	HE better % (on placebo)
Barbaro [3]	Flumazenil	III	265	6 days	HR, RF,	97.3	>90
		IV	262		acidosis	91.3	>90
Kircheis [4]	Ornithine-aspartate	MHE	27	7 days	GI bleed,	100	0
		I	19		HR, RF	100	22
		II	27			100	44
Stauch [5]	Ornithine-asparate	MHE I + II	20	14 days	Unstable patients	100	0
						100	40
Marchesini [6]	BCAA oral	I	34	3 mth	Unstable patients	100	38
Michel [7]	L-Dopa	I–III	38	7 days	None	61	37
Michel [8]	BCAA iv	I–III	24	5 days	Unstable patients	74	26
Wahren [9]	BCAA iv	II–IV	25	5 days	None	80	48
Blanc [10]	Neomycin + lactulose	II–IV	40	5 days	?	85	70
Strauss [11]	Neomycin	II–IV	19	5 days	MOF	89.5	89.5

[a] All patients were on neomycin.
HR, hepatorenal syndrome; RF, respiratory failure; MOF, multiorgan failure; BCAA, branched chain amino acids; MHE, minimal hepatic encephalopathy.

function than either conventional clinical assessment or the EEG [16]. However, the tests are cumbersome, and when applied repeatedly the reliability of most of them is adversely affected by the learning effect. Few are useful in routine practice. The most frequently applied test is the number connection test [14, 16]. This test is easily administered and the results can be quickly quantified. One important consequence of the application of psychometric tests in cirrhotic patients was the finding that even patients with apparently normal mental status have a measurable deficit in their intellectual performance [13]. These patients are usually referred to as suffering from "minimal HE" or "stage 0 HE". However, psychometric tests may overdiagnose minimal HE, because scores are usually not corrected for age [14, 18]. Furthermore, it is unknown whether abnormalities of test results correlate with impaired quality of life or performance in daily life [18]. On the contrary, the driving ability of patients with test results classifying them as "unable to drive a car" [15] was not different from that of healthy controls. A quality-of-life questionnaire (sickness impact profile (SIP)) detects the extent and frequency of deficits in daily functioning in patients without clinically apparent HE. From the 136 statements, five were selected as predictive of minimal HE [18].

A standardized prospectively developed test battery that includes the NCT A and B, the line tracing test, the serial dotting test and the digit symbol test was recommended by the working party to be used in future studies [2]. This test (PHES) can be applied at the bedside and performed within 10–20 minutes and examines visual perception, visuo-spatial orientation, visual construction, motor speed and accuracy, and is also sensitive against disturbances of concentration, attention and working memory. Each individual test and the whole battery has been standardized in a large group of healthy controls (including all ages). A composite score of the single test results was calculated. Each of the individual test results was scored 0 points in the ± 1 SD range from the mean. Thereby, subjects can achieve between +6 and −18 points. When a cutoff between normal and pathological results was set at −4 points, only 1 (0.9%) of the controls, 25% of cirrhotic patients without clinical evidence of HE, but all patients with grade I HE achieved pathological results. **B2** The test has a high specificity for HE as compared with other metabolic encephalopathies [19, 20].

Electrophysiological tests

The simplest EEG assessment of HE is to grade the degree of abnormality of the conventional EEG trace. A more refined assessment by computer assisted techniques allows variables in the EEG such as the mean dominant EEG frequency and the power of a particular EEG rhythm to be quantified. Evoked responses (by visual, somatosensory, or acoustic stimuli) or event related responses, like the P300 peak after auditory stimuli, are sensitive to detect subtle changes of brain function and can be used for diagnosis of minimal HE [20].

Critical flicker frequency

Retinal glial cells are involved in ammonia detoxification by glutamine synthesis. In patients with liver failure, they exhibit morphological changes similar to those observed in brain astrocytes, suggesting that retinal gliopathy could serve as a marker of cerebral gliopathy in patients with hepatic encephalopathy. These observations provided the rationale for the development of a visual test (the critical flicker/fusion frequency) for determining whether hepatic encephalopathy is present. Initial experience suggests that the critical flicker/fusion frequency may be a highly objective and sensitive measure of minimal hepatic encephalopathy [21, 22, 23].

Diagnosis of minimal hepatic encephalopathy

One important consequence of the application of psychometric tests in patients with cirrhosis was the finding that even patients with apparently normal mental status have some form of a measurable deficit in their intellectual performance, long-term memory, and learning capability [15, 24]. These patients are usually referred to as "minimal HE" or "stage 0 HE". Up to 15% of patients with cirrhosis have minimal HE when defined by the presence of a prolonged NCT or an abnormal EEG [25]. Several approaches are being studied to evaluate for minimal hepatic encephalopathy. At present, none is used routinely in clinical practice.

One study comparing the Psychometric Hepatic Encephalopathy Score (PHES) with an EEG in 100 patients with cirrhosis found agreement in detection of MHE in only 73% [26]. The poor correlation may reflect differences in how these tests detect various features of MHE.

The Inhibitory Control Test (ICT) is a computerized test of attention and response inhibition that has been used to characterize attention deficit disorder, schizophrenia and traumatic brain injury. The subject is instructed only to respond to two alternating letters (X/Y) (called "targets") and not to respond when they are not alternating (called "lures"). Lower lure responses, higher target responses, and shorter lure and target reaction times indicate good psychometric performance. A study comparing ICT to a psychometric battery of tests for MHE diagnosis in 136 patients estimated sensitivity for MHE to be 88% [27]. Patients with MHE had significantly higher ICT lures and lower targets compared to patients without MHE.

The PHES was compared with a comprehensive computerized assessment (Cognitive Drug Research [CDR]) of cognitive function in 89 patients with cirrhosis [28]. There was a high correlation between the two assessment methods. The MELD score correlated with PHES. In contrast, the CDR domains Continuity of Attention and Quality of Episodic Memory were significantly related to venous blood ammonia levels. There were marked deteriorations in the CDR composite scores representing Accuracy of Working and Episodic Memory after amino acid challenge to increase blood ammonia. Both PHES and CDRS returned to the control range after liver transplantation.

The Repeatable Battery for the Assessment of Neuropsychological Status (RBANS) measures a wide range of neurocognitive functions relevant to MHE. The test has been used in multiple clinical trials in the USA for a variety of neurologic disorders and in patients with advanced cirrhosis [29]. The RBANS has not yet been compared directly with the PHES, and its responsiveness to hepatic encephalopathy treatment is unknown.

A concern in patients with minimal hepatic encephalopathy is whether they are at increased risk for driving accidents. Studies evaluating this question have produced disparate conclusions. At least three reports concluded that 44–60% of patients with advanced liver disease (but without overt clinical signs of HE) were unfit to drive based upon the results of extensive batteries of neuropsychologic tests

[1, 21, 22]. In one study, for example, 40 patients with chronic liver disease and portal hypertension without clinical signs of portasystemic encephalopathy were given the same extensive psychometric tests typically used for expert reports on driving capacity [15]. Sixty percent of patients were considered to be unfit to drive, and 25% were considered to be questionable. The total driving score of patients with minimal hepatic encephalopathy was significantly reduced compared with controls or cirrhotic patients without minimal hepatic encephalopathy [30]. A later report found that patients with minimal hepatic encephalopathy had poor insight into their driving skills [31].

Evidence-based medicine and hepatic encephalopathy

Evidence based medicine is a process of systematically finding, appraising, and using research findings as the basis for clinical decisions [32] based on the formulation of relevant questions concerning a patient's problem.

The answer to the question "Does treatment with specific drugs, compared to placebo, improve HE?" should be addressed separately for overt and subclinical HE. In the following sections we have identified the studies that attempt to answer this question and we have critically appraised the evidence for the most important treatment regimens. The magnitude of the treatment effect of various interventions has been assessed. This assessment is difficult in HE because of the use of different methods which are not readily comparable for quantifying the severity of this disease. The question of the clinical applicability and generalizability of the findings of randomized controlled studies in HE must be addressed in the context of the treatment and the grade of encephalopathy studied.

To identify all randomized controlled trials in HE, a Medline search was conducted using several terms. A total of 50 randomized trials had the endpoint "improvement of HE" and included more than ten patients per study group (see Table 39.5). In addition, two meta-analyses have been published [33, 34].

Treatment of hepatic encephalopathy

Clinically overt he (grade I–IV) in patients with cirrhosis

Supportive care and treatment of precipitating causes of HE

It is important to recognize that HE, acute and chronic, is reversible and that a precipitating cause rather than worsening of hepatocellular function can be identified in the majority of patients [1, 2]. These causes include gastrointestinal bleeding, increased protein intake, hypokalemic alkalosis, infection, and constipation (all of which increase arterial ammonia levels), hypoxia, and the use of sedatives and tranquilizers. Patients with advanced cirrhosis may be particularly sensitive to benzodiazepines.

Treatment of these precipitating events is typically associated with a prompt and permanent improvement of HE. As a result, every attempt should be made to identify and to treat such precipitating events. This approach has never been tested formally but is based on common clinical experience. As judged from the outcomes observed in placebo groups of controlled studies (see Table 39.3) standard medical care is highly effective.

Enemas

Cleansing of the colon by enemas is a rapid and effective procedure to remove ammoniagenic substrates. The efficacy of enemas of 1–3 liters of 20% lactulose or lactitol solutions was proven in randomized controlled trials; a favorable response was noted in 78–86% of patients (ARR 0.4%, NNT = 2.5) [35, 36]. **A1d** Interestingly, enemas with tap water were ineffective, raising the possibility that colonic acidification rather than bowel cleansing was the effective therapeutic mechanism.

Nutrition

Patients with grade III–IV HE usually do not receive oral nutrition. In general, there is no need for parenteral nutrition if patients improve within two days.

Based on the "false neurotransmitter hypothesis", total parenteral nutrition with specific amino acid solutions has been proposed. A number of randomized controlled studies have evaluated the use of solutions with a high content of branched chain amino acids (BCAA) and a low content of aromatic amino acids (AAA). These studies differ with respect to the amino acid solutions used, the study protocols, patient selection and the duration of treatment, and are difficult to compare. The results have been conflicting, but most studies did not find any improvement in HE or any reduction in mortality in patients treated with BCAA [37, 38]. Although a meta-analysis revealed a significant trend toward improvement in these outcomes, it was concluded that further randomized controlled trials are needed [34]. At present, infusions of modified amino acid solutions should not be used in the standard treatment of patients with HE. **A1c**

There is no proven need for a specific diet for patients with HE. Although mentioned in all textbooks, the recommendation of a low protein diet in patients with advanced liver disease is not supported by good clinical or experimental evidence. On the contrary, in patients with alcoholic hepatitis, low protein intake is associated with worsening HE, while a higher protein intake correlates with improvement in HE [39]. The recommendations of the

Table 39.5 Randomized trials with endpoint "improvement of HE".

Test drug	Control				Total
	Placebo	**Standard therapy**[a]	**Lactulose/lactitol**	**Neomycin**	
Flumazenil	7	—	—	—	7
BCAA IV	4	2	—	—	6
BCAA oral	2	—	—	—	2
Lactulose	5	1	—	3	9
Lactitol	—	—	—	3	3
Neomycin	1	—	—	—	1
Lactulose + neomycin	1	—	—	—	1
Lactulose/lactose enemas	1	—	—	1	2
LOLA	2	—	1		3
Zinc	—	2	—		2
Benzoate	—	—	1		1
L-Dopa	1	—	—		1
Rifaximine	—	—	2	2	4 + 1 dose finding study
SF-68	—	—	1	—	1
Acarbose	1	—	—	—	1
L-Carnitin	1	1	1		3
Probiotics	1	1	—		2
Total	27	7	6	9	49 + 1

[a] Usually includes lactulose or neomycin.

European Society of Parenteral and Enteral Nutrition (ESPEN) are that oral protein intake should not exceed 70 g/day in a patient with a history of HE; a level below 70 g/day is rarely necessary and minimum intake should not be lower than 40 g/day to avoid negative nitrogen balance [40]. **C5**

Pharmacotherapy

Flumazenil

Based upon the GABA-benzodiazepine hypothesis of the pathogenesis of HE, the benzodiazepine receptor antagonist flumazenil has been tested for treatment of HE in five randomized placebo controlled trials involving over 600 patients. Four were crossover trials, and one used a parallel group design. Flumazenil was superior to placebo in four of these studies (Table 39.5). In the only large double-blind, placebo controlled crossover trial 537 cirrhotic patients with grade III (265 patients) or IVa (262 patients) hepatic encephalopathy were randomized to receive intravenous flumazenil or a placebo over a 3–5 minute period [3]. Patients subsequently received the other study medication if they were still in grade III or IVa encephalopathy after the first study period. Treatment was begun within 15 minutes of randomization. Outcome measures included both a neurological score and a grading derived from con-

tinuous EEG recordings. Table 39.6 shows the results obtained by combining the scores from the initial and crossover period. Improvement of the neurological score was documented in 46 of grade III and in 39 of grade IVa patients during the combined flumazenil treatment periods and in 10 (Grade III) and 3 (Grade IVa) of the patients during placebo treatment periods. Improvement of the EEG score occurred in 73 (Grade III) and 57 (Grade IVa) patients during flumazenil treatment and 13 (Grade III) and 9 (Grade IVa) patients during placebo treatment. The effects of flumazenil were statistically significant (p < 0.01). **A1d** In the second study [41], 24 of 49 randomized patients were excluded from the final analysis, mainly due to inadequate benzodiazepine screening. However, flumazenil was superior to placebo even when the data were evaluated by intention-to-treat analysis; among the 25 patients who were not excluded, clinically relevant improvement was seen in 35% compared to 0% in patients given placebo. **A1d** In the Canadian trial, very strict exclusion criteria resulted in the rejection of 56 of 77 potential patients [42]. Improvement in neurological symptoms was observed in 6 of 11 flumazenil treatment periods compared to 0 of 10 placebo periods; a few patients showed improvement in the EEG during both treatments. The beneficial effect of flumazenil was not related to the presence of identifiable benzodiazepines in the blood. **A1d** In the fourth positive study, drug effects were evaluated on continuous EEG recordings obtained before, during and ten minutes after a

Table 39.6 Randomized controlled trials of flumazenil for hepatic encephalopathy.

	Study design	No. of pats.	Dose (mg)	Outcome measure	HE grade	Number improved/number of treatment periods (%)			
						Flumazenil		Placebo	
						clinical	EEG	clinical	EEG
Barbaro [3]	Crossover RCT	527	1	Neurological EEG and	3	46/262[f] (17.6)	73/262[f] (27.9)	10/262 (3.8)	13/262 (5)
				Score	4	39/265[f] (14.7)	57/265[f] (21.5)	3/265 (1.1)	9/265 (3.4)
Gyr [41]	RCT	49[a]	1/hr ×3hr	PSE score dependent on neurologic symptoms	2–4	5/14[f] (35) (28)[bf]	0/11 (0) (0)		
Pomier-Layrargues [42]	Crossover RCT	21	2	HE grade EEG	2–4	6/13[f] (46)	4/12 (33)	0/15 (0)	2/13 (15)
Cadranel [43]	Crossover RCT	14[c]	1	HE grade EEG	2–4	d	12/18[f] (67)	0/8 (17)	
Van der Rijt [44]	Crossover RCT	18	0.25/h for 3 d	HE grade EEG	0–4	6/18[g] (35)	0/18	2/18 (12)	0/18
Lacetti [45]	RCT[e]	54	2	Glasgow coma scale	3–4	22/28[f] (79)		16/26 (61)	

[a] 24 Patients excluded from analysis (see text).
[b] Intent to treat analysis.
[c] 18 episodes of HE in 14 patients.
[d] "Modest improvement".
[e] All patients received BCAA, IV fluids and lactulose.
[f] $p < 0.05$.
[g] $p = 0.06$.

bolus dose of the drug [43]. No patient improved on placebo; on flumazenil the EEG recording improved in 12 out of 18 cases (66%) and was associated with a short-lasting modest clinical improvement. **A1d** In the fifth study the response rate with flumazenil was greater than that observed with placebo, but the result was not statistically significant [44].

A meta-analysis of all published trials involving a total of 641 patients showed that flumazenil induces clinical and electroencephalographic improvement of HE in patients with cirrhosis [46]. Taken together, these studies suggest that some patients with severe HE will experience clinical improvement when flumazenil is added to standard treatment. **A1c**

Antibiotics

Neomycin has been used as standard treatment of HE for almost 40 years. Surprisingly, there is no evidence that neomycin is effective. The only randomized placebo controlled study found no benefit of neomycin compared to standard treatment alone [12]. Based on this negative study and the potential for serious adverse effects of this drug, neomycin should not be prescribed for this condition. **A1d** The combination of neomycin with lactulose was not superior to placebo [33]. **A1d** Other antibiotics including paromomycin, metronidazole, vancomycin [47] but there is no evidence supporting their efficacy but are better tolerated. Rifaximin was introduced for treatment of HE about 15 years ago [48, 49]. In a prospective randomized controlled trial two doses of rifaximin were compared for treatment of HE, but this prospective trial unfortunately did not include a control group. A dose of 1200 mg/d appeared to be most effective [50]. Rifaximin was than compared to lactitol in a prospective randomized, double-blind, double-dummy, controlled trial. The overall efficacy of both drugs in episodic HE type was similar (81.6 and 80.4% improved on rifaximin and lactitol, respectively) but rifaximin was associated with a more profound decrease of serum ammonia levels [51]. In a metaanalyis rifaximin was at least equally effective as and in some studies superior to nonabsorbable disaccharides and antimicrobials in relieving signs or symptoms observed in patients with mild-to-moderately severe hepatic encephalopathy [52]. A recently published randomized controlled trial showed rifaximin 550 mg tablets significantly reduced the risk of overt hepatic encephalopathy (HE) recurrence over a six month period, maintaining remission more effectively than placebo [53]. Additionally in this study, treatment significantly reduced the risk of hospitalization for HE. Future clinical trials should focus on using standardized methods of evaluating mental status and limiting enrollment to patients with mild-to-moderate, episodic, persistent, or minimal hepatic encephalopathy. **A1c** Well-designed studies are needed to fully delineate the efficacy of rifaximin and other pharmacologic treatments for patients with hepatic encephalopathy.

Disaccharides

Synthetic disaccharides (lactulose, lactitol, lactose in lactase deficiency) are currently the mainstay of therapy of HE. The dose of lactulose (45–90 g/day) should be titrated in every patient to achieve two to three soft stools with a pH below 6 per day. Lactitol has been evaluated in a number of clinical trials. It appears to be as effective as lactulose, is more palatable, and may have fewer adverse effects [33, 54]. **A1d** In patients with lactase deficiency, lactose has

most of the same effects as the synthetic disaccharides in the colon [55, 56].

The efficacy of these disaccharides is considered to be beyond doubt, although only one a properly conducted placebo controlled trial has been performed [12, 55]. Approximately 70–80% of patients with HE improve on lactulose treatment, a response rate comparable to that observed in patients treated with neomycin [10, 11]. Treatment is usually well tolerated, and the principal toxicity is abdominal cramping, diarrhea, and flatulence. Nevertheless, in view of the questionable efficacy of neomycin, the efficacy of oral lactulose or lactitol for treatment of clinically overt HE has to be questioned. The first placebo controlled trial (with a crossover design) involved just seven patients, of whom [57] only two had clinical symptoms. One patient improved on lactulose. This result is clearly not significant, and the trial lacked adequate power. The second trial reported only the outcome of 14 of the 26 randomized patients [58]. In another prospective trial 90 patients with cirrhosis and minimal hepatic encephalopathy (MHE) were randomly assigned in a 1:1 ratio to receive treatment (lactulose) for 3 months (n = 31) or no treatment (n = 30) in a nonblinded design. Psychometric performance by number and figure connection tests parts A and B, picture completion, and block design tests and HRQOL by the Sickness Impact Profile (SIP). The mean number of abnormal neuropsychological tests decreased significantly in patients in the treated group compared with patients in the untreated group (multivariate analysis of variance for time and treatment, P = 0.001). The mean total SIP score improved among patients

Table 39.7 Randomized controlled trials of lactulose for hepatic encephalopathy.

	N	design	Lactulose (g/day)	Control	standard Tx	Outcome measures	Baseline characteristics	result
Elkington [56]	7	crossover	67	sorbitol	40 g protein	NH₃,PSE, EEG	not given, 2 pts. overt HE	no difference
Simmons [57]	26	RCT	60	glucose	40 g protein	HE grade	not given, all overt HE	? no difference, data of 12 pats not given
Dhiman [59]	26	RCT	30–60	—		N abnormal ψ-tests	Only MHE control group worse	L better than control group, no difference to baseline!
Watanabe [60]	36	RCT	27	—	40 g protein	N abnormal ψ-tests	Only MHE	?
Horsmans [61]	14	RCT	60	lactose	60 g protein	N abnormal ψ-tests	Only MHE control group worse	L better than control group, no difference to baseline!
Sharma [72]	140	RCT	30–60			Recurrent HE	Pts-recovered from HE	L better than no Tx
Prasad [58]	90	RCT	90			N abnormal ψ-tests	Only MHE	L better than no Tx

MHE: minimal HE; ψ-tests: psychometric tests.

in the treated group compared with patients in the untreated group. [59] The interpretation of the three new studies [60, 90, 91] performed within the last five years is difficult due to the definitions used to document the effect of therapy. A recent trial studied consecutive cirrhotic patients who recovered from HE. Patients were randomized to receive lactulose or placebo [61]. Of 300 patients with HE who recovered, 140 (46.6%) met the inclusion criteria and were included. Primary end point was development of overt HE. All patients were assessed by psychometry (number connection test A and B, figure connection test if illiterate, digit symbol test, and object assembly test), critical flicker frequency test, and blood ammonia level at inclusion. Twelve (19.6%) of 61 patients in the lactulose group and 30 (46.8%) of 64 in the placebo group ($P < 0.001$) developed HE over a median follow-up of 14 months (range, 1–20 months). Readmission rate due to causes other than HE (lactulose vs placebo: 9 vs 6) and deaths (5 vs 11) in 2 groups were similar. This is the first RCT which proves that lactulose is more effective than placebo. In contrast to oral lactulose administration, the efficacy of lactulose or lactose enemas is beyond any doubt (see above).

L-ornithine-L-aspartate

Ornithine and aspartate increase ammonia removal. In cirrhotics, ornithine aspartate infusions prevented hyperammonemia after an oral protein load in a dose-dependent fashion [62]. In a randomized, placebo-controlled trial of patients with HE, ornithine aspartate (20 g/day given intravenously over four hours for seven days) improved fasting and postprandial blood ammonia levels compared to placebo treated patients [4]. There was also symptomatic improvement (assessed by psychometric tests and the PSE index) in patients with grade I or II HE, but no effect was observed in those with minimal HE. A smaller placebo-controlled study also found benefits of oral ornithine-aspartate (18 g/day) with no adverse effects [63]. In a randomized controlled study from Mexico oral administration of lactulose or L-ornithine-L-aspartate to Mexican patients with cirrhosis and hyperammonemic encephalopathy significantly reduced serum ammonia levels in study groups and additionally improved mental status parameters, number connection test, asterixis scores, and EEG activity in the group receiving L-ornithine-L-aspartate [64].The results of this study are encouraging, and a confirmatory trial is needed. A recent meta-analysis came to the same conclusions [65]. **A1c** In patients with acute liver failure, L-ornithine-L-aspartate was ineffective [66].

L-Carnitine

L-carnitine is a natural substance involved in regulating substrate flux and energy balance across cell membranes. Carnitine has beneficial effects in different pathologies and prevents acute ammonia toxicity [67–69]. Several mechanisms have been suggested to explain its efficacy on ammonia toxicity, most importantly the interaction with NMDA-receptors [70]. A recent randomized, placebo-controlled trial in 150 patients with minimal to mild HE showed that on a 90-d treatment with 2 g L-carnitine/BID fasting serum ammonia levels decreased and psychometric tests improved with a significant difference to patients receiving placebo [71]. In a continuation of their studies arandomized, double-blind, placebo-controlled study administering Acetyl-L-carnitine (ALC) in 125 cirrhotic patients with MHE was conducted [72]. Patients in group A were treated with ALC and in group B with placebo for 90 days. Minimal hepatic encephalopathy was diagnosed with the Trail Making Test (TMT), Symbol Digit Modalities Test (SDMT) and Auditory Verbal Learning Test (AVL) and cognitive function with the Mini Mental State Examination (MMSE). After 90 days in group A treated with ALC, there were decreases in prothrombin time, bilirubin serum levels, AST, fasting, and psychometric tests improved. No significant differences were observed in EEG in either group of patients treated with ALC or placebo. The benefits of ALC in comparison with placebo are demonstrated in greater reductions in serum ammonia levels, as well as in improvements of neuropsychological functioning. A systematic review of the literature assessing the use of carnitine in the treatment of HE identified three high-quality human trials for review. Analysis of the selected carnitine trials compared to currently accepted therapies suggests that L-acyl-carnitine is promising as a safe and effective treatment for HE, and further trials of this drug are warranted [73]. **A1c**

Benzoate

A different approach to elimination of ammonia is the use of benzoate. Benzoate reacts with glycine to form hippurate. For each mole of benzoate, one mole of waste nitrogen is excreted into the urine. In a prospective, randomized double-blind study of 74 patients with acute HE, sodium benzoate (5 g bid) was compared with lactulose [74]. Treatment effects were evaluated using the PSE index, visual, auditory and somatosensory evoked potentials, and a battery of psychometric tests. The improvement in encephalopathy parameters and the incidence of adverse effects were similar in the two treatment groups. **A1d** In view of the unknown efficacy of lactulose, a confirmatory placebo controlled trial is needed.

Acarbose

Theoretically, the inhibition of intestinal disaccharidases should induce malabsorption of disaccharides and increase delivery of undigested carbohydrates to the colon. Acarbose (AO-128, an inhibitor of alpha glycosidase that is approved for treatment of diabetes mellitus) inhibits alpha-glucosidases that convert carbohydrates into monosaccharides. It also promotes the proliferation of intestinal saccharolytic bacterial flora at the expense of proteolytic bacterial flora producing mercaptans, benzodiazepine-like substances and ammonia. Their reduction could improve HE. A double-blind, randomized, controlled trial was performed in 35 cirrhotic patients with PSE. Patients were given a two-week treatment consisting of AO-128 (2 mg three times daily) or an identical placebo. Efficacy of treatment was assessed by the PSE index (PSEI) in weekly intervals. More patients receiving AO-128 than patients receiving placebo showed >40% improvement in the PSEI (83% vs 35%; p < 0.05). The mean stool pH decreased from 5.8+/−0.3 to 5.5+/−0.3 (p < 0.004) after AO-128 treatment, whereas no changes were observed in the placebo group. The EEG and nitrogen balance did not show changes in any of the two groups. An improvement was seen in the NCT performance after AO-128 (from grade 2.0+/−1.04 to grade 1.25+/−0.87; p < 0.05). Seven patients treated with AO-128 developed diarrhea, as compared with none in the placebo group (p < 0.05) [75]. To further test this hypothesis a randomized controlled crossover trial involving 107 cirrhotic patients with diabetes mellitus and grade 1 to 2 HE was performed [76]. Treatment was associated with a reduction in blood ammonia blood levels and improvement in HE. **A1d**

Modification of colonic flora (probiotics and prebiotics)

Alteration of gut flora (either with probiotics or with prebiotics such as fermentable fiber) has been associated with improvement in HE in pilot studies [77–79]. Such therapy appears to lower blood ammonia concentrations possibly by favoring colonization with acid-resistant, non-urease producing bacteria associated with MHE in 50% of patients [78]. Treatment with fermentable fibres alone was also of benefit in a substantial proportion of patients. A small trial demonstrated a significant rate of MHE reversal and excellent adherence in cirrhotics after probiotic yogurt supplementation with potential for long-term adherence [80]. In an open label randomized controlled study in patients with MHE, probiotics and lactulose were equally effective to improve the test employed to measure MHE [81]. **A1d** In a further study in 125 patients with cirrhosis and HE were randomized either to a treatment with Bifidobacterium+fructo-oligosaccharides (FOS) or lactulose for 60 days.

Bifidobacterium+FOS-treated patients compared with lactulose-treated patients showed a significant improvement of psychometric tests and a decrease of fasting ammonia levels at end of the study (82).

Molecular adsorbent recirculating system (MARS)

Extracorporeal albumin dialysis (ECAD) using molecular adsorbent recirculating system (MARS) may improve severe HE in patients with advanced cirrhosis via the removal of protein or non-protein-bound toxins. A prospective, randomized, controlled, multicenter trial of the efficacy, safety and tolerability of ECAD was conducted in such patients [83]. Patients were randomized to ECAD and standard medical therapy (SMT) or SMT alone. ECAD was provided daily for six hours for five days or until the patient had a two-grade improvement in HE. HE grades (West Haven criteria) were evaluated every 12 hours using a scoring algorithm. The primary endpoint was the difference in improvement proportion of HE between the two groups. A total of 70 subjects (median age, 53; 56% male; 56% HE grade III; 44% HE grade IV; median model for end-stage liver disease (MELD) 32 (11–50) and CPT 13 (10–15)) were enrolled in eight tertiary centers. Patients were randomized to ECAD + SMT (n = 39) or SMT alone (n = 31). Groups were matched in demographics and clinical variables. The improvement proportion of HE was higher in ECAD (mean, 34%; median, 30%) versus the SMT group (mean, 18.9%; median, 0%) (p = 0.044) and was reached faster and more frequently than in the SMT group (p = 0.045). Subjects receiving ECAD tolerated treatment well, with no unexpected adverse events. The conclusion was that the use of ECAD may be associated with an earlier and more frequent improvement of HE (grade III/IV). Because this five-day study was not designed to examine the impact of MARS on survival, a full assessment of the role of albumin dialysis awaits the results of additional controlled trials. The shortcomings of this trial do not allow us to recommend its general use [84].

Persistent HE type C

Patients with HE that is refractory to standard therapy are rare. Most have surgical shunts or a large diameter transjugular intrahepatic portosystemic shunt (TIPS). Due to the small number of such patients, there are no controlled studies. Case reports on individual patients describe successful approaches by narrowing or closure of the shunt, protein restriction together with BCAA supplementation, supplementation of zinc and thiamin, and the use of bromocriptin and oral flumazenil. The only controlled study was performed in 37 hospitalized patients with documented severe protein intolerance [85]. Addition of BCAA to the diet enabled the daily protein intake to be increased to up to 80 g without worsening of cerebral function. **B4** Many control patients who received casein as a protein source deteriorated after increasing dietary protein intake. No benefit of BCAA supplementation was observed in protein-tolerant patients.

In protein-intolerant patients vegetable proteins appear to be better tolerated than proteins derived from fish, milk or meat. In three controlled studies a vegetable diet was better tolerated than a diet which also included meat [86, 87]. **A1d** Other studies did not show these favorable effects [88]. **B4** The beneficial effects of a vegetable diet on the protein tolerance of patients with HE cannot be explained by the amino acid compositions of the proteins alone [89].

Minimal HE

Although the number of patients with minimal HE is large, good clinical studies are rare. Even among experts, there is no agreement on how to define minimal HE or whether minimal HE even exists. Efficacy of treatment is judged by the improvement of psychometric tests or of electrophysiological measurements (see Table 39.6). The clinical relevance of these outcomes is uncertain. Substances that improved responses in psychometric tests in randomized trials include lactulose [59, 90, 91], modification of colonic flora to increase lactobacilli [79, 80], ornithin aspartate [5], and oral BCAA [92, 93].

Prevention of HE

The occurrence of HE is a problem after TIPS insertion [94]. Although most clinicians administer prophylactic treatments after TIPS placement, the frequency of episodes of overt HE was about 10% per month. **B4** The manifestation of HE before TIPS and/or reduced liver function were identified as independent risk factors.

Summary of recommended treatment of hepatic encephalopathy in clinical practice

Treatment of episodic he type C

Treatment of episodic HE type C involves two steps. The first is to identify and to correct precipitating causes:
- gastrointestinal bleeding
- sedatives or tranquilizers
- infections

- hypovolemia, hypoxia, electrolyte imbalance, hypoglycemia

The second step is initiation of measures to lower blood ammonia concentrations using:
- lactulose enemas
- ornithine aspartate IV
- parenteral or enteral nutrition, if patient is unable to eat
- flumazenil if the patient has been given benzodiazepines

Chronic therapy

Chronic management of the patient with recurrent episodic HE type C requires individual adjustment of treatment. The titration of protein tolerance after an episode of HE should permit the design of an individual diet for each patient. Limitation of protein intake is reasonable in some patients, but protein restriction should be avoided if possible, since it will lead to negative nitrogen balance. In protein-intolerant patients, vegetable proteins are better tolerated than proteins derived from fish, milk, or meat. The supplementation of a low protein diet with branched chain amino acids should be considered. Additionally, patients may benefit from zinc and thiamin supplementation. The long-term benefit of all other treatments (including lactulose and neomycin) is uncertain. The need for treatment of minimal HE is not established and unproven therapy should be administered in the context of randomized controlled clinical trials.

References

1 Ferenci P, Püspök A, Steindl P. Current concepts in the pathophysiology of hepatic encephalopathy. *Eur J Clin Invest* 1992; **22**: 573–581.

2 Ferenci P, Lockwood A, Mullen K, Tarter R, Weissenborn K, Blei AT. Hepatic encephalopathy: definition, nomenclature, diagnosis and quantification. Final report of the Working Party at the 11th World Congresses of Gastroenterology, Vienna 1998. *Hepatology* 2002; **35**: 716–721.

3 Barbaro G, Di Lorenzo G, Soldini M *et al.* Flumazenil for hepatic encephalopathy grade III and IVa in patients with cirrhosis: an Italian multicenter double-blind, placebo-controlled, cross-over study. *Hepatology* 1998; **28**: 374–378.

4 Kircheis G, Nilius R, Held C *et al.* Therapeutic efficacy of l-ornithine-l-aspartate infusions in patients with cirrhosis and hepatic encephalopathy: results of a placebo-controlled, double-blind study. *Hepatology* 1997; **25**: 1351–1360.

5 Stauch S, Kircheis G, Adler G *et al.* Oral L-ornithine-L-aspartate therapy of chronic hepatic encephalopathy: results of a placebo-controlled double-blind study. *J Hepatol* 1998; **28**: 856–864.

6 Marchesini G, Dioguardi FS, Bianchi GP *et al.* Long-term oral branched-chain amino acid treatment in chronic hepatic encephalopathy. A randomized double-blind casein-controlled trial. The Italian Multicenter Study Group. *J Hepatol* 1990; **11**: 92–101.

7 Michel H, Solere M, Granier P *et al.* Treatment of cirrhotic hepatic encephalopathy with l-dopa. A controlled trial. *Gastroenterology* 1980; **79**: 207–211.

8 Michel H, Pomier-Layrargues G, Aubin JP *et al.* Treatment of hepatic encephalopathy by infusion of a modified amino acid solution: results of a study in 47 cirrhotic patients. In: Capocaccia L, Fischer JE, Rossi-Fanelli F, eds. *Hepatic Encephalopathy and Chronic Liver Failure.* Plenum Press, New York/London, 1984: 301–310.

9 Wahren J, Denis J, Desurmont P *et al.* Is intravenous administration of branched chain amino acids effective in the treatment of hepatic encephalopathy? A multicenter study. *Hepatology* 1983; **3**: 475–480.

10 Blanc P, Daures JP, Liautard J *et al.* Lactulose-neomycin combination versus placebo in the treatment of acute hepatic encephalopathy. Results of a randomized controlled trial. *Gastroenterol Clin Biol* 1994; **18**: 1063–1068.

11 Strauss E, Tramote R, Silva EP *et al.* Double-blind randomized clinical trial comparing neomycin and placebo in the treatment of exogenous hepatic encephalopathy. *Hepatogastroenterology* 1992; **39**: 542–545.

12 Conn HO, Lieberthal MM. *The Hepatic Coma Syndromes and Lactulose.* Williams & Wilkins, Baltimore, MD, 1979.

13 Conn HO, Leevy CM, Vlahcevic ZR *et al.* Comparison of lactulose and neomycin in the treatment of chronic portalsystemic encephalopathy. *Gastroenterology* 1977; **72**: 573–583.

14 Weissenborn K, Ruckert N, Hecker H *et al.* The number connection tests A and B: interindividual variability and use for the assessment of early hepatic encephalopathy. *J Hepatol* 1998; **28**: 646–653.

15 Schomerus H, Hamster W, Blunck H *et al.* Latent portosystemic encephalopathy I. Nature of cerebral functional defects and fitness to drive. *Dig Dis Sci* 1981; **26**: 622–630.

16 Rikkers L, Jenko P, Rudman D *et al.* Subclinical hepatic encephalopathy: detection, prevalence and relationship to nitrogen metabolism. *Gastroenterology* 1978; **75**: 462–469.

17 Quero JC, Hartmann IJ, Meulstee J *et al.* The diagnosis of subclinical hepatic encephalopathy in patients with cirrhosis using neuropsychological tests and automated electroencephalogram analysis. *Hepatology* 1996; **24**: 556–560.

18 Groeneweg M, Quero JC, De Bruijn I *et al.* Subclinical hepatic encephalopathy impairs daily functioning. *Hepatology* 1998; **28**: 45–49.

19 Weissenborn K, Ennen JC, Schomerus H, Rückert N, Hecker H. Neuropsychological characterization of hepatic encephalopathy. *J Hepatol* 2001; **34**: 768–773.

20 Kullmann F, Hollerbach S, Holstege A *et al.* Subclinical hepatic encephalopathy: the diagnostic value of evoked potentials. *J Hepatol* 1995; **22**: 101–110.

21 Kircheis G, Wettstein M, Timmermann L *et al.* Critical flicker frequency for quantification of low-grade hepatic encephalopathy. *Hepatology* 2002; **35**: 357.

22 Romero-Gomez M, Cordoba J, Jover R *et al.* Value of the critical flicker frequency in patients with minimal hepatic encephalopathy. *Hepatology* 2007; **45**: 879.

23 Sharma, P, Sharma BC, Puri, V, Sarin SK. Critical flicker frequency: diagnostic tool for minimal hepatic encephalopathy. *J Hepatol* 2007 **47**: 67.

24 Ortiz M, Cordoba J, Jacas C *et al.* Neuropsychological abnormalities in cirrhosis include learning impairment. *J Hepatol* 2006; **44**: 104.

25 Amodio P, Marchetti P, Del Piccolo F *et al.* Study on the Sternberg paradigm in cirrhotic patients without overt hepatic encephalopathy. *Metab Brain Dis* 1998; **13**: 159.

26 Amodio P, Campagna F, Olianas S, *et al.* Detection of minimal hepatic encephalopathy: normalization and optimization of the Psychometric Hepatic Encephalopathy Score. A neuropsychological and quantified EEG study. *J Hepatol* 2008; **49**: 346.

27 Bajaj JS, Hafeezullah M, Franco J *et al.* Inhibitory control test for the diagnosis of minimal hepatic encephalopathy. *Gastroenterology* 2008; **135**: 1591–1600.

28 Mardini H, Saxby BK, Record CO. Computerized psychometric testing in minimal encephalopathy and modulation by nitrogen challenge and liver transplant. *Gastroenterology* 2008; **135**: 1582–1590.

29 Mooney S, Hasssanein TI, Hilsabeck RC *et al.* Utility of the Repeatable Battery for the Assessment of Neuropsychological Status (RBANS) in patients with end-stage liver disease awaiting liver transplant. *Arch Clin Neuropsychol* 2007; **22**: 175.

30 Wein C, Koch H, Popp B *et al.* Minimal hepatic encephalopathy impairs fitness to drive. *Hepatology* 2004; **39**: 739.

31 Bajaj JS, Saeian K, Hafeezullah M *et al.* Patients with minimal hepatic encephalopathy have poor insight into their driving skills. *Clin Gastroenterol Hepatol* 2008; **6**: 1135–1139.

32 Rosenberg W, Donald A. Evidence based medicine: an approach to clinical problem-solving. *Br Med J* 1995; **310**: 1122–1126.

33 Blanc P, Daures JP, Rouillon JM *et al.* Lactitol or lactulose in the treatment of chronic hepatic encephalopathy: results of a meta-analysis. *Hepatology* 1992; **15**: 222–228.

34 Naylor CD, O'Rourkee K, Detsky AS *et al.* Parenteral nutrition with branched-chain amino acids in hepatic encephalopathy. A meta-analysis. *Gastroenterology* 1989; **97**: 1033–1042.

35 Uribe M, Campollo O, Vargas-F *et al.* Acidifying enemas (lactitol and lactose) vs nonacidifying enemas (tap water) to treat acute portal-systemic encephalopathy: a double-blind, randomized clinical trial. *Hepatology* 1987; **7**: 639–643.

36 Uribe M, Berthier J, Lewis H *et al.* Lactose enemas plus placebo tablets vs. neomycin tablets plus starch enemas in acute portal systemic encephalopathy. A double-blind randomized controlled study. *Gastroenterology* 1981; **81**: 101–106.

37 Ferenci P. Critical evaluation of the role of branched chain amino acids in liver disease. In: Thomas JC, Jones EA, eds, *Recent Advances in Hepatology 2.* Churchill Livingstone, New York, 1986: 137–154.

38 Fabbri A, Magrini N, Bianchi G *et al.* Overview of randomized clinical trials of oral branched-chain amino acid treatment in chronic hepatic encephalopathy. *J Parent Ent Nutr* 1996; **20**: 159–164.

39 Morgan TR, Moritz TE, Mendenhall CL *et al.* Protein consumption and hepatic encephalopathy in alcoholic hepatitis. VA Cooperative Study Group 275. *J Am Coll Nutr* 1995; **14**: 152–158.

40 Plauth M, Merli M, Kondrup J *et al.* ESPEN Guidelines for nutrition in liver disease and transplantation. *Clin Nutr* 1997; **16**: 43–55.

41 Gyr K, Meier R, Haussler J *et al.* Evaluation of the efficacy and safety of flumazenil in the treatment of portal systemic encepha-

lopathy: a double blind, randomized, placebo controlled multi-center study. *Gut* 1996; **39**: 319–325.

42 Pomier-Layrargues G, Giguere JF, Lavoie J *et al.* Flumazenil in cirrhotic patients in hepatic coma: a randomized double-blind placebo-controlled crossover trial. *Hepatology* 1994; **19**: 32–37.

43 Cadranel JF, el Younsi M, Pidoux B *et al.* Flumazenil therapy for hepatic encephalopathy in cirrhotic patients: a double-blind pragmatic randomized, placebo study. *Eur J Gastroenterol Hepatol* 1995; **7**: 325–329.

44 Van der Rijt CC, Schalm SW, Meulstee J *et al.* Flumazenil therapy for hepatic encephalopathy. A double-blind cross over study. *Gastroenterol Clin Biol* 1995; **19**: 572–580.

45 Laccetti M, Manes G, Uomo G, Lioniello M, Rabitti PG, Balzano A. Flumazenil in the treatment of acute hepatic encephalopathy in cirrhotic patients: a double blind randomized placebo controlled study. *Dig Liver Dis* 2000; **32**: 335–338.

46 Goulenok C, Bernard B, Cadranel JF *et al.* Flumazenil vs placebo in hepatic encephalopathy in patients with cirrhosis: a meta-analysis. *Aliment Phamacol Ther* 2002; **16**: 361–372.

47 Tarao K, Ikeda T, Hayashi K *et al.* Successful use of vancomycin hydrochloride in the treatment of lactulose resistant chronic hepatic encephalopathy. *Gut* 1990; **31**: 702–706.

48 Bucci L, Palmieri GC. Double-blind, double-dummy comparison between treatment with rifaximin and lactulose in patients with medium to severe degree hepatic encephalopathy. *Curr Med Res Opin* 1993; **13**: 109–118.

49 Miglio F, Valpiani D, Rossellini SR, Ferrieri A. Rifaximin, a non-absorbable rifamycin, for the treatment of hepatic encephalopathy. A double-blind, randomised trial. *Curr Med Res Opin* 1997; **13**: 593–601.

50 Williams R, James OF, Warnes TW, Morgan MY Evaluation of the efficacy and safety of rifaximin in the treatment of hepatic encephalopathy: a double-blind, randomized, dose-finding multi-centre study. *Eur J Gastroenterol Hepatol* 2000; **12**: 203–208.

51 Mas A, Rodes J, Sunyer L *et al.* Comparison of rifaximin and lactitol in the treatment of acute hepatic encephalopathy: results of a randomized, double-blind, double-dummy, controlled clinical trial. *J Hepatol* 2003; **38**: 51–58.

52 Lawrence KR, Klee JA. Rifaximin for the treatment of hepatic encephalopathy. *Pharmacotherapy* 2008; **28**: 1019–1032.

53 Bass NM, Mullen KD, Sanyal A *et al.* Rifaximin for treatment of hepatic encephalopathy. *NEJM* 2010; **362**: 1071–1081.

54 Morgan MY, Hawley KE. Lactitol vs lactulose in the treatment of acute hepatic encephalopathy in cirrhotic patients: a double blind, randomized trial. *Hepatology* 1987; **7**: 1278–1284.

55 Orlandi F, Freddara U, Candelaresi MT *et al.* Comparison between neomycin and lactulose in 173 patients with hepatic encephalopathy: a randomized clinical study. *Dig Dis Sci* 1981; **26**: 408–506.

56 Uribe-Esquivel M, Moran S, Poo JL *et al.* In vitro and in vivo lactose and lactulose effects on colonic fermentation and portal-systemic encephalopathy parameters. *Scand J Gastroenterol* 1997; **222** (Suppl.): 49.

57 Elkington SG, Floch MH, Conn HO. Lactulose in the treatment of chronic portal-systemic encephalopathy. A double-blind clinical trial. *N Engl J Med* 1969; **281**: 498–412.

58 Simmons F, Goldstein H, Boyle JD. A controlled clinical trial of lactulose in hepatic encephalopathy. *Gastroenterology* 1970; **59**: 827–832.

59 Prasad S, Dhiman RK, Duseja A, Chawla YK, Sharma A, Agarwal R. Lactulose improves cognitive functions and health-related quality of life in patients with cirrhosis who have minimal hepatic encephalopathy. *Hepatology* 2007; **45**: 549–559.

60 Dhiman RK, Sawhney MS, Chawla YK, Das G, Ram S, Dilawari JB. Efficacy of lactulose in cirrhotic patients with subclinical hepatic encephalopathy. *Dig Dis Sci* 2000; **45**: 1549–1552.

61 Sharma BC, Sharma P, Agrawal A, *et al.* Secondary prophylaxis of hepatic encephalopathy: an open-label randomized controlled trial of lactulose versus placebo. *Gastroenterology* 2009; **137**: 885.

62 Staedt U, Leweling H, Gladisch R *et al.* Effects of ornithine aspartate on plasma ammonia and plasma amino acids in patients with cirrhosis. A double-blind, randomized study using a four-fold crossover design. *J Hepatol* 1993; **19**: 424–430.

63 Stauch, S, Kircheis, G, Adler, G *et al.* Oral L-ornithine L-aspartate therapy of chronic hepatic encephalopathy: Results of a placebo-controlled double-blind study. *J Hepatol* 1998; **28**: 856.

64 Poo JL, Góngora J, Sánchez-Avila F *et al.* Efficacy of oral L-ornithine-L-aspartate in cirrhotic patients with hyperammonemic hepatic encephalopathy. Results of a randomized, lactulose-controlled study. *Ann Hepatol* 2006; **5**: 281–288.

65 Jiang Q, Jiang XH, Zheng MH, Chen YP. L-Ornithine-l-aspartate in the management of hepatic encephalopathy: a meta-analysis. *J Gastroenterol Hepatol* 2008 (epub).

66 Acharya SK, Bhatia V, Sreenivas V, *et al.* Efficacy of L-Ornithine L-aspartate in acute liver failure: a double-blind, randomized, placebo-controlled study. *Gastroenterology* 2009; **136**: 2159.

67 Therrien G, Rose C, Butterworth J, Butterworth RF. Protective effect of L-carnitine in ammonia-precipitated encephalopathy in the portacaval shunted rat. *Hepatology* 1997; **25**: 551–556.

68 Matsuoka M, Igisu H, Kohriyama K, Inoue N. Suppression of neurotoxicity of ammonia by L-carnitine. *Brain Res* 1991; **567**: 328–331.

69 Siciliano M, Annicchiarico BE, Lucchese F, Bombardieri G. Effects of a single, short intravenous dose of acetyl-L-carnitine on pattern-reversal visual-evoked potentials in cirrhotic patients with hepatic encephalopathy. *Clin Exp Pharmacol Physiol* 2006; **33**: 76–80.

70 Llansola M, Erceg S, Hernandez-Viadel M, Felipo V. Prevention of ammonia and glutamate neurotoxicity by carnitine: molecular mechanisms. *Metab Brain Dis* 2002; **17**: 389–397.

71 Malaguarnera M, Pistone G, Elvira R, Leotta C, Scarpello L, Liborio R. Effects of L-carnitine in patients with hepatic encephalopathy. *World J Gastroenterol* 2005; **11**: 7197–7202.

72 Malaguarnera M, Gargante MP, Cristaldi E *et al.* Acetyl-L-carnitine treatment in minimal hepatic encephalopathy. *Dig Dis Sci* 2008; **53**: 3018–3025.

73 Shores NJ, Keeffe EB. Is oral L-acyl-carnitine an effective therapy for hepatic encephalopathy? Review of the literature. *Dig Dis Sci* 2008; **53**: 2330–2333.

74 Sushma S, Dasarathy S, Tandon RK *et al.* Sodium benzoate in the treatment of acute hepatic encephalopathy: a double-blind randomized trial. *Hepatology* 1992; **16**: 138–144.

75 Uribe M, Moran S, Poo JL, Mendez-Sanchez N, Guevara L, Garcia-Ramos G. Beneficial effect of carbohydrate maldigestion induced by a disaccharidase inhibitor (AO-128) in the treatment of chronic portal-systemic encephalopathy. A double-blind, randomized, controlled trial. *Scand J Gastroenterol* 1998; **33**: 1099–1106.

76 Gentile S, Guarino G, Romano M *et al.* A randomized controlled trial of acarbose in hepatic encephalopathy. *Clin Gastroenterol Hepatol* 2005; **3**: 184.

77 Macbeth WA, Kass EH, Mcdermott WV Jr. Treatment of hepatic encephalopathy by alteration of intestinal flora with lactobacillus acidophilus. *Lancet* 1965; **191**: 399.

78 Liu Q, Duan ZP, Ha da K *et al.* Synbiotic modulation of gut flora: effect on minimal hepatic encephalopathy in patients with cirrhosis. *Hepatology* 2004; **39**: 1441.

79 Loguercio C, Abbiati R, Rinaldi M *et al.* Long-term effects of enterococcus faecium SF68 versus lactulose in the treatment of patients with cirrhosis and grade 1–2 hepatic encephalopathy. *J Hepatol* 1995; **23**: 39.

80 Bajaj JS, Saeian K, Christensen KM *et al.* Probiotic yogurt for the treatment of minimal hepatic encephalopathy. *Am J Gastroenterol* 2008; **103**: 1707–1715.

81 Sharma P, Sharma BC, Puri V, Sarin SK. An open-label randomized controlled trial of lactulose and probiotics in the treatment of minimal hepatic encephalopathy. *Eur J Gastroenterol Hepatol* 2008; **20**: 506–511.

82 Malaguarnera M, Gargante MP, Malaguarnera G *et al.* Bifidobacterium combined with fructo-oligosaccharide versus lactulose in the treatment of patients with hepatic encephalopathy. *Eur J Gastroenterol Hepatol.* 2010; **22**: 199–206.

83 Hassanein TI, Tofteng F, Brown RS Jr *et al.* Randomized controlled study of extracorporeal albumin dialysis for hepatic encephalopathy in advanced cirrhosis. *Hepatology* 2007; **46**: 1853–1862.

84 Ferenci P, Kramer L. MARS and the failing liver – any help from the outer space? *Hepatology* 2007; **46**: 1682–1684.

85 Horst D, Grace ND, Conn HO *et al.* Comparison of dietary protein with an oral, branched chain-enriched amino acid supplement in chronic portal-systemic encephalopathy: a randomized controlled trial. *Hepatology* 1984; **4**: 279–287.

86 Uribe M, Marquez MA, Ramos GG *et al.* Treatment of chronic portal-systemic encephalopathy with vegetable and animal protein diets. *Dig Dis Sci* 1982; **27**: 1109–1116.

87 Bianchi GP, Marchesini G, Fabbri A *et al.* Vegetable versus animal protein diet in cirrhotic patients with chronic encephalopathy. A randomized cross-over comparison. *J Intern Med* 1993; **233**: 385–392.

88 Greenberger NJ, Carley J, Schenker S *et al.* Effect of vegetable and animal protein diets in chronic hepatic encephalopathy. *Dig Dis* 1977; **22**: 845–855.

89 Keshavarzian A, Meek J, Sutton C *et al.* Dietary protein supplementation from vegetable sources in the management of chronic portal systemic encephalopathy. *Am J Gastroenterol* 1984; **79**: 945–949.

90 Watanabe A, Sakai T, Sato S *et al.* Clinical efficacy of lactulose in cirrhotic patients with and without subclinical hepatic encephalopathy. *Hepatology* 1997; **26**: 1410–1414.

91 Horsmans Y, Solbreux PM, Daenens C *et al.* Lactulose improves psychometric testing in cirrhotic patients with subclinical encephalopathy. *Aliment Pharmacol Ther* 1997; **11**: 165–170.

92 Egberts EH, Schomerus H, Hamster W *et al.* Branched chain amino acids in the treatment of latent portosystemic encephalopathy. A double-blind placebo-controlled crossover study. *Gastroenterology* 1985; **88**: 887–895.

93 Plauth M, Egberts EH, Hamster W *et al.* Long-term treatment of latent portosystemic encephalopathy with branched-chain amino acids. A double-blind placebo-controlled crossover study. *J Hepatol* 1993; **17**: 308–314.

94 Nolte W, Wiltfang J, Schindler C *et al.* Portosystemic hepatic encephalopathy after transjugular intrahepatic portosystemic shunt in patients with cirrhosis: clinical, laboratory, psychometric, and electroencephalographic investigations. *Hepatology* 1998; **28**: 1215–1225.

40 Hepatocellular carcinoma

Massimo Colombo and Massimo Iavarone

Department of Medicine, First Division of Gastroenterology, Fondazione IRCCS Cà Granda Ospedale Maggiore Policlinico, Università degli Studi di Milano, Milan, Italy

Introduction

Hepatocellular carcinoma (HCC) is the fifth most common cancer worldwide and the third most common cause of cancer mortality, with an estimated worldwide prevalence of 632,000 cases [1]. Accounting for about 90% of all primary liver cancers, HCC is unique in that it develops in the background of well-recognized risk factors that are responsible for marked variations of the tumor prevalence and clinical presentation, worldwide. Sequential scrutiny of the cancer registries has demonstrated important variations in the temporal trends of HCC incidence, with some evidence for an increase in incidence in resource-rich countries [1]. In these regions molecular epidemiology investigations have predicted a further rise in HCC incidence and mortality rates in the next decades due to the accumulation of patients with chronic liver diseases who are expected to develop HCC.

Early diagnosis

Early diagnosis of HCC is feasible through surveillance of patients at risk, who are readily identifiable. Surveillance is feasible since the test adopted, abdominal ultrasound (US), is user friendly and acceptable to the population, while it has high diagnostic accuracy. Moreover, the diagnostic tests and recall procedures have been standardized, while early cancer definition also incorporates suitability for potentially curative treatments [2, 3]. The term "very early tumor" has been recently defined to indicate a <2 cm nodule with an indistinct nodular pattern and a hypoattenuated vascular pattern on contrast imaging; this has a better prognosis than same size nodules which have a distinct nodular pattern but are hypervascular on imaging and infiltrating at histology [4]. The disparity in outcomes between patients diagnosed with an early HCC compared to those with a more advanced tumor strongly supports screening for HCC.

Population to be screened

Patients with cirrhosis and carriers of hepatitis B virus (HBV) and hepatitis C virus (HCV) are the target population for screening (see Table 40.1) [2, 3, 5, 6].

Cirrhosis is the leading cause of HCC worldwide, the risk of HCC increasing in parallel with disease severity. The annual rate of conversion of virus-related cirrhosis to liver cancer is approximately 3%, but with important regional variations (from 1.5–2% in Europe to 3–8% in Asia) [2]. HCC risk can further increase in the presence of co-factors known to accelerate progression of HCC like aflatoxin B_1 in HBV carriers, and alcohol consumption, iron and obesity in HCV carriers [5]. In many developed countries diabetes and non-alcoholic steato-hepatitis have emerged as important risk factors for cryptogenic cirrhosis and HCC in patients lacking HBV or HCV, while transition from cirrhosis to HCC is accelerated in livers expressing histopathological markers of increased cell proliferation or cell dysplasia, independently of etiology. Age cutoffs have been indicated for starting surveillance of African and Asian patients, since the risk of HCC increases in parallel with ageing, viremia and severity of the underlying liver disease [7]. It is still uncertain whether surveillance programs are improved by patients' stratification by clinical and histological scores. By combining sex, age and serum alfafetoprotein (AFP) levels, patients with compensated cirrhosis can be stratified in categories at increasing risk for the tumor. The lowest risk group (1.5% rate per year) included women younger than 53 years of age with normal AFP levels compared to men older than 53 year of age with

Evidence-Based Gastroenterology and Hepatology, 3rd edition.
J. McDonald, A.K. Burroughs, B. Feagan, and M.B. Fennerty. © 2010 Blackwell Publishing Ltd

Table 40.1 Groups of patients for whom surveillance is recommended by the European (EASL), American (AASLD) and Japanese (JSH) Associations for the Study of the Liver.

Guidelines	Target population	
	Chronic hepatitis B or C	Cirrhosis
EASL 2001[3]	HBV: not specified HCV: histological	Child-Pugh A and B Child-Pugh C if liver transplant available
AASLD 2005 [2]	HBV, non cirrhotics: ALT + DNA + and specific age cut-offs for ethnic groups	All etiologies A$_1$AT, AIH, NASH (?)
JSH 2008 [5]	Increased HCC risk: sex, age, alcohol	Very high risk: HBV/ HCV

high AFP levels who are at the highest risk (10%) for developing HCC [8]. In cirrhotic patients with mixed etiology, sex, age, disease severity and liver cell dysplasia identified a subset of patients with an exceedingly high (72%) risk of developing HCC during a follow-up of three years [9]. In Spain, similar criteria of disease severity (excluding cell dysplasia) led to the identification of cirrhotic patients at high risk (30.1%) and those at low risk (2.3%) of developing HCC during four years of surveillance [10]. Patients with severe co-morbidities and those with advanced liver disease (Child-Pugh C class patients), who do not have criteria for curative therapies, should not enter surveillance programs. Moreover, surveillance programs should be restricted to individuals >30 years and those <75 years of age, due to the low risk of cancer in younger people, while the older ones would not have significant benefit if diagnosed with a HCC. However, these criteria for selection are not evidence-based and may not be appropriate for all geographical areas. Importantly, patient stratification by risk level does not change selection of patients for surveillance, since the growth rate of tumors is the only variable which influences the outcome of screening. **B4**

Epidemiological, clinical and experimental studies have established a strong link between chronic infection with HBV virus and HCC. This virus agent, in fact, is responsible for both genotoxic lesions of the liver cells and tumor promotion through increased liver cell proliferation associated with persisting hepatitis. Importantly from a clinical point of view, HBV does not necessarily require the step to cirrhosis to be oncogenic [11]. In a prospective cohort study in Taiwan, the risk of HCC in 3454 HBsAg carriers was 102 times greater than in 19,253 non-carriers [12]. **B4** However, the carriers at especially high risk for developing HCC were those with actively replicating HBV (HBsAg$^+$/HBV

DNA$^+$) and those with cirrhosis, thus underlying the pathogenic relevance of virus persistence, liver inflammation and long duration of infection. The important role of virus replication in HCC has a solid basis: HBeAg seropositive carriers have six-fold greater risk of HCC (60.2 vs 9.6) than HBeAg negative carriers, after adjustment for age, sex, infection with hepatitis C, cigarette smoking and alcohol use [7]. In the HBeAg negative carriers, the risk of HCC is higher in patients with serum HBV-DNA >13 pg/ml than in those with undetectable (<2.5 pg) HBV-DNA [7]. In a prospective study of 3653 infected Chinese patients followed for more than ten years, a strict correlation was demonstrated between ≥10,000 copies/ml HBV-DNA at baseline and increased risk of HCC, again after adjusting for sex, age, cigarette smoking, alcohol consumption, HBeAg, ALT levels and cirrhosis at study entry. **B4** The study also provided evidence of reduced HCC risk in patients with spontaneous reduction of HBV-DNA levels during follow-up, though several concerns were raised on the methodology and conduct of the investigations [13]. In another prospective study in Taiwan, the risk of HCC correlated in an additive manner with HBV viremia and the genotype C of HBV, the latter being associated with higher levels of viremia [14]. **B4** In two studies in mainland China, an association was demonstrated between increased risk of HCC, viremia, cirrhosis, core promoter and precore mutations, and genotype C of HBV, all thought to reflect independent predictors of HCC that ultimately may interact to boost hepatocarcinogenesis [15, 16]. The potential pathogenic role of genotype C was also confirmed in Japanese patients with HCC [17]. In certain geographical areas, however, environmental factors play a more important co-carcinogenetic role in HCC than host or virus factors. In China and Africa, development of HCC in HBV carriers is strongly boosted by exposure to dietary aflatoxin, which cooperates with HBV in causing irreversible genetic damage to the infected liver cells [18, 19]. In Qidong, China, even modest levels of aflatoxin exposure tripled the risk of HCC in HBV infected men [20]. Aflatoxin does not seem to play any appreciable role in the West, but systematic investigations on this risk factor are lacking. Finally, the frequent report of family clusters of HCC has suggested the possible existence of increased susceptibility to the carcinogenetic effect of HBV in family members, after adjustment for relevant environmental risk factors for HCC [21]. The identification of the above predictors of HCC in HBV carriers has been instrumental in the definition of the epidemiological profile of the HBV population to be targeted by screening programs aimed at early diagnosis of HCC [2]. Healthy carriers may develop HCC, but are at substantially lower risk, and often distinguishing between clinical subsets of HBsAg carriers may be difficult unless the patients are periodically assessed with laboratory or histological investigations [22]. The strong link between HBV and HCC has been further confirmed by the decrease of HCC that has been observed among Taiwanese children since the start of mass vaccination of all newborns against HBV [23]. The AASLD indicates surveillance for non-cirrhotic HBV-carriers with signs of liver inflammation, like elevated serum ALT values and >10^3 HBV-DNA, following the demonstration of the pathogenetic importance of HBV replication in HCC.

Patients with porphyria cutanea tarda, genetic hemochromatosis, α-1-antitrypsin deficiency, tyrosinemia and hypercitrullinemia are also at high risk for HCC. Patients with glycogenosis types I and III, Wilson's disease and hereditary fructose intolerance may also develop HCC, but are at substantially lower risk [24]. HCC has also developed in patients with autoimmune hepatitis and primary biliary cirrhosis, probably reflecting treatment-related improvement in patient survival. HCC was also found in 64% of 160 Japanese patients and in 48% of 101 South African black people with Budd-Chiari syndrome [25, 26]. However, in these studies the possible role of other unidentified carcinogens could not be excluded.

Screening tests

Ultrasound is the method of choice for screening, since it has adequate sensitivity, specificity, positive and negative predictive values [3]. Based upon studies of tumor volume doubling time, six months has been selected by most experts in the West as the ideal interval of screening with US, whereas in the Far East, the three-month interval for screening is largely adopted. In Italy, a study in hemophiliacs chronically infected with hepatitis C virus demonstrated similar efficacy of 6-month and 12-month intervals of screening in the identification of potentially curable HCC [27]. In France, a multicenter study in patients with compensated cirrhosis showed that increasing the frequency of US examinations every three months did not increase the accuracy of screening whereas it resulted in increased costs to treat patients with false-positive results [28].

The serum assay AFP is no longer considered for screening by AASLD and EASL due to the high rates of false positive and false negative results in patients with chronic liver disease. Whether other serum markers like des-gamma carboxy-prothrombin (DCP) and fucosylated AFP (AFP-L3) should be incorporated into surveillance for HCC, is debatable [2]. A DCP value of 150 mAU/ml had a better positive predictive value for differentiating early HCC from cirrhosis than an AFP value of 13 ng/ml (92% vs 54%) [29]. The AFP-L3 variant with high affinity to lens-culinaris, is more specific for HCC than total AFP too, but differences among studies in assay methods, cutoff values chosen as diagnostic for HCC, and case mix with respect

to early tumors, do not allow for a definitive evaluation of the accuracy of this marker [29].

The recall policy

An abnormal screening test needs to be confirmed by either a US-guided liver biopsy or imaging-studies [3]. In patients with cirrhosis and a liver nodule detected during screening/surveillance, HCC can be diagnosed by imaging techniques without the need for a histological examination (see Table 40.2) [30]. CT scan, MRI and contrast-enhanced US serve the purpose whenever arterial enhancement of the nodule is demonstrated and followed by wash-out of contrast in the delayed venous phase [31]. The accuracy of radiological diagnosis, however, is tumor size dependent: the diagnosis is attained in all nodules >2 cm in diameter with one imaging technique only, whereas nodules between 5 and 20 mm in size escape diagnosis in two-thirds of the cases despite application of two imaging techniques [30]. Liver nodules not accurately diagnosed by imaging will require histological examination with a liver biopsy or close monitoring with US carried out at three-month intervals (enhanced follow-up). The risk of seeding should be considered as a complication of biopsy: in 41 papers specifying the total number of patients biopsied, the median risk of seeding was 2.9% (range 0–11%) for biopsy group, being lower (0.61–1.4%) in therapeutic percutaneous procedures [32]. The radiological diagnosis of HCC is complicated by false positive results in the presence of artero-venous shunts and macroregenerative nodules with dysplastic liver cells. Currently, dysplastic macronodules can be discriminated from early tumors by morphological criteria based on exclusion of microscopic stromal invasion [33].

Table 40.2 Radiological diagnosis of hepatocellular carcinoma in patients with cirrhosis according to the guidelines of EASL and AASLD [2, 3, 29].

Imaging techniques	Contrast-enhanced US, contrast-enhanced spiral CT and gadolinium-enhanced MRI
1–2 cm nodule	Two imaging techniques showing hyperenhanced nodule in the arterial phase and hypoenhanced nodule in the portal phase (wash-out)
>2 cm nodule	one imaging technique
Prospective validation	89 patients with a 5–20 mm nodule
Sensitivity	33%
Specificity	100%
Pos Pred Value	100%
Neg Pred Value	42%

Immunostaining for GPC-3, and structural and functional analysis of the genetic profile of the nodules may also distinguish between macronodules and tumors [4, 34]. Falsely negative nodules at contrast imaging are also a problem when searching for very early tumors, accounting for approximately 20% of all 1–2 cm in size HCCs [33].

Is liver-related mortality reduced by screening?

In the last decade, more than 50% of all patients in Japan have been diagnosed with a TNM I/II tumor compared to the 1980s, when only a minority of the patients with a HCC were diagnosed in the early stage [35]. In a national survey of 554 members of the AASLD, the vast majority of responders indicated that patients with cirrhosis were routinely screened using US [36].

A surveillance program of semi-annual determinations of AFP in HBV carriers in Alaska led to the identification of curable HCC in 40% of the affected patients, a fact that was perceived as beneficial since prior to AFP screening programs the case-fatality rate for HCC in Alaskan natives was 100%, with an average survival of three months [37]. **B4** A randomized controlled study conducted in Shanghai area using abdominal US and serum AFP every six months among individuals with chronic hepatitis and other risks for HCC, showed a reduction in the mortality rates in the screened versus unscreened population (83.2 vs 131.5 per 100,000 inhabitants) [38]. **A1d** The study, however, has limitations in the design and conduct, because the proportion of patients with cirrhosis is unknown, transplantation was not included among the radical therapies and the compliance of the population to the program was suboptimal (58%) (see Table 40.3). Notwithstanding all these limitations, the RCT in Shanghai confirms the importance of early diagnosis for improving HCC-related mortality in the community.

In cirrhotic patients attending hospital facilities, the HCC-specific mortality rates were reduced in patients with HCC detected during surveillance, most likely due to improvements in both detection and treatment. In a re-analysis of 112 cirrhotic patients with HCC detected during a hospital-based surveillance program, the survival rates were improved in patients who were treated for a liver cancer which had developed during the previous five years of surveillance compared to previous intervals (90% vs 55%, p = 0.0009) (see Table 40.4) [7]. **B3** Increased survival was attributed to a significant reduction in the mortality rates of treated patients (from 34% to 5%, p = 0.003), due to wider application of curative treatments and improved selection of patients undergoing surgical or ablative treatments. In Taiwan between 1989 and 1998, there was a significant increase in survival among 3345 patients with a HCC during the previous five years (from 29% to 35%), that was only in part (34%) due to advancement in medical care, but mostly (66%) attributable to early detection [39]. **B4**

Is surveillance in patients with cirrhosis cost-effective?

The economic consequences of HCC surveillance strategy are poorly appreciated, due to the lack of randomized trials evaluating moderators of treatment outcome, like compliance, heterogeneity and etiology of liver disease and treatment effectiveness that may impact on cost-effectiveness of surveillance. Patient compliance is an important variable of surveillance, as 1–15% of all patients failed to comply with clinic-based surveillance programs in Europe and

Table 40.3 A population-based screening for HCC: the importance of early diagnosis for improving HCC-related mortality[38].

Findings	Screened group (pp x yr = 38,444)	Control group (pp x yr = 41,077)
HCC occurrence		
Cases	86	67
Early cancer	39	0
Total incidence (per 100,000)	223.7	163.1
Rate ratio (95% CI)	1.37 (0.99, 1.89)	reference
Deaths from HCC		
Deaths	32	54
Total mortality (per 100,000)	83.2	131.5
Rate ratio (95% CI)	0.63 (0.41, 0.98)	reference

Table 40.4 A clinic-based surveillance of 447 cirrhotics: the importance of treatment refinement for improving HCC-related mortality[7].

Outcomes	1987–91	1992–96	1997–2001	p
HCC, No.	52	37	23	
HCC size, cm	3.7 (1.5–8)	3.0 (1.5–6)	2.2 (1.4–3.1)	0.02
Radical treatments	28%	38%	43%	0.02
Mortality in treated	34%	28%	5%	0.024
Mortality in untreated	69%	100%	92%	ns
Overall mortality	45%	37%	10%	0.0009

Japan (reviewed by Thompson Coon 2007 *et al.*) [40], compared to the 42% of the population enrolled in a study in Shanghai [38]. Cost-effectiveness of screening is largely influenced also by the heterogeneity of the natural history of tumor disease, the annual risk of HCC ranging from 1% in HBV patients to 5–8% in some patients with compensated cirrhosis due to HCV [5]. Since the cost for tumor detected is inversely proportional to the tumor incidence, screening is considered worthwhile in populations with equal or greater than 1.5% incidence of HCC. In population-based screening programs with HCC incidence lower than 1.5%, the low cost-effectiveness of surveillance is counterbalanced by the high numbers of targeted individuals with a preserved liver function, who have more chances of receiving curative treatments compared to patients enrolled in clinic-based surveillance programs. Finally, since cost-effectiveness of surveillance largely depends upon the outcome of treatments, studies like the Shanghai program which lack access to liver transplantation, do not inform about cost-effectiveness of surveillance in the West, where liver transplantation is a first option for selected patients with cirrhosis and a small tumor. In the absence of randomized trials, decision analysis (Markov modeling) has provided the best means to estimate cost-effectiveness of HCC surveillance in this patient population. A cost-effectiveness ratio represents the cost for life-year saved compared to a cost-utility ratio, which describes the cost per quality-adjusted life-year (QALY) saved. Surveillance programs in which cost-utility ratios are measured at less than US$ 50,000 x QALY are thought to be cost-effective (see Table 40.5) [41].

Table 40.5 Markov decision models to simulate cost-utility ratio of surveillance according to AASLD/EASL guidelines [40, 41].

Study	Etiology of cirrhosis	Incremental cost utility ratio (US$/ QALY)	Prerequisite
Sarasin et al. 1996[a]	Mixed	48,293	60 % survival 3-yr after resection
Everson et al. 2000[a]	Mixed	35,000	2.5% HCC x year
Saab et al. 2003[a]	Wait list	74,000	
Arguedas et al. 2003[a]	HCV	26,689	50-yr old eligible to OLT
Lin et al. 2004[a]	HCV	73,789	
Patel et al. 2005[a]	HCV	26,100 46,700 50,400	Hepatic resection Cadaveric liver transplant Living donor liver transplant
Thompson Coon 2007	Mixed	£ 31,900	Most alcohol-related
Anderson et al. 2008	Mixed	30,700	US alone

[a] Referenced by Thompson Coon 2007 [40].

Treatment of patients with cirrhosis and HCC

The success of HCC treatment largely depends on staging accuracy, that is, the clinical classification of disease severity aimed to establish prognosis and select the adequate treatment for the best candidates. The Barcelona Clinic Liver Center (BCLC) classification for HCC has been endorsed by EASL and AASLD as standard of care for patients with cirrhosis, since it links tumor stage with treatment strategies (see Table 40.6). The compelling evidence that surveillance improves treatment of HCC is due to its ability to improve detection of small, treatable tumors.

Early HCC

Survival of patients with compensated cirrhosis and an early HCC reaches up to 70–75% at five years after resection, transplantation or percutaneous interstitial treatments in carefully selected candidates (see Tables 40.7, 40.8, 40.9). Patients with a very early tumor, that is, well differenti-

ated, less than 2 cm in size with an ill-defined nodular pattern at US, show the best survival rates and the lowest recurrence rates after either resection or percutaneous ablation [51]. While percutaneous ablation of HCC with alcohol (PEI) or radiofrequency (RF) likely are equally effective for treating ≤2 cm tumors, patients with 3–4 cm tumors, who are at increased risk of local recurrence, benefit more from RF than from PEI [47–53]. **A1d** However, most studies comparing RF to PEI are underpowered, lack estimates of overall survival at five years and do not account for patients unfit for RF who could receive PEI only. Further, RF had greater reported mortality (0.5%) and complication rates (8.9%) than PEI. Overall, limited hepatic resection is superior to local ablative therapies in cirrhotic patients with 2–5 cm HCC who have moderate portal hypertension (<10 mmHg HVPG) [46]. The database of the Liver Cancer Study Group of Japan, including 8010 patients with compensated cirrhosis treated by resection and 4037 patients treated by PEI, all with a less than 5 cm HCC, showed survival figures at five years of 58% vs 39% respectively [54]. Recently, acetic acid demonstrated a higher necrotizing power than ethanol and percutaneous acetic acid injec-

Table 40.6 The Barcelona Clinic Liver Cancer (BCLC) staging classification for hepatocellular carcinoma.

Stage	Performance status	Tumor volume number and invasiveness	Child-Pugh	Expected survival
(A) Early[a]	0	Single <5 cm or 3 nodules <3 cm each	A and B	50–75% at 5 yr
(B) Intermediate	0	Large/multinodular	A and B	16 months
(C) Advanced	1–2	Vascular invasion and/or extrahepatic spread	A and B	6 months
(D) End stage	3–4	Any of the above	C	<3 months

[a] The early stage is further stratified in: (A1) performance status (PS) 0, single <5 cm, no portal hypertension (HTN) and normal bilirubin; (A2) PS 0, single <5 cm, portal HTN and normal bilirubin; (A3) PS 0, single <5 cm, portal HTN and elevated bilirubin; (A4) PS 0, up to 3 <3 cm Child-Pugh class A–B.

Table 40.7 Outcomes of liver transplantation in cirrhotic patients with a single small tumor or less than three small tumors (Milan criteria).

Center	Selection	Cases	5-year survival	Recurrence	Reference
Milan	Single ≤5 cm ≤three ≤3 cm	48	75%[a]	8%	Mazzaferro et al. (1996) [42]
Barcelona	Single ≤5 cm	79	75%	4%	Llovet et al. (1998) [43]
Paris	Three ≤3 cm	45	74%	11%	Bismuth et al. (1999) [44]
Berlin	Single ≤5 cm three ≤3 cm	120	71%	16%	Jonas et al. (2001) [45]

[a] Four-year survival rates.

Table 40.8 Five-year survival of 77 Spanish patients with Child-Pugh A cirrhosis and a less than 5 cm tumor treated by resection.

Overall 5-year survival	50%	
Median survival (months)	(a) 91 <1 mg bilirubin	p = 0.03
	(b) 30 ≥1 mg bilirubin	
	(c) 80 <10 mmHg HVPG	P = 0.02
	(d) 69 ≥10 mmHg HVPG	
5-year survival	74% a + c	
	50% a + d	
	15% b + d	

From Bruix J et al. Gastroenterology 1996; **111**: 1018–1023 [46].
HVPG: hepatic venous pressure gradient.

tion (PAI) seemed to have a better local control and improved survival rate than PEI in two randomized trials [55, 56]. However, two other studies found similar outcome of PEI vs PAI for treating small HCC [57, 58].

In principle, orthotopic liver transplantation is the treatment of choice for a patient with either a small HCC or patients with multiple nodules, as long as they are within the so-called Milan criteria (single nodule ≤5 cm or 3 nodules ≤3 cm without portal invasion) and have no contraindications for liver transplantation [42]. **B2** While liver transplantation cures both the tumor and the underlying cirrhosis, it is limited by the paucity of donors, the risk of severe recurrence of HCV and the lack of validated adjuvant treatments to prevent the risk of HCC recurrence.

Indeed, both resection and ablation of HCC are almost invariably complicated by tumor recurrence, which may reach up to 75% at five years. Early recurrence refers to HCC occurring in the first two years after partial/total resection or local ablation as a consequence of pre-treatment spread of neoplastic cells, while late recurrence (>2 years) are *de novo* primary tumors developing in the cirrhotic liver [59]. In patients with cirrhosis and a <5 cm HCC treated with hepatic resection or local ablation early recurrence is predicted by non-anatomical resection of the tumor, microscopic vascular invasion by tumor cells and high pre-therapy levels of serum AFP. In these patients, late recurrence (>24 months) is predicted by the grade of hepatitis activity, number of tumor nodules and gross tumor classification [59]. Unfortunately, preoperative prediction of early recurrence is difficult due to sampling errors with needle-biopsy and the lack of universally accepted cutoff values of serum AFP for selecting patients to hepatic resection. Since the clinical heterogeneity of HCC is governed by heterogeneity of the molecular pathways, transcription analysis of HCC cells has been applied to the prognosis in patients undergoing hepatic resection.

Table 40.9 Radiofrequency ablation and ethanol injection for the treatment of HCC 3–4 cm in size.

Author	Selection	Treatment	2-year local recurrence	3-year survival
Lencioni 2003 [47]	1 nodule ≤5 cm	PEI (n = 50)	38%	73%
	≤3 nodules ≤3 cm	RF ablation (n = 52)	**4%**	81%
Lin 2004 [48]	3 nodules ≤4 cm	PEI low dose (n = 52)	45%	50%
		PEI high dose (n = 53)	33%	55%
		RF ablation (n = 52)	**18%**	74%
Shiina 2005 [49]	3 nodules ≤3 cm	PEI (n = 114)	11%	63%
		RF ablation (n = 118)	**2%**	80%
Lin 2005 [50]	3 nodules ≤3 cm	PEI (n = 62)	34%	51%
		PAI[a] (n = 63)	31%	53%
		RF ablation (n = 62)	**14%**	74%
Brunello 2008 [51]	≤3 nodules ≤3 cm	PEI (n = 69)	NA	57%
		RF ablation (n = 70)		60%

[a] PAI: Percutaneous acetic acid injection.

At least three HCC subsets have been identified linked to chromosome stability/instability and progenitor cell-like molecular signature, the latter having a very high risk of recurrence and short survival after resection compared to patients with molecular signatures predictive of less invasive tumor phenotype [60, 61].

The effectiveness of adjuvant therapies in reducing HCC recurrence following resection or local ablation is not evidence-based [62]. In the transplantation setting, the adoption of stringent criteria for listing (Milan criteria) and prioritization of patients to liver transplant have resulted in a satisfactory balance between survival and recurrence rates. Because restricting priority to HCC candidates within Milan criteria (TNMI and II) only, may impose an unreasonable "punishment" on some patients with larger tumors who may benefit from liver transplantation, transplantation of patients with a tumor beyond Milan criteria has been attempted, but with uncertain cost-effectiveness ratio despite accurate preoperative selection with imaging. The recurrence rates in patients with a radiological preoperative tumor exceeding TNM I/II are invariably higher than those in patients within Milan criteria, whereas expanding listing to include patients exceeding Milan criteria with better tumor grading, is challenged by the high risk of sampling errors with preoperative liver biopsy [63, 64]. Major obstacles to new guidelines for expanding listing beyond Milan, are that the analysis of the explanted livers has invariably demonstrated tumor understaging by preoperative imaging, lack of intention-to-treat data on survival and limited (<20%) incremented number of patients beyond Milan criteria selected by expanded criteria. This,

together with the lack of studies comparing the outcome of liver transplantation in patients within Milan versus those beyond Milan, makes the issue of expanded criteria for transplantation still unsolved. A recent multicenter retrospective study enrolling 1112 patients transplanted with HCC exceeding Milan criteria, showed a five-year overall survival of 71.2% for those patients who fell within the up-to-seven criteria (HCC with seven as the sum of the size of the largest tumor and the number of tumors) without microvascular invasion [65]. Bridge treatments with chemoembolization (TACE) or RF are likely to reduce the risk of drop-outs from the waiting list due to tumor progression and the risk of post-transplant recurrence, as well. Cost-effectiveness analysis using a Markov model suggested a survival advantage for neoadjuvant bridge therapy, that is, between listing and grafting, in patients within Milan criteria with waiting times exceeding six months [66]. However, a meta-analysis of 12 studies provided no evidence for a benefit with bridge TACE [67], while treatment response to repeat TACE could be a selection criterion for transplant candidacy independently of tumor stage at presentation [68]. There are controversial results in published studies; however, in those centers where the waiting-list time is longer than six months, the RFTA is usually adopted to reduce the risk of HCC progression [69].

Intermediate HCC

These patients have a heterogeneous clinical condition, ranging from multiple small tumors to a single >5 cm nodule in size or a combination of nodules exceeding Milan criteria. The standard of care is arterial chemoembolization with doxorubicin, mitomycin or cisplatin as antitumoral drugs, which achieves partial responses in up to 50% of patients and significantly delays tumor progression. The best candidates are patients with better preserved liver function (Child-Pugh A) and small esophageal varices. In a meta-analysis of seven trials including a total of 516 patients, comparing embolization versus conservative management, survival benefits were obtained in two studies, the median survival for intermediate HCC cases treated with chemoembolization being 20 months as compared to the 16 months of the untreated patients (see Figure 40.1) [70–76]. **A1c** It is noteworthy that the two randomized studies showing greater survival for patients treated with chemoembolization versus untreated patients, enrolled patients with advanced stage of HCC, too. One major issue with this loco-regional treatment of HCC is the lack of standardization in the schedule of treatments, particles used for embolization, the selectivity of embolization and the antineoplastic drugs, as well as the lack of clear-cut criteria for patient selection [77]. Indeed RCT of chemoembolization (TACE) versus embolization alone (TAE) show no difference [77]. A preliminary study suggests that TACE with drug-eluting beads containing doxorubicin provides objective response rates of approximately 70%, with negligible systemic toxicity [78]. Internal radiation with ^{131}I-labelled lipiodol or Y-90 is under investigation following promising results in patients with advanced HCC [79, 80]. An international study of adjuvant therapy with the multikinase inhibitor Sorafenib in patients with intermediate HCC treated with chemoembolization, is planned.

Advanced HCC

After many years of unsuccessful clinical trials demonstrating a lack of efficacy for standard anticancer chemotherapy and hormones the multikinase inhibitor Sorafenib, blocking tumor cell proliferation and angiogenesis, was shown to possess anti-tumor activity in patients with advanced HCC [62, 81]. In a multicenter study in the USA, Europe and Oceania, Sorafenib at oral daily doses of 800mg, improved patients' survival from 7.9 months to 10.7 months, with a prolongation of the median time to progression to 5.5 months from 2.8 months of placebo-treated patients [82]. In a similar trial conducted in Asia–Pacific Sorafenib was superior to placebo in terms of both overall survival and time to progression [83]. **A1d** Efficacy and tolerability of treatment with Sorafenib are guaranteed in patients with well preserved hepatic function (Child-Pugh A), whereas limited data exists in patients with Child-Pugh B status. One major problem in the management of patients receiving targeted anti-cancer therapy with Sorafenib is that only a minority (3%) of the treated patients ultimately achieved a significant (partial) tumor shrinkage as defined by the Response Evaluation Criteria in Solid Tumors (RECIST) criteria, thus emphasizing the need for new response markers to direct therapy in clinical practice.

End-stage HCC

These patients have a dismal course (less than three months' survival) requiring best supportive care only, including

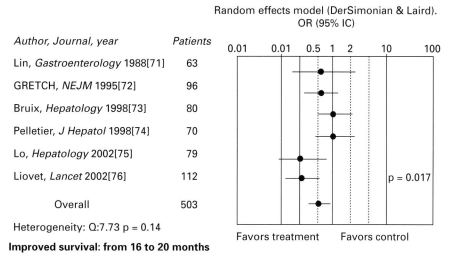

Figure 40.1 Chemoembolization in the treatment of intermediate HCC two-year survival vs conservative management.

analgesics, steroids and antibiotics when spontaneous bacterial peritonitis occurs.

Treatment of patients with normal livers

Hepatic resection is the primary option for the few patients with an HCC which develops in normal livers with well-preserved function. In two case series, the cumulative five-year survival for 128 such patients in two centers treated with hepatic resection was approximately 45%, compared with 12–26% for the 51 treated with orthotopic liver transplantation [84, 85]. The good results with hepatic resection probably depended on the absence of cirrhosis, which allowed for extensive resection of the liver without affecting survival. The poor results with liver transplantation probably reflected bias in patient selection, for example transplantation may have been done in patients with advanced HCC who were judged to be unsuitable candidates for resection.

Acknowledgement

This work was supported by a grant from Fondazione Italiana Ricerca Cancro.

The author thanks Caterina M. Puricelli for her expert secretarial assistance.

References

1 Parkin DM. Global cancer statistics in the year 2000. *Lancet Oncol* 2001; **2**: 533–543.

2 Bruix J, Sherman M. Management of hepatocellular carcinoma. *Hepatology* 2005; **42**: 1208–1236.

3 Bruix J, Sherman M, Llovet JM *et al.* Clinical management of hepatocellular carcinoma. conclusions of the Barcelona – 2000 EASL Conference. *J Hepatol* 2001; **35**: 421–430.

4 Kojiro M, Roskams T. Early hepatocellular carcinoma and dysplastic nodules. *Sem Liver Dis* 2005; **25**: 133–142.

5 Makuuchi M, Kokudo N, Arii S *et al.* Development of evidence-based clinical guidelines for the diagnosis and treatment of hepatocellular carcinoma in Japan. *Hepatol Res* 2008; **38**: 37–51.

6 Fattovich G, Stroffolini T, Zagni I *et al.* Hepatocellular carcinoma in cirrhosis: incidence and risk factors. *Gastroenterology* 2004; **127**: S35–50.

7 Yang HI, Lu SN, Liaw YF *et al.* Hepatitis B e antigen and the risk of hepatocellular carcinoma. *N Engl J Med* 2002; **347**: 168–174.

8 Sangiovanni A, Del Ninno E, Fasani P *et al.* Increased survival of cirrhotic patients with a hepatocellular carcinoma detected during surveillance. *Gastroenterology* 2004; **126**: 1005–1014.

9 Ganne-Carrié N, Chastang C, Chapel F *et al.* Predictive score for the development of hepatocellular carcinoma and additional value of liver large cell dysplasia in Western patients with cirrhosis. *Hepatology* 1996; **23**: 1112–1118.

10 Velazquez RF, Rodriguez M, Navascues CA *et al.* Prospective analysis of risk factors for hepatocellular carcinoma in patients with liver cirrhosis. *Hepatology* 2003; **37**: 520–527.

11 Rogler CE. Cellular and molecular mechanisms of hepatocarcinogenesis associated with hepadnavirus infection. In: Mason WS, Seager C, eds. *Hepadnavirus Molecular Biology and Pathogenesis.* Springer-Verlag, Berlin, 1991: 102–140.

12 Beasley RP. Hepatitis B virus. The major etiology of hepatocellular carcinoma. *Cancer* 1988; **61**: 1842–1856.

13 Chen CJ, Yang HI, Su J *et al.* Risk of hepatocellular carcinoma across a biological gradient of serum hepatitis B virus DNA level. *JAMA* 2006; **295**: 65–73.

14 Yu MW, Yeh SH, Chen PJ *et al.* Hepatitis B virus genotype and DNA level and hepatocellular carcinoma: a prospective study in men. *J Natl Cancer Inst* 2005; **97**: 265–272.

15 Chan HLY, Hui AY, Wong ML *et al.* Genotype C hepatitis B virus infection is associated with an increased risk of hepatocellular carcinoma. *Gut* 2004; **53**, 1494–1498.

16 Yuen MF, Lai CL. Combination therapy for chronic hepatitis B: simultaneous or sequential? *Am J Gastroenterol* 2007; **102**: 105–106.

17 Fujie H, Moriya K, Shintani Y *et al.* Hepatitis B virus genotypes and hepatocellular carcinoma in Japan. *Gastroenterology* 2001; **120**; 1564–1565.

18 Ozturk M. p53 mutation in hepatocellular carcinoma after aflatoxin exposure. *Lancet* 1991; **338**: 1356–1359.

19 Wogan GN. Aflatoxins as risk factors for hepatocellular carcinoma in humans. *Cancer Res* 1992; **52**: 2114S–2118S.

20 Ming L, Thorgeirsson S, Gail MH *et al.* Dominant role of hepatitis B virus and cofactor role of aflatoxin in hepatocarcinogenesis in Qidong, China. *Hepatology* 2002; **36**: 1214–1220.

21 Lok AS, Lai CL. (1988) Factors determining the development of hepatocellular carcinoma in hepatitis B surface antigen carriers. A comparison between families with clusters and solitary cases. *Cancer* 1998; **61**: 1287–1291.

22 de Franchis R, Meucci G, Vecchi M *et al.* The natural history of asymptomatic hepatitis B surface antigen carriers. *Ann Intern Med* 1993; **118**: 191–194.

23 Chang MH, Chen CJ, Lai MS *et al.* Universal hepatitis B vaccination in Taiwan and the incidence of hepatocellular carcinoma in children. *N Engl J Med* 1997; **336**: 1855–1859.

24 Colombo M. Hepatocellular carcinoma in cirrhotics. *Semin Liv Dis* 1993; **13**: 374–383.

25 Nakamura T, Nakamura S, Aikawa T *et al.* Obstruction of the inferior vena cava in the hepatic portion and the hepatic vein: report of eight cases and review of the Japanese literature. *Angiology* 1968; **19**: 479–498.

26 Kew MC, McKnight A, Hodkingson H *et al.* The role of membranous obstruction of the inferior vena cava in the etiology of hepatocellular carcinoma in Southern African Blacks. *Hepatology* 1989, **9**: 121–125.

27 Santagostino E, Colombo M, Rivi M *et al.* Six-month versus 12-month surveillance for hepatocellular carcinoma in 559 hemophiliacs infected with the hepatitis C virus. *Blood* 2003; **102**: 78–82.

28 Trinchet JC, Beaugrand M, Cooperative Groups GRETCH. A randomized trial comparing 3-month vs 6-month screening for HCC by ultrasonography in cirrhosis. *Proceedings of the ILCA First*

Annual Conference 2007, Barcelona 5–7 October 2007 2007; Abstract no. 23: 11.

29 Marrero JA, Lok AS. Newer markers for hepatocellular carcinoma. *Gastroenterology* 2004; **127**: S113–119.

30 Forner A, Vilana R, Ayuso C *et al.* Diagnosis of hepatic nodules 20 mm or smaller in cirrhosis: prospective validation of the non-invasive diagnostic criteria for hepatocellular carcinoma. *Hepatology* 2008; **47**, 97–104.

31 Marrero JA, Hussain HK, Nghiem HV *et al.* Improving the prediction of hepatocellular carcinoma in cirrhotic patients with an arterially-enhancing liver mass. *Liver Transplant* 2005; **11**: 281–289.

32 Stigliano R, Marelli L, Yu D *et al.* Seeding following percutaneous diagnostic and therapeutic approaches for hepatocellular carcinoma. What is the risk and the outcome? Seeding risk for percutaneous approach of HCC. *Cancer Treatment Reviews* 2007; **33**: 437–447.

33 Bolondi L, Gaiani S, Celli N *et al.* Characterization of small nodules in cirrhosis by assessment of vascularity: the problem of hypovascular hepatocellular carcinoma. *Hepatology* 2005; **42**: 27–34.

34 Llovet JM, Chen Y, Wurmbach E *et al.* A molecular signature to discriminate dysplastic nodules from early hepatocellular carcinoma in HCV cirrhosis. *Gastroenterology* 2006; **131**: 1758–1767.

35 Toyoda H, Kumada T, Kiriyama S *et al.* Impact of surveillance on survival of patients with initial hepatocellular carcinoma: a study from Japan. *Clin Gastroenterol Hepatol* 2006; **4**: 1170–1176.

36 Chalasani N, Said A, Ness R *et al.* Screening for hepatocellular carcinoma in patients with cirrhosis in the United States: results of a national survey. *Am J Gastroenterol* 1999; **94**: 2224–2229.

37 Heyward WL, Lanier AP, McMahon BJ *et al.* Early detection of primary hepatocellular carcinoma: screening for primary hepatocellular carcinoma among persons infected with hepatitis B virus. *JAMA* 1985; **254**: 3052–3054.

38 Zhang BH, Yang BH, Tang ZY. Randomized controlled trial of screening for hepatocellular carcinoma. *J Cancer Res Clin Oncol* 2004; **130**: 417–422.

39 Chie WC, Chang YH, Chen HH. A novel method for evaluation of improved survival trend for common cancer: early detection or improvement of medical care. *J Eval Clin Pract* 2007; **13**: 79–85.

40 Thompson Coon J, Rogers G, Hewson P *et al.* Surveillance of cirrhosis for hepatocellular carcinoma: systematic review and economic analysis. *Health Technol Assess* 2007; **11**: no. 34.

41 Andersson KL, Salomon JA, Chung RT *et al.* Cost-effectiveness of alternative surveillance strategies for hepatocellular carcinoma in patients with cirrhosis. *Clin Gastroenterol Hepatol* 2008; **6**(12): 1418–1424.

42 Mazzaferro V, Regalia E, Doci R *et al.* Liver transplantation for the treatment of small hepatocellular carcinomas in patients with cirrhosis. *N Engl J Med* 1996; **334**: 693–699.

43 Llovet JM, Bruix J, Fuster J *et al.* Liver transplantation for small hepatocellular carcinoma: the tumor-node-metastasis classification does not have prognostic power. *Hepatology* 1998; **27**: 1572–1577.

44 Bismuth H, Majno PE, Adam R. Liver transplantation for hepatocellular carcinoma. *Semin Liv Dis* 1999; **19**: 311–322.

45 Jonas S, Bechstein WO, Steinmüller T *et al.* Vascular invasion and histopathologic grading determine outcome after liver transplantation for hepatocellular carcinoma in cirrhosis. *Hepatology* 2001; **33**: 1080–1086.

46 Bruix J, Castells A, Bosch J *et al.* Surgical resection of hepatocellular carcinoma in cirrhotic patients: prognostic value of preoperative portal pressure. *Gastroenterology* 1996; **111**: 1018–1023.

47 Lencioni RA, Allgaier HP, Cioni D *et al.* Small hepatocellular carcinoma in cirrhosis: randomized comparison of radio-frequency thermal ablation versus percutaneous ethanol injection. *Radiology* 2003; **228**: 235–240.

48 Lin OS, Keeffe EB, Sanders GD *et al.* Cost-effectiveness of screening for hepatocellular carcinoma in patients with cirrhosis due to chronic hepatitis C. *Aliment Pharmacol Ther* 2004; **19**: 1159–1172.

49 Shiina S, Teratani T, Obi S *et al.* A randomized controlled trial of radiofrequency ablation with ethanol injection for small hepatocellular carcinoma. *Gastroenterology* 2005; **129**: 122–130.

50 Lin SM, Lin CJ, Lin CC *et al.* Randomised controlled trial comparing percutaneous radiofrequency thermal ablation, percutaneous ethanol injection, and percutaneous acetic acid injection to treat hepatocellular carcinoma of 3 cm or less. *Gut* 2005; **54**: 1151–1156.

51 Brunello F, Veltri A, Carucci P *et al.* Radiofrequency ablation versus ethanol injection for early hepatocellular carcinoma: A randomized controlled trial. *Scand J Gastroenterol* 2008; **43**: 727–735.

52 Nakashima O, Sugihara S, Kage M *et al.* Pathomorphologic characteristics of small hepatocellular carcinoma: a special reference to small hepatocellular carcinoma with indistinct margins. *Hepatology* 1995; **22**: 101–105.

53 Sala M, Llovet JM, Villana R *et al.* Initial response to percutaneous ablation predicts survival in patients with hepatocellular carcinoma. *Hepatology* 2004; **40**: 1352–1360.

54 Arii S, Yamaoka Y, Futagawa S *et al.* Results of surgical and nonsurgical treatment for small-sized hepatocellular carcinomas: a retrospective and nationwide survey in Japan. *Hepatology* 2000; **32**: 1224–1229.

55 Ohnishi K, Yoshioka H, Ito S *et al.* Prospective randomized controlled trial comparing percutaneous acetic acid injection and percutaneous ethanol injection for small hepatocellular carcinoma. *Hepatology* 1998; **27**: 67–72.

56 Tsai WL, Cheng JS, Lai KH *et al.* Clinical trial: percutaneous acetic acid injection vs percutaneous ethanol injection for small hepatocellular carcinoma – a long-term follow-up study. *Aliment Pharmacol Ther* 2008; **28**: 304–311.

57 Huo TI, Huang YH, Wu JC *et al.* Comparison of percutaneous acetic acid injection and percutaneous ethanol injection for hepatocellular carcinoma in cirrhotic patients: a prospective study. *Scand J Gastroenterol* 2003; **38**: 770–778.

58 Lin SM, Lin CJ, Lin CC *et al.* Randomised controlled trial comparing percutaneous radiofrequency thermal ablation, percutaneous ethanol injection, and percutaneous acetic acid injection to treat hepatocellular carcinoma of 3 cm or less. *Gut* 2005; **54**: 1151–1156.

59 Imamura H, Matsuyama Y, Tanaka E *et al.* Risk factors contributing to early and late phase intrahepatic recurrence of hepatocellular carcinoma after hepatectomy. *J Hepatol* 2003; **38**: 200–207.

60 Lee JS, Chu IS, Heo J *et al.* Classification and prediction of survival in hepatocellular carcinoma by gene expression profiling. *Hepatology* 2004; **40**: 667–676.

61 Yamashita T, Forgues M, Wang W *et al.* EpCAM and a-fetoprotein expression defines novel prognostic subtypes of hepatocellular carcinoma. *Cancer Res* 2008; **68**: 1451–1461.

62 Llovet JM, Bruix J. Novel advancements in the management of hepatocellular carcinoma in 2008. *J Hepatol* 2008; **48**: S20–37.

63 Decaens T, Roudot-Thoraval F, Hadni-Bresson S *et al.* Impact of UCSF criteria according to pre- and post-OLT tumor features: analysis of 479 patients listed for HCC with a short waiting time. *Liver Transpl* 2006; **12**: 1761–1769.

64 Cillo U, Vitale A, Bassanello M *et al.* Liver transplantation for the treatment of modearately of well-differentiated hepatocellular carcinoma. *Ann Surg* 2004; **239**: 150–159.

65 Mazzaferro V, Llovet JM, Miceli R *et al.* Metroticket Investigator Study Group Predicting survival after liver transplantation in patients with hepatocellular carcinoma beyond the Milan criteria: a retrospective, exploratory analysis. *Lancet Oncol* 2009; **10**: 35–43.

66 Llovet JM, Mas X, Aponte JJ *et al.* Cost-effectiveness of adjuvant therapy for hepatocellular carcinoma during the waiting list for liver transplantation. *Gut* 2002; **50**: 123–128.

67 Lesurtel M, Mullhaupt B, Pestalozzi BC *et al.* Transarterial chemoembolization as a bridge to liver transplantation for hepatocellular carcinoma: an evidence-based analysis. *Am J Transplant* 2006; **6**: 2644–2650.

68 Millonig G, Graziadei IW, Freund MC *et al.* Response to preoperative chemoembolization correlates with outcome after liver transplantation in patients with hepatocellular carcinoma. *Liver Transplant* 2007: **13**: 272–279.

69 Mazzaferro V, Battiston C, Perrone S *et al.* Radiofrequency ablation of small hepatocellular carcinoma in cirrhotic patients awaiting liver transplantation a prospective study. *Ann Surg* 2004; **240**: 900–909.

70 Llovet JM, Bruix J. Systematic review of randomized trials for unresectable hepatocellular carcinoma: chemoembolization improves survival. *Hepatology* 2003; **37**: 429–442.

71 Lin DY, Liaw YF, Lee TY *et al.* Hepatic arterial embolization in patients with unresectable hepatocellular carcinoma – a randomized controlled trial. *Gastroenterology* 1988; **94**: 453–456.

72 Groupe d'Etude et de Traitement du Carcinome Hépatocellulaire A comparison of lipiodol chemoembolization and conservative treatment for unresectable hepatocellular carcinoma. *N Engl J Med* 1995; **332**: 1256–1261.

73 Bruix J, Llovet JM, Castells A *et al.* Transarterial embolization versus symptomatic treatment in patients with advanced hepatocellular carcinoma: results of a randomized controlled trial in a single institution. *Hepatology* 1998; **27**: 1578–1583.

74 Pelletier G, Ducreux M, Gay F *et al.* Treatment of unresectable hepatocellular carcinoma with lipiodol chemoembolization: a multicenter randomized trial. *J Hepatol* 1998; **28**: 129–134.

75 Lo CM, Ngan H, Tso WK *et al.* Randomized controlled trial of transarterial lipiodol chemoembolization for unresectable hepatocellular carcinoma. *Hepatology* 2002; **35**: 1164–1171.

76 Llovet JM, Real MI, Montana X *et al.* Arterial embolisation or chemoembolization versus symptomatic treatment in patients with unresectable hepatocellular carcinoma: a randomised controlled trial. *Lancet* 2002; **359**: 1734–1739.

77 Marelli L, Stigliano R, Triantos C *et al.* Transarterial therapy for hepatocellular carcinoma: which technique is more effective? A systematic review of cohort and randomized studies. *Cardiovasc Intervent Radiol* 2007; **30**: 6–25.

78 Varela M, Real MI, Burrel M *et al.* Chemoembolization of hepatocellular carcinoma with drug eluting beads: efficacy and doxorubicin pharmacokinetics. *J Hepatol* 2007; **46**: 474–481.

79 Raoul JL, Guyader D, Bretagne JF *et al.* Prospective randomized trial of chemoembolization versus intra-arterial injection of 131I-labeled-iodized oil in the treatment of hepatocellular carcinoma. *Hepatology* 1997; **26**: 1156–1161.

80 Kulik LM, Carr BI, Mulcahy MF *et al.* Safety and efficacy of 90Y radiotherapy for hepatocellular carcinoma with and without portal vein thrombosis. *Hepatology* 2008; **47**: 71–81.

81 Abou-Alfa GK, Schwartz L, Ricci S *et al.* Phase II study of sorafenib in patients with advanced hepatocellular carcinoma. *J Clin Oncol* 2006; **24**: 4293–4300.

82 Llovet J, Ricci S, Mazzaferro V *et al.* Sorafenib in advanced hepatocellular carcinoma. *N Engl J Med* 2008; **359**: 378–390.

83 Cheng A, Kang Y, Chen C *et al.* Efficacy and safety of sorafenib in patients in the Asia-Pacific region with advanced hepatocellular carcinoma: a phase III randomised, double-blind, placebo-controlled trial. *Lancet Oncol* 2009; **10**(1): 25–34.

84 Ringe B, Pichlmayr R, Wittekind C *et al.* Surgical treatment of hepatocellular carcinoma: experience with liver resection and transplantation in 198 patients. *World J Surg* 1991; **15**: 270–285.

85 Iwatsuki S, Starzl TE, Sheahan DG *et al.* Hepatic resection versus transplantation for hepatocellular carcinoma. *Ann Surg* 1991; **214**: 221–229.

41 Fulminant hepatic failure: Treatment

James O'Beirne[1], Nicholas Murphy[2] and Julia Wendon[3]

[1] Royal Free Hospital, London, UK
[2] Queen Elizabeth Hospital (Birmingham), Birmingham, UK
[3] Liver Intensive Care, King's College Hospital, London, UK

Introduction

Intensive care medicine has developed as a specialty over the last 50 years since the introduction of positive pressure ventilation. Major growth in the size and scope of the specialty has occurred in the last few decades in response to the need to support failing organ systems in critically ill patients and many new techniques and methods have been introduced into routine practice. However, due to the relatively small numbers and heterogeneity of patients and conditions in single centers, the majority of methods used have been introduced without the evidence of benefit from controlled clinical trials.

The same problems have hindered the development of an evidence base for the management of fulminant liver failure and much of the current management of this condition has derived from current practice in general and neuro-intensive care. Recently, the development of collaborative groups in the USA and Europe has lead to the performance of multicenter randomized trials specifically designed to address the major deficiencies in the current evidence base.

The management of fulminant hepatic failure can be split into two main headings: (1) general supportive care and (2) therapies aimed at managing the failing liver and its complications.

Definition

In 1970 Trey and Davidson introduced the term fulminant hepatic failure (FHF) to describe a syndrome of rapidly progressing liver failure in which encephalopathy follows the onset of symptoms within eight weeks in someone without previous liver disease [1]. This definition is still used today; however, it has become clear that this definition is too broad and that subgroups exist. Both etiology and speed of progression to encephalopathy from the onset of jaundice can be used to define subgroups. This is important, as both factors have been shown to be independent predictors of prognosis (Figure 41.1) [2]. Interestingly, it is the hyperacute group that have the best chance for spontaneous recovery, although it also carries the highest risk of cerebral edema [2, 3].

Etiology

FHF has many causes, worldwide, viral hepatitis is by far the most common cause. Within the UK, paracetamol (acetaminophen) self-poisoning has been the most frequent cause of FHF over the last fifteen years. However, recent epidemiological data from the major UK liver units suggest that the incidence of paracetamol induced FHF is falling. In 1998 legislation was introduced in the UK limiting the amount of paracetamol that could be sold over the counter. This appears to have reduced the morbidity and mortality associated with paracetamol self-poisoning [4], more so the most serious paracetamol self-poisoning. However, this effect has not been noticed in all areas of the country and some studies have shown no effect of legislation on the incidence and outcome of paracetamol poisoning [5, 6].

The reduction in presentation following paracetamol hepatotoxicity in the UK is at odds with recent data from the USA. Once thought to be a rare cause of FHF in the USA, recent data show an increasing incidence of paracetamol hepatotoxicity, which now accounts for 42% of all cases of FHF prospectively reported to the US Acute Liver Failure Study Group [7]. Within this cohort the majority of cases were unintentional overdoses. In both the UK and the USA the second most common cause of FHF is seronegative or FHF of indeterminate cause [8]. Despite intensive

Evidence-Based Gastroenterology and Hepatology, 3rd edition.
J. McDonald, A.K. Burroughs, B. Feagan, and M.B. Fennerty. © 2010 Blackwell Publishing Ltd

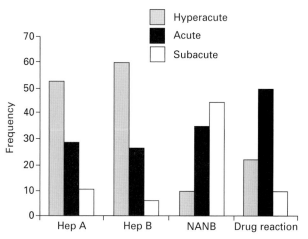

Figure 41.1 Speed of onset according to etiology (note that the majority of paracetamol poisoning would appear in the hyperacute group [2].

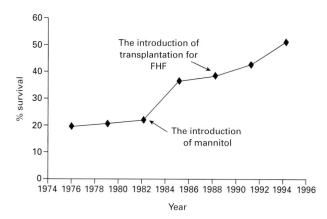

Figure 41.2 Improving survival in FHF.

research in this area the etiology or etiologies in this group, as the name suggests, remain unknown.

Pathogenesis

FHF is not a disease but a syndrome, with a severity proportional to the degree of hepatic necrosis and the degree of the systemic response to this injury. FHF causes profound physiological derangement, characterized by encephalopathy, vasoparesis [9], and coagulopathy. As the syndrome progresses, cerebral edema [10] and renal failure are prominent and there is impaired immunity, with increased susceptibility to infection and subsequent multiple organ failure [11].

The rate of progression of FHF can be unpredictable in the hyperacute group. The syndrome typically evolves over several days, but deep coma can occur within hours. The mainstay of treatment in FHF is supportive while the decision to proceed to hepatic transplantation is being considered.

The cause of death in FHF can be split into two main groups; those with cerebral edema who die of brain ischemia or brain stem herniation, and those who succumb to sepsis and multiple organ failure. In a recent study of FHF patients listed for transplantation the major cause of death was multiple organ failure, with only 5% of patients succumbing to death directly related to intracranial hypertension [12]. This is at variance with previous surveys of cause of death in ALF, which showed a much higher incidence of cerebral deaths [13]. The reasons for this change are not clear, but better general ICU care and specifically the use of osmotherapy are likely to have been responsible for this change.

Intensive care management versus ward management

There have been no controlled clinical trials comparing intensive care with ward management, but considering the almost 100% mortality before the adoption of modern intensive care units, it seems likely that intensive care management reduces mortality [14]. Patients with grade III and IV encephalopathy should be intubated, ventilated and managed within an intensive care unit. The use of high-dependency areas for patients with liver failure and lower levels of coma is to be encouraged [15].

Management in a liver unit

Survival rates for FHF have increased markedly since the introduction of liver transplantation as a therapeutic modality for patients predicted to have a low rate of survival with medical management alone. Survival rates for FHF with medical therapy alone in cases that progress to grade III or IV encephalopathy are poor, varying between 10 and 40% depending on etiology. With the introduction of orthotopic liver transplantation (OLT) as a therapeutic option for patients with FHF, survival rates have increased to 80% at one year [16], and although not subjected to a randomized controlled trial it stands to reason, therefore, that the optimal management of patients with FHF should occur in liver units with ready access to a liver transplant program (see Figure 41.2).

FHF is a rare syndrome which can evolve rapidly; it is therefore crucial that patients predicted to have a severe course are identified early to allow safe and timely transfer to a liver unit. Criteria have therefore been developed to help advise peripheral hospitals when patients with FHF should be transferred to a liver unit (see Box 41.1) [17]. These criteria are based on clinical judgment and have not been subjected to a controlled clinical trial.

General supportive management

Fluid resuscitation and circulatory management

Patients with FHF develop marked hemodynamic changes. Vasodilatation can be profound and is invariably accompanied by a compensatory increase in cardiac output [18]. This distributive shock, with relative hypovolemia, causes hypotension despite the increased cardiac output. Prognostic criteria such as acidosis, serum lactate and renal function should therefore only be assessed following adequate resuscitation, as there can be marked improvement in these following fluids.

The choice of resuscitation fluid in FHF is not clear. As yet there have been no randomized studies performed to specifically address this question. Colloid solutions provide greater volume expansion for a given volume transfused compared to crystalloids and were traditionally favored for resuscitation in critically ill patients until the publication of a meta-analysis of 30 randomized controlled trials in 1998, which suggested that albumin may increase mortality [19]. This publication led to a change in practice in many centers, although the methodology of the review was heavily criticized. A large randomized controlled clinical trial has since been performed in 7000 patients, comparing 4% human albumin solution and normal saline for the resuscitation of critically ill patients. This study found no difference in the primary endpoint of mortality between albumin and saline, but in subgroup analysis there was an increase in mortality in brain-injured patients receiving albumin, which needs to be subjected to further study [20]. **A1a** Despite the apparent safety of albumin, it is clear that its use has declined as a resuscitation fluid, with only 7% of units in a large European survey using albumin for resuscitation [21]. In practice, most patients will receive a mixture of colloid and crystalloid for resuscitation and no clear evidence-based recommendation can be given as to which crystalloid or colloid is appropriate in FHF patients. Balanced salt solutions are associated with less risk of hyperchloremia, may have an advantage over saline and are recommended for patients undergoing surgery. Recent data suggests that starch-based colloids may increase the incidence of renal failure and need for renal replacement therapy, especially with increasing doses and it would seem logical to limit the use of this colloid [22].

The hemodynamic changes associated with FHF are fairly predictable. As stated above, profound systemic vasodilatation is followed by a compensatory increase in cardiac output. Blood pressure is often low despite aggressive fluid resuscitation. Endpoints in resuscitation are difficult to define and so the use of some sort of monitor of both cardiac preload and cardiac output can be used to observe response to interventions. There is little evidence to suggest any technique is superior to any other and so local experience should dictate which techniques are used. The use of static measures of preload and therefore adequacy of resuscitation, such as central venous pressure (CVP) and pulmonary artery occlusion pressure (PAOP) can be unreliable and are better supplemented by dynamic measurements, which are better at predicting the response to volume resuscitation in the critically ill. Measurement of stroke volume variation (SVV), pulse pressure variation (PPV) and even the cardiac output response to passive leg raising have all been found to be useful in predicting the response to transfused volume [23–25].

Despite 20 years of clinical trials, the role of the pulmonary artery catheter (PAC) in the management of the critically ill patient is still not settled and remains controversial. In 1996 Connors found in a retrospective case control study that the use of PAC in the initial management of critically ill patients during the first 24 hours appeared to increase mortality and costs [26]. Since that study, two randomized trials examining the clinical utility of PAC have been published. The first study (PAC-Man) reported the outcome of critically ill patients randomized to management with a PAC or no PAC/other cardiac output monitor. There were no differences in hospital mortality between the groups and the conclusion of the study was that PAC did not affect survival in critically ill patients. However, in the PAC group there was a 10% incidence of non-fatal complications [27]. **A1d** In a *post hoc* analysis of the same study, no difference could be found between PAC and other forms of cardiac output monitoring: suggesting that this form of invasive hemodynamic monitoring was either ineffective or that the information produced was not being interpreted correctly [28]. The use of PAC within a rigid treatment algorithim was examined in a recent randomized trial in patients with acute lung injury. In this randomized study of 1000 patients, the role of PAC compared to a central venous catheter within a fluid liberal or conservative management strategy was assessed. No overall mortality difference was seen in any of the groups and in particular no benefit of PAC insertion was seen [29]. **A1c** Taken together, data from these trials suggest that the PAC has no role in the routine management of critically ill patients and the decision to insert a PAC must be made on a case-by-case basis.

During the early 1970s, it was first suggested that during critical illness a pathological supply-dependency line is seen (see Figure 41.2) [30]. This was proposed because of markedly increased resting oxygen consumption noted in critical illness associated with systemic inflammation. Oxygen delivery increases to meet the demand and it was noted that survivors had higher oxygen transport parameters than non-survivors did. It was also noted that if oxygen delivery was increased, by fluid resuscitation and/or inotropic drugs, oxygen consumption increased as well, suggesting that covert tissue hypoxia exists and that this may be the cause of multiple organ failure.

Work by Bihari and Gimson in the 1980s suggested the presence of a pathological supply-dependency for oxygen in patients with FHF. The patients with FHF who failed to survive had both a lower baseline VO_2 than survivors and greater increases in VO_2 following infusion of epoprosternol, suggesting a greater oxygen debt [18]. However, since then the whole premise of this argument, that there exists a pathological supply dependency in critical illness, has been questioned because of the inevitable increase in calculated oxygen consumption when delivery is increased due to mathematical coupling [31]. Furthermore, it is clear that not all patients with critical illness have pathological oxygen supply dependency. Early studies evaluating the use of strategies to increase oxygen delivery to supranormal levels in an attempt to decrease organ failure did not succeed and in some reports were actually harmful [32]. From other studies done earlier in the course of septic shock, however, it appears that the early (i.e. less than six hours) institution of a protocol to increase oxygen delivery reduces mortality [33]. The interpretation of the above data with relevance to FHF must be cautious. However, given the similarities between FHF and septic shock it would seem reasonable to assume that early vigorous volume resuscitation is appropriate, but routine targeting of supranormal oxygen delivery should be avoided.

Adrenaline and noradrenaline are effective agents and are frequently employed to improve MAP in FHF, commencing at 0.1 μg/kg/min. Both of these agents have been shown to improve MAP, significantly the addition of epoprosternol (a microcirculatory vasodilator) to noradrenaline increases oxygen delivery while maintaining MAP [34]. Epinephrine, like other beta agonists has deleterious effects on intermediary metabolism if used over a period of time. These effects include hyperlactemia and hyperglycemia. This is related partly to the effect of epinephrine on glycolysis within skeletal muscles [35]. Norepinephrine does not have these effects and so is recommended on current evidence.

Blood pressure is important in maintaining flow to essential organs. What pressure is acceptable in FHF is unknown. However, cerebral autoregulation is disturbed in FHF, making cerebral blood flow directly proportional to cerebral perfusion pressure [36]. This implies that hypotension will result in cerebral ischemia, which may be a factor precipitating brain swelling in FHF [37], and that hypertension will result in cerebral hyperemia and increased ICP. Although, as discussed later, targeting a specific blood pressure to maintain cerebral perfusion in the face of cerebral edema is often futile and probably unnecessary [38]. **B4**

Alternatives to norepinephrine or epinephrine to maintain blood pressure, such as terlipressin or vasopressin, have not been systematically evaluated in FHF. Terlipressin is widely used in patients with chronic liver disease and hepatorenal syndrome and has been used in cathecholamine refractory septic shock [39–41]. Whilst it is evident that terlipressin is effective at reducing the need for cathecholamines in septic shock states its use in patients with FHF may be compromised by its effects on cerebral blood flow and intracranial pressure. Shawcross et al. showed in a small study of six FHF patients with grade 4 encephalopathy, that a single dose of terlipressin (0.25 mg) caused a significant increase in cerebral blood flow (CBF) from a median of 69 (range 48–83) ml/100 g/min to 81 (range 62–97) ml/100 g/min (p = 0.016) accompanied by a significant increase in intracranial pressure (ICP) from a median of 15 mmHg (13–18) to 20 mmHg (16–23), which was sustained for three hours post terlipressin administration. There was no significant change in systemic hemodynamincs to explain these findings and the authors hypothesized that terlipressin affected CBF via an interaction with cerebral V2 receptors [42]. In a separate study, the effect of terlipressin (1 mg bolus) was examined in ten patients with FHF. The effects on intracranial pressure, cerebral blood flow and cerebral perfusion pressure were compared to norepinephrine. Surprisingly, given the findings of the previous study, the authors found that a 1 mg dose of terlipressin did not increase ICP or CBF despite increasing cerebral perfusion pressure (CPP) through increases in mean arterial pressure. **B4** When the effect of increasing the rate of norepinephrine infusion was studied, there were significant increases in both CBF and ICP. The findings of this study show that terlipressin can increase CPP without increasing CBF, suggesting that terlipressin restored cerebral blood flow autoregulation through an unknown mechanism [43]. The reason for these disparate findings is not clear and highlights the need for further studies in this area.

Mechanical ventilation

Intubation of the trachea and mechanical ventilation is indicated for several reasons in FHF but not usually for hypoxemia [18]. As patients progress from grade II to grade III encephalopathy, decreasing consciousness can lead to airway compromise with the risk of aspiration. Grade III encephalopathy is often characterized by agitation and aggressive behaviour. Sedation in these patients is required to allow appropriate monitoring and treatment, but requires intubation and ventilation. In patients at risk of intracranial hypertension it is common practice to target a partial pressure of CO_2 of between 4 and 5 kPA; this minimizes the risk of increased cerebral blood flow due to increases in CO_2. Controlled trials have shown there to be no benefit from routine hyperventilation in FHF in terms of prevention of intracranial hypertension [44]. **A1d**

As opposed to other causes of systemic inflammatory response syndrome, the lungs are *relatively* spared early in the course of FHF. However, a proportion of patients progress to multiple organ dysfunction in which lung disease is prominent [45].

The normal lung can tolerate "conventional" ventilation with physiological tidal volumes and low levels of positive end expiratory pressure (PEEP) for extended periods without apparent harm. The situation is different for damaged lungs and particularly so in patients with acute respiratory distress syndrome (ARDS). There is increasing evidence that mechanical ventilation in the setting of ARDS can increase lung injury and negatively impinge on outcome. Ventilator induced lung injury (VILI) encompasses a wide spectrum of damage, consisting of conventional barotrauma, pneumothorax, pneumomediastinum and alveolar damage, and increasing pulmonary edema [46]. Recent controlled clinical trials have shown improvements in mortality with a protective ventilatory strategy [47, 48]. **A1d** A recent consensus conference has recommended certain steps to minimize damage to the lungs during mechanical ventilation [49]. **A1c**

• Minimize the inspired oxygen level and take aggressive steps to do this if the inspired fraction is greater than 0.65.
• Recruit alveoli by increasing PEEP. The amount of PEEP necessary to prevent cyclic opening and closure of alveoli is approximately 10–15 cmH$_2$O.
• Minimize high airway pressures. Transalveolar pressures should not exceed 25–30 cmH$_2$O. This corresponds to an end inspiratory static (plateau) pressure of 30–40 cmH$_2$O.
• Prevent atelectasis by employing larger breaths periodically to re-expand collapsed units during tidal ventilation with small tidal volumes.

Patients who spontaneously recover from FHF or who are transplanted may need mechanical ventilation for a prolonged period of time and often require tracheostomy to facilitate weaning from the ventilator. A recent prospective study has shown that the percutaneous approach is safe in patients with liver disease, even with refractory coagulopathy and should be the method of choice [50]. **B4**

Sedation and paralysis

Patients with acute hepatic failure requiring mechanical ventilation are deeply encephalopathic. The need for sedation varies between patients and should be tailored individually, the primary aim being relief from pain and tolerance of the ICU environment and interventions. Mechanical ventilation is usually tolerated with minimum amounts of opiate and little if any hypnotic agent. The effect of sedation should be continuously evaluated to ensure that aims are achieved and over sedation avoided, although it should be noted that scoring systems, for example the six-point Ramsay scale have not been validated in FHF and are difficult to interpret in the setting of hepatic encephalopathy [51]. Deep sedation is unnecessary and will only add to cardiovascular depression and prolong recovery in patients with impaired liver function. There are no randomized data to support the use of one sedative agent over another in the routine management of FHF, but Propofol may have some advantage over benzodiazeopines as it has been used to reduce ICP in brain-injured patients and may reduce cerebral blood flow through the reduction in cerebral metabolic rate for oxygen [52, 53]. These considerations, however, have to be contrasted with the need to prevent surges in intracranial pressure during routine nursing care; supplemental sedation or small doses of nondepolarizing neuromuscular blocker may be useful during suctioning of the patient's trachea.

The issue of paralysis in FHF should be considered. It had been common practice to paralyze all ventilated patients with FHF whilst at risk from cerebral edema. However, there have not been any controlled clinical trials comparing paralysis or not in FHF, and, for that matter, in any other branch of intensive care medicine. A recent retrospective review of 1030 patients with acute traumatic brain injury showed that ICU stay and infectious complications were higher in the group who received routine paralysis [54]. **B4** Anecdotal reports have also suggested an association between long-term paralysis and a necrotizing myopathy, in patients with asthma, that may prolong ICU stay and impinge adversely on outcome [55]. Thus, there is no indication for routine paralysis in FHF. **B4**

Nutrition in FHF

There are no randomized trials concerning nutrition in FHF, but in common with other critical illnesses FHF is characterized by increased energy requirements and given that the majority of patients will be sedated and ventilated, this energy must come from supplemental feeding [56]. Initially, the majority of FHF patients will be fed nasogastrically with standard enteral formulae as per international guidelines [57]. **A1c** The enteral route, if available, is always superior to the parenteral route, assuming that adequate feed can be given. There is no difference between gastric and post-duodenal feeding in terms of adequacy of feeding or infectious complications and therefore, if tolerated, nasogastric feeding is appropriate [58, 59]. In patients who fail gastric feeding and have residual feed volumes, consideration can be given to prokinetic agents, such as metoclopramide or erythromycin. These drugs are highly effective at stimulating gastric motility and reducing nasogastric aspirates, but the effect can be short-lived and placement of feeding tubes beyond the pylorus is often required [60]. Feeding should be instituted within 24 hours of admission to the intensive care unit and in the initial phases of the illness should be no more than 20–25 kcal/Kg BW/day increasing to 25–30 kcal/Kg BW/day in the recovery phase [57]. **A1c** Despite a theoretical risk of worsening encephalopathy in FHF, due to the administration of protein, there is no data to support routine protein restriction. In practice, most patients will tolerate protein intake of 1–1.5 g/kg/day without complication. Renal failure is a common complication of FHF and the majority of patients will require renal replacement therapy (RRT) during the course of the illness. RRT can cause reductions in important trace elements and vitamins such as copper, selenium, thiamine and vitamin E, and therefore consideration should be given to trace element and vitamin supplementation during FHF, especially if complicated by renal failure requiring RRT [61]. Some vitamins such as vitamin C and vitamin E have important antioxidant properties and supplementation with these vitamins has been studied in general critical care populations with some benefits [62, 63]. The use of immuno nutrition (feeds supplemented by compounds such as arginine, glutamine and fish oil) has not been studied in FHF. Individual trials have shown benefit in some subsets of critical care patients and glutamine supplementation is considered a standard of care in parenterally fed patients [64]. **B4** Further studies are needed in this area, particularly in relation to FHF.

Hypoglycemia is a feature of advanced liver failure due to lack of gluconeogenesis from the failing liver. Whilst it is not uncommon for FHF patients to require administration of glucose containing solutions to maintain blood glucose levels, many patients will need insulin to control elevated blood glucose levels. In 2001, Van den Berghe reported a reduction in mortality in surgical ICU patients treated with intensive insulin therapy to maintain blood glucose levels between 4.4 and 6.1 mmol/l [65]. This approach has not been evaluated in FHF patients and there is concern that such tight glycemic control may predispose to adverse events related to hypoglycemia. A larger study has recently been published concerning blood glucose levels in critically ill patients. This study actually showed a significantly increased mortality in patients with tight glucose control compared to a more liberal regimen [66]. **A1c**

Stress ulcer prophylaxis

Many small randomized controlled clinical trials over the past 20 years have looked at the prevention of stress ulceration. While the incidence of stress ulcer has fallen over this period, the cause of this decline is unclear. It is probably the result of both improved resuscitation and the widespread use of stress ulcer prophylaxis. The most recent large study estimates the incidence of clinically important stress ulcer bleeding to be about 3% in general ICU patients [67].

Stress ulceration is probably the result of ischemic injury to the gastric mucosa, and adequate resuscitation is the single most important factor in its prevention. Apart from good general ICU care, there have been two broad approaches to reducing the incidence of stress ulceration: decreasing the acidity of the stomach with the use of antacids, H$_2$-blockers, or proton pump inhibitors; and the use of sucralfate, a cytoprotective agent. The role of acid suppression in encouraging an increase in bacterial overgrowth and the ensuing micro-aspiration of colonized pharyngeal fluid, thus promoting the development of hospital-acquired pneumonia, has led to the comparison of the ulcer, pneumonia and mortality rates between the two methods.

Recently, several meta-analyses have attempted to resolve the uncertainty regarding efficacy on one hand and adverse effects of the drugs on the other [68, 69]. After combining their efforts, the two main groups of investigators published a meta-analysis which included all relevant published and unpublished randomized clinical trials [70]. The meta-analysis demonstrated similar efficacy for H$_2$-blockers and sucralfate for the outcome of reduction in stress ulceration bleeding, but an increase in the incidence of pneumonia and an excess mortality in the H$_2$-blocker group. **A1a** A more recent trial conducted by some of the same authors suggests a significantly higher rate of stress ulceration with sucralfate compared to ranitidine, without any difference in pneumonia or mortality rates [70]. **A1d**

The aim of stress ulcer prophylaxis is to increase the pH of the gastric lumen and therefore reduce acid related damage. Therefore, it would seem logical that proton pump inhibitors would be more efficacious in preventing bleeding. In randomized controlled trials proton pump inhibitors appear to cause more durable increases in gastric pH, but evidence that they are more effective in preventing clinically significant GI bleeding than H$_2$ receptor antagonists is lacking, although adverse events were similar between groups [71, 72]. **A1c**

FHF was excluded in most of the trials comparing sucralfate to pH-altering drugs and was not included in the meta-analysis. It is therefore difficult to make firm conclusions. Patients with FHF tend to fall into the high-risk group by virtue of both being ventilated and having a coagulopathy.

The balance of evidence suggests that pH-altering drugs such as H$_2$-blockers or proton pump inhibitors provide the best defense against stress ulceration, but that this may be offset by an increased incidence of pneumonia. Current guidelines on the management of septic shock advise the use of either H$_2$ RA or proton pump inhibitors for the prevention of bleeding and it would appear reasonable to extrapolate this guidance to patients with FHF [73]. **B4**

Infection, prophylactic antibiotics and selective decontamination of the digestive tract

Patients with FHF are prone to infection. Early studies of FHF patients reported an incidence of bacterially proven infection in 80% of patients and fungal infection in 30% [11]. Initial analysis of isolates from infected FHF patients showed that the most frequently cultured organism was coagulase negative staphylococcal species [74]. However, it is clear from more recent studies that the epidemiology of infection in FHF patients has changed. In a recent retrospective review of over 200 patients with FHF Karvellas *et al.* have reported that whilst 34% of patients will at some point develop bacteremia during ICU admission, this occurred later in the course of the illness (median time to bacteremia ten days) than in the original studies. Moreover, the most frequently cultured organisms were Gram-negative organisms such as *E. Faecium*, *Klebsiella* spp. and Vancomycin resistant enterococcus [75]. The underlying reasons for this change in epidemiology are not clear, but the widespread use of prophylactic antibiotics in patients with advanced liver failure must have an impact on the timing of the development of infection and the prevalence of resistant strains such as *Acinetobacter* spp.

The predisposition to infection displayed by FHF patients is multifactorial. These patients often have multiple vascular access devices and may undergo prolonged ventilation and renal replacement therapy, all of which are well-known risk factors for the development of bacteremias in the critically ill [75, 76]. In addition to risk factors related to interventions, patients with FHF also appear to have important immunological defects which predispose to infection and have a prognostic importance. Neutrophils from patients with FHF have been shown to be deficient in killing and phagocytic ability; defects which are reversed *in vitro* by the administration of G-CSF [77, 78]. Recently, Antoniades *et al.* have characterized the function of monocytes from patients with acetaminophen induced liver failure. Monocytes are important orchestrators of the immune response, (and) have a critical role in protection from infection and show marked deactivation in patients with FHF from acetaminophen [79]. In particular, the density of surface HLA-DR on monocytes was shown to have prognostic ability in reference to acetaminophen induced FHF patients [80].

Inflammation induced by infection also appears to impact upon the severity of hepatic encephalopathy. The presence of components of the systmemic inflammatory response syndrome (SIRS) appears to predict the severity of HE. The mechanism for this interaction is incompletely understood but it appears to be due to increased cerebral blood flow [81].

Because of the high incidence of infection and the underlying immunological defects in FHF, the use of prophylactic antimicrobial agents has been investigated. Both parenteral antibiotics and the use of selective decontamination of the digestive tract (SDD), in combination and individually, have been studied.

Intravenous antibiotics, if given prophylactically will reduce the incidence of infection in patients with FHF to approximately 20% [82, 83]. **B4** However, the use of prophylactic antibiotics has not been shown to improve outcome or reduce the length of stay in patients with FHF [83]. The role of SDD is less clear and has not been evaluated in controlled trials compared with placebo or intravenous antibiotics alone in FHF. Rolando reported that SDD used in combination with intravenous antibiotics provided no additional benefit [82–84]. **B4**

The most recent systematic review of randomized controlled trials of antibiotic prophylaxis in intensive care units was published in the Cochrane database of systematic reviews [85]. This systematic review evaluated 32 RCTs, which included 5639 unselected general ICU patients. Selected groups, for example patients with FHF, were excluded from the review. Pooled estimates of the 16 RCTs testing the effect of the SDD and systemic antibiotic combination indicate a significant reduction of both respiratory tract infections (OR 0.35; 95% CI: 0.29–0.41) and total mortality (OR 0.80; 95% CI: 0.68–0.93) (Figure 41.3). **A1a** The number needed to treat to prevent one infection is five, and the NNT to prevent one death is 23. When the data on the effect of SDD alone compared to control were pooled from the 16 available trials, a marked reduction in respiratory tract infections was demonstrated (OR 0.56; 95% CI: 0.46–0.68) but no corresponding effect on overall mortality (OR 1.01; 95% CI: 0.84–1.22) was found (Figure 41.4).

Although prophylactic intravenous antibiotics have been shown to reduce the number of proven infections in FHF, improvements in outcome have not been demonstrated. SDD on its own has not been shown to reduce infection or improve outcome in FHF. **B4** There is also a risk of promoting the emergence of multiply resistant organisms within intensive care units by the blanket use of broad spectrum antimicrobials. SDD selects for an increase in Gram-positive organisms, especially methicillin resistant staphylococcus (MRSA) and vancomycin resistant enterococcus (VRE). In a large single center randomized trial the use of SDD was not associated with the development of resistant strains such as VRE and MRSA. However, a follow-up study

Antibiotics for preventing respiratory tract infection in adults receiving intensive care
Comparison: topical plus systemic vs no prophylaxis
Outcome: RTIs

Study	Expl n/N	Ctrl n/N	Peto OR (95% CI fixed)	Weight (%)	Peto OR (95% CI fixed)
Abele-Horn	13/58	23/30		3·9	0·11 (0·04 to 0·27)
Aerdts	1/28	29/60		3·5	0·14 (0·05 to 0·36)
Blair	12/161	38/170		8·5	0·31 (0·17 to 0·57)
Boland	14/32	17/32		3·3	0·69 (0·26 to 1·83)
Cockerill	4/75	12/75		2·9	0·33 (0·12 to 0·92)
Finch	4/20	7/24		1·7	0·62 (0·16 to 2·40)
Jacobs 1	0/45	4/46		0·8	0·13 (0·02 to 0·95)
Kerver	5/49	31/47		4·6	0·09 (0·04 to 0·22)
Palomar	10/50	25/49		4·6	0·26 (0·11 to 0·59)
Rocha	7/47	25/54		4·4	0·24 (0·10 to 0·55)
Sanchez-Garcia	32/131	60/140		12·2	0·44 (0·27 to 0·73)
Stoutenbeek 2	61/202	99/200		19·4	0·45 (0·30 to 0·67)
Ulrich	7/55	26/57		4·7	0·21 (0·09 to 0·47)
Verwaest a	22/193	40/185		10·4	0·48 (0·28 to 0·82)
Verwaest b	31/200	40/185		11·6	0·67 (0·40 to 1·12)
Winter	3/91	17/92		3·6	0·21 (0·08 to 0·54)
Total (95% CI)	226/1437	493/1446		100·0	0·35 (0·29 to 0·41)

Chi-square 37·10 (df = 15) Z = 11·88

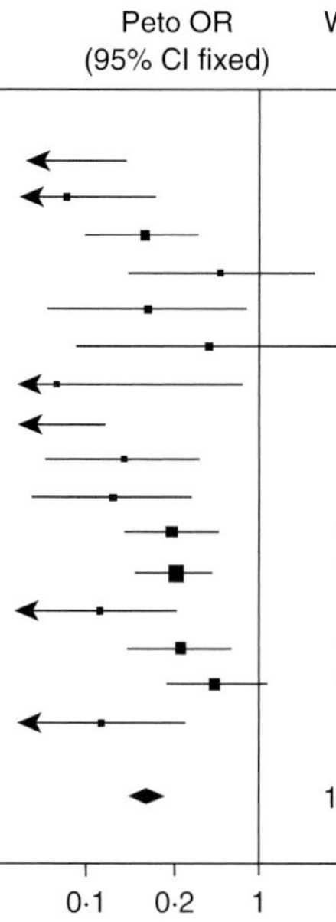

(a)   0·1   0·2   1   5   10

Review: antibiotics for preventing respiratory tract infection in adults receiving intensive care
Comparison: topical plus systemic vs no prophylaxis
Outcome: overall mortality

Study	Expl n/N	Ctrl n/N	Peto OR (95% CI Fixed)	Weight (%)	Peto OR (95% CI Fixed)
RCTs with individual patient data available					
Aerdts	4/28	12/60		1·8	0·68 (0·22 to 2·17)
Blair	24/161	32/170		7·3	0·76 (0·43 to 1·34)
Boland	2/32	4/32		0·9	0·48 (0·09 to 2·57)
Cockerill	11/75	16/75		3·5	0·64 (0·28 to 1·46)
Finch	15/24	10/25		2·0	2·42 (0·80 to 7·32)
Palomar	14/50	14/49		3·2	0·97 (0·41 to 2·32)
Rocha	27/74	40/77		5·9	0·54 (0·28 to 1·02)
Sanchez-Garcia	51/131	65/140		10·4	0·74 (0·46 to 1·19)
Stoutenbeek 2	42/201	44/200		10·6	0·94 (0·58 to 1·51)
Ulrich	22/55	33/57		4·4	0·49 (0·24 to 1·03)
Verwaest a	47/220	40/220		10·9	1·22 (0·76 to 1·95)
Verwaest b	45/220	40/220		10·7	1·16 (0·72 to 1·86)
Winter	33/91	40/92		6·9	0·74 (0·41 to 1·34)
Subtotal (95% CI)	337/1362	390/1417		78·3	0·86 (0·72 to 1·02)
Chi-square 13·41 (df = 12) Z = 1·75					
RCTs with individual patient data not available					
Jacobs 1	14/45	23/46		3·5	0·46 (0·20 to 1·06)
Kerver	14/49	15/47		3·2	0·85 (0·36 to 2·03)
Lenhart	52/265	75/262		15·1	0·61 (0·41 to 0·91)
Subtotal (95% CI)	80/359	113/355		21·7	0·61 (0·44 to 0·86)
Chi-square 1·02 (df = 2) Z = 2·87					
Total (95% CI)	417/1721	503/1772		100·0	0·80 (0·68 to 0·93)

Chi-square 17·41 (df = 15) Z = 2·88

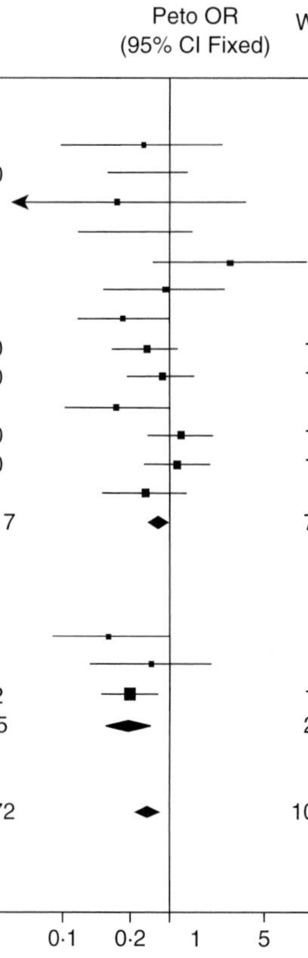

(b)   0·1   0·2   1   5   10

Figure 41.3 (a) and (b) Antibiotics for preventing respiratory tract infections (source: (Cochrane Review). In: *The Cochrane Library*, issue 2, 1999. Oxford: Update Software).

Review: antibiotics for preventing respiratory tract infection in adults receiving intensive care
Comparison: topical vs control
Outcome: RTIs

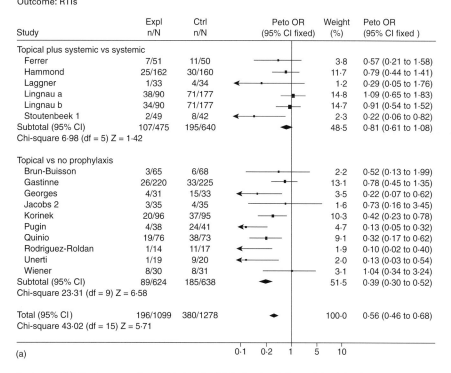

(a)

Review: antibiotics for preventing respiratory tract infection in adults receiving intensive care
Comparison: topical vs control
Outcome: overall mortality

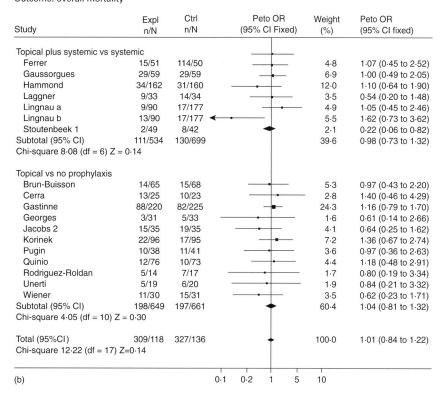

(b)

Figure 41.4 (a) and (b) Antibiotics for preventing respiratory tract infections (source: Cochrane Review) *The Cochrane Library*, issue 2, 1999. Oxford: Update Software).

suggested that SDD promoted the development of extended spectrum beta-lactamase producing strains [86, 87]. Future research should be aimed at determining the cost-effectiveness of SDD, with inclusion of estimates of the effects of the emergence of resistant microorganisms. However, for the individual patient the evidence in favor of the use of prophylactic antimicrobials is compelling.

Management of cerebral edema

Hepatic encephalopathy (HE) is always present in FHF and although the pathogenesis has not been fully elucidated, considerable evidence points to a central role for ammonia as a major factor. The ammonia hypothesis is supported by extensive animal data and clinical studies correlating the level of ammonia with onset and severity of intracranial hypertension (ICH) [88–90]. Recent studies have suggested a role for infection and inflammation in the pathogenesis of HE, with evidence that the molecular mediators of infection and inflammation may act synergistically with ammonia to produce HE [81, 91–93].

Infection is a common precipitant of HE in both chronic liver disease and FHF. Large studies have demonstrated the role of the systemic inflammatory response syndrome (SIRS) and infection in the progression and severity of HE and other complications of liver failure [75, 92–94]. ALF is an inflammatory state and increased levels of the pro-inflammatory cytokines TNF-α, IL-6 and IL-1 β can be demonstrated, especially in patients with raised ICP. The generation of these pro-inflammatory cytokines may be due to activation of the immune system by infection and also release from the necrotic liver [91].

The generation of cerebral edema in HE is dependent on blood ammonia, with entry into the brain increased in ALF, and serum levels > 150–200 μmol/l found to predict intracranial hypertension [89, 90]. Ammonia is detoxified in the brain by formation of glutamine in astrocytes from amidation of glutamate. Glutamine accumulation in the astrocyte causes osmotic swelling, and cellular dysfunction through induction of oxidative stress and mitochondrial permeability transition [95, 96]. Indeed inhibition of glutamine synthetase ameliorates brain edema and improves the survival in animal models of ALF [97]. Astrocytic swelling thus contributes to the elevation of ICP in addition to the other component of intracranial hypertension in FHF, which is increased cerebral blood flow (CBF), although this has not been consistently demonstrated. Vascular autoregulation within the brain is defective in patients with ALF, with uncoupling of blood flow and cerebral metabolic rate [36, 98]. Cerebral hyperemia has been shown to be contributory to an increase in ICP in animal models based on porto-caval anastomosis and ammonia infusions [99], and an increase in cerebral blood flow has been shown in some

human studies in ALF [100], but not in others [37, 101]. Indeed, studies have shown a wide variation in cerebral blood flow in patients with ALF and an increase in cerebral lactate production has been shown, indicating possible ischemia that may induce cerebral swelling [37]. Recent work has shown that in patients with elevated ICP, CBF was increased and associated with the presence of SIRS criteria, markers of inflammation (C-reactive protein, white cell count) and elevated levels of the pro-inflammatory cytokines TNF-α and IL-6. Moreover, patients who developed surges in ICP also had associated increases in CBF and inflammatory markers [102]. The blood brain barrier is thought to remain intact in ALF and thus it seems unlikely that circulating cytokines can have a direct effect on cerebral function, although a recent small series has shown net efflux of inflammatory cytokines from the brain, suggesting that the blood brain barrier may be impaired in some way as has been shown in experimental animals [91, 103].

The above studies lead to the proposal of a "two hit" hypothesis, whereby the initial event in the precipitation of HE is raised ammonia levels consequent upon liver failure, which causes astrocyte swelling and cellular dysfunction, setting the stage for the worsening of ICP via increased cerebral blood flow in the setting of a concurrent inflammatory state.

Intracranial pressure monitoring

The use of intracranial pressure (ICP) monitors in FHF has not been subjected to a randomized controlled trial. As with any monitor used in critical illness, finding a positive outcome related to their use is difficult. At best, studies have suggested they may help with the management of patients with raised ICP. One study using historical controls suggested greater interventions associated with their use, and assuming the interventions were appropriate, this may be of benefit. The duration of survival from the onset of grade IV encephalopathy was significantly greater in the ICP monitored group (median 60 vs 10 hours, p < 0.01), although overall survival was unchanged [104]. Blei *et al.* performed a postal survey of complications in 262 patients from liver transplant centers across the USA [105]. Epidural transducers were the most commonly used devices and had the lowest complication rate (3.8%); subdural bolts and parenchymal monitors (fiberoptic pressure transducers in direct contact with brain parenchyma and intraventricular catheters) were associated with complication rates of 20% and 22% respectively. Fatal hemorrhage occurred in 1% of patients undergoing epidural ICP monitoring, whereas subdural and intraparenchymal devices had fatal hemorrhage rates of 5% and 4% respectively. They concluded that epidural transducers were the safest form of monitoring even if not the most accurate. A similar survey of 25 centers contributing to the US Acute Liver Failure Study Group was recently performed by Vaquero et al. [106]. In this study, only 27.7% of patients with grade III or IV encephalopathy had an ICP monitor placed. Patients with ICP monitoring were more likely to be younger and be listed for liver transplantation. There was considerable heterogeneity amongst centers regarding the frequency of use and the type of monitor used. In this study subdural monitors were used most commonly. Similar to the earlier study by Keays et al. the use of ICP monitoring was associated with more interventions such as mannitol, barbiturate and vasopressor administration. There was no difference in survival or neurological outcome between the two groups, although only patients who underwent transplantation were compared. Complications of insertion were seen in 10% of patients, all of these events being related to intracranial bleeding. In three patients intracranial bleeding was clinically insignificant, but in two patients bleeding may have contributed to mortality. Whilst the complication rate appears to be lower than the previous study by Blei et al. (10% vs 20% bleeding rate), the use of recombinant factor VII was more frequent, suggesting that aggressive control of coagulation does not protect from bleeding when using subdural or parenchymal monitors. The issue of coagulation is highlighted in a recent report of a protocolized approach to FHF management, which reported intrancranial bleeding in 3 of 22 patients treated with platelet, fresh frozen plasma and cryoprecipitate infusions, in addition to recombinant factor VII and desmopressin administration prior to insertion [107]. Another use of ICP monitoring is to determine if transplantation may be rendered futile by a poor neurological outcome. A cerebral perfusion pressure (mean arterial pressure minus intracranial pressure) of less than 50 mmHg has in the past been considered a contraindication for OLT [108]. This was because of concern regarding cerebral ischemia resulting in poor neurological outcome. Recent reports of patients with CPPs of less than 50 mmHg in which full neurological recovery has taken place have called this practice into question. Davies reported four patients with fulminant hepatic failure who developed prolonged intracranial hypertension (>35 mmHg for 24–38 h) that was refractory to standard therapy and associated with impaired cerebral perfusion pressure (<50 mmHg for 2–72 h) [38]. All survived with complete neurological recovery.

In the absence of randomized trial evidence showing benefit of ICP monitor insertion, the decision to use this form of monitoring must be taken on a case-by-case basis. There are currently multiple interventions that can be used to lower a raised ICP and only with knowledge of the ICP can the cerebral perfusion pressure (MAP-ICP) be calculated and manipulated. However, the risk of monitor insertion is not insubstantial and not all patients will develop intracranial hypertension. Risk factors for the development of intracranial hypertension are now well described and it would seem appropriate to offer this form of monitoring to those most at risk, such as those with sustained high ammonia levels, renal failure or high vasopressor requirements, especially if young and hyperacute in presentation [89]. **B4**

Radiological assessment

CT scanning, since its introduction into routine clinical practice, has become a standard investigation in any patient with suspected intracranial pathology. In FHF, correlation between ICP measurements and pressures predicted by CT imaging have been generally poor [109]. As little information is gained in relation to the difficulty associated with transporting these very sick patients to the CT scanner, a decision regarding the need for a CT must be carefully considered. CT may be of help if there is any diagnostic difficulty as to the cause of the coma or if a complication of ICP bolt insertion is suspected.

Functional radiology with single photon emission tomography SPECT scanning has been used to assess regional cerebral blood flow in patients with FHF, but it is difficult to see this being used clinically [110].

Monitoring of cerebral oxygenation

ICP and CPP monitoring are used to infer the adequacy of cerebral perfusion and oxygenation. The direct monitoring of cerebral oxygenation and blood flow are appealing. Instead of inferring the adequacy of cerebral perfusion and oxygenation from clinical signs and pressure measurements they provide direct evidence for the ongoing viability of the brain.

Methods used for the estimation of cerebral oxygenation include the sampling of jugular venous blood for oxygen saturation and products of metabolism such as lactate. A brain that is affected by limitation of supply will extract more oxygen from the arterial blood. This will result in a reduction in venous oxygen saturation. Jugular venous saturation of less than 55% suggests an ischemic brain, and steps can be made to improve the blood flow to the brain, either by increasing blood flow, decreasing ICP or reducing the metabolic demands of the brain. High JV saturation >85% may represent a hyperemic brain and steps can be made to reduce cerebral blood volume if ICP is raised. Very high JV saturation is often seen as a terminal event and may represent a complete loss of oxygen extraction by the brain.

Direct estimates of cerebral oxygenation can be achieved by the insertion of a probe into the brain parenchyma to either measure the partial pressure of oxygen or, if a microdialysis is used, to measure extracellular metabolic products [111]. Microdialysis has produced data that offers insights into the pathogenesis of hepatic encephalopathy, but as yet can only be considered a research tool [112–114]. Non-invasive methods of measuring cerebral oxygenation and blood flow include near infrared spectroscopy, transcranial Doppler and SPECT scanning. A small study of FHF patients showed that near infrared spectroscopy can detect changes in cerebral blood flow, but further work comparing to conventional monitoring is needed [115]. A study of transcranial Doppler measurements of the middle cerebral artery in FHF showing detectable changes in Doppler signals in relation to changes in MAP, and CPP has recently been reported, but as yet appears to lack the precision for decision making in this critical area [116].

Validation of non-invasive methods of monitoring cerebral function are ongoing, but controlled trials showing improvement in outcome are lacking.

Treatment of intracranial hypertension

Current guidelines recommend the reduction of intracranial pressure when it exceeds 20–25 mmHg [117]. Apart from adjuvant therapies, such as optimizing patient position to facilitate venous drainage via the jugular vein [118], two approaches can be used to facilitate reductions in ICP: namely osmotherapy and modulation of cerebral blood flow. Osmotherapy initially with urea and then mannitol has been used for many years to treat cerebral edema associated with traumatic brain injury. Canalese *et al.* showed that 1 g/kg of mannitol was an effective treatment for established intracranial hypertension in FHF and that dexamethasone was ineffective for prevention [119]. Since then, the same workers have shown that 0.5 g/kg of mannitol is as effective [120]. **B4** They suggest that boluses should be delivered rapidly to achieve maximum effect. Hypertonic saline has been used for many years in neurosurgical and trauma patients as osmotherapy of raised ICP [121–123]. A study of hypertonic saline as osmotherapy in FHF has been conducted. In this small randomized trial patients with FHF and grade III or IV encephalopathy received standard medical therapy or standard medical therapy plus an infusion of 30% saline to maintain serum sodium levels between 145–155 mmol/l. All patients were undergoing ICP monitoring. There was a significant reduction in ICP in treated patients compared to controls and more control patients had episodes of ICH characterized by elevations of ICP > 25 mmHg. This study was not powered to show differences in outcomes such as survival, but establishes the efficacy and safety of moderate induced hypernatremia to control ICP [124]. **A1d**

Hyperventilation decreases ICP by inducing cerebrovascular vasoconstriction; this reduces cerebral blood volume. It has not been shown to be any advantage in the long term in controlling ICP in FHF [44]. **B4** A short-term period of

hyperventilation in patients with raised ICP unresponsive to osmotherapy may be tried, while monitoring jugular venous saturation to assess cerebral oxygenation.

Barbiturates decrease cerebral metabolic rate via their anesthetic action and cause cerebral vasoconstriction. They have been used as agents to prevent secondary brain damage in traumatic brain injury. However, myocardial depression and hypotension with a possible compromise in cerebral perfusion pressure have limited the enthusiasm for routine use. There have not been any randomized controlled clinical trials evaluating barbiturate infusions in FHF. Forbes *et al.* investigated the role of thiopentone infusions in 13 patients with FHF in an uncontrolled study [125]. The overall survival rate of 5 out of 13 was claimed to be better than expected, but it is difficult to come to any conclusions from these data. Prolonged recovery and hypotension limit the use of thiopentone in FHF, although it may be tried when all else fails. A study in traumatic brain injury found barbiturate infusion to be of no additional benefit to acute hyperventilation [126].

Hypothermia has been investigated extensively in patients with traumatic brain injury. Initial enthusiasm for the technique in small trials was tempered with the publication of a large multi-center trial that failed to show an improved outcome, but also demonstrated an increase in complications, including bleeding and infections [127]. This is in contrast to ischemic injury following cardiac arrest, where improved survival has been shown [128]. Recently, moderate hypothermia has been reported as a rapid effective measure in reducing ICP in ALF, although there are no controlled trials [129]. **B4** Hypothermia may have a beneficial effect on the ICP in ALF by multiple mechanisms, such as decreasing ammonia extraction and reducing the cerebral metabolic rate. However, the main mechanism responsible seems to be modulation of CBF and the restoration of cerebral autoregulation to arterial pressure [130]. Hypothermia, however, may have deleterious effects on coagulation and infection and therefore cannot be recommended as routine therapy at the current time; however, a currently ongoing multicenter study will clarify the role of hypothermia.

Indomethacin is a non-steroidal anti-inflammatory drug which is also a potent cerebral arteriolar vasoconstrictor and has been used to treat sustained intracranial hypertension in patients with traumatic brain injury [131, 132]. Experimental and clinical studies indicate that indomethacin reduces ICP primarily by decreasing CBF and therefore, it may have value in the management of patients with elevated ICP in FHF with evidence of hyperemia. The use of indomethacin to control ICP in FHF has been reported in case reports and a small series [133]. Twelve patients with FHF and intracranial hypertension were studied with microdialysis, jugular venous oximetry and transcranial Doppler before and after the administration of a single bolus of indomethacin. ICP was reduced from 30 (7 to 53) to 12 (4 to 33) mmHg (p < 0.05) and there were improvements in CPP. Importantly, there was no evidence of brain ischemia as evidenced by unchanged jugular venous oxygen saturation and brain lactate concentration [134]. Further studies on the role of indomethacin for ICP treatment in FHF appear warranted.

N-acetylcysteine (NAC) has been shown to reduce clinical signs of intracranial hypertension in patients with FHF following paracetamol hepatotoxicity [135]. NAC treated patients had a lower incidence of cerebral edema (10/25, 40%) than was observed in control patients (17/25, 68%; p = 0.047; 95% CI for difference in incidence: 2–54) [135]. **A1d**

Anticonvulsant therapy

The incidence of clinical seizure activity in FHF has not been reported but it is likely that sedative and paralysing agents mask it during mechanical ventilation. Ellis and colleagues recently reported the incidence of subclinical seizure activity and the effect of the anticonvulsant phenytoin in FHF. With the use of a cerebral function monitor they found an incidence of 32% in the control group. The occurrence of seizure activity likely increases the risk of developing cerebral edema. The use of phenytoin reduced the incidence of subclinical seizure activity although not significantly. The incidence of cerebral edema in the patients that received an autopsy was significantly higher in the control group [136]. **A1d**

Renal failure

The incidence of acute renal failure associated with FHF is high; up to 70% of all patients develop renal failure (defined as urine output of less than 300 ml/24 hours and a serum creatinine of greater than 300 mmol/l in the presence of adequate intravascular filling) [10]. The etiology of renal failure in FHF is multifactorial, with both pre-renal and renal components. Relative hypovolemia and hypotension contribute to pre-renal causes. Disordered renal vascular autoregulation, present in sepsis, may also exist in the hyperdynamic circulatory failure of FHF, making renal blood flow directly dependent on blood pressure. Direct renal toxicity in patients with FHF secondary to paracetamol poisoning contributes to the very high incidence of renal failure in this group of patients [10]. The contribution of the hepatorenal syndrome, or functional renal failure in the presence of FHF, is difficult to quantify and it probably represents one end of a continuum of disordered renal function from the hepatorenal syndrome to acute tubular necrosis [137].

Renal protection

There is no proven preventative strategy against the development of renal failure, or treatment, that will shorten the duration of established renal dysfunction in FHF.

Dopamine has agonist activity at all adrenergic receptors, depending on concentration. Dopamine at a so-called "renal dose" (<5 μg/kg/min) augments renal blood flow and increases urine volume and sodium excretion in animals and healthy humans. In FHF and other forms of distributive circulatory failure an increase in renal blood flow has been difficult to show [138]. There is now good evidence that dopamine does not prevent renal failure in critically ill patients [139]. **A1d** It has been suggested that dopamine may exacerbate renal dysfunction by delivering a sodium load to an already ischemic renal medulla [140]. The term "low-dose" dopamine has been questioned because of the wide variation in plasma concentration in critically ill patients [141], and because of significant effects on other organ systems, specifically anterior pituitary and immune function [142].

Other strategies, including frusemide, aminophyline and fenoldopam infusions have not been shown to prevent renal failure in the critically ill. Atrial natriuretic peptide, while showing promise in animal models, has not been shown to be useful in the clinical setting in early human trials [143].

The magic bullet in the prevention of renal failure in FHF remains elusive and so what is left is the maintenance of intravascular volume and an adequate perfusion pressure. Despite this, extra-corporeal support is common.

Renal replacement therapy

While the incidence of renal failure in FHF remains high and attempts to prevent or treat it remain poor, renal replacement therapy has become a major part of the routine management. Proving that renal replacement therapy improves outcome is difficult as no randomized controlled trials have been done, but it can be assumed that it has contributed in part to the improvement in mortality figures over the last 30 years.

The type of replacement has been investigated in critically ill patients. It has been shown that intermittent forms of therapy cause more hemodynamic compromise than continuous forms of therapy. This has been examined in FHF. Davenport *et al.* investigated the effect of various modes of renal replacement therapy in 30 consecutive patients referred with both fulminant hepatic and acute renal failure [144]. Continuous forms of therapy were associated with more hemodynamic stability during the first hour of treatment [145]. **B4** Intracranial pressure remained stable during the continuous modes but increased significantly during intermittent machine hemofiltration [146].

The adequacy of renal replacement therapy must be considered. Patients with FHF often have severe metabolic acidosis and rapidly progress to anuria. They are markedly catabolic and serum concentrations of creatinine rise rapidly. Urea is notably low in FHF. The rate of ultrafiltration in critically ill patients has been investigated recently. It has been shown that, in general, modest increases in ultrafiltration rates are associated with an improved outcome overall [147]. **B4**

There is no evidence base for recommendations on when to start renal replacement therapy RRT in FHF. In general, conventional indications for the institution of RRT in critically ill patients should be adhered to, but given that hemofiltration and dialysis both reduce serum ammonia levels there may be a role for the early institution of RRT in patients with very high ammonia levels who may be at risk of ICH [148, 149]. Most liver centers use bicarbonate based buffers as replacement fluid, as lactate containing fluids may elevate the serum lactate causing interference with prognostication. Anticoagulation of the extracorporeal circuit could predispose to bleeding and in coagulopathic patients the use of epoprostenol or no anticoagulation can be considered.

Critical illness related corticosteroid insufficiency

Critical illness related corticosteroid insufficiency (CIRCI) appears to be common in heterogenous populations of critically ill patients. Low levels of cortisol and inadequate response to adrenocortical stimulation have identified patients with a poor prognosis. The mechanism of CIRCI is not completely understood and may be due to decreased production of cortisol, corticotrophin releasing hormone or due to increased resistance to the cellular effects of cortisol [150]. Studies of the effect of corticosteroid replacement in the critically ill have produced conflicting results, but use of moderate doses of hydrocortisone (200–300 mg/day) appears to show benefit in ARDS, community acquired pneumonia and caused quicker resolution of shock in vasopressor dependent patients [151–153]. **B4** Recently, Harry and colleagues [154] investigated the serum cortisol levels and the response to SST in 45 patients with acute hepatic dysfunction (AHD). Abnormal tests were common, occurring in 62% of patients. Those who required noradrenaline (NA) for blood pressure support had a significantly lower increment (median, 161 vs 540 nmol/l; p < 0.001) following synacthen compared with patients who did not. The increase was significantly lower in those who fulfilled liver transplant criteria compared with those who did not. There was an inverse correlation between increment and severity of illness (Sequential Organ Failure Assessment, r 0.63; p < 0.01) [154]. The same authors also investigated the effect of corticosteroid therapy (300 mg hydrocortisone/

day) in 20 vasopressor dependent patients with acute liver failure (ALF) or acute chronic liver failure (ACLF) and compared these to a historical control group of patients not treated with steroids. The use of steroids was associated with reduction in vasopressor doses but no survival benefit. Notably, the incidence of infection was higher in the corticosteroid treated group, especially with resistant organisms such as methicillin resistant staphylococcus aureus (MRSA) [155]. **B4**

Further controlled trials are needed and it remains to be seen if there will be any benefit from the replacement of steroids in patients with FHF.

Specific therapies

N-acetylcysteine (NAC) in paracetamol poisoning and other etiologies

Paracetamol poisoning is the single largest cause of FHF in the UK, accounting for between 50 and 60% of cases seen [156]. NAC can prevent hepatic damage following paracetamol poisoning. Smilkstein *et al.* evaluated the time interval from poisoning to treatment with NAC in relation to the incidence of hepatic damage as defined by increased transaminase values. NAC was found to be most effective when given during the first eight hours following ingestion. More recent data suggest that NAC is effective when given up to 72 hours after ingestion with a decrease in the occurrence of grade III/IV encephalopathy, cerebral edema, hypotension requiring inotropic support, and mortality, when compared to untreated controls [135, 157]. **A1d**

The mechanism of action of NAC in patients with established hepatic necrosis is unclear. Improvements in oxygen transport parameters have been shown with its use in patients with FHF due to paracetamol poisoning and FHF due to other etiology [158]. This, however, has been questioned recently [159]. A benefit in terms of a hemodynamic effect of this agent is seen when it is used in conjunction with epoprostenol. The beneficial effects may be attributable to a repletion of glutathione status and/or the antioxidant properties of NAC. NAC is also a sulphydryl donor and this may be beneficial in patients in whom sulphydryl groups may be oxidized, impairing microcirculatory function. Infusion of NAC has been shown to increase serum cGMP with no change in atrial natriuretic peptide, suggesting it may indeed have a role in the nitric oxide pathway in patients with acute liver failure [160].

Recently, a randomized controlled multicenter from the US acute liver failure study group examining the role of NAC in non-paracetamol ALF has been reported. This placebo-controlled study of 173 patients found no difference in overall survival between the two groups (70% survival NAC vs 66% placebo). However, there was significant benefit for NAC in terms of transplant-free survival compared to placebo (40% vs 27%), but this benefit was only seen in patients with lower grades of encephalopathy (grade I and II) [161]. **A1d**

Blood purification: dialysis, plasmapheresis, hemofiltration, sorbant hemoperfusion and artificial hepatic support

To support the acutely failing liver effectively there has to be a thorough understanding of the functional role of the liver in body homeostasis. The liver is a complex organ with many functions, in addition to the metabolic functions of the hepatocyte, which make up two-thirds of its mass. The remaining third is made up of other cell types including the Kupffer cells and endothelial cells. These other cells are important in many of its functions, including the immunological activity of the liver.

There two main components to the pathophysiology of FHF. The metabolic mass theory, which states that there is a functioning mass of hepatocytes under which end organ dysfunction will occur, leading to the manifestations of FHF and ultimately death. The toxic liver hypothesis states that it is the toxins produced by the failing liver itself that are the cause of the syndrome of FHF. The truth probably lies somewhere in between and so any extracorporeal system has to both clear the serum of any toxins produced by the failing liver and maintain the metabolic and, if possible, the other functions of the native liver. Established FHF will lead inexorably to multiple organ failure and ultimately death in the majority of patients managed with medical therapy alone and so some kind of liver support, to maintain organ function is very attractive while waiting for definitive surgical treatment or regeneration and recovery. There are two main types of blood purification systems available. These are either biological or non-biological approaches.

Experience with extracorporeal systems designed to clear the blood through physiochemical means alone consist of dialysis, sorbent hemoperfusion, hemofiltration and plasmpharesis, and combinations of the above. More recently, extracorporeal dialysis against 20% albumin has been employed with the commercially available MARS (molecular absorbent recirculation system) [162].

Early work with hemodialysis showed improved coma scores in patients with chronic liver disease. With increasing pore size and improving biocompatibility with polyacrylonitrile (PAN) membranes the hope was to improve middle-molecule clearance. No improvement mortality in FHF was shown [163]. Hemoperfusion involves the adsorption of lipophilic chemicals onto activated charcoal or synthetic resins. Again, early studies suggested an improvement in coma scores [164], but controlled studies failed to show an improved outcome with treatment [10]. **A1d**

Plasmapheresis or the exchange of plasma by fresh-frozen-plasma (FFP) has theoretical advantages over other forms of blood cleansing regimens in that it removes both low molecular weight molecules and the higher molecular weight middle-molecules both bound and unbound. The Copenhagen group have been studying high volume plasmapharesis with exchanges of 11/hour for three consecutive days [165]. Their studies suggest an improvement in hemodynamics and improved CPP but no reduction in ICP. They also noted a decrease in Glasgow Coma Score, decreased INR and reduced serum bilirubin [165]. Improvement in mortality has yet to be shown with the technique although the results of a randomized clinical trial are awaited with interest. The MARS system is an extracorporeal circuit in which 20% human albumin solution is dialyzed against the patient's blood. The albumin within the circuit binds protein bound molecules, including bilirubin and bile acids, from the patient [162]. MARS therapy has been proposed as a liver support device in the management of FHF. The evidence for effect is limited to case reports and small case series with heterogeneous patients, but some success has been reported, including the improvement of coma scores [166]. A recent report of the use of MARS in 113 FHF patients showed increased survival without transplantation (66%) compared to historical controls (40%), but the retrospective design of the study and the differing baseline characteristics of the patients make interpretation of this data difficult [167]. In contrast, in a center which used MARS routinely for the management of FHF the majority of patients died in the absence of liver transplantation despite the use of MARS for extended periods of time [168]. **B4** The results from a French multicenter study of MARS in FHF are eagerly awaited.

Bioreactors containing hepatocytes have been the basis for biological extracorporeal support systems. These remain experimental and confined to clinical trials. Experience with the systems so far suggests few problems with biocompatibility, but there are few data to suggest an improvement in clearance or synthesis by the artificial liver. The systems at the present time are divided into those utilizing porcine hepatocytes or immortalized hepatoblastoma cell lines. The ELAD system comprises a continuous system using a hepatoblastoma cell line. A randomized study utilizing this system, assessing biocompatibility, showed an improvement in galactose clearance at six hours, but no other measured variables were significantly different between the treatment and control groups [169]. **A1d**

Recently, a randomized multicenter study has been published reporting the effects of the Hepatassist® bio artificial liver (BAL) support device in ALF and primary non-function of hepatic allografts [170]. This device incorporates a bioreactor comprising 7×10^6 cryopreserved porcine hepatocytes housed within hollow fibres. The extracorporeal circuit includes an oxygenator and a charcoal column. The circuit is perfused with plasma generated by a conventional plasmapheresis machine. This study enrolled 171 patients, 24 with primary non-function and 147 with acute or sub-acute liver failure. Patients were randomized to standard of care or treatment with the bio artificial liver, with treated patients receiving an average of 2.9 treatments. The commonest reason for the cessation of treatment was a liver becoming available for transplantation. The overall survival between the treated and non-treated groups was not significantly different, although when the data was analyzed to account for the impact of transplantation upon survival there appeared to be a survival benefit for acute and sub-acute liver failure patients at 30 days. [161] **A1d**

Temporizing hepatectomy

The toxic liver theory of FHF has led to the introduction of temporizing hepatectomy in an attempt to regain hemodynamic control or a reduction in ICP in patients on the super-urgent transplant list. There have been several published case reports of successful liver transplantation following a prolonged anhepatic state. Ringe *et al.* presented the results of 30 patients who underwent hepatectomy (and temporary portacaval shunting to provide an outflow of the transected portal vein) between 1986 and 1993 [171]. Improvement in hemodynamic parameters was seen in 17 of the 30 patients following hepatectomy, with liver transplantation occurring 6–41 hours later (the effect on ICP was not stated). It is impossible to draw conclusions from these anecdotal data. Temporizing hepatectomy has been criticized because of removing the option to perform an auxiliary transplant. Temporizing hepatectomy may have a role in severe liver trauma, with uncontrollable bleeding and primary graft non-function where there is no hope of recovery.

Liver transplantation

Prognostic factors in fulminant hepatic failure and orthoptic liver transplantation

Hepatic transplantation in FHF has not been and never will be subjected to a controlled clinical trial. However, patients with FHF due to causes other than paracetamol poisoning who undergo transplantation have a 65% two-month survival rate [16], compared to 20–25% for patients managed with maximal medical therapy alone [172]. **B4** The survival without transplantation after paracetamol poisoning is higher than with FHF from other causes.

The task for the medical staff looking after patients with FHF is to decide which of these patients will not survive without liver transplantation. The decision needs to be made as early as possible because there exists a "window period" during which a successful outcome can be expected [173]. Following paracetamol poisoning, time from ingestion to transplant was significantly longer in non-survivors following transplantation [16].

In order to make an informed decision regarding the likelihood of spontaneous recovery from FHF an understanding of the natural history of the disease is necessary. Because FHF is a rare syndrome, these data have only become available over the past 20 years, since the introduction of liver failure units around the world.

Poor prognostic markers developed from analysis of large databases from these liver units have been refined into clinically usable indications for transplantation. O'Grady *et al.* developed criteria from a database of 588 patients presenting to King's College Hospital liver unit (see Box 41.2) [156]. The time course of the illness is important. It has been known for many years that the time to encephalopathy from the onset of symptoms is important prognostically, the "hyperacute" patients having a better prognosis than the "sub-acute". Etiology and age are important in that different criteria were developed for FHF caused by paracetamol poisoning. The extremes of age are associated with a poor prognosis. A high serum creatinine and bilirubin were associated with a poor prognosis, as were prolongation of coagulation parameters [156]. Following paracetamol poisoning no particular prognostic cutoff level of INR has been found, but it has been noted that a rise of the INR from day three to day four is associated with a 7% survival as compared to a 79% survival in those whose INR fell from day three to four [157]. Metabolic acidosis following fluid resuscitation was found to be

---

BOX 41.2 King's College Hospital prognostic criteria

In *non-paracetamol induced* liver failure
Prothombin time > 100 seconds (INR > 6.5)
Or
pH < 7.3
Or any three of the following:
Age < 10 years
Age > 40 years
Seronegative hepatitis (non A, B, C, E, F), halothane or
  other drug reaction
Duration of jaundice > 7 days before encephalopathy
Prothrombin time > 50 seconds (INR > 3.5)
Bilirubin > 300 μmol/l
In *paracetamol induced* FHF
pH < 7.3 (following fluid resuscitation)
Or the coexistence of:
Prothrombin time > 100 (INR > 6.5), creatinine > 300 μmol/l
  and grade III or worse encephalopathy

highly specific for a poor outcome in paracetamol poisoning. A serum pH persistently less than 7.3 has become an independent transplant criterion regardless of grade of encephalopathy [156]. **B4** The metabolic acidosis seen in FHF is often associated with a raised whole blood lactate concentration. This hyperlactatemia is caused by both an increased production, but also by decreased clearance by the liver [174, 175]. Prolonged high blood lactate concentration in critical illness other than FHF is associated with poor prognosis. The relationship between whole blood lactate and prognosis in FHF has been investigated recently. Bernal and colleagues showed that a post-resuscitation lactate concentration of greater than 3.0 mmol/l can predict death with similar accuracy to the King's criteria, but earlier in the course of the illness. The addition of post-resuscitation lactate concentration to the KCH criteria increased sensitivity from 76% to 91% and lowered the negative likelihood ratio from 0.25 to 0.10 [176]. **B4**

The importance of lactate in the prognosis of ALF secondary to paracetamol overdose has been reflected by its inclusion as a criteria for registration on the UK superurgent liver transplant scheme. Other recent variations to the classic King's criteria have recently been adopted in the UK. Patients who are deteriorating in terms of mean arterial pressure, ICP or oxygenation can be listed for urgent liver transplantation if they fulfill two out of the three classical criteria in an attempt to increase the sensitivity of the King's criteria. The level of pH as the sole criteria at which a patient can be listed has been reduced to 7.25, reflecting improved and earlier renal support, whilst at the same time a lactate of greater than 3.5 mmol/l has become a single criterion for urgent registration.

A French group performed multivariate analysis of data from 115 patients with fulminant hepatitis B and found that a low factor V following the onset of grade III encephalopathy was the strongest predictor of a poor outcome (see Box 41.3) [177].

Both the King's and the Clichy criteria are in common use around the world. Following the publication of the King's College Hospital data the criteria were evaluated retrospectively in a French liver unit. Eighty-one non-transplanted patients with non-paracetamol induced acute liver failure were studied. The mortality rate was 0.81. The predictive accuracies, respectively on admission and 48 hours

before death, were 0.80 and 0.79 for the King's criteria and 0.60 and 0.73 for the Clichy criteria. The positive and negative predictive values, 48 hours before death, were 0.89 and 0.47 for the King's criteria and 0.89 and 0.36 for the Clichy criteria respectively. The low negative predictive values (0.36 and 0.47) indicated that neither of these could identify a subgroup with a low risk of death [178]. The additions to the King's criteria have yet to be subjected to external validation but these studies are ongoing.

While the above study compared prognostic criteria in non-paracetamol induced FHF, two recent studies compared general ICU scoring systems, the Acute Physiology and Chronic Health Evaluation (APACHE) scores, and the King's criteria for urgent liver transplantation [16, 179]. Mitchell *et al.* prospectively evaluated the APACHE II system in patients with FHF due to paracetamol poisoning. The study aimed to see whether the APACHE system is able to provide an accurate risk of hospital death in patients with paracetamol induced FHF or identify those patients needing transfer for possible hepatic transplantation and compared this to the King's College Hospital transplant criteria. A total of 102 patients were studied. An APACHE II score of >15 had the ability to predict death, which was similar to that of the King's criteria (sensitivity 82% and 65% respectively; specificity 98% and 99% respectively) when evaluating those patients who were transplanted as "deaths". An APACHE II score of >15 was able to identify four more patients than the King's criteria on the first day of admission. The calculated risk of death according to the APACHE II score, using the original drug overdose coefficient, was poorly calibrated. This is probably due to the lower incidence of potentially life-threatening drug overdoses in the original calibration population. From these data the crude APACHE II score may be able to identify non-survivors at an earlier stage than the King's College Hospital criteria.

Delays in listing patients for transplantation and in organ procurement result in further patient deterioration. This altered status results in the withdrawal of patients from the urgent list. Withdrawal of patients is based on clinical experience. However, several authors have analyzed the outcome from transplantation in FHF to help define contraindications to transplantation on the basis of poor outcome after transplantation. Devlin *et al.* used APACHE III data to look at 100 patients transplanted for FHF [16]. They found that in the paracetamol group at the time of transplantation, APACHE III score and serum bilirubin were significantly higher in the non-survivors. In the non-paracetamol group, serum creatinine, organ system failure scores, and APACHE III scores were significantly higher in the non-survivors. Bernal *et al.* studied the use of liver transplantation and the application of King's College Hospital transplant criteria in 548 patients presenting to the liver failure unit with severe paracetamol poi-

---

BOX 41.3 The Clichy criteria in viral FHF

Coma or confusion
and
Factor V < 20% if under 30 years of age
or
Factor V < 30% if over 30 years of age

soning [180]. Of 424 patients who did not fulfill criteria, 28 (7%) died. Of 124 who fulfilled the criteria, 68 (55%) were listed for transplant, and 44 underwent transplantation. Thirty-three of the transplanted patients left hospital. Of the 80 patients who satisfied criteria but were not transplanted, nine survived to leave hospital. The reasons why patients who satisfied criteria were not listed were multiple organ failure and cerebral edema. These reasons also applied to the patients listed but withdrawn before a graft was available. In contrast to the report of Devlin et al., the authors were unable to identify any preoperative factors predictive of death in the transplanted group. This suggests that patients unlikely to survive with a transplant are recognized and subsequently removed from the list. However, graft factors (identified by early markers of graft function, INR and AST) were also significantly worse in the non-survivors.

Auxiliary OLT and regeneration

Auxiliary partial orthotopic liver transplantation holds potential advantages over conventional orthotopic liver transplantation in the setting of FHF. It has been known for many years that survivors from FHF often return to full health with normal or only slightly abnormal livers. The liver has great powers of regeneration and this has led to the introduction of partial liver transplantation in the hope of native liver regeneration and the eventual withdrawal of immunosuppression. A multicenter European study reported the results of 30 patients who underwent auxiliary transplantation for FHF [181]. After 3 months, 19 of the 30 patients survived; 13 had resumed normal native liver function with interruption of immunosuppression. The indications are not well defined, but the survivors of immunosuppression were aged less than 40 years and had FHF secondary to viral hepatitis and paracetamol poisoning.

A more recent study reported the outcomes of patients who underwent auxiliary grafting for FHF at a single center, 49 patients received an auxiliary graft, overall survival was 77% and over 50% of patients were able to be weaned from immunosuppression. Sequential post-transplant biopsies of native livers showed excellent regeneration, especially in patients transplanted for acteminophen hepatotoxicity, where 100% native liver recovery was noted in survivors [182].

References

1 Trey C, Davidson CS. The management of fulminant hepatic failure. *Progress in Liver Diseases* 1970; **3**: 282–298.

2 O'Grady JG, Schalm SW, Williams R. Acute liver failure: redefining the syndromes. *Lancet* 1993; **342**(8866): 273–275.

3 Gimson AE, O'Grady J, Ede RJ, Portmann B, Williams R. Late onset hepatic failure: clinical, serological and histological features. *Hepatology* (Baltimore, Md) 1986; **6**(2): 288–294.

4 Hawton K, Townsend E, Deeks J *et al.* Effects of legislation restricting pack sizes of paracetamol and salicylate on self poisoning in the United Kingdom: before and after study. *BMJ* (Clinical research ed.) 2001; **322**(7296): 1203–1207.

5 Newsome PN, Bathgate AJ, Henderson NC *et al.* Referral patterns and social deprivation in paracetamol-induced liver injury in Scotland. *Lancet* 2001; **358**(9293): 1612–1613.

6 Hawkins LC, Edwards JN, Dargan PI. Impact of restricting paracetamol pack sizes on paracetamol poisoning in the United Kingdom: a review of the literature. *Drug Saf* 2007; **30**(6): 465–479.

7 Larson AM, Polson J, Fontana RJ *et al.* Acetaminophen-induced acute liver failure: results of a United States multicenter, prospective study. *Hepatology* (Baltimore, Md) 2005; **42**(6): 1364–1372.

8 Ostapowicz G, Fontana RJ, Schiodt FV *et al.* Results of a prospective study of acute liver failure at 17 tertiary care centers in the United States. *Annals of Internal Medicine* 2002; **137**(12): 947–954.

9 Trewby PN, Williams R. Pathophysiology of hypotension in patients with fulminant hepatic failure. *Gut* 1977; **18**(12): 1021–1026.

10 O'Grady JG, Gimson AE, O'Brien CJ, Pucknell A, Hughes RD, Williams R. Controlled trials of charcoal hemoperfusion and prognostic factors in fulminant hepatic failure. *Gastroenterology* 1988; **94**(5 Pt 1): 1186–1192.

11 Rolando N, Harvey F, Brahm J *et al.* Prospective study of bacterial infection in acute liver failure: an analysis of fifty patients. *Hepatology* (Baltimore, Md) 1990; **11**(1): 49–53.

12 Bernal W, Cross TJ, Auzinger G *et al.* Outcome after wait-listing for emergency liver transplantation in acute liver failure: a single centre experience. *Journal of Hepatology* 2009; **50**(2): 306–313.

13 Makin AJ, Wendon J, Williams R. A 7-year experience of severe acetaminophen-induced hepatotoxicity (1987–1993). *Gastroenterology* 1995; **109**(6): 1907–1916.

14 Lucke B. Studies on epidemic hepatitis and its sequelae. *Transactions & Studies of the College of Physicians of Philadelphia* 1948; **16**(1): 32–41.

15 McQuillan P, Pilkington S, Allan A *et al.* Confidential inquiry into quality of care before admission to intensive care. *BMJ* (Clinical research ed.) 1998; **316**(7148): 1853–1858.

16 Devlin J, Wendon J, Heaton N, Tan KC, Williams R. Pretransplantation clinical status and outcome of emergency transplantation for acute liver failure. *Hepatology* (Baltimore, Md) 1995; **21**(4): 1018–1024.

17 O'Grady J. Acute liver failure. *Journal of the Royal College of Physicians of London* 1997; **31**(6): 603–607.

18 Bihari DJ, Gimson AE, Williams R. Cardiovascular, pulmonary and renal complications of fulminant hepatic failure. *Seminars in Liver Disease* 1986; **6**(2): 119–128.

19 Human albumin administration in critically ill patients: systematic review of randomised controlled trials. Cochrane Injuries Group Albumin Reviewers. *BMJ* (Clinical research ed.) 1998; **317**(7153): 235–240.

20 Finfer S, Bellomo R, Boyce N, French J, Myburgh J, Norton R. A comparison of albumin and saline for fluid resuscitation in the intensive care unit. *The New England Journal of Medicine* 2004; **350**(22): 2247–2256.

21 Schortgen F, Deye N, Brochard L. Preferred plasma volume expanders for critically ill patients: results of an international survey. *Intensive Care Medicine* 2004; **30**(12): 2222–2229.

22 Brunkhorst FM, Engel C, Bloos F *et al.* Intensive insulin therapy and pentastarch resuscitation in severe sepsis. *The New England Journal of Medicine* 2008; **358**(2): 125–139.

23 Marx G, Cope T, McCrossan L *et al.* Assessing fluid responsiveness by stroke volume variation in mechanically ventilated patients with severe sepsis. *European Journal of Anaesthesiology* 2004; **21**(2): 132–138.

24 Monnet X, Rienzo M, Osman D *et al.* Passive leg raising predicts fluid responsiveness in the critically ill. *Critical Care Medicine* 2006; **34**(5): 1402–1407.

25 Huang CC, Fu JY, Hu HC *et al.* Prediction of fluid responsiveness in acute respiratory distress syndrome patients ventilated with low tidal volume and high positive end-expiratory pressure. *Critical Care Medicine* 2008; **36**(10): 2810–2816.

26 Connors AF, Jr., Speroff T, Dawson NV *et al.* The effectiveness of right heart catheterization in the initial care of critically ill patients. SUPPORT Investigators. *JAMA* 1996; **276**(11): 889–897.

27 Harvey S, Harrison DA, Singer M *et al.* Assessment of the clinical effectiveness of pulmonary artery catheters in management of patients in intensive care (PAC-Man): a randomised controlled trial. *Lancet* 2005; **366**(9484): 472–477.

28 Harvey SE, Welch CA, Harrison DA, Rowan KM, Singer M. Post hoc insights from PAC-Man – the UK pulmonary artery catheter trial. *Critical Care Medicine* 2008; **36**(6): 1714–1721.

29 Wheeler AP, Bernard GR, Thompson BT *et al.* Pulmonary-artery versus central venous catheter to guide treatment of acute lung injury. *The New England Journal of Medicine* 2006; **354**(21): 2213–2224.

30 Powers SR, Jr., Mannal R, Neclerio M *et al.* Physiologic consequences of positive end-expiratory pressure (PEEP) ventilation. *Annals of Surgery* 1973; **178**(3): 265–272.

31 Gasman JD, Ruoss SJ, Fishman RS, Rizk NW, Raffin TA. Hazards with both determining and utilizing oxygen consumption measurements in the management of critically ill patients. *Critical Care Medicine* 1996; **24**(1): 6–9.

32 Gattinoni L, Brazzi L, Pelosi P *et al.* A trial of goal-oriented hemodynamic therapy in critically ill patients. SvO2 Collaborative Group. *The New England Journal of Medicine* 1995; **333**(16): 1025–1032.

33 Rivers E, Nguyen B, Havstad S *et al.* Early goal-directed therapy in the treatment of severe sepsis and septic shock. *The New England Journal of Medicine* 2001; **345**(19): 1368–1377.

34 Wendon JA, Harrison PM, Keays R, Gimson AE, Alexander GJ, Williams R. Effects of vasopressor agents and epoprostenol on systemic hemodynamics and oxygen transport in fulminant hepatic failure. *Hepatology* (Baltimore, Md) 1992; **15**(6): 1067–1071.

35 James JH, Luchette FA, McCarter FD, Fischer JE. Lactate is an unreliable indicator of tissue hypoxia in injury or sepsis. *Lancet* 1999; **354**(9177): 505–508.

36 Larsen FS, Ejlersen E, Hansen BA, Knudsen GM, Tygstrup N, Secher NH. Functional loss of cerebral blood flow autoregulation in patients with fulminant hepatic failure. *Journal of Hepatology* 1995; **23**(2): 212–217.

37 Wendon JA, Harrison PM, Keays R, Williams R. Cerebral blood flow and metabolism in fulminant liver failure. *Hepatology* (Baltimore, Md) 1994; **19**(6): 1407–1413.

38 Davies MH, Mutimer D, Lowes J, Elias E, Neuberger J. Recovery despite impaired cerebral perfusion in fulminant hepatic failure. *Lancet* 1994; **343**(8909): 1329–1330.

39 Morelli A, Ertmer C, Lange M *et al.* Effects of short-term simultaneous infusion of dobutamine and terlipressin in patients with septic shock: the DOBUPRESS study. *British Journal of Anaesthesia* 2008; **100**(4): 494–503.

40 Sanyal AJ, Boyer T, Garcia-Tsao G *et al.* A randomized, prospective, double-blind, placebo-controlled trial of terlipressin for type 1 hepatorenal syndrome. *Gastroenterology* 2008; **134**(5): 1360–1368.

41 Umgelter A, Reindl W, Schmid RM, Huber W. Continuous terlipressin infusion in patients with persistent septic shock and cirrhosis of the liver. *Intensive Care Medicine* 2008; **34**(2): 390–391.

42 Shawcross DL, Davies NA, Williams R, Jalan R. Systemic inflammatory response exacerbates the neuropsychological effects of induced hyperammonemia in cirrhosis. *Journal of Hepatology* 2004; **40**(2): 247–254.

43 Eefsen M, Dethloff T, Frederiksen HJ, Hauerberg J, Hansen BA, Larsen FS. Comparison of terlipressin and noradrenalin on cerebral perfusion, intracranial pressure and cerebral extracellular concentrations of lactate and pyruvate in patients with acute liver failure in need of inotropic support. *Journal of Hepatology* 2007; **47**(3): 381–386.

44 Ede RJ, Gimson AE, Bihari D, Williams R. Controlled hyperventilation in the prevention of cerebral oedema in fulminant hepatic failure. *Journal of Hepatology* 1986; **2**(1): 43–51.

45 Baudouin SV, Howdle P, O'Grady JG, Webster NR. Acute lung injury in fulminant hepatic failure following paracetamol poisoning. *Thorax* 1995; **50**(4): 399–402.

46 Dreyfuss D, Saumon G. Ventilator-induced lung injury: lessons from experimental studies. *American Journal of Respiratory and Critical Care Medicine* 1998; **157**(1): 294–323.

47 Amato MB, Barbas CS, Medeiros DM *et al.* Effect of a protective-ventilation strategy on mortality in the acute respiratory distress syndrome. *The New England Journal of Medicine* 1998; **338**(6): 347–354.

48 Ventilation with lower tidal volumes as compared with traditional tidal volumes for acute lung injury and the acute respiratory distress syndrome. The Acute Respiratory Distress Syndrome Network. *The New England Journal of Medicine* 2000; **342**(18): 1301–1308.

49 Artigas A, Bernard GR, Carlet J *et al.* The American-European Consensus Conference on ARDS, part 2. Ventilatory, pharmacologic, supportive therapy, study design strategies and issues related to recovery and remodeling. *Intensive Care Medicine* 1998; **24**(4): 378–398.

50 Auzinger G, O'Callaghan GP, Bernal W, Sizer E, Wendon JA. Percutaneous tracheostomy in patients with severe liver disease and a high incidence of refractory coagulopathy. *Critical Care* (London, England) 2007; **11**(5): R110.

51 Ramsay MA, Savege TM, Simpson BR, Goodwin R. Controlled sedation with alphaxalone-alphadolone. *BMJ* 1974; **2**(5920): 656–659.

52 Adembri C, Venturi L, Pellegrini-Giampietro DE. Neuroprotective effects of propofol in acute cerebral injury. *CNS Drug Reviews* 2007; **13**(3): 333–351.

53 Herregods L, Verbeke J, Rolly G, Colardyn F. Effect of propofol on elevated intracranial pressure. Preliminary results. *Anaesthesia* 1988; **43** Suppl: 107–109.

54 Hsiang JK, Chesnut RM, Crisp CB, Klauber MR, Blunt BA, Marshall LF. Early, routine paralysis for intracranial pressure control in severe head injury: is it necessary? *Critical Care Medicine* 1994; **22**(9): 1471–1476.

55 Road J, Mackie G, Jiang TX, Stewart H, Eisen A. Reversible paralysis with status asthmaticus, steroids, and pancuronium: clinical electrophysiological correlates. *Muscle & Nerve* 1997; **20**(12): 1587–1590.

56 Walsh TS, Wigmore SJ, Hopton P, Richardson R, Lee A. Energy expenditure in acetaminophen-induced fulminant hepatic failure. *Critical Care Medicine* 2000; **28**(3): 649–654.

57 Kreymann KG, Berger MM, Deutz NE *et al.* ESPEN Guidelines on Enteral Nutrition: Intensive care. *Clinical Nutrition* (Edinburgh, Scotland) 2006; **25**(2): 210–223.

58 Montejo JC, Grau T, Acosta J *et al.* Multicenter, prospective, randomized, single-blind study comparing the efficacy and gastrointestinal complications of early jejunal feeding with early gastric feeding in critically ill patients. *Critical Care Medicine* 2002; **30**(4): 796–800.

59 Ho KM, Dobb GJ, Webb SA. A comparison of early gastric and post-pyloric feeding in critically ill patients: a meta-analysis. *Intensive Care Medicine* 2006; **32**(5): 639–649.

60 Nguyen NQ, Chapman MJ, Fraser RJ, Bryant LK, Holloway RH. Erythromycin is more effective than metoclopramide in the treatment of feed intolerance in critical illness. *Critical Care Medicine* 2007; **35**(2): 483–489.

61 Story DA, Ronco C, Bellomo R. Trace element and vitamin concentrations and losses in critically ill patients treated with continuous venovenous hemofiltration. *Critical Care Medicine* 1999; **27**(1): 220–223.

62 Crimi E, Liguori A, Condorelli M *et al.* The beneficial effects of antioxidant supplementation in enteral feeding in critically ill patients: a prospective, randomized, double-blind, placebo-controlled trial. *Anesthesia and Analgesia* 2004; **99**(3): 857–863, Table of contents.

63 Heyland DK, Dhaliwal R, Suchner U, Berger MM. Antioxidant nutrients: a systematic review of trace elements and vitamins in the critically ill patient. *Intensive Care Medicine* 2005; **31**(3): 327–337.

64 Wernerman J. Clinical use of glutamine supplementation. *The Journal of Nutrition* 2008; **138**(10): 2040S–2044S.

65 Van den Berghe G, Wouters P, Weekers F *et al.* Intensive insulin therapy in the critically ill patients. *The New England Journal of Medicine* 2001; **345**(19): 1359–1367.

66 Finfer S, Chittock DR, Su SY *et al.* Intensive versus conventional glucose control in critically ill patients. *The New England Journal of Medicine* 2009; **360**(13): 1283–1297.

67 Cook D, Heyland D, Griffith L, Cook R, Marshall J, Pagliarello J. Risk factors for clinically important upper gastrointestinal bleeding in patients requiring mechanical ventilation. Canadian Critical Care Trials Group. *Critical Care Medicine* 1999; **27**(12): 2812–2817.

68 Tryba M. Prophylaxis of stress ulcer bleeding. A meta-analysis. *Journal of Clinical Gastroenterology* 1991; **13**(Suppl. 2): S44–S55.

69 Cook DJ, Reeve BK, Guyatt GH *et al.* Stress ulcer prophylaxis in critically ill patients. Resolving discordant meta-analyses. *JAMA* 1996; **275**(4): 308–314.

70 Cook D, Guyatt G, Marshall J *et al.* A comparison of sucralfate and ranitidine for the prevention of upper gastrointestinal bleeding in patients requiring mechanical ventilation. Canadian Critical Care Trials Group. *The New England Journal of Medicine* 1998; **338**(12): 791–797.

71 Somberg L, Morris J, Jr., Fantus R *et al.* Intermittent intravenous pantoprazole and continuous cimetidine infusion: effect on gastric pH control in critically ill patients at risk of developing stress-related mucosal disease. *The Journal of Trauma* 2008; **64**(5): 1202–1210.

72 Kantorova I, Svoboda P, Scheer P *et al.* Stress ulcer prophylaxis in critically ill patients: a randomized controlled trial. *Hepatogastroenterology* 2004; **51**(57): 757–761.

73 Dellinger RP, Levy MM, Carlet JM *et al.* Surviving Sepsis Campaign: international guidelines for management of severe sepsis and septic shock: 2008. *Critical Care Medicine* 2008; **36**(1): 296–327.

74 Wade J, Rolando N, Philpott-Howard J, Wendon J. Timing and aetiology of bacterial infections in a liver intensive care unit. *The Journal of Hospital Infection* 2003; **53**(2): 144–146.

75 Karvellas CJ, Pink F, McPhail M *et al.* Predictors of bacteraemia and mortality in patients with acute liver failure. *Intensive Care Medicine* 2009; **35**(8, August): 1390–1396.

76 Garrouste-Orgeas M, Chevret S, Mainardi JL, Timsit JF, Misset B, Carlet J. A one-year prospective study of nosocomial bacteraemia in ICU and non-ICU patients and its impact on patient outcome. *The Journal of Hospital Infection* 2000; **44**(3): 206–213.

77 Rolando N, Clapperton M, Wade J, Panetsos G, Mufti G, Williams R. Granulocyte colony-stimulating factor improves function of neutrophils from patients with acute liver failure. *European Journal of Gastroenterology & Hepatology* 2000; **12**(10): 1135–1140.

78 Clapperton M, Rolando N, Sandoval L, Davies E, Williams R. Neutrophil superoxide and hydrogen peroxide production in patients with acute liver failure. *European Journal of Clinical Investigation* 1997; **27**(2): 164–168.

79 Antoniades CG, Berry PA, Davies ET *et al.* Reduced monocyte HLA-DR expression: a novel biomarker of disease severity and outcome in acetaminophen-induced acute liver failure. *Hepatology* (Baltimore, Md) 2006; **44**(1): 34–43.

80 Antoniades CG, Berry PA, Wendon JA, Vergani D. The importance of immune dysfunction in determining outcome in acute liver failure. *Journal of Hepatology* 2008; **49**(5): 845–861.

81 O'Beirne JP, Chouhan M, Hughes RD. The role of infection and inflammation in the pathogenesis of hepatic encephalopathy and cerebral edema in acute liver failure. *Nature Clinical Practice* 2006; **3**(3): 118–119.

82 Rolando N, Wade JJ, Stangou A *et al.* Prospective study comparing the efficacy of prophylactic parenteral antimicrobials, with or without enteral decontamination, in patients with acute liver failure. *Liver Transpl Surg* 1996; **2**(1): 8–13.

83 Rolando N, Philpott-Howard J, Williams R. Bacterial and fungal infection in acute liver failure. *Seminars in Liver Disease* 1996; **16**(4): 389–402.

84 Rolando N, Gimson A, Wade J, Philpott-Howard J, Casewell M, Williams R. Prospective controlled trial of selective parenteral and enteral antimicrobial regimen in fulminant liver failure. *Hepatology* (Baltimore, Md) 1993; **17**(2): 196–201.

85 Liberati A, D'Amico R, Pifferi, Torri V, Brazzi L. Antibiotic prophylaxis to reduce respiratory tract infections and mortality in adults receiving intensive care. *Cochrane Database of Systematic Reviews* (online) 2004(1):CD000022.

86 de Jonge E, Schultz MJ, Spanjaard L et al. Effects of selective decontamination of digestive tract on mortality and acquisition of resistant bacteria in intensive care: a randomised controlled trial. *Lancet* 2003; **362**(9389): 1011–1016.

87 Al Naiemi N, Heddema ER, Bart A et al. Emergence of multidrug-resistant Gram-negative bacteria during selective decontamination of the digestive tract on an intensive care unit. *The Journal of Antimicrobial Chemotherapy* 2006; **58**(4): 853–856.

88 Bhatia V, Singh R, Acharya SK. Predictive value of arterial ammonia for complications and outcome in acute liver failure. *Gut* 2006; **55**(1): 98–104.

89 Bernal W, Hall C, Karvellas CJ, Auzinger G, Sizer E, Wendon J. Arterial ammonia and clinical risk factors for encephalopathy and intracranial hypertension in acute liver failure. *Hepatology* (Baltimore, Md) 2007; **46**(6): 1844–1852.

90 Clemmesen JO, Larsen FS, Kondrup J, Hansen BA, Ott P. Cerebral herniation in patients with acute liver failure is correlated with arterial ammonia concentration. *Hepatology* (Baltimore, Md) 1999; **29**(3): 648–653.

91 Wright G, Shawcross D, Olde Damink SW, Jalan R. Brain cytokine flux in acute liver failure and its relationship with intracranial hypertension. *Metabolic Brain Disease* 2007; **22**(3–4): 375–388.

92 Rolando N, Wade J, Davalos M, Wendon J, Philpott-Howard J, Williams R. The systemic inflammatory response syndrome in acute liver failure. *Hepatology* (Baltimore, Md) 2000; **32**(4 Pt 1): 734–739.

93 Vaquero J, Polson J, Chung C et al. Infection and the progression of hepatic encephalopathy in acute liver failure. *Gastroenterology* 2003; **125**(3): 755–764.

94 Leithead JA, Ferguson JW, Bates CM et al. The systemic inflammatory response syndrome is predictive of renal dysfunction in patients with non-paracetamol-induced acute liver failure. *Gut* 2009; **58**(3): 443–449.

95 Reddy PV, Murthy Ch R, Reddanna P. Fulminant hepatic failure induced oxidative stress in nonsynaptic mitochondria of cerebral cortex in rats. *Neuroscience letters* 2004; **368**(1): 15–20.

96 Norenberg MD, Jayakumar AR, Rama Rao KV, Panickar KS. New concepts in the mechanism of ammonia-induced astrocyte swelling. *Metabolic Brain Disease* 2007; **22**(3–4): 219–234.

97 Blei AT, Olafsson S, Therrien G, Butterworth RF. Ammonia-induced brain edema and intracranial hypertension in rats after portacaval anastomosis. *Hepatology* (Baltimore, Md) 1994; **19**(6): 1437–1444.

98 Strauss G, Hansen BA, Knudsen GM, Larsen FS. Hyperventilation restores cerebral blood flow autoregulation in patients with acute liver failure. *Journal of Hepatology* 1998; **28**(2): 199–203.

99 Larsen FS, Gottstein J, Blei AT. Cerebral hyperemia and nitric oxide synthase in rats with ammonia-induced brain edema. *Journal of Hepatology* 2001; **34**(4): 548–554.

100 Aggarwal S, Kramer D, Yonas H et al. Cerebral hemodynamic and metabolic changes in fulminant hepatic failure: a retrospective study. *Hepatology* (Baltimore, Md)1994; **19**(1): 80–87.

101 Strauss G, Hansen BA, Kirkegaard P, Rasmussen A, Hjortrup A, Larsen FS. Liver function, cerebral blood flow autoregulation, and hepatic encephalopathy in fulminant hepatic failure. *Hepatology* (Baltimore, Md) 1997; **25**(4): 837–839.

102 Jalan R, Olde Damink SW, Hayes PC, Deutz NE, Lee A. Pathogenesis of intracranial hypertension in acute liver failure: inflammation, ammonia and cerebral blood flow. *Journal of Hepatology* 2004; **41**(4): 613–620.

103 Gove CD, Hughes RD, Ede RJ, Williams R. Regional cerebral edema and chloride space in galactosamine-induced liver failure in rats. *Hepatology* (Baltimore, Md) 1997; **25**(2): 295–301.

104 Keays RT, Alexander GJ, Williams R. The safety and value of extradural intracranial pressure monitors in fulminant hepatic failure. *Journal of Hepatology* 1993; **18**(2): 205–209.

105 Blei AT, Olafsson S, Webster S, Levy R. Complications of intracranial pressure monitoring in fulminant hepatic failure. *Lancet* 1993; **341**(8838): 157–158.

106 Vaquero J, Fontana RJ, Larson AM et al. Complications and use of intracranial pressure monitoring in patients with acute liver failure and severe encephalopathy. *Liver Transpl* 2005; **11**(12): 1581–1589.

107 Raschke RA, Curry SC, Rempe S et al. Results of a protocol for the management of patients with fulminant liver failure. *Critical Care Medicine* 2008; **36**(8): 2244–2248.

108 Donovan JP, Shaw BW, Jr., Langnas AN, Sorrell MF. Brain water and acute liver failure: the emerging role of intracranial pressure monitoring. *Hepatology* (Baltimore, Md) 1992; **16**(1): 267–268.

109 Munoz SJ, Robinson M, Northrup B et al. Elevated intracranial pressure and computed tomography of the brain in fulminant hepatocellular failure. *Hepatology* (Baltimore, Md) 1991; **13**(2): 209–212.

110 Strauss GI, Hogh P, Moller K, Knudsen GM, Hansen BA, Larsen FS. Regional cerebral blood flow during mechanical hyperventilation in patients with fulminant hepatic failure. *Hepatology* (Baltimore, Md) 1999; **30**(6): 1368–1373.

111 Tofteng F, Larsen FS. Monitoring extracellular concentrations of lactate, glutamate, and glycerol by in vivo microdialysis in the brain during liver transplantation in acute liver failure. *Liver Transpl* 2002; **8**(3): 302–305.

112 Hutchinson PJ, Gimson A, Al-Rawi PG, O'Connell MT, Czosnyka M, Menon DK. Microdialysis in the management of hepatic encephalopathy. *Neurocritical Care* 2006; **5**(3): 202–205.

113 Larsen FS. Is it worthwhile to use cerebral microdialysis in patients with acute liver failure? *Neurocritical Care* 2006; **5**(3): 173–175.

114 Tofteng F, Hauerberg J, Hansen BA, Pedersen CB, Jorgensen L, Larsen FS. Persistent arterial hyperammonemia increases the concentration of glutamine and alanine in the brain and correlates with intracranial pressure in patients with fulminant hepatic failure. *J Cereb Blood Flow Metab* 2006; **26**(1): 21–27.

115 Nielsen HB, Tofteng F, Wang LP, Larsen FS. Cerebral oxygenation determined by near-infrared spectrophotometry in patients

with fulminant hepatic failure. *Journal of Hepatology* 2003; **38**(2): 188–192.

116 Aggarwal S, Brooks DM, Kang Y, Linden PK, Patzer JF, 2nd. Noninvasive monitoring of cerebral perfusion pressure in patients with acute liver failure using transcranial doppler ultrasonography. *Liver Transpl* 2008; **14**(7): 1048–1057.

117 Stravitz RT, Kramer AH, Davern T *et al.* Intensive care of patients with acute liver failure: recommendations of the US Acute Liver Failure Study Group. *Critical Care Medicine* 2007; **35**(11): 2498–2508.

118 Davenport A, Will EJ, Davison AM. Effect of posture on intracranial pressure and cerebral perfusion pressure in patients with fulminant hepatic and renal failure after acetaminophen self-poisoning. *Critical Care Medicine* 1990; **18**(3): 286–289.

119 Canalese J, Gimson AE, Davis C, Mellon PJ, Davis M, Williams R. Controlled trial of dexamethasone and mannitol for the cerebral oedema of fulminant hepatic failure. *Gut* 1982; **23**(7): 625–629.

120 Ede RJ, Williams RW. Hepatic encephalopathy and cerebral edema. *Seminars in Liver Disease* 1986; **6**(2): 107–118.

121 Horn P, Munch E, Vajkoczy P *et al.* Hypertonic saline solution for control of elevated intracranial pressure in patients with exhausted response to mannitol and barbiturates. *Neurological Research* 1999; **21**(8): 758–764.

122 Schatzmann C, Heissler HE, Konig K *et al.* Treatment of elevated intracranial pressure by infusions of 10% saline in severely head injured patients. *Acta Neurochirurgica* 1998; **71**: 31–33.

123 De Vivo P, Del Gaudio A, Ciritella P, Puopolo M, Chiarotti F, Mastronardi E. Hypertonic saline solution: a safe alternative to mannitol 18% in neurosurgery. *Minerva Anestesiologica* 2001; **67**(9): 603–611.

124 Murphy N, Auzinger G, Bernel W, Wendon J. The effect of hypertonic sodium chloride on intracranial pressure in patients with acute liver failure. *Hepatology* (Baltimore, Md) 2004; **39**(2): 464–470.

125 Forbes A, Alexander GJ, O'Grady JG *et al.* Thiopental infusion in the treatment of intracranial hypertension complicating fulminant hepatic failure. *Hepatology* (Baltimore, Md) 1989; **10**(3): 306–310.

126 Louis PT, Goddard-Finegold J, Fishman MA, Griggs JR, Stein F, Laurent JP. Barbiturates and hyperventilation during intracranial hypertension. *Critical Care Medicine* 1993; **21**(8): 1200–1206.

127 Clifton GL, Miller ER, Choi SC *et al.* Lack of effect of induction of hypothermia after acute brain injury. *The New England Journal Of Medicine* 2001; **344**(8): 556–563.

128 Bernard SA, Gray TW, Buist MD *et al.* Treatment of comatose survivors of out-of-hospital cardiac arrest with induced hypothermia. *The New England Journal Of Medicine* 2002; **346**(8): 557–563.

129 Jalan R, Olde Damink SW, Deutz NE, Hayes PC, Lee A. Moderate hypothermia in patients with acute liver failure and uncontrolled intracranial hypertension. *Gastroenterology* 2004; **127**(5): 1338–1346.

130 Jalan R, Olde Damink SW, Deutz NE, Hayes PC, Lee A. Restoration of cerebral blood flow autoregulation and reactivity to carbon dioxide in acute liver failure by moderate hypothermia. *Hepatology* (Baltimore, Md) 2001; **34**(1): 50–54.

131 Nilsson F, Bjorkman S, Rosen I, Messeter K, Nordstrom CH. Cerebral vasoconstriction by indomethacin in intracranial hypertension. An experimental investigation in pigs. *Anesthesiology* 1995; **83**(6): 1283–1292.

132 Imberti R, Fuardo M, Bellinzona G, Pagani M, Langer M. The use of indomethacin in the treatment of plateau waves: effects on cerebral perfusion and oxygenation. *Journal of Neurosurgery* 2005; **102**(3): 455–459.

133 Clemmesen JO, Hansen BA, Larsen FS. Indomethacin normalizes intracranial pressure in acute liver failure: a twenty-three-year-old woman treated with indomethacin. *Hepatology* (Baltimore, Md) 1997; **26**(6): 1423–1425.

134 Tofteng F, Larsen FS. The effect of indomethacin on intracranial pressure, cerebral perfusion and extracellular lactate and glutamate concentrations in patients with fulminant hepatic failure. *J Cereb Blood Flow Metab* 2004; **24**(7): 798–804.

135 Keays R, Harrison PM, Wendon JA *et al.* Intravenous acetylcysteine in paracetamol induced fulminant hepatic failure: a prospective controlled trial. *BMJ* (Clinical research ed.) 1991; **303**(6809): 1026–1029.

136 Ellis AJ, Wendon JA, Williams R. Subclinical seizure activity and prophylactic phenytoin infusion in acute liver failure: a controlled clinical trial. *Hepatology* (Baltimore, Md) 2000; **32**(3): 536–541.

137 Arroyo V. Review article: hepatorenal syndrome – how to assess response to treatment and nonpharmacological therapy. *Alimentary pharmacology & therapeutics* 2004; **20**(Suppl. 3): 49–54; discussion 5–6.

138 Bersten AD, Holt AW. Vasoactive drugs and the importance of renal perfusion pressure. *New Horizons* (Baltimore, Md) 1995; **3**(4): 650–661.

139 Bellomo R, Chapman M, Finfer S, Hickling K, Myburgh J. Low-dose dopamine in patients with early renal dysfunction: a placebo-controlled randomised trial. Australian and New Zealand Intensive Care Society (ANZICS) Clinical Trials Group. *Lancet* 2000; **356**(9248): 2139–2143.

140 Weisberg LS, Kurnik PB, Kurnik BR. Risk of radiocontrast nephropathy in patients with and without diabetes mellitus. *Kidney International* 1994; **45**(1): 259–265.

141 Juste RN, Moran L, Hooper J, Soni N. Dopamine clearance in critically ill patients. *Intensive Care Medicine* 1998; **24**(11): 1217–1220.

142 Van den Berghe G, de Zegher F. Anterior pituitary function during critical illness and dopamine treatment. *Critical Care Medicine* 1996; **24**(9): 1580–1590.

143 Brenner RM, Chertow GM. The rise and fall of atrial natriuretic peptide for acute renal failure. *Current Opinion in Nephrology and Hypertension* 1997; **6**(5): 474–476.

144 Davenport A, Will EJ, Davison AM. Effect of renal replacement therapy on patients with combined acute renal and fulminant hepatic failure. *Kidney International* 1993; **41**: S245–S251.

145 Davenport A, Will EJ, Davidson AM. Improved cardiovascular stability during continuous modes of renal replacement therapy in critically ill patients with acute hepatic and renal failure. *Critical Care Medicine* 1993; **21**(3): 328–338.

146 Davenport A, Will EJ, Davison AM *et al.* Changes in intracranial pressure during machine and continuous haemofiltration. *The International Journal of Artificial Organs* 1989; **12**(7): 439–444.

147 Ronco C, Bellomo R, Homel P *et al.* Effects of different doses in continuous veno-venous haemofiltration on outcomes of acute

renal failure: a prospective randomised trial. *Lancet* 2000; **356**(9223): 26–30.

148 Braun MC, Welch TR. Continuous venovenous hemodiafiltration in the treatment of acute hyperammonemia. *American Journal of Nephrology* 1998; **18**(6): 531–533.

149 Lai YC, Huang HP, Tsai IJ, Tsau YK. High-volume continuous venovenous hemofiltration as an effective therapy for acute management of inborn errors of metabolism in young children. *Blood Purification* 2007; **25**(4): 303–308.

150 Marik PE. Critical illness-related corticosteroid insufficiency. *Chest* 2009; **135**(1): 181–193.

151 Confalonieri M, Urbino R, Potena A *et al.* Hydrocortisone infusion for severe community-acquired pneumonia: a preliminary randomized study. *American Journal of Respiratory and Critical Care Medicine* 2005; **171**(3): 242–248.

152 Meduri GU, Tolley EA, Chrousos GP, Stentz F. Prolonged methylprednisolone treatment suppresses systemic inflammation in patients with unresolving acute respiratory distress syndrome: evidence for inadequate endogenous glucocorticoid secretion and inflammation-induced immune cell resistance to glucocorticoids. *American Journal of Respiratory and Critical Care Medicine* 2002; **165**(7): 983–991.

153 Sprung CL, Annane D, Keh D *et al.* Hydrocortisone therapy for patients with septic shock. *The New England Journal of Medicine* 2008; **358**(2): 111–124.

154 Harry R, Auzinger G, Wendon J. The clinical importance of adrenal insufficiency in acute hepatic dysfunction. *Hepatology* (Baltimore, Md) 2002; **36**(2): 395–402.

155 Harry R, Auzinger G, Wendon J. The effects of supraphysiological doses of corticosteroids in hypotensive liver failure. *Liver Int* 2003; **23**(2): 71–77.

156 O'Grady JG, Alexander GJ, Hayllar KM, Williams R. Early indicators of prognosis in fulminant hepatic failure. *Gastroenterology* 1989; **97**(2): 439–445.

157 Harrison PM, O'Grady JG, Keays RT, Alexander GJ, Williams R. Serial prothrombin time as prognostic indicator in paracetamol induced fulminant hepatic failure. *BMJ* (Clinical research ed.) 1990; **301**(6758): 964–966.

158 Harrison PM, Wendon JA, Gimson AE, Alexander GJ, Williams R. Improvement by acetylcysteine of hemodynamics and oxygen transport in fulminant hepatic failure. *The New England Journal of Medicine* 1991; **324**(26): 1852–1857.

159 Walsh TS, Hopton P, Philips BJ, Mackenzie SJ, Lee A. The effect of N-acetylcysteine on oxygen transport and uptake in patients with fulminant hepatic failure. *Hepatology* (Baltimore, Md) 1998; **27**(5): 1332–1340.

160 Harrison P, Wendon J, Williams R. Evidence of increased guanylate cyclase activation by acetylcysteine in fulminant hepatic failure. *Hepatology* (Baltimore, Md) 1996; **23**(5): 1067–1072.

161 Lee WM, Hynan LS, Rossaro L *et al.* Intravenous N-acetylcysteine improves transplant-free survival in early stage non-acetaminophen acute liver failure. *Gastroenterology* 2009; **137**: 856–864.

162 Stange J, Hassanein TI, Mehta R, Mitzner SR, Bartlett RH. The molecular adsorbents recycling system as a liver support system based on albumin dialysis: a summary of preclinical investigations, prospective, randomized, controlled clinical trial, and clinical experience from 19 centers. *Artificial Organs* 2002; **26**(2): 103–110.

163 Logsen Hea. *Correction of Increased Plasma Amino Acid Levels by Dialysis with Amino-Acid-Electrolyte Glucose Solutions.* Springer-Verlag, New York, 1981.

164 Gimson AE, Braude S, Mellon PJ, Canalese J, Williams R. Earlier charcoal haemoperfusion in fulminant hepatic failure. *Lancet* 1982; **2**(8300): 681–683.

165 Tygstrup NLF, Hansen BA. *Treatment of acute liver failure by high volume plasmapheresis.* Cambridge University Press, Cambridge, 1997.

166 Novelli G, Rossi M, Pretagostini R *et al.* MARS (Molecular Adsorbent Recirculating System): experience in 34 cases of acute liver failure. *Liver* 2002; **22**(Suppl. 2): 43–47.

167 Kantola T, Koivusalo AM, Hockerstedt K, Isoniemi H. The effect of molecular adsorbent recirculating system treatment on survival, native liver recovery, and need for liver transplantation in acute liver failure patients. *Transpl Int* 2008; **21**(9): 857–866.

168 Wai CT, Lim SG, Aung MO *et al.* MARS: a futile tool in centres without active liver transplant support. *Liver Int* 2007; **27**(1): 69–75.

169 Ellis AJ, Hughes RD, Wendon JA *et al.* Pilot-controlled trial of the extracorporeal liver assist device in acute liver failure. *Hepatology* (Baltimore, Md) 1996; **24**(6): 1446–1451.

170 Demetriou AA, Brown RS, Jr., Busuttil RW *et al.* Prospective, randomized, multicenter, controlled trial of a bioartificial liver in treating acute liver failure. *Annals of Surgery* 2004; **239**(5): 660–667; discussion 667–670.

171 Ringe B, Lubbe N, Kuse E, Frei U, Pichlmayr R. Management of emergencies before and after liver transplantation by early total hepatectomy. *Transplantation Proceedings* 1993; 25(1 Pt 2): 1090.

172 Benhamou JP. *Fulminant and Sub-Fulminant Hepatic Failure – Definitions and Causes.* Mitre Press, London, 1991.

173 O'Grady JG, Wendon J, Tan KC *et al.* Liver transplantation after paracetamol overdose. *BMJ* (Clinical research ed.) 1991; **303**(6796): 221–223.

174 Walsh TS, McLellan S, Mackenzie SJ, Lee A. Hyperlactatemia and pulmonary lactate production in patients with fulminant hepatic failure. *Chest* 1999; **116**(2): 471–476.

175 Murphy ND, Kodakat SK, Wendon JA *et al.* Liver and intestinal lactate metabolism in patients with acute hepatic failure undergoing liver transplantation. *Critical Care Medicine* 2001; **29**(11): 2111–2118.

176 Bernal W, Donaldson N, Wyncoll D, Wendon J. Blood lactate as an early predictor of outcome in paracetamol-induced acute liver failure: a cohort study. *Lancet* 2002; **359**(9306): 558–563.

177 Bernuau J, Goudeau A, Poynard T *et al.* Multivariate analysis of prognostic factors in fulminant hepatitis B. *Hepatology* (Baltimore, Md) 1986; **6**(4): 648–651.

178 Pauwels A, Mostefa-Kara N, Florent C, Levy VG. Emergency liver transplantation for acute liver failure. Evaluation of London and Clichy criteria. *Journal of Hepatology* 1993; **17**(1): 124–127.

179 Mitchell I, Bihari D, Chang R, Wendon J, Williams R. Earlier identification of patients at risk from acetaminophen-induced acute liver failure. *Critical Care Medicine* 1998; **26**(2): 279–284.

180 Bernal W, Wendon J, Rela M, Heaton N, Williams R. Use and outcome of liver transplantation in acetaminophen-induced

acute liver failure. *Hepatology* (Baltimore, Md) 1998; **27**(4): 1050–1055.

181 Chenard-Neu MP, Boudjema K, Bernuau J *et al.* Auxiliary liver transplantation: regeneration of the native liver and outcome in 30 patients with fulminant hepatic failure – a multicenter European study. *Hepatology* (Baltimore, Md) 1996; **23**(5): 1119–1127.

182 Quaglia A, Portmann BC, Knisely AS *et al.* Auxiliary transplantation for acute liver failure: histopathological study of native liver regeneration. *Liver Transpl* 2008; **14**(10): 1437–1448.

42 Liver transplantation: Prevention and treatment of rejection

Maria Pleguezuelo, Giacomo Germani and Andrew K Burroughs
The Royal Free Sheila Sherlock Liver Centre, Royal Free Hospital *and* University College London, London, UK

Introduction

Liver transplantation (LT) has evolved rapidly over the past four decades. It may seem logical to consider LT recipients as a homogeneous group of patients who should be managed using universally applicable protocols, but they are a heterogeneous group of individuals, with different predisposing factors and co-factors for the development of rejection [1]. However, appropriate therapeutic approaches should be generated on the basis of evidence. In this chapter we attempt to elucidate the following:

• Do the severity, timing and number of episodes of acute cellular rejection affect prognosis?
• Is it possible to predict which patients will develop clinically significant acute rejection?
• Can immunosuppression be tailored to the individual patient?
• What is the evidence from randomized controlled trials that supports the choice of an immunosuppressive agent?
• Is it possible to withdraw immunosuppression or to change to less toxic immunosuppression?
• What is the influence of immunosuppression on HCV (hepatitis C virus) recurrence after LT?
• Does immunnosuppression have a role in preventing HCC recurrence after LT?

During the past 25 years LT has become the standard therapy for acute and chronic liver failure of all etiologies. Nowadays most patients and liver grafts survive beyond the perioperative period, achieving one-year and ten-year survival rates of 90% and 65–80% respectively [2, 3]. In addition to longer survival, most LT recipients experience improved quality of life, including resumption of active employment and reproductive capacity [4–8]. Despite these advances, LT faces several major challenges. Long-term outcome of patients is becoming the main concern for clinicians who have to deal with the side effects of immunosuppressant drugs in the long term. These include opportunistic infections that affect up to 50% of recipients, contributing to mortality in approximately 10%, and an increased incidence of *de novo* malignancy as a consequence of immunosuppression. In addition, complications arise from direct drug toxicity such as hypertension, renal dysfunction, induction of diabetes and dyslipidemias and rarely nodular regenerative hyperplasia of the liver, in patients receiving azathioprine [9–12]. The most important complication is the development of nephrotoxicity due to calcineurin inhibitors. In a series from Birmingham, 4% of patients surviving one year or more developed severe chronic renal failure, with a mortality of 44% in this group [13]. In a study on 36,849 LT recipients the cumulative incidence of chronic renal failure after LT at 12, 36 and 60 months was 8.0 ± 0.1, 13.9 ± 0.2 and 18.1 ± 0.2 percent respectively [14]. In another series 6.9% had renal dysfunction within one year and 4.7% after one year, defined as a creatinine $>1.8\,mg/dl$ for two weeks or more [15]. Moreover, the nephrotoxic effects, hypertension and hyperlipidemia of some immunosuppressive agents have been implicated in the pathogenesis of chronic allograft loss [16]. These problems have stimulated the re-evaluation of the ability of some patients to tolerate their liver graft without the need for long-term immunosuppression (operational tolerance), or with greatly reduced immunosuppression (prope tolerance) with the benefits derived from the return of natural immunity and reduction in drug-related toxicity [17–22].

However, at present the "manipulation" of the immune system to induce tolerance and thus significantly reduce or eliminate immunosuppression is not yet clinically viable [23–25]. Therefore, the vast majority of LT recipients need to take lifelong immunosuppressive therapy and this situation will not change until more reliable methods for

Evidence-Based Gastroenterology and Hepatology, 3rd edition.
J. McDonald, A.K. Burroughs, B. Feagan, and M.B. Fennerty. © 2010
Blackwell Publishing Ltd

predicting and monitoring tolerance in individual patients are developed [21, 22].

Acute allograft rejection

Definition of rejection

Viewed from a biological perspective, the recipient's immune system is activated after transplantation but, because of the baseline immunosuppressive therapy, only some recipients will have clinical manifestations of this [26]. An important distinction has to be made between histological changes of cellular rejection, which may be seen in the absence of any significant clinical or biochemical abnormalities (biological rejection), and those accompanied by clinical signs of graft dysfunction (clinical rejection). However, abnormalities of liver function tests are almost universally present, and symptoms absent, so in the vast majority of the cases, the distinction between clinical and biological rejection, as defined above, can rarely be made in clinical practice.

Acute cellular rejection

Cellular rejection was defined in 1995, by an international panel of experts, as "inflammation of the allograft elicited by genetic disparity between the donor and recipient, primarily affecting interlobular bile ducts and vascular endothelia, including portal veins and hepatic venules and occasionally the hepatic artery and its branches" [26].

Clinical and laboratory findings

Most cases occur in the early postoperative period within 30 days. Late cases are usually associated with non-compliance of immunosuppressive therapy. A major problem is that the incidence varies according to whether rejection is defined on the basis of *clinically significant* rejection or simply on the basis of *histological abnormalities* or a *combination* of the two.

Clinically significant rejection occurs in approximately 50% of patients, whereas histological abnormalities can be seen in up to 80% of protocol biopsies performed at the end of the first week following transplantation [27].

Several reports have clearly indicated that standard liver tests, when elevated, have a low sensitivity and specificity for rejection and show only a weak correlation with the severity of histopathological findings [28, 29]. Various markers have been studied in an attempt to seek a specific indicator of graft rejection [30]. However, although markers of immune activation, such as peripheral eosinophilia, serum intercellular adhesion molecule (ICAM)-1 and interleukin (IL)-2 receptor are elevated, there is considerable overlap with other conditions (including sepsis and reper-

fusion injury) and none of these markers has been adopted into routine clinical practice.

Graft eosinophilia has been identified as an independently associated feature of acute cellular rejection in LT [31]. The absence of peripheral eosinophilia predicted the absence of moderate/severe histological rejection in one study [32]. However, as yet this has not been validated in other centers. Eosinophilia cannot be used to predict or to assess the response to corticosteroids for the treatment of acute rejection [32]. Therefore, liver histology remains the gold standard for the diagnosis of acute rejection [33–35].

Histopathological features

The three main histopathological features are:
• A predominantly mononuclear but mixed portal inflammation, containing blast-like or activated lymphocytes, neutrophils and eosinophils (graded 1 to 3).
• Subendothelial inflammation of portal or terminal hepatic veins (or both) (graded 1 to 3).
• Bile duct inflammation and damage (graded 1 to 3).

In general, at least two of the above histopathological findings and biochemical evidence of liver damage constitutes the minimal diagnostic criteria for hepatic rejection. The diagnosis is strengthened if >50% of the ducts are damaged or if unequivocal endothelitis of the portal vein branches or terminal hepatic venules can be identified (see Table 42.1).

Early studies of the liver allograft rejection were focused mainly on inflammatory changes occurring in portal tracts,

Table 42.1 Banff schema for grading of acute liver allograft rejection.

Overall grade[a]	Criterion
Indeterminate	Portal inflammatory infiltrate that fails to meet the criteria for the diagnosis of acute rejection
Mild	Rejection infiltrate in a minority of the triads that is generally mild and confined within the portal spaces
Moderate	Rejection infiltrate that expands most or all of the triads
Severe	As for "moderate" but with spillover into periportal areas and moderate to severe perivenular inflammation that extends into the hepatic parenchyma and is associated with perivenular hepatocyte necrosis

[a]Verbal descriptions of mild, moderate and severe acute rejection could also be labeled as grades 1, 2 and 3 respectively.

but also recognized the presence of inflammation involving hepatic venous endothelium and surrounding liver parenchyma [36–38]. During the Eighth Banff Conference on Allograft Pathology in 2005, the term *central perivenulitis* emerged to describe a spectrum of inflammatory regions of the liver that are in most cases thought to be a manifestation of liver allograft rejection. In cases in which perivenular inflammation occurrs within the first weeks of LT and is associated with characteristic portal tract changes, the diagnosis of rejection is straightforward [39]. However in cases where portal inflammation lacks typical features of ACR the term *isolated central perivenulitis* should be used [40]. Krasinkas *et al.* demonstrated that isolated central perivenulitis is a common finding in late post-transplant biopsies and that most cases are probably related to rejection and are associated with a worse outcome compared to cases of purely portal-based rejection [40]. In 2004 Lovell *et al.* found that patients with centrilobular alterations in their first post-transplant biopsy (n = 15) developed chronic rejection more frequently (60% vs 30%; p < 0.04) and subsequent episodes of acute rejection (53% vs 25%; p < 0.04) when compared to patients who did not have centrilobular alterations (n = 20) [41].

Grading and staging

In 1997, an international consensus on a common grading system for acute allograft rejection was achieved and subsequently it has been prospectively tested and proved to be simple, reliable and clinically relevant [42–44].

According to this Banff schema, which represents a merger and simplification of many previously published studies (see Table 42.1), there are two main components: the first is a global assessment of the overall rejection grade (indeterminate, mild, moderate, severe), the second involves scoring the three specific features of rejection semiquantitatively to produce an overall Rejection Activity Index (RAI) [45].

Datta-Gupta *et al.* showed that graft eosinophilia was an independent diagnostic marker of acute cellular rejection and it was included in the scoring system developed at the Royal Free Hospital [31].

Role of liver biopsy and indication for treatment

The use of liver biopsy in the early post-transplant setting depends on each center's policy. Nowadays there is less uniformity regarding the use of protocol liver biopsies. This is mainly for two reasons: risks associated with the procedure and doubts about the usefulness of these biopsies to guide therapy, particularly amongst patients with normalizing transaminase values and other biochemical values [46]. However, to date, no large series has described a substantial risk associated with percutaneous liver biop-

sies in transplant recipients [46–48], and greater use of transjugular liver biopsies improves the applicability and does not increase the complication rate compared to percutaneous biopsies [49, 50].

Although it is accepted that liver histology is the gold standard and is essential for the diagnosis of acute cellular rejection, controversy continues to arise over the indications for treatment of rejection. The implication of this is that if treatment is not going to be given, why do a liver biopsy? Specifically, there is the question of the patient who has histological features of acute cellular rejection on protocol liver biopsy, with static or improving graft dysfunction. Some studies suggest that there is spontaneous resolution of mild rejection without biochemical dysfunction [51, 52]. However, abnormal liver function is more usual, and liver function tests are seldom normal at 5–7 days post-transplantation when protocol biopsies are usually done.

Bartlett *et al.* reviewed the literature concerning the natural history of acute cellular rejection, comprising 1566 patients, all of whom had protocol biopsies: 331 (21%) patients had evidence of acute histologic rejection with "normal or normalizing liver function tests" [53]. The majority (91%) of these patients did not receive adjuvant immunosuppression, and only 4% developed chronic rejection. **B3** Given these results, the authors concluded that withholding adjuvant immunosuppression from patients with histologic acute cellular rejection with "normal or normalizing liver function tests" is safe, thus not supporting the practice of protocol liver biopsies. However, the study has several limitations: the retrospective nature of the analysis of a heterogeneous group of studies, the lack of definition of "normal or normalizing liver function tests" and the lack of evaluation of histological severity of acute cellular rejection in patients without "biochemical graft dysfunction". Before abandoning protocol biopsies, a hard look needs to be given to the evidence supporting this approach, and well designed prospective studies are necessary [54].

A further issue is that even severe histological rejection, and not only mild rejection, may resolve spontaneously and only rarely does this lead to graft loss [1, 55]. There is now evidence that the development of early rejection which responds to treatment has no negative long-term effects and may even be associated with lower risk for later immunological complications [44, 56]. Thus, the more fundamental question is how much rejection is not harmful, and therefore complete suppression of rejection is not a goal in managing immunosuppression.

Prognostic factors

Do the severity, timing and number of episodes of acute cellular rejection affect prognosis?

Number of episodes

In an abstract, Wiesner et al. evaluating a LT database with 870 patients followed for a median of three years, showed that the number of episodes of acute rejection and the histological severity were significantly associated with chronic rejection (p < 0.001) [57]. Dousset et al. prospectively evaluated 170 LT patients and showed that there was no difference in graft function between patients with a single episode of acute rejection (n = 56) and those without rejection (n = 84) [58]. Among patients treated for a single episode of acute rejection, late hepatic function was not influenced by the severity of acute rejection, or by the response to corticosteroids. In contrast, patients with more than one acute rejection episode (n = 30) had significant impairment of liver function tests (aspartate aminotransferase (AST) p < 0.05; alanine aminotransferase (ALT), p < 0.001; alkaline phosphatase, p < 0.01), lower dye clearances (p < 0.01), and more severe histological damage (p < 0.001). The authors concluded that a single episode of acute rejection does not impair long-term hepatic function, whereas recurrent episodes can lead to damage to the liver allograft.

Severity

McVicar et al. described a group of patients who had focal rejection in the hepatic allograft biopsy defined as lymphocytic infiltration involving less than 20% of portal tracts [59]. In the follow-up of patients showing focal or mild rejection, only six (15%) patients subsequently developed abnormal liver function tests and required treatment with additional immunosuppression for acute cellular rejection, suggesting additional immunosuppression is not needed in these patients, and close follow-up would identify the small number requiring therapy [56]. **B4**

In Birmingham, during follow-up of 151 patients to assess the effect of not treating mild acute rejection (protocol seven-day biopsies), 97 had histologically mild rejection, 50 had biochemical dysfunction and received prednisone for three days, while the remaining 47 cases with stable biochemistry had no additional treatment. Fifty-four patients with no rejection were included for comparison. The outcome at three months in all three groups was similar [27]. **B4**

Wiesner et al., using the Liver Transplantation Database in a cohort study of 762 consecutive adult LT recipients, examined the association of histological severity of acute rejection and overall patient outcome [44]. They showed, using univariate analysis, that acute rejection overall, including mostly the milder grades, was significantly associated with an increased patient survival (relative risk (RR) 0.71, p = 0.05) and a trend toward improved graft survival. Moreover, adjusting for other risk factors such as age and renal insufficiency revealed no significant decrease in survival among patients who had rejection. These findings

were similar to those of Fisher et al. who analyzed nine studies (comprising a total of 1473 patients), and found that there was no correlation between mortality and incidence of treated acute cellular rejection [60]. **B4**

These findings in LT are in contrast to renal transplantation in which acute rejection is significantly associated with decreased patient and graft survival. Why acute cellular rejection in LT recipients is not associated with decreased patient and graft survival remains unexplained. It is possible that acute rejection in the setting of controlled alloreactivity exerts a tolerizing effect, making the graft less susceptible to further immunological attack. However, it should be noted that successful treatment for cellular rejection occurs in nearly all cases. Thus, the correct interpretation of the finding reported above is that the occurrence and successful treatment of acute cellular rejection does not influence survival in LT patients, but it does imply that abolishing early cellular rejection need not, and indeed, should not be a goal of initial immunosuppression. This may eliminate the WOFIE period to provide some tolerance to the graft [17, 21, 22].

Timing

As regards timing of acute cellular rejection, there is no firm consensus to define what is early or late rejection. In three different studies the timing and the outcome varied according to the definition of each center.

In a retrospective multi-center analysis of 623 LT, the cumulative incidence of biopsy proved rejection was 59% for early episodes (<6 months) and 21% for late episodes (= 6 months). Patient and graft survival did not differ significantly between those who experienced an early acute rejection episode and those who did not (p = 0.49 and p = 0.13 respectively). Furthermore, these parameters did not differ significantly between recipients who experienced a late acute rejection episode and those who did not (patient survival p = 0.18 and graft survival p = 0.20) [57].

Wiesner et al. analyzed 762 consecutive adult LT recipients (Liver Transplantation Database) and found 367 (48%) who developed at least one acute cellular rejection episode within the first six weeks post-transplantation (occurring at a median time of eight days) [44]. Multivariate analysis indicated that acute cellular rejection was not significantly associated with mortality but there was a trend to better survival (RR 0.78, p = 0.25) and re-transplantation free survival (RR 0.86, p = 0.44). **B4** However, severe rejection doubled the risk of death or re-transplantation compared to mild rejection. Using proportional hazards modelling, in the same study, seven factors were identified as independently associated with an increased incidence of early acute hepatic allograft rejection: younger recipient age, lack of renal impairment, lack of edema, higher AST levels, fewer human leukocyte antigen (HLA) DR matches, longer cold ischemic times and older donors.

Mor *et al.* retrospectively reviewed 375 LT, and defined late onset acute cellular rejection as that which occurred after six months [61]. There were 315 episodes of early acute cellular rejection in 226 patients, and 31 episodes of late acute cellular rejection in 26 patients. Low cyclosporine levels appeared to account for 58% of these late episodes. Most episodes of rejection responded to pulse corticosteroids, and chronic ductopenic rejection arose in only two patients. There was no difference in survival between patients experiencing early and late rejection.

Anand *et al.* reviewed late onset acute cellular rejection, defining it as rejection recognized after the first 30 days post-transplantation [62]. They evaluated 717 patients who had undergone transplantation in Birmingham between 1982 and 1994: 59 (8%) patients had 71 episodes of late rejection. They, too, found that the most common precipitating event was low levels of calcineurin antagonists, and that most acute episodes of rejection in this timeframe were responsive to standard therapy. However, in contrast to Mor *et al.* [61], Anand found that 16 (27%) of 59 patients developing late onset rejection progressed to chronic ductopenic rejection and graft loss. Delayed response to an earlier episode of acute rejection, and centrilobular necrosis or bile duct loss at the time of diagnosis of late rejection, were associated with high risk of progression to chronic rejection and graft loss.

These results regarding timing, severity and number of episodes of early acute cellular rejection indicate that attempts to reduce the incidence of early acute rejection to very low levels in LT is neither necessary nor appropriate. Second, knowledge of the pathways of rejection and tolerance suggest that increased immunosuppression will inhibit the development of donor-specific tolerance, increase the incidence of immunosuppressive-related complications and result in poorer outcome [21, 22, 24]. Indeed, it is probably better not to treat certain mild, acute or other rejection episodes, and this practice is commonplace in some centers. However, randomized controlled trials are needed to provide evidence supporting this approach and to define thresholds for treatment.

Prediction of acute rejection

Is it possible to predict which patients will develop clinically significant acute rejection?

Data from Birmingham show that there is a lower incidence of acute rejection when there is no evidence of immune involvement in the pathogenesis of the original liver disease, for example fulminant hepatic failure from paracetamol [1, 63]. In contrast, in patients transplanted for primary biliary cirrhosis and sclerosing cholangitis, in which immune-mediated damage of bile ducts is a feature of the original disease, acute rejection occurs more frequently and there is more frequent progression to ducto-

penic rejection. **B4** In 63 patients reported by Hayashi *et al.* patients with autoimmune hepatitis had more acute rejection than patients with alcoholic cirrhosis (81% vs 46.8%, p < 0.001) regardless of the type of immunosuppression, and steroid-resistant rejection also occurred more frequently in patients with autoimmune liver disease than in patients with alcoholic liver disease (38.1% vs 12.8%; p = 0.003) with a trend towards more chronic rejection (11.1% vs 2.1%) [64]. **B4** However, there was no difference in allograft or patient survival at one and three years. Berlakovich *et al.* evaluated 252 LT patients: those who had undergone LT for alcoholic cirrhosis (n = 60), hepatoma (n = 91) and posthepatitic cirrhosis (n = 59) had less acute rejection and less need of rescue therapy than patients who had received LT for cholestatic disease (n = 42) [65]. The cumulative rates of acute rejection episodes per patient per month at six months, when 94% of all acute rejection episodes occurred, were: 0.45 for alcoholic cirrhosis, 0.55 for post-hepatitic cirrhosis, 0.65 for hepatoma and 1.0 for cholestatic disease. **B4**

The group which has been consistently shown to have a lower incidence of acute and chronic rejection is chronic hepatitis B. This might reflect the underlying defect in cell-mediated immunity, which allowed the patients to become chronically infected with the virus in the first place [66, 67].

Farges *et al.*, in a retrospective analysis of 330 patients who were LT recipients for chronic liver disease, found that acute rejection (48% at one year) and chronic rejection (10% at three years) were comparable in patients who had undergone LT for primary biliary cirrhosis, sclerosing cholangitis, autoimmune cirrhosis and hepatitis C cirrhosis [66]. However, the incidence of acute (but not chronic) rejection was significantly lower in patients who had undergone LT for alcoholic cirrhosis (29% at one year), or hepatitis B virus (HBV) cirrhosis (21% at one year) and the latter also had lower chronic rejection (0% at three years). **B4** Thus, some groups of patients can receive less immunosuppresion. In particular, as HBV replication is potentiated by immunosuppression, it is also beneficial to reduce immunosuppression in these patients. However, Wiesner *et al.*, using multivariate analysis, showed that the six-week incidence of acute rejection in a cohort of 762 consecutive adult LT recipients was not dependent on the underlying disease [44].

Neuberger *et al.* showed that the percentage of patients with severe acute rejection at the liver biopsy performed seven days after the transplantation was higher among patients transplanted for HCV-related liver disease (69%) compared to other etiologies [1].

Although it is difficult to draw firm recommendations from these studies, most centers tend to lessen maintenance immunosuppression for HBV, HCV cirrhosis, alcoholic liver disease and hepatoma and/or use early steroid withdrawal, from the outset. Conversely, patients with autoimmune hepatitis, primary biliary cirrhosis, or primary sclerosing cholangitis may need steroid maintenance and heavier initial immunosuppression.

Gomez-Manero et al. reviewed 133 transplanted recipients to identify predisposing factors for early (≤45 days after LT) acute rejection [68]. No protocol liver biopsies were performed. Younger recipients, those with better hepatocellular liver function (Child A) and those who underwent transplantation for liver disease other than alcoholic cirrhosis, had a greater risk for early acute rejection. Combining these three variables, they developed a mathematical model to allow prediction of the individual risk of each patient. **B4** In our center we retrospectively evaluated a cohort of 470 LT patients who received protocol biopsies, looking at the presence of predictive factors for the absence of acute cellular rejection, during the first three months after LT. We found that the absence of rejection was associated with pre-transplant need of renal support, higher INR (International Normalized Ratio) level and a "healthy" appearance of the graft [69].

In summary, different studies have aimed to identify patients with a greater risk for developing acute rejection, but with some exceptions, they have been limited to a small number of patients and focused on a limited number of risk factors, and the results have been frequently contradictory. For this reason there is no consensus about the majority of factors predisposing to the occurrence of acute rejection after LT.

Immunosuppression in liver transplant recipients

Choice of an immunosuppressive agent

What evidence is there from randomised controlled trials to support the choice of an immunosuppressive agent?

Calcineurin inhibitors

Calcineurin inhibitors are still the cornerstone of immunosuppressive regimens. Both cyclosporine (CsA) and tacrolimus (Tac) bind to cytoplasmic receptors (cyclophilin and FK-binding protein 12 respectively), and the resulting complexes inactivate calcineurin, a pivotal enzyme in T cell receptor signaling. Calcineurin inhibition prevents IL-2 gene transcription, thereby inhibiting T cell IL production [70].

Regimens based on CsA resulted in one-year graft survival rates that exceeded 70%, but graft rejection still remained a cause of re-transplantation and death. Tac was superior to the old formulation of CsA (Sandimmune) for preventing acute rejection in three RCTs [71–73]. However, no significant benefits in mortality or graft loss were found. Thereafter, the microemulsion formulation of CsA (CsA-

ME) (Neoral) was developed improving absorption, generating new trials versus Tac [74]. Monitoring two-hour post-dose CsA levels (C_2) has advantages over conventional trough CsA blood levels (pre-dose) (C_0) [75].

The best evidence for comparison of the two CNI is derived from a meta-analysis of 16 RCT (nine multi-centers), including 3813 patients (1899 randomized to Tac and 1914 to CsA) (see Table 42.2) [71–73, 76–90]. The earliest three trials compared Tac with the original oil-based formulation of CsA, in the other studies CsA-ME was used [71–73]. C_0 was used in all RCT but one, which used C_2 monitoring [89]. Prednisone was used as concomitant medication in all trials except one [83]; azathioprine (AZA) was used in nine trials (it was given only in the CsA group in four) and mycophenolate mofetil was used in four trials. The duration of the studies reached 12 months in 14 trials, and in the other two only six (77), and three months [85]. Immunosuppression with Tac reduced mortality by 15% at one-year post-LT (RR 0.85; 95% CI: 0.73–0.99), reduced graft loss by 22% (RR 0.78; 95% CI: 0.68–0.79), rejection by 18% (RR 0.82; 95% CI: 0.76–0.88) and steroid-resistant rejection by 43% (RR 0.57; 95% CI: 0.49–0.66). **A1a** New-onset diabetes occurred at a 27% higher rate with Tac (RR 1.27; 95% CI: 1.12–1.44).

The reduction in mortality associated with Tac was maintained when subanalyses of HCV patients were performed (RR 0.85; 95% CI: 0.73–0.99). **A1c** No significant differences were found in need for dialysis, or serum creatinine levels one year after LT or in the incidence of lymphoproliferative disorders. Thus, treating 100 patients post-LT with Tac instead of CsA would avoid death in two patients, graft loss in five, rejection in nine and steroid-resistant rejection in seven. Discontinuation of treatment was more frequent in patients with CsA than with Tac (RR 0.57; 95% CI: 0.49–0.66). **A1a** Neither the formulation of CsA (oil-based vs microemulsion) nor the method to guide its dose (C_0 vs C_2), affected the outcomes, although only one study used C_2 monitoring.

The updated TMC study, giving data three years after randomization reported that 23.6% of patients in the Tac group and 26.2% in the CsA group had died [91]. Re-transplantation rates were 4.6% (Tac group) and 12.1% (CsA group). The primary endpoint (combined frequency, whichever occurred first, of death, re-transplantation or treatment failure for immunological reasons), was still significantly less frequent in the Tac group than in the CsA-ME (RR 0.75; 95% CI: 0.60–0.95). However, the combined endpoint of death or re-transplantation rate was not statistically different between groups. Discontinuation of CsA was more frequent than Tac (56.4% vs 33.9%, p < 0.01). In the Tac group, a total of 62.1% of patients were alive at three years, with the original graft and still on their allocated medication, compared with 41.6% in the CsA group (p < 0.001).

Table 42.2 Randomized trials of tacrolimus vs cyclosporin included in the meta-analysis.

Author	Year	Groups	n	Immunosuppression Dose	Blood levels to maintain	Other agents	Results Minimum follow-up (months)	BPACR (%)	Patient mortality (%)
Fung	1991	Tac CsA-OB (C$_0$)	41 40	0.1 mg/kg → 0.15 mg/kg 4 mg/kg → 8 mg/kg		Steroids Steroids	12	9.8 30	7.3 17.5
US study	1994	Tac CsA-OB (C$_0$)	263 266	0.05 mg/kg → 0.15 mg/kg 1–2 mg/kg → 5 mg/kg		Steroids Steroids ± AZA	12	18.2[a] 20.7	11.8 12.4
European study	1994	Tac CsA-OB (C$_0$)	264 265	0.075 mg/kg → 0.3 mg/kg 1–6 mg/kg → 8–15 mg/kg		Steroids Steroids ± AZA ± ATG	12	24.6 27.9	17.4 23.1
Stegall	1997	Tac CsA-ME (C$_0$)	35 36	6 mg 600 mg	10–15 ng/ml 300–350 ng/ml	Steroids + MMF Steroids + MMF	6	14.3 8.3	11.4 5.6
Fisher	1998	Tac CsA-ME (C$_0$)	49 50	0.15 mg/kg 8–10 mg/kg	10–15 ng/ml → 5–10 ng/ml 300–400 ng/ml → 200–300 ng/ml	Steroids + MMF Steroids + MMF	60	6.1[a] 10.0	2.0 4.0
Zervos	1998	Tac CsA-ME (C$_0$)	25 24	0.05 mg/kg 3 mg/kg	15 ng/ml 200–300 ng/ml	Steroids Steroids	14	32.0[a] 50.0	28.0 33.3
Klupp	1999	Tac CsA-ME (C$_0$)	40 40	According to protocol centre According to protocol centre		Steroids + MMF Steroids + MMF	26	0 10.0	5.0 7.5
Rolles	1999	Tac CsA-ME (C$_0$)	30 34	0.05 mg/kg/d 5 mg/kg	5–15 ng/ml 100–300 ng/ml	None None	12	26.7[a] 38.2	16.7 20.6
Muehlbacher	1991	Tac CsA-ME (C$_0$)	313 307	0.15 mg/kg 8–15 mg/kg	10–20 ng/ml → 5–15 ng/ml 150–300 ng/ml	Steroids Steroids ± AZA	12	16. 16.9	15.1 12.1
O'Grady (tmc)	2002	Tac CsA-ME (C$_0$)	301 305	0.1 mg/kg 10 mg/kg	5–15 ng/ml 200–300 ng/ml → 150–250 ng/ml	Steroids + AZA Steroids + AZA	12	19.3 28.9	16.6 23.6
Therapondos	2002	Tac CsA-ME (C$_0$)	20 20	0.1 mg/kg 10 mg/kg	5–15 ng/ml 150–200 nmol/L	Steroids + AZA Steroids + AZA	12	10.0[a] 5.0	10.0 5.0
Timmermann	2002	Tac CsA-ME (C$_0$)	72 71	0.1 mg/kg According to protocol centre	5–15 ng/ml According to protocol centre	Steroids ± ALG Steroids ± AZA ± ALG	3	13.9 18.3	9.7 9.7
Greig	2003	Tac CsA-ME (C$_0$)	71 72	0.1–0.15 mg/kg 10–15 mg/kg	10–20 ng/ml → 5–15 ng/ml 300–400 ng/ml → 100–250 ng/ml	Steroids + AZA Steroids + AZA	12	2.8 13.9	2.8 11.1
Grazi	2004	Tac CsA-ME (C$_2$)	245 250	0.1–0.15 mg/kg 10–15 mg/kg	5–15 ng/ml → 5–12 ng/ml 0.8–1.2 ug/ml → 0.7–0.9 ug/ml	Steroids ± AZA Steroids ± AZA	12	11.8 10.8	13.9 14.8
Kelly	2004	Tac CsA-ME (C$_0$)	92 93 (pediat)	0.3 mg/kg 10 mg/kg	10–20 ng/ml → 5–10 ng/ml 250–350 mg/L → 100–150 mg/L	Steroids Steroids + AZA	12	7.6 13.9	7.6 9.7
Martin	2004	Tac CsA-ME (C$_0$)	38 41	0.1–0.15 mg/kg 6–10 mg/kg	5–10 ng/ml → 5–10 ng/ml 200–250 ng/ml → 100–250 ng/ml	Steroids + AZA Steroids + AZA	12	18.4[a] 24.4	15.8 19.5

[a]Trials in which protocol biopsies were performed after transplantation: US study: days 7–28–360; Fisher et al.; only in HCV positive patients: month 12–24–36; Zervos et al.; month 12–18; Rolles et al.: days 5–10; Therapondos et al.: day 7; Martin et al.: month 3–12.

Tac: tacrolimus; CsA: cyclosporin; CsA-OB: cyclosporin, oily-based formulation; CsA-ME: cyclosporin, microemulsion formulation; AZA: azathioprine; MMF: mycophenolate mofetil; ATG: antithymocyte globulin; ALG: antilymphocyte globulin; BPACR: biopsy proven acute cellular rejection.

The five-year post-randomization surveillance of the Spanish multicenter RCT demonstrated no differences in overall survival (CsA-ME 76% vs Tac 66%, p = 0.18), re-transplantation (CsA-ME 8% vs Tac 10%, p = 0.73) or acute rejection rates (CsA-ME 33% vs Tac 26%, p = 0.8) [92]. However, the proportion of patients switched from CsA-ME to Tac was significantly higher (CsA-ME to Tac 29% vs Tac to CsA-ME 8%, p = 0.01), mainly due to lack of efficacy of allocated therapy. Both groups had similar occurrence of side effects, except for hyperglycemia, which was more frequent in the Tac group (CsA-ME 9.8% vs Tac 26.5%, p = 0.04), while CsA-ME had a higher rate of severe adverse events or prolongation of hospitalization (CsA-ME 94% vs Tac 64%, p < 0.05). In this study C_0 monitoring was used.

However, in some of these trials, methodological aspects such as risk of bias in the sequence generation, baseline imbalance of the clinical factors, as well as the additional use of AZA in the CsA group and not Tac group, and the absence of defining diagnosis of rejection, suggest some caution in interpreting the magnitude of the difference between CsA and Tac.

In addition, several changes have occurred in the clinical practice since the design of these trials, such as the adoption of the C_2 monitoring for CsA and the fact that AZA is now rarely used in primary immunosuppression regimens.

CNI-induced nephrotoxicity has a component of reversible renal vasoconstriction. Eventually tubulointerstitial chronic fibrosis and irreversible change result, but the interval between reversible and irreversible changes is variable [93]. Withdrawal of CNI during early stages of renal dysfunction results in improvement of renal function, but the optimal moment for conversion is not clear, although it is likely to be within six months of LT [94].

Therapeutic drug monitoring of cyclosporine Therapeutic monitoring of CNI is essential. CsA has a narrow therapeutic index, and an extremely variable pharmacokinetic profile and a strong pharmacodynamic linkage between desired and adverse effects.

An expert group has recommended C_2 monitoring of CsA as optimal single-time point for monitoring [95]. LIS2T is an RCT that compared CsA-ME with C_2 monitoring vs Tac [96], stratifying patients according to HCV status. Patients received either CsA-ME (n = 250) or Tac (n = 245) with steroids and some with AZA (41% CsA and 43% Tac). The primary outcome was the incidence of biopsy proven acute rejection within three months after LT: 26% CsA-ME vs 24% Tac (p = ns). The six-month survival rate was 89% (CsA-ME) vs 88% (Tac) (p = ns); the six-month graft loss rate was 4% (CsA-ME) vs 5% (Tac) (p = ns). The sub-analysis of patients receiving dual or triple therapy with AZA whether with CsA-ME or Tac showed similar acute rejection rates, also between HCV-positive and HCV-negative recipients. However, among HCV-positive patients death or graft loss at six months was significantly higher in the Tac group (15%) than in the CsA-ME group (6%) (p < 0.05). Tolerability and safety were comparable, other than a higher incidence of diabetes mellitus (14% vs 7%, p < 0.02) and diarrhea (29% vs 14%, p < 0.001) in patients treated with Tac. Patients undergoing living-donor transplantation (n = 39) in the LIS2T study showed similar results in terms of acute rejection, overall survival and graft loss between both treatments [97].

Thereafter, further surveillance in the LIS2T study with follow-up data available in 90% of patients, confirmed equivalent outcomes in trial groups as regards patient survival (85% CsA-ME vs 86% Tac), graft survival and rejection at 12 months after LT [98]. In HCV-positive patients, death or graft loss were more frequent in Tac patients (16% Tac vs 6% CsA-ME, p < 0.03), despite HCV recurrence being similar. However, the mean time to histological diagnosis of HCV recurrence was significantly longer with CsA-ME than with Tac (100 ± 50 days vs 70 ± 40 days; p < 0.05). More patients required medication for hyperglycemia in the Tac group, regardless of diabetic status at baseline.

Annual costs were lower for CsA-ME with C_2 monitoring than for Tac ($5432 ± 2091 vs $8291 ± 3948 respectively, p = 0.001) in an RCT [99]. However, the annual pre-transplant and one-year post-transplant drug costs, and costs of concomitant medications were similar. Interestingly, this trial found no significant differences between Tac and CsA-ME-C_2 therapies in terms of one-year patient survival, early acute rejection and incidence of metabolic disorders (diabetes mellitus, hypertension and hyperlipidemia). Opposite to the previous study, Shenoy *et al.* found that recurrent HCV occurred less frequently in Tac treated patients than in CsA-ME treated ones (21% vs 61%; p = 0.04), despite earlier recurrence (Tac 72 ± 42 days vs CsA-ME 145 ± 43 days, p = 0.006) [99]. These data from a single industry sponsored study show that CsA-ME-C_2 provides at least equivalent immunosuppression to Tac, with similar costs, but the beneficial effects on HCV shown in the first study have not been substantiated [98].

Dosage of cyclosporine CsA is usually administered orally as two doses every 12 hours in LT patients. However, some patients have difficulty in achieving therapeutic C_0 or C_2 levels. To address this and to minimize adverse effects, conversion to once daily dosing of CsA-ME (75 ± 15 mg/day) was evaluated in 68 maintenance LT patients (4 ± 1.3 year after LT) with abnormal renal function [100]. The C_2 levels ranged 748 ± 105 ng/ml, without rejection episodes (although protocol biopsies were not done) and with improvement in renal function. Similar results were obtained in a non-randomized trial including 14 patients who underwent living-donor LT [101].

A randomized trial evaluated 60 post-LT patients with renal dysfunction to receive twice-daily CsA-ME vs conversion to once-daily equal dose vs conversion to once-daily reduced dose (to yield a C_2 level 25–35% lower than the post-conversion C_2) [102]. After conversion, C_0 did not change, whereas C_2 nearly doubled and the AUC increased by 29%. Moreover, once-daily dosing was associated with a trend to lower nocturnal mean arterial blood pressure. Thus, it has been suggested that reduction of 25–30% in the dose should be considered when conversion to once-daily dose is performed.

Therapeutic drug monitoring of tacrolimus   Tac whole-blood trough concentration (C_0) is routinely used to monitor therapy in most centres. As for CsA, C_0 does not accurately reflect systemic exposure over the first 12 hours after dosing, for example patients with similar C_0 Tac concentrations can have very different AUC due to the wide intra- and inter-subject variability in Tac pharmacokinetics [103]. Moreover, as for CsA there is no clear association between C_0 concentrations and clinical outcomes. Clearance of Tac in patients in the early post-LT period is influenced by hematocrit and serum albumin, as well as concurrent medications such as diltiazem and fluconazole [104]. Thus, hypoalbuminemia and anemia, two of the most frequent clinical conditions in liver recipients, may increase the Tac clearance.

The relationship between the dose of Tac, trough concentration (enzyme linked immunosorbent assay, ELISA) and selected clinical endpoints (acute rejection, nephrotoxicity and other toxicities) were examined in a prospective multicenter study, which confirmed a poor correlation between the daily dose (mg/kg per day) and the steady-state whole-blood concentration. It suggested that to minimize nephrotoxicity without increasing the risk of rejection, it is necessary to maintain trough Tac blood concentration below 15 ng/ml [105].

In a recent study in which C_0 was confirmed to be suboptimal to monitor Tac therapy, C_4 or C_6 were found the best single timepoints [106]. However this study was developed and validated in patients more than six months post-LT, and thus it cannot be extrapolated to the early post-LT period when the risk of rejection is greatest and when Tac pharmacokinetics may fluctuate widely.

To improve Tac monitoring, measurement of calcineurin activity (CNA) has been proposed, and evaluated in peripheral blood mononuclear cells from 14 patients at 0, 2, 3, 4, 6 and 9 hours after Tac intake on days 8, 21 and 90, post-LT [107]. The time of maximal inhibition of CNA was reached four hours after Tac intake; this could be a means to improve Tac monitoring during the early phase post-LT, but it is difficult to envisage widespread applicability.

Dosage of tacrolimus   A multicenter four-period crossover study showed that conversion from Tac twice a day to a modified extended release (XL) formulation administered once-daily in the morning, led to equivalent exposure at a steady state [108]. There was less intrasubject variability with XL compared to Tac. The two-year post-conversion surveillance showed that the mean Tac whole blood trough concentration ranged from 6.2 to 6.6 ng/ml over the two years after conversion and most patients did not require dose adjustment; patient and graft survival at was 98.6% with an acute rejection rate of 5.8% [109]. Adverse effects were similar to those observed in historical cohorts with twice-a-day Tac.

Tacrolimus rescue for acute cellular rejection   Two studies have demonstrated that Tac at levels of 15–20 mg/dl are effective as rescue therapy for steroid-resistant acute rejection in patients on CsA-based therapy [75, 110]. Moreover, a pilot study suggested that increasing Tac dosage (increments of 1–2 mg every one or two days with trough Tac blood levels of 15–20 ng/ml), and continued low doses of steroids could be considered as treatment for early acute rejection episodes (biopsy proven), including severe grades of rejection [111]. **B4** However, these higher doses of Tac (>15 ng/ml) are associated with renal dysfunction in the long-term, so that the cost-benefit of this strategy versus steroid therapy requires evaluation [105].

In summary, CNI-based immunosuppression, particularly Tac, improves the long-term graft survival in post-LT patients but renal dysfunction is frequent (9.5%) and this can worsen survival and lead to renal transplantation [13]. Reduction in CNI dosage often does not resolve this problem and suspension of CNI is often associated with increased rejection. Better use of CNI, and/or substitution with effective immunosuppressive agents without nephrotoxicity is required. The use of AZA, mycophenolate mofetil (MMF) and sirolimus with lower doses of CsA or Tac is the most commonly used strategy, as use of these agents as single drugs increases rates of rejection and graft loss [112].

Antimetabolites: azathioprine and mycophenolate mofetil

Azathioprine is a prodrug form of 6-mercaptopurine which inhibits T cell activation, reduces antibody synthesis and decreases the circulating monocytes and granulocytes [113]. AZA alone is relatively effective in the prevention of rejection but has very little effect upon an established immune response [114].

Mycophenolate mofetil is a selective inhibitor of the *de novo* pathway of purine biosynthesis, thereby providing more specific and potent inhibition of T cell and B cell proliferation than AZA. It has been used for both treatment and prevention of rejection in combination with CNI (see Table 42.3) [115].

Table 42.3 Randomized trials on MMF in liver transplanted patients.

Author	Year	Groups	Immunosuppression				n
			Dose MMF	Interval since LT	Other agents	BPACR (%)	
Fischer	2000	MMF	1 g bid	No interval	CsA + Ster + ATG	19.4	31
		AZA			CsA + Ster + ATG	40.6	32
Wiesner	2001	MMF	1.5 g bid	No interval	CsA + Ster	38.5	278
		AZA			CsA + Ster	47.7	287
Schlitt	2001	MMF + CNI withdrawal	1 g bid	76 m (median)	± Ster	21.4	14
		CNI		90 m (median)	± Ster	0	14
Reich	2005	MMF + CNI discontinuation	1.5 g/d	16.5 m (mean)	Ster	30.0	20
		MMF + reduction 50% CNI dose		12.9 m (mean)	Ster	11.1	18
Reggiani	2005	MMF	0.75 g/d followed by 0.5 mg/d	No interval	Tac	75[a]	12
		MMF + steroids			Tac	16.7	7
Pageaux	2006	MMF + reduction ≥50% CNI dose	2–3 g/d	62.4 m (median)	± Ster	0	27
		MMF + standard CNI		68.4 m (median)	± Ster ± AZA	3.4	29
Ciccinati (Beckebaum)	2007 (2004)	MMF + low dose CNI	1 g bid	67.2 (mean)	± Ster	0	21
		MMF + full dose CNI		64.8 (mean)		0	11

[a] Only trial in which protocol biopsies were performed (at day 7 after transplantation). This trial was stopped due to a high incidence of acute rejection in the study group.

MMF: mycophenolate mofetil; Ster: steroids; CNI: calcineurin inhibitors; Tac: tacrolimus; CsA: cyclosporin; AZA: azathioprine; ATG: antithimocyte globulin; BPACR: biopsy proven acute cellular rejection; LT: liver transplantation.

MMF (1–1.5 g twice daily) was superior to AZA (1–2 mg/kg/d) in preventing biopsy proven acute rejection in the first six months post-LT in two RCTs, but patient and graft overall was not improved [115, 116]. **Ald** Compared with AZA, MMF has fewer myelotoxic and hepatotoxic adverse effects, but has more gastrointestinal upset including diarrhea, which affects 30% of patients but usually resolves with reducing the dose [117]. The two agents should never be used together. MMF is teratogenetic and 3% of patients develop neutropenia [114]. Opportunistic infections are not significantly increased in comparison to AZA treatment. Monitoring of blood levels is not usually required. Retrospective analysis of large series of liver recipients (n = 15,133) reported better patient and graft survival, as well reduced late acute rejection rates in patients treated with MMF in addition to Tac and steroids, compared with Tac and steroids alone, again just showing that increased immunopotency results in less rejection [118, 119].

An enteric-coated formulation of mycophenolate sodium (EC-MPS) has been developed to reduce the gastrointestinal side effects by delaying mycophenolic acid (MPA, the active metabolite of MMF) release until the small intestine. Bioequivalence has been shown in renal transplantation for both pharmacokinetics [120–122], and RCT [123]. In LT EC-MPS use is limited [124, 125].

MMF has been successfully used as rescue therapy in 38 of 47 (80.9%) liver recipients with acute steroid resistant rejection, in 5 of 8 (62.5%) patients with chronic rejection, in 52 of 60 (86.7%) patients with chronic graft dysfunction and in 46 of 59 (77.9%) patients with CNI-related nephrotoxicity [126]. An RCT including 30 liver recipients who received Tac plus MMF vs Tac plus MMF plus steroids (MMF 750 mg bd for all), showed a higher rate of biopsy proven acute rejection in the former group (75% vs 17%, p < 0.002), with similar toxicity [127]. However early acute rejection did not affect graft or patient survival. As previously mentioned, this study unfortunately did not evaluate equipotent regimes in terms of immunosuppression and just showed that more immunosuppression results in less rejection.

To date there is no clear evidence that combination of MMF with CNI improves graft or patient survival compared to CNI and steroids or AZA. Its role may be more as a renal-sparing agent. When administered to reduce the CNI dose in patients with impaired renal function or as monotherapy, acute rejection episodes occurred in 9–38% of cases after CNI withdrawal [128–130], which was more frequent when withdrawal occurred within six months [131] or 12 months [132] after LT in two RCTs, with rates of 50% [131] and 60% [132]. Later withdrawal was safe in a retrospective review of 45 patients with renal dysfunction, treated at a median of 45 months after LT, either with MMF as monotherapy (n = 16), or in combination with low dose of CNI [133]. Therapeutic trough levels were deliberately kept < 5 ng/ml or CsA < 50 ng/ml. Acute cellular rejection was documented in only 6% with MMF monotherapy, and serum creatinine values decreased, more so in the monotherapy group compared to the combination group. Similarly, another non-controlled but prospective study introduced MMF 7.7 ± 4.3 years after LT in 49 patients with CNI-associated chronic renal failure (14 Tac, 35 CsA) [134]. Creatinine clearance increased significantly after CNI reduction (from the baseline level of 42.9 ± 14 ml/min to 48.8 ± 17 ml/min after one year and 58.4 ± 20 ml/minute after three years, p < 0.0001). No acute or chronic rejection was reported. **B4**

A trial randomized 28 post-LT patients on CNI treatment (CsA or Tac) with impaired renal function (defined as >20% decline in renal function with creatinine level 1.8–4 mg/dl and/or creatinine clearance 20–60 ml/min) either to discontinuation or 50% reduction of CNI dose [129]. Both groups received MMF 1.5 g twice daily and steroids. Improvement of 15% or more in glomerular filtration rate (GFR) occurred in 64% of patients with CNI suspension and in 50% of patients with CNI dose reduction, and GFR remained stable in 36% and 37% respectively in a *per protocol* analysis. Mild or moderate rejection occurred in 30% with CNI discontinuation and in 11% with CNI dose reduction. However, no comparison was made with full dose of CNI. The same strategy was evaluated in an RCT in 32 post-LT patients who received MMF followed by stepwise reduction of CNI (n = 21) or continued CNI therapy (n = 11) [135]. Serum creatinine levels and BUN decreased significantly with MMF at three months (p < 0.01) and GFR increased (p < 0.001), and the lipid profile, blood pressure and transaminase levels also improved after introduction of MMF. No rejection episodes were observed. **A1d** However, the follow-up for some patients was very short.

Pharmacokinetic data have shown that peak concentrations and bioavailability with IV MMF are more than twice those of oral MMF, which may provide immunological advantage, but this has not been evaluated [136, 137].

Therapeutic drug monitoring of MMF is effective in preventing acute rejection in kidney and heart transplantation [138, 139]. Some evidence suggests that MPA concentrations (its active metabolite) could be used for predicting acute rejection in LT recipients [140]. However, routine monitoring of MMF has not been widely performed and dose adjustments are usually performed based on adverse effects. It is common practice to use 2 g/day or less in some LT studies rather than the 3 g/day in the renal transplant registration studies. There is great inter-individual variability of MPA pharmacokinetics, and as in the case of CsA and Tac, measurement after dosing of MMF may have a stronger correlation with AUC, than C_0 monitoring [141–144]. Subtherapeutic values of MPA measured as C_0 and AUC have been found in approximately two-thirds of patients during the first days after LT and in one-third at months 3 and 6 post-LT, but the clinical associations with this are unclear [145].

mTOR inhibitors: sirolimus and everolimus

These are inhibitors of the mammalian target of rapamycin (mTOR). Their immunosuppressive activity is primarily related to the blockade of interleukin-2 and interleukin-15 induction of proliferation of T and B cells, and their synergism with other drugs such as CsA, Tac or MMF allows new combinations of therapy (see Table 42.4).

Cell growth and angiogenesis are also linked with mTOR activity; mTOR inhibition decreases HCC growth [146]. Recurrence of HCC after LT has become an important problem due to a longer recipient survival under chronic immunosuppression. Data from uncontrolled clinical studies and case reports suggest mTOR inhibitors may delay onset or reduce recurrent HCC [147–149]. A large randomized trial is taking place to clarify this issue (clinicaltrials.gov identifier NCT 00328770).

Sirolimus Sirolimus (rapamycin) is a macrocyclic lactone with similar structure to Tac, but its mechanism of action and adverse effect profiles are quite different. Sirolimus (SRL) blocks signal transduction in T-lymphocytes and inhibits cell-cycle progression from G1 to S phase, but does not inhibit calcineurin [150, 151].

While AZA and MMF often are used in conjunction with CNI inhibitors, since their use as single agents increases rates of rejection and graft loss [112], SRL is a promising alternative that may be equivalent to CNI in preventing graft rejection [152–154]. The adverse effects of SRL include dose-dependent hyperlipidemia, thrombocytopenia, anemia, leukopenia, with the absence of neurotoxicity, nephrotoxicity and diabetogenesis, but it has adverse effects on wound healing [155]. Risk of oligospermia in young male patients has also been reported [156].

Sirolimus as primary immunosuppression An international trial comparing SRL with Tac and steroids (n = 110) vs Tac and steroids alone (n = 112) in LT patients was suspended in phase II due to an increase of hepatic artery thrombosis in the SRL group (5.5% vs 0.9%) [157]. This has not been seen in non-randomized studies, but a formal warning remains on the drug information sheet [158, 159].

The first report only comprised 15 patients treated with SRL alone, or SRL plus CsA-ME, or SRL plus CsA-ME plus steroids [160]. Patients on triple therapy had no rejection, while 28% and 75% of those with dual and monotherapy, respectively had rejection. A retrospective study compared three groups: SRL alone (n = 28), SRL plus CIN (n = 56)

Table 42.4 RCT on mTOR inhibitors in liver recipients.

Author	Year	Groups	n	mTOR inhibitor			Other agents	ACR (%)
				Dose	Blood levels at 12 months	Time from LT (months)		
Shenoy	2007	SRL conversion	20	3 mg/d (5 mg load)	6.7 ± 3 mg/dL (mean ± SD)	6–132	± AZA ± MMF ± Ster	5
		Continued CIN	20			12–144 (range)	± AZA ± MMF ± Ster	5
Watson	2007	SRL conversion	13	2 mg/d (no loading dose)	7.3 (3.8–9.9) ng/mL (median – range)	36	± AZA ± Ster	15.4
		Continued CIN	14			60 (median)	± AZA ± Ster	0
Levy	2006	Everol 1 g	28		N/A		CsA + Ster	32.1
		Everol 2 g/d	30				CsA + Ster	26.7
		Everol 4 g/d	31				CsA + Ster	25.8
		Placebo	30				CsA + Ster	40.0

Protocol biopsies were not performed in any of the three trials. In the Levy *et al.* trial, histological diagnosis of rejection was required, but not in the Shenoy *et al.* trial. The definition of ACR was not stated in the Watson *et al.* trial.
SRL: sirolimus; Everol: everolimus; MMF: mycophenolate mofetil; Ster: steroids; CNI: calcineurin inhibitors; CsA: cyclosporin; AZA: azathioprine; ACR: acute cellular rejection; LT: liver transplantation.

and CNI alone (n = 101) [161]. One-year patient and graft survival rates and histologically proven acute cellular rejection rates (no protocol liver biopsies) were not significantly different. The mean creatinine at one month was similar despite being higher in the SRL group at the time of transplantation.

Trotter *et al.* reported that low dose SRL plus CNI and minimal dose of steroids (three-day taper), resulted in less acute rejection rates than historical controls (treated with CNI plus 14-day tapered prednisone (30% vs 70%; p < 0.01) [162]. Steroid-resistant rejection decreased by 90%. **B4** However, as in many studies the interpretation of these data is difficult as no protocol biopsies were done. McAlister *et al.* reported 56 patients who received low-dose Tac and SRL (target: trough levels, 5 and 7 ng/ml respectively) with prednisone up to six months after transplantation [159]. The biopsy proven acute cellular rejection rate was 14%, approximately 50% lower than historical controls. No patient had steroid-resistant rejection. Pridohl *et al.* reported patients transplanted for acute liver failure with triple immunosuppression (SRL, Tac and steroids); acute rejection and steroid-resistant rates were 14% and 0% respectively [163]. Some authors have suggested that SRL should be used in combination with low dose Tac to minimize adverse effects from either drug, whilst avoiding an increased risk of rejection [164, 165].

Dunkelberg *et al.* reported 170 LT recipients treated with SRL (2 mg/day) as part of primary immunosuppression [158]. One-year patient (93%) and graft survival rates (92%) were not different from historical controls (95% and 89%

respectively). The acute rejection rate and use of OKT3 (monoclonal antibody against CD3, muromonabCD3) was significantly lower in SRL-treated patients (14%) versus controls (39%), similar to a previous report [162]. However, the proportion of patients needing OKT3 was very high, both in the controls and SRL-treated groups, so that the precise immunosuppressive endpoints are difficult to compare with other publications. Hepatic artery and wound complications in SRL-treated patients were similar to historical controls.

Further studies are needed to assess the value of SRL as primary immunosuppression after LT, either as a single agent or in combination with other agents.

Conversion from CNI to sirolimus Chronic renal dysfunction occurs in approximately 18% of LT recipients by five-year post-LT and several patients develop end-stage renal disease which shortens patient survival [14]. In contrast to CNI, neither nephrotoxicity nor neurotoxicity has been described with SRL [155], so that it has been used in liver recipients with renal dysfunction, in order reduce or stop CNI, as well as for neurotoxicity or chronic rejection.

The first RCT assessing CNI withdrawal and replacement with SRL allocated 40 liver recipients with CrCl between 40–80 ml/min, to receive either SRL or continued CNI [166]. The mean SRL concentrations at one, three and twelve months were 9 ± 3.1; 7.7 ± 1.9 and 6.7 ± 3 mg/dl respectively, with a mean dose throughout of 3 mg/day. Early improvement in CrCl was seen at one and three months in SRL patients: 75 ml/min SRL vs 61 ml/min controls, p = 0.024 at one month and 75 ml/min SRL vs 56 ml/min controls, p = 0.012 at three months. However, at 12 months the difference was not significant: 72 ml/min SRL vs 58 ml/min controls, p = 0.09. **Ald** This could be because the conversion was too late, at a mean of 4.4 years after LT. The incidence of acute rejection was 5% in both groups and there was no significant difference in lipid profile.

Similarly, another RCT allocated 27 liver recipients with GFR < 65 ml/min, to remain on CNI therapy (86% Tac, 14% CsA) or to switch to SRL based immunosuppression [94]. Renal function was measured by the change in 51Cr-ethylenediaminetetraaceticacid GFR (delta GFR). The median time from LT to randomization was three years (0.88–7.4). The median whole blood SRL concentrations were 6.3 ng/ml at three months and 7.3 ng/ml at 12 months. Tac median 12-hour trough concentrations were 7.7 at three months and 7 ng/ml at 12 months. Mean CsA concentrations at three and twelve months were 86 and 107 and 147 ng/ml. Conversion to SRL led to a modest but significant improvement in renal function at three months after conversion, but the difference was not significant at one year. **Ala** No significant differences in serum creatinine were found. No acute rejection was diagnosed in patients with CNI, while it occurred in two patients (15%) on SRL. Adverse effects were similar except for rash and hypercholesterolemia requiring new statin therapy in the SRL group.

These data suggest that conversion to SRL can be done safely and provide adequate immunosuppression without increased incidence of rejection, graft loss or infection in LT recipients. However, there is no evidence as yet for long-lasting renal improvement. Moreover it is not clear if Tac dosing was reduced to a minimum as therapeutic concentrations could still be measured in blood. Multicenter randomized trials including larger groups, in particular, with much earlier conversion intervals, minimal Tac dosing, as well as longer follow-up, are needed to address the benefit of conversion to SRL. Lastly, the hypercholesterolemia induced by SRL may affect cardiovascular risk despite use of statin agents.

Everolimus Everolimus is a rapamycin derived compound with improved bioavailability and shorter half-life than SRL (18–35 hours vs 60 hours). Experience with everolimus in liver recipients is more limited than that with SRL. It has lower rates of acute rejection than those seen with AZA in heart transplants and similar to MMF in kidney transplants and may result in less cytomegalovirus infection [167, 168]. It inhibits the growth of human Epstein-Barr virus-transformed B lymphocytes *in vitro* and *in vivo*, so it may be optimal when treating post-transplant lymphoproliferative diseases or for prevention [169]. CsA increases exposure to everolimus.

Levy *et al.* performed a randomized placebo-controlled trial evaluating everolimus combined with CsA (target trough level of 150–400 ng/ml) and prednisone in liver recipients [170]. Three different doses of everolimus were compared: 0.5 mg bid (n = 28) vs 1 mg bid (n = 30) vs 2 mg bid (n = 31) vs placebo (n = 30). Biopsy proven acute rejection episodes were: 39.3% (0.5 mg); 30% (1.0 mg); 29% (2 mg) vs 40% placebo, all non-significant. Rejection was three-fold higher when levels were = 3 ng/ml. Overall graft and patient survival rates and renal dysfunction and its severity were similar across groups. However, the small sample size and high drop-out rates prevent robust conclusions. Larger RCTs are required.

Anti-CD3 pan-T cell (orthoclone OKT3)

Muromonab–CD3 (OKT3) is a monoclonal antibody with defined specificity to the CD3 receptor of T cells, thus inactivating both naive and activated cytotoxic T cells. It has been used to prevent acute rejection and to reduce CNI dosage [171, 172]. It was the first monoclonal antibody preventing liver graft rejection. Re-exposure to OKT3 can result in lower efficacy due to the development of antimurine antibodies. There is increased risk of developing post-LT lymphoproliferative disorders and its use is associated with worse recurrence of HCV.

Randomization of 52 LT patients to receive either CsA + AZA + steroids or AZA + steroids + OKT3 followed by conversion to CsA at 14 days, showed lower incidence of acute rejection within two weeks after LT (41% vs 72%, p < 0.02) as well as better renal function in the OKT3 group [173]. Nevertheless, long-term follow-up showed similar rejection rates at 30 days post-LT and similar renal function at 6, 12 and 24 months [174]. **Ald** A trial comparing OKT3 (n = 44) vs a IL-2 receptor antibody (LO-Tact-1) (n = 43) vs no induction (n = 42) in liver recipients on treatment with CsA, AZA and steroids, showed that both agents significantly reduced acute rejection with fewer CMV infections in the LO-Tact-1 group [175]. These results, as well as improved use of current immunosuppressives, make OKT3 less likely to be used as induction therapy.

Interleukin-2 receptor blockers: daclizumab and basiliximab

T-lymphocytes play a central role in the initiation and progression of the rejection response. Activated T-lymphocytes secrete IL-2 that acts in an autocrine and paracrine fashion to drive the response forward, and produces more IL-2 receptors (IL-2R). As only activated T-lymphocytes express IL-2R, blocking this receptor with a monoclonal antibody provides a highly selective approach to prevent rejection [176]. Daclizumab and basiliximab are chimeric and humanized antibodies that act on a receptorial subunit, which is expressed only on activated T-lymphocytes, thus selectively inhibiting their proliferation. However, due to

Table 42.5 Randomized trials on IL-2 blocker in liver transplanted patients.

Author	Year	Groups	n	Dose IL-2 blocker	BPACR (%)
Boillot	2005	Daclizumab + Tac	351	2 × 2 mg/kg IV pre-reperfusion – 1 mg/kg between day 7–10	25.4
		Tac + Ster	347		26.5
Yoshida	2005	Daclizumab + Low Tac + MMF + Ster	72	2 mg/kg IV 4 h post-LT – 1 mg/kg IV day 4	23.2
		Full Tac + MMF + Ster	76		27.7
Neuhaus	2002	Basiliximab + CsA + Ster	188	40 mg IV day 0 and 4	35.1
		Placebo + CsA + Ster	193		43.5
Pageaux	2004	Basiliximab + CsA + Placebo	84	20 mg IV day 0 and 4	24.4[a]
		Basiliximab + CsA + Ster	90		38.1
Llado	2006	Basiliximab + CsA	96	20 mg IV day 0 and 4	18
		Basiliximab + CsA + Ster	102		13

[a] Only trial in which protocol biopsies were performed (at month 12 after transplatation).
MMF: mycophenolate mofetil; Ster: steroids; CsA: cyclosporin; AZA: azathioprine; BPACR: biopsy proven acute cellular rejection; LT: liver transplantation.

some redundancy within the IL-2R complex, which permits the IL-2R signalling despite the use of these antibodies, they have to be used together with other agents, such as CNI (see Table 42.5).

A pilot study evaluated the daclizumab (1 mg/kg IV, immediately pre- and post-operatively and four more doses at two-week intervals), combined with MMF and steroids, without use of CNI [177]. The study was stopped after the first seven liver recipients due to a 100% incidence of acute rejection, with 57% being steroid resistant. In contrast, retrospective analysis of 25 patients receiving the same therapy but with CNI had a rejection rate of 36% [24].

Considering the sequence of events in graft rejection in LT [24], immunosuppression with IL-2R blockers could play a role at the very beginning, leaving the introduction of CNI to a point when these agents can be introduced without excessive risk of infection or renal dysfunction, that is, monotherapy with IL-2R blockade for the first to second week and then monotherapy with CNI or other drugs.

Daclizumab A multicenter randomized trial assessed daclizumab as a steroid avoiding agent in 347 patients receiving Tac plus steroids against 351 patients on steroid-free regimen with Tac following daclizumab induction (follow-up three months) [178]. Acute rejection proven by biopsy that required treatment was similar, as well as graft and patient survival. The daclizumab group had less corticosteroid-resistant acute rejection (6.3 vs 2.8% respectively, p = 0.027), less diabetes mellitus and CMV infection, without increased renal toxicity. **A1d**

In a multicenter, pilot study, 102 liver recipients were treated with daclizumab (2 mg/kg within six hours follow-ing transplant and 1 mg/kg on day 7), MMF and Tac [179]. Acute rejection proven by biopsy was 9.8% at six months (none graded as severe) and 11.8% after 12 months. Patient and graft survival rates at six months were 96% and 95% respectively. Infections, hypertension, diabetes mellitus and hypercholesterolemia occurred in 22%, 37%, 14% and 2% of patients respectively. **B4** Thus, a steroid-free regimen using daclizumab, MMF, and Tac may prevent the occurrence of acute rejection without decreasing safety.

An RCT compared renal function in liver recipients treated with daclizumab (2 mg/kg IV within four hours postoperatively and 1 mg/kg IV on day 4 postLT) and delayed low-dose Tac (starting day 4–6) (n = 72), vs those treated with standard Tac regimen without induction (n = 76) [180]. Both groups also received MMF and tapering steroids. The GFR was significantly better in the daclizumab group during the first week after LT, but this was not maintained during the 12 months follow-up. **A1d** Patient survival and acute rejection rates were similar. Therapy with daclizumab and delayed CNI may not have long-term benefits.

A large series of 209 LT patients receiving daclizumab induction (2 mg/kg intraoperatively and 1 mg/kg on day 5 post-LT) was compared with 115 patients without induction therapy [181]. Despite the delayed initiation of CNI in the daclizumab group, there was less acute rejection within six months (25% vs 39%; p = 0.01). Moreover, patients on daclizumab with pre-LT creatinine levels >1.5 mg/dl showed sustained improvement of renal function, while it worsened in those without daclizumab. However patient and graft survival and the chronic rejection rates were not significantly different, again questioning whether long-term benefit accrues. **B4** Currently, daclizumab has been withdrawn from the market.

Basiliximab Calmus *et al.* evaluated 101 patients treated with basiliximab (20 mg dose on day 0 and 4) in conjunction with CsA (adjusted according to therapeutic levels), AZA (1.5 mg/kg per day), and steroids (tapering from 200 mg/day to 5 mg/day) [182], and compared these with a historical cohort derived from Multicentre International Study in Liver Transplantation of Neoral (MILTON) [183]. One-year patient and graft survival rates were 90.1% and 88.1% respectively. Biopsy-confirmed ACR with basiliximab was 22.8% and none was severe. Malignancies, infections or other adverse effects were not increased. Rejection episodes were more frequent in HCV positive compared to HCV negative patients (29% vs 20%, p = ns). **B3** Basiliximab in association with Tac and steroids similarly prevented ACR in live donor liver recipients, with a rejection-free probability of 93.5% within three months and 93.8% patient survival rate at three years [184, 185]. Neuhaus *et al.* reported an RCT comparing basiliximab (n = 188) or placebo (n = 193) in addition to CsA and steroids [186]. There were no protocol biopsies, but clinically suspected rejection was confirmed by liver biopsy. Within six months, acute rejection rates were 35.1% basiliximab and 43.5% placebo (p = ns). Rejection rates in HCV positive patients were slightly more in basiliximab treated patients (39.1% vs 36.2%, p = ns). Complications including infections were similar. **A1d** The greater rejection rates in HCV positive patients might result from false positive reporting linked to histological similarities between recurrent hepatitis C and acute rejection [187]. However, caution is needed in HCV infection, as adjuvant IL-2R antibodies combined with MMF in the early peritransplantation period was associated with early recurrence of hepatitis C and more rapid histological progression of disease in another study [188].

An RCT evaluated 198 liver recipients (45% HCV-positive) treated with basiliximab as induction therapy with CsA as maintenance immunosuppression, 102 of whom received steroids and 96 were steroid-free [189]. Biopsy-proven ACR, patient and graft survival, and infection rates were similar, including in HCV versus non-HCV subgroups. Diabetic patients in the steroid group had significantly more bacterial infections. The incidence of *de novo* hypertension and hypercholesterolemia was comparable at six months. **A1d**

In another multicenter trial treated initially with basiliximab, CsA and steroids were allocated to receive maintenance therapy either with CsA and steroids (n = 90) or steroid withdrawal at day 14 (n = 84) [190]. Biopsy-confirmed rejection and treated acute rejection by six months was higher in the steroid-free group (38.1% vs 24.4%, p = 0.03). Metabolic complications were similar.

These results were also similar at 12 months follow-up. Acute rejection was easily controlled in most patients and did not affect graft survival. **A1d**

Non-randomized studies suggest basiliximab induction may allow delay in introducing CNI and reduced CNI dosage, thus improving renal function as well as reducing acute rejection. A prospective study included adult living donor LT (LDLT) recipients assigned to either basiliximab induction (Tac delayed until renal function improved; n = 27) or conventional immunosuppression without basiliximab (Tac started on the first day post-LT; n = 18) [191]. Patients in the induction group were in worse condition pre-LT and had a higher blood loss and transfusion. The serum creatinine levels at the second and third months post-LT were lower in the induction group (p < 0.05). Renal insufficiency (an increase of = 0.5 mg/dl in serum creatinine over the baseline value, or an increase of >50% over baseline, or a reduction of 50% in calculated creatinine clearance, or need for dialysis) at the third month post-LT was lower in the induction group (26% vs 67%, p = 0.007). Acute rejection at six months, as well as infections and diabetes mellitus were similar, and the median cholesterol level was lower in the induction group (152 mg/dl vs 196 mg/dl, p = 0.03). **B3** However, the lack of randomization, the small number of patients and the short follow-up, negate robust conclusions. The same considerations pertain to 31 patients (94% chronic hepatitis B carriers) treated with basiliximab with steroid withdrawal 24 hours after LT and reduction of Tac dosage, which showed similar findings compared to historical controls [192].

Anti-thymocyte globulin

Anti-thymocyte globulins are heterologous preparations consisting of polyclonal anti-lymphocyte antibodies. A rabbit derived polyclonal antibody (RATG) was shown to be an effective immunosuppressive agent in LT [193]. The role of RATG in LT has been evaluated as a CNI sparing agent [194], or to delay CNI administration in patients with renal dysfunction [195], to reduce or eliminate steroid use [196], or to avoid maintenance immunosuppression [197]. Moreover, its ability to selectively deplete T cells has been used for both prophylaxis and treatment of acute cellular rejection *per se*.

In conjunction with steroids, RATG reduced rejection without increasing infectious complications or malignancy [193, 198]. Eason and colleagues randomized 71 liver recipients to induction therapy with either RATG (n = 36) or steroids (n = 3 5) with maintenance Tac and MMF, with or without prednisone [196]. The rate of biopsy proven rejection was not significantly different: 20.5% RATG vs 32% steroids. However, the RATG group had less rejection needing steroids (p = 0.01), without increased complications, in particular cytomegalovirus infection, diabetes and HCV recurrence. A follow-up of these patients and data on additional patients undergoing steroid-free OLT confirmed these results [199]. **A1d**

Starzl *et al.* reported using RATG (5 mg/kg) as pre-treatment therapy in 82 solid organ transplant recipients (17 LT) followed by minimum use of post-transplant immunosuppression (Tac monotherapy during the first four months, then spaced Tac therapy) [198]. Graft survival rates were 89% at one year and 88% at 13–18 months. RATG enabled 57.5% of recipients with surviving grafts to be maintained with spaced doses of Tac monotherapy from four months. **B4**

A retrospective analysis of 198 liver recipients, 118 receiving RATG and delayed initiation of CNI, and 80 receiving no antibody and early initiation of CNI, showed that delayed CNI initiation with RATG significantly improved serum creatinine levels and GFR, with similar patient and graft survival [200]. Overall infection and cytomegalovirus infection rates were significantly lower with RATG, with less early biopsy-proven acute rejection (16% vs 26%, p = 0.08). Another comparison between 129 liver recipients with CNI immediately after LT vs 262 with CNI after initial short-term RATG induction, showed that by one year acute rejection rates were significantly lower in RATG treated patients (14.5% vs 31.8%, p = 0.0008) [201]. Again, serum creatinine levels and GFR were better in the RATG group, with no additional harmful effects. Undesired side effects occurred at a similar rate in both groups. **B3**

Use of a three-day ATG induction therapy regimen after LT has been promoted as it results in no more rejection than a ten-day course, while reducing the adverse effects, especially lethal infection [202].

Anti-CD52 (alemtuzumab)

New protocols of tolerogenic preconditioning have been developed using alentuzumab (Campath-1H) and low doses of CNI. Alentuzumab is a humanized monoclonal antibody directed against the CD52 antigen, a pan T, B and natural killer cell, and monocyte markers [203]. It rapidly depletes lymphocytes, monocytes and other cells without affecting neutrophils and hematopoietic stem cells. The depleted cells begin to re-emerge gradually during a period of six months without returning to baseline levels. This activity is believed to prevent an aggressive lymphocytic immune response after transplantation and allow a more gradual engagement of the host immune system under low conventional immunosuppression. This regimen of host conditioning prior to transplantation, followed by minimum post-transplant immunosuppression could increase the chance of developing tolerance [21, 22, 204–207].

The most extensive experience with the use of alemtuzumab in solid organ transplantation has been done in kidney transplantation [17, 208], as well as intestinal and multivisceral transplantation [209], in which treatment with Campath-1H and low dose of CNI has shown encouraging results.

The outcome of 77 liver recipients treated with Campath-1H and low dose Tac, with steroid-free maintenance, compared with 50 patients treated with Tac and steroids (HCV patients excluded), showed no differences in patient and graft survival, while rejection-free survival was higher in the Campath-1 group: 51% vs 65% at 12 months, p = 0.009 [23, 210]. Tac-related nephrotoxicity and mean creatinine levels were higher in the control group (p = 0.0001 and p < 0.05 respectively). **B3** No differences in viral infection rates were found. Thus, Campath-1 may be at least as effective, as Tac and steroid regimens, with less renal toxicity, but long-term follow-up is needed, especially with regard to risk of malignancy.

A similar study evaluated 76 liver recipients (50% HCV positive) treated with Campath-1 induction and low-dose Tac compared to 84 patients (31% HCV positive) receiving standard immunosuppression [211]. No differences in rejection or patient and graft survival were found at one year. However, HCV positive patients did significantly worse than those who were HCV negative, both in the induction and the control group. Moreover increased HCV viral replication was worse with Campath-1. **B3** Until now, optimal dose of Campath-1 and ideal combinations of maintenance immunosuppression remain to be determined and the effect on HCV recurrence documented. Its use as a primary treatment for rejection has not been studied. Randomized-controlled trials addressing these issues need to be performed.

Ursodeoxycolic acid

Ursodeoxycholic acid (UDCA) is a hydrophilic bile acid which may improve parenchymal function in cholestatic states and possibly slow the progression of primary biliary cirrhosis [212, 213]. Additionally, UDCA reduces the expression of major histocompatibility complex (MHC) class I antigens in patients with primary biliary cirrhosis and therefore may have immunomodulatory effects on T cell-dependent liver damage [212–214]. During acute cellular rejection, MHC class I and II antigens are expressed on hepatocytes, although these are not primary target cells. Cholestasis itself may induce an increased expression of MHC class I antigens on hepatocytes, which can lead to lymphocyte CD8+-dependent cytotoxicity [215]. Based on these theoretical considerations, UDCA might decrease acute cellular rejection episodes in LT patients.

There are seven randomized controlled trials involving 335 liver recipients which evaluated UDCA or tauro-UDCA for prevention of acute allograft rejection (see Table 42.6) [216–222].

All seven trials failed to demonstrate that UDCA prevented the occurrence of acute rejection, confirmed by a

Table 42.6 Randomized trials on ursodeoxycholic acid in liver transplanted patients included in the meta-analysis.

Author	Year	Groups	n	Immunosuppression			Results	
				Dose UDCA	**Duration UDCA (First dose- Maintenance)**	**Other agents**	**ACR (%)**	**Patient Mortality (%)**
Sama	1991	UDCA	20	600 mg/kg	5–7 d after LT – 6 months	Steroids + CsA	65.0	25.0
		No treatment	20			Steroids + CsA	65.0	30.0
Koneru	1993	UDCA	16	900 mg/d	3–5 d after LT – 3 months	Steroids + AZA + CNI	18.7	N/A
		No treatment	16			Steroids + AZA + CNI	56.2	
Pageaux	1995	UDCA	26	600 mg/d	3–5 d after LT – 2 months	Steroids + AZA + CNI	34.6	N/A
		Placebo	24			Steroids + AZA + CNI	37.5	
Keiding	1997	UDCA	54	15 mg/kg	3–5 d after LT – 3 months	Steroids + AZA + CNI	64.8[a]	25.9
		Placebo	48			Steroids + AZA + CNI	66.7	20.8
Barnes	1997	UDCA	28	10–15 mg/kg	3–5 d after LT – 3 months	Steroids + AZA + CNI	60.7[a]	7.1
		Placebo	24			Steroids + AZA + CNI	70.8	29.2
Fleckenstein	1998	UDCA	14	15 mg/kg	3–5 d after LT – 3 months	Steroids + AZA + CNI	57.1	14.3
		Placebo	16			Steroids + AZA + CNI	56.3	25.0
Angelico	1999	TUDCA	14	500 mg/d	3–5 d after LT – 12 months	Steroids + AZA + CNI	50.0	18.7
		No treatment	15			Steroids + AZA + CNI	58.8	11.8

[a] Trials in which protocol biopsies were performed after liver transplantation: Keiding *et al.*: days 7–21–90–365; Barnes *et al.*: day 7 and month 3. UDCA: ursodeoxycholic acid; TUDCA: tauro-ursodeoxycholic acid; CNI: calcineurin inhibitors; CsA: cyclosporin; AZA: azathioprine; ACR: acute cellular rejection.

meta-analysis of six trials [223]: acute cellular rejection (RR 0.89; 95% CI: 0.74–1.08), mortality, re-transplantation or steroid-resistant rejection were not improved. **A1a**

Assy *et al.* [224] performed a further RCT evaluating whether UDCA decreased rejection after total immunosuppressant withdrawal, in 26 liver recipients, free of rejection while on immunosuppressive agents for a minimum of two years after LT. They were randomized to UDCA (15 mg/kg) (n = 14) or placebo (n = 12) followed by sequential withdrawal of their immunosuppression over several months. Rejection and its severity were no different: UDCA 43% vs control 75% (p = 0.09) nor in the severity of the rejection. **A1d**

Granulocyte-colony stimulating factor

Studies in animal models as well as clinical trials have demonstrated significant benefits of human recombinant granulocyte-colony stimulating factor (G-CSF) for the treatment of infections in bone marrow recipients, while the experience in solid organ transplantation is more limited. G-CSF used for the first 7–10 days resulted in less acute rejection in 37 liver transplant recipients, compared with historical controls (n = 49) receiving the same immunosuppressive protocol (22% vs 51%). This could be related to a significant reduction in serum TNF levels, which may

be a key player in allograft rejection [225, 226]. However, a subsequent multicenter randomized placebo-controlled trial comprising 194 patients did not confirm reduced infection rates and biopsy proven rejection was more common in the G-CSF treated group compared with placebo (30% vs 19%) [227]. **A1d**

New immunosuppressive agents

Leflunomide is a member of malononitrilamide family which targets the *de novo* pathway of pyrimidine biosynthesis and thus inhibits T and B cell proliferation. A retrospective review of the use of leflunomide was carried out in 8 liver and 45 kidney transplant recipients [228]. CNI were stopped completely in four liver recipients and reduced by 65% in another patient. No evidence of acute rejection developed in any of these liver (or kidney) transplant patients.

FK778, a synthetic derived from leflunomide, has been developed to reduce the extended half-life of leflunomide (6–45 hours vs 15–18 days) [229]. Studies in LT are awaited.

FTY 720 is a unique immunosuppressive agent that not only inhibits lymphocyte proliferation, but also results in a redistribution of lymphocytes into lymph nodes and out of circulation. This ability of FTY 720 to impair effector T cell homing is achieved without affecting induction or expansion of memory responses, suggesting that it may leave tolerizing interactions intact [230]. Studies in human LT are awaited.

Janus kinases (JAK) are intermediaries between cytokine receptors and STAT, which result in activation of the immune cells. JAK-3 may be an excellent target for clinical immunosuppression due to its requirement for signaling by multiple cytokines. JAK3/STAT inhibitors in animal models lead to immunosuppression to prevent rejection, without inducing many of the side effects observed with other current therapies [231]. Human studies are awaited.

The future immunosuppression in liver transplantation

Future immunosuppressive strategies will be designed to help the development of tolerance of the allograft, selectively stimulating and/or minimally suppressing the recipient's immune reaction. Studies of the current immunosuppressive agents suggest two ways in which this goal might be attained. First, CNI dosage minimization or even avoidance will continue to be the focus of future studies, to avoid adverse effects and too much rejection. Second, use of new selective immunosuppresive agents which do not depress tolerizing mechanisms or even enhance them, while avoiding side effects, need to be developed [21, 22]. Both approaches need an easy method to assess immunopotency of the immunosuppressive agents and/or a measure of tolerance. The surrogate markers of blood concentrations of immunosuppressives in current use relate more to avoiding toxicity than to issues of rejection or tolerance. These new assays would allow personalized medicine, by individual tailoring doses of immunosuppressive therapy, depending on "day-to-day" immune status.

Weaning immunosuppression

Steroid withdrawal and steroid avoidance

Steroids have been the cornerstone of immunosuppressive regimens since the inception of solid organ transplantation. In the past two decades immunosuppressive protocols have evolved driven by a deeper understanding of immunological events after transplantation, and more focus has been placed on minimizing the multitude of side effects and toxicities associated with a long-term therapy with steroids (renal function, infectious risk, loss of bone density, diabetes, hypertension, hyperlipidemia, etc.). The trend has been to use fewer steroids for maintenance therapy. In 2000, a series showed safe withdrawal from the third postoperative month, but the duration of steroid use after LT and the potential role of complete steroid avoidance remain uncertain [232].

Studies evaluating steroid-withdrawal and steroid avoidance in LT are heterogeneous, especially with regards to the interval at withdrawal (1 day–9 months). The major-

ity of protocols utilize regimens based on MMF in conjunction with Tac and the proportion of studies using CsA is lower compared to those using Tac. However, many protocols utilize antibody induction agents such as daclizumab, basiliximab and rabbit-derived antithymocyte globulin, thus increasing immunopotency.

Steroid withdrawal   Steroid withdrawal based on Tac-containing regimens showed comparable patient and graft survival to protocols using maintenance immunosuppression with steroids; one study found that histology-proven acute rejection was less with steroid withdrawal compared to a steroid regimen (6% vs 27%; p = 0.001) [192, 233, 234]. Infection was less amongst patients who underwent steroid withdrawal (0% vs 18%; p = 0.001) and two studies showed significant reduction in the onset of diabetes mellitus amongst patients who stopped steroids (Table 42.7) [192, 234]. **B3**

Pageaux *et al.* evaluated the impact of steroid withdrawal based on a CsA-based regimen in 174 patients, randomized to receive CsA and prednisolone (n = 90) or CsA and placebo (n = 84) [190]. Histologically proven acute rejection at six months was significantly more frequent among patients without steroids than patients on prednisolone (38.1% vs 24.4%; p = 0.03). However, patient and graft survival were similar between the two group, as well as infection rate, diabetes and hypertension. **A1d**

Greig *et al.* evaluated the safety and efficacy of early steroid withdrawal, comparing 71 patients treated with Tac to 72 patients treated with CsA-ME. They found that patients on Tac had a statistically significant better patient and graft survival (97% and 97%) compared to patients on micro-CsA (89% and 86% respectively) [86]. Acute rejection occurring during the first year was similar (35% with Tac and 43% with micro-CsA), and no chronic rejection developed during this period, presumably because of the short follow-up. **B4**

Steroid avoidance   Several studies have evaluated the safety and efficacy of steroid avoidance in liver transplanted patients (see Table 42.8) [127, 178, 189, 196, 235–247].

No study found statistically significant differences in patient and graft survival comparing steroid-free and steroid inclusive regimens, but these studies are heterogeneous with a range of evaluation time between three months and five years, and often evaluated increased immunosuppression in the steroid free groups. **B4**

Two studies found statistical differences in biopsy-confirmed acute rejection rates [127, 235]: 24.3% with steroids vs 39.4% without (p = 0.04) [235], and 16.7% steroids vs 75% no steroids (p = 0.002) by Reggiani *et al.* [127]. In contrast, Varo *et al.* reported patients on steroids having a higher acute rejection rate compared to patients on steroid-free regimen (11.5% vs 26.6%; p = 0.01) [240].

Table 42.7 Steroid withdrawal in clinical trial (RCT and non-RCT) in the last five years.

Author	Year	No. of patients	Immunosuppression IS regimens	Interval at withdrawal	Mean follow-up (months)	Survival Patient (%)	Graft (%)	Rejection[a] Acute (%)	Chronic (%)	Complications Infections (%)	Diabetes (%)	Hypertension (%)
Greig	2003	71	Tac + AZA + (steroids)	4–9 months	12	97	97	35	0	NS	NS	NS
		72	CsA + AZA + (steroids)			89	86	43	0			
						p = 0.05	p = 0.01					
Pageaux	2004	90	Bas + CsA + steroids	14 days	12	97.8	100	24.4	NS	13.3	22	33.3
		84	Bas + CsA + (steroids)			91.7	98.8	38.1	NS	8.3	14.3	28.6
								p = 0.03				
Liu	2004	31	Bas + Tac + MMF + (steroids)	1 day	10.8	94	94	6	NS	0	0	NS
		49	Tac + steroids		21.6	96	94	27	NS	18	28	
								p = 0.001		p = 0.001	p = 0.001	
Junge	2005	14	Tac + steroids	3 months	24	93[b]	NS[a]	NS[a]	NS	NS[a]	42.8	NS
		16	Tac + MMF + (steroids)			100[b]			NS		12.5	
Moench	2007	54	Tac + steroids	14 days	12	88.8[c]	NS	35.2	0/54	33	53	52
		56	Tac + (steroids)			85.7[c]	NS	48.2	2/56	25	30	39
											p = 0.02	

[a] Data non specified, but no difference between the two group was reported.
[b] Two-year survival.
[c] One-year survival.
All studies considered biopsy-proven acute rejection except from Junge et al. and Moench et al. in which this data is not specified.

Table 42.8 Steroid avoidance in clinical trials (RCT and non-RCT) in the last five years.

Author	Year	IS regimens	No. of patients	Mean follow-up (months)	Survival patient (%)	Survival Graft (%)	Rejection[i] acute (%)	Complications infections (%)	Complications Diabetes (%)	Hypertension (%)
Eason	2003	Tac + MMF + steroids	59	18.5	85[c]	80[c]	31	25	14	NS
		Tac + MMF + RATG	60		85[c]	82[c]	25	22	2	NS
Mogl	2004	Tac + steroids	27	28	78.8	NS	30	NS	NS	NS
		Tac + MMF	26		85.7		31			
Filipponi	2004	Bas + CsA + AZA + steroids	74	12	72.9[c]	84.8[c]	23	86.5	NS	NS
		Bas + CsA + AZA	66		81.5[c]	89[c]	39	81.8	NS	NS
							p = 0.002			
Reggiani	2005	Tac + MMF + steroids	18	31	100	88.9	16.7[e]	27.8	27.8	27.8
		Tac + MMF	12		91.7	91.7	75[e]	50	16.7	16.7
							p = 0.002			
Boillot	2005	Tac + steroids	347	3	94.5[a]	92.2[a]	26.5	11.5	15.3	14.4
		Dac + Tac	351		93.7[a]	90.5[a]	25.4	5.1	5.7	12.8
Margarit	2005	Tac + steroids	32	44	84–78–73[d]	75–60–60[d]	32.3	30[g]	18.7	9.6
		Tac	28		85–81–66[d]	84–78–73[d]	39	26[g]	7.1	3.5
Kato	2005	Tac + MMF + steroids	20	15	NS	NS	28–6–20[e]	37	43	58
		Dac + Tac + MMF	19	8			0–0–13[e]	14	7	36
Studenik	2005	Dac + Tac + MMF + steroids	19	13	NS[h]	NS[h]	16	20	11	37
		Dac + Tac + MMF	20				35	5	5	15
									p = 0.02	
Varo	2005	Tac + steroids	79	NS (0–12)	NS[h]	NS[h]	26.6	NS[h]	NS[h]	NS
		Dac + Tac + MMF	78				11.5			
							p = 0.01			
Jensen	2006	Tac + MMF + steroids	15	67	85.7	78.5	20	NS	13.3	
		Tac + Dac + MMF	15		91.6	91.6	13.3		13.3	
Pelletier	2006	Bas/Tac + MMF + steroids	36	13.7	83[c]	81[c]	14	28	NS	NS
		Bas/Tac + MMF	36		90[c]	90[c]	25	52		
								p = 0.03		

Author	Year	Regimen	n							
Fasola	2006	Tac + steroids	80	NS (0–12)	89.5	84.8	18	NS	NS	NS
		Tac + MMF + steroids	79		89.4	88.1	13			
		Dac + Tac + MMF	153		92.5	89.9	7			
Lladò	2006	Bas + CsA + MMF + steroids	102	6	89[b]	88[b]	13	51	29	44
		Bas + Csa + MMF	96		94[b]	90[b]	18	47	18	25
										p = 0.006
Samonakis	2006	Tac + AZA + steroids	29	21.7	93.2	89.7	86[f]	NS	NS[h]	NS
		Tac	27		77.8	88.9	70[f]			
Lerut	2008	Tac + steroids	156	12	93.6	92.3	19.2[f]	NS	NS	NS
		Tac	(total)		85.9	83.3	23[f]			
Gras[i]	2008	Tac + steroids	34	36	91	88	53	NS	NS	NS
		Bas + Tac	50		96	94	26			

Patient and graft survival: [a] 3 months, [b] 6 months, [c] 1 year, [d] 1, 3 and 5 years.
[e] Acute rejection at these interval times: 0–3 months, 3–6 months and 6–12 months;
[f] treated acute rejection.
[g] Infection episodes.
[h] Data non-specified, but no difference between the two group was reported.
[i] Study on pediatric patients.
[j] All studies considered biopsy-proven acute rejection except from Mogl et al., Varo et al. and Gras et al. in which this data is not specified.

Patients following regimens without steroids experienced a lower incidence of infections (28% vs 52%; p = 0.03) [242], a lower diabetes mellitus rate (7% vs 43%; p = 0.02) [237], and a lower incidence of hypertension (25% vs 44%; p = 0.006) [189] after LT compared to those using steroids. **B4** Segev *et al.* performed a systematic review of 19 individual studies and 11 updates of these, comparing steroid-free to steroids-based protocols in liver transplanted recipients [248]. There was no difference in survival, graft loss or infection rates. There was a significant reduction in serum cholesterol, risk of CMV infection and HCV recurrence in the steroid-free group. However, the heterogeneity, short-term follow-up and relatively small size of many randomized controlled trials included in this meta-analysis and the lack of evaluating steroid dosage make the conclusions less robust. **A1c** Moreover, since in 19 individual studies, nine had replaced steroids with another immunosuppressive agent (one basiliximab, five daclizumab, one thymoglobulin and two MMF) and six studies had administered perioperative steroids (one or two doses) to the steroid-free arm, the real impact of steroid-free regimens on outcome after LT has not been evaluated properly.

However the data available on steroid withdrawal and/or steroid avoidance in LT recipients, do show at least comparable results to maintenance immunosuppressive protocols including steroids. **B3** Thus, steroids can be either avoided completely or withdrawn without significant sequelae. However, the long-term consequences of steroid avoidance remain unclear. Long-term follow-up studies are needed to explore more fully the benefits of steroid withdrawal and/or steroid avoidance in liver transplanted patients, particularly those transplanted for HCV related cirrhosis.

Total withdrawal of immunosuppression

The main aspiration of transplant clinicians is the acceptance of the graft by the recipient without any long-term pharmacological help [17, 21, 22]. Long-term survivors following LT recipients are often systematically and excessively immunosuppressed. Consequently, drug weaning is an important management strategy, providing it is done gradually under careful physician surveillance. Only a few studies have reported cohorts with total withdrawal (see Table 42.9).

In 1998 Devlin *et al.* evaluated 18 adults with uneventful post-LT follow-up and showed that it was possible to either completely withdraw (5/18 patients) or significantly reduce (9/18 patients) maintenance immunosuppression to levels previously considered subtherapeutic [18]. Parameters associated with successful drug withdrawal were transplantation for non-immune-mediated liver disorders, fewer donor-recipient HLA A, B and DR mismatches, and low incidence of early rejection. In 13/18 immunosuppression was recommended due to elevated

liver function tests, but only 4 out of these 13 patents had a histologically proven acute rejection. In a recent update of this study one patient out of the five successfully withdrawn from immunosuppression, developed chronic rejection and required re-transplantation, while in another patient immunosuppression was restarted due to low-grade rejection [249]. **B4**

Takatsuki *et al.* described 63 living donor LT recipients receiving Tac: 26 were entered in an elective program of withdrawal, while in the remaining 37 withdrawal was due to serious complications of immunosuppression [250]. In 24 patients, 6 from the elective cohort, Tac was stopped with a median drug-free period of 23.5 months. Rejection occurred in 16 patients (25.4%) after a median interval of 9.5 months, but all episodes were treated by reintroducing Tac or with short courses of steroids. In a later update of this study, the number of patients included in elective weaning increased to 67, with almost similar results (23.8% success and 12% acute rejection) [251]. **B4**

Contrasting with previous results, Eason *et al.* only achieved immunosuppression withdrawal in 1 of 18 patients (5.5%) but 11 of 18 (61%) had rejection [252]. These poor results were probably due to weaning immunosuppression just six months after transplantation, much earlier than in other studies. **B4**

UDCA did not prevent rejection after total immunosuppression withdrawal [224].

The role of liver cell chimersim and the role of donor bone marrow cell (DBMC) infusion were evaluated in immunosuppression withdrawal programs [253, 254]. Pons *et al.* achieved complete immunosuppression withdrawal in 3 out of 9 (33%) liver recipient patients [253]. Liver endothelial cell chimerism was studied in five patients and it was not associated with immunosuppression withdrawal.

Tryphonopoulos *et al.* reported similar patient and graft survival, comparing patients who received DBMC and patients who did not [254]. Rejection episodes were significantly lower in the DBMC group in the first two years, but overall there was no significant difference. Successful weaning was achieved in 20 patients out of 104 (19%), without difference between groups. **B4** Two patients developed chronic rejection and one required re-transplantation. These data confirmed previous results by Rolles *et al.*, who showed, in a randomized controlled study, that donor-specific bone marrow infusion has no benefit in inducing tolerance in patients undergoing LT [255]. **A1d**

Tisone *et al.* evaluated weaning immunosuppression in 34 HCV positive patients with recurrent allograft disease [256]. Complete and permanent immunossuppression withdrawal was achieved in 23.5%, with 35.2% rejecting during tapering, and another 41.2% developed rejection within eight months. Weaned patients showed stabilization or improvement of histological fibrosis, lower necroin-

Table 42.9 Complete elective imunosuppression withdrawal in liver transplantation.

| Author | Year | No. of patients | Selection criteria | | Immunosuppression | Time between LT and weaning (years) | Follow-up after IS withdrawal (months) | Complete withdrawal (%) | Rejection[c] / Graft loss | | |
			Months after LT	Other	Maintenance IS				Acute	Chronic	Graft loss due to rejection
Takatsuki/Oike	2001/2002	26[a]	>24	>1 year rejection-free Normal LFTs	Tac	>2	Median: 21.9 Range: 3–69	23.8	12	0	0
Pons	2003	9	> 24		CsA	Median: 5.2 Range: 2–8.8	Range: 17–24	33	22	0	0
Eason	2005	18	>6	Normal LFTs	Tac	>0.5	12	5.6	61	0	0
Devlin/Girlanda	1998/2005		>60	Side effects of IS	CsA + AZA	Median: 7 Range: 5–11	120	16.7	28	5.6	5.6
Tryphonopoulos	2005	104	>36	>1 year rejection-free No autoimmune disease	Tac (85%) CsA (14%)	Mean: 4 Range: 3.6–4.6	Mean: 25.8 Range: 11–36	19	67[b]	1.9	0.96
Tisone	2006	34	>12	HCV-RNA positive No rejection or cirrhosis on basal biopsy	CsA	Mean: 5.25	Mean: 45.5 Range: 15–44	23.4	76.4	0	0
Assy	2007	26	>24	>2 years rejection free History of compliance	CsA + AZA (54%) CsA + steroids (19%) CsA (27%)	>2	12	8	58	0	0

[a] LDLT recipients.
[b] Treated acute rejection.
[c] All studies considered biopsy-proven acute rejection except from Takatsuki et al. and Oike et al. in which this data is not specified.
Table modified by Lerut J, Sanchez-Fueyo A. An appraisal of tolerance in liver transplantation. Am J Transplatation 2006; **6**(8): 1774–1780.

flammation and improved liver function after a mean follow-up of 45 months. Low blood CSA trough levels during the first post-transplant week and initial steroid-free immunosuppression were found to be independent predictors of sustained weaning, suggesting this subgroup had less propensity for rejection. **B4**

Immunosuppression in recipients with HCV related cirrhosis

Hepatitis C (HCV)-induced cirrhosis is a leading indication for LT [257]. HCV re-infection after LT occurs in virtually all patients transplanted for HCV-related liver disease [258, 259]. Histological evidence of chronic HCV infection develops in 50% to 90% of patients by 12 months after LT [260], and cirrhosis occurs in about 20% of patients within five years after transplant [257, 258, 261]. Several studies have evaluated host and viral factors that might be associated with the severity of HCV recurrence. Among host factors, immunosuppression is one of the major factors that accounts for accelerated HCV recurrence and it has been an area of extensive research and controversy [262].

In a recent multi-center international survey, the prevalent immunosuppressive strategies in LT for hepatitis C were evaluated among 81 LT programs worldwide. The most common regimen used (41%) was based on triple therapy (Tac, MMF and steroids). Concerning the use of steroids, 7.4% of programs used steroid-free protocols, 11% discontinued steroids within a week, 56% within three months and 98% within the first year. When US-programs and non-US programs were compared, CsA was used significantly more among non-US programs (35.6% vs 2.8%) and the duration of steroid therapy was significantly shorter in US programs (10.8 vs 29.4 weeks) [263].

Steroids

Although the data on increase of HCV viral loads due to steroid boluses are convincing, the effects of steroid maintenance are still controversial [264, 265]. The link between steroid therapy and viral replication after LT in HCV recipients prompted many centres to advocate steroid therapy withdrawal. However, robust data are limited as to the efficacy of this approach. A rapid reduction in steroid dosage may be harmful for HCV recurrence [266]. **B4**

The direct effect of dexamethasone and prednisolone on HCV replication has been investigated using an *in vitro* replicon model. At clinically relevant concentrations (1–10 nM) treatment with both dexamethasone and prednisolone did not enhance, but resulted in a slight reduction of HCV replication. This minor reduction of HCV replication was confirmed by RT-PCR, showing more than 41% reduction in HCV-RNA levels [267].

In a recent study HCV patients transplanted between 2001 and 2004 (n = 90) were compared to a historical group

of HCV patients transplanted before the introduction of dual initial immunosuppression (CsA or Tac plus steroids) and slow steroid tapering (1999–2000) (n = 52) [266]. The historical cohort showed a significantly higher rate of severe disease (48%) compared to patients transplanted between 2001 and 2004 (29%). Among patients more recently transplanted the proportion on triple or quadruple regimens (10% vs 25%; p = 0.001) and the number of boluses of methyl-prednisolone were less (4 vs 11; p = 0.002) and the duration of maintenance prednisone was longer (350 days vs 249 days; p < 0.0001) [266]. **B4** These data confirm a previous study by Samonakis *et al.*, who found that short-term maintenance steroids (≤6 months) and AZA were associated with less fibrosis progression [268]. **B4** This was further suggested by Vivarelli *et al.*, who compared rapid tapering of steroid (from 25 mg (day 6 to day 30 post-LT) to 15 mg (day 31 to 45), 10 mg (day 46 to 60) 5 mg (day 61 to 75), 2.5 mg (day 76 to 90)) and withdrawal at day 91 after LT (group A) to slow tapering (from 25 mg (day 6 to day 30 post-LT) to 15 mg (day 31 to 90), 10 mg (day 91 to 180), 7.5 mg (day 181 to 270), 5 mg (day 271 to the end of first year), 2.5 mg) and withdrawal 25 months after LT (group B) [269]. At 12 months after LT the rate of advanced fibrosis was higher in the group A compared to group B (42.1% vs 7.6%). Moreover, one and two-year advanced fibrosis-free survivals were 65.2% and 60.8% in group A and 93.7% in group B (p = 0.03 and p = 0.02 respectively). **B4**

In a recent randomized trial 103 liver transplanted patients for HCV cirrhosis were randomized to Tac (0.1 mg/kg/day) either alone or with AZA (1 mg/kg) and prednisolone (20 mg daily tailing off to zero by 3–6 months) [270]. There were no differences in short-term or overall survival between the two treatment arms and, despite more rejection episodes, the group that had maintenance low dose steroids for between three and six months had slower progression to Ishak stage 4 (23% vs 44%; p = 0.044). **A1d**

Filipponi *et al.* compared patients on steroid maintenance versus steroid-free regimens in HCV liver transplanted patients [235]. At 12 months after LT there was no significant difference with regard to liver fibrosis and viral loads. However, in patients treated with steroids the antiviral treatment failure rate was significantly higher, but the biopsy proven acute rejection rate was significantly lower. **B4** Steroid avoidance was also evaluated in a prospective, randomized, multicenter trial comparing 312 patients randomized to three arms: (1) Tac and steroids; (2) Tac, steroids and MMF; and (3) daclizumab induction, Tac and MMF. Patient and graft survival did not differ significantly among treatment arms; freedom from HCV recurrence at one year was 62%, 60% and 67% in the three groups respectively; freedom from rejection was significantly higher in patients treated with corticosteroid-free immunosuppression compared to those exposed to steroids. Long-term follow-up is not yet available [271]. Kato *et al.* randomized HCV positive liver transplanted patients to receive Tac and daclizumab, or Tac and steroids during 1999–2001 and Tac plus MMF and daclizumab or Tac plus MMF and steroids during 2002–2005 [272]. No statistically significant difference was found in mean fibrosis stage between the various treatment arms, either averaging across the two time periods or during these periods themselves. Patients on steroid free-regimens experienced a lower rate of diabetes mellitus (10% vs 45%; p = 0.01) and wound infections (6% vs 31%; p = 0.01). In a recent meta-analysis on steroid avoidance in LT, HCV recurrence was assessed heterogeneously (biopsy-proven (Ishak score) n = 1; biopsy-proven (Ishak ≥ 8) n = 1; biopsy proven (fibrosis, score NS) n = 2; biopsy-proven reinfection n = 2; biopsy-proven n = 2; biopsy-proven and biochemical abnormalities n = 1; biopsy-proven with high LFTs and HCV-RNA n = 1; biopsy-proven and HCV-RNA n = 1; not specified n = 1), HCV recurrence was lower with steroid avoidance and although no individual trial reached statistical significance, meta-analysis demonstrated this effect (RR 0.90; 95% CI: 0.82–0.99, p = 0.03). However, there was considerable clinical heterogeneity. Data on fibrosis progression and on steroid dose and withdrawal were not reported [248].

Calcineurine inhibitors

In a recent meta-analysis by Berenguer *et al.* including five randomized control trials (1995–2006) comparing Tac based vs CsA-based immunosuppression in HCV-infected liver transplant recipients, no statistically significant differences for mortality, graft survival, biopsy proven acute rejection, corticoresistant acute rejection or fibrosis cholestatic hepatitis were found [273]. These data confirm previous single center evaluations of differences between CsA and Tac showing no histological differences in HCV recurrence at 12 months nor overall survival rates (90) and no differences in HCV-RNA levels, serum transaminases, histological grading of portal inflammation and fibrosis [274]. **A1a**

CsA has recently been found to have an antiviral effect on HCV [275–281]. CsA has been shown to have a suppressive effect on the HCV replicon RNA level and HCV protein expression in an HCV sub-genomic replicon cell culture system. CsA also inhibited multiplication of HCV genome in a cultured human hepatocyte cell line infected with HCV [275]. This anti-HCV activity is independent of its immunosuppressive and cytotoxic function. Moreover Nakagawa *et al.* found that Tac does not suppress HCV replication [276]. However, despite the clear antiviral effect of CsA *in vitro*, there is still controversy about the effect of CsA on HCV-replication *in vivo*, in the setting of clinical organ transplantation. In a study, ten patients with chronic hepatitis C who did not respond to IFN therapy and who had elevated serum ALT values for at least six months

were treated with CsA for three months (dose increased at one month intervals from 1.5–2 to 2–3 and 3–4 mg/kg/day). Serum ALT levels gradually decreased in all but one patient; however, serum HCV-RNA titers did not change in any patient throughout the study period [282].

On the basis of current data, it is not possible to conclude that CsA by itself has a profound effect on viral replication or on the course of HCV recurrence after transplantation [283].

In contrast, there are also cohort studies that show advantages using CsA-based regimen compared to Tac-based ones [98, 266, 277, 284–286]. Berenguer *et al.* found that the interval from LT to acute hepatitis was shorter in patients on Tac regimen compared to those on CsA (59 days vs 92 days; p = 0.02) [266], and that one of the variables associated with a higher probability of developing cirrhosis was induction therapy with Tac [284]. Levy *et al.* found that the mean time to histological diagnosis of hepatitis C recurrence was significantly longer with CsA-based regimen (100 ± 50 days) than with Tac (70 ± 40 days) even if the rate of histologically-proven HCV recurrence rate was similar between the two groups [98]. In an update study based on the same cohort of patients Shenoy *et al.* confirmed earlier recurrence in the Tac group (72 ± 42 days vs 145 ± 43 days, p = 0.006) but found that recurrent HCV occurred less frequently in Tac treated patients than in CsA-ME treated ones (21% vs 61%; p = 0.04) [99]. Median time from LT to initiation of antiviral therapy was longer in CsA group compared to Tac group (4.9 ± 1.1 year vs 2.6 ± 1.2 years) [277].

In another study, three-year actuarial risk of fibrosis stage 2 (METAVIR scoring system) was 66% with CsA and 90% with Tac [285]. The relationship between progression of liver fibrosis and histological necroinflammation in HCV recipients was evaluated in 55 patients transplanted for HCV liver disease between 1993 and 2002, retrospectively stratified in three different 40-month periods of transplantation. In a multiregression analysis, Tac at dose to maintain serum concentration of 5–10 ng/ml) was a major factor associated with three-year fibrosis progression rate in HCV-transplanted patients [286]. However this was based on only ten patients.

A more interesting set of data is the potential influence of CsA on the efficacy of antiviral therapy in transplant recipients. Firpi *et al.* reported 115 patients in whom co-treatment of CsA with low-dose IFNα resulted in greater inhibition of HCV replication in comparison with the effects of CsA or IFNα alone [277]. A higher SVR rate was achieved in CsA based immunosuppression compared to Tac based regimens (46% vs 27%; p = 0.03) when evaluated retrospectively. Inoue *et al.* observed higher SVR rate among patients with chronic HCV treated with IFN-α2b in combination with CsA compared to the group with IFN alone (55% vs 32%; p = 0.01) [287]. **B4**

CsA taper in association with MMF compared to unchanged immunosuppression with CsA was associated with a marked progression of allograft fibrosis (66% vs 0%), a slight increase of aminotranferases and HCV viral loads ($372 \pm 280 \times 10^3 \, IU/ml$ vs $124 \pm 245 \times 10^3 \, IU/ml$). On the other hand renal function improved significantly in the group with MMF and CsA taper [288].

Margarit *et al.* randomized 35 HCV-positive liver transplanted patients to Tac monotherapy (n = 20) and dual therapy (Tac and steroids) (n = 15) [238]. HCV recurrence, diagnosed as elevation of liver enzymes together with histologic confirmation from liver biopsy, was seen in 17/20 (85%) patients on Tac-monotherapy and in 14/15 (93%). No difference in fibrosis score (Ishak classification) (2.77 ± 2 vs 3.27 ± 1.8) and survival rate at one, three and five years after LT (89%, 83% and 61% vs 81%, 61% and 61%) was seen between the two groups. A comparison was also made between the 12 HCV patients who received no steroids at all (only-Tac) and the 23 patients who received steroids either from the beginning or to treat rejection (only-Tac-Ster). Fibrosis score (Ishak classification) was significantly lower in only-Tac group compared to the only-Tac-steroid group (1.78 ± 1 vs 3.73 ± 1.94; p = 0.005). Patient survival rate at one, three and five years after LT was no different between groups (92%, 92% and 73% only-Tac vs 78%, 61% and 51% only-Tac-steroids). **A1d**

Tac monotherapy (n = 27) in a randomized comparison with triple therapy (Tac, AZA and steroids tapered with six months) (n = 29), resulted in less severe graft hepatitis C with Tac triple therapy (p = 0.0044), despite a higher histological rejection rate (70% vs 86%) and more steroid resistant rejection episodes (10% vs 18.5%) [245, 270]. **A1d**

Azathioprine and mycophenolate mofetil

Antimetabolite immunosuppressants such as AZA and MMF have some common features with ribavirin, an antiviral drug which has been shown to enhance the activity of interferon in the treatment of HCV. Both ribavirin and MMF inhibit the inosine monophosphate deydrogenase that has been shown to have *in vitro* antiviral properties against flaviviruses [289]. Moreover, ribavirin and three metabolites of AZA are processed to monophosphate nucleotides by inosine monophosphate deydrogenase [290]. These data suggested the possibility that these immunosuppressive agents might also inhibit the hepatitis C virus replication. However, potential beneficial effects of MMF and AZA on HCV recurrence have not been documented in the literature [291].

Azathioprine Stangl *et al.* used the Bovine viral diarrhea virus (BDVD), a *Flaviviridae* virus closely related to HCV, to test the potential antiviral effects of AZA and MMF [292]. At doses that achieved similar cytotoxicity, AZA decreased BVDV replication ten times more than MMF. The inhibi-

tion of BVDV by AZA was not related to its cytotoxicity and the effect of AZA on a HCV replicon was at least as large as that of ribavirine.

Several studies (1996–2008) have reported on the impact of AZA on the severity of HCV recurrence [268, 284, 286, 293–299]. Most (70%) found that severity of HCV recurrence was decreased using AZA [268, 284, 294–296, 298, 299], whereas three studies showed similar severity in HCV recurrence whether AZA was used or not [286, 293, 297]. **B4** However, no study showed that AZA was associated with increased severity of recurrent HCV.

Patients treated with AZA containing immunosuppressive regimens reported by Hunt *et al.* experienced less recurrence (35.2% vs 77%; p < 0.005) and fibrosis progression (5.8% vs 37.5%; p = 0.014) than those without AZA [294]. Berenguer *et al.* evaluating pre-transplantation and early post-transplantation variables associated with a high risk for severe HCV related disease post-transplantation, found that one of the risk factors associated with severe disease was a short duration induction (<6 months) with AZA (RH 2.22; 95% CI: 1.37–3.60; p = 0.001) [284, 295]. In other studies, the use of AZA was associated with a lower risk of allograft failure and lower mortality (OR 0.3; 95% CI: 0.16–0.64; OR 0.32; 95% CI: 0.12–0.79) [268, 298].

A randomized, multicenter and prospective clinical trial randomized 180 liver transplanted patients to dual therapy (Tac and steroids, n = 92) and triple therapy (Tac, steroids and AZA, n = 88). Considering the HCV-positive subpopulation (n = 85) the use of AZA was associated with a lower rate of acute rejection (20% vs 48%; p = 0.008), but with no difference in graft and patient survival. Data on recurrent HCV was not reported [300].

A direct comparison between MMF and AZA in HCV-positive liver transplanted patients was evaluated by Wiesner *et al.* [115]. In 565 randomized patients, 278 (HCV+, n = 27) received CsA, steroids and MMF (1 g twice daily IV for four to ten days, followed by oral 1.5 g twice daily) and 287 (HCV-, n = 27) CsA, steroids and AZA (1.0 to 2.0 mg/kg/d IV followed by oral administration). A significant reduction in the incidence of acute hepatic allograft rejection or graft loss in the MMF group compared with the AZA group (30.6% vs 41.4%; p < 0.04) was seen at six months after LT. The incidence of HCV recurrence, defined histologically and in the presence of HCV-RNA, was 18.5% in the MMF group and 29.1% in the AZA group at six months after LT, but no long-term data is available.

However, a prospective crossover study reported that MMF, used as a substitute of AZA, led to an increase in viral load but it was not associated with an increase in ALT level [301]. Recently Kornberg *et al.* performed a prospective study revealing contrasting early and delayed results [302]. Twenty-one patients received quadruple induction CsA-based immunosuppression, augmented by MMF (n = 12) or by AZA (n = 9). In the MMF group recurrent disease was diagnosed earlier than in the AZA group (50 ± 35 vs 35 ± 35 weeks), but patients under MMF had less severe allograft fibrosis at diagnosis of disease recurrence (Ishak-Knodell) (1.5 ± 0.5 vs 2.2 ± 1.2). However, stage of fibrosis significantly increased in the MMF-group during six months of antiviral treatment compared to the AZA-group (1.5 ± 0.5 vs 2.3 ± 0.5; p = 0.04).

Mychophenolate mofetil Firpi *et al.* randomized 30 patients to four mycophenolate dose regimens (1000 mg twice daily, 500 mg twice daily, 250 mg twice daily or a matched oral placebo twice daily) for eight weeks, and showed that no subject became virus negative or had a one-log decrease in virus level [291]. The mean change in HCV-RNA level at week 4 and 8 compared with baseline was +19% and +10% respectively.

Wiesner *et al.* evaluated retrospectively 3463 patients who underwent LT for HCV-related liver disease, and assessed the impact of MMF on long-term outcomes comparing patients who were discharged from the hospital on Tac-based immunosuppression with or without MMF [119]. Patients treated at discharge with MMF, Tac and steroids had significantly increased four-year survival (79.5% vs 73.8%; p = 0.002) and graft survival (74.9% vs 69.5%; p = 0.024) and lower rate of acute rejection after discharge (defined as treatment for acute rejection or acute rejection as the cause of graft failure) (27.3% vs 32.1%; p = 0.047). However, MMF did not show convincing histological improvement of HCV recurrence. **B4** The combination of MMF (500–2000 mg/day) and Tac taper (target level 50% starting) over two months, was assessed in a retrospective case-control study comparing 40 patients with histologically proven HCV recurrence after LT to 40 non-MMF HCV positive liver transplanted patients (Tac n = 29, CsA n = 8, Tac + AZA n = 1, CsA + steroids n = 1). MMF in combination with CNI taper showed a positive effect on fibrosis progression, graft inflammation and ALT levels [296].

Anti-lymphocyte preparations

Anti-lymphocyte antibody preparations such as OKT3 to treat steroid-resistant acute rejection impact on the progression of HCV recurrence. Cholestatic hepatitis is associated with very high serum viral load, and a strongly associated risk factor is associated with high levels of immunosuppression, mainly pulses of methylprednisolone and/or OKT3 therapy [295, 303–306]. **B4**

Induction immunosuppression has not been a common practice in LT but is now being used in recipients with compromised renal function as it can diminish the need to delay introduction of calcineurin inhibitor and as part of partly tolerizing regimens [21, 22, 197]. De Ruvo *et al.* compared thymoglobulin induction plus Tac monotheapy

(n = 22) to Tac plus steroid immunosuppression without induction (n = 30) [307]. Patient survival and acute rejection rates did not differ. HCV recurrence was similar (54.5% vs 60%), but in the thymoglobulin group mean time to histologic recurrence was shorter (121 ± 54.3 days vs 205 ± 127 days; p = 0.04), despite lower HCV-RNA loads (mean peak: 12.4 ± 14.1 MEq/ml vs 19.2 ± 14.3 MEq/ml; p = 0.02). The fibrosis score (Ishak score) was not significantly different between the two groups (0.85 ± 0.8 vs 1.54 ± 1.3). **B3**

Induction therapy with either anti-CD25 monoclonal antibodies or rabbit antithymocyte globulins (RATG) resulted in good patient and graft survival, with acute rejection in 37.5% of patients treated with RATG and 20% in patients treated with anti-CD25. The rates of HCV recurrence, as defined on virological and biological criteria and confirmed by liver histology, were 80% in the anti-CD25 group and 56.25% in the RATG group, but with no reporting on severity or timing of recurrence [308]. Ramirez *et al.* compared induction with an anti-IL2 receptor inhibitor basiliximab to a historical group of 46 recipients on Tac-based immunosuppression [309]. In those with basiliximab induction, 43 of 46 patients (93.4%) remained rejection free during follow-up and the patient and graft survival rate at two years was 93.5%; histological HCV recurrence rate was 24%. The historical controls had a rejection rate of 31%, with lower patient and graft survival (71.7% and 69.5%) and a higher histological HCV recurrence rate (71%). Alemtuzumab (anti-CD25) was used by Marcos *et al.* in 38 HCV positive recipients, patient and graft survival at one year after LT were 71% and 70% versus 65% and 54% under conventional treatment [211]. Only 6% of the HCV positive recipients pre-treated with alemtuzumab developed first rejection during first four months after transplantation compared to 30% in the conventional group. However, HCV positive patients did significantly worse than those who were HCV negative, both in the induction and the control group. **B4** Moreover increased HCV viral replication was worse with alemtuzumab, but there was no data on histological recurrence.

In conclusion, studies on impact of immunosuppression regimens on post-transplantation outcome in HCV positive recipients support the idea that any dramatic change in immunosuppression as rapid withdrawal or alteration in the level or type of suppression (i.e. corticosteroids boluses and OKT3 use) are deleterious for recurrence. There may be a beneficial effect of low dose slow tapering of steroids and maintenance AZA. More randomized studies are needed to confirm these findings. A possible mechanism for these effects is that rapid change in immunosuppresion enables a vigorous immune response and killing of HCV-infected hepatocytes, which despite lowering the overall HCV load in the liver, results in extensive fibrosis [305, 310].

Chronic ductopenic rejection

Definition

Chronic or ductopenic rejection is mainly an immunologic injury to the allograft and can result in irreversible damage to the bile ducts, arteries and veins. The pathogenetic mechanism is obscure and the role of histocompatibility and viral agents is unclear. Mast cells seem to be important effector cells [311]. Its incidence at five years after transplantation has decreased from 10–15% in the 1980s to 3–5% in current recipients [312]. This may be due to a better recognition and control of acute and early phases of chronic rejection, but there may be other reasons, such as improvements in preservation solutions.

Clinical and laboratory findings

The natural history is poorly understood. Many cases occur following unresolved acute cellular rejection episodes. Chronic rejection in liver allografts shares risk factors and morphological characteristics with chronic rejection seen in other solid organ transplants, but there are also substantial differences. It has a relatively rapid onset, usually within several months, but it can occur weeks after transplantation, often following a progressive course. The peak incidence of graft failure from chronic rejection is 2–6 months post-transplantation and it progressively decreases with time [313]. Most cases require re-transplantation within the first year. Chronic rejection presenting after one year post-transplantation is "late onset chronic rejection" which presents more insidiously and may have different histological features [314].

However, despite its progressive course, in some cases it is potentially reversible, a quality that has been attributed to apparently unique immunologic properties and remarkable regenerative capabilities of the liver [315].

The diagnosis is clinically suspected when a patient develops progressive cholestasis and an increase in canalicular enzymes [26]. The early transition from acute to chronic rejection may be associated with an elevation in AST levels, which along with bilirubin concentrations, are associated with graft failure from chronic rejection. As with acute rejection, the clinical and biochemical manifestations of chronic rejection are non-specific and therefore the diagnosis also requires histological confirmation.

Theruvath et al. evaluated 924 liver transplants (median follow-up of 66 months), in whom histologically proven chronic rejection occurred in 2.1% [316]. Primary sclerosing cholangitis and a history of acute rejection were variables associated with an increased risk for development of chronic rejection. **B4** Wiesner et al. evaluated 870 consecutive primary liver transplant recipients and found that autoimmune liver disease was an independent risk factor for developing chronic rejection [44]. **B4**

Histopathological features

Two main histologic features are considered diagnostic: damage or loss of small ducts (less than $60 < \mu m$ in diameter) in more than 50% of the portal tracts, (there needs to be specific cytokeratin staining of biliary epithelium) and foam cell obliterative arteriopathy of large and medium sized arteries [26]. Recently it has been recognized that distinct early histopathological changes presage disappearance of bile ducts in the form of a parenchymal inflammatory reaction. The early recognition of this "hepatitic" phase may be of fundamental importance. It could indicate the need for increased or altered immunosuppressive therapy [317]. In the past it may have been mistakenly diagnosed as superimposed hepatitis leading to an inappropriate reduction of immunosuppression, which could exacerbate the chronic rejection.

Bile duct loss in more than 50% of portal tracts and absence of necroinflammatory activity, represent late histopathologic changes, the classic textbook description, but these changes are late in the evolution of the process and are likely to be irreversible. Diagnosis at this stage may be useful in deciding when to list a patient for re-transplantation; additional immunosuppressive therapy is unlikely to be of any benefit and may do harm by increasing the risk of infection prior to transplantation.

Grading and staging

There is a tentative scheme for grading chronic rejection proposed by the National Institute of Diabetes, Digestive, and Kidney Disease (see Box 42.1) [318].

Treatment

Treatment is dependent on the stage at which the process is diagnosed. Cases of early chronic rejection may respond to increased dosage of Tac, which is the only effective rescue therapy, documented by different centers, resulting in a 70% graft survival at one-year follow-up. Patients who have a serum bilirubin level less than 10 mg/dl at the time of conversion to Tac and who develop chronic rejection more than 90 days after transplantation, have the best response [319]. **B4** The combination of mycophenolate mofetil with sirolimus has also been reported in an animal model to be effective in chronic rejection. Sirolimus may help to reduce arterial intimal thickening which is believed to be a pathophysiological root cause of chronic rejection [320]. **C5** However, the safety and benefit of sirolimus alone for chronic rejection is currently unknown.

BOX 42.1 NIDDK definitions of grades far chronic rejection, and for rejection uncertain for chronicity (indefinite for bile duct loss)

Rejection, uncertain for chronicity (indefinite bile duct loss)
No complicating lobular changes
Lobular changes, including one of the three findings:
• Centrilobular cholestasis
• Perivenular sclerosis
• Hepatocellular ballooning
• Necrosis and dropout
Chronic rejectiona
Early or mild
Bile duct loss, without centrilobular cholestasis, perivenular sclerosis, or hepatocyte ballooning or necrosis and dropout
Intermediate/moderate
Bile duct loss, with one of the following four findings:
• Centrilobular cholestasis
• Perivenular sclerosis
• Hepatocellular ballooning
• Necrosis and dropout
Late or severe
Bile duct loss, with at least two of the four following findings:
• Centrilobular cholestasis
• Perivenular sclerosis
• Hepatocellular ballooning
• Necrosis and dropout

a Bile duct loss >50% of triads.
NIDDK, National Institute of Diabetes, Digestive and Kidney disease.

Neff *et al.* in a retrospective review of 21 transplant recipients with clinical and histological diagnosis of chronic rejection treated with sirolimus (0.07 mg/kg) and Tac (serum level 8–14 ng/dl), showed an improvement in the bile duct to hepatic artery ratio and total bilirubin levels. However, a large number of patients experienced drug-related side effects and were unable to tolerate therapy [321]. **B4**

Re-transplantation remains the best treatment for chronic rejection associated with severe biochemical cholestasis and advanced bile duct loss, which is usually unresponsive to immunosuppression. The recurrence rate of chronic rejection is as high as 90%, although it is not clear if some characteristics, for example early re-transplantation, are predictive factors for recurrence [322].

Recently it has been recognized that some cases of advanced chronic rejection have recovered spontaneously, or with the use of additional immunosuppression. In some of these cases, follow-up liver biopsies have shown a per-sistent paucity of bile ducts without other histological features of chronic rejection. Ductopenia has also been noted as an incidental finding in protocol biopsies taken at annual review from patients who are clinically well, with no previous biopsies suggesting chronic rejection. These findings suggest that some patients may suffer permanent duct loss as a result of rejection, but that sufficient ducts remain to allow the graft to function normally. Because of these observations and the risks associated and logistical difficulties with a second transplantation, the decision to re-transplant should only be made when a confident diagnosis of irreversible and progressive graft damage is established.

Acknowledgements

Dr Maria Pleguezuelo is supported by the Liver Research Unit, University Hospital Reina Sofia, Cordoba, Spain; Dr Giacomo Germani is supported by University Hospital of Padua, Department of Surgical and Gastroenterological Sciences, Gastroenterology Section, University of Padua, Italy.

References

1 Neuberger J, Adams DH. What is the significance of acute liver allograft rejection? *J Hepatol* 1998; **29**(1): 143–150.

2 Burroughs AK, Sabin CA, Rolles K *et al.* Three-month and 12-month mortality after first liver transplant in adults in Europe: predictive models for outcome. *Lancet* 2006; **367**(9506): 225–232.

3 Abbasoglu O. Liver transplantation: yesterday, today and tomorrow. *World J Gastroenterol* 2008; **14**(20): 3117–3122.

4 Gross CR, Malinchoc M, Kim WR *et al.* Quality of life before and after liver transplantation for cholestatic liver disease. *Hepatology* 1999; **29**(2): 356–364.

5 Jain AB, Reyes J, Marcos A *et al.* Pregnancy after liver transplantation with tacrolimus immunosuppression: a single center's experience update at 13 years. *Transplantation* 2003; **76**(5): 827–832.

6 Ratcliffe J, Longworth L, Young T, Bryan S, Burroughs A, Buxton M. Assessing health-related quality of life pre- and post-liver transplantation: a prospective multicenter study. *Liver Transpl* 2002; **8**(3): 263–270.

7 Gane E, Portmann B, Saxena R, Wong P, Ramage J, Williams R. Nodular regenerative hyperplasia of the liver graft after liver transplantation. *Hepatology* 1994; **20**(1 Pt 1): 88–94.

8 UNOS website. 2000. www.unos.org

9 Abouljoud MS, Levy MF, Klintmalm GB. Hyperlipidemia after liver transplantation: long-term results of the FK506/cyclosporine a US Multicenter trial. US Multicenter Study Group. *Transplant Proc* 1995; **27**(1): 1121–1123.

10 Jindal RM, Sidner RA, Milgrom ML. Post-transplant diabetes mellitus. The role of immunosuppression. *Drug Saf* 1997; **16**(4): 242–257.

11 Mor E, Facklam D, Hasse J *et al.* Weight gain and lipid profile changes in liver transplant recipients: long-term results of the American FK506 Multicenter Study. *Transplant Proc* 1995; **27**(1): 1126.

12 Pham H, Lemoine A, Salvucci M *et al.* Occurrence of gammopathies and lymphoproliferative disorders in liver transplant recipients randomized to tacrolimus (FK506) or cyclosporine-based immunosuppression. *Liver Transpl Surg* 1998; **4**(2): 146–151.

13 Fisher NC, Nightingale PG, Gunson BK, Lipkin GW, Neuberger JM. Chronic renal failure following liver transplantation: a retrospective analysis. *Transplantation* 1998; **66**(1): 59–66.

14 Ojo AO, Held PJ, Port FK *et al.* Chronic renal failure after transplantation of a nonrenal organ. *N Engl J Med* 2003; **349**(10): 931–940.

15 Schmitz V, Laudi S, Moeckel F *et al.* Chronic renal dysfunction following liver transplantation. *Clin Transplant* 2008; **22**(3): 333–340.

16 Pelletier SJ, Orosz CG, Cosio FG, Ferguson RM. Risk factors in chronic rejection. *Current Opinion in Organ Transplantation* 1996; **4**: 28–40.

17 Calne R, Friend P, Moffatt S *et al.* Prope tolerance, perioperative campath 1H, and low-dose cyclosporin monotherapy in renal allograft recipients. *Lancet* 1998; **351**(9117): 1701–1702.

18 Devlin J, Doherty D, Thomson L *et al.* Defining the outcome of immunosuppression withdrawal after liver transplantation. *Hepatology* 1998; **27**(4): 926–933.

19 Mazariegos GV, Reyes J, Marino IR *et al.* Weaning of immunosuppression in liver transplant recipients. *Transplantation* 1997; **63**(2): 243–249.

20 Ramos HC, Reyes J, bu-Elmagd K *et al.* Weaning of immunosuppression in long-term liver transplant recipients. *Transplantation* 1995; **59**(2): 212–217.

21 Starzl TE. Acquired immunologic tolerance: with particular reference to transplantation. *Immunol Res* 2007; **38**(1–3): 6–41.

22 Starzl TE. Immunosuppressive therapy and tolerance of organ allografts. *N Engl J Med* 2008; **358**(4): 407–411.

23 Adams DH, Neuberger JM. Patterns of graft rejection following liver transplantation. *J Hepatol* 1990; **10**(1): 113–119.

24 Rosen HR. Transplantation immunology: what the clinician needs to know for immunotherapy. *Gastroenterology* 2008; **134**(6): 1789–1801.

25 Isaacs JD. T cell immunomodulation – the Holy Grail of therapeutic tolerance. *Curr Opin Pharmacol* 2007; **7**(4): 418–425.

26 Terminology for hepatic allograft rejection. International Working Party. *Hepatology* 1995; **22**(2): 648–654.

27 Hubscher S. Diagnosis and grading of liver allograft rejection: a European perspective. *Transplant Proc* 1996; **28**(1): 504–507.

28 Prieto M, Berenguer M, Rayon JM *et al.* High incidence of allograft cirrhosis in hepatitis C virus genotype 1b infection following transplantation: relationship with rejection episodes. *Hepatology* 1999; **29**(1): 250–256.

29 Slapak GI, Saxena R, Portmann B *et al.* Graft and systemic disease in long-term survivors of liver transplantation. *Hepatology* 1997; **25**(1): 195–202.

30 Neuberger J. Liver allograft rejection – current concepts on diagnosis and treatment. *J Hepatol* 1995; **23**(Suppl. 1): 54–61.

31 Datta GS, Hudson M, Burroughs AK *et al.* Grading of cellular rejection after orthotopic liver transplantation. *Hepatology* 1995; **21**(1): 46–57.

32 Barnes EJ, bdel-Rehim MM, Goulis Y *et al.* Applications and limitations of blood eosinophilia for the diagnosis of acute cellular rejection in liver transplantation. *Am J Transplant* 2003; **3**(4): 432–438.

33 Aran PP, Bissel MG, Whitington PF, Bostwick DG, Adamac T, Baker AL. Diagnosis of hepatic allograft rejection: role of liver biopsy. *Clin Transplant* 1993; **7**(5): 475–481.

34 Neuberger J, Wilson P, Adams D. Protocol liver biopsies: the case in favour. *Transplant Proc* 1998; **30**(4): 1497–1499.

35 Wiesner RH. Is hepatic histology the true gold standard in diagnosing acute hepatic allograft rejection? *Liver Transpl Surg* 1996; **2**(2): 165–167.

36 Porter KA. Pathology of liver transplantation. *Transplant Rev* 1969; **2**: 129–170.

37 Snover DC, Sibley RK, Freese DK *et al.* Orthotopic liver transplantation: a pathological study of 63 serial liver biopsies from 17 patients with special reference to the diagnostic features and natural history of rejection. *Hepatology* 1984; **4**(6): 1212–1222.

38 Demetris AJ, Lasky S, Van Thiel DH, Starzl TE, Dekker A. Pathology of hepatic transplantation: a review of 62 adult allograft recipients immunosuppressed with a cyclosporine/steroid regimen. *Am J Pathol* 1985; **118**(1): 151–161.

39 Hubscher SG. Central perivenulitis: a common and potentially important finding in late posttransplant liver biopsies. *Liver Transpl* 2008; **14**(5): 596–600.

40 Krasinskas AM, Demetris AJ, Poterucha JJ, Abraham SC. The prevalence and natural history of untreated isolated central perivenulitis in adult allograft livers. *Liver Transpl* 2008; **14**(5): 625–632.

41 Lovell MO, Speeg KV, Halff GA, Molina DK, Sharkey FE. Acute hepatic allograft rejection: a comparison of patients with and without centrilobular alterations during first rejection episode. *Liver Transpl* 2004; **10**(3): 369–373.

42 Demetris AJ, Ruppert K, Dvorchik I *et al.* Real-time monitoring of acute liver-allograft rejection using the Banff schema. *Transplantation* 2002; **74**(9): 1290–1296.

43 Ormonde DG, de Boer WB, Kierath A *et al.* Banff schema for grading liver allograft rejection: utility in clinical practice. *Liver Transpl Surg* 1999; **5**(4): 261–268.

44 Wiesner RH, Demetris AJ, Belle SH *et al.* Acute hepatic allograft rejection: incidence, risk factors, and impact on outcome. *Hepatology* 1998; **28**(3): 638–645.

45 Banff schema for grading liver allograft rejection: an international consensus document. *Hepatology* 1997; **25**(3): 658–663.

46 Bubak ME, Porayko MK, Krom RA, Wiesner RH. Complications of liver biopsy in liver transplant patients: increased sepsis associated with choledochojejunostomy. *Hepatology* 1991; **14**(6): 1063–1065.

47 Garcia-Tsao G, Boyer JL. Outpatient liver biopsy: how safe is it? *Ann Intern Med* 1993; **118**(2): 150–153.

48 Larson AM, Chan GC, Wartelle CF *et al.* Infection complicating percutaneous liver biopsy in liver transplant recipients. *Hepatology* 1997; **26**(6): 1406–1409.

49 Papatheodoridis GV, Patch D, Watkinson A, Tibballs J, Burroughs AK. Transjugular liver biopsy in the 1990s: a 2-year audit. *Aliment Pharmacol Ther* 1999; **13**(5): 603–608.

50 Kalambokis G, Manousou P, Vibhakorn S et al. Transjugular liver biopsy – indications, adequacy, quality of specimens, and complications – a systematic review. J Hepatol 2007; **47**(2): 284–294.

51 Klintmalm GB, Nery JR, Husberg BS, Gonwa TA, Tillery GW. Rejection in liver transplantation. Hepatology 1989; **10**(6): 978–985.

52 Williams JW, Peters TG, Vera SR, Britt LG, van Voorst SJ, Haggitt RC. Biopsy-directed immunosuppression following hepatic transplantation in man. Transplantation 1985; **39**(6): 589–596.

53 Bartlett AS, Ramadas R, Furness S, Gane E, McCall JL. The natural history of acute histologic rejection without biochemical graft dysfunction in orthotopic liver transplantation: a systematic review. Liver Transpl 2002; **8**(12): 1147–1153.

54 Burroughs AK, Patch DW, Stigliano R, Cecilioni L. Protocol biopsies in liver transplantation. Liver Transpl 2003; **9**(7): 780–781.

55 Tisone G, Orlando G, Vennarecci G et al. Spontaneous resolution of severe acute rejection in liver transplantation. Transplant Proc 1999; **31**(8): 3164–3166.

56 Tippner C, Nashan B, Hoshino K et al. Clinical and subclinical acute rejection early after liver transplantation: contributing factors and relevance for the long-term course. Transplantation 2001; **72**(6): 1122–1128.

57 Wiesner RH, Goldstein RM, Donovan JP, Miller CM, Lake JR, Lucey MR. The impact of cyclosporine dose and level on acute rejection and patient and graft survival in liver transplant recipients. Liver Transpl Surg 1998; **4**(1): 34–41.

58 Dousset B, Conti F, Cherruau B et al. Is acute rejection deleterious to long-term liver allograft function? J Hepatol 1998; **29**(4): 660–668.

59 McVicar JP, Kowdley KV, Bacchi CE et al. The natural history of untreated focal allograft rejection in liver transplant recipients. Liver Transpl Surg 1996; **2**(2): 154–160.

60 Fisher LR, Henley KS, Lucey MR. Acute cellular rejection after liver transplantation: variability, morbidity, and mortality. Liver Transpl Surg 1995; **1**(1): 10–15.

61 Mor E, Gonwa TA, Husberg BS, Goldstein RM, Klintmalm GB. Late-onset acute rejection in orthotopic liver transplantation – associated risk factors and outcome. Transplantation 1992; **54**(5): 821–824.

62 Anand AC, Hubscher SG, Gunson BK, McMaster P, Neuberger JM. Timing, significance, and prognosis of late acute liver allograft rejection. Transplantation 1995; **60**(10): 1098–1103.

63 Neuberger J. Incidence, timing, and risk factors for acute and chronic rejection. Liver Transpl Surg 1999; **5**(4 Suppl. 1): S30–S36.

64 Hayashi M, Keeffe EB, Krams SM et al. Allograft rejection after liver transplantation for autoimmune liver diseases. Liver Transpl Surg 1998; **4**(3): 208–214.

65 Berlakovich GA, Rockenschaub S, Taucher S, Kaserer K, Muhlbacher F, Steiniger R. Underlying disease as a predictor for rejection after liver transplantation. Arch Surg 1998; **133**(2): 167–172.

66 Farges O, Saliba F, Farhamant H et al. Incidence of rejection and infection after liver transplantation as a function of the primary disease: possible influence of alcohol and polyclonal immunoglobulins. Hepatology 1996; **23**(2): 240–248.

67 Adams DH, Hubscher SG, Neuberger JM, McMaster P, Elias E, Buckels JA. Reduced incidence of rejection in patients undergoing liver transplantation for chronic hepatitis B. Transplant Proc 1991; **23**(1 Pt 2): 1436–1437.

68 Gomez-Manero N, Herrero JI, Quiroga J et al. Prognostic model for early acute rejection after liver transplantation. Liver Transpl 2001; **7**(3): 246–254.

69 Cecilioni L, Stigliano R, Patch D, Quaglia A, Burroughs AK. Predictive factors for the absence of cellular rejection after liver transplantation in a protocol biopsy population (Abstract). Hepatology 2003; **38**(Suppl. 1): A379.

70 Margarit C, Rimola A, Gonzalez-Pinto I et al. Efficacy and safety of oral low-dose tacrolimus treatment in liver transplantation. Transpl Int 1998; **11**(Suppl. 1): S260–S266.

71 The US Multicenter FK506 Liver Study Group. A comparison of tacrolimus (FK 506) and cyclosporine for immunosuppression in liver transplantation. The US Multicenter FK506 Liver Study Group. N Engl J Med 1994; **331**(17): 1110–1115.

72 European FK506 Multicentre Liver Study Group. Randomised trial comparing tacrolimus (FK506) and cyclosporin in prevention of liver allograft rejection. European FK506 Multicentre Liver Study Group. Lancet 1994; **344**(8920): 423–428.

73 Fung JJ, Eliasziw M, Todo S et al. The Pittsburgh randomized trial of tacrolimus compared to cyclosporine for hepatic transplantation 447. J Am Coll Surg 1996; **183**(2): 117–125.

74 Belli LS, De Carlis L, Rondinara GF et al. Sandimmun-Neoral in liver transplantation: a remarkable improvement in long-term immunosuppression. Transplant Proc 1994; **26**(5): 2983–2984.

75 Levy G, Burra P, Cavallari A et al. Improved clinical outcomes for liver transplant recipients using cyclosporine monitoring based on 2-hr post-dose levels (C2). Transplantation 2002; **73**(6): 953–959.

76 McAlister VC, Haddad E, Renouf E, Malthaner RA, Kjaer MS, Gluud LL. Cyclosporin versus tacrolimus as primary immunosuppressant after liver transplantation: a meta-analysis. Am J Transplant 2006; **6**(7): 1578–1585.

77 Stegall MD, Wachs ME, Everson G et al. Prednisone withdrawal 14 days after liver transplantation with mycophenolate: a prospective trial of cyclosporine and tacrolimus. Transplantation 1997; **64**(12): 1755–1760.

78 Fisher RA, Ham JM, Marcos A et al. A prospective randomized trial of mycophenolate mofetil with neoral or tacrolimus after orthotopic liver transplantation. Transplantation 1998; **66**(12): 1616–1621.

79 Zervos XA, Weppler D, Fragulidis GP et al. Comparison of tacrolimus with microemulsion cyclosporine as primary immunosuppression in hepatitis C patients after liver transplantation. Transplantation 1998; **65**(8): 1044–1046.

80 Klupp J, Glanemann M, Bechstein WO et al. Mycophenolate mofetil in combination with tacrolimus versus Neoral after liver transplantation. Transplant Proc 1999; **31**(1–2): 1113–1114.

81 Rolles K, Davidson BR, Burroughs AK. A pilot study of immunosuppressive monotherapy in liver transplantation: tacrolimus versus microemulsified cyclosporin. Transplantation 1999; **68**(8): 1195–1198.

82 Muhlbacher F. Tacrolimus versus cyclosporin microemulsion in liver transplantation: results of a 3-month study. Transplant Proc 2001; **33**(1–2): 1339–1340.

83 O'Grady JG, Burroughs A, Hardy P, Elbourne D, Truesdale A. Tacrolimus versus microemulsified ciclosporin in liver transplantation: the TMC randomised controlled trial. *Lancet* 2002; **360**(9340): 1119–1125.

84 Therapondos G, Flapan AD, Dollinger MM, Garden OJ, Plevris JN, Hayes PC. Cardiac function after orthotopic liver transplantation and the effects of immunosuppression: a prospective randomized trial comparing cyclosporin (Neoral) and tacrolimus. *Liver Transpl* 2002; **8**(8): 690–700.

85 Timmermann W, Erhard J, Lange R et al. A randomised trial comparing the efficacy and safety of tacrolimus with microemulsified cyclosporine after liver transplantation. *Transplant Proc* 2002; **34**(5): 1516–1518.

86 Greig P, Lilly L, Scudamore C et al. Early steroid withdrawal after liver transplantation: the Canadian tacrolimus versus microemulsion cyclosporin A trial: 1-year follow-up. *Liver Transpl* 2003; **9**(6): 587–595.

87 Kelly D, Jara P, Rodeck B et al. Tacrolimus and steroids versus ciclosporin microemulsion, steroids, and azathioprine in children undergoing liver transplantation: randomised European multicentre trial. *Lancet* 2004; **364**(9439): 1054–1061.

88 Levy G, Villamil F, Samuel D et al. Results of LIS2T, a multicenter, randomized study comparing cyclosporine microemulsion with C2 monitoring and tacrolimus with C0 monitoring in de novo liver transplantation. *Transplantation* 2004; **77**(11): 1632–1638.

89 Levy G, Grazi GL, Sanjuan F et al. 12-month follow-up analysis of a multicenter, randomized, prospective trial in de novo liver transplant recipients (LIS2T) comparing cyclosporine microemulsion (C2 monitoring) and tacrolimus. *Liver Transpl* 2006; **12**(10): 1464–1472.

90 Martin P, Busuttil RW, Goldstein RM et al. Impact of tacrolimus versus cyclosporine in hepatitis C virus-infected liver transplant recipients on recurrent hepatitis: a prospective, randomized trial. *Liver Transpl* 2004; **10**(10): 1258–1262.

91 O'Grady JG, Hardy P, Burroughs AK, Elbourne D. Randomized controlled trial of tacrolimus versus microemulsified cyclosporin (TMC) in liver transplantation: poststudy surveillance to 3 years. *Am J Transplant* 2007; **7**(1): 137–141.

92 Gonzalez-Pinto IM, Rimola A, Margarit C et al. Five-year follow-up of a trial comparing tacrolimus and cyclosporine microemulsion in liver transplantation. *Transplant Proc* 2005; **37**(4): 1713–1715.

93 de Mattos AM, Olyaei AJ, Bennett WM. Nephrotoxicity of immunosuppressive drugs: long-term consequences and challenges for the future. *Am J Kidney Dis* 2000; **35**(2): 333–346.

94 Watson CJ, Gimson AE, Alexander GJ et al. A randomized controlled trial of late conversion from calcineurin inhibitor (CNI)-based to sirolimus-based immunosuppression in liver transplant recipients with impaired renal function 451. *Liver Transpl* 2007; **13**(12): 1694–1702.

95 Levy G, Thervet E, Lake J, Uchida K. Patient management by Neoral C(2) monitoring: an international consensus statement. *Transplantation* 2002; **73**(9 Suppl.): S12–18.

96 Levy G, Villamil F, Samuel D et al. Results of LIS2T, a multicenter, randomized study comparing cyclosporine microemulsion with C2 monitoring and tacrolimus with C0 monitoring in de novo liver transplantation. *Transplantation* 2004; **77**(11): 1632–1638.

97 Tanaka K, Lake J, Villamil F et al. Comparison of cyclosporine microemulsion and tacrolimus in 39 recipients of living donor liver transplantation. *Liver Transpl* 2005; **11**(11): 1395–1402.

98 Levy G, Grazi GL, Sanjuan F et al. 12-month follow-up analysis of a multicenter, randomized, prospective trial in de novo liver transplant recipients (LIS2T) comparing cyclosporine microemulsion (C2 monitoring) and tacrolimus. *Liver Transpl* 2006; **12**(10): 1464–1472.

99 Shenoy S, Hardinger KL, Crippin J et al. A randomized, prospective, pharmacoeconomic trial of neoral 2-hour postdose concentration monitoring versus tacrolimus trough concentration monitoring in de novo liver transplant recipients. *Liver Transpl* 2008; **14**(2): 173–180.

100 Levy G, Lilly LB, Grant DR et al. Once daily dosing with Neoral C2 monitoring in maintenance liver transplant patients (Abstract). *Am J Transplant* 2003; **3**(Suppl. 5): 422.

101 Fukudo M, Yano I, Masuda S et al. Cyclosporine exposure and calcineurin phosphatase activity in living-donor liver transplant patients: twice daily vs once daily dosing. *Liver Transpl* 2006; **12**(2): 292–300.

102 Kovarik JM, Villamil F, Otero A et al. Cyclosporine pharmacokinetics and blood pressure responses after conversion to once-daily dosing in maintenance liver transplant patients. *Clin Transplant* 2008; **22**(1): 68–75.

103 chi-Andanson M, Charpiat B, Jelliffe RW, Ducerf C, Fourcade N, Baulieux J. Failure of traditional trough levels to predict tacrolimus concentrations. *Ther Drug Monit* 2001; **23**(2): 129–133.

104 Zahir H, McLachlan AJ, Nelson A, McCaughan G, Gleeson M, Akhlaghi F. Population pharmacokinetic estimation of tacrolimus apparent clearance in adult liver transplant recipients. *Ther Drug Monit* 2005; **27**(4): 422–430.

105 Venkataramanan R, Shaw LM, Sarkozi L et al. Clinical utility of monitoring tacrolimus blood concentrations in liver transplant patients. *J Clin Pharmacol* 2001; **41**(5): 542–551.

106 Langers P, Press RR, den Hartigh J et al. Flexible limited sampling model for monitoring tacrolimus in stable patients having undergone liver transplantation with samples 4 to 6 hours after dosing is superior to trough concentration. *Ther Drug Monit* 2008; **30**(4): 456–461.

107 Blanchet B, Duvoux C, Costentin CE et al. Pharmacokinetic-pharmacodynamic assessment of tacrolimus in liver-transplant recipients during the early post-transplantation period. *Ther Drug Monit* 2008; **30**(4): 412–418.

108 Florman S, Alloway R, Kalayoglu M et al. Conversion of stable liver transplant recipients from a twice-daily Prograf-based regimen to a once-daily modified release tacrolimus-based regimen. *Transplant Proc* 2005; **37**(2): 1211–1213.

109 Florman S, Alloway R, Kalayoglu M et al. Once-daily tacrolimus extended release formulation: experience at 2 years postconversion from a Prograf-based regimen in stable liver transplant recipients. *Transplantation* 2007; **83**(12): 1639–1642.

110 Klintmalm GB, Gibbs JF, McMillan R et al. Rejection: FK 506 for rescue or maintenance. *Transplant Proc* 1993; **25**(2): 1914–1915.

111 Millis JM, Woodle ES, Piper JB et al. Tacrolimus for primary treatment of steroid-resistant hepatic allograft rejection. *Transplantation* 1996; **61**(9): 1365–1369.

112 Schmeding M, Neumann UP, Neuhaus R, Neuhaus P. Mycophenolate mofetil in liver transplantation – is monotherapy safe? *Clin Transplant* 2006; **20**(Suppl. 17): 75–79.

113 Nielsen OH, Vainer B, Rask-Madsen J. Review article: the treatment of inflammatory bowel disease with 6-mercaptopurine or azathioprine. *Aliment Pharmacol Ther* 2001; **15**(11): 1699–1708.

114 Mueller XM. Drug immunosuppression therapy for adult heart transplantation. Part 1: immune response to allograft and mechanism of action of immunosuppressants. *Ann Thorac Surg* 2004; **77**(1): 354–362.

115 Wiesner R, Rabkin J, Klintmalm G *et al.* A randomized double-blind comparative study of mycophenolate mofetil and azathioprine in combination with cyclosporine and corticosteroids in primary liver transplant recipients. *Liver Transpl* 2001; **7**(5): 442–450.

116 Fischer L, Sterneck M, Gahlemann CG, Malago M, Rogiers X, Broelsch CE. A prospective study comparing safety and efficacy of mycophenolate mofetil versus azathioprine in primary liver transplant recipients. *Transplant Proc* 2000; **32**(7): 2125–2127.

117 Fulton B, Markham A. Mycophenolate mofetil. A review of its pharmacodynamic and pharmacokinetic properties and clinical efficacy in renal transplantation. *Drugs* 1996; **51**(2): 278–298.

118 Wiesner RH, Steffen BJ, David KM, Chu AH, Gordon RD, Lake JR. Mycophenolate mofetil use is associated with decreased risk of late acute rejection in adult liver transplant recipients. *Am J Transplant* 2006; **6**(7): 1609–1616.

119 Wiesner RH, Shorr JS, Steffen BJ, Chu AH, Gordon RD, Lake JR. Mycophenolate mofetil combination therapy improves long-term outcomes after liver transplantation in patients with and without hepatitis C. *Liver Transpl* 2005; **11**(7): 750–759.

120 Salvadori M, Holzer H, de Mattos A *et al.* Enteric-coated mycophenolate sodium is therapeutically equivalent to mycophenolate mofetil in de novo renal transplant patients. *Am J Transplant* 2004; **4**(2): 231–236.

121 Budde K, Curtis J, Knoll G *et al.* Enteric-coated mycophenolate sodium can be safely administered in maintenance renal transplant patients: results of a 1-year study. *Am J Transplant* 2004; **4**(2): 237–243.

122 Ciancio G, Burke GW, Gaynor JJ *et al.* Randomized trial of mycophenolate mofetil versus enteric-coated mycophenolate sodium in primary renal transplant recipients given tacrolimus and daclizumab/thymoglobulin: one year follow-up. *Transplantation* 2008; **86**(1): 67–74.

123 Johnston A, He X, Holt DW. Bioequivalence of enteric-coated mycophenolate sodium and mycophenolate mofetil: a meta-analysis of three studies in stable renal transplant recipients. *Transplantation* 2006; **82**(11): 1413–1418.

124 Miras M, Carballo F, Egea J *et al.* Clinical evolution in the first 3 months of patients after liver transplantation in maintenance phase converted from mycophenolate mofetil to mycophenolate sodium due to gastrointestinal complications. *Transplant Proc* 2007; **39**(7): 2314–2317.

125 Cantisani GP, Zanotelli ML, Gleisner AL, de Mello BA, Marroni CA. Enteric-coated mycophenolate sodium experience in liver transplant patients. *Transplant Proc* 2006; **38**(3): 932–933.

126 Pfitzmann R, Klupp J, Langrehr JM *et al.* Mycophenolatemofetil for immunosuppression after liver transplantation: a follow-up study of 191 patients. *Transplantation* 2003; **76**(1): 130–136.

127 Reggiani P, Arru M, Regazzi M *et al.* A "steroid-free" tacrolimus and low-dose mycophenolate mofetil primary immunosuppression does not prevent early acute rejection after liver transplantation. *Transplant Proc* 2005; **37**(4): 1697–1699.

128 Herrero JI, Quiroga J, Sangro B *et al.* Conversion of liver transplant recipients on cyclosporine with renal impairment to mycophenolate mofetil. *Liver Transpl Surg* 1999; **5**(5): 414–420.

129 Reich DJ, Clavien PA, Hodge EE. Mycophenolate mofetil for renal dysfunction in liver transplant recipients on cyclosporine or tacrolimus: randomized, prospective, multicenter pilot study results. *Transplantation* 2005; **80**(1): 18–25.

130 Koch RO, Graziadei IW, Schulz F *et al.* Long-term efficacy and safety of mycophenolate mofetil in liver transplant recipients with calcineurin inhibitor-induced renal dysfunction. *Transpl Int* 2004; **17**(9): 518–524.

131 Schlitt HJ, Barkmann A, Boker KH *et al.* Replacement of calcineurin inhibitors with mycophenolate mofetil in liver-transplant patients with renal dysfunction: a randomised controlled study. *Lancet* 2001; **357**(9256): 587–591.

132 Stewart SF, Hudson M, Talbot D, Manas D, Day CP. Mycophenolate mofetil monotherapy in liver transplantation. *Lancet* 2001; **357**(9256): 609–610.

133 Raimondo ML, Dagher L, Papatheodoridis GV *et al.* Long-term mycophenolate mofetil monotherapy in combination with calcineurin inhibitors for chronic renal dysfunction after liver transplantation. *Transplantation* 2003; **75**(2): 186–190.

134 Creput C, Blandin F, Deroure B *et al.* Long-term effects of calcineurin inhibitor conversion to mycophenolate mofetil on renal function after liver transplantation. *Liver Transpl* 2007; **13**(7): 1004–1010.

135 Beckebaum S, Cicinnati VR, Klein CG *et al.* Impact of combined mycophenolate mofetil and low-dose calcineurin inhibitor therapy on renal function, cardiovascular risk factors, and graft function in liver transplant patients: preliminary results of an open prospective study. *Transplant Proc* 2004; **36**(9): 2671–2674.

136 Jain A, Venkataramanan R, Kwong T *et al.* Pharmacokinetics of mycophenolic acid in liver transplant patients after intravenous and oral administration of mycophenolate mofetil. *Liver Transpl* 2007; **13**(6): 791–796.

137 Jain A, Sharma R, Ryan C *et al.* Potential immunological advantage of intravenous mycophenolate mofetil with tacrolimus and steroids in primary deceased donor liver transplantation and live donor liver transplantation without antibody induction. *Liver Transpl* 2008; **14**(2): 202–209.

138 Meiser BM, Pfeiffer M, Schmidt D *et al.* Combination therapy with tacrolimus and mycophenolate mofetil following cardiac transplantation: importance of mycophenolic acid therapeutic drug monitoring. *J Heart Lung Transplant* 1999; **18**(2): 143–149.

139 van Gelder T, Hilbrands LB, Vanrenterghem Y *et al.* A randomized double-blind, multicenter plasma concentration controlled study of the safety and efficacy of oral mycophenolate mofetil for the prevention of acute rejection after kidney transplantation. *Transplantation* 1999; **68**(2): 261–266.

140 Tredger JM, Brown NW, Adams J *et al.* Monitoring mycophenolate in liver transplant recipients: toward a therapeutic range. *Liver Transpl* 2004; **10**(4): 492–502.

141 Mardigyan V, Tchervenkov J, Metrakos P, Barkun J, Deschenes M, Cantarovich M. Best single time points as surrogates to the

tacrolimus and mycophenolic acid area under the curve in adult liver transplant patients beyond 12 months of transplantation. *Clin Ther* 2005; **27**(4): 463–469.

142 Chen H, Peng C, Yu Z *et al.* Pharmacokinetics of mycophenolic acid and determination of area under the curve by abbreviated sampling strategy in Chinese liver transplant recipients. *Clin Pharmacokinet* 2007; **46**(2): 175–185.

143 Hao C, Erzheng C, Anwei M *et al.* Validation of limited sampling strategy for the estimation of mycophenolic acid exposure in Chinese adult liver transplant recipients. *Liver Transpl* 2007; **13**(12): 1684–1693.

144 Hao C, Anwei M, Bing C *et al.* Monitoring mycophenolic acid pharmacokinetic parameters in liver transplant recipients: prediction of occurrence of leukopenia. *Liver Transpl* 2008; **14**(8): 1165–1173.

145 Brunet M, Cirera I, Martorell J *et al.* Sequential determination of pharmacokinetics and pharmacodynamics of mycophenolic acid in liver transplant patients treated with mycophenolate mofetil. *Transplantation* 2006; **81**(4): 541–546.

146 Rizell M, Andersson M, Cahlin C, Hafstrom L, Olausson M, Lindner P. Effects of the mTOR inhibitor sirolimus in patients with hepatocellular and cholangiocellular cancer. *Int J Clin Oncol* 2008; **13**(1): 66–70.

147 Zhou J, Fan J, Wang Z *et al.* Conversion to sirolimus immunosuppression in liver transplantation recipients with hepatocellular carcinoma: Report of an initial experience. *World J Gastroenterol* 2006; **12**(19): 3114–3118.

148 Kneteman NM, Oberholzer J, Al Saghier M *et al.* Sirolimus-based immunosuppression for liver transplantation in the presence of extended criteria for hepatocellular carcinoma. *Liver Transpl* 2004; **10**(10): 1301–1311.

149 Elsharkawi M, Staib L, Henne-Bruns D, Mayer J. Complete remission of posttransplant lung metastases from hepatocellular carcinoma under therapy with sirolimus and mycophenolate mofetil. *Transplantation* 2005; **79**(7): 855–857.

150 Neuhaus P, Klupp J, Langrehr JM. mTOR inhibitors: an overview. *Liver Transpl* 2001; **7**(6): 473–484.

151 Sehgal SN. Rapamune (RAPA, rapamycin, sirolimus): mechanism of action immunosuppressive effect results from blockade of signal transduction and inhibition of cell cycle progression. *Clin Biochem* 1998; **31**(5): 335–340.

152 Backman L, Reisaeter AV, Wramner L, Ericzon BG, Salmela K, Brattstrom C. Renal function in renal or liver transplant recipients after conversion from a calcineurin inhibitor to sirolimus. *Clin Transplant* 2006; **20**(3): 336–339.

153 Maheshwari A, Torbenson MS, Thuluvath PJ. Sirolimus monotherapy versus sirolimus in combination with steroids and/or MMF for immunosuppression after liver transplantation. *Dig Dis Sci* 2006; **51**(10): 1677–1684.

154 Nair S, Eason J, Loss G. Sirolimus monotherapy in nephrotoxicity due to calcineurin inhibitors in liver transplant recipients. *Liver Transpl* 2003; **9**(2): 126–129.

155 Murgia MG, Jordan S, Kahan BD. The side effect profile of sirolimus: a phase I study in quiescent cyclosporine-prednisone-treated renal transplant patients. *Kidney Int* 1996; **49**(1): 209–216.

156 Bererhi L, Flamant M, Martinez F, Karras A, Thervet E, Legendre C. Rapamycin-induced oligospermia. *Transplantation* 2003; **76**(5): 885–886.

157 Wyeth Ayerst Pharmaceuticals. Data File 2002.

158 Dunkelberg JC, Trotter JF, Wachs M *et al.* Sirolimus as primary immunosuppression in liver transplantation is not associated with hepatic artery or wound complications. *Liver Transpl* 2003; **9**(5): 463–468.

159 McAlister VC, Peltekian KM, Malatjalian DA *et al.* Orthotopic liver transplantation using low-dose tacrolimus and sirolimus. *Liver Transpl* 2001; **7**(8): 701–708.

160 Watson CJ, Friend PJ, Jamieson NV *et al.* Sirolimus: a potent new immunosuppressant for liver transplantation. *Transplantation* 1999; **67**(4): 505–509.

161 Zaghla H, Selby RR, Chan LS *et al.* A comparison of sirolimus vs calcineurin inhibitor-based immunosuppressive therapies in liver transplantation. *Aliment Pharmacol Ther* 2006; **23**(4): 513–520.

162 Trotter JF, Wachs M, Bak T *et al.* Liver transplantation using sirolimus and minimal corticosteroids (3-day taper). *Liver Transpl* 2001; **7**(4): 343–351.

163 Pridohl O, Heinemann K, Hartwig T *et al.* Low-dose immunosuppression with FK 506 and sirolimus after liver transplantation: 1-year results. *Transplant Proc* 2001; **33**(7–8): 3229–3231.

164 McAlister VC, Gao Z, Peltekian K, Domingues J, Mahalati K, MacDonald AS. Sirolimus-tacrolimus combination immunosuppression. *Lancet* 2000; **355**(9201): 376–377.

165 Pridohl O, Heinemann K, Hartwig T *et al.* Low-dose immunosuppression with FK 506 and sirolimus after liver transplantation: 1-year results. *Transplant Proc* 2001; **33**(7–8): 3229–3231.

166 Shenoy S, Hardinger KL, Crippin J *et al.* Sirolimus conversion in liver transplant recipients with renal dysfunction: a prospective, randomized, single-center trial. *Transplantation* 2007; **83**(10): 1389–1392.

167 Nashan B. Review of the proliferation inhibitor everolimus. *Expert Opin Investig Drugs* 2002; **11**(12): 1845–1857.

168 Nashan B. Early clinical experience with a novel rapamycin derivative. *Ther Drug Monit* 2002; **24**(1): 53–58.

169 Majewski M, Korecka M, Kossev P *et al.* The immunosuppressive macrolide RAD inhibits growth of human Epstein-Barr virus-transformed B lymphocytes *in vitro* and *in vivo*: a potential approach to prevention and treatment of posttransplant lymphoproliferative disorders. *Proc Natl Acad Sci USA* 2000; **97**(8): 4285–4290.

170 Levy G, Schmidli H, Punch J *et al.* Safety, tolerability, and efficacy of everolimus in *de novo* liver transplant recipients: 12 and 36-month results. *Liver Transpl* 2006; **12**(11): 1640–1648.

171 Fung JJ, Demetris AJ, Porter KA *et al.* Use of OKT3 with cyclosporin and steroids for reversal of acute kidney and liver allograft rejection. *Nephron* 1987; **46**(Suppl. 1): 19–33.

172 Farges O, Ericzon BG, Bresson-Hadni S *et al.* A randomized trial of OKT3-based versus cyclosporine-based immunoprophylaxis after liver transplantation. Long-term results of a European and Australian multicenter study. *Transplantation* 1994; **58**(8): 891–898.

173 Millis JM, McDiarmid SV, Hiatt JR *et al.* Randomized prospective trial of OKT3 for early prophylaxis of rejection after liver transplantation. *Transplantation* 1989; **47**(1): 82–88.

174 McDiarmid SV, Busuttil RW, Levy P, Millis MJ, Terasaki PI, Ament ME. The long-term outcome of OKT3 compared with

cyclosporine prophylaxis after liver transplantation. *Transplantation* 1991; **52**(1): 91–97.

175 Reding R, Feyaerts A, Vraux H *et al.* Prophylactic immunosuppression with anti-interleukin-2 receptor monoclonal antibody LO-Tact-1 versus OKT3 in liver allografting. A two-year follow-up study. *Transplantation* 1996; **61**(9): 1406–1409.

176 Kupiec-Weglinski JW, Diamantstein T, Tilney NL. Interleukin 2 receptor-targeted therapy–rationale and applications in organ transplantation. *Transplantation* 1988; **46**(6): 785–792.

177 Hirose R, Roberts JP, Quan D *et al.* Experience with daclizumab in liver transplantation: renal transplant dosing without calcineurin inhibitors is insufficient to prevent acute rejection in liver transplantation. *Transplantation* 2000; **69**(2): 307–311.

178 Boillot O, Mayer DA, Boudjema K *et al.* Corticosteroid-free immunosuppression with tacrolimus following induction with daclizumab: a large randomized clinical study. *Liver Transpl* 2005; **11**(1): 61–67.

179 Figueras J, Prieto M, Bernardos A *et al.* Daclizumab induction and maintenance steroid-free immunosuppression with mycophenolate mofetil and tacrolimus to prevent acute rejection of hepatic allografts. *Transpl Int* 2006; **19**(8): 641–648.

180 Yoshida EM, Marotta PJ, Greig PD *et al.* Evaluation of renal function in liver transplant recipients receiving daclizumab (Zenapax), mycophenolate mofetil, and a delayed, low-dose tacrolimus regimen vs. a standard-dose tacrolimus and mycophenolate mofetil regimen: a multicenter randomized clinical trial. *Liver Transpl* 2005; **11**(9): 1064–1072.

181 Sellers MT, McGuire BM, Haustein SV, Bynon JS, Hunt SL, Eckhoff DE. Two-dose daclizumab induction therapy in 209 liver transplants: a single-center analysis. *Transplantation* 2004; **78**(8): 1212–1217.

182 Calmus Y, Scheele JR, Gonzalez-Pinto I *et al.* Immunoprophylaxis with basiliximab, a chimeric anti-interleukin-2 receptor monoclonal antibody, in combination with azathioprine-containing triple therapy in liver transplant recipients. *Liver Transpl* 2002; **8**(2): 123–131.

183 Otto MG, Mayer AD, Clavien PA, Cavallari A, Gunawardena KA, Mueller EA. Randomized trial of cyclosporine microemulsion (neoral) versus conventional cyclosporine in liver transplantation: MILTON study. Multicentre International Study in Liver Transplantation of Neoral. *Transplantation* 1998; **66**(12): 1632–1640.

184 Gruttadauria S, Cintorino D, Piazza T, Mandala L, Doffria E, Musumeci A, *et al.* A safe immunosuppressive protocol in adult-to-adult living related liver transplantation. *Transplant Proc* 2006; **38**(4): 1106–1108.

185 Vigano J, Gruttadauria S, Mandala L *et al.* The role of basiliximab induction therapy in adult-to-adult living-related transplantation and deceased donor liver transplantation: a comparative retrospective analysis of a single-center series. *Transplant Proc* 2008; **40**(6): 1953–1955.

186 Neuhaus P, Clavien PA, Kittur D *et al.* Improved treatment response with basiliximab immunoprophylaxis after liver transplantation: results from a double-blind randomized placebo-controlled trial. *Liver Transpl* 2002; **8**(2): 132–142.

187 Petrovic LM, Villamil FG, Vierling JM, Makowka L, Geller SA. Comparison of histopathology in acute allograft rejection and recurrent hepatitis C infection after liver transplantation. *Liver Transpl Surg* 1997; **3**(4): 398–406.

188 Nelson DR, Soldevila-Pico C, Reed A *et al.* Anti-interleukin-2 receptor therapy in combination with mycophenolate mofetil is associated with more severe hepatitis C recurrence after liver transplantation. *Liver Transpl* 2001; **7**(12): 1064–1070.

189 Llado L, Xiol X, Figueras J *et al.* Immunosuppression without steroids in liver transplantation is safe and reduces infection and metabolic complications: results from a prospective multicenter randomized study. *J Hepatol* 2006; **44**(4): 710–716.

190 Pageaux GP, Calmus Y, Boillot O *et al.* Steroid withdrawal at day 14 after liver transplantation: a double-blind, placebo-controlled study. *Liver Transpl* 2004; **10**(12): 1454–1460.

191 Lin CC, Chuang FR, Lee CH *et al.* The renal-sparing efficacy of basiliximab in adult living donor liver transplantation. *Liver Transpl* 2005; **11**(10): 1258–1264.

192 Liu CL, Fan ST, Lo CM *et al.* Interleukin-2 receptor antibody (basiliximab) for immunosuppressive induction therapy after liver transplantation: a protocol with early elimination of steroids and reduction of tacrolimus dosage. *Liver Transpl* 2004; **10**(6): 728–733.

193 Wall WJ. Use of antilymphocyte induction therapy in liver transplantation. *Liver Transpl Surg* 1999; **5**(4 Suppl. 1): S64–S70.

194 Tector AJ, Fridell JA, Mangus RS *et al.* Promising early results with immunosuppression using rabbit anti-thymocyte globulin and steroids with delayed introduction of tacrolimus in adult liver transplant recipients. *Liver Transpl* 2004; **10**(3): 404–407.

195 Tchervenkov JI, Tzimas GN, Cantarovich M, Barkun JS, Metrakos P. The impact of thymoglobulin on renal function and calcineurin inhibitor initiation in recipients of orthotopic liver transplant: a retrospective analysis of 298 consecutive patients. *Transplant Proc* 2004; **36**(6): 1747–1752.

196 Eason JD, Loss GE, Blazek J, Nair S, Mason AL. Steroid-free liver transplantation using rabbit antithymocyte globulin induction: results of a prospective randomized trial. *Liver Transpl* 2001; **7**(8): 693–697.

197 Starzl TE, Murase N, bu-Elmagd K *et al.* Tolerogenic immunosuppression for organ transplantation. *Lancet* 2003; **361**(9368): 1502–1510.

198 Langrehr JM, Nussler NC, Neumann U *et al.* A prospective randomized trial comparing interleukin-2 receptor antibody versus antithymocyte globulin as part of a quadruple immunosuppressive induction therapy following orthotopic liver transplantation. *Transplantation* 1997; **63**(12): 1772–1781.

199 Eason JD, Nair S, Cohen AJ, Blazek JL, Loss GE, Jr. Steroid-free liver transplantation using rabbit antithymocyte globulin and early tacrolimus monotherapy. *Transplantation* 2003; **75**(8): 1396–1399.

200 Bajjoka I, Hsaiky L, Brown K, Abouljoud M. Preserving renal function in liver transplant recipients with rabbit anti-thymocyte globulin and delayed initiation of calcineurin inhibitors. *Liver Transpl* 2008; **14**(1): 66–72.

201 Soliman T, Hetz H, Burghuber C *et al.* Short-term induction therapy with anti-thymocyte globulin and delayed use of calcineurin inhibitors in orthotopic liver transplantation. *Liver Transpl* 2007; **13**(7): 1039–1044.

202 Soliman T, Hetz H, Burghuber C *et al.* Short-term versus long-term induction therapy with antithymocyte globulin in orthotopic liver transplantation. *Transpl Int* 2007; **20**(5): 447–452.

203 Tzakis AG, Tryphonopoulos P, Kato T *et al.* Preliminary experience with alemtuzumab (Campath-1H) and low-dose tacrolimus immunosuppression in adult liver transplantation. *Transplantation* 2004; **77**(8): 1209–1214.

204 Calne R. "Almost tolerance" in the clinic. *Transplant Proc* 1998; **30**(7): 3846–3848.

205 Alexander SI, Smith N, Hu M *et al.* Chimerism and tolerance in a recipient of a deceased-donor liver transplant. *N Engl J Med* 2008; **358**(4): 369–374.

206 Kawai T, Cosimi AB, Spitzer TR *et al.* HLA-mismatched renal transplantation without maintenance immunosuppression. *N Engl J Med* 2008; **358**(4): 353–361.

207 Scandling JD, Busque S, Dejbakhsh-Jones S *et al.* Tolerance and chimerism after renal and hematopoietic-cell transplantation. *N Engl J Med* 2008; **358**(4): 362–368.

208 Knechtle SJ, Pirsch JD, Fechner H *et al.* Campath-1H induction plus rapamycin monotherapy for renal transplantation: results of a pilot study. *Am J Transplant* 2003; **3**(6): 722–730.

209 Tzakis AG, Kato T, Nishida S *et al.* Alemtuzumab (Campath-1H) combined with tacrolimus in intestinal and multivisceral transplantation. *Transplantation* 2003; **75**(9): 1512–1517.

210 Tryphonopoulos P, Madariaga JR, Kato T *et al.* The impact of Campath 1H induction in adult liver allotransplantation. *Transplant Proc* 2005; **37**(2): 1203–1204.

211 Marcos A, Eghtesad B, Fung JJ *et al.* Use of alemtuzumab and tacrolimus monotherapy for cadaveric liver transplantation: with particular reference to hepatitis C virus. *Transplantation* 2004; **78**(7): 966–971.

212 Angulo P, Batts KP, Therneau TM, Jorgensen RA, Dickson ER, Lindor KD. Long-term ursodeoxycholic acid delays histological progression in primary biliary cirrhosis. *Hepatology* 1999; **29**(3): 644–647.

213 Lindor KD, Therneau TM, Jorgensen RA, Malinchoc M, Dickson ER. Effects of ursodeoxycholic acid on survival in patients with primary biliary cirrhosis. *Gastroenterology* 1996; **110**(5): 1515–1518.

214 Calmus Y, Gane P, Rouger P, Poupon R. Hepatic expression of class I and class II major histocompatibility complex molecules in primary biliary cirrhosis: effect of ursodeoxycholic acid. *Hepatology* 1990; **11**(1): 12–15.

215 Calmus Y, Arvieux C, Gane P *et al.* Cholestasis induces major histocompatibility complex class I expression in hepatocytes. *Gastroenterology* 1992; **102**(4 Pt 1): 1371–1377.

216 Sama C, Mazziotti A, Grigioni W *et al.* Ursodeoxycolic acid administration does not prevent rejection after OLT. *J Hepatol* 1991; **13**(Suppl. 2): 68.

217 Koneru B, Tint GS, Wilson DJ, Leevy CB, Salen F. Randomised prospective trial of ursodeoxycholic acid in liver trasplant recipients. *Hepatology* 1993; **18**: 336A.

218 Pageaux GP, Blanc P, Perrigault PF *et al.* Failure of ursodeoxycholic acid to prevent acute cellular rejection after liver transplantation. *J Hepatol* 1995; **23**(2): 119–122.

219 Keiding S, Hockerstedt K, Bjoro K *et al.* The Nordic multicenter double-blind randomized controlled trial of prophylactic ursodeoxycholic acid in liver transplant patients. *Transplantation* 1997; **63**(11): 1591–1594.

220 Barnes D, Talenti D, Cammell G *et al.* A randomized clinical trial of ursodeoxycholic acid as adjuvant treatment to prevent liver transplant rejection. *Hepatology* 1997; **26**(4): 853–857.

221 Fleckenstein JF, Paredes M, Thuluvath PJ. A prospective, randomized, double-blind trial evaluating the efficacy of ursodeoxycholic acid in prevention of liver transplant rejection. *Liver Transpl Surg* 1998; **4**(4): 276–279.

222 Angelico M, Tisone G, Baiocchi L *et al.* One-year pilot study on tauroursodeoxycholic acid as an adjuvant treatment after liver transplantation. *Ital J Gastroenterol Hepatol* 1999; **31**(6): 462–468.

223 Chen W, Gluud C. Bile acids for liver-transplanted patients. *Cochrane Database of Systematic Reviews* 2005, Issue 3. Art. No.: CD005442. DOI: 10.1002/14651858.CD005442.

224 Assy N, Adams PC, Myers P *et al.* Randomized controlled trial of total immunosuppression withdrawal in liver transplant recipients: role of ursodeoxycholic acid. *Transplantation* 2007; **83**(12): 1571–1576.

225 Foster PF, Kociss K, Shen J *et al.* Granulocyte colony-stimulating factor immunomodulation in the rat cardiac transplantation model. *Transplantation* 1996; **61**(7): 1122–1125.

226 Imagawa DK, Millis JM, Olthoff KM *et al.* The role of tumor necrosis factor in allograft rejection. I. Evidence that elevated levels of tumor necrosis factor-alpha predict rejection following orthotopic liver transplantation. *Transplantation* 1990; **50**(2): 219–225.

227 Winston DJ, Foster PF, Somberg KA *et al.* Randomized, placebo-controlled, double-blind, multicenter trial of efficacy and safety of granulocyte colony-stimulating factor in liver transplant recipients. *Transplantation* 1999; **68**(9): 1298–1304.

228 Williams JW, Mital D, Chong A *et al.* Experiences with leflunomide in solid organ transplantation. *Transplantation* 2002; **73**(3): 358–366.

229 Jin MB, Nakayama M, Ogata T *et al.* A novel leflunomide derivative, FK778, for immunosuppression after kidney transplantation in dogs. *Surgery* 2002; **132**(1): 72–79.

230 Pinschewer DD, Ochsenbein AF, Odermatt B, Brinkmann V, Hengartner H, Zinkernagel RM. FTY720 immunosuppression impairs effector T cell peripheral homing without affecting induction, expansion, and memory. *J Immunol* 2000; **164**(11): 5761–5770.

231 Changelian PS, Flanagan ME, Ball DJ *et al.* Prevention of organ allograft rejection by a specific Janus kinase 3 inhibitor. *Science* 2003; **302**(5646): 875–878.

232 Reding R. Steroid withdrawal in liver transplantation: benefits, risks, and unanswered questions. *Transplantation* 2000; **70**(3): 405–410.

233 Junge G, Neuhaus R, Schewior L *et al.* Withdrawal of steroids: a randomized prospective study of prednisone and tacrolimus versus mycophenolate mofetil and tacrolimus in liver transplant recipients with autoimmune hepatitis. *Transplant Proc* 2005; **37**(4): 1695–1696.

234 Moench C, Barreiros AP, Schuchmann M *et al.* Tacrolimus monotherapy without steroids after liver transplantation – a prospective randomized double-blinded placebo-controlled trial. *Am J Transplant* 2007; **7**(6): 1616–1623.

235 Filipponi F, Callea F, Salizzoni M *et al.* Double-blind comparison of hepatitis C histological recurrence Rate in HCV+ Liver transplant recipients given basiliximab + steroids or basiliximab + placebo, in addition to cyclosporine and azathioprine. *Transplantation* 2004; **78**(10): 1488–1495.

236 Mogl MT, Neumann U, Langrehr JM, Neuhaus P. A prospective randomized trial comparing steroid-free immunosuppression

induction with tacrolimus and MMF versus tacrolimus and steroids in patients with HCV (Abstract). *Am J Transplant* 2004; **4**: 364.

237 Kato T, Yoshida H, Sadfar K *et al.* Steroid-free induction and preemptive antiviral therapy for liver transplant recipients with hepatitis C: a preliminary report from a prospective randomized study. *Transplant Proc* 2005; **37**(2): 1217–1219.

238 Margarit C, Bilbao I, Castells L *et al.* A prospective randomized trial comparing tacrolimus and steroids with tacrolimus monotherapy in liver transplantation: the impact on recurrence of hepatitis C. *Transpl Int* 2005; **18**(12): 1336–1345.

239 Studenik P, Mejzlik V, Stouracova M, Ondrasek J, Cerny J. Steroid free tacrolimus and mychophenolate mofetil based immunosuppression in liver transplant (Abstract). *Liver Transpl* 2005; **11**: C42.

240 Varo E, Otero A, Ortiz de UJ, Martin-Vivaldi R, Cuervas-Mons V, Gonzalez-Pinto I. Steroid-free regimen versus standrad treatment in liver transplant recipients (Abstract). *Transpl Int* 2008; **18**: 116.

241 Jensen A.C., Maxwell PR. Six-year follow-up of steroid elimination 24 hours after liver transplantation using daclizumab, tacrolimus and mycophenolate mofetil (Abstract). *Am J Transplant* 2006; **6**: 210.

242 Pelletier SJ, Vanderwall K, Debroy MA *et al.* Preliminary analysis of early outcomes of a prospective, randomized trial of complete steroid avoidance in liver transplantation. *Transplant Proc* 2005; **37**(2): 1214–1216.

243 Nair S, Loss GE, Cohen AJ, Eason JD. Induction with rabbit antithymocyte globulin versus induction with corticosteroids in liver transplantation: impact on recurrent hepatitis C virus infection. *Transplantation* 2006; **81**(4): 620–622.

244 Fasola C, Klintmalm GB. Hepaptitis C recurrence after liver transplantation: in search of the optimal immunosuppression to improve outcome. *Current Opinion in Organ Transplantation* 2006; **11**: 637–642.

245 Samonakis DN, Mela M, Quaglia A *et al.* Rejection rates in a randomised trial of tacrolimus monotherapy versus triple therapy in liver transplant recipients with hepatitis C virus cirrhosis. *Transpl Infect Dis* 2006; **8**(1): 3–12.

246 Gras JM, Gerkens S, Beguin C *et al.* Steroid-free, tacrolimus-basiliximab immunosuppression in pediatric liver transplantation: clinical and pharmacoeconomic study in 50 children. *Liver Transpl* 2008; **14**(4): 469–477.

247 Lerut J, Mathys J, Verbaandert C *et al.* Tacrolimus monotherapy in liver transplantation: one-year results of a prospective, randomized, double-blind, placebo-controlled study. *Ann Surg* 2008; **248**(6): 956–967.

248 Segev DL, Sozio SM, Shin EJ *et al.* Steroid avoidance in liver transplantation: meta-analysis and meta-regression of randomized trials. *Liver Transpl* 2008; **14**(4): 512–525.

249 Girlanda R, Rela M, Williams R, O'Grady JG, Heaton ND. Long-term outcome of immunosuppression withdrawal after liver transplantation. *Transplant Proc* 2005; **37**(4): 1708–1709.

250 Takatsuki M, Uemoto S, Inomata Y *et al.* Weaning of immunosuppression in living donor liver transplant recipients. *Transplantation* 2001; **72**(3): 449–454.

251 Oike F, Yokoi A, Nishimura E *et al.* Complete withdrawal of immunosuppression in living donor liver transplantation. *Transplant Proc* 2002; **34**(5): 1521.

252 Eason JD, Cohen AJ, Nair S, Alcantera T, Loss GE. Tolerance: is it worth the risk? *Transplantation* 2005; **79**(9): 1157–1159.

253 Pons JA, Yelamos J, Ramirez P *et al.* Endothelial cell chimerism does not influence allograft tolerance in liver transplant patients after withdrawal of immunosuppression. *Transplantation* 2003; **75**(7): 1045–1047.

254 Tryphonopoulos P, Tzakis AG, Weppler D *et al.* The role of donor bone marrow infusions in withdrawal of immunosuppression in adult liver allotransplantation. *Am J Transplant* 2005; **5**(3): 608–613.

255 Rolles K, Burroughs AK, Davidson BR, Karatapanis S, Prentice HG, Hamon MD. Donor-specific bone marrow infusion after orthotopic liver transplantation. *Lancet* 1994; **343**(8892): 263–265.

256 Tisone G, Orlando G, Cardillo A *et al.* Complete weaning off immunosuppression in HCV liver transplant recipients is feasible and favourably impacts on the progression of disease recurrence. *J Hepatol* 2006; **44**(4): 702–709.

257 Berenguer M, Lopez-Labrador FX, Wright TL. Hepatitis C and liver transplantation. *J Hepatol* 2001; **35**(5): 666–678.

258 Gane E. The natural history and outcome of liver transplantation in hepatitis C virus-infected recipients. *Liver Transpl* 2003; **9**(11): S28–S34.

259 Forman LM, Lewis JD, Berlin JA, Feldman HI, Lucey MR. The association between hepatitis C infection and survival after orthotopic liver transplantation. *Gastroenterology* 2002; **122**(4): 889–896.

260 Feray C, Gigou M, Samuel D *et al.* The course of hepatitis C virus infection after liver transplantation. *Hepatology* 1994; **20**(5): 1137–1143.

261 Kalambokis G, Manousou P, Samonakis D *et al.* Clinical outcome of HCV-related graft cirrhosis and prognostic value of hepatic venous pressure gradient. *Transpl Int* 2009; **22**: 172–181.

262 Teixeira R, Menezes EG, Schiano TD. Therapeutic management of recurrent hepatitis C after liver transplantation. *Liver Int* 2007; **27**(3): 302–312.

263 Gedaly R, Clifford TM, McHugh PP, Jeon H, Johnston TD, Ranjan D. Prevalent immunosuppressive strategies in liver transplantation for hepatitis C: results of a multi-center international survey. *Transpl Int* 2008; **21**(9): 867–872.

264 Berenguer M, Lopez-Labrador FX, Greenberg HB, Wright TL. Hepatitis C virus and the host: An imbalance induced by immunosuppression? *Hepatology* 2000; **32**(2): 433–435.

265 Neumann UP, Berg T, Bahra M *et al.* Fibrosis progression after liver transplantation in patients with recurrent hepatitis C. *J Hepatol* 2004; **41**(5): 830–836.

266 Berenguer M, Aguilera V, Prieto M *et al.* Significant improvement in the outcome of HCV-infected transplant recipients by avoiding rapid steroid tapering and potent induction immunosuppression. *J Hepatol* 2006; **44**(4): 717–722.

267 Henry SD, Metselaar HJ, Van DJ, Tilanus HW, Van Der Laan LJ. Impact of steroids on hepatitis C virus replication in vivo and in vitro. *Ann N Y Acad Sci* 2007; **1110**: 439–447.

268 Samonakis DN, Triantos CK, Thalheimer U *et al.* Immunosuppression and donor age with respect to severity of HCV recurrence after liver transplantation. *Liver Transpl* 2005; **11**(4): 386–395.

269 Vivarelli M, Burra P, La Barba G et al. Influence of steroids on HCV recurrence after liver transplantation: A prospective study. *J Hepatol* 2007; **47**(6): 793–798.

270 Manousou P, Samonakis D, Cholongitas E et al. Outcome od recurrent HCV after liver transplantation in a randomized trial of tacrolimus monotherapy versus triple therapy. *Liver Transpl* 2009; **15**(12): 1783–1791.

271 Klintmalm GB, Washburn WK, Rudich SM et al. Corticosteroid-free immunosuppression with daclizumab in HCV(+) liver transplant recipients: 1-year interim results of the HCV-3 study. *Liver Transpl* 2007; **13**(11): 1521–1531.

272 Kato T, Gaynor JJ, Yoshida H et al. Randomized trial of steroid-free induction versus corticosteroid maintenance among ortho-topic liver transplant recipients with hepatitis C virus: impact on hepatic fibrosis progression at one year. *Transplantation* 2007; **84**(7): 829–835.

273 Berenguer M, Royuela A, Zamora J. Immunosuppression with calcineurin inhibitors with respect to the outcome of HCV recurrence after liver transplantation: results of a meta-analysis. *Liver Transpl* 2007; **13**(1): 21–29.

274 Hilgard P, Kahraman A, Lehmann N et al. Cyclosporine versus tacrolimus in patients with HCV infection after liver transplantation: effects on virus replication and recurrent hepatitis. *World J Gastroenterol* 2006; **12**(5): 697–702.

275 Watashi K, Hijikata M, Hosaka M, Yamaji M, Shimotohno K. Cyclosporin A suppresses replication of hepatitis C virus genome in cultured hepatocytes. *Hepatology* 2003; **38**(5): 1282–1288.

276 Nakagawa M, Sakamoto N, Enomoto N et al. Specific inhibition of hepatitis C virus replication by cyclosporin A. *Biochem Biophys Res Commun* 2004; **313**(1): 42–47.

277 Firpi RJ, Zhu H, Morelli G et al. Cyclosporine suppresses hepatitis C virus in vitro and increases the chance of a sustained virological response after liver transplantation. *Liver Transpl* 2006; **12**(1): 51–57.

278 Goto K, Watashi K, Murata T, Hishiki T, Hijikata M, Shimotohno K. Evaluation of the anti-hepatitis C virus effects of cyclophilin inhibitors, cyclosporin A, and NIM811. *Biochem Biophys Res Commun* 2006; **343**(3): 879–884.

279 Henry SD, Metselaar HJ, Lonsdale RC et al. Mycophenolic acid inhibits hepatitis C virus replication and acts in synergy with cyclosporin A and interferon-alpha. *Gastroenterology* 2006; **131**(5): 1452–1462.

280 Ishii N, Watashi K, Hishiki T et al. Diverse effects of cyclosporine on hepatitis C virus strain replication. *J Virol* 2006; **80**(9): 4510–4520.

281 Paeshuyse J, Kaul A, De Clercq E et al. The non-immunosuppressive cyclosporin DEBIO-025 is a potent inhibitor of hepatitis C virus replication in vitro. *Hepatology* 2006; **43**(4): 761–770.

282 Kakumu S, Takayanagi M, Iwata K et al. Cyclosporine therapy affects aminotransferase activity but not hepatitis C virus RNA levels in chronic hepatitis C. *J Gastroenterol Hepatol* 1997; **12**(1): 62–66.

283 Watashi K, Metselaar HJ, Van Der Laan LJ. Interfering with interferon: re-igniting the debate on calcineurin inhibitor choice and antiviral therapy for hepatitis C virus recurrence. *Liver Transpl* 2008; **14**(3): 265–267.

284 Berenguer M, Prieto M, San JF et al. Contribution of donor age to the recent decrease in patient survival among HCV-infected liver transplant recipients. *Hepatology* 2002; **36**(1): 202–210.

285 Villamil F, Levy G, Grazi GL et al. Long-term outcomes in liver transplant patients with hepatic C infection receiving tacrolimus or cyclosporine. *Transplant Proc* 2006; **38**(9): 2964–2967.

286 Baiocchi L, Angelico M, Petrolati A et al. Correlation between liver fibrosis and inflammation in patients transplanted for HCV liver disease. *Am J Transplant* 2008; **8**(3): 673–678.

287 Inoue K, Sekiyama K, Yamada M, Watanabe T, Yasuda H, Yoshiba M. Combined interferon alpha2b and cyclosporin A in the treatment of chronic hepatitis C: controlled trial. *J Gastroenterol* 2003; **38**(6): 567–572.

288 Kornberg A, Kupper B, Wilberg J et al. Conversion to mycophe-nolate mofetil for modulating recurrent hepatitis C in liver transplant recipients. *Transpl Infect Dis* 2007; **9**(4): 295–301.

289 Neyts J, Meerbach A, McKenna P, De CE. Use of the yellow fever virus vaccine strain 17D for the study of strategies for the treatment of yellow fever virus infections. *Antiviral Res* 1996; **30**(2–3): 125–132.

290 Nelson JA, Carpenter JW, Rose LM, Adamson DJ. Mechanisms of action of 6-thioguanine, 6-mercaptopurine, and 8-azagua-nine. *Cancer Res* 1975; **35**(10): 2872–2878.

291 Firpi RJ, Nelson DR, Davis GL. Lack of antiviral effect of a short course of mycophenolate mofetil in patients with chronic hepa-titis C virus infection. *Liver Transpl* 2003; **9**(1): 57–61.

292 Stangl JR, Carroll KL, Illichmann M, Striker R. Effect of antime-tabolite immunosuppressants on Flaviviridae, including hepa-titis C virus. *Transplantation* 2004; **77**(4): 562–567.

293 Singh N, Gayowski T, Ndimbie OK, Nedjar S, Wagener MM, Yu VL. Recurrent hepatitis C virus hepatitis in liver transplant recipients receiving tacrolimus: association with rejection and increased immunosuppression after transplantation. *Surgery* 1996; **119**(4): 452–456.

294 Hunt J, Gordon FD, Lewis WD et al. Histological recurrence and progression of hepatitis C after orthotopic liver transplantation: influence of immunosuppressive regimens. *Liver Transpl* 2001; **7**(12): 1056–1063.

295 Berenguer M, Crippin J, Gish R et al. A model to predict severe HCV-related disease following liver transplantation. *Hepatology* 2003; **38**(1): 34–41.

296 Bahra M, Neumann UI, Jacob D et al. MMF and calcineurin taper in recurrent hepatitis C after liver transplantation: impact on histological course. *Am J Transplant* 2005; **5**(2): 406–411.

297 Belli LS, Burroughs AK, Burra P et al. Liver transplantation for HCV cirrhosis: improved survival in recent years and increased severity of recurrent disease in female recipients: results of a long term retrospective study. *Liver Transpl* 2007; **13**(5): 733–740.

298 Eid AJ, Brown RA, Paya CV, Razonable RR. Association between toll-like receptor polymorphisms and the outcome of liver transplantation for chronic hepatitis C virus. *Transplantation* 2007; **84**(4): 511–516.

299 Walter T, Dumortier J, Guillaud O et al. Rejection under alpha interferon therapy in liver transplant recipients. *Am J Transplant* 2007; **7**(1): 177–184.

300 Gonzalez MG, Madrazo CP, Rodriguez AB et al. An open, ran-domized, multicenter clinical trial of oral tacrolimus in liver

allograft transplantation: a comparison of dual vs. triple drug therapy. *Liver Transpl* 2005; **11**(5): 515–524.

301 Zekry A, Gleeson M, Guney S, McCaughan GW. A prospective cross-over study comparing the effect of mycophenolate versus azathioprine on allograft function and viral load in liver transplant recipients with recurrent chronic HCV infection. *Liver Transpl* 2004; **10**(1): 52–57.

302 Kornberg A, Kupper B, Tannapfel A, Hommann M, Scheele J. Impact of mycophenolate mofetil versus azathioprine on early recurrence of hepatitis C after liver transplantation. *Int Immunopharmacol* 2005; **5**(1): 107–115.

303 Papatheodoridis GV, Davies S, Dhillon AP *et al.* The role of different immunosuppression in the long-term histological outcome of HCV reinfection after liver transplantation for HCV cirrhosis. *Transplantation* 2001; **72**(3): 412–418.

304 McCaughan GW, Zekry A. Impact of immunosuppression on immunopathogenesis of liver damage in hepatitis C virus-infected recipients following liver transplantation. *Liver Transpl* 2003; **9**(11): S21–S27.

305 McCaughan GW, Zekry A. Mechanisms of HCV reinfection and allograft damage after liver transplantation. *J Hepatol* 2004; **40**(3): 368–374.

306 Berenguer M, Aguilera V, Prieto M *et al.* Effect of calcineurin inhibitors on survival and histologic disease severity in HCV-infected liver transplant recipients. *Liver Transpl* 2006; **12**(5): 762–767.

307 De Ruvo N, Cucchetti A, Lauro A *et al.* Preliminary results of a "prope" tolerogenic regimen with thymoglobulin pretreatment and hepatitis C virus recurrence in liver transplantation. *Transplantation* 2005; **80**(1): 8–12.

308 Kamar N, Borde JS, Sandres-Saune K *et al.* Induction therapy with either anti-CD25 monoclonal antibodies or rabbit anti-thymocyte globulins in liver transplantation for hepatitis C. *Clin Transplant* 2005; **19**(1): 83–89.

309 Ramirez CB, Doria C, di Francesco F, Iaria M, Kang Y, Marino IR. Basiliximab induction in adult liver transplant recipients with 93% rejection-free patient and graft survival at 24 months. *Transplant Proc* 2006; **38**(10): 3633–3635.

310 Lake JR. The role of immunosuppression in recurrence of hepatitis C. *Liver Transpl* 2003; **9**(11): S63–S66.

311 O'Keeffe C, Baird AW, Nolan N, McCormick PA. Mast cell hyperplasia in chronic rejection after liver transplantation. *Liver Transpl* 2002; **8**(1): 50–57.

312 Demetris AJ, Murase N, Lee RG *et al.* Chronic rejection. A general overview of histopathology and pathophysiology with emphasis on liver, heart and intestinal allografts. *Ann Transplant* 1997; **2**(2): 27–44.

313 Lowes JR, Hubscher SG, Neuberger JM. Chronic rejection of the liver allograft. *Gastroenterol Clin North Am* 1993; **22**(2): 401–420.

314 Kemnitz J, Gubernatis G, Bunzendahl H, Ringe B, Pichlmayr R, Georgii A. Criteria for the histopathological classification of liver allograft rejection and their clinical relevance. *Transplant Proc* 1989; **21**(1 Pt 2): 2208–2210.

315 Blakolmer K, Seaberg EC, Batts K *et al.* Analysis of the reversibility of chronic liver allograft rejection implications for a staging schema. *Am J Surg Pathol* 1999; **23**(11): 1328–1339.

316 Theruvath TP, Neumann UP, Langrehr JM *et al.* Risk factors for chronic rejection after liver transplantation. *Liver transpl* 2003; **9**(6): C4 [abstract].

317 Quaglia AF, Del Vecchio BG, Greaves R, Burroughs AK, Dhillon AP. Development of ductopaenic liver allograft rejection includes a "hepatitic" phase prior to duct loss. *J Hepatol* 2000; **33**(5): 773–780.

318 Demetris AJ, Seaberg EC, Batts KP *et al.* Reliability and predictive value of the National Institute of Diabetes and Digestive and Kidney Diseases Liver Transplantation Database nomenclature and grading system for cellular rejection of liver allografts. *Hepatology* 1995; **21**(2): 408–416.

319 Sher LS, Cosenza CA, Michel J *et al.* Efficacy of tacrolimus as rescue therapy for chronic rejection in orthotopic liver transplantation: a report of the U.S. Multicenter Liver Study Group. *Transplantation* 1997; **64**(2): 258–263.

320 Gregory CR, Huang X, Pratt RE *et al.* Treatment with rapamycin and mycophenolic acid reduces arterial intimal thickening produced by mechanical injury and allows endothelial replacement. *Transplantation* 1995; **59**(5): 655–661.

321 Neff GW, Montalbano M, Slapak-Green G *et al.* A retrospective review of sirolimus (Rapamune) therapy in orthotopic liver transplant recipients diagnosed with chronic rejection. *Liver Transpl* 2003; **9**(5): 477–483.

322 van Hoek B, Wiesner RH, Ludwig J, Gores GJ, Moore B, Krom RA. Combination immunosuppression with azathioprine reduces the incidence of ductopenic rejection and vanishing bile duct syndrome after liver transplantation. *Transplant Proc* 1991; **23**(1 Pt 2): 1403–1405.

43 Liver transplantation: Prevention and treatment of infection

Antoni Rimola and Miquel Navasa

Liver Unit, Institut de Malalties Digestives i Metaboliques, Hospital Clinic, IDIBAPS, CIBEREHD, Barcelona, Spain

Early studies reported that 50–80% of patients developed infection after liver transplantation and that this complication was a major cause of death, especially during the first postoperative year, with a rate of infection-related mortality of around 20% [1–6]. Little information is available on the incidence of infection after liver transplantation in more recent years. However, due to progressively implemented preventive strategies against infection, especially opportunistic infections, it is likely that infectious complications have become less frequent. As an example, in our institution the incidence of infection decreased from 83% in the period 1988–1990 to 42% in the period 2001–2003 [7]. This, coupled with the improvement in the diagnosis of infection, has reduced the mortality secondary to infection, as shown in several recent prospective clinical trials on the efficacy and safety of different immunosuppressive regimens in which the short and mid-term infection-related mortality was less than 10% [8–10]. Nonetheless, infection remains a common and relevant complication in liver transplantation, requiring appropriate prophylactic and therapeutic measures, as summarized in this chapter. Since the rationale for these measures not only arises from the particular characteristics of each infection but also from the risk factors for and the time of occurrence of the different types of infection, these two aspects are also addressed in this chapter. As the spectrum of infection and its prevention and treatment have experienced important changes over time, this chapter is mainly focused on current practice.

Risk factors for infection

All liver transplant recipients have two risk factors for infection: the major abdominal surgical procedure of trans-

plantation and the administration of immunosuppressive treatment. In most cases powerful immunosuppression is administered during the early postoperative period, the phase with the greatest risk of rejection. Subsequently, immunosuppression is gradually reduced until the end of the first or second postoperative year, when immunosuppression is stabilized at a low grade of immune suppression. Other circumstances common in liver transplant recipients are also risk factors for infection by increasing the so-called "net state of immunosuppression" [11]. The most relevant of these circumstances are listed in Table 43.1. Apart from these general risk factors, there are also specific risk factors for the different types of infection, which will be addressed in the sections dealing with these infections.

Time of infection occurrence

Classically, three different periods have been defined according to the predominant types of infection in each period: the first postoperative month, from month two to month six, and beyond six months (see Figure 43.1) [11–15].

During the first postoperative month, the most frequent infectious complications are bacteremia, pneumonia and surgical site infection, predominantly caused by nosocomial bacteria and recipient colonizing bacteria. Fungal infections are also relatively common. Despite the high grade of immunosuppression during this period, opportunistic infections are infrequent, with the exception of herpes simplex, probably because immunosuppression requires some time to promote the clinical expression of most opportunistic infections. Infections derived from the graft donor, although potentially serious, are also uncommon [16].

Characteristically, opportunistic infections and reactivated latent infections emerge during the intermediate period, from months two to six. Classical pathogens in this

Evidence-Based Gastroenterology and Hepatology, 3rd edition.
J. McDonald, A.K. Burroughs, B. Feagan, and M.B. Fennerty. © 2010
Blackwell Publishing Ltd

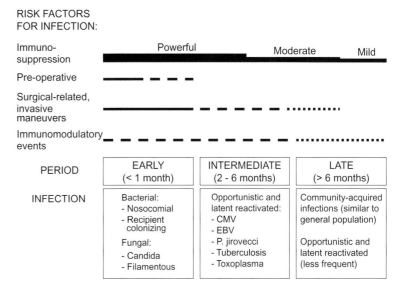

RISK FACTORS
FOR INFECTION:

Figure 43.1 Occurrence of the most frequent infections in liver transplant recipients according to time after transplantation and to the main risk factors for infection. Continuous or broken lines indicate the relative importance (strong or less intense, respectively) of the different risk factors in each period.

Table 43.1 Circumstances affecting the net state of immunosuppression in liver transplant recipients (adapted from reference 11).

Pharmacological immunosuppression

Invasive manoeuvres compromising muco-cutaneous barrier integrity:
Intravenous lines
Tracheal intubation
Reoperation
Bladder catheterization

Underlying immunomodulatory conditions (pre- and/or post-operative):
Very advanced liver disease
Metabolic:
Renal failure
Diabetes mellitus
Malnutrition
Multiple organ failure

Viral infection:
Cytomegalovirus
Epstein-Barr virus
Hepatitis C virus

period include cytomegalovirus (CMV) and other herpes group viruses, *Pneumocystis jirovecii* (formerly, *P. carinii*), other fungi (variable according to fungal geographical distribution), and protozoa (mainly *Toxoplasma* and *Leishmania*). Infections caused by mycobacteria, *Listeria* spp. and *Nocardia* spp. can also be observed. Although beyond the scope of this chapter, recurrence of hepatitis C virus should also be mentioned because this complication represents a major problem in liver transplantation.

Beyond month six post-transplantation, and coincidentally with a progressive reduction of immunosuppression

and little requirement of re-hospitalization, the risk of infection drastically decreases, becoming similar to that in the general population. During this late period, most infections are community acquired, although opportunistic infections can also occur.

This spectrum of infection occurrence can be altered due to a variety of reasons, with important overlap between the periods. For example, biliary and graft vascular problems can persist beyond the early postoperative period, with the subsequently prolonged risk of infection related to these surgical complications. The need to maintain long-term immunosuppression due to late-onset or persisting rejection is associated with an increased risk of opportunistic infections and latent infection reactivation throughout the time under potent pharmacological immunosuppression. Finally, the persistence or *de novo* appearance of immunomodulatory events, such as chronic renal failure or severe recurrence of pre-transplant liver disease (particularly, hepatitis C), can modify the risk of infection during the intermediate and late post-transplant periods.

Bacterial infection

Incidence and special risk factors

Bacterial infections are the most frequent infectious complications in liver transplant recipients and predominantly occur during the early postoperative period. The commonest bacterial infections in this period are surgical site infection, bacteremia and pneumonia. In most studies, the development of bacteremia and pneumonia has been associated with increased risk of mortality [17–22]. Surgical site infection, although not greatly influencing survival, increases hospital resource utilization and cost [23, 24]. In recent reports, the mean incidence of surgical site infection, involving the incision wound and intra-abdominal organ-space infections (namely, localized or diffuse peritonitis, cholangitis, infected biloma and hepatic abscess), is approximately 25%, ranging from 5% to 40% [23–33]. Bacteremia has also been reported with variable frequency, between 9% and 36% [19, 28–30, 33–36]. In a recent prospective, multicenter study involving 16 Spanish centers and including 1012 liver transplantations followed up to two years, the incidence of the bloodstream infections (caused by bacteria in 96% of the cases) was 10% [22]. In this study, most bloodstream infection episodes were catheter-related (30%), secondary to surgical site infection (24%) and, to a lesser extent, to pneumonia (6%), whereas the primary source of bacteremia was not identified in 34% of cases. Similar sources of bacteremia have been found by other authors [18, 36, 37]. A 7–28% incidence of pulmonary infections has been reported in recent series [17, 19, 21, 28–30, 33, 35, 38–42]. Other types of infection, such as urinary tract or central nervous system infections, are much less frequently observed [13].

Aside from the general risk factors for infection previously mentioned, other factors specifically favor bacterial infection in liver transplant recipients. Prolonged surgery or reoperation, increased perioperative transfusion, living donor liver transplantation and biliary anastomosis with choledochojejunostomy predispose to surgical site infections [25, 26, 43, 44]. Specific risk factors for bacterial pneumonia are prolonged mechanical ventilation, persistent non-infectious pulmonary alterations and living donor transplantation [19–20, 39]. Rejection and prolonged hospital stay are risk factors for bacterial infections in general [35, 37, 40, 45]. In children, low weight and low age have been associated with increased risk of bacterial infection

[30]. The type and intensity of pharmacological immunosuppression does not clearly influence the risk of bacterial infection, although mTOR inhibitors (sirolimus and everolimus; also called proliferation signal inhibitors, PSIs) may favor surgical-site infections by impairing wound healing [46].

In later post-transplant periods, bacterial infections are much less frequent and are mainly limited to community-acquired infections, especially pneumonia and urinary tract infections [16, 47–49], and to infections related to persisting biliary and arterial complications [32, 33, 50, 51]. Liver transplant patients are slightly more susceptible to some intracellular bacteria, such as *Listeria* spp., *Legionella* spp., and *Nocardia* spp. [47, 52]. The negative impact of late bacterial complications on the survival of liver transplant patients is low or very modest [53–58].

Causative organisms

Organisms causing bacterial infections in liver transplant patients during the early postoperative period correspond to environmental bacteria (transmitted from contaminated persons or equipment) and recipient endogenous bacteria [2, 3, 12, 13, 15, 17, 19–22, 24–28, 34, 36, 45, 59–61], summarized in Table 43.2.

Occasionally, other pathogens, such as *Legionella* spp., can transiently acquire special relevance [62–64]. Anaerobes are a rare cause of infection in liver transplant patients [35, 29, 30, 61], although *Clostridium difficile* colitis has been reported as being relatively prevalent in some centers [2, 43]. A substantial proportion of surgical-site and, to a lesser extent, pulmonary infections are polymicrobial. In pneumonia, the isolation of different organisms can correspond to either true polymicrobial infections or subsequent super-

Table 43.2 The commonest microorganisms responsible for major bacterial infections in the early postoperative period following liver transplantation. Only data from recent studies (published from 2000 onwards) are included [17, 19–22, 24–26, 28, 34, 36, 59–61].

Surgical-site infections		Bacteremia		Pulmonary infections	
General type	**Most frequent[a]**	**General type**	**Most frequent[a]**	**General type**	**Most frequent**
Gram+ cocci: 40–56%	*Enterococcus* spp. *Staph. aureus* CN staphylococcus	Gram+ cocci: 32–75%	CN staphylococcus *Enterococcus* spp. *Staph. aureus*	Gram+ cocci: 0–42%	*Staph. aureus* *Streptococcus* spp.
Aerobic Gram– bacilli: 44–53%	*E. coli* *Klebsiella* spp. *Pseudomonas* spp.	Aerobic Gram– bacilli: 25–59%	*E. coli* *Klebsiella* spp *Pseudomonas* spp.	Aerobic Gram– bacilli: 48–100%	*Pseudomonas* spp. *Klebsiella* spp. *S. maltophilia*
Polymicrobial: 17–48%		Polymicrobial: 4%		Polymicrobial: 10%	
				Unidentified: 30%	

[a]In some institutions, *Acinetobacter baumanii* is also very prevalent.
CN: coagulase-negative.

infections by pathogens resistant to the current antibiotic therapy [17, 20]. As expected, causative organisms in pneumonia cannot be identified in a significant percentage of cases because the microbiological diagnosis frequently requires bronchoscopy with bronchoalveolar lavage, which is not always performed before starting antibiotic therapy [20, 38, 40, 62].

In late periods of liver transplantation, the most frequent bacterial complications are community-acquired pneumonia, mainly caused by *Streptococcus. pneumoniae*, *Haemophilus influenza* and *Mycoplasma*, and urinary tract infections, mainly caused by Gram-negative bacilli [47, 13, 35, 49]. Other late bacterial infections are cholangitis related to persistent biliary complications, mainly caused by enterobacteria and *Pseudomonas* spp. [33], and hepatic abscess secondary to vascular complications, caused by a variety of organisms including Gram-positive cocci, Gram-negative bacilli and anaerobes [51]. Liver transplant patients can also develop tuberculosis. However, since this complication has special characteristics, its prevention and treatment will be addressed separately at the end of this section.

Multi-drug resistant bacteria

A world-wide problem during the last decades has been the progressive emergence of bacteria resistant to multiple antibiotics. The most relevant multi-resistant bacteria in liver transplant patients are shown in Table 43.3 [19, 22, 24, 26, 29, 33, 59, 60, 65–67].

Methicillin-resistant *Staphylococcus aureus* (MRSA) is a frequent cause of early postoperative infection following liver transplantation. Nasal carriage of MRSA (acquired pre- or postoperatively) is associated with an increased risk of MRSA infection [68–72]. MRSA strains are usually susceptible to the glycopeptide antibiotics vancomycin and teicoplanin.

The prevalence of vancomycin-resistant enterococci (VRE) follows a variable geographical distribution, being high in most centers from the USA [65, 71, 73], and low in most European countries [29, 74, 75]. Bowel colonization, acquired pre- or post-transplant, is the major source of VRE infection [71, 76]. Linezolid and daptomycin are active against most VRE [77, 78].

Among the enteric Gram-negative bacilli, *Escherichia coli* and *Klebsiella pneumoniae* are the organisms most commonly producing extended-spectrum beta-lactamase (ESBL), although other enterobacteriaceae strains can also express ESBL [79]. In general, ESBL-producing enterobacteria are susceptible to carbapenems (imipenem, meropenem and ertapenem) [80, 81].

Pseudomonas spp. are the most relevant multi-resistant non-fermentative Gram-negative bacilli in liver transplant patients. Other multi-resistant members of this family with increasing importance for liver transplant patients are *Acinetobacter baumanii* and *Stenotrophomonas maltophilia*. Tigecycline is habitually active against *A. baumanii* and *S. maltophilia* [82]. *S. maltophilia* is also highly susceptible to cotrimoxazole [83].

Several authors have found a direct association between mortality and VRE colonization and infection by some multi-resistant organisms [22, 65, 71, 76].

Prevention

In theory, infection can be prevented by strategies reducing risk factors for infection and those reducing the infective capacity of potentially pathogenic organisms. However, risk factors for infection are either not susceptible to improvement (i.e. the severity of pre-transplant liver disease) or have experienced little change over the last years. Only two surgical and anesthetic approaches should be mentioned. One is the attempt to decrease the operative hemorrhage, an important risk factor for early bacterial complications, by the use of temporary portocaval shunting [84], the reduction of both central venous pressure and plasma transfusion [85], or the administration of aprotinin [86]. The other is the immediate tracheal extubation after

Table 43.3 Multi-resistant bacteria in liver transplant patients with bacterial infections.

Bacteria	Mechanisms of multi-resistance	Percentage of multi-resistant organisms (average and range)	References
Staphylococcus aureus	Methicillin resistance	67% (16–100%)	19, 22, 26, 33, 60, 65, 66
Enterococcus spp.	Vancomycin resistance	10% (0–50%)	26, 29, 33, 60, 65, 67
Enteric Gram-negative bacilli	ESBL production[a]	27% (9–60%)	22, 24, 33, 60, 65, 67
Nonfermentative Gram-negative bacilli	Multiple mechanisms[b]	15% (10–47%)	22, 65

[a] ESBL (extended-spectrum beta-lactamase) producing organisms resistant to penicillins, cephalosporins and aztreonam.
[b] *Pseudomonas* spp. (the most representative organisms of this group) resistant to at least three of the following antibiotics: beta-lactams, carbapenems, aminoglycosides, or quinolones. Other relevant pathogens are *Acinetobacter baumanii* and *Stenotrophomonas maltophilia*.

surgery ("fast track" policy) to reduce the risk for pneumonia [87]. Nevertheless, the impact of these strategies on the incidence of bacterial infection is uncertain. At present, therefore, prevention of bacterial complications in liver transplant patients is almost exclusively based on interventions on the microbial flora.

Peri-operative antibiotic prophylaxis

Although controlled studies on this topic are lacking (namely, prophylaxis versus no prophylaxis), peri-operative antibiotic prophylaxis is the standard practice to prevent surgical-site infections as well as other bacterial infections during the very early post-operative period. However, due to the marked differences from one center to another regarding the predominant causative organisms, no specific prophylaxis can be universally recommended. Furthermore, the paucity of prospective, comparative studies on different antibiotic regimens adds important difficulties. The only exception is a study comparing cefazolin and amoxicillin-clavulanate, in which no difference in the rate of surgical-site infection was observed between the two regimes [24]. Unfortunately, these two antibiotic regimes were suboptimal because around 40% of isolated organisms were resistant to the administered agents. **A1d** Thus, only general rules for peri-operative antibacterial prophylaxis can be made.

The appropriate antibiotic agents must be selected according to the local microbial epidemiology and the susceptibility of the most prevalent organisms at each center [88]. The most currently used antibiotics are third and fourth generation cephalosporins, frequently administered in association with other agents, especially those active against *Enterococcus* spp., such as ampicillin or amoxicillin (with or without clavulanate) [20, 25, 33, 65, 70, 75, 89, 90]. Other antibiotic combinations involve quinolones, antipseudomonal penicillins, or aztreonam [25]. One dilemma is the prophylactic use of antibiotics active against multiresistant bacteria, because it seems judicious to reserve these often last-line antimicrobial agents for treatment [91]. In this setting, only the prophylactic administration of vancomycin or teicoplanin could be reasonable in centers with a high prevalence of MRSA [70, 91–93]. In contrast, the prophylactic administration of antibiotics active against VRE, such as linezolid, or ESBL-producing enterobacteria, such as carbepenems, is uncommon even at institutions with a high prevalence of these microorganisms.

Peri-operative antibiotic prophylaxis is routinely initiated immediately prior to transplantation and prolonged throughout the operation, although in some centers prophylaxis is extended to the first postoperative 24 hours or longer [33, 65, 70, 88, 89, 93].

Although the risk of donor-derived bacterial infection is low and the impact on patient and graft survival is usually negligible, the antibiotic prophylaxis in the recipient is usually adapted to the organisms responsible for the donor infection and its duration prolonged for five to ten days [17, 94–96].

Selective bowel decontamination and administration of probiotics and prebiotics

Since a high proportion of early infections are caused by bacteria of intestinal origin, selective decontamination of the digestive tract with nonabsorbable antibiotics has been used in different centers. However, few randomized, prospective, controlled trials have properly assessed the efficacy of this strategy [97–101]. Decontaminating regimens in these studies included gentamicin or tobramycin, polymyxin or colistin, and amphotericin or nystatin, administered orally for a variable period of time. In one study an oral paste with antimicrobial agents was also administered [100]. A reduction of infections caused by Gram-negative bacilli was attained in most treated groups, although the global rate of early bacterial infection was not significantly different, as emphasized in a recent meta-analysis [102]. **A1a** Survival was not influenced by the use of selective digestive decontamination. Therefore, the potential benefit of this type of prophylaxis is uncertain and it cannot be routinely recommended [45]. **A1a**

In two randomized trials, a marked reduction was achieved in the incidence of early infection caused by enteric bacteria with the prophylactic administration of a combination of living lactic acid bacteria (probiotics) and bioactive fibers (prebiotics), but clinical outcomes were not significantly different [103, 104]. **A1d**

Prophylactic measures for multi-drug resistant bacteria

General measures include hand hygiene and barrier precautions, which are applicable for all these organisms [45, 105, 106]. Based on the association of nasal carriage of MRSA with infection by this organism [68–72], periodical pre- and post-operative screening for MRSA and nares decolonization with mupirocin application have been proposed in liver transplant candidates and recipients [69–71, 107]. Unfortunately, one study showed that this policy was not effective as it did not prevent postoperative MRSA infection and was followed by a frequent recurrence of nasal MRSA colonization [108]. **B4** Since other sites of colonization may be important, skin cleansing with chlorhexidine has also been postulated for a better control of MRSA [109, 110], as well as for VRE [111], but no study has evaluated these measures in liver transplant patients.

Antibiotic prophylaxis for invasive procedures

The diagnosis and treatment of biliary complications, especially stenosis, frequently require endoscopic cholangiography. Bactobilia, that is, the bacterial colonization of bile, has been found with a very high incidence in liver transplant patients with biliary stenosis, stents or previous papillotomy [112]. **B4** On the other hand, in a large series of patients undergoing ERCP, the only factor predisposing to cholangitis was liver transplantation [113]. Based on these data, antibiotic prophylaxis for ERCP is recommended in liver transplant patients [114]. Piperacillin-tazobactam and impenem provide adequate coverage [112]. Although, to the knowledge of the authors of this chapter, there are no studies on the risk of cholangitis in patients undergoing percutaneous cholangiography, it seems advisable to follow the same recommendation as for ERCP.

In one study, liver biopsy was associated with sepsis when this procedure was performed in liver transplant patients with choledochojejunostomy [115]. For the authors of this study, antibiotic prophylaxis at the time of liver biopsy may be appropriate in this high-risk subgroup of patients, but biliary obstruction was not categorically excluded at the time of biopsy.

For surgical re-intervention very early after transplantation, the same peri-operative antibiotic prophylaxis as for liver transplantation appears adequate. For surgical interventions in later periods, the general guidelines for non-transplant patients undergoing surgery [116] seem sufficient, although the type of antibiotics to be administered should be adapted to the liver transplant patient condition (i.e. grade of immunosuppression) and local microbial epidemiology. **B4**

Treatment

Antibiotic treatment should be started whenever a liver transplant patient develops either signs strongly suggesting infection (mainly significant fever), signs of sepsis or a well documented localized infection. Nevertheless, it is important to note that not all febrile episodes in liver transplant recipients correspond to infection [18]. When the need for treatment is defined, and after blood and other relevant site cultures are taken, antibiotic therapy is empirically initiated, without knowledge of the causative organisms and their *in vitro* susceptibility. Empirical therapy should be selected on the basis of different factors, particularly the site of the suspected infection and the local predominant pathogens and their susceptibility patterns. Other important factors are the time since transplantation, recent antibiotic administration, and the colonization status of the patient, if known. At each institution, protocols for empirical treatment of bacterial complications should be periodically revised and adapted to the changes in epidemiology and *in vitro* susceptibility of predominant organisms.

According to the commonest pathogens during the early period after transplantation (see Table 43.2), the most frequently used agents in the empiric therapy are third and fourth-generation cephalosporins, piperacilli-tazo-

bactam and quinolones [13, 117–119]. The administration of glycopeptides (vancomycin or teicoplanin) and carbapenems (imipenem, meropenem or ertapenem) can be justified in patients with sepsis and hospitalized in centers with a high incidence of MRSA and ESLB-producing Gram-negative bacilli, respectively [66, 118]. Once the responsible bacteria are identified and susceptibility tests are available, further adjustments may be required, consisting of either the withdrawal of superfluous antibiotics or the adequate antimicrobial changes if resistant organisms are isolated. Information on the adequacy of the initial empirical treatment is scarce in liver transplant patients with bacterial infection, although some authors have reported around 20% of failure [20, 61, 117]. However, the effectiveness of the initial empiric therapy does not seem to influence the final outcome provided the antibiotic therapy is rapidly modified according to the microbiological results, as also described in non-transplant populations [120–122]. **B4**

In later periods after transplantation, community-acquired pnemonia and urinary tract infection, the commonest bacterial infections in this postoperative phase [16, 47–49], are treated according to standard protocols in each center for immunosuppressed patients. Specific antibiotic therapy is administered for infections caused by infrequent but characteristic organisms, such as *Listeria* spp. and *Nocardia* spp. [47, 52].

Special considerations

Surgical or percutaneous drainage is often required for the treatment of infections arising in devitalized anatomic sites, such as infected abdominal cavity collections or hepatic abscess [32, 36, 51]. Treatment of cholangitis secondary to biliary stenosis must include the endoscopic, radiological or surgical resolution of the stenosis [50]. The removal of IV lines is mandatory in catheter-related bacteremia [66].

Antibiotic treatment of pneumonia, especially in early stages following liver transplantation and in patients with mechanical ventilation, can be difficult because the responsible organisms are not identified in approximately 50% of episodes [20, 38]. Polymicrobial pneumonia, caused by more than one bacteria or bacteria combined with non-bacterial microbes, such as fungi, cytomegalovirus or *P. jirovecii* may represent an added difficulty for treatment [17, 20]. Although the empiric treatment of pneumonia attains a positive response in a relatively high proportion of patients, in patients who impair regardless of this therapy, invasive diagnostic procedures, such as fiberoptic bronchoscopy with bronchoalvelar lavage or lung biopsy, must be performed [20, 38, 62]. **B4** In spite of an aggressive diagnostic approach, the etiology of pneumonia can only be established on necropsy basis in some patients.

Since most liver transplant patients receive calcineurin inhibitors (tacrolimus or cyclosporine) as immunosuppressive drugs, the potential capacity of different antibiotics to increase the risk of toxicity of calcineurin inhibitors must be taken into consideration [14]. Aminoglycosides can increase the risk of nephrotoxicity, and they should be avoided if possible [123]. Since imipenem may enhance the risk of seizures, particularly in patients with renal function or neurological impairment [124], the administration of other carbapenems (meropenem or ertapenem) may be more appropriate in patients treated with calcineurin inhibitors. Pharmacokinetic interactions of several antibiotics with calcineurin inhibitors metabolized by the hepatic cytochrome P-450 have been described [125, 126]. Rifampicin and nafcillin induce the metabolism of calcineurin inhibitors, with risk of rejection due to low levels of these immunosuppressants, whereas macrolides reduce their metabolism, with the consequent increased risk of toxicity. In patients who necessarily have to receive these antibiotics, a careful monitoring of blood levels of calcineurin inhibitors is mandatory. Since proliferation signal inhibitors (PSIs, also named mTOR inhibitors: sirolimus and everolimus) are also metabolized by the cytochrome P-450 [127, 128], it is likely that similar drug interactions can also occur.

Tuberculosis

The incidence of tuberculosis in liver transplant recipients is around 1–2% in developed countries and 10–15% in endemic regions, which is much higher than that in the general population in the respective countries [129]. Reactivation of latent tuberculosis is considered the main mechanism for active tuberculosis in transplant recipients, which predominantly occurs within the first postoperative year [130, 131]. Approximately half of the patients have pulmonary disease, whereas the other half present with extrapulmonary or disseminated tuberculosis [130, 131]. Aggressive investigations are often required for the diagnosis, and, in some patients, the definitive diagnosis can only be established after a positive response to empiric treatment.

Prevention

In patients receiving kidney transplantation, and, by extension, in patients with extra-renal transplantation, there is the general recommendation to administer antituberculous chemoprophylaxis with isoniazid for the first 9–12 postoperative months in transplant recipients with a past history of tuberculosis and/or pre-operative positive tuberculin test [88, 132–134]. **B4** However, regardless of the excellent efficacy of this strategy [130], prophylaxis with isoniazid in liver transplant patients with a positive tuberculin test is challenging for two reasons. First, a positive skin test without other additional risk factors is rarely associated

with latent infection reactivation [88]. As an example, in a study by our group, none of 73 patients with a pre-transplant positive tuberculin test developed post-transplant tuberculosis regardless of not receiving isoniazid prophylaxis [135]. In contrast, in the same study, tuberculosis was diagnosed in 2% of 279 patients with a negative tuberculin test; the incidence was especially high (10%) in patients with a past history of tuberculosis and untreated with isoniazid prophylaxis, thus suggesting that anergic patients with possible latent tuberculosis were very prone to develop latent infection reactivation. Second, an important concern for generalized isoniazid prophylaxis in liver transplant recipients with a pre-transplant tuberculin skin positive test is the high incidence of isoniazid hepatotoxicity, ranging from 17% to 41%, which can outweigh the possible benefit of this strategy [130, 135]. For these reasons, although there are no controlled studies on this issue, the general feeling is to limit isoniazid prophylaxis to patients with a history or chest X-ray evidence of past tuberculosis, particularly if it has been inadequately treated, or to patients with a positive skin test and additional risk factors (recent tuberculin conversion, non-Caucasian ethnicity or regional endemicity, and excessive immunosuppression) [88, 134]. **B4** In the remaining cases, surveillance and treatment of active tuberculosis, if it develops, seem sufficient. Alternative prophylactic regimes, particularly the combination of a quinolone and ethambutol, can be administered in the case of previous isoniazid administration forming part of inadequate antituberculous therapies or in the case of liver graft alterations precluding isoniazid treatment or making it hazardous. Another possibility is to administer prophylaxis while patients are on the waiting list for liver transplantation, although this strategy has been rarely explored [136].

Treatment

The most recommended standard treatment for active tuberculosis in the general population is the combination of rifampicin, isoniazid, pyrazinamid and ethambutol for two months, followed by an additional four-month therapy with rifampicin and isoniazid [137, 138]. In transplant recipients, the length of treatment is extended up to 12 months in pulmonary disease and up to 18 months in extrapulmonary disease [139–143]. **B4** However, this therapeutic regime cannot be accomplished in a substantial proportion of patients due to hepatotoxicity, with an average incidence of around 30–40% [131, 130, 141, 144]. In patients with hepatoxicity or significant liver graft alterations, the most hepatotoxic combination of rifampicin with isoniazid and/or pyrazinamide is usually withdrawn or avoided, and non-hepatotoxic or less hepatotoxic regimes, including ethambutol, quinolones, and rifabutin combined with isoniazid or pyrazinamide, are administered with satisfactory results [140, 142, 145].

Viral infections

Cytomegalovirus

Cytomegalovirus (CMV) belongs to the human herpesvirus family and is a significant opportunistic pathogen in liver transplantation. Infection by CMV is defined as the isolation of CMV or the detection of viral proteins or nuclear acids in whatever fluid or tissue of the organism [146, 147].

The clinical spectrum of CMV infection is very wide, from an asymptomatic infection to a lethal disease [147, 148]. Infection with CMV is classified as asymptomatic or symptomatic. An asymptomatic infection is defined by the detection of either the antigen pp65 of CMV in the leucocytes or the DNA of CMV in plasma, blood or leucocytes by PCR, without symptoms of the infection and without affecting organs [143, 149]. Symptomatic infection or CMV disease may manifest as a febrile viremic illness often associated with leukopenia and thrombocytopenia (CMV syndrome) or as an organ-specific disease, such as colitis, hepatitis and pneumonia. In case of organ involvement, the diagnosis can be established by histopathologic or cytological changes suggestive of CMV disease, particularly intranuclear inclusions and positive immunohistochemistry. In most cases, CMV disease occurs at weeks four to six after transplantation.

Risk factors

CMV infection can be primarily acquired from the graft or from transfused blood products in patients lacking pre-existent CMV-specific immunity or can result from reactivation of latent virus or superinfection with a new strain [146, 150–152]. The risk of developing CMV infection and disease after liver transplantation is related to the donor and recipient CMV serostatus. Seronegative recipients of grafts from seropositive donors (D+/R−) are at the highest risk, with an incidence of infection of up to 80% and an incidence of disease of up to 60% in the absence of anti-CMV prophylaxis [151]. Seronegative patients who receive an organ from a seronegative donor (D−/R−) are considered at the lowest risk, although CMV infection can still develop from blood products, particularly if they receive unscreened pool of platelets [150]. Seropositive recipients have an intermediate risk, with an incidence of CMV disease of approximately 20% when the donor is also seropositive (D+/R+) and 10% when the donor is seronegative (D−/R+) [151]. Re-transplantation, antilymphocytic antibodies, and high levels of immunosuppressants are also risk factors for CMV infection.

Prophylaxis

Prophylaxis of CMV infection is the administration of anti-CMV treatment prior to the detection of active CMV replication, usually for the first three post-operative months. There are two strategies of prophylaxis: universal prophylaxis, when it is administered to all transplant recipients, and targeted prophylaxis, when it is only administered to high-risk patients [153]. Oral valganciclovir is the most commonly used antiviral agent for prophylaxis of CMV in liver transplant patients. A number of reports have documented the efficacy of this strategy [153–159], with CMV disease development in only 15–30% of the D+/R− patients who received valganciclovir prophylaxis [160, 161]. **B4** The other potential benefit is the reduction of the indirect effects of CMV infection, including graft loss, fungal infection and even bacterial infection [160–163]. Potential risks are cost, toxicity, CMV resistance to ganciclovir, and the possible development of late onset CMV disease [164]. These risks have questioned universal prophylaxis and even targeted prophylaxis in favour of pre-emptive therapy. Prolonged prophylaxis beyond the month three and CMV infection monitoring after prophylaxis cessation have been proposed [162].

Preemptive therapy

Preemptive therapy is the administration of anti-CMV treatment after the detection of active CMV infection but prior to the development of symptomatic disease. With this strategy, transplant recipients are carefully monitored for early evidence of viral replication by using CMV antigenemia assay or PCR for detection of viral DNA, followed by preemptive therapy at the first positive result. Some authors use a specific quantitative threshold value as an indicator for the initiation of antiviral medication in seropositive transplant recipients, but begin treatment in high risk recipients whenever any level of CMV antigenemia or viral DNA becomes detectable [159]. Valganciclovir is also the drug of choice for preemptive therapy. Recent studies have shown its efficacy in D+/R−, pointing again to the advantages of preemptive therapy over targeted prophylaxis [161, 162, 164]. **B4** However, more studies are needed to validate these findings.

Therapy

The recommended treatment of a proven or suspected CMV infection is the IV administration of ganciclovir, an inhibitor of the CMV DNA polymerase [165]. In mild to moderate CMV disease, the duration of treatment is usually 14–21 days, although the best strategy is to stop the therapy when two weekly negative CMV tests (antigenemia or PCR) are achieved [151]. In many cases, oral valganciclovir can be used to complete the treatment after an initial period of IV administration of ganciclovir and when clinical symptoms have resolved. In a recent trial, oral valganciclovir has been as effective as IV ganciclovir in the treatment of non-severe CMV disease [166]. **A1d** The duration of the treatment in compartmentalized disease, that is, organ involvement with minimally detectable or undetectable viremia, is more challenging. The most important adverse effect of ganciclovir and valganciclovir is bone marrow suppression. In case of severe bone marrow toxicity or ganciclovir resistance (very rare in liver transplant recipients), foscarnet is the best alternative treatment. Nephrotoxicity is the most important adverse effect of foscarnet [165].

Epstein-Barr (EBV) virus

In liver transplantation, EBV infection is usually primary in children, whereas reactivation is the predominant mechanism for infection in adults [167]. Symtomatic EBV infection mainly consists of fever, leukopenia, lympho-monocytosis or thrombocytopenia, although approximately the half of patients present with atypical symptoms and signs [146]. However, the most important consequence of EBV infection in solid organ transplant recipients is its association with the development of post-transplantation lymphoproliferative disease.

Post-transplantation lymphoproliferative disease

The association between EBV and post-transplant lymphoproliferative disease (PTLD) has been recognized since the early days of transplantation, although not all cases can be attributed to EBV [168–171]. The major pathogenic mechanism for PTLD is the insufficient EBV-specific cytotoxic T-cell control on EBV-driven B-cell proliferation [171]. PTLD, a systemic process involving both nodal and extra-nodal tissues, ranges from an infectious mononucleosis-like reactive plasmacytic hyperplasia to a lymphoma [172]. The incidence of PTLD in liver transplant recipients is around 2%, although children are particularly exposed, with an incidence approximately three times as high [173]. Poly- and monoclonal anti-lymphocyte antibodies and maintenance immunosuppression with azathioprine are major risk factors for PTLD, although doses of maintenance azathioprine used in liver transplantation are lower than in other solid organ transplants [174]. High EBV load may also be a risk factor, and this has led some authors to postulate that preemptive antiviral therapy and reduction of immunosuppression on the basis of viral load monitoring could be indicated to prevent EBV-associated PTLD [174, 175]. However, the efficacy of such a prophylaxis strategy is uncertain. Treatment of PTLD includes reduction of immunosuppression if possible, chemotherapy and anti-B-cell antibodies (rituximab) when PTLD has evolved to lymphoma, and surgical resection and radiotherapy in patients with tumor masses. Administration of interferon, immune globulin and anti-EBV treatment with acyclovir or ganciclovir are other potential therapies, although their efficacy is unproven [143, 174].

Other herpesvirus

Herpes simplex virus

Herpes simplex virus (HSV) infection, commonly caused by reactivation of a latent infection, predominantly involves mucosal surfaces [13]. Disseminated forms are rare. Treatment and prophylaxis is based on the administration of acyclovir or valacyclovir.

Varicella zoster virus

Localized cutaneous zoster, secondary to a reactivation of latent varicella zoster virus infection, occurs with an incidence of approximately 5–10% in solid-organ transplant recipients [143]. Primary infection, although very rare in adults, can be more aggressive with severe organ involvement. Acyclovir and valacyclovir are the most used agents for treatment of varicella zoster virus infection [143].

Human herpesvirus 6 and 7

After the primary infection, human herpesvirus (HHV) type 6 and type 7 remain latent in the host and can reactivate after transplantation and cause varied clinical manifestations, such as fever, cutaneous rash, pneumonitis, encephalitis, hepatitis and myelosuppression [176]. Although the incidence of HHV 6 and 7 infection is low [177], the interest for these pathogens or copathogens in transplant recipients is increasing due to the possibility of indirect effects: association with CMV disease, increased risk of opportunistic infections, and graft dysfunction and rejection [171, 176, 178]. Antiviral agents active against CMV are also active against HHV-6.

Human herpesvirus 8

Human herpesvirus 8 (HHV-8) causes Kaposi's sarcoma, as well as primary effusion lymphoma (PEL) and many cases of multicentric Castleman disease (MCD) [179, 180]. Other co-factors, mainly immunosuppression, are also necessary. Current treatment options of Kaposi's sarcoma are limited to reduction in immunosuppression and chemotherapy [146]. Although an important reduction in HHV-8 replication by valganciclovir has been recently reported in non-transplanted patients [181], antiviral medication in combination with chemotherapy has been rarely investigated in the setting of organ transplantation [180, 182]. Interestingly, the conversion to PSI immunosuppressive drugs has been followed by regression of Kaposi's sarcoma in kidney transplant patients [183, 184]. **B4** Therefore, PSIs provide a potential treatment option in the management of post-transplant Kaposi's sarcoma.

Fungal infections

Systemic fungal infections are a significant cause of morbidity and mortality in solid organ transplant recipients.

Table 43.4 Specific risk factors for fungal infections (in addition to the general factors for infection shown in Table 43.1).

Pre-transplant period:
 Steroid therapy
 Hemodyalisis, hemofiltration
 Fungal colonization (*Aspergillus*)
 Re-transplantation

Intra-operative period:
 Prolonged and difficult surgical intervention
 Important blood product transfusion
 Combined liver-kidney transplantation

Early post-operative period (<30 days):
 Hemodialysis, hemofiltration

In all periods:
 Broad-spectrum antibacterial therapy
 Prolonged stay at the intensive care unit
 Prolonged mechanical ventilation
 Parenteral nutrition

The incidence of fungal infections after liver transplantation has been reported in the range of 7–42%, with *Candida* spp. and *Aspergillus* spp. as the most common pathogens [185, 186]. Other fungi (i.e. *Cryptococcus neoformans* or spp.) are much less frequently detected. Mortality rate has been reported as high as 92–100% for invasive aspergillosis and 70% for invasive candidiasis. The incidence of invasive fungal infection (but, unfortunately, not its related mortality) has decreased over time in most transplant centers due to the improvement in surgical technique and postoperative care, the use of low-dose steroid or even steroid-free immunosuppressive regimes, and the identification of risk factors for invasive fungal infection which has led to antifungal preemptive therapy [185–187]. Table 43.4 shows the specific risk factors for fungal infection, which should be taken into consideration to indicate antifungal prophylaxis [185–189].

Antifungal prophylaxis

Both universal and preemptive strategies have been attempted in the prevention of fungal infection. Nystatin was initially used to prevent *Candida* mucositis, and fluconazole or other azole agents are routinely administered in most centers. Furthermore, targeted or preemptive antifungal prophylaxis has been increasingly used once risk factors for fungal infection became known. A recent meta-analysis of six studies on antifungal prophylaxis (study drugs: fluconazole, itraconazole and liposomal amphotericin B, alone or in combination, for five days to ten weeks) showed a beneficial effect of such a prophylaxis on morbidity and mortality attributable to fungal infections [188]. Compared to controls, patients who received prophylaxis had fewer fungal infection episodes, due to a decrease in both invasive and superficial infections (69% and 73% relative risk reduction respectively). Fungal infection-related mortality also experienced a 72% relative risk reduction in the prophylaxis groups. In contrast, antifungal prophylaxis did not affect the need of empiric treatment for suspected fungal infections, the incidence of invasive *Aspergillus* infection and overall mortality. Patients receiving prophylaxis showed an increased proportion of episodes of non-*albicans* *Candida*, mainly *Candida glabrata*. Overall, the conclusion of this meta-analysis is that the benefits of universal antifungal prophylaxis are evident but limited and should be balanced with the disadvantages, particularly the selection of azole-resistant *Candida* spp.

In a recent study, liposomal amphotericin B versus fluconazole prophylaxis targeted to high-risk liver transplant subjects (two or more risk factors) attained similar rates of invasive fungal infection [189]. However, the incidence of invasive fungal infection in both arms was lower than that previously reported in untreated high-risk patients. The two antifungal prophylactic regimes were well tolerated. Another recent, prospective, multicenter, noncomparative, open-label trial, evaluating the prophylactic use of caspofungin in adult liver transplant recipients at high risk for invasive fungal infection [190], showed that only 2 out of 71 patients developed mucor and *Candida albicans* surgical infections, and this occurred 41 and 19 days after the end of prophylaxis, thus indicating that caspofungin was higly effective. Caspofungin was well tolerated in general, but it was associated with drug-related altered liver function requiring therapy discontinuation in 8% of patients.

Universal prevention against *Pneumocystis jirovecci* is followed at most centers, with excellent results since infection by this fungus has been virtually eradicated [45, 143]. In liver transplantation, the administration of low-dose cotrimoxazole for the first six to nine postoperative months is the first-option prophylaxis. Beyond this period, prophylaxis could be indicated in patients receiving powerful immunosuppression. Cotrimoxazole prophylaxis is also effective against *Toxoplasma gondii*, a protozoa which can also cause infection in liver transplant recipients [45]. In patients in whom cotrimoxazole cannot be given or is discontinued early due to toxicity, aerosolized pentamidine or oral dapsone are adequate alternatives.

Treatment of invasive fungal infections

Invasive fungal infection is associated with a poor outcome, especially when the infection is diagnosed late. Therefore, early diagnosis and treatment are highly recommended. Microbiological, histological, radiological and molecular tests are necessary for the diagnosis [191, 192]. Antifungal treatment can be empirically initiated in patients with signs of infection not responding to adequate antibacterial treatment, provided appropriate tests to detect fungal infection are performed, but results are not available yet [192].

Invasive *Candida* spp. infection is treated with fluconazole or itraconazole, unless the patient was receiving azole prophylaxis or azole-resistant non- *Candida albicans* is isolated (i.e. *Candida glabrata*). In these cases, amphotericin B or caspofungin are the recommended drugs [193]. Invasive aspergillosis is usually treated with amphotericin B, voriconazole or caspofungin, alone or in combination, mainly according to the severity of the infection and the response to the initial therapy [192, 194]. However, the management of invasive aspergillosis is a challenging issue. Reduction in immunosuppression, if possible, is also recommended.

Acknowledgment

CIBEREHD is funded by the Instituto de Salud Carlos III, Ministerio de Ciencia e Innovación, Spain.

References

1 Cuervas-Mons V, Julio Martinez A, Dekker A *et al.* Adult liver transplantation: an analysis of the early causes of death in 40 consecutive cases. *Hepatology* 1986; **6**: 495–501.

2 Kusne S, Dummer JS, Singh N *et al.* Infections after liver transplantation: an analysis of 101 consecutive cases. *Medicine* (Baltimore) 1986; **67**: 132–143.

3 Paya CV, Hermans PE, Washington JA 2nd *et al.* Incidence, distribution, and outcome of episodes of infection in 100 orthotopic liver transplantations. *Mayo Clin Proc* 1989; **64**: 555–564.

4 Barkholt L, Ericzon BG, Tollemar J *et al.* Infections in human liver recipients: different patterns early and late after transplantation. *Transpl Int* 1993; **6**: 77–84.

5 Singh N, Gayowski T, Wagener M *et al.* Infectious complications in liver transplant recipients on tacrolimus. Prospective analysis of 88 consecutive liver transplants. *Transplantation* 1994; **58**: 774–778.

6 Hadley S, Samore MH, Lewis WD *et al.* Major infectious complications after orthotopic liver transplantation and comparison of outcomes in patients receiving cyclosporine or FK506 as primary immunosuppression. *Transplantation* 1995; **59**: 851–859.

7 Amador A, Charco R, Martí J *et al.* One thousand liver transplants: the Hospital Clinic experience. *Transplant Proc* 2005; **37**: 3916–3918.

8 Wiesner R, Rabkin J, Klintmalm G *et al.* A randomized double-blind comparative study of mycophenolate mofetil and azathioprine in combination with cyclosporine and corticosteroids in primary liver transplant recipients. *Liver Transpl* 2001; **7**: 442–450.

9 Neuhaus P, Clavien PA, Kittur D *et al.* Improved treatment response with basiliximab immunoprophylaxis after liver trans-

10 Neuberger JM, Mamelok RD, Neuhaus P *et al.* Delayed introduction of reduced-dose tacrolimus, and renal function in liver transplantation: the ReSpECT study. *Am J Transplant* 2009; **9**: 327–336.

11 Fishman JA, Rubin RH. Infection in organ-transplant recipients. *N Engl J Med* 1998; **338**: 1741–1751.

12 Kwak EJ, Kusne S. Risk and epidemiology of infections after liver transplantation. In: Bowden RA, Ljungman P, Paya CV (eds) *Transplant Infections*, 2nd edn. Lippincott, Williams & Wilkins. Philadelphia, 2003: 120–131.

13 Holt CD, Winston DJ. Infections after liver transplantation. In: Busuttil RW, Klintmalm GK (eds) *Transplantation of the Liver*, 2nd edn. Elsevier Saunders, Philadelphia, 2005: 963–994.

14 Marty FM, Rubin RH. The prevention of infection post-transplant: the role of prophylaxis, preemptive and empiric therapy. *Transpl Int* 2006; **19**: 2–11.

15 Fishman JA. Infection in solid-organ transplant recipients. *N Engl J Med* 2007; **357**: 2601–2614.

16 Angelis M, Cooper JT, Freeman RB. Impact of donor infections on outcome of orthotopic liver transplantation. *Liver Transpl* 2003; **9**: 451–462.

17 Xia D, Yan LN, Xu L *et al.* Postoperative severe pneumonia in adult liver transplant recipients. *Transplant Proc* 2006; **38**: 2974–2978.

18 Singh N, Paterson DL, Gayowski T *et al.* Predicting bacteremia and bacteremic mortality in liver transplant recipients. *Liver Transpl* 2000; **6**: 54–61.

19 Saner FH, Damink SWO, Pavlakovic G *et al.* Pulmonary and blood stream infections in adult living donor and cadaveric liver transplant patients. *Transplantation* 2008; **85**: 1564–1568.

20 Torres A, Ewig S, Insausti J *et al.* Etiology and microbial patterns of pulmonary infiltrates in patients with orthotopic liver transplantation. *Chest* 2000; **117**: 494–502.

21 Aduen JF, Hellinger WC, Kramer DJ *et al.* Spectrum of pneumonia in the current era of liver transplantation and its effect on survival. *Mayo Clin Proc* 2005; **80**: 1303–1306.

22 Moreno A, Cervera C, Gavaldá J *et al.* Bloodstream infections among transplant recipients: results of a nationwide surveillance in Spain. *Am J Transplant* 2007; **7**: 2579–2586.

23 Hollenbeak CS, Alfrey EJ, Souba WW. The effect of surgical site infections on outcomes and resource utilization after liver transplantation. *Surgery* 2001; **130**: 388–395.

24 García-Prado ME, Cordero-Matía E, Pareja-Ciuro F *et al.* Surgical site infection in liver transplant recipients: impact of the type of perioperative prophylaxis. *Transplantation* 2008; **85**: 1849–1854.

25 Asensio A, Ramos A, Cuervas-Mons V *et al.* Effect of antibiotic prophylaxis on the risk of surgical site infection in orthotopic liver transplant. *Liver Transpl* 2008; **14**: 799–805.

26 Iinuma Y, Senda K, Fujihara N *et al.* Surgical site infection in living-donor liver transplant recipients: a prospective study. *Transplantation* 2004; **78**: 704–709.

27 Arnow PM, Zachary KC, Thistlethwaite JR *et al.* Pathogenesis of early operative site infections after orthotopic liver transplantation. *Transplantation* 1998; **65**: 1500–1503.

28 Garbino J, Romand JA, Pittet D *et al.* Infection and rejection in liver transplant patients: a 10-year Swiss single-centre experience. *Swiss Med Wkly* 2005; **135**: 587–593.

29 Losada I, Cuervas-Mons V, Millán I *et al.* Early infection in liver transplant recipients: incidence, severity, risk factors and antibiotic sensitivity of bacterial isolates. *Enferm Infecc Microbiol Clin* 2002; **20**, 422–430.

30 Bouchut JC, Stamm D, Boillot O *et al.* Postoperative infectious complications in paediatric liver transplantation: a study of 48 transplants. *Paediatr Anaesth* 2001; **11**: 93–98.

31 Hollenbeak CS, Alfrey EJ, Sheridan K *et al.* Surgical site infections following pediatric liver transplantation: risks and costs. *Transpl Infect Dis* 2003; **5**: 72–78.

32 Rabkin JM, Orloff SL, Corless CL *et al.* Hepatic allograft abscess with hepatic arterial thrombosis. *Am J Surg* 1998; **175**: 354–359.

33 Kim YJ, Kim SI, Wie SH *et al.* (2008) Infectious complications in living-donor liver transplant recipients: a 9-year single-center experience. *Transpl Infect Dis* 2008; **10**: 316–324.

34 Singh N, Wagener MM, Obman A *et al.* (2004) Bacteremias in liver transplant recipients: shift toward Gram-negative bacteria as predominant pathogens. *Liver Transpl* 2004; **10**: 844–849.

35 Cubiella J, Sala M, Fernández J *et al.* Complicaciones infecciosas asociadas al trasplante hepático: análisis de 104 pacientes. *Gastroenterol Hepatol* 2001; **24**: 186–190.

36 Hashimoto M, Sugawara Y, Tamura S *et al.* Bloodstream infection after living donor liver transplantation. *Scand J Infect Dis* 2008; **40**: 509–516.

37 Wade JJ, Rolando N, Hayllar K *et al.* Bacterial and fungal infections after liver transplantation: an analysis of 284 patients. *Hepatology* 1995; **21**: 1328–1336.

38 Durán FG, Piqueras B, Romero M *et al.* Pulmonary complications following orthotopic liver transplant. *Transpl Int* 1998; **11**(suppl. 1): S255–259.

39 Pellegrino CM, Codeluppi M, Assenza S *et al.* Incidence and clinical outcomes of ventilator-associated pneumonia in liver transplant and non-liver transplant surgical patients. *Transplant Proc* 2008; **40**: 1986–1988.

40 Hong SK, Hwang S, Lee SG *et al.* Pulmonary complications following adult liver transplantation. *Transplant Proc* 2006; **38**: 2979–2981.

41 Golfieri R, Giampalma E, Morselli Labate AM *et al.* Pulmonary complications of liver transplantation: radiological appearance and statistical evaluation of risk factors in 300 cases. *Eur Radiol* 2000; **10**: 1169–1183.

42 Mack CL, Millis JM, Whitington PF *et al.* Pulmonary complications following liver transplantation in pediatric patients. *Pediatr Transplant* 2000; **4**: 39–44.

43 George DL, Arnow PM, Fox AS *et al.* Bacterial infection as a complication of liver transplantation: epidemiology and risk factors. *Rev Infect Dis* 1991; **13**: 387–396.

44 García-Valdecasas JC, Prados M, Rimola A *et al.* Risk factors for severe bacterial infection after liver transplantation. *Transplant Proc* 1995; **27**: 2334–2335.

45 Blair JE, Kusne S. Bacterial, mycobacterial, and protozoal infections after liver transplantation – part I. *Liver Transpl* 2005; **11**: 1452–1459.

46 Everson GT. Everolimus and mTOR inhibitors in liver transplantation: opening the "box". *Liver Transpl* 2006; **12**: 1571–1573.

47 Del Pozo JL. Update and actual trends on bacterial infections following liver transplantation. *World J Gastroenterol* 2008; **14**: 4977–4983.

48 Their M, Holmberg C, Lautenschlager I *et al.* Infections in pediatric kidney and liver transplant patients after perioperative hospitalization. *Transplantation* 2000; **69**: 1617–1623.

49 Trzeciak S, Sharer R, Piper D *et al.* Infections and severe sepsis in solid-organ transplant patients admitted from a university-based ED. *Am J Emerg Med* 2004; **22**: 530–533.

50 Verdonk RC, Buis CI, Van der Jagt EJ *et al.* Nonanastomotic biliary strictures after liver transplantation, part 2: Management, outcome, and risk factors for disease progression. *Liver Transpl* 2007; **13**: 725–732.

51 Tachopoulou OA, Vogt DP, Henderson JM *et al.* Hepatic abscess after liver transplantation: 1990–2000. *Transplantation* 2003; **75**: 79–83.

52 Mizuno S, Zendejas IR, Reed AI *et al.* Listeria monocytogenes following orthotopic liver transplantation: central nervous system involvement and review of the literature. *World J Gastroenterol* 2007; **13**: 4391–4393.

53 Abbasoglu O, Levy MF, Brkic BB *et al.* Ten years of liver transplantation: an evolving understanding of late graft loss. *Transplantation* 1997; **64**: 1801–1807.

54 Raakow R, Bechstein WO, Kling N *et al.* The importance of late infections for the long-term outcome after liver transplantation. *Transpl Int* 1996; **9**(suppl. 1): S155–S156.

55 Lukes DJ, Herlenius G, Rizell M *et al.* Late mortality in 679 consecutive liver transplant recipients: the Gothenburg liver transplant experience. *Transplant Proc* 2006; **38**: 2671–2672.

56 Soltys KA, Mazariegos GV, Squires RH *et al.* Late graft loss or death in pediatric liver transplantation: an analysis of the SPLIT database. *Am J Transplant* 2007; **7**: 2165–2171.

57 Pruthi J, Medkiff KA, Esrason KT *et al.* Analysis of causes of death in liver transplant recipients who survived more than 3 years. *Liver Transpl* 2001; **7**: 811–815.

58 Rabkin JM, de la Melena V, Orloff SL *et al.* Late mortality after orthotopic liver transplantation. *Am J Surg* 2001; **181**: 475–479.

59 Bellier C, Bert F, Durand F *et al.* Risk factors for *Enterobacteriaceae* bacteremia after liver transplantation. *Transpl Int* 2008; **21**: 755–763.

60 Bedini A, Codeluppi M, Cocchi S *et al.* Gram-positive bloodstream infections in liver transplant recipients: incidence, risk factors, and impact on survival. *Transplant Proc* 2007; **39**: 1947–1949.

61 Candel FJ, Grima E, Matesanz M *et al.* Bacteremia and septic shock after solid-organ transplantation. *Transplant Proc* 2005; **37**: 4097–4099.

62 Singh N, Gayowski T, Wagener M *et al.* Pulmonary infections in liver transplant recipients receiving tacrolimus. Changing pattern of microbial etiologies. *Transplantation* 1996; **61**: 396–401.

63 Chow JW, Yu VL. Legionella: a major opportunistic pathogen in transplant recipients. *Semin Respir Infect* 1998; **13**: 132–139.

64 Prodinger WM, Bonatti H, Allerberger F *et al.* Legionella pneumonia in transplant recipients: a cluster of cases of eight years' duration. *J Hosp Infect* 1994; **26**: 191–202.

65 Singh N, Gayowski T, Rihs JD *et al.* Evolving trends in multiple-antibiotic-resistant bacteria in liver transplant recipients: a longitudinal study of antimicrobial susceptibility patterns. *Liver Transpl* 2001; **7**: 22–26.

66 Torre-Cisneros J, Herrero C, Cañas E *et al.* High mortality related with Staphylococcus aureus bacteremia after liver

transplantation. *Eur J Clin Microbiol Infect Dis* 2002; **21**: 385–388.

67 Zhou JD, Guo JJ, Zhang Q *et al*. Drug resistance of infectious pathogens after liver transplantation. *Hepatobiliary Pacreat Dis Int* 2006; **5**: 190–194.

68 Bert F, Galdbart JO, Zarrouk V *et al*. Association between nasal carriage of *Staphylococcus aureus* and infection in liver transplant recipients. *Clin Infect Dis* 2000; **31**: 1295–1299.

69 Desai D, Desai N, Nightingale P *et al*. Carriage of methicillin-resistant *Staphylococcus aureus* is associated with an increased risk of infection after liver transplantation. *Liver Transpl* 2003; **9**: 754–759.

70 Hashimoto M, Sugawara Y, Tamura S *et al*. Methicillin-resistant *Staphylococcus aureus* infection after living-donor liver transplantation in adults. *Transpl Infect Dis* 2008; **10**: 110–116.

71 Russell DL, Flood A, Zaroda TE *et al*. Outcomes of colonization with MRSA and VRE among liver transplant candidates and recipients. *Am J Transplant* 2008; **8**: 1737–1743.

72 Chang FY, Singh N, Gayowski T *et al*. Staphylococcus aureus nasal colonization and association with infections in liver transplant recipients. *Transplantation* 1998; **65**: 1169–1172.

73 Bakir M, Bova JL, Newell KA *et al*. Epidemiology and clinical consequences of vancomycin-resistant enterococci in liver transplant patients. *Transplantation* 2001; **72**: 1032–1037.

74 Werner G, Coque TM, Hammerum AM *et al*. Emergence and spread of vancomycin resistance among enterococci in Europe. *Euro Surveill* 2008; **13**: ii19046.

75 Gouvêa EF, Branco RC, Monteiro RCM *et al*. Outcome of infections caused by multiple drug-resistant bacteria in liver transplant recipients. *Transplant Proc* 2004; **36**: 958–960.

76 McNeil SA, Malani PN, Chenoweth CE *et al*. Vancomycin-resistant enterococcal colonization and infection in liver transplant candidates and recipients: a prospective surveillance study. *Clin Infect Dis* 2006; **42**: 195–203.

77 Linden PK. Treatment options for vancomycin-resistant enterococcal infections. *Drugs* 2002; **62**: 425–441.

78 Levine DP. Clinical experience with daptomycin: bacteraemia and endocarditis. *J Antimicrob Chemother* 2008; **62**(suppl. 3): iii35–39.

79 Shah AA, Hasan F, Ahmed S *et al*. Characteristics, epidemiology and clinical importance of emerging strains of Gram-negative bacilli producing extended-spectrum beta-lactamases. *Res Microbiol* 2004; **155**: 409–421.

80 Rupp ME, Fey PD. Extended spectrum beta-lactamase (ESBL)-producing Enterobacteriaceae: considerations for diagnosis, prevention and drug treatment. *Drugs* 2003; **63**: 353–365.

81 Pitout JD, Laupland KB. Extended-spectrum beta-lactamase-producing Enterobacteriaceae: an emerging public-health concern. *Lancet Infect Dis* 2008; **8**: 159–166.

82 Insa R, Cercenado E, Goyanes MJ *et al*. In vitro activity of tigecycline against clinical isolates of *Acinetobacter baumannii* and *Stenotrophomonas maltophilia*. *J Antimicrob Chemother* 2007; **59**: 583–585.

83 Gales AC, Jones RN, Forward KR *et al*. Emerging importance of multidrug-resistant *Acinetobacter* species and *Stenotrophomonas maltophilia* as pathogens in seriously ill patients: geographic patterns, epidemiological features, and trends in the SENTRY Antimicrobial Surveillance Program (1997–1999). *Clin Infect Dis* 2001; **32**(suppl. 2): S104–S113.

84 Davila D, Bartlett A, Heaton N. Temporary portocaval shunt in orthotopic liver transplantation: need for a standardized approach? *Liver Transpl* 2008; **14**: 1414–1419.

85 Massicotte L, Lenis S, Thibeault L *et al*. Effect of low central venous pressure and phlebotomy on blood product transfusion requirements during liver transplantations. *Liver Transpl* 2006; **12**: 117–123.

86 Liu CM, Chen J, Wang XH. Requirements for transfusion and postoperative outcomes in orthotopic liver transplantation: a meta-analysis on aprotinin. *World J Gastroenterol* 2008; **14**: 1425–1429.

87 Glanemann M, Busch T, Neuhaus P *et al*. Fast tracking in liver transplantation. Immediate postoperative tracheal extubation: feasibility and clinical impact. *Swiss Med Wkly* 2007; **137**: 187–191.

88 Soave R. Prophylaxis strategies for solid-organ transplantation. *Clin Infect Dis* 2001; **33**(suppl. 1): S26–S31.

89 Grazi GL, Mazziotti A, Fisichella S *et al*. Antimicrobial prophylaxis with ceftriaxone for prevention of early postoperative infections after 49 liver transplantations. *J Chemother* 2000; **12**(suppl. 3): 10–16.

90 Gridelli B, Panarello G, Salvatore G *et al*. Infections after living-donor liver transplantation. *Surg Infect (Larchmt)* 2006; **7**(suppl. 2): S105–S108.

91 Aguado JM, San Juan R. Surgical prophylaxis in liver transplantation: is it necessary but not enough? *Transplantation* 2008; **85**: 1715–1716.

92 Calleja Kempin JI, Bañares R, Polo JR *et al*. Effect of antibiotic prophylaxis with vancomycin on methicillin-resistant Staphylococcus aureus infection following liver transplantation. *Rev Esp Enferm Dig* 1993; **84**: 22–25.

93 Kusne S. Regarding the risk for development of surgical site infections and bacterial prophylaxis in liver transplantation. *Liver Transpl* 2008; **14**: 747–749.

94 Cerutti E, Stratta C, Romagnoli R *et al*. Bacterial- and fungal-positive cultures in organ donors: clinical impact in liver transplataton. *Liver Transpl* 2006; **12**: 1253–1259.

95 Mattner F, Kola A, Fischer S *et al*. Impact of bacterial and fungal donor organ contamination in lung, heart-lung, heart and liver transplantation. *Infection* 2008; **36**: 207–212.

96 Len O, Gavaldà J, Blanes M *et al*. Donor infection and transmission to the recipient of a solid allograft. *Am J Transplant* 2008; **8**: 2420–2425.

97 Bion JF, Badger I, Crosby HA *et al*. Selective decontamination of the digestive tract reduces gram-negative pulmonary colonization but not systemic endotoxemia in patients undergoing elective liver transplantation. *Crit Care Med* 1994; **22**: 40–49.

98 Smith SD, Jackson RJ, Hannakan CJ *et al*. Selective decontamination in pediatric liver transplants. A randomised prospective study. *Transplantation* 1993; **55**: 1306–1309.

99 Arnow PM, Carandang GC, Zabner R *et al*. Randomized controlled trial of selective bowel decontamination for prevention of infections following liver transplantation. *Clin Infect Dis* 1996; **22**: 997–1003.

100 Zwaveling JH, Maring JK, Klompmaker IJ *et al*. Selective decontamination of the digestive tract to prevent postoperative infection: a randomized placebo-controlled trial in liver transplant patients. *Crit Care Med* 2002; **30**: 1204–1209.

101 Hellinger WC, Yao JD, Alvarez S *et al.* A randomized, prospective, double-blinded evaluation of selective bowel decontamination in liver transplantation. *Transplantation* 2002; **73**: 1904–1909.

102 Safdar N, Said A, Lucey MR. The role of selective digestive decontamination for reducing infection in patients undergoing liver transplantation: a systematic review and meta-analysis. *Liver Transpl* 2004; **10**: 817–827.

103 Rayes N, Seehofer D, Theruvath T *et al.* Supply of pre- and probiotics reduces bacterial infection rates after liver transplantation – a randomized, double-blind trial. *Am J Transplant* 2005; **5**: 125–130.

104 Rayes N, Seehofer D, Hansen S *et al.* Early enteral supply of lactobacillus and fiber versus selective bowel decontamination: a controlled trial in liver transplant recipients. *Transplantation* 2002; **74**: 123–127.

105 Muto CA, Jernigan JA, Ostrowsky BE *et al.* SHEA guideline for preventing nosocomial transmission of multidrug-resistant strains of *Staphylococcus aureus* and *enterococcus*. *Infect Control Hosp Epidemiol* 2003; **24**: 362–386.

106 Siegel JD, Rhinehart E, Jackson M *et al.* Management of multidrug-resistant organisms in health care settings, 2006. *Am J Infect Control* 2007; **35**(suppl. 2): S165–S193.

107 Santoro-Lopes G, de Gouvêa EF, Monteiro RC *et al.* Colonization with methicillin-resistant *Staphylococcus aureus* after liver transplantation. *Liver Transpl* 2005; **11**: 203–209.

108 Paterson DL, Rihs JD, Squier C *et al.* Lack of efficacy of mupirocin in the prevention of infections with *Staphylococcus aureus* in liver transplant recipients and candidates. *Transplantation* 2003; **75**: 194–198.

109 Patel R. Association between nasal methicillin-resistant *Staphylococcus aureus* carriage and infection in liver transplant recipients. *Liver Transpl* 2001; **7**: 752–753.

110 Simor AE, Phillips E, McGeer A *et al.* Randomized controlled trial of chlorhexidine gluconate for washing, intranasal mupirocin, and rifampin and doxycycline versus no treatment for the eradication of methicillin-resistant *Staphylococcus aureus* colonization. *Clin Infect Dis* 2007, **44**: 178–185.

111 Vernon MO, Hayden MK, Trick WE *et al.* Chlorhexidine gluconate to cleanse patients in a medical intensive care unit: the effectiveness of source control to reduce the bioburden of vancomycin-resistant *enterococci*. *Arch Intern Med* 2006; **166**: 306–312.

112 Millonig G, Buratti T, Graziadei IW *et al.* Bactobilia after liver transplantation: frequency and antibiotic susceptibility. *Liver Transpl* 2006; **12**: 747–753.

113 Cotton PB, Connor P, Rawls E *et al.* Infection after ERCP, and antibiotic prophylaxis: a sequential quality-improvement approach over 11 years. *Gastrointest Endosc* 2008; **67**: 471–475.

114 ASGE Standards of Practice Committee. Antibiotic prophylaxis for GI endoscopy. *Gastrointest Endosc* 2008; **67**: 791–798.

115 Bubak ME, Porayko MK, Krom RA *et al.* Complications of liver biopsy in liver transplant patients: increased sepsis associated with choledochojejunostomy. *Hepatology* 1991; **14**: 1063–1065.

116 Bratzler DW, Houck PM Antimicrobial prophylaxis for surgery: an advisory statement from the National Surgical Infection Prevention Project. *Am J Surg* 2005; **189**: 395–404.

117 Philpott-Howard J, Burroughs A, Fisher N *et al.* Piperacillin-tazobactam versus ciprofloxacin plus amoxicillin in the treatment of infective episodes after liver transplantation. *J Antimicrob Chemother* 2003; **52**: 993–1000.

118 Bellier C, Bert F, Durand F *et al.* Risk factors for *Enterobacteriaceae* bacteremia after liver transplantation. *Transpl Int* 2008; **21**: 755–763.

119 Gearhart M, Martin J, Rudich S *et al.* Consequences of vancomycin-resistant *Enterococcus* in liver transplant recipients: a matched control study. *Clin Transplant* 2005; **19**: 711–716.

120 Anderson DJ, Engemann JJ, Harrell LJ *et al.* Predictors of mortality in patients with bloodstream infection due to ceftazidime-resistant *Klebsiella pneumoniae*. *Antimicrob Agents Chemother* 2006; **50**; 1715–1720.

121 Tumbarello M, Sanguinetti M, Montuori E *et al.* Predictors of mortality in patients with bloodstream infections caused by extended-spectrum-beta-lactamase-producing *Enterobacteriaceae*: importance of inadequate initial antimicrobial treatment. *Antimicrob Agents Chemother* 2007; **51**: 1987–1994.

122 Blot S. Limiting the attributable mortality of nosocomial infection and multidrug resistance in intensive care units. *Clin Microbiol Infect* 2008; **14**: 5–13.

123 Vidal L, Gafter-Gvili A, Borok S *et al.* Efficacy and safety of aminoglycoside monotherapy: systematic review and meta-analysis of randomized controlled trials. *J Antimicrob Chemother* 2007; **60**: 247–257.

124 Balfour JA, Bryson HM, Brogden RN. Imipenem/cilastatin: an update of its antibacterial activity, pharmacokinetics and therapeutic efficacy in the treatment of serious infections. *Drugs* 1996; **51**: 99–136.

125 Iwasaki K. Metabolism of tacrolimus (FK506) and recent topics in clinical pharmacokinetics. *Drug Metab Pharmacokinet* 2007; **22**: 328–335.

126 Campana C, Regazzi MB, Buggia I *et al.* Clinically significant drug interactions with cyclosporin. An update. *Clin Pharmacokinet* 1996; **30**: 141–1479.

127 Sattler M, Guengerich FP, Yun CH *et al.* Cytochrome P-450 3A enzymes are responsible for biotransformation of FK506 and rapamycin in man and rat. *Drug Metab Dispos* 1992; **20**: 753–761.

128 Kirchner GI, Meier-Wiedenbach I, Manns MP. Clinical pharmacokinetics of everolimus. *Clin Pharmacokinet* 2004; **43**: 83–95.

129 Singh N. Inching closer towards optimization of treatment for latent tuberculosis in liver transplant recipients. *Transplantation* 2007; **83**: 1536–1537.

130 Singh N, Paterson DL. Mycobacterium tuberculosis infection in solid-organ transplant recipients: impact and implications for management. *Clin Infect Dis* 1998; **27**: 1266–1277.

131 Aguado JM, Herrero JA, Gavaldá J *et al.* Clinical presentation and outcome of tuberculosis in kidney, liver, and heart transplant recipients in Spain. Spanish Transplantation Infection Study Group, GESITRA. *Transplantation* 1997; **63**: 1278–1286.

132 EBPG Expert Group on Renal Transplantation. European best practice guidelines for renal transplantation. Section IV: Long-term management of the transplant recipient. IV.7.2. Late infections. Tuberculosis. *Nephrol Dial Transplant* 2002; **17**(suppl. 4): 39–43.

133 American Thoracic Society (ATS) and the Centers for Disease Control and Prevention (CDC). Targeted tuberculin testing and

treatment of latent tuberculosis infection. *Am J Respir Crit Care Med* 2000; **161**(4 part 2): S221–S247.

134 Rubin RH. Management of tuberculosis in the transplant recipient. *Am J Transplant* 2005; **5**: 2599–2600.

135 Benito N, Sued O, Moreno A *et al.* Diagnosis and treatment of latent tuberculosis infection in liver transplant recipients in an endemic area. *Transplantation* 2002; **74**: 1381–1386.

136 Jahng AW, Tran T, Bui L *et al.* Safety of treatment of latent tuberculosis infection in compensated cirrhotic patients during transplant candidacy period. *Transplantation* 2007; **83**: 1557–1562.

137 Horsburgh CR Jr, Feldman S, Ridzon R *et al.* Practice guidelines for the treatment of tuberculosis. *Clin Infect Dis* 2000; **31**: 633–639.

138 Blumberg HM, Burman WJ, Chaisson RE *et al.* American Thoracic Society/Centers for Disease Control and Prevention/ Infectious Diseases Society of America: treatment of tuberculosis. *Am J Respir Crit Care Med* 2003; **167**: 603–662.

139 Malhotra KK. Challenge of tuberculosis in renal transplantation. *Transplant Proc* 2007; **39**: 756–758.

140 Muñoz P, Rodriguez C, Bouza E. Mycobacterium tuberculosis infection in recipients of solid organ transplants. *Clin infect Dis* 2005; **40**, 581–587.

141 Clemente WT, Faria LC, Lima SS *et al.* Tuberculosis in liver transplant recipients: a single Brazilian center experience. *Transplantation* 2009; **87**: 397–401.

142 Meyers BR, Papanicolaou GA, Sheiner P *et al.* Tuberculosis in orthotopic liver transplant patients: increased toxicity of recommended agents; cure of disseminated infection with nonconventional regimens. *Transplantation* 2000; **69**: 64–69.

143 Patel R, Paya CV. Infections in solid-organ transplant recipients. *Clin Microbiol Rev* 1997; **10**: 86–124.

144 Schluger LK, Sheiner PA, Jonas M *et al.* Isoniazid hepatotoxicity after orthotopic liver transplantation. *Mt Sinai J Med* 1996; **63**: 364–369.

145 Zhang XF, Lv Y, Xue WJ *et al.* Mycobacterium tuberculosis infection in solid organ transplant recipients: experience from a single center in China. *Transplant Proc* 2008; **40**: 1382–1385.

146 Kusne S, Blair JE. Viral and fungal infections after liver transplantation – Part II. *Liver Transpl* 2006; **12**: 2–11.

147 Levitsky J, Freifeld AG, Bargenquast K *et al.* The clinical value to quantitative polymerase chain reaction in cytomegalovirus infection after solid organ transplantation. *Am J Transplant* 2004; **4**(suppl. 8): 339.

148 Kanj SS, Sharara AI, Clavien PA *et al.* Cytomegalovirus infection following liver transplantation: review of the literature. *Clin Infect Dis* 1996; **22**: 537–549.

149 Gaeta A, Nazzari C, Angeletti S *et al.* Monitoring for cytomegalovirus infection in organ transplant recipients: analysis of pp65 antigen, DNA and late mRNA in peripheral blood leukocytes. *J Med Virol* 1997; **53**: 189–195.

150 Narvios AB, de Lima M, Shah H *et al.* Transfusion of leukoreduced cellular blood components from cytomegalovirus-unscreened donors in allogeneic hematopoietic transplant recipients: analysis of 72 recipients. *Bone Marrow Transplant* 2005; **36**: 499–501.

151 Razonable RR. Cytomegalovirus infection after liver transplantation: current concepts and challenges. *World J Gastroenterol* 2008; **14**: 4849–4860.

152 Falagas ME, Snydman DR, Ruthazer R *et al.* Primary cytomegalovirus infection in liver transplant recipients: comparison of infections transmitted via donor organs and via transfusions. *Clin Infect Dis* 1996; **23**: 292–297.

153 Kusne S, Shapiro R, Fung J. Prevention and treatment of cytomegalovirus infection in organ transplant recipients. *Transpl Infect Dis* 1999; **1**: 187–203.

154 Singh N, Paterson DL, Gayowski T *et al.* Cytomegalovirus antigenemia directed pre-emptive prophylaxis with oral versus IV ganciclovir for the prevention of cytomegalovirus disease in liver transplant recipients. *Transplantation* 2000; **70**: 717–722.

155 Limaye A, Bakthavatsalam R, Kim HW *et al.* Impact of cytomegalovirus in organ transplant recipients in the era of antiviral prophylaxis. *Transplantation* 2006; **81**: 1645–1652.

156 Diaz-Pedroche C, Lumbreras C, San Juan R *et al.* Valganciclovir preemptive therapy for the prevention of cytomegalovirus disease in high risk seropositive solid-organ transplant recipients. *Transplantation* 2006; **82**: 30–35.

157 Jain A, Orloff M, Kashyap R *et al.* Does valganciclovir hydrochloride (Valcyte) provide effective prophylaxis against cytomegalovirus infection in liver transplant recipients? *Transplant Proc* 2005; **37**: 3182–3186.

158 Paya C, Humar A, Dominguez E *et al.* Efficacy and safety of valganciclovir vs. oral ganciclovir for prevention of cytomegalovirus disease in solid organ transplant recipients. *Am J Transplant* 2004; **4**: 611–620.

159 Singh N, Gayowski T, Wagener MM *et al.* Efficacy of valganciclovir administered as preemptive therapy for cytomegalovirus disease in liver transplant recipients: impact on viral load and late-onset CMV disease. *Transplantation* 2005; **79**: 85–90.

160 Kalil AC, Levitsky J, Lyden E *et al.* Metaanalysis: the efficacy of strategies to prevent organ disease by cytomegalovirus in solid organ transplant recipients. *Ann Intern Med* 2005; **143**, 870–880.

161 Small L, Lau J, Snydman D. Preventing post-organ transplantation cytomegalovirus disease with ganciclovir: a meta-analysis comparing prophylactic and preemptive therapies. *Clin Infect Dis* 2006; **43**: 869–880.

162 Snydman DR. The case for cytomegalovirus prophylaxis in solid organ transplantation. *Rev Med Virol* 2006; **16**: 289–295.

163 Singh N, Wannstedt C, Keyes L *et al.* Valganciclovir as preemptive therapy for cytomegalovirus in cytomegalovirus-seronegative liver transplant recipients of cytomegalovirus-seropositive donor allografts. *Liver Transpl* 2008; **14**: 240–244.

164 Singh N. Cytomegalovirus infection in solid organ transplant recipients: new challenges and their implications for preventive strategies. *J Clin Virol* 2006; **35**: 474–477.

165 Biron KK. Antiviral drugs for cytomegalovirus diseases. *Antiviral Res* 2006; **71**: 154–163.

166 Asberg A, Humar A, Rollag H *et al.* Oral valganciclovir is noninferior to intravenous ganciclovir for the treatment of cytomegalovirus disease in solid organ transplant recipients. *Am J Transplant* 2007; **7**: 2106–2113.

167 Compston LI, Sarkobie F, Li C *et al.* Multiplex real-time PCR for the detection and quantification of latent and persistent viral genomes in cellular or plasma blood fractions. *J Virol Methods* 2008; **15**: 47–54.

168 Paya CV, Fung JJ, Nalesnik MA *et al.* ASTS/ASTP EBV-PTLD Task Force and The Mayo Clinic Organized International

Consensus Development Meeting: Epstein-Barr virus-induced posttransplant lymphoproliferative disorders. *Transplantation* 1999; **68**: 1517–1525.

169 Jain A, Nalesnik M, Reyes J *et al.* Posttransplant lymphoproliferative disorders in liver transplantation: a 20-year experience. *Ann Surg* 2002; **236**: 429–436.

170 Avolio AW, Agnes S, Barbarino R *et al.* Posttransplant lymphoproliferative disorders after liver transplantation: analysis of early and late cases in a 255 patients series. *Transplant Proc* 2007; **39**: 1956–1960.

171 Humar A, Washburn K, Freeman R *et al.* An assessment of interactions between hepatitis C virus and herpesvirus reactivation in liver transplant recipients using molecular surveillance. *Liver Transpl* 2007; **13**: 1422–1427.

172 Harris NL, Ferry JA, Swerdlow SH. Posttransplant lymphoproliferative disorders: summary of Society for Hemopathology workshop. *Semin Diagn Pathol* 1997; **14**: 8–14.

173 Cockfield SM. Identifying the patient at risk for post-transplant lymphoproliferative disorder. *Transpl Infect Dis* 2001; **3**: 70–78.

174 Everly MJ, Bloom RD, Tsai DE *et al.* Posttransplant lymphoproliferative disorder. *Ann Pharmacother* 2007; **41**: 1850–1858.

175 Green M. Management of Epstein-Barr virus-induced posttransplant lymphoproliferative disease in recipients of solid organ transplantation. *Am J Transplant* 2001; **1**: 103–108.

176 Benito N, Moreno A, Pumarola T *et al.* Human herpesvirus type 6 and type 7 in transplant recipients. *Enf Infecc Microbiol Clin* 2003; **21**: 424–432.

177 Cervera C, Marcos MA, Linares L *et al.* A prospective survey of human herpesvirus-6 primary infection in solid organ transplant recipients. *Transplantation* 2006; **82**: 979–982.

178 Humar A, Asberg A, Kumar D *et al.* An assessment of herpesvirus co-infections in patients with CMV disease: correlation with clinical and virologic outcomes. *Am J Transplant* 2009; **9**: 374–381.

179 Di Benedetto F, Di Sandro S, De Ruvo N *et al.* Kaposi's sarcoma after liver transplantation. *J Cancer Res Clin Oncol* 2008; **134**: 653–658.

180 Casper C. New approaches to the treatment of human herpesvirus 8-associated disease. *Rev Med Virol* 2008; **18**: 321–329.

181 Casper C, Krantz EM, Corey L *et al.* Valganciclovir for suppression of human herpesvirus-8 replication: a randomized, double-blind, placebo-controlled, crossover trial. *J Infect Dis* 2008; **198**: 23–30.

182 Verucchi G, Calza L, Trevisani F *et al.* Human herpesvirus-8-related Kaposi's sarcoma after liver transplantation successfully treated with cidofovir and liposomal daunorubicin. *Transpl Infect Dis* 2005; **7**: 34–37.

183 Campistol JM, Schena FP. Kaposi's sarcoma in renal transplant recipients – the impact of proliferation signal inhibitors. *Nephrol Dial Transplant* 2007; **22**(suppl. 1): i17–i22.

184 Monaco AP. The role of mTOR inhibitors in the management of posttransplant malignancy. *Transplantation* 2009; **87**: 157–163.

185 Husain S, Tollemar J, Dominguez EA *et al.* Changes in the spectrum and risk factors for invasive candidiasis in liver transplant recipients: prospective, multicenter, case-controlled study. *Transplantation* 2003; **75**: 2023–2029.

186 Fortun J, Martin-Davila P, Moreno S *et al.* Risk factors for invasive aspergillosis in liver transplant recipients. *Liver Transpl* 2002; **8**: 1065–1070.

187 Singh N, Avery RK, Munoz P *et al.* Trends in risk profiles for and mortality associated with invasive aspergillosis among liver transplant recipients. *Clin Infect Dis* 2003; **36**: 46–52.

188 Cruciani M, Mengoli C, Malena M *et al.* Antifungal prophylaxis in liver transplant patients: A systematic review and meta-analysis. *Liver Transpl* 2006; **12**: 850–858.

189 Hadley S, Huckabee C, Pappas PG *et al.* Outcomes of antifungal prophylaxis in high-risk liver transplant recipients. *Transpl Infect Dis* 2009; **11**: 40–48.

190 Fortun J, Martín-Davila P, Montejo M *et al.* Prophylaxis with caspofungin for invasive fungal infections in high-risk liver transplant recipients. *Transplantation* 2009; **87**: 424–435.

191 Wheat LJ. Antigen detection, serology, and molecular diagnosis of invasive mycoses in the immunocompromised host. *Transpl Infect Dis* 2006; **8**: 128–139.

192 De Pauw BE, Picazo JJ. Present situation in the treatment of invasive fungal infection. *Int J Antimicrob Agents* 2008; **32**(suppl. 2): S167–S171.

193 Pappas PG, Kauffman CA, Andes D *et al.* Clinical practice guidelines for the management of candidiasis: 2009 update by the Infectious Diseases Society of America. *Clin Infect Dis* 2009; **48**: 503–535.

194 Candel FJ, Matesanz M, Mensa J. Sequential prescription of antifungals in invasive fungal infection: the importance of mechanism of action. *Int J Antimicrob Agents* 2008; **32**(suppl. 2): S133–S135.

44 Management of HCV infection and liver transplantation

Brett E Fortune, Hugo R Rosen and James R Burton, Jr
University of Colorado, Denver, Colorado, USA

Introduction

Hepatitis C virus (HCV) is the leading indication for liver transplantation (LT) worldwide. With recurrence of HCV being universal and a significant percentage developing severe allograft fibrosis, recurrent HCV infection represents one of the most significant issues facing the transplant physician today. HCV in the transplant setting is most challenging given the limited applicability and reduced tolerability of antivival therapy and lower rates of response in comparison to the non-transplant setting.

Natural history of recurrent HCV

Recurrence is immediate and universal with viral levels after 1–3 months post-LT, often being twenty-fold greater than in the pre-LT period [1]. The natural history of recurrent HCV after LT is accelerated compared to HCV infection in the non-transplant setting. Between 20–40% of patients transplanted for HCV develop allograft cirrhosis in five years compared to less than 5–20% at 20 years in the non-transplant setting [2–4]. Once cirrhosis develops, decompensation (variceal bleeding, ascites, hepatic encephalopathy) occurs in 25–67% within three years, compared to ~10% in immunocompetent HCV patients with cirrhosis [3–5]. Once decompensation develops after LT, outcome is very poor, with <10% surviving three years. Despite this accelerated course, a third of patients will demonstrate minimal fibrosis at five years [6]. Although short-term studies have shown patient and graft survival is similar for patients undergoing LT for HCV compared to other indications, analysis of the United Network for Organ Sharing (UNOS) database revealed significantly diminished sur-

vival five years after LT in HCV-positive patients compared to HCV-negative patients (56.7% vs 65.6%; p < 0.05) [7].

Fibrosing cholestatic HCV infection occurs in approximately 5% of patients transplanted for HCV diagnoses. It is characterized by a rapidly progressive cholestatic hepatitis which typically develops one to three months post-LT, resulting in graft failure in three to nine months [8]. Typically very high HCV RNA levels are seen with serum bilirubin levels >6g/dl and alkaline phosphatase levels greater than five times the upper limit of normal with normal cholangiogram. The pathogenesis is likely immunologically different from typical HCV-induced allograft failure with preferential Th2 cytokine production by intrahepatic lymphocytes being implicated [9, 10]. Treatment focuses on minimizing immunosuppression and viral suppression with indefinite use of interferon based antiviral therapy [11].

Factors associated with severe HCV recurrence

A number of factors have been associated with severe HCV recurrence that affects both patient and graft survival. Table 44.1 outlines these donor, viral and transplant factors. Given the detrimental effects of treating acute cellular rejection with corticosteroids [12–14], suspicion for rejection in HCV patients should always be confirmed with liver biopsy. Differentiating recurrent HCV alone from recurrent HCV and rejection can be challenging [15]. Mild rejection may be treated without steroids by increasing calcineurin inhibitors or addition/increase of mycophenolate mofetil [16, 17]. The long-term effects of this approach are unknown. How best to handle maintenance immunosuppression is a hotly debated topic. Despite numerous pieces of literature on the role of immunosuppression and the effects on recurrent HCV, no clear conclusions can be drawn.

Evidence-Based Gastroenterology and Hepatology, 3rd edition.
J. McDonald, A.K. Burroughs, B. Feagan, and M.B. Fennerty. © 2010
Blackwell Publishing Ltd

Treatment of recurrent HCV

The treatment of HCV after LT has improved significantly over the past decade, with the best results obtained with utilizing pegylated interferon (peginterferon) with ribavirin, which this review will focus on primarily [18, 19]. Trials utilizing standard interferon and ribavirin have been reviewed separately [20]. The timing of antiviral therapy has played a major variable in studies investigating efficacy of treatment. Several treatment strategies have been proposed for managing recurrent HCV, with goals to prevent or slow disease progression (see Table 44.2). Rates of sustained virological response (SVR; HCV RNA undetectable six months after stopping therapy) are far less than those achieved in immunocompetent HCV-infected patients (overall 20–30%). There are a number of factors contributing to lower virological response rates to antiviral therapy in liver transplant patients (see Table 44.3) with similar

predictors of virological response as in non-transplant HCV infection. Possible predictors of SVR include early virological response (EVR, >2 log drop in HCV RNA at 12 weeks), infection with genotype 2, adherence to therapy and baseline viremia [18]. Primary treatment endpoints include histological response, graft survival and patient survival. While typically the major indication for treatment is driven largely by allograft damage, significant psychological and social factors of the patient play a role in withholding antiviral therapy in some cases.

Pre-transplant antiviral therapy

Pre-transplant antiviral therapy is an attractive approach in which those with undetectable HCV RNA going into transplant may eliminate the risk of developing recurrent HCV. In some cases when patients achieve SVR from this regimen, they may completely avoid transplantation altogether. A recent review shows that up to two-thirds of patients who obtain SVR prior to liver transplantation will remain free of HCV in the post-transplant setting. This rate is lower for patients without achievement of SVR [21].

Table 44.1 Risk factors associated with severe HCV recurrence.

Category	Factor
Donor factors	Donor age >40 yrs Prolonged cold ischemia time Female sex Living donor liver transplant experience (<20 cases)
Viral factors	HCV genotype 1 in some studies High viral load at liver tansplantation

Transplant factors	CMV infection
	Diabetes mellitus
	Higher average daily steroid use
	Treatment of acute cellular rejection with:
	   Corticosteroid boluses
	   OKT3 use

Table 44.3 Contributing factors leading to lower response rates to antiviral therapy in liver transplant patients.

- High HCV RNA levels post-LT
- High prevalence of genotype 1, previous non-responders to antiviral therapy
- Presence of immunosuppression
- Poor clinical status and tolerability, especially early post-LT
- Cytopenias as result of immunosuppression requiring dose reduction and use of growth factors
- Renal insufficiency limiting dose of ribavirin on account of its associated risk of hemolytic anemia

Table 44.2 Antiviral treatment strategies for recurrent HCV.

Treatment strategy	Timing of antiviral therapy	Advantage	Disadvantage
Pre-transplant	Prior to LT	Eliminate or reduce risk of recurrent HCV Potential to avoid LT	Low virological response Limited tolerability and potential for serious adverse effects
Preemptive	Early post-LT	Relatively low HCV RNA levels Minimal or no histological disease	Maximal immunosuppression Higher risk of rejection and infection
Established disease	Diagnosis of acute hepatitis or established and/or severe disease	Lower immunosuppression Improved clinical status and better tolerance Lower risk of rejection	High HCV RNA levels More advanced fibrosis

Unfortunately, this is a difficult group to treat given low response rates due to the high prevalence of genotype 1 and underlying cirrhosis and its associated side effects (e.g. leukopenia, thrombocytopenia).

One of the largest studies of pre-transplant antiviral therapy by Everson *et al.* described their experience with a low accelerating dose regimen (LADR) of primarily non-pegylated interferon and ribavirin and its efficacy for HCV clearance prior to transplant [22]. A total of 124 patients (70% genotype 1 and 63% having Child-Pugh class B or C) were treated, with 24% achieving SVR (13% genotype 1 and 50% non-genotype 1). Twelve out of 15 (80%) of patients who were HCV RNA negative going into transplant remained HCV RNA negative at least six months after LT.

Three comparative studies of peginterferon in liver transplant candidates (although included patients were not necessarily already considered or placed on transplant listing) have been reported [23–25]. DiMarco *et al.* reported results of 102 patients (67% treatment naive) randomized to receive peginterferon α-2b monotherapy or peginterferon plus ribavirin (800 mg) for up to 52 weeks (treatment was stopped if HCV RNA was not undetectable at 24 weeks) [23]. Overall, SVR was 19.6% in the peginterferon and ribavirin group and 9.8% in peginterferon monotherapy group (p = 0.06). Not surprising, response rates for non-genotype 1 were higher than for genotype 1 (66% vs 11%, p = 0.001). Discontinuation was 27% in the peginterferon and ribavirin group and 41% in the peginterferon group. Helbling *et al.* randomized 124 naive patients to either peginterferon α-2a plus standard dose ribavirin (1000–1200 mg) or peginterferon plus low dose ribavirin (600–800 mg) for 48 weeks [24]. SVR was 50% with the standard dose ribavirin group compared to 38% for the lower dose group (p = 0.153). Both groups had similar rates of treatment discontinuation. Finally, in a nonrandomized controlled trial, the first to specifically assess the effect of antiviral therapy on liver function in patients with decompensated HCV cirrhosis, Iacobellis *et al.* compared 66 patients treated with peginterferon α-2b and ribavirin (800–1000 mg) to 63 controls (no treatment). Twenty percent of the treatment group achieved SVR [25]. The study had similar discontinuation rates for the treatment group as observed in prior studies and survival was not different between the two groups, but a *post hoc* analysis showed a survival benefit in the treated group. An important finding in this study was a decreased incidence of decompensation (ascites, hepatic encephalopathy) in the treated group compared to the controls during follow-up. However it did not translate into increased survival in the treated patients.

In summary, pre-transplant antiviral therapy should be strongly considered in patients with cirrhosis who have Child-Pugh scores ≤ 7 or Model for End-Stage Liver Disease (MELD) scores ≤ 18 [8]. (MELD score = 10 [0.957 Ln (serum creatinine) + 0.378 Ln (total bilirubin) + 1.12 Ln

(INR) + 0.643].) **B2** A special group that should be strongly considered for antiviral therapy while awaiting transplantation are patients with well compensated liver disease upgraded on the transplant list solely for an indication of hepatocellular carcinoma, especially if they are non-genotype 1. **B4** Our program attempts to make these patients HCV RNA negative on treatment for at least two months before proceeding with either cadaveric or living donor transplantation. However, it is important to emphasize that the majority of HCV-infected patients without hepatocellular carcinoma will not be optimal candidates for antiviral therapy by the time they have moved up on the transplant list, due to their disease severity.

Preemptive antiviral treatment

Preemptive treatment refers to early antiviral therapy days to weeks after LT, before the development of histological recurrence. A number of theoretical advantages exist with this approach in that patients have lower HCV RNA levels and lack histological disease. However, from a clinical standpoint, treatment at this time is most challenging due to poor clinical status, cytopenias from maximal immunosuppression, and higher rates of rejection and infection in the early transplant period. Only about 60% of LT recipients are eligible for preemptive therapy, with the need for dose reduction occurring in up to 50% of treated patients [26]. A recent meta-analysis found no studies of preemptive therapy that satisfied inclusion for analysis [19]. In summary, the efficacy of preemptive anti-viral therapy remains to be defined and should only be considered in patients undergoing retransplantation for rapidly progressive HCV recurrence [8].

Treatment of established disease

Given the lack of efficacy and limitations of preemptive therapy, many transplant centers have opted to delay treatment until significant recurrent disease is verified. By taking this approach, treatment is focused on those likely to achieve benefit with antiviral therapy, avoiding unnecessary toxicity and side effects in those without significant disease recurrence. Two general approaches have been used to treat established disease. One approach initiates antiviral treatment at the diagnosis of acute recurrent hepatitis utilizing liver biopsy to exclude other causes for elevated liver enzymes, such as rejection. The second approach followed by most transplant centers is to initiate antiviral therapy when clinically significant evidence of recurrence exists. This latter approach utilizes protocol and/or clinically indicated liver biopsies reporting both the grade and stage of recurrent disease.

Table 44.4 Published of controlled trials utilizing peginterferon and ribavirin for treating recurrent HCV vs no treatment.

Author year	Type of Study	# of Patients	Antiviral Regimen	Duration (weeks)	SVR	Histological Response[a]	Genotype 1 (%)
Castells, 2005	NRT	48	(1) PEG-IFN (1.5 mcg/kg/wk) + Riba (600–800 mg/d) for 24 wks + 24 wks if RNA neg	24–48	(1) 33%	NR	100
			(2) No treatment		(2) 0%		
Bizollon, 2007	NRT	48	(1) PEG-IFN (1.5 mcg/kg/wk) + Riba (800–1000 mg/d)	48	(1) 30%	(1) 100%	85
			(2) No treatment		(2) 0%	(2) 24%	
Carrion, 2007	RCT	54	(1) PEG-IFN (1.5 mcg/kg/wk) + Riba (800–1200 mg/d)	48	(1) 48%	(1) 74%	79
			(2) No treatment		(2) 0%	(2) 30%	

NRT: nonrandomized trial; RCT: randomized controlled trial; Riba: ribavirin; SVR: sustained virological response; NR: not reported.
[a] Defined as fibrosis stabilization (same fibrosis stage) or fibrosis improvement (reduction of >/= 1 fibrosis stage).

Protocol liver biopsies in patients transplanted for HCV may be useful given the potential for significant fibrosis progression and has largely become standard of care [8]. Since fibrosis progression is not linear over time, possibly progressing more rapidly in the first post-LT year, the 12-month liver biopsy has the ability to stratify fibrosis progression. Those developing severe disease recurrence within the first transplant year are at a high likelihood of progressing to cirrhosis and should be considered for antiviral therapy [14, 27]. Furthermore, the absence of fibrosis 12 months post-LT is associated with excellent cirrhosis-free survival [14]. The measurement of hepatic venous pressure gradients (HVPG; wedged hepatic vein pressure minus free hepatic vein pressure) appears to be a useful tool in assessing disease severity in recurrent HCV [28]. HVPG measurements ≥6 mm Hg in one study [29], or ≥10 mm Hg in another study [5], at one year post-LT have been shown to be extremely accurate in predicting clinical decompensation over liver biopsy. The same group has also shown good correlation between HVPG measurements and histological response with antiviral therapy [30]. In summary, patients with fibrosis stage ≥ 2 out of 4, severe inflammation (grade 3 or 4), evidence of significant hepatic dysfunction (elevated bilirubin, prolonged prothrombin time), or HPVG gradients ≥6 should be strongly considered for antiviral therapy [5, 8] **B4**

Controlled trials of peginterferon and ribavirin

The current standard of care for treating established recurrent HCV is pegylated interferon and ribavirin therapy. Multiple studies using various study designs and endpoints have been performed to evaluate the efficacy of established disease therapy after transplantation, with endpoints consisting of SVR, histological improvement, and allograft and patient survival. It appears that there is no significant correlation between success of antiviral therapy and the interval of time from transplant and start of antiviral therapy. There are only three comparative studies of peginterferon and ribavirin in treatment of established recurrent HCV (see Table 44.4 and Figure 44.1) with only one randomized study [30–32].

Castells *et al.* studied 24 patients receiving peginterferon α2b (1.5 mcg/kg/wk) and ribavirin (600–800 mg/day) for 48 weeks (if HCV RNA undetectable at 24 weeks) and 24 consecutive untreated controls [30]. All patients were genotype 1 and treatment was initiated for acute recurrent HCV confirmed on biopsy (mean four months after LT). Growth factors (filgrastim and darbepoetin alpha) were given and anemia and leukopenia occurred in 71% and 96% of cases respectively. Overall SVR was 33% in the treatment group and 0% in controls. One patient developed acute cellular rejection in the treatment group (two in the control group) that resolved with adjusting immunosuppression. No histological follow-up was reported in this study. On univariate analysis, SVR was associated with absence of corticosteroid administration to treat rejection (p = 0.01), presence of early virological response (EVR > 2 log drop in HCV RNA at week 12) (p = 0.002) and absence of cytomegalovirus infection (p = 0.001). **B2**

Bizollon *et al.* studied 27 patients with established recurrent HCV (median ten months after LT) receiving peginterferon α2b (1.5 mg/kg/wk) and ribavirin (800–1000 mg/d) for 48 weeks and compared them to 21 consecutive untreated controls [31]. Seventy nine percent were genotype 1 and some had previous treatment post-LT with non-pegylated interferon and ribavirin. Filgrastim was not used, but erythropoietin alpha was given. SVR was 30% in

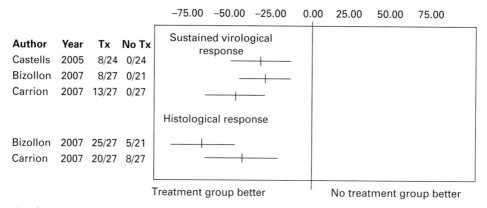

Figure 44.1 Forest Plot of sustained virological response and histological response rates in comparative studies of pegylated interferon and ribavirin versus no therapy in patients transplanted for HCV related cirrhosis with recurrent disease.
Tx: treatment.
Adapted from Xirouchakis E *et al*. Pegylated-interferon and ribavirin in transplant candidates and recipients with HCV cirrhosis: systemic review and meta-analysis of prospective controlled studies. *J Viral Hep* 2008; **15**: 699–709.

treatment group and 0% in controls. Two patients in the treatment group and one in the control group had acute cellular rejection. Patients completing treatment had improvement (65%) or stabilization (35%) of fibrosis 24 weeks after completing treatment. All eight patients achieving SVR had improvement in histology. Based on univariate analysis, the use of cyclosporine (p = 0.03) and early virological response (p = 0.02) were associated with SVR. **B2**

Carrion *et al*. have published the only randomized study to date [32]. In this study, 54 patients with mild HCV recurrence (F0-F2) at least six months post-LT were randomized to either peginterferon α2b (1.5 mcg/kg/wk) and ribavirin (800–1200 mg/day) for 48 weeks or no treatment. Filgrastim and darbepoetin were used to treat neutropenia and anemia respectively. Eighty-five percent were genotype 1 and treatment was initiated a mean of 16 months post-LT. Overall SVR in the treatment group was 48%. Histological response (improvement or stabilization six months after completing antiviral therapy) was seen in 74% of the treated compared to 30% of controls with all patients achieving SVR having a histological response. Biochemical response (normalization of ALT) on multivariate analysis independently predicted fibrosis improvement or stabilization. Hepatic venous pressure gradient also correlated with progression of fibrosis. **A1d**

Graft survival

Bizollon *et al*. in a retrospective study analyzed the effect of SVR on graft survival in 80 patients treated for recurrent HCV at least six months after transplant with nonpegylated interferon and ribavirin [33]. Erythropoietin was utilized. Overall SVR was 42%. In those achieving SVR, 82% had either stabilization or improvement in fibrosis compared to

26% in those not achieving SVR (p < 0.001). Among responders without cirrhosis at inclusion, none developed cirrhosis at the end of follow-up. In the one patient with cirrhosis at inclusion, no decompensation or hepatocellular carcinoma occurred. In nonresponders, 9 of 48 (19%) developed cirrhosis after a mean of 32 months. Four of the nine developed decompensation, with three being retransplanted a mean of seven months following diagnosis of cirrhosis.

Veldt *et al*. performed a larger study to investigate treatment benefits on graft survival [34]. In this retrospective cohort study, 78 patients treated predominately with peginterferon (n = 61) in combination with ribavirin (n = 69) were compared to 81 contemporary untreated patients, to assess graft survival. As treated patients may have been selected on the basis of medical compliance, mean immunosuppression levels were compared during the first month after transplant, between treated and untreated patients, as a measure for previous treatment compliance; no statistical differences were seen. Patients with severe recurrence resulting in graft failure or death within six months of transplant were not evaluated. Erythropoietin was utilized in this study. Seventy-four percent of treated patients had stage <2 compared to 82% in control group (p = 0.82). Overall SVR was 34%. A difference in graft survival was shown for patients treated within six months of HCV recurrence (n = 40) compared to those not treated within this time period (log rank p = 0.002). **B2**

Patient survival

Two studies specifically focused on the effect of antiviral therapy on overall survival [35, 36]. Picciotto *et al*. prospectively analyzed the long-term effect of SVR on survival in 61 patients naive to treatment receiving peginterferon

(1 mcg/kg/wk) with ribavirin (600–800 mg) [35]. No patients received erythropoietin or filgrastim. Overall SVR was 28%. The group achieving SVR had an improved survival compared to those not achieving SVR ($x2 = 6.9$; $p < 0.01$). **B4** Berenguer *et al.* performed a larger study to investigate effect of antiviral therapy on survival by comparing those receiving antiviral treatment (n = 89; 31 treated with interferon and ribavirin and 58 treated with peginterferon and ribavirin) with untreated contemporary controls (n = 75) [36]. Overall SVR was 37%. At seven years after transplant, 74% of the treatment group were alive versus 62% in the control group (p = 0.04). They also saw higher five-year survival among the SVR group versus the nonresponder group, 93% versus 69%, p = 0.032). **B2**

Risk of acute cellular rejection and alloimmune hepatitis

A potentially serious and controversial complication of antiviral therapy in transplant patients is rejection. Concern exists that pegylated interferon may be associated with an increased risk of rejection because of its extended half-life. Three uncontrolled studies of pegylated interferon and ribavirin yield conflicting results, with no cases of rejection in two studies, and a rate of 25% in another [37–39]. Although rates of rejection were not significantly different in these trials, the trend for acute rejection was observed and cannot be dismissed [40]. However, controlled trials of pegylated interferon monotherapy as prophylactic therapy and for treatment of established disease showed no difference in rejection rates between treated and control patients [41]. Additionally, a recent randomized controlled trial of peginterferon and ribavirin for established disease reported no significant risk of rejection with treatment [32]. No clear association with antiviral therapy and development of chronic rejection exists. Moreover, data from the University of Colorado and other centers suggest that close monitoring of calcineurin inhibitor levels are necessary during antiviral therapy as a greater proportion of antiviral responders experienced a greater reduction in immunosuppression levels than nonresponders [42]. This is presumably due to improved hepatic function leading to enhanced biotransformation and lower immunosuppression levels [43]. This decrease in immunosuppression levels may play a key role in predisposing these patients to rejection.

Another potential complication from antiviral therapy is *de novo* autoimmune (or more appropriately alloimmune) hepatitis (AIH). Several case reports have observed patients with the development of worsening allograft function and found to have biopsy findings consistent with AIH [44–46]. The theory for this occurrence is based on the immunomodulary properties of peginterferon/interferon therapy. One case series found a positive predictive factor to be the use of anti-lymphocyte antibodies as induction for immunosuppression and protection from AIH with the use of G-CSF [45]. Unfortunately, due to small populations, it is difficult to determine the clinical significance of these findings, but AIH as a potential complication of peginterferon-based therapy cannot be dismissed. There should be a high suspicion for this condition in patients on antiviral therapy who have worsening liver enzymes in the setting of an undetectable HCV RNA. Treatment revolves around stopping antiviral therapy and modification to immunosuppression regimen.

Retransplantation for allograft cirrhosis

For patients who either fail or do not tolerate antiviral therapy, the only option for those developing allograft failure from recurrent HCV is retransplantation. Retransplantation, regardless of indication may conflict with the mandate to avoid futile transplantation in that retransplantation is associated with a 20–30% reduction in survival and 40–50% higher costs compared to primary transplantation [47]. A recent US multicenter study of retransplantation for HCV found that 30% of patients with graft failure from recurrent HCV are not considered for retransplantation and only half of those who are evaluated are eventually relisted [48]. Furthermore, of those who are eventually listed, 80% die while waiting for retransplantation. The current MELD allocation system designed to transplant the "sickest first" may not favor patients needing retransplantation [49]. In the above mentioned multicenter study, MELD scores greater than 30 were associated with poor survival following retransplantation [47].

Summary

Based on available data, treatment of established disease recurrence (moderate fibrosis; stage ≥ 2) appears to be the most efficacious approach to managing recurrent HCV. **A1d B2** The primary goal of therapy should be SVR using full dose combination therapy with peginterferon and ribavirin and utilizing growth factors if necessary to minimize dose reduction and discontinuation. If SVR is not attainable, histological and overall graft and survival benefit appears to correlate with antiviral treatment. A number of unanswered questions remain in the management of recurrent HCV. The optimal basal immunosuppressive regimen for HCV patients remains to be defined. The optimal length of antiviral therapy post-LT and role of maintenance peginterferon is not known. Given the accelerated natural history of recurrent HCV, limitations of antiviral therapy and poor outcome with retransplantation, there is an urgent need for safer and more effective therapies. New antiviral therapies currently under investigation may have a promising role in managing these difficult patients by shortening treatment course and/or improving antiviral response rates. Unfortunately these new drugs will be used in combination with peginterferon and ribavirin, thus not avoiding many of the potential side effects seen in treating patients post-transplant. Additionally, the interactions of these new medications with current immunosuppressive medication remain to be defined.

References

1 Chazouilleres O, Kim M, Combs C et al. Quantitation of hepatitis C virus RNA in liver transplant recipients. *Gastroenterology* 1994; **106**: 994–999.

2 Gane EJ, Portmann BC, Naoumov NV et al. Long-term outcome of hepatitis C infection after liver transplantation. *N Engl J Med* 1996; **334**: 815–820.

3 Berenguer M, Prieto M, Rayon JM et al. Natural history of clinically compensated HCV-related graft cirrhosis following liver transplantation. *Hepatology* 2000; **32**: 852–858.

4 Fattovich G, Giustina G, Degos F et al. Morbidity and mortality in compensated cirrhosis type C: a retrospective study of 384 patients. *Gastroenterology* 1997; **112**: 463–472.

5 Kalambokis G, Manousou P, Samonakis D et al. Clinical outcome of HCV-related graft cirrhosis and prognostic value of hepatic venous pressure gradient. *Transplant Intern* 2009; **22**: 172–181.

6 Charlton M, Wiesner RH. Natural history and management of hepatitis C infection after liver transplantation. *Semin Liver Dis* 2004; **24**: 79–88.

7 Forman LM, Lewis JD, Berlin JA et al. The association between hepatitis C infection and survival after orthotopic liver transplantation. *Gastroenterology* 2002; **122**: 889–896.

8 Wiesner RH, Sorrell M, Villamil F, International Liver Transplant Society Expert Panel. Report of the first International Liver Transplant Society expert panel consensus conference on liver transplantation and hepatic C. *Liver Transpl* 2003; **9**: S1–9.

9 Zekry A, Bishop GA, Bowen DG et al. Interhepatic cytokine profiles associated with posttransplantation hepatitis C virus-related liver injury. *Liver Transpl* 2002; **8**: 292–301.

10 McCaughan GW and Zekry A. Mechanisms of HCV Reinfection and allograft damage after liver transplantation. *J Hepatol* 2004; **40**: 368–374.

11 Gopal DV, Rosen HR. Duration of antiviral therapy for cholestatic HCV recurrence may need to be indefinite. *Liver Transpl* 2003; **9**: 348–353.

12 Charlton M, Seaberg E, Wiesner R et al. Predictors of patient and graft survival following liver transplantation for hepatitis C. *Hepatology* 1998; **28**(3): 823–830.

13 Prieto M, Berenguer M, Rayón JM et al. (1999) High incidence of allograft cirrhosis in hepatitis C virus genotype 1b infection following relationship with rejection episodes. *Hepatology* **29**(1), 250–256.

14 Neumann UP, Berg T, Bahra M et al. Long-term outcome of liver transplants for chronic hepatitis C: a 10-year follow-up. *Transplantation* 2004; **77**(2): 226–231.

15 Burton JR Jr, Rosen HR. Acute rejection in HCV-infected liver transplant recipients: The great conundrum. *Liver Transpl* 2006; **12**(11 Suppl. 2); S38–47.

16 Klintmalm GB, Washburn WK, Rudich SM et al. Corticosteroid-free immunosuppression with daclizumab in HCV(+) liver transplant recipients: 1-year interim results of the HCV-3 study. *Liver Transpl* 2007; **13**(11): 1521–1531.

17 Bahra M, Neumann UI, Jacob D et al. MMF and calcineurin taper in recurrent hepatitis C after liver transplantation: impact on histological course. *Am J Transplant* 2005; **5**(2): 406–411.

18 Berenguer M. Systematic review of the treatment of established recurrent hepatitis C with pegylated interferon in combination with ribavirin. *J Hepatol* 2008; **49**: 274–287.

19 Xirouchakis E, Triantos C, Manousou P et al. Pegylated-Interferon and ribavirin in liver transplant candidates and recipients with HCV cirrhosis: systematic review and meta-analysis of prospective controlled studies. *J Viral Hepat* 2008; **15**: 699–709.

20 Triantos C, Samonakis D, Stigliano R et al. Liver transplantation and hepatitis C virus: systematic review of antiviral therapy. *Transplantation* 2005; **79**: 261–268.

21 Terrault NA. Hepatitis C therapy before and after transplantation. *Liver Transpl* 2008; **14**(Suppl. 2): S58–66.

22 Everson GT, Trotter J, Forman L et al. Treatment of advanced hepatitis C with a low accelerating dose regimen of antiviral therapy. *Hepatology* 2005; **42**(2): 255–262.

23 Di Marco V, Almasia PL, Ferraro D et al. Peg-interferon alone or combined with ribavirin in HCV cirrhosis with portal hypertension: a randomized controlled trial. *J Hepatol* 2007; **47**(4): 484–491.

24 Helbing B, Jochum W, Stamenic I et al. HCV-related advanced fibrosis/cirrhosis: randomized controlled trial of pegylated interferon alpha-2a and ribavirin. *J Viral Hepat* 2006; **13**(11): 762–769.

25 Iacobellis A, Siciliano M, Perri F et al. Peginterferon alpha-2b and ribavirin in patients with hepatitis C virus and decompensated cirrhosis: a controlled study. *J Hepatol* 2007; **46**(2): 206–212.

26 Terrault NA. Prophylactic and preemptive therapies for hepatitis C virus-infected patients undergoing liver transplantation. *Liver Transpl* 2003; **9**: S95–100.

27 Firpi RJ, Abdelmalek MF, Soldevila-Pico C et al. One-year protocol liver biopsy can stratify fibrosis progression in liver transplant recipients with recurrent hepatitis C infection. *Liver Transpl* 2004; **10**: 1240–1247.

28 Samonakis D, Cholongitas E, Thalheimer U et al. Hepatic venous pressure gradient to assess fibrosis and its progression after liver transplantation for HCV cirrhosis. *Liver Transpl* 2007; **13**: 1305–1311.

29 Blasco A, Forns X, Carrion JA et al. Hepatic venous pressure gradient identified patients at risk of severe hepatic C recurrence after liver transplantation. *Hepatology* 2006; **43**: 492–499.

30 Castells L, Vargas V, Allende H et al. Combined treatment with pegylated interferon (alpha-2b) and ribavirin in the acute phase of hepatitis C virus recurrence after liver transplantation. *J Hepatol* 2005; **43**(1): 53–59.

31 Bizollon T, Pradat P, Mabrut JY et al. Histological benefit of retreatment by pegylated interferon alpha-2b and ribavirin in patients with recurrent hepatitis C virus infection post-transplantation. *Am J Transplant* 2007; **7**(2): 448–453.

32 Carrion JA, Navasa M, Garcia-Retortillo M *et al*. Efficacy of antiviral therapy on hepatitis C recurrence after liver transplantation: a randomized controlled study. *Gastroenterology* 2007; **132**(5): 1746–1756.

33 Bizollon T, Pradat P, Mabrut JY *et al*. Benefit of sustained virological response to combination therapy on graft survival of liver transplanted patients with recurrent chronic hepatitis C. *Am J Transplant* 2005; **5**: 1909–1913.

34 Veldt BJ, Poterucha JJ, Watt KD *et al*. Impact of pegylated interferon and ribavirin treatment on graft survival in liver transplant patients with recurrent hepatitis C infection. *Am J Transplant* 2008; **8**: 679–687.

35 Picciotto FP, Tritto G, Lanza AG *et al*. Sustained virological response to antiviral therapy reduces mortality in HCV reinfection after liver transplantation. *J Hepatol* 2007; **46**: 459–465.

36 Berenguer M, Palau A, Aguilera V *et al*. Clinical benefits of antiviral therapy in patients with recurrent hepatitis C following liver transplantation. *Am J Transplant* 2008; **8**: 679–687.

37 Oton E, Barcena R, Garcia-Garzon S *et al*. Pegylated interferon and ribavirin for the recurrence of chronic hepatitis C genotype 1 in transplant patients. *Transpl Proc* 2005; **37**: 3963–3964.

38 Biselli M, Andreone P, Gramenzi A *et al*. Pegylated interferon plus ribavirin for recurrent hepatitis C infection after liver transplantation in naïve and non-responder patients on a stable immunosuppressive regimen. *Dig Liver Dis* 2006; **38**(1): 27–32.

39 Dumortier J, Scoazec JY, Chevallier P *et al*. Treatment of recurrent hepatitis C after liver transplantation; a pilot study of peginterferon alfa-2b and ribavirin combination. *J Hepatol* 2004; **40**(4): 669–674.

40 Samuel D. Antiviral treatment of recurrent hepatitis C after liver transplantation: The need for a multifaceted approach. *Hepatol* 2005; **41**(3); 436–438.

41 Chalasani N, Manzarbeitia C, Ferenci P *et al*. Peginterferon alfa-2a for hepatitis C after liver transplantation: two randomized, controlled trials. *Hepatology* 2005; **41**: 289–298.

42 Oo YH, Dudley T, Nightingale P *et al*. Tacrolimus and cyclosporine doses and blood levels in hepatitis C and alcoholic liver disease patients after liver transplantation. *Liver Transpl* 2008; **14**: 81–87.

43 Kugelmas M, Osgood MJ, Trotter JF *et al*. Hepatitis C virus therapy, hepatocyte drug metabolism, and risk for acute cellular rejection. *Liver Transpl* 2003; **9**: 1159–1165.

44 Cholongitas E, Samonakis D, Patch D *et al*. (2006) Induction of autoimmune hepatitis by pegylated interferon in a liver transplant patient with recurrent hepatitis C virus. *Transplant* 2006; **81**(3): 488–490.

45 Berardi S, Lodato F, Gramenzi A *et al*. High incidence of allograft dysfunction in liver transplanted patients treated with pegylated-interferon alpha-2b and ribavirin for hepatitis C recurrence: possible de novo autoimmune hepatitis? *Gut* 2007; **56**: 237–242.

46 Fiel MI, Agarwal K, Stanca C *et al*. Post-transplant plasma cell hepatitis (de novo autoimmune hepatitis) is a variant of rejection and may lead to a negative outcome in patients with hepatitis C virus. *Liver Transpl* 2008; **14**(6): 861–871.

47 Azoulay D, Linhares MM, Guguet E *et al*. Decision for retransplantation of the liver: an experience- and cost-based analysis. *Ann Surg* 2002; **236**: 713–721.

48 McCashland T, Watt K, Lyden E *et al*. (2007) Retransplantation for hepatitis C: results of a U.S. multicenter retransplant study. *Liver Transpl* 2007; **13**: 1247–1253.

49 Burton JR Jr, Sonnenberg A, Rosen HR. Retransplantation for recurrent hepatitis C in the MELD era: maximizing utility. *Liver Transpl* 2004; **10**: S59–64.

45 Management of HBV infection and liver transplantation

Evangelos Cholongitas[1] *and George V Papatheodoridis*[2]

[1] The Royal Free Sheila Sherlock Liver Centre, Royal Free Hospital *and* University College London, London, UK
[2] Department of Internal Medicine, Athens University Medical School, Hippokration General Hospital, Athens, Greece

Hepatitis B virus (HBV) related chronic liver disease is a frequent indication for orthotopic liver transplantation (LT) in the Far East and the Mediterranean countries. Post-transplant HBV recurrence, which was almost universal in the era of no immunoprophylaxis or its short-term use, usually has an aggressive course resulting in graft loss, if left untreated [1–3]. Therefore, the HBV management is crucial for a satisfactory long-term outcome of HBV transplant patients.

HBV related liver disease was considered to be a relative or even absolute contraindication for LT in many centers, until the introduction of long-term hepatitis B immune globulin (HBIG) use in the early 1990s, which significantly decreased the post-transplant HBV recurrence rate and improved prognosis in this setting [4]. During the last decade, new antivirals, mainly nucleos(t)ide analogues, have been used, either as monotherapy or in combination with HBIG, in an effort to further improve the post-transplant outcome, treat HBIG failures, and/or reduce the need for the expensive HBIG preparations [5]. The HBV management in transplant patients can be divided into the pre-transplant, prophylactic post-transplant and therapeutic post-transplant approach [5]. In addition, the management of recipients who receive grafts from anti-HBc positive donors is discussed, as these recipients are at risk of iatrogenic HBV infection.

Pre-transplant approach

The pre-transplant approach is based on antiviral therapy in order to lower the viral load and achieve serum HBV-DNA undetectability by sensitive assays at the time of LT and thus to prevent post-transplant HBV recurrence [5]. Sometimes, the clinical improvement of HBV patients on the waiting list during or following effective antiviral therapy may even result in postponement or obviate the need for LT. Only two oral agents, lamivudine and adefovir dipivoxil, are currently licensed for use in patients with either chronic hepatitis B (CHB) or HBV decompensated cirrhosis, while three additional oral agents, entecavir, telbivudine and tenofovir disoproxil fumarate have been licensed for the treatment of CHB but not of HBV decompensated cirrhosis as yet. Interferon-alfa, which was the only available anti-HBV therapeutic option until the late 1990s, is usually contraindicated or causes intolerance and therefore cannot be used in patients with decompensated cirrhosis. The pre-transplant approach is usually combined with prophylactic post-transplant therapy [5].

Lamivudine

Lamivudine, a cytosine analogue, was the first agent that could be widely used in the pre-transplant period revolutionizing the management of such patients. Lamivudine is generally well tolerated even in severely ill cirrhotics and has a good safety profile with rare and generally mild side effects. Lamivudine, at a daily dose of 100 mg, has been shown to stabilize or even improve liver function sometimes resulting in withdrawal of patients from transplant lists [6, 7]. **B4** Unfortunately, the improvement or stabilization of liver function is often not sustained over time, since the prolongation of lamivudine therapy is associated with progressively increasing rates of lamivudine resistance often followed by virologic and biochemical breakthroughs [6, 7]. **B4** Lamivudine resistance is usually associated with the emergence of a mutation at position 204 within the YMDD motif of the major catalytic region C of the HBV polymerase gene (substitution of methionine with valine (rtM204V) or with isoleucine (rtM204I)), often in combination with another mutation at position 180 within the region B (substitution of leucine with methionine (rtL180M))

Evidence-Based Gastroenterology and Hepatology, 3rd edition.
J. McDonald, A.K. Burroughs, B. Feagan, and M.B. Fennerty. © 2010
Blackwell Publishing Ltd

[8]. Lamivudine resistance usually emerges after the first six months with cumulative rates of 15–25% at the end of first year and >60–65% at the end of fourth year of lamivudine therapy [9].

Breakthroughs during lamivudine therapy have a risk for severe exacerbation of liver disease, which may result in rapid development of liver failure and patient death [10]. Moreover, pre-transplant HBV viremia even when due to YMDD mutants has been associated with increased probability of post-transplant HBV recurrence [11, 12], poorer outcome after LT and lower hepatocellular carcinoma (HCC) recurrence-free post-transplant survival in patients with HCC before LT [13]. Thus, transplant centers may be reluctant to perform LT in HBV cirrhotics with viremia irrespective of the type of HBV strains [14]. Another important issue is that the emergence of lamivudine resistance may have a negative impact on the efficacy of and the probability of resistance to other anti-HBV agents [9]. For all these reasons, lamivudine monotherapy is no longer considered an appropriate first-line therapy for pre-transplant HBV patients. **B4**

Adefovir

The availability of adefovir, an acyclic nucleotide analogue of adenosine esterified with two pivalic acid molecules that is effective against both wild and lamivudine resistant HBV strains, was initially used in order to ameliorate the consequences of lamivudine resistance [9]. The use of adefovir monotherapy as first-line treatment in HBV-pretransplant patients has not been adequately evaluated. In CHB, adefovir monotherapy is associated with lower rates of resistance compared to lamivudine, but resistance may emerge in the second year and develop in up to 30% of cases treated with adefovir for five years [15]. Adefovir resistance is related to the emergence of a mutation at position 236 (substitution of asparagine with threonine, (rtN236T)) and/or at position 181 (substitution of alanine with valine or threonine (rtA181V or rtA181T)) of the HBV polymerase gene [16]. Another issue with adefovir monotherapy is that this agent, at least in the licensed 10 mg daily dose, is not very potent, resulting in residual viremia in approximately 80% of HBeAg-positive and 50% of HBeAg-negative CHB patients [9]. In addition, it may have some potential for nephrotoxicity. For these reasons, adefovir monotherapy was not considered as an attractive option for patients with HBV decompensated cirrhosis, in whom complete inhibition of viral replication should be achieved [17]. Because of the suboptimal profile of both lamivudine and adefovir monotherapy in HBV pre-transplant patients, *ab initio* use of lamivudine and adefovir combination has been recommended for such cases in several guidelines, despite the lack of strong data on efficacy and safety for such a strategy [18]. **B4**

Entecavir

Entecavir, a carboxylic analogue of guanosine, is a potent and selective anti-HBV agent that has been approved relatively recently for the treatment of CHB [9]. In nucleos(t)ide naive patients with HBeAg-positive or HBeAg-negative CHB, entecavir (0.5 mg daily) has greater potency than lamivudine and adefovir and a very good resistance profile with <2% cumulative five-year resistance rate [9, 19]. Entecavir was also reported to have the same good efficacy and safety profile in the subgroup of naive patients with advanced fibrosis or cirrhosis [20]. Given the absence of nephrotoxicity and its overall good safety profile in combination with the high efficacy and low resistance risk, entecavir is expected to be a first-line option for the treatment of nucleos(t)ide naive patients with HBV decompensated cirrhosis. It should be noted, however, that entecavir is not yet approved for the treatment of such patients, as relevant data are lacking.

Telbivudine

Telbivudine, another nucleoside analogue (L-deoxythymidine) that was approved recently for the treatment of CHB, is more potent than lamivudine but it also selects for mutations in the YMDD motif similar to those conferring lamivudine resistance (mainly rtM204I) [9]. In nucleos(t)ide naive CHB patients, telbivudine resistance starts to emerge within the first year (sixth to twelfth month) and increases during the second year of therapy. The telbivudine resistance rates were 4.4% and 2.7% at the end of first year and 21.6% and 8.6% at the end of the second year of therapy in HBeAg-positive and HBeAg-negative CHB respectively [21]. The absence of residual viremia (HBV-DNA < 400 copies/ml) at six months of telbivudine therapy is associated with low two-year probability of resistance [9]. Given its unfavourable resistance profile compared to other anti-HBV agents such as entecavir and tenofovir, the place of telbivudine monotherapy in the treatment of HBV pre-transplant patients will be unclear, even if the agent is approved for use in this setting.

Tenofovir

Tenofovir, the second acyclic nucleotide analogue of adenosine, is the most recently approved agent for the treatment of CHB. It is administered orally as tenofovir disoproxil fumarate, which is a prodrug with good oral availability and is a potent agent for the treatment of both nucleos(t)ide naive and lamivudine resistant CHB [22–24]. Tenofovir has not been licensed for treatment of decompensated cirrhosis, but there are a few case reports with successful tenofovir use in such cases [25]. However, since tenofovir may be potentially nephrotoxic, both its efficacy and safety should be tested in proper trials before its wide use in pre-transplant patients. To date, there is no evidence of resistance in CHB patients treated with tenofovir for 72 weeks, but more long-term data are lacking [22–24]. **B4** Due to the great potency and the possible high genetic barrier of this agent, long-term tenofovir resistance rates are expected to be low. If its safety in decompensated cirrhosis is confirmed, tenofovir will be a first-line option for the treatment of nucleos(t)ide naive patients with HBV decompensated cirrhosis. Thus, the results of a current trial, in which tenofovir, entecavir and tenofovir plus emtricitabine are compared in patients with HBV decompensated cirrhosis, are awaited.

Management of HBV resistance

Patients with decompensated cirrhosis under antivirals should be monitored carefully for virologic response and possible virologic breakthroughs, with serum HBV-DNA testing at least every three months [18]. In CHB, any virologic breakthrough (increase in serum HBV-DNA by $\geq 1 \log_{10}$ iu/ml above nadir after an early virological response) is considered in practice as viral resistance, if drug compliance is confirmed [18]. **B4** In decompensated cirrhosis, however, stricter criteria of response should be applied and any detectable viremia should be considered as a treatment failure, regardless of resistance and breakthroughs, signalling the need for treatment modification.

Lamivudine resistance represents the most common problem of HBV resistance because of the longer use and the poor resistance profile of lamivudine. Adefovir was the first agent used as rescue therapy for lamivudine resistance. The addition of adefovir to ongoing lamivudine therapy instead of the substitution of lamivudine with adefovir is the preferred option for lamivudine resistant CHB [9]. In pre-transplant HBV cirrhotic patients with lamivudine resistance, the addition of adefovir results in biochemical, virologic and liver function improvement [26, 27]. In particular, in a large study with 226 HBV patients on the waiting list with lamivudine resistance, the addition of adefovir achieved HBV-DNA undetectability in 59% of cases, without adefovir resistance during the first 48 weeks [27]. **B4** Moreover, alanine aminotransferase (ALT), albumin, bilirubin and prothrombin time normalized in 77%, 76%, 60% and 84% of the 226 patients respectively [27]. Despite the addition of adefovir, however, a significant proportion of patients (41% at 48 weeks and 35% at 96 weeks) maintained detectable serum HBV-DNA, which is not an acceptable result for current day practice.

Entecavir monotherapy (1 mg daily ≥ 2 hours before or after meals) has worse potency and higher resistance rates in lamivudine resistant than naive patients [9]. In particular, the cumulative entecavir resistance rate has been reported to be 6%, 15%, 36%, 46% and 51% at year 1, 2, 3,

4 and 5 years of entecavir therapy respectively [19]. **B4** Entecavir resistance requires selection of two lamivudine resistant mutations (rtM204V/I and rtL180M) and at least one additional substitution at positions 169, 173, 184, 202 or 250 of the HBV polymerase gene (rtI169T, rtV173L, rtT184G, rtS202I or rtM250V) [28]. Thus, entecavir resistance requires three mutations in nucleoside naive patients and only one additional mutation in patients with pre-existing lamivudine resistance. These findings have made entecavir a less attractive long-term therapeutic option for HBV patients with lamivudine resistance [9]. As there is cross-resistance between lamivudine and telbivudine, telbivudine is not expected to be effective in lamivudine resistant patients.

Tenofovir is effective against lamivudine resistant strains and is a more potent anti-HBV agent compared to adefovir [29]. Therefore, it is currently expected to become the treatment of choice for patients with lamivudine resistance. Whether switching to tenofovir or addition of tenofovir to ongoing lamivudine is the optimal and the more cost-effective approach for using tenofovir in patients with lamivudine resistance is not yet clear [29]. However, it seems safer to add in tenofovir considering the experience gained with adefovir, particularly in patients with decompensated cirrhosis.

There are no clear data for the treatment of patients with resistance to other anti-HBV agents, particularly in pre-transplant patients. Generally, resistance to an agent of one class (nucleosides: lamivudine, entecavir, telbivudine; nucleotides: adefovir, tenofovir) usually eliminates or reduces the activity of other agents of the same class due to partial or complete cross-resistance. This is well documented for lamivudine, telbivudine and entecavir, but it seems to be also the case, at least partly, for adefovir and tenofovir. Thus, in case of resistance to a nucleoside, a reasonable approach would be to add a nucleotide and vice versa. In particular in pre-transplant patients, in whom complete inhibition of HBV replication is absolutely desirable, entecavir and tenofovir (the most potent agent of each class) are expected to become the agents of choice, whenever approved. Of course, the most effective treatment of resistance is its prevention by starting treatment with agents that are potent and have a high genetic barrier [28].

Prophylactic post-transplant approach

Immunoprophylaxis alone

The efficacy of HBIG is associated with the pre-transplant type of liver disease (e.g. fulminant HBV infection, HBV and HDV co-infection) [30], viremic status and dose and duration of HBIG treatment, while the most widely accepted recommendations for HBIG prophylaxis depend mainly on the pre-transplant viremic status [31]. Patients with detectable HBV-DNA by conventional hybridization assays, who may be transplanted only after clearance of HBV-DNA by lamivudine, are treated with more aggressive HBIG protocols compared to non-viremic patients [31, 32]. **B4** However, several practical questions about the ideal duration, but also about dosage, frequency and mode of HBIG administration remain to be answered [5].

HBIG may only rarely lead to eradication of HBV and therefore there is need for indefinite HBIG prophylaxis, which is an extremely expensive approach. The most cost-effective approach seems to be the individual tailoring of HBIG administration according to serum anti-HBs levels [5, 31], which is time-consuming [30]. Cheaper HBIG preparations for intramuscular administration have also been tried [33–35], as they have similar pharmacokinetic properties with intravenous preparations [36]. Interestingly, subcutaneous HBIG administration is under investigation, but no relevant long-term data are currently available [37].

Besides the high cost, long-term HBIG administration may also have some local or systemic side effects, while there is a progressively increasing risk of escape HBV mutants [8, 31]. Since the clinical significance of such HBV escape mutants has not been clarified, there is no consensus about continuation of HBIG therapy, or not, after their emergence [31], but most centers probably stop HBIG administration [5].

Another strategy aiming at cost reduction has been the substitution of HBIG with HBV vaccination. However, data on the efficacy of vaccination are rather conflicting and therefore greater numbers of patients and longer follow-up periods are required before definite conclusions can be drawn [38–42].

Prophylactic post-transplant monotherapy with nucleos(t)ides analogues

Lamivudine monotherapy, before and prophylactically after LT, gave promising short-term results [5]. However, it was subsequently shown that the efficacy of such a policy declines over time with frequent development of virologic breakthroughs and HBV recurrence in 35–50% of cases at two years post-transplant and severe clinical outcomes in some patients [43–48]. Thus, such an approach has been abandoned not only in liver transplant but also in HBsAg-positive renal allograft recipients.

There are no studies on the efficacy of monoprophylaxis with the newer nucleos(t)ides analogues. However, based on the data in pre-transplant setting, it is expected that adefovir monoprophylaxis will also be associated with emergence of adefovir-resistant mutants in post-transplant patients. Entecavir, which is a more potent agent with very

low resistance rates in nucleoside naive cases and without risk for nephrotoxicity, seems to be a more attractive option for monoprophylaxis in post-transplant patients. However, entecavir should be avoided in patients with previous lamivudine resistance, which should preferably be treated with adefovir or tenofovir. Tenofovir is more potent and cheaper than adefovir having better resistance profile, but its use may also have a risk for renal dysfunction, particularly in patients receiving nephrotoxic immunosuppressive therapy. Finally, telbivudine monotherapy has moderate resistance rate and therefore does not seem to be a good option for post-transplant patients. Thus, entecavir seems the most attractive monoprophylaxis option in the post-LT HBV setting, followed by tenofovir, particularly in cases with previous lamivudine resistance. However, well-designed studies are needed to determine the optimal monoprophylaxis approach, if any. For now, the combination of HBIG (at least for a short period) and one nucleos(t)ide appears to be the most reasonable post-transplant approach, but monoprophylaxis with one of the new nucleos(t)ide analogues cannot be excluded in the future, particularly in patients with low risk of recurrence.

Prophylactic post-transplant combined approach

Post-transplant prophylactic combination of HBIG and lamivudine was tried in order to improve the efficacy of post-transplant prophylaxis and/or reduce cost. The efficacy of such a combined regimen has been shown to be superior compared to the efficacy of prophylaxis with any of the two agents alone. A recent meta-analysis of six studies showed that HBIG plus lamivudine, compared to HBIG alone, was associated with 12-fold, 12-fold and 5-fold reduction of HBV recurrence, HBV-related death and all-cause post-transplant mortality respectively [49]. **A1a** In 36 studies of HBIG and lamivudine combination identified in the literature, post-transplant HBV recurrence was observed in only 95 (6.3%) of 1493 patients during a mean follow-up of 6–96 months (see Table 45.1) [12, 13, 32–34, 48, 50–79]. It should be noted that 11 of the 95 patients with post-transplant HBV recurrence had developed YMDD mutants during pre-transplant lamivudine therapy [12, 48, 57, 64, 68, 69, 76], while HBIG and/or LAM had been discontinued when HBV recurrence occurred in another 19 patients [51, 54, 57, 71, 75]. One particularly important aspect in favor of the combined HBIG and lamivudine prophylaxis is that such an approach was used in patients with high pre-transplant viremia levels (>50% of cases had HBV-DNA detectable by hybridization assays) and achieved low HBV reinfection rates at a reduced cost. Moreover, a relatively low HBIG dosage [12, 33, 34, 58, 63, 66, 67], similar to the recommended dosage for non-viremic HBV transplant patients [31], and/or intramuscular HBIG

Table 45.1 Published studies using combination of hepatitis B immune globulin (HBIG) and lamivudine (LAM) for prevention of hepatitis B virus (HBV) recurrence after liver transplantation (LT) for HBV related chronic liver disease.

Study First author, year	Patients, n	Post-LT HBIG dose (IU), (cumulative within first month (mo)) – after the first mo	Mean follow-up, mos	HBV recurrence, n (%)	Survival (%)
Markowitz, 1998 [66]	14	(80,000) – 10,000/mo IV	13	0	93
Yao, 1999 [33]	10	(15,555[a]) – 1111/3 weeks (wks) IM	16	1 (10)	90
Yoshida, 1999 [34]	7	(34,720) – 2170/1–4 wks IM	18	1 (14)	86
McCaughan, 1999 [65]	9	Low dose (no details)	17	0	89
Roche, 1999 [64]	15	No details-anti-HBs > 500 iu/l	16	1 (7)	93
Angus, 2000 [63]	32	(3200–6400) – 400 or 800/mo IM	18	1 (3)	100[b]
Han, 2000 [62]	59	(80,000) – 10,000/mo IV	15	0	98
Lee, 2000 [61]	5	(26,000) – 2000/mo IV[c]	11	0	80
Andreone, 2000 [60]	19	(45,000) – 5000/mo IV	17	1 (5)	95
Rosenau, 2001 [12]	21	(40,000-anti-HBs > 500 iu/l) – anti-HBs > 100 iu/l IV	20	2 (10)	90
Machicao, 2001 [59]	30	High dose	22	0	97
Choi, 2002 [58]	56	(10,000) – 10,000/mo IV x mos[d] – 2000/2 mos IM	26	4 (7)	NA
Kim, 2002 [57]	51	(80,000) – 10,000/mo IV x 6/12 mos	21	4 (8)	NA.
Chu, 2002 [56]	8	(10,000) – 10,000/mo IV x 43 mos – 1000/mo IM x 12 mos	16[e]	0	100
Honaker, 2002 [55]	9	(80,000–100,000 IV) – 10,000–40,000/1 – 2 mos IV	50	0	100
Anselmo, 2002 [54]	89	(80,000 IV) – 10000/mo IV after 1998: (22,000 IV) – 1560 iu IM – anti-HBs	NA	10 (11)	94 (1 year)
Sousa, 2003 [53]	10	(70,000 IV) – 10,000/mo IV first year (10,000 IV every 2 mos second to third year, then 10,000 IV every 3–4 mos)	30.1	0	100
Dumortier, 2003 [52]	17	(100,000 IV) – 10,000 IM/1 – 2 mos – anti-HBs	30	0	80 (5 years)
Ferretti, 2004 [51]	28	(40,000–80,000 IV) – 1200 IM/2–6 wks	20	1 (3.5)	83
Karasu, 2004 [50]	80	(4000 IV – 2000–8000 IM) – IM (anti-HBs)	21	3 (4%)	85 (1 year)
Neff , 2004 [32]	41	(130,000 IV) – 10,000 IV/mo x 6 mos	49[f]	5 (12)[f]	80[f]
Marzano, 2005 [67]	77	(50,000 IV) – 6000 IV/mo	39	4 (5)	96
Zheng, 2006 [48]	114	(7200 IM) – 800 IM/mo	54	16 (14)	95
Karaderim, 2006 [68]	35	(4000 IV + 2000 IM/day for anti-HBs > 200–100 iu/ml)	15	2 (20)	86
Nath, 2006 [69]	14	(80,000 IV (within first 7 days))	14	1 (7)[g]	100
Gane, 2006 [70]	147[h]	(5600 IM within first wk) – 800 IM/mo	62	5 (4)	92 (1 year)
Yoshida, 2007 [71]	34	(120,000 IV) – 10,000 IV/mo x ≥ 6 mos	54	3 (9)	68
Jiao, 2007 [72]	56	(10,000 IM) – 400–1200/1–4 wks IM	32	3 (5)	91
Neff, 2007 [73]	10	(140,000 IV) – 10,000 IV/mo x ≥ 6 mos	6.5	0	100
Zimmerman, 2007 [13]	77	Before 1998: (80,000 IV (within 7 days)) – 10,000 IV/mo After 1998: (22,000 IV (within 6 days)) – IM (anti-HBs)	48	12 (15)	75
Akyildiz, 2007 [74]	209	(8000–36,000 IV/IM) – anti-HBs	18	11 (5)	100

Table 45.1 Continued

Study First author, year	Patients, n	Post-LT HBIG dose (IU), (cumulative within first month (mo)) – after the first mo	Mean follow-up, mos	HBV recurrence, n (%)	Survival (%)
Buti, 2007 [75]	29	(62,000 IV) – 2000/mo IV (x1 mo)/IM	83	4 (13)	90
Takaki, 2007 [76]	23	(10,500 IV within first wk) – anti-HBs > 100 iu/ml for first 6 mos – anti-HBs > 10 iu/l	30	0[i]	NA
Freshwater, 2008 [77]	24	(25,000 IV (within 3 days)) – 5000 IV for anti-HBs > 100 IU/ml	32	0[j]	NA
Yilmaz, 2008 [78]	16	(17,500–20,500 IV (within 5–7 days) – 1500 IM/3–5 wks	96	0	85
Angus, 2008 [79]	18	(2100–5600 IM) – 400 or 800/mo IM	21.8	0	100

NA: not available.

[a] Plus 70,000 IV during the first seven days in two HBV-DNA positive patients.

[b] Five patients, who died within one month after LT from unrelated to HBV causes, were not included in this survival estimation.

[c] One patient received 80,000 IU of HBIG during the first month, while another patient received only 2000 IU of HBIG during the anhepatic phase and four IM injections of 650 iu each within the first six months after LT.

[d] Thirteen patients received higher HBIG dosage (10,000 IU IV daily for seven days, 10,000 IU IV weekly for one month, and then 10,000 iu IV monthly for several years before conversion to IM HBIG.

[e] Post-transplant LAM was added when HBIG administration changed from IV to IM (16 months median follow-up after the onset of LAM).

[f] No HBV recurrence in 18 patients with undetectable pre-LT HBV-DNA during 70 months of follow-up.

[g] All patients received LAM plus adefovir (10 mg/day) from day 8.

[h] No patient with YMDD mutants.

[i] Two patients had transiently positive HBsAg (one was under adefovir due to LAM resistance pre-LT).

[j] One patient had detectable HBV-DNA (YMDD mutants), but none had clinical HBV recurrence.

preparations were usually used [13, 33, 34, 48, 50, 51, 58, 70, 72, 75, 79], or HBIG was even discontinued after a certain period [56, 57, 69, 73]. Therefore, the prophylactic post-transplant combination of HBIG and lamivudine preceded by short-term pre-transplant anti-HBV therapy is the currently recommended approach [5]. **B4** In the near future, the newer nucleos(t)ides analogues are expected to replace lamivudine in the post-transplant prophylaxis as well, probably leading to use even less HBIG.

The optimal post-transplant prophylaxis for patients who develop YMDD mutants in the pre-transplant period might be different than that for patients without such HBV strains. In total, seven studies have focused on patients with YMDD mutans pre-LT showing that only 4.2% (6/143) of patients developed post-OLT HBV recurrence during a mean follow-up of 19–36 months (see Table 45.2) [27, 67, 77, 80–83]. **B4** The triple combination of HBIG, lamivudine and adefovir was used in most patients (55% of 134 cases) with available data [73], while fewer (45%) were treated with HBIG plus lamivudine or HBIG plus adefovir or adefovir plus lamivudine. Of the six cases with post-LT HBV recurrence, two developed in patients under HBIG plus lamivudine and adefovir and four in patients under HBIG plus lamivudine (two had stopped HBIG and two did not receive adefovir pre-transplant and transplanted with

HBV-DNA > 5 $\log_{10}$ copies/ml) [27, 67]. Tenofovir instead of adefovir is expected to offer better results in this setting. The *ab initio* use of potent antivirals with a high genetic barrier is definitely preferred in the transplant setting and particularly in cases with pre-existing evidence of viral resistance, as the risk of multi-drug resistance is higher than in non-transplant cases [84].

One relatively recent strategy of the prophylactic combined approach has been the withdrawal of HBIG administration after a certain period followed by maintenance lamivudine alone [85]. The first results of two small randomized trials were encouraging, with no HBV recurrence after 12–17 months under lamivudine monoprophylaxis [86, 87]. However, longer follow-up showed that 20% of patients eventually experienced recurrence of HBV at seven years [75], which might have been related to poor compliance [75], or premature discontinuation of HBIG [86]. **B4** Indeed, HBV recurrence was not observed in any of 16 patients who continuously received HBIG for two years and then switched over to lamivudine monotherapy for an additional period of up to 27 months [88]. The latter findings were confirmed by a more recent retrospective study with median follow-up of 40 months after HBIG discontinuation [89]. These data suggest that the combination of HBIG plus lamivudine might be replaced by

Table 45.2 Published studies using combination of adefovir (ADV) and lamivudine (LAM) and hepatitis B immune globulin (HBIG) for prevention of hepatitis B virus (HBV) recurrence after liver transplantation (LT) for HBV related chronic liver disease in patients who had developed lamivudine resistance pre-LT.

Study First author, year	Patients, n	Patients under HBIG, n	Patients under LAM/ LAM+ADV, n/n	Mean follow-up, months (mos)	HBV recurrence, n (%)	Survival (%)
Marzano, 2005 [67]	22	22[a]	11/11[b]	35	4 (18)[c]	96
Lo, 2005 [80]	16	8[d]	0/16	21	0	94
Caccamo, 2005 [81]	17	17	17/0	32	0	91 (1 year)
Schiff, 2007 [27]	57	34	0/57	9	2 (3.5)[e]	87
Yang, 2007 [82]	16	16	0/16	19	0[f]	94
Osborn, 2007 [83]	9	9	NA/NA	25	0	78
Freshwater, 2008 [77]	6	6	0/6	7	0	NA

NA: not available.

[a] Two patients discontinued HBIG.

[b] HBIG+ADV+LAM in 11/13 patients with phenotypic LAM-resistance (HBV-DNA > 10^5 copies/ml) and HBIG+LAM in 9/9 with genotypic LAM resistance (detected retrospectively) and 2/13 with phenotypic LAM-resistance.

[c] 2/13 patients under HBIG+LAM (transplanted with HBV-DNA > 10^5 copies/ml and without ADV pre-LT) and 2/9 patients under HBIG+LAM (the two cases who discontinued HBIG).

[d] HBIG for 9–59 mos post-LT.

[e] 2/34 patients under HBIG+LAM+ADV.

[f] One patient had detectable HBV-DNA but negative HBsAg at six months post-LT. not available.

lamivudine monotherapy after ≥ 24 months post-transplant in selected HBV transplant patients with low risk of HBV recurrence, although stronger data are needed before the wide use of such a strategy. **B4**

Given the poor resistance profile of lamivudine monotherapy, the replacement of HBIG and lamivudine combination with lamivudine and adefovir combination after the first few post-OLT months was also evaluated [73, 79, 90]. In the first relevant randomized study, 34 patients under low-dose intramuscular HBIG plus lamivudine for ≥12 months were randomized to continue the same treatment or switch to adefovir plus lamivudine [79]. At a median of 21 months post-switch, there was no case of disease recurrence (one patient in the switch group became HBsAg positive but remained HBV-DNA negative), while the switch approach was associated with substantially lower cost and better patient quality of life [79]. **A1d** In another recent study, 19 patients who were under adefovir plus lamivudine before LT, received low dose intramuscular HBIG, lamivudine and adefovir for only one week post-LT, followed by adefovir plus lamivudine without any case of HBV recurrence after 12 months of follow-up [90]. However, larger studies with longer follow-up are needed for definitive conclusions about this approach. Finally, the use of newer, more potent antivirals, such as entecavir or tenofovir, in order to early and safely discontinue HBIG certainly deserves to be evaluated.

Therapeutic post-transplant approach

Therapeutic post-transplant approach is used in cases with HBV recurrence despite previous post-transplant prophylaxis. Given the immunosuppressive therapy taken by all post-transplant patients, the high levels of HBV replication and the risk for rapid progression of liver disease in such cases, the primary targets of treatment of post-transplant HBV recurrence are the control of liver disease and stabilization of graft function [5]. Generally, the principles of treatment in post-transplant HBV recurrence resemble those in the pre-transplant setting. In the pre-lamivudine era, interferon-alfa was a common option, but now its role has almost disappeared due to both low efficacy and low but possible theoretic risk of graft rejection [5]. Lamivudine has been frequently used in cases with recurrence despite HBIG prophylaxis, but it will be inactive in cases with lamivudine resistance [5]. Again, the main disadvantage of long-term lamivudine monotherapy is the progressively increasing rates of resistance exceeding 50% at three-years of therapy in transplant patients [91–95]. The emergence of such HBV mutants is associated with rapid development of advanced histologic lesions and even liver failure and death in some HBV transplant patients [94, 96, 97]. Thus, lamivudine is not an appropriate option for the treatment of HBV transplant patients. **B4**

Table 45.3 Published studies of adefovir (ADV) therapy for hepatitis B virus (HBV) recurrence HBV infection after liver transplantation (LT) in patients who developed LAM resistance post-LT.

Study First author, year	Patients, n	Baseline serum HBV-DNA (+), n (%)	Baseline HBeAg (+), n (%)	Mean duration of ADV (mos)	Clearance of serum HBV-DNA, n (%) Hybridization-PCR	Clearance of HBeAg, n (%)	Clearance of HBsAg, n (%)
Beckebaum, 2003 [98]	1	1 (100)	1 (100)	15[a]	0	0	0
Chan, 2004 [47]	6	6 (100)	NA	20[b]	NA	NA	NA
Akay, 2004 [99]	2	2 (100)	NA	4[a]	2 (100)	NA	1 (50)
Neff, 2004 [32]	9	9 (100)	7 (77)	30.8[a]	3 (33)	4 (44)	3 (33)
Wai, 2004 [100]	4	4 (100)	NA	24[c]	0.	NA	NA
Toniutto, 2004 [101]	1	1 (100)	0	2[a]	1	NA	NA
Bacerna, 2005 [102]	42	42 (100)	30 (71.4)	21.5	27 (64)	6 (14)	4 (9.5)
Akyildiz, 2006 [74]	11	9 (81)	NA	14[c]	7 (77)	NA	NA
Schiff, 2007 [27]	241	NA	132 (69)	36[a]	35/45 (78)	29/50 (58) (8 months)	NA

NA: not available.

[a] LAM plus ADV.

[b] ADV plus LAM in 1, LAM plus famiciclovir followed by ADV in one, LAM plus famiciclovir in one and LAM alone in three patients.

[c] ADV monotherapy.

Adefovir added to ongoing lamivudine therapy has been shown to be effective in transplant patients with lamivudine resistance, achieving significant improvements of serum HBV-DNA and transaminases levels (see Table 45.3) [27, 32, 47, 74, 98–102]. In the largest study, including 241 patients with lamivudine-resistant recurrent HBV infection, the addition of adefovir achieved HBV-DNA undetectability in >95% of cases (94% with HBIG and 100% without HBIG administration) with a cumulative resistance probability of 2% at 144 weeks (see Table 45.3) [27]. **B4** Tenofovir has also been reported to be effective in patients with post-transplant HBV re-infection and lamivudine resistance [32]. Since tenofovir is more potent and has a better therapeutic ratio compared to adefovir, it is expected to become the nucleotide of choice for such post-transplant patients. Entecavir might be also used in patients with post-transplant HBV re-infection because of its great potency, high genetic barrier and absence of nephrotoxicity, particularly in cases without lamivudine resistance. Entecavir has been tried in some transplant patients with adefovir [103] and lamivudine resistance [104], but the high probability of resistance with long-term entecavir in non-transplant patients with lamivudine resistance discourages its use in similar post-transplant cases [19].

Anti-HBc positive donors

The current efforts to overcome the organ shortage include the use of marginal liver grafts, such as those from anti-

HBc positive donors. Unfortunately, the "occult" HBV infection in the donor liver may be reactivated in the recipient due to post-LT immunosuppressive therapy leading to *de novo* HBV infection. The most reasonable approach is to direct anti-HBc positive grafts to recipients with HBV related liver disease, as they will require life-long anti-HBV prophylaxis anyway. However, due to organ shortage, HBsAg-negative patients may also receive these grafts. The post-LT outcome of HBsAg-negative recipients of grafts from anti-HBc donors has been evaluated in 30 studies published as full papers (see Table 45.4) [105–134]. *De novo* HBV infection developed in 27% (82/300) of HBsAg-negative recipients who received no anti-HBV prophylaxis, this being significantly more frequent in HBV naive than anti-HBc positive recepients (12/123 or 10% vs 70/177 or 40%, p < 0.001). In the anti-HBc positive group, *de novo* infection developed less frequently in cases with anti-HBs positivity compared to no anti-HBs positivity (1/67 or 1% vs 5/37 or 14%, p = 0.021) [105, 106, 109–111, 113, 114, 121, 124–128, 130, 132, 133]. Anti-HBV prophylaxis reduced *de novo* HBV infection rates in both anti-HBc positive (4%) and HBV naive recipients (9%) [108, 112, 114–116, 118–125, 127, 128, 130, 131, 134]. In particular, *de novo* HBV infection rate was 23%, 5% and 0% in HBsAg-negative recipients under HBIG, lamivudine and their combination, respectively [105, 108, 112, 114–116, 120, 121, 124, 125, 128, 130, 131, 134].

Whether HBIG may be safely discontinued after a certain period or monoprophylaxis with a new nucleos(t)ide analogue with low resistance rates, are effective strategies in

Table 45.4 Published studies* with liver transplantation from anti-HBc positive donors to HBsAg negative recipients.

First author, year	anti-HBc (+), anti-HBs (−) recipients				anti-HBc (+), anti-HBs (+) recipients				HBV naïve recipients			
	Patients, N	Anti-HBV prophylaxis	F-up, months	De novo HBV, n	Patients, N	Anti-HBV prophylaxis	F-up, months	De novo HBV, n	Patients, N	Anti-HBV prophylaxis	F-up, months	De novo HBV, n
Chazouilleres, 1994 [109]									8	None	22	7
Wachs, 1995 [133]									6	None	NA	3
Dickson, 1997 [111]	2	None	22	0					18	None	22	15
Dodson, 1997 [113]	15	None	56	2	7	None	56	0	25	None	56	16
Crespo, 1999 [110]									2	None	51	2
Dodson, 1999 [112]	8	HBIG+LAM	46	0					8	HBIG+LAM: 7, HBIG: 1	46	1
Rokuhara, 2000 [127]	1	None	15	1	3	HBIG: 1 None: 2	11	1	3	None	51	1
Prieto, 2001 [126]	3	None	29	0	2	None	29	0	25	None	29	15
Yu, 2001a [134]	NA	LAM	NA	NA	NA	LAM	NA	NA	5	LAM	17	0
Nery, 2001 [123]	NA	None or HBIG+LAM	23	0	NA	None or HBIG+LAM	23	0	8	LAM or HBIG+LAM	19	0
Manzabeita, 2002 [121]	11	None	26	2	13	None	26	0	2	HBIG	26	2
Roque-Afonso, 2002 [128]	4	HBIG	26	0					12	None: 4, HBIG: 8	22	5
Bacerna 2002 [106]	13	HBIG+LAM:4, LAM: 9	22	1	19	None	NA	0	64	NA	NA	10
Nery, 2003 [124]					23	HBIG+LAM: 7, None: 6	21	0	8	HBIG+LAM: 2, LAM: 6	37	1
Loss, 2003 [120]									11	HBIG (bolus)+ LAM+Vaccination	33	0
Fabrega, 2003 [115]									6	HBIG+LAM	23	0
Villamil, 2004 [132]	2	None	44	0					8	None	63	2
Suehiro, 2005 [130]	4	HBIG+LAM	39	0	3	NA	39	0	15	HBIG+LAM	39	0
Donataccio, 2006b [114]	NA	HBIG	NA	NA	NA	HBIG	NA	NA	11	HBIG+LAM: 1, HBIG: 6, None: 4	57	7
Pracoso, 2006 [125]					4	LAM: 3, None: 1	19	0	3	LAM: 1, None: 2	30	0
Bacerna, 2006 [105]	3	None	40	0	6	None	45	0				
Lin, 2007c [119]					5	LAM+Vaccination	57	0				
Celebi-Kobak, 2007 [108]	4	LAM	17	0	3	LAM	28	0	4	LAM	23	0
Takemura, 2007 [131]	2	HBIG	31	0	5	HBIG	31	1	9	HBIG	31	1

F-up: follow-up; HBIG: hepatitis B immunoglobulin; LAM: lamivudine, NA: not available.

* Six studies with insufficient data on the serological HBV status of donors and/or recipients are not included [107, 116–118, 122, 129]. De novo HBV infection developed in (1) one case under no anti-HBV prophylaxis among 18 recipients with past HBV infection or HBV naïve under HBIG±LAM or no prophylaxis [122]; (2) 0/1 anti-HBc positive recipient (unknown anti-HBs status) under HBIG+LAM [116]; (3) 2/12 recipients with past HBV infection or HBV naïve under no anti-HBV prophylaxis [107]; (4) 15/16 anti-HBc positive recipients (unknown anti-HBs status) under no anti-HBV prophylaxis during 12 (5–26) months of follow-up [129]; (5) 3/28 recipients with unknown HBV status under HBIG+LAM [117]; (6) 2/14 recipients with unknown HBV status under HBIG plus vaccination [118].

De novo HBV infection also developed in (1) 0/3 anti-HBc positive recipients (unknown anti-HBs status) under LAM during 20 months of follow-upa [134];

(2) 0/1 anti-HBc positive recipient (unknown anti-HBs status) under HBIG during 11 months of follow-upb [114];

(3) 1/25 anti-HBc negative and anti-HBs positive recipients under LAM plus vaccination during 57 (33–85) months of follow-upc [119].

all, or in subsets, of such transplant patients remains to be determined. Pre- and post-transplant HBV vaccination has also been evaluated in this setting [105, 106, 108, 114–116, 118–121, 124, 125, 128, 131, 134], but further studies are required before safe conclusions can be drawn. For now, successful pre-LT vaccination does not appear to provide satisfactory protection from *de novo* post-LT HBV infection [105, 106, 108, 114–116, 121, 124, 125, 128, 131, 134]. However, HBV vaccination should be offered to all naive HBV LT candidates, even though additional anti-HBV prophylaxis might be required in cases of LT with anti-HBc positive grafts. If *de novo* post-LT HBV infection develops, antiviral treatment (see therapeutic post-transplant approach) is mandatory.

References

1 Todo S, Demetris AJ, Van Thiel D *et al.* Orthotopic liver transplantation for patients with hepatitis B virus-related liver disease. *Hepatology* 1991; **13**: 619–626.

2 O'Grady JG, Smith HM, Davies SE *et al.* Hepatitis B virus reinfection after orthotopic liver transplantation. Serological and clinical implications. *J Hepatol* 1992; **14**: 104–111.

3 Davies SE, Portmann BC, O'Grady JG *et al.* Hepatic histological findings after transplantation for chronic hepatitis B virus infection, including a unique pattern of fibrosing cholestatic hepatitis. *Hepatology* 1991; **13**: 150–157.

4 Samuel D, Muller R, Alexander G *et al.* Liver transplantation in European patients with the hepatitis B surface antigen. *N Engl J Med* 1993; **329**: 1842–1847.

5 Papatheodoridis GV, Sevastianos V, Burroughs AK. Prevention of and treatment for hepatitis B virus infection after liver transplantation in the nucleoside analogues era. *Am J Transpl* 2003; **3**: 250–258.

6 Villeneuve JP, Condreay LD, Willems B *et al.* Lamivudine treatment for decompensated cirrhosis resulting from chronic hepatitis B. *Hepatology* 2000; **31**: 207–210.

7 Kapoor D, Guptan RC, Wakil SM *et al.* Beneficial effects of lamivudine in hepatitis B virus-related decompensated cirrhosis. *J Hepatol* 2000; **33**: 308–312.

8 Hunt CM, McGill JM, Allen ML *et al.* Clinical relevance of hepatitis B virus mutations. *Hepatology* 2000; **31**: 1037–1044.

9 Papatheodoridis GV, Manolakopoulos S, Dusheiko G *et al.* Therapeutic strategies in the management of patients with chronic hepatitis B. *Lancet Infect Dis* 2008; **8**: 167–178.

10 Papatheodoridis GV, Dimou E, Laras A *et al.* Course of virologic breakthroughs under long-term lamivudine in HBeAg-negative precore mutant HBV liver disease. *Hepatology* 2002; **36**: 219–226.

11 Merle P, Trepo C. Therapeutic management of hepatitis B-related cirrhosis. *J Viral Hepat* 2001; **8**: 391–399.

12 Rosenau J, Bahr MJ, Tillmann HL *et al.* Lamivudine and low-dose hepatitis B immune globulin for prophylaxis of hepatitis B reinfection after liver transplantation possible role of mutations in the YMDD motif prior to transplantation as a risk factor for reinfection. *J Hepatol* 2001; **34**: 895–902.

13 Zimmerman MA, Ghobrial RM, Tong MJ *et al.* (2007) Antiviral prophylaxis and recurrence of hepatocellular carcinoma following liver transplantation in patients with hepatitis B. *Transplant Proc* 2007; **39**: 3276–3280.

14 Samuel D. Liver transplantation and hepatitis B virus infection: the situation seems to be under control, but the virus is still there. *J Hepatol* 2001; **34**: 943–945.

15 Hadziyannis SJ, Tassopoulos NC, Heathcote EJ *et al.* Long-term therapy with adefovir dipivoxil for HBeAg-negative chronic hepatitis B for up to 5 years. *Gastroenterology* 2006; **131**: 1743–1751.

16 Bartholomeusz A, Locarnini S. Hepatitis B virus mutations associated with antiviral therapy. *J Med Virol* 2006; **78**(Suppl. 1): S52–55.

17 Tan J, Lok AS. Antiviral therapy for pre- and post-liver transplantation patients with hepatitis B. *Liver Transpl* 2007; **13**: 323–326.

18 Lok ASF, McMahon BJ. Chronic hepatitis B. *Hepatology* 2007; **45**: 507–539.

19 Tenney D, Pokorowski KA, Rose RE *et al.* Entecavir at five years shows long-term maintenance of high genetic barrier to hepatitis B virus resistance. *Hepatol Int* 2008; **2**: S77.

20 Schiff E, Simsek H, Lee WM *et al.* Efficacy and safety of entecavir in patients with chronic hepatitis B and advanced hepatic fibrosis or cirrhosis. *Am J Gastroenterol* 2008; **103**: 2776–83.

21 Lai CL, Gane E, Liaw YF *et al.* Telbivudine versus lamivudine in patients with chronic hepatitis B. *N Engl J Med* 2007; **357**: 2576–2588.

22 Heathcote J, George J, Gordon S *et al.* Tenofovir disoproxil fumarate (TDF) for the treatment of HBeAg-positive chronic hepatitis B: week 72 TDF data and week 24 adefovir dipivoxil switch data (Study 103). *J Hepatol* 2008; **48**(Suppl. 2): S32.

23 Marcellin P, Jacobson I, Habersetzer F *et al.* Tenofovir disoproxil fumarate (TDF) for the treatment of HBeAg-negative chronic hepatitis B: week 72 TDF data and week 24 adefovir dipivoxil switch data (Study 102). *J Hepatol* 2008; **48**(Suppl. 2): S26.

24 Van Bommel F, de Man R, Stein K *et al.* A multicenter analysis of antiviral response after one year of tenofovir mono-therapy in HBV-monoinfected patients with prior nucleos(t)ide analog experience. *J Hepatol* 2008; **48**(Suppl. 2): S32.

25 Taltavull TC, Chahri N, Verdura B *et al.* Successful treatment with tenofovir in a child C cirrhotic patient with lamivudine-resistant hepatitis B virus awaiting liver transplantation. Post-transplant results. *Transpl Int* 2005; **18**: 879–883.

26 Schiff ER, Lai CL, Hadziyannis S *et al.* Adefovir dipivoxil therapy for lamivudine-resistant hepatitis B in pre- and post-liver transplantation patients. *Hepatology* 2003; **38**: 1419–1427.

27 Schiff E, Lai CL, Hadziyannis S *et al.* Adefovir dipivoxil for wait-listed and post-liver transplantation patients with lamivudine-resistant hepatitis B: final long-term results. *Liver Transpl* 2007; **13**: 349–360.

28 Bartholomeusz A, Locarnini SA. Antiviral drug resistance: clinical consequences and molecular aspects. *Semin Liver Dis* 2006; **26**: 162–170.

29 Berg T, Moller B, Trinh H *et al.* Tenofovir disoproxil fumarate (TDF) versus emtricitabine plus TDF for treatment of chronic hepatitis B (CHB) in subjects with persistent viral replication receiving adefovir dipivoxil (ADV). *J Hepatol* 2008; **48**(Suppl. 2): S34.

30 Lake J. Do we really need long-term hepatitis B hyperimmune globulin? What are the alternatives? *Liver Transpl* 2008; **14**: S23–26.

31 Shouval D, Samuel D. Hepatitis B immune globulin to prevent hepatitis B virus graft reinfection following liver transplantation: a concise review. *Hepatology* 2000; **32**: 1189–1195.

32 Neff GW, O'Brien CB, Nery J *et al.* Outcomes in liver transplant recipients with hepatitis B virus: resistance and recurrence patterns from a large transplant center over the last decade. *Liver Transpl* 2004; **10**: 1372–1378.

33 Yao FY, Osorio RW, Roberts JP *et al.* Intramuscular hepatitis B immune globulin combined with lamivudine for prophylaxis against hepatitis B recurrence after liver transplantation. *Liver Transpl Surg* 1999; **5**: 491–496.

34 Yoshida EM, Erb SR, Partovi N *et al.* Liver transplantation for chronic hepatitis B infection with the use of combination lamivudine and low-dose hepatitis B immune globulin. *Liver Transpl Surg* 1999; **5**: 520–525.

35 van Hoek B, Kroes AC, Ringers J *et al.* Switching intravenous to out-of-hospital fixed-dose intramuscular hepatitis B immunoglobulin after liver transplantation for HBsAg-positive HBV-DNA negative cirrhosis is feasible and reduces cost. *Hepatology* 2000; **32**: 242A.

36 Hooman N, Rifai K, Hadem J *et al.* Antibody to hepatitis B surface antigen trough levels and half-lives do not differ after intravenous and intramuscular hepatitis B immunoglobulin administration after liver transplantation. *Liver Transpl* 2008; **14**: 435–442.

37 Powell JJ, Apiratpracha W, Partovi N *et al.* Subcutaneous administration of hepatitis B immune globulin in combination with lamivudine following orthotopic liver transplantation: effective prophylaxis against recurrence. *Clin Transplant* 2006; **20**: 524–525.

38 Sanchez-Fueyo A, Rimola A, Grande L *et al.* Hepatitis B immunoglobulin discontinuation followed by hepatitis B virus vaccination: a new strategy in the prophylaxis of hepatitis B virus recurrence after liver transplantation. *Hepatology* 2000; **31**: 496–501.

39 Angelico M, Di Paolo D, Trinito MO *et al.* Failure of a reinforced triple course of hepatitis B vaccination in patients transplanted for HBV-related cirrhosis. *Hepatology* 2002; **35**: 176–181.

40 Bienzle U, Gunther M, Neuhaus R *et al.* Successful hepatitis B vaccination in patients who underwent transplantation for hepatitis B virus-related cirrhosis: preliminary results. *Liver Transpl* 2002; **8**: 562–564.

41 Di Paolo D, Lenci I, Trinito MO *et al.* Extended double-dosage HBV vaccination after liver transplantation is ineffective, in the absence of lamivudine and prior wash-out of human hepatitis B immunoglobulins. *Dig Liver Dis* 2006; **38**: 749–754.

42 Lo CM, Liu CL, Chan SC *et al.* Failure of hepatitis B vaccination in patients receiving lamivudine prophylaxis after liver transplantation for chronic hepatitis B. *J Hepatol* 2005; **43**: 283–287.

43 Mutimer D, Dusheiko G, Barrett C *et al.* Lamivudine without HBIg for prevention of graft reinfection by hepatitis B: long-term follow-up. *Transplantation* 2000; **70**: 809–815.

44 Malkan G, Cattral MS, Humar A *et al.* Lamivudine for hepatitis B in liver transplantation: a single-center experience. *Transplantation* 2000; **69**: 1403–1407.

45 Wai CT, Lim SG, Tan KC. Outcome of lamivudine resistant hepatitis B virus infection in liver transplant recipients in Singapore. *Gut* 2001; **48**: 581.

46 Fontana RJ, Keefe EB, Han S *et al.* (1999) Prevention of recurrent hepatitis B infection following liver transplantation: experience in 112 North American patients. *Hepatology* 1999; **30**: 301A.

47 Chan HL, Chui AK, Lau WY *et al.* Outcome of lamivudine resistant hepatitis B virus mutant post-liver transplantation on lamivudine monoprophylaxis. *Clin Transplant* 2004; **18**: 295–300.

48 Zheng S, Chen Y, Liang T *et al.* Prevention of hepatitis B recurrence after liver transplantation using lamivudine or lamivudine combined with hepatitis B Immunoglobulin prophylaxis. *Liver Transpl* 2006; **12**: 253–258.

49 Loomba R, Rowley AK, Wesley R *et al.* Hepatitis B immunoglobulin and lamivudine improve hepatitis B-related outcomes after liver transplantation: meta-analysis. *Clin Gastroenterol Hepatol* 2008; **6**: 696–700.

50 Karasu Z. Low-dose hepatitis B immune globulin and higher-dose lamivudine combination to prevent hepatitis B virus recurrence after liver transplantation. *Antivir Ther* 2004; **9**: 921–927.

51 Ferretti G, Merli M, Ginanni CS *et al.* Low-dose intramuscular hepatitis B immune globulin and lamivudine for long-term prophylaxis of hepatitis B recurrence after liver transplantation. *Transplant Proc* 2004; **36**: 535–538.

52 Dumortier J, Chevallier P, Scoazec JY *et al.* Combined lamivudine and hepatitis B immunoglobulin for the prevention of hepatitis B recurrence after liver transplantation: long-term results. *Am J Transplant* 2003; **3**: 999–1002.

53 Sousa JM, Pareja F, Serrano J *et al.* Comparison between levels of anti-HBS with a fixed administration dose of HBIG and a combination of HBIG and lamivudine for the prophylaxis of hepatitis B after liver transplantation. *Transplant Proc* 2003; **35**: 723–724.

54 Anselmo DM, Ghobrial RM, Jung LC *et al.* New era of liver transplantation for hepatitis B: a 17-year single-center experience. *Ann Surg* 2002; **235**: 611–619.

55 Honaker MR, Shokouh-Amiri MH, Vera SR *et al.* Evolving experience of hepatitis B virus prophylaxis in liver transplantation. *Transpl Infect Dis* 2002; **4**: 137–143.

56 Chu C-J, Fontana RJ, Moore C *et al.* Efficacy of HBIG weaning in the long-term prophylaxis of HBV reinfection following liver transplantation. *Hepatology* 2002; **36**: 221A.

57 Kim DD, Heffernan DJ, Bass NM *et al.* Comparison of 6 versus 12 months hepatitis B immune globulin in combination with lamivudine as prophylaxis in liver transplant recipients with hepatitis B. *Hepatology* 2002; **36**: 221A.

58 Choi J, Bae S, Yoon S *et al.* Intramuscular hepatitis B immune globulin and lamivudine for prophylaxis against hepatitis B recurrence after liver transplantation. *Hepatology* 2002; **36**: 184A.

59 Machicao VI, Soldevilla-Pico C, Devarbhavi HC *et al.* Hepatitis B liver transplant patients on combination of lamivudine and high dose IV immune globulin have less significant histological progression than hepatitis C transplanted patients. *Hepatology* 2001; **34**: 411A.

60 Andreone P, Grazi GL, Gramenzi A *et al.* Lamivudine (LAM) plus HBIg combination therapy compared to HBIg or no therapy in preventing hepatitis B (HBV) recurrence after liver transplantation (LT). *J Hepatol* 2000; **32**(Suppl. 2): 51.

61 Lee PH, Hu RH, Tsai MK *et al.* Liver transplantation for patients with hepatitis B: prevention of hepatitis B recurrence by intravenous antihepatitis B immunoglobulin and lamivudine. *Transplant Proc* 2000; **32**: 2245–2247.

62 Han SH, Ofman J, Holt C *et al.* An efficacy and cost-effectiveness analysis of combination hepatitis B immune globulin and lamivudine to prevent recurrent hepatitis B after orthotopic liver transplantation compared with hepatitis B immune globulin monotherapy. *Liver Transpl* 2000; **6**: 741–748.

63 Angus PW, McCaughan GW, Gane EJ *et al.* Combination low-dose hepatitis B immune globulin and lamivudine therapy provides effective prophylaxis against posttransplantation hepatitis B. *Liver Transpl* 2000; **6**: 429–433.

64 Roche B, Samuel D, Roque AM *et al.* Intravenous anti HBs Ig combined with oral lamivudine for prophylaxis against HBV recurrence after liver transplantation. *J Hepatol* 1999; **30**(Suppl. 1): 80.

65 McCaughan GW, Spencer J, Koorey D *et al.* Lamivudine therapy in patients undergoing liver transplantation for hepatitis B virus precore mutant-associated infection: high resistance rates in treatment of recurrence but universal prevention if used as prophylaxis with very low dose hepatitis B immune globulin. *Liver Transpl Surg* 1999; **5**: 512–519.

66 Markowitz JS, Martin P, Conrad AJ *et al.* Prophylaxis against hepatitis B recurrence following liver transplantation using combination lamivudine and hepatitis B immune globulin. *Hepatology* 1998; **28**: 585–589.

67 Marzano A, Lampertico P, Mazzaferro V *et al.* (2005) Prophylaxis of hepatitis B virus recurrence after liver transplantation in carriers of lamivudine-resistant mutants. *Liver Transpl* 2005; **11**: 532–538.

68 Karademir S, Astarcioglu H, Akarsu M *et al.* Prophylactic use of low-dose, on-demand, intramuscular hepatitis B immunoglobulin and lamivudine after liver transplantation. *Transplant Proc* 2006; **38**: 579–583.

69 Nath DS, Kalis A, Nelson S *et al.* Hepatitis B prophylaxis post-liver transplant without maintenance hepatitis B immunoglobulin therapy. *Clin Transplant* 2006; **20**: 206–210.

70 Gane EJ, Angus PW, Strasser S *et al.* Lamivudine plus low-dose hepatitis B immunoglobulin to prevent recurrent hepatitis B following liver transplantation. *Gastroenterology* 2007; **132**: 931–937.

71 Yoshida H, Kato T, Levi D. Lamivudine monoprophylaxis for liver transplant recipients with non-replicating hepatitis B virus infection. *Clin Transplant* 2007; **21**: 166–171.

72 Jiao ZY, Jiao Z. Prophylaxis of recurrent hepatitis B in Chinese patients after liver transplantation using lamivudine combined with hepatitis B immune globulin according to the titer of antibody to hepatitis B surface antigen. *Transplant Proc* 2007; **39**: 1533–1536.

73 Neff GW, Kemmer N, Kaiser TE *et al.* Combination therapy in liver transplant recipients with hepatitis B virus without hepatitis B immune globulin. *Dig Dis Sci* 2007; **52**: 2497–2500.

74 Akyildiz M, Karasu Z, Zeytunlu M *et al.* Adefovir dipivoxil therapy in liver transplant recipients for recurrence of hepatitis B virus infection despite lamivudine plus hepatitis B immunoglobulin prophylaxis. *J Gastroenterol Hepatol* 2007; **22**: 2130–2134.

75 Buti M, Mas A, Prieto M *et al.* Adherence to lamivudine after an early withdrawal of hepatitis B immune globulin plays an important role in the long-term prevention of hepatitis B virus recurrence. *Transplantation* 2007; **84**: 650–654.

76 Takaki A, Yagi T, Iwasaki Y *et al.* Short-term high-dose followed by long-term low-dose hepatitis B immunoglobulin and lamivudine therapy prevented recurrent hepatitis B after liver transplantation. *Transplantation* 2007; **83**: 231–233.

77 Freshwater DA, Dudley T, Cane P *et al.* Viral persistence after liver transplantation for hepatitis B virus: a cross-sectional study. *Transplantation* 2008; **85**: 1105–1111.

78 Yilmaz N, Shiffman ML, Todd SR *et al.* Prophylaxis against recurrence of hepatitis B virus after liver transplantation: a retrospective analysis spanning 20 years. *Liver Int* 2008; **28**: 72–78.

79 Angus P, Patterson SJ, Strasser S *et al.* A randomized study of adefovir dipivoxil in place of HBIG in combination with lamivudine as post-liver transplant hepatitis B prophylaxis. *Hepatology* 2008; **48**: 1460–1466.

80 Lo CM, Liu CL, Lau GK *et al.* Liver transplantation for chronic hepatitis B with lamivudine-resistant YMDD mutant using add-on adefovir dipivoxil plus lamivudine. *Liver Transpl* 2005; **11**: 807–813.

81 Caccamo L, Romeo R, Rossi G *et al.* No hepatitis recurrence using combination prophylaxis in HBV-positive liver transplant recipients with YMDD mutants. *Transpl Int* 2005; **18**: 186–192.

82 Yang Y, Zhang Q, Cai CJ *et al.* Prophylaxis of hepatitis B recurrence in post-liver transplantation patients with lamivudine-resistant YMDD mutant. *Chin Med J (Engl)* 2007; **120**: 1400–1403.

83 Osborn MK, Han SH, Regev A *et al.* Outcomes of patients with hepatitis B who developed antiviral resistance while on the liver transplant waiting list. *Clin Gastroenterol Hepatol* 2007; **5**: 1454–1461.

84 Villet S, Pichoud C, Villeneuve JP *et al.* Selection of a multiple drug-resistant hepatitis B virus strain in a liver-transplanted patient. *Gastroenterology* 2006; **131**: 1253–1261.

85 Terrault NA, Wright TL. Combined short-term hepatitis B immunoglobulin (HBIG) and long-term lamivudine (LAM) versus HBIG monotherapy as hepatitis B virus (HBV) prophylaxis in liver transplant recipients. *Hepatology* 1998; **28**: 389A.

86 Buti M, Mas A, Prieto M *et al.* A randomized study comparing lamivudine monotherapy after a short course of hepatitis B immune globulin (HBIg) and lamivudine with long-term lamivudine plus HBIg in the prevention of hepatitis B virus recurrence after liver transplantation. *J Hepatol* 2003; **38**: 811–817.

87 Naoumov NV, Lopes AR, Burra P *et al.* Randomized trial of lamivudine versus hepatitis B immunoglobulin for long-term prophylaxis of hepatitis B recurrence after liver transplantation. *J Hepatol* 2001; **34**: 888–894.

88 Dodson SF, de Vera ME, Bonham CA *et al.* Lamivudine after hepatitis B immune globulin is effective in preventing hepatitis B recurrence after liver transplantation. *Liver Transpl* 2000; **6**: 434–439.

89 Wong SN, Chu CJ, Wai CT *et al.* Low risk of hepatitis B virus recurrence after withdrawal of long-term hepatitis B immunoglobulin in patients receiving maintenance nucleos(t)ide analogue therapy. *Liver Transpl* 2007; **13**: 374–381.

90 Gane EJ, Strasser S, Patterson SJ *et al.* A prospective study on the safety and efficacy of lamivudine and adefovir prophylaxis in HBsAg positive liver transplantation candidates. *Hepatology* 2007; **46**: 479A.

91 Perrillo R, Rakela J, Dienstag J *et al.* Multicenter study of lamivudine therapy for hepatitis B after liver transplantation. Lamivudine Transplant Group. *Hepatology* 1999; **29**: 1581–1586.

92 Seehofer D, Rayes N, Bechstein WO *et al.* Therapy of recurrent hepatitis B infection after liver transplantation. A retrospective analysis of 200 liver transplantations based on hepatitis B associated liver diseases. *Z Gastroenterol* 2000; **38**: 773–783.

93 Fontana RJ, Hann HW, Wright T *et al.* A multicenter study of lamivudine treatment in 33 patients with hepatitis B after liver transplantation. *Liver Transpl* 2001; **7**: 504–510.

94 Ben-Ari Z, Mor E, Shapira Z *et al.* Long-term experience with lamivudine therapy for hepatitis B virus infection after liver transplantation. *Liver Transpl* 2001; **7**: 113–117.

95 Rayes N, Seehofer D, Hopf U *et al.* Comparison of famciclovir and lamivudine in the long-term treatment of hepatitis B infection after liver transplantation. *Transplantation* 2001; **71**: 96–101.

96 Ben-Ari Z, Pappo O, Zemel R *et al.* Association of lamivudine resistance in recurrent hepatitis B after liver transplantation with advanced hepatic fibrosis. *Transplantation* 1999; **68**: 232–236.

97 Peters MG, Singer G, Howard T *et al.* Fulminant hepatic failure resulting from lamivudine-resistant hepatitis B virus in a renal transplant recipient: durable response after orthotopic liver transplantation on adefovir dipivoxil and hepatitis B immune globulin. *Transplantation* 1999; **68**: 1912–1914.

98 Beckebaum S. Efficacy of combined lamivudine and adefovir dipivoxil treatment for severe HBV graft reinfection after living donor liver transplantation. *Clin Transplant* 2003; **17**: 554–559.

99 Akay S, Karasu Z, Akyildiz M *et al.* Adefovir treatment in post-transplant hepatitis B virus infection resistant to lamivudine plus hepatitis B virus immunoglobulin. *Transplant* 2004; *Proc* **36**: 2768–2770.

100 Wai CT, Prabhakaran K, Wee A *et al.* Adefovir dipivoxil as the rescue therapy for lamivudine-resistant hepatitis B post liver transplant. *Transplant Proc* 2004; **36**: 2313–2314.

101 Toniutto P, Fumo E, Caldato M *et al.* Favourable outcome of adefovir-dipivoxil treatment in acute de novo hepatitis B after liver transplantation. *Transplantation* 2004; **77**: 472–473.

102 Barcena R. Study on the efficacy and safety of adefovir dipivoxil treatment in post–liver transplant patients with hepatitis B virus infection and lamivudine-resistant hepatitis B virus. *Transpl Proc* 2005; **37**: 3960–3962.

103 Kamar N, Milioto O, Alric L *et al.* Entecavir therapy for adefovir-resistant hepatitis B virus infection in kidney and liver allograft recipients. *Transplantation* 2008; **86**: 611–614.

104 Shakil OA, Lilly L, Angus P *et al.* Entecavir significantly reduces viral load in liver transplant recipients failing lamivudine therapy for chronic hepatitis B infection. *J Hepatol* 2002; **36**(Suppl. 1): 122.

105 Bacerna R, Moraleda G, Moreno J *et al.* Prevention of de novo HBV infection by the presence of anti-HBs in transplanted patients receiving core antibody-positive livers. *World J Gastroenterol* 2006; **12**: 2070–2074.

106 Barcena Marugan R, Garcia-Hoz F, Vazquez Romero M *et al.* (2002) Prevention of de novo hepatitis B infection in liver allograft recipients with previous hepatitis B infection or hepatitis B vaccination. *Am J Gastroenterol* 2002; **97**: 2398–2401.

107 Castells L, Vargas V, Rodrygez F *et al.* Transmission of hepatitis B virus by transplantation of livers from donors positive for antibody to hepatitis B core antigen. *Transplant Proc* 1999; **31**: 2464–2465.

108 Celebi Kodak A, Karasu Z, Kilic M *et al.* (2007) Living donor liver transplantation from hepatitis b core antibody positive donors. *Transplant Proc* 2007; **39**: 1488–1490.

109 Chazouilleres O, Mamish D, Kim M *et al.* "Occult" hepatitis B virus as source of infection in liver transplant recipients. *Lancet* 1994; **343**: 142–146.

110 Crespo J, Fabrega E, Casafont F *et al.* Severe clinical course of de novo hepatitis B infection after liver transplantation. *Liver Transpl Surg* 1999; **5**: 175–183.

111 Dickson RC, Everhart JE, Lake JR *et al.* Transmission of hepatitis B by transplantation of livers from donors positive for antibody to hepatitis B core antigen. The National Institute of Diabetes and Digestive and Kidney Diseases Liver Transplantation Database. *Gastroenterology* 1997; **113**: 1668–1674.

112 Dodson F, Bonham C, Geller D *et al.* Prevention of de novo hepatitis B infection in recipients of hepatic allografts from anti-HBc positive donors. *Transplantation* 1999; **68**: 1058–1061.

113 Dodson SF, Issa S, Araya V *et al.* Infectivity of hepatic allografts with antibodies to hepatitis B virus. *Transplantation* 1997; **64**: 1582–1584.

114 Donataccio D, Roggen F, De Reyck C *et al.* Use of anti- HBc positive allografts in adult liver transplantation: toward a safer way to expand the donor pool. *Transpl Int* 2006; **19**: 38–44.

115 Fabrega E, Garcia-Suarez C, Guerra A *et al.* Liver transplantation with allografts from hepatitis B core antibody-positive donors: a new approach. *Liver Transplant* 2003; **9**: 916–920.

116 Holt CD, Thomas R, van Thiel DH *et al.* Use of hepatitis B core antibody-positive donors in orthotopic liver transplantation. *Arch Surg* 2002; **137**: 572–575.

117 Jain A, Orloff M, Abt P *et al.* Use of hepatitis B core antibody positive liver allograft in hepatitis C virus-positive and -negative recipients with use of short course of hepatitis B immunoglobulin and lamivudine. *Transplant Proc* 2005; **37**; 3187–3189.

118 Kwon C, Suh K, Yi N *et al.* Long-term protection against hepatitis B in pediatric liver recipients can be achieved effectively with vaccination after transplantation. *Pediatr Transplant* 2006; **10**: 479–486.

119 Lin CC, Chen CL, Concejero A *et al.* Active immunization to prevent *de novo* hepatitis B virus infection in pediatric live donor liver recipients. *Am J Transplant* 2007; **7**: 195–200.

120 Loss Jr G, Mason A, Nair S *et al.* (2003) Does lamivudine prophylaxis eradicate persistent HBV DNA from allografts derived from anti-HBc-positive donors? *Liver Transplant* 2003; **12**: 1258–1264.

121 Manzarbeitia C, Reich DJ, Ortiz JA *et al.* Safe use of livers from donors with positive hepatitis B core antibody. *Liver Transplant* 2002; **8**: 556–561.

122 Montalti R, Nardo B, Bertelli R *et al.* Donor pool expansion in liver transplantation. *Transplant Proc* 2002; **36**: 520–522.

123 Nery JR, Gedaly R, Vianna R *et al.* Are liver grafts from hepatitis B surface antigen negative/anti-hepatitis B core antibody positive donors suitable for transplantation? *Transplant Proc* 2001; **33**: 1521–1522.

124 Nery JR, Nery-Avila C, Reddy KR *et al.* Use of liver grafts from donors positive for antihepatitis B-core antibody (anti-HBc) in the era of prophylaxis with hepatitis-B immunoglobulin and lamivudine. *Transplantation* 2003; **75**: 1179–1186.

125 Prakoso E, Strasser SI, Koorey DJ *et al.* (2006) Long-term lamivudine monotherapy prevents development of hepatitis B virus infection in hepatitis B surface-antigen negative liver transplant recipients from hepatitis B core-antibody-positive donors. *Clin Transplant* 2006; **20**: 369–373.

126 Prieto M, Gomez MD, Berenguer M *et al.* De novo hepatitis B after liver transplantation from hepatitis B core antibody-positive donors in an area with high prevalence of anti-HBc positivity in the donor population. *Liver Transplant* 2001; **7**: 51–58.

127 Rokuhara A, Tanaka E, Yagi S *et al.* De novo infection of hepatitis B virus in patients with orthotopic liver transplantation: analysis by determining complete sequence of the genome. *J Med Virol* 2000; **62**: 471–478.

128 Roque-Afonso AM, Feray C, Samuel D *et al.* Antibodies to hepatitis B surface antigen prevent viral reactivation in recipients of liver grafts from anti-HBC positive donors. *Gut* 2002; **50**: 95–99.

129 Shinji U, Kohachiro S, Hiroyuki M *et al.* Transmission of hepatitis B virus from hepatitis B core antibody-positive donors in living related liver transplants. *Transplantation* 1998; **65**: 494–499.

130 Suehiro T, Shimada M, Kishikawa K *et al.* Prevention of hepatitis B virus infection from hepatitis B core antibody-positive donor graft using hepatitis B immune globulin and lamivudine in living donor liver transplantation. *Liver International* 2005; **25**: 1169–1174.

131 Takemura N, Sugawara Y, Tamura S *et al.* Liver transplantation using hepatitis B core antibody-positive grafts: review and university of Tokyo experience. *Dig Dis Sci* 2007; **52**: 2472–2477.

132 Villamil I, Gonzalez-Quintela A, Aguilera A *et al.* Truly de novo HBV infection after liver transplantation. *Am J Gastroenterol* 2004; **99**: 767–768.

133 Wachs ME, Amend WJ, Ascher NL *et al.* The risk of transmission of hepatitis B from HBsAg(−), HBcAb(+), HBIgM(−) organ donors. *Transplantation* 1995; **59**: 230–234.

134 Yu AS, Vierling JM, Colquhoun SD *et al.* Transmission of hepatitis B infection from hepatitis B core antibody-positive liver allografts is prevented by lamivudine therapy. *Liver Transplant* 2001; **7**: 513–517.

46 Liver biopsy

Evangelos Cholongitas[1], Andrew K Burroughs[1] and Amar P Dhillon[2]

[1]The Royal Free Sheila Sherlock Liver Centre, Royal Free Hospital, *and* University College London, London, UK
[2]Histopathology Department, Royal Free Hospital, London, UK

Introduction

Since the introduction of the 1-sec Menghini needle technique in the early 1950s, liver biopsy (LB) has become the commonest procedure performed in clinical hepatology and remains an important tool in the differential diagnosis and therapeutic decision-making in patients with clinically diagnosed acute and chronic liver disease. Other indications include the evaluation of cholestatic liver disease (primary biliary cirrhosis, primary sclerosing cholangitis), the diagnosis and follow-up of treatment of heritable disorders (hemochromatosis, Wilson's disease), and LB may be helpful in identification of systemic inflammatory or granulomatous disorders [1–5]. LB is useful in evaluating otherwise unexplained abnormalities of liver function tests, particularly in patients with fever of unknown origin [1–5]. In patients with non-alcoholic fatty liver disease (NAFLD), imaging techniques are sensitive for detecting fatty liver (especially moderate to severe steatosis) [6–9], but they cannot distinguish simple steatosis from steatohepatitis and they cannot measure the degree of fibrosis [8, 10–12]. Thus, LB can confirm the diagnosis of NAFLD and identify the severity and the extent of fibrosis. Other indications for LB include the diagnosis of drug-induced liver damage and the diagnosis of neoplastic and other mass lesions, as well as conditions such as sarcoidosis and hematologic diseases. Finally, in the liver transplantation setting, LB is essential for diagnosis of acute or chronic rejection, recurrence of the primary disease, and characterization of additional intercurrent disease.

However, LB only represents approximately 1/50000 of the total liver mass [13] and several studies have stressed this limitation, evaluating the optimal size of a liver specimen and the impact of heterogeneity and intra- and inter-observer variation on the histopathological interpretation of LB.

The status of LB is being challenged by non-invasive markers for the evaluation of fibrosis, both serum markers and types of transient elastography [14], but in reality LB and non-invasive surrogates are complementary investigations [15]. Furthermore, recent studies have tried to determine optimal standards for length and number of complete portal tracts for accurate evaluation of grading and staging in chronic viral hepatitis [16, 17].

Percutaneous (PLB) and transjugular (TJLB) liver biopsy are the two main techniques. Laparoscopic LB is more invasive [18]. The needles used can be considered large, that is, an external diameter ≥1.0 mm (14–19 G) and thin when <1.0 mm (≥20 G)) [19]. Suction (Menghini) or cutting (Trucut) needles are the most used.

Liver biopsy and its histological interpretation in chronic viral hepatitis

Although LB is an invasive procedure and should only be performed if it can offer significant and accurate diagnostic information, it is considered a key component during the initial work up of patients with chronic hepatitis C (CHC), and histopathology is the "gold standard" for assessing changes after antiviral therapy [20]. Although serological markers (anti-HCV) and HCV-RNA are very reliable for CHC diagnosis, LB is considered mandatory for grading (necroinflammatory activity) and staging (fibrosis) in most CHC patients [21, 22]. LB can also reveal unsuspected additional diagnoses, complications of treatment and progression/regression of CHC. LB is useful for evaluation of steatosis and siderosis, which may affect both the natural history and response to antiviral therapy [23–27]. However, LB is not considered necessary before starting antiviral therapy in CHC patients with genotype 2 [21], and is currently being debated in CHC patients with persistently

Evidence-Based Gastroenterology and Hepatology, 3rd edition.
J. McDonald, A.K. Burroughs, B. Feagan, and M.B. Fennerty. © 2010
Blackwell Publishing Ltd

normal aminotransferase levels [28–31]. In chronic hepatitis B (CHB), LB is also a useful tool, because it provides important information concerning the severity of liver damage and the decision to treat [32]. In patients with e-antigen positive CHB, LB is recommended for those with elevated ALT/AST twice the upper limit of normal, while it is considered mandatory in the majority of patients with e-antigen negative CHB [32]. Regardless of the accepted utility of LB in identifying active HBV disease, the distinction between histologically inactive/active levels of inflammation and insignificant/significant fibrosis for the purposes of making therapeutic decisions has never been formally investigated.

Several histopathological scoring systems have been developed in order to facilitate the comparison between different trials and to standardize histopathological observations of hepatitis. Although there are many such systems [33–36], all of them produce values for various categories of inflammation (grade) and fibrosis/architectural disruption (stage), and in fact they "score" (i.e. categorize) similar histological features. In the Knodell "histological activity index" system (HAI) [33], each of four histopathological axes of assessment (piecemeal/bridging necrosis, lobular inflammation, portal inflammation and fibrosis/architectural change) is assessed separately and assigned a "score", which is in fact a "numerical" shorthand symbol for a descriptive category. None of the scores, in any of the scoring systems is actually a measurement, or a real number in the arithmetical sense. Currently, the most widely used histopathological scoring system is the "Ishak" [34], which assesses fibrosis in seven categories ranging from normal to cirrhosis and so has potentially more discriminant descriptive power than the "Knodell". The METAVIR scoring system was designed for HCV chronic hepatitis specifically [36]. All of the histological stage scoring systems are a composite evaluation, and attempt to describe architectural changes as well as fibrosis, and all of the systems have several drawbacks [37]. The most common error in evaluating fibrosis is to use the stage scores as numerical data, such that stage 2 is considered to comprise twice the amount of fibrosis as stage 1. In fact fibrosis measurement is the only way to quantitate collagen (e.g. different cirrhotic livers would all score 6 in the Ishak staging system, but might contain vastly different amounts of collagen) [37]. The proper measurement of collagen may be essential in some studies (e.g. to establish the effects of antifibrotic therapy), and then appropriate methodology (e.g. with image analysis rather than histological scoring) must be used [37]. On the other hand, specific measurement of LB collagen alone cannot address the issue of hepatic architectural disruption and nodularity per se, so that for routine diagnostic purposes histopathological examination may not only be sufficient, but is superior. If both evaluations can be performed, additional diagnostic and prognostic

benefits may ensue [38]. Collagen proportionate area measured using Sirius red stained sections, with digital image analysis computerizsed techniques, correlates with hepatic venous pressure gradient and allows histological gradation of fibrosis in cirrhotic liver [38].

Different approaches of liver biopsy

Percutaneous liver biopsy

Percutaneous liver biopsy (PLB) is the commonest and quickest LB procedure [39]. It is commonly undertaken as a day case procedure. It is performed under local anesthesia with lidocaine, with the patient holding breath in expiration and it lasts just a few seconds [19, 40]. After biopsy, many physicians use a short observation period because most of the complications occur during the first few hours after the procedure [39, 41, 42].

Although PLB is considered a safe procedure, major and minor complications occur in up to 6% of patients and in 0.04–0.11% can be life threatening [13, 42, 43]. The most common complications include pain, hemorrhage (intraperitoneal bleeding, hematoma (intrahepatic or subcapsular) and hemobilia), infection, pneumothorax and inadvertent puncture of other intraabdominal organs. The complication rate is related to technical and patient factors. **B4** Technical factors include: (1) the experience of the operator who performs the procedure (less complications especially for those units performing more than 100 biopsies per year) [44–46]; (2) the use of ultrasonography (US) either before or the time of LB [47–49]; (3) the size of biopsy needle (less complications for the fine-needle); and (4) the use of more than one pass [46, 50–54]. Patient factors (high risk group) include: (1) the nature of the underlying liver disease (the presence of cirrhosis and tumor increase the complication rate) [54]; and (2) impaired coagulation beyond current safe limits [42], that is, platelet counts less than 60000/mm^3 and INR > 1.6. Patients with chronic renal insufficiency (serum creatinine greater than 1.5 mg/dl) are also considered at high risk: they usually receive desmopressin 15–30 minutes prior to the procedure [42].

Pre-liver biopsy US helps to detect focal hepatic tumors (benign or malignant), cysts, ascites, intrahepatic biliary dilatation or hepatic anatomical variation. Regarding the impact of US guidance on complication rate, recent evidence suggests that real time US guidance, compared to US guidance in order only to identify the puncture site, does not give any advantage regarding safety or size of liver specimen [55]. Both approaches decrease minor and major complications [47–49], particularly the risk of hemorrhage [56], but there is no clear evidence of this benefit [57, 58], compared to the blind approach, where the liver is percussed. Routine use of US for diffuse liver disease is still debated and has not been established to be cost-effective related to time in hospital [48, 56, 59]. The lower bleeding rate under US guidance may be related to the use of fewer passes used to obtain an adequate sample [46, 51]. US does help the operator to avoid puncture of adjacent important structures [60, 61]; US changed the biopsy site in 21 (12.7%) of 165 patients in a prospective study [60]. The use of US may be especially important in obese patients, those with cirrhosis and patients with chronic obstructive pulmonary disease [56]. Although blind PLB is more commonly performed, it was found that US guidance was used by 56% of gastroenterologists and hepatologists in France [53]. In addition, Angtuaco et al. randomly sent questionnaires involving 260 members of the American Association for the Study of Liver Diseases and found that 75% had performed liver biopsies under US guidance [62]. Post-biopsy US is not routinely needed; usually it is performed in the presence of possible complications.

Although fine-needle PLB should be avoided for grading and staging in chronic viral hepatitis patients, guidance fine-needle PLB (via US or computed tomography) is considered particularly useful for diagnosis of hepatocellular carcinoma (HCC) [18, 54]. Indeed, histopathology is often the only way to establish or exclude HCC and to differentiate malignant from dysplastic or benign (degenerative) lesions arising from a background of cirrhosis [63, 64]. Using current guidelines for diagnosis of HCC [65], biopsy is limited to tumors between 1–2 cm diameter [66, 67], which do not have both arterial hypervascularity and portal venous washout. However, there is the risk of malignant seeding [68]. A recent review showed the median seeding rate to be 2.29% for biopsy alone and 0.95% when associated with ablation techniques [69]. **B4** This was confirmed by another review, where the risk of malignant seeding with biopsy alone was estimated at up to 2.7% [70]. **B4**

Plugged PLB is performed through a sheath following embolization of the biopsy track and it is used in patients with impaired blood coagulation. Plugged PLB is easier and quicker than TJLB (15 min vs 41 min respectively) and thus, it is recommended in cases of coagulopathy when TJLB approach is not available or has been performed unsuccessfully [71].

Menghini versus Tru-cut technique in PLB

It is considered that the Tru-cut needle produces larger and less fragmented samples compared to the suction needle [4, 47, 54], particularly in patients with advanced fibrosis or cirrhosis [72], but in our recent systematic review on the quality of PLB, we found that the Menghini technique yielded significantly longer samples (19.9 ± 6.6 mm) compared to Tru-cut (14.3 ± 3.2 mm, p = 0.016), but without a significant difference in the mean number of complete portal tracts (CPT) (7.3 vs 6.9, p = 0.8). **B4** This could be

explained by the fact that the Tru-cut needle provides a maximum length of sample determined by the notch in the needle shaft (usually 20–25 mm) whereas with Menghini needle the length depends on the force of aspiration and operator experience. Finally, there are conflicting results regarding the relative safety of these two techniques: a retrospective study reported a higher rate of major complications with the Tru-cut needle as a result of its longer intrahepatic phase [18, 54], but another prospective study found no significant difference in complication rates related to the type of needle used [73]. **B4**

Quality of PLB for accurate histological interpretation

Diagnostically, PLB of ≥15 mm length has been considered necessary for accurate diagnosis in chronic liver disease [74]; a review also concluded that six to eight complete portal tracts (CPT) should be present for precise diagnosis [13]. However, with the increasing need to assess fibrosis in chronic viral hepatitis, larger liver samples are needed to reliably assess grading and staging. Holund et al. [75] were the first to study the optimal specimen size for accurate assessment of necroinflammation and fibrosis. The studies of Colloredo et al. [16] and Bedossa et al. [17] established the minimum size for reliable scoring of LB for chronic viral hepatitis. In the first study 161 LB from CHC and CHB patients were evaluated, finding that a specimen of at least 20 mm long (of a 1.4 mm diameter, that is, 17 gauge biopsy) and/or containing ≥11 CPT was necessary for reliable assessment of grading and staging in chronic viral hepatitis [16]. Inadequate small samples tend to underestimate the degree of disease grade and stage. **B2** In the second study the adequacy of LB samples was assessed using image analysis in 17 surgical specimens taken from CHC patients [17]. A 25 mm long specimen (of a "virtual" 1 mm diameter biopsy) was the minimum length for reliable staging [17]. **B4** Indeed, the CPT number is the most suitable parameter to compare different kinds of liver biopsy specimens (e.g. percutaneous versus transjugular, or Menghini versus Tru-cut, or using different needle sizes) [76].

Although the recommendation that an adequate LB should have 11 or more CPT, or be longer than 20–25 mm for the assessment of chronic viral hepatitis, has been accepted rapidly as the optimal standard, there are several additional considerations. An important implication of these studies is that more than one pass is likely for most PLB, in order to achieve an adequate liver sample size [16, 17]. Indeed, the mean length and number of CPT in series of PLB reported in the literature was 17.7 ± 5.8 mm and 7.5 ± 3.4 respectively, which are less than the optimal standard [76]. Interestingly, in the same review, US guidance and more experienced operators were important factors for the length of PLB, but not for the number of CPT [76]. Thus, based on documented series of PLB in the literature, the average length and number of CPT of PLB are both below the current optimal criteria for accurate histological interpretation [16, 17]. Therefore, more than one pass is likely to be needed, but this increases the risk of complications with PLB, making the minimum requirement for optimal PLB unrealistic and potentially more dangerous for the patient [46, 50, 51, 53]. **B4**

Evaluation of heterogeneity and inter-observer variation in histopathological hepatitis scores in PLB using the new sampling standard

The minimum requirements for a LB reported above in relation to sampling heterogeneity in diffuse liver disease and inter-observer variability, are very important [16, 17]. Interestingly, there was no significant sample variability (that is, no there was significant difference in stage or grade between synchronous R and L lobe samples) in only one study in which the liver samples were on average >20 mm long and thus adequate [77]. Conversely, Siddique *et al.* found a ≥2 point difference in Knodell scores of paired (two separate R lobe samples, via the same puncture site, with 4–5 portal tracts in each) HCV liver biopsies in 69% (total necroinflammatory score) and 21% (fibrosis score) of the pairs of biopsies [78]. Clearly inadequate samples are likely to give variable results, while adequate samples will give more reproducible results.

Regarding intra- and inter-observer variability, Rousselet *et al.* confirmed the influence of length and number of portal tracts on inter-observer agreement, at least between academic versus non-academic histopathologists and the available data from the literature shows that the agreement between histopathologists increases with the length and number of portal tracts in PLB [79]. **B2**

Transjugular liver biopsy

Transjugular liver biopsy (TJLB) was first described experimentally in 1964 and it has been used in clinical practice since 1970. TJLB is usually used when there are contraindications to PLB, that is, in patients with massive obesity, gross ascites and severe coagulopathy [13, 45, 80]. However, in recent years, the use of TJLB has expanded to other patient groups, such as liver transplant recipients in the early post transplantation period [81, 82], patients with acute liver failure [83, 84], and those with congenital clotting disorders [85, 86]. The main advantage of TJLB is that there is no penetration of Glisson's capsule and, therefore, bleeding is extremely rare [13, 18, 45, 87]. Moreover, hepatic venography, hepatic venous pressure gradient (HVPG) measurements and portography with CO_2 can be performed concomitantly [18, 45]. Interestingly, HVPG might be a better endpoint than histology for the assessment of

therapeutic benefit of antiviral therapy and thus the transjugular approach may be the first choice in these cases [88].

The mean procedure time of TJLB is estimated to be 40.6 (15.5–48) minutes [80]. Initially, TJLB was performed by aspiration technique (Menghini); this resulted in excessive fragmentation and small specimens making diagnosis difficult [89, 90]. The development of a standard and, later, automated Tru-cut needle improved its effectiveness without increasing complications [91, 92]. At our center we use a quick-core 19 G Tru-cut needle. Indeed, minor complications may be more frequent with Menghini TJLB needle, possibly related to the difficulty in controlling the depth of puncture [80]. **B2** Tru-cut needles give better samples (longer and more adequate for histological diagnosis) than Menghini needles (median length: 14.5 mm vs 9.5 mm respectively, p = 0.008) [80]. **B2**

The total complication rate is 7.1% [80]. Minor complications are reported in 6.6% and include abdominal pain, supraventricular arrhythmias and complications from the neck. The latter are significantly less under ultrasound guidance [80]. Major complications occurred in 0.6% and include hepatic hematoma and intra-peritoneal hemorrhage. The latter is the most common major complication (0.2%) as a result of capsular perforation. This occurs particularly in patients with small livers, but it can be detected and treated during the procedure by injecting gelatin or coils at the site of leakage [93]. Death occurred in 0.09% of TJLBs due to intraperitoneal hemorrhage (0.06%) or ventricular arrhythmia (0.03%). Pediatric compared to adult series showed significantly higher total complication rates [81]. **B4**

Quality of TJLB for accurate histological interpretation

Adequate biopsy specimens are crucial for accurate histological interpretation [16, 17], but TJLB specimens have been said to give smaller and more fragmented specimens, compared to PLB [13, 94]. However, a review of TJLB series reported in the literature showed that the mean length and number of CPT with TJLB after an average 2.5 passes were 12.8 ± 4.5 mm and 6.8 ± 2.3 respectively [80]. **B2** In addition, TJLB with three passes using Tru-cut needle gives comparable liver biopsy specimens to PLB (mean length and number of CPT were 22 ± 7 mm and 8.7 ± 5 respectively) without any serious complications [82]. **B2** TJLB with four passes provided liver specimens with a significantly greater number of CPT, compared to three passes TJLB (median: 9 vs 8, p = 0.04) [95], without an increase in complications compared to a previous series [93]. **B2** In addition, four passes, compared to three passes, more often produced specimens of adequate length (≥25 mm: 50% vs 35%, p = 0.026) with more CPT (≥11: 40% vs 26%, p = 0.027) [95]. **B2** Thus, at least four passes with TJLB should be performed when liver specimens are needed for histopathological hepatitis grading and staging.

These data showed that TJLB gives comparable specimens to PLB, but as for PLB, optimal quality criteria for grading and staging are not universally obtained. However, in contrast to the risks of percutaneous biopsy with multiple passes, TJLB allows multiple passes (to obtain adequate samples) [46, 50, 51, 96], with far less likelihood of increasing complications [93, 97]. Therefore, TJLB could be an alternative and safe approach to obtain an adequate size of samples for reliable assessment of liver histology.

Heterogeneity of liver disease and inter- or intra-observer variation have been evaluated in only one study [98]: three cores of TJLB allowed a more accurate histological interpretation, compared to one or two cores of TJLB. **A1d**

Another advantage of TJLB is the opportunity to measure hepatic venous pressure gradient. This is particularly useful if the patient has cirrhosis, as it has prognostic significance [99], but it can also be used as an indirect marker of fibrosis [81, 88, 100].

Laparoscopic and endoscopic liver biopsy

Diagnostic laparoscopy with LB is a safe and very efficient procedure, which can be performed under local anesthesia with conscious sedation and allows the visualization of the liver surface and can yield a larger amount of tissue (wedge biopsy) compared to the other techniques [18]. However, wedge biopsy in patients with diffuse liver disease, may overestimate the extent of fibrosis (staging) because of the exaggerated tissue changes that are observed in subcapsular tissue [101]. Therefore, during laparoscopy, needle biopsy samples of deeper tissue should be obtained for accurate staging. Laparoscopic LB should also be considered when both coagulation abnormalities and focal liver lesions are present [45], as well as for tumor staging and diagnosis of peritoneal disease. Laparotomy has the same advantages with laparoscopy, but is a more invasive procedure and with a higher rate of complications. In fact, the surgical approach is usually performed after accidental discovery of a focal or diffuse liver lesion during routine surgery [46].

Finally, in a recent study, De Witt *et al.* have proposed the endoscopic US-guided fine needle biopsy as an alternative, safe and sensitive procedure for the diagnosis and staging of liver metastases and mass lesions, since it was able to detect the presence of liver malignancy in 41% of patients with a previously negative evaluation [102].

"Histological" assessment without liver biopsy

LB is an invasive procedure, requires hospitalization for at least a few hours and it is associated with low but significant morbidity and mortality rates. Thus, it is not suitable for repeat testing to assess progression of liver disease. In addition, to achieve the new standards for optimal LB (20–25 mm length and 11 CPT) the patients will require more than one pass using a standard PLB, increasing the risk of complications. The question has been asked as to whether LB can be regarded as "the gold standard" for staging and grading of diffuse liver diseases when risks of biopsy, inadequate sampling, intra- and inter-observer error are taken into account [103].

Many studies have evaluated non-invasive markers (NIM). There are two types of NIM [104]. The first is based on serum markers: direct and indirect [105]. The indirect NIM may be simple, such as Fibroindex (AST, platelet count, gamma globulin) [106], and APRI index (AST/platelet count) [107], or more complex and expensive such as Fibrotest (a2-macroglobulin, haptoglobin, gamma globulin, apolipoprotein, bilirubin) [108], and PGAA index (a2-macroglobulin, γGT, apolipoprotein A1, prothrombin time) [109]. Direct NIM are more expensive and are based on measurement of extracellular matrix in serum [110]. The second category of NIM are methodologies related to liver imaging techniques [105], such as transient elastography (FibroScan), which is based on ultrasound technology [111]. Some scores combine direct and indirect NIM (e.g. Fibrometer), while the accuracy of single NIM has been increased using them in algorithms (e.g. Fibrotest with Fibroscan) [110, 112].

Unfortunately, all these non-invasive tests are currently unable to distinguish different stages of fibrosis and are considered less reliable, compared to LB [113, 114]. The non-invasive tests are not measurements of fibrosis, and the studies that attempt to validate non-invasive tests generally compare them to histopathological stage scores, which are not liver fibrosis measurements either. Initially, studies had compared NIM with sub-optimal LB (<20–25 mm length and/or containing <11 CP), but more recent studies have overcome this drawback [115]. Furthermore, all NIM have been compared with categorical variables, that is, the stage scores, and only one study has evaluated NIM with histological digital analysis of collagen, which is a quantitative measurement of liver fibrosis [116]. Finally, several issues are as yet not clear, such as the effect of necroinflammation on NIM measurements [115], the role of NIM in the liver transplantation setting [117], and in liver diseases other than chronic viral hepatitis, such as NAFLD and PBC/PSC [118].

NIMs may become an important tool for follow-up of fibrosis, using LB as the initial diagnostic assessment. The latter should be performed to obtain optimal LB specimens. TJLB techniques offer the possibility of safely obtaining ideal liver biopsy samples on repeated occasions, which is very important, particularly in clinical trials, where the efficacy of antiviral therapies is being assessed.

References

1 Sherlock S, Dick R, Van Leeuwen D. Liver biopsy: the Royal Free experience. *J Hepatol* 1984; **1**: 75–85.

2 Alberti A, Morsica G, Chemello L *et al.* Hepatitis C viraemia and liver disease in symptom-free individuals with anti-HCV. *Lancet* 1992; **340**: 697–698.

3 Caldironi MW, Mazzucco M, Aldinio MT *et al.* Echo-guided fine-needle biopsy for the diagnosis of hepatic angioma. A report on 114 cases. *Minerva Chir* 1998; **53**: 505–509.

4 Gilmore IT, Burroughs A, Murray-Lyon IM *et al.* Indications, methods, and outcomes of percutaneous liver biopsy in England and Wales: an audit by the British Society of Gastroenterology and the Royal College of Physicians of London. *Gut* 1995; **36**: 437–441.

5 Holtz T, Moseley RH, Scheiman JM. Liver biopsy in fever of unknown origin. A reappraisal. *J Clin Gastroenterol* 1993; **17**: 29–32.

6 Sorbi D, McGill DB, Thistle JL *et al.* An assessment of the role of liver biopsies in asymptomatic patients with chronic liver test abnormalities. *Am J Gastroenterol* 2000; **95**: 3206–3210.

7 Bacon BR, Farahvash MJ, Janney CG *et al.* Nonalcoholic steatohepatitis: an expanded clinical entity. *Gastroenterology* 1994; **107**: 1103–1109.

8 Angulo P, Keach JC, Batts KP *et al.* Independent predictors of liver fibrosis in patients with nonalcoholic steatohepatitis. *Hepatology* 1999; **30**: 1356–1562.

9 Powell EE, Cooksley WG, Hanson R *et al.* The natural history of nonalcoholic steatohepatitis: a follow-up study of forty-two patients for up to 21 years. *Hepatology* 1990; **11**: 74–80.

10 Campbell MS, Reddy KR. Review article: the evolving role of liver biopsy. *Aliment Pharmacol Ther* 2004; **20**: 249–259.

11 Hubscher SG. Role of liver biopsy in the assessment of non-alcoholic fatty liver disease. *Eur J Gastroenterol Hepatol* 2004; **16**: 1107–1115.

12 Clark JM, Diehl AM. Nonalcoholic fatty liver disease: an under-recognized cause of cryptogenic cirrhosis. *JAMA* 2003; **289**: 3000–3004.

13 Bravo AA, Sheth SG, Chopra S. Liver biopsy. *N Engl J Med* 2001; **344**: 495–500.

14 Burroughs AK, Cholongitas E. Non-invasive tests for liver fibrosis: encouraging or discouraging results? *J Hepatol* 2007; **46**: 751–755.

15 Van Leeuwen DJ, Balabaud C, Crawford JM *et al.* A clinical and histopathologic perspective on evolving noninvasive and invasive alternatives for liver biopsy. *Clin Gastroenterol Hepatol* 2008; **6**: 491–496.

16 Colloredo G, Guido M, Sonzogni A *et al.* Impact of liver biopsy size on histological evaluation of chronic viral hepatitis: the smaller the sample, the milder the disease. *J Hepatol* 2003; **39**: 239–244.

17 Bedossa P, Dargere D, Paradis V. Sampling variability of liver fibrosis in chronic hepatitis C. *Hepatology* 2003; **38**: 1449–1457.

18 Tobkes AI, Nord HJ. Liver biopsy: review of methodology and complications. *Dig Dis* 1995; **13**: 267–274.

19 Sherlock S, Dooley J. *Diseases of the Liver and Biliary System*. Blackwell Science, London, 1997.

20 Lee SS. Review article: indicators and predictors of response to anti-viral therapy in chronic hepatitis C. *Aliment Pharmacol Ther* 2003; **17**: 611–621.

21 Strader DB, Wright T, Thomas DL *et al.* Diagnosis, management, and treatment of hepatitis C. *Hepatology* 2004; **39**: 1147–1171.

22 Saadeh S, Cammell G, Carey WD *et al.* The role of liver biopsy in chronic hepatitis C. *Hepatology* 2001; **33**: 196–200.

23 Fontaine H, Nalpas B, Poulet B *et al.* Hepatitis activity index is a key factor in determining the natural history of chronic hepatitis C. *Hum Pathol* 2001; **32**: 904–909.

24 Lagging LM, Westin J, Svensson E *et al.* Progression of fibrosis in untreated patients with hepatitis C virus infection. *Liver* 2002; **22**: 136–144.

25 McCaughan GW, George J. Fibrosis progression in chronic hepatitis C virus infection. *Gut* 2004; **53**: 318–321.

26 Ryder SD, Irving WL, Jones DA *et al.* Progression of hepatic fibrosis in patients with hepatitis C: a prospective repeat liver biopsy study. *Gut* 2004; **53**: 451–455.

27 Koukoulis GK. Chronic hepatitis C: grading, staging, and searching for reliable predictors of outcome. *Hum Pathol* 2001; **32**: 899–903.

28 Pradat P, Alberti A, Poynard T *et al.* Predictive value of ALT levels for histologic findings in chronic hepatitis C: a European collaborative study. *Hepatology* 2002; **36**: 973–977.

29 Hui CK, Belaye T, Montegrande K *et al.* A comparison in the progression of liver fibrosis in chronic hepatitis C between persistently normal and elevated transaminase. *J Hepatol* 2003; **38**: 511–517.

30 Poynard T, Yuen MF, Ratziu V *et al.* Viral hepatitis C. *Lancet* 2003; **362**: 2095–2100.

31 Alberti A, Noventa F, Benvegnu L *et al.* Prevalence of liver disease in a population of asymptomatic persons with hepatitis C virus infection. *Ann Intern Med* 2002; **137**: 961–964.

32 Papatheodoridis GV, Hadziyannis SJ. Review article: current management of chronic hepatitis B. *Aliment Pharmacol Ther* 2004; **19**: 25–37.

33 Knodell RG, Ishak KG, Black WC *et al.* Formulation and application of a numerical scoring system for assessing histological activity in asymptomatic chronic active hepatitis. *Hepatology* 1981; **1**: 431–435.

34 Ishak K, Baptista A, Bianchi L *et al.* Histological grading and staging of chronic hepatitis. *J Hepatol* 1995; **22**: 696–699.

35 Dufour JF, DeLellis R, Kaplan MM. Regression of hepatic fibrosis in hepatitis C with long-term interferon treatment. *Dig Dis Sci* 1998; **43**: 2573–2576.

36 Bedossa P, Poynard T. An algorithm for the grading of activity in chronic hepatitis C. The METAVIR Cooperative Study Group. *Hepatology* 1996; **24**: 289–293.

37 Standish R, Cholongitas E, Dhillon A *et al.* An appraisal of the histopathological assessment of liver fibrosis. *Gut* 2005; **55**: 569–578.

38 Calvaruso V, Burroughs AK, Standish R, *et al.* Computer-assisted image analysis of liver collagen: relationship to Ishak scoring and hepatic venous pressure gradient. *Hepatology* 2009; **49**: 1236–1244.

39 Actis GC, Olivero A, Lagget M *et al.* The practice of percutaneous liver biopsy in a gastrohepatology day hospital: a retrospective study on 835 biopsies. *Dig Dis Sci* 2007; **52**: 2576–2579.

40 Kugelmas M. Liver biopsy. *Am J Gastroenterol* 2004; **99**: 1416–1417.

41 Montalto G, Soresi M, Carroccio A *et al.* Percutaneous liver biopsy: a safe outpatient procedure? *Digestion* 2001; **63**: 55–60.

42 Gunneson TJ, Menon KV, Wiesner RH *et al.* Ultrasound-assisted percutaneous liver biopsy performed by a physician assistant. *Am J Gastroenterol* 2002; **97**: 1472–1475.

43 Mayoral W, Lewis JH. Percutaneous liver biopsy: what is the current approach? Results of a questionnaire survey. *Dig Dis Sci* 2001; **46**: 118–127.

44 Thampanitchawong P, Piratvisuth T. Liver biopsy: complications and risk factors. *World J Gastroenterol* 1999; **5**: 301–304.

45 Lebrec D. Various approaches to obtaining liver tissue–choosing the biopsy technique. *J Hepatol* 1996; **25**(Suppl. 1): 20–24.

46 Grant A, Neuberger J. Guidelines on the use of liver biopsy in clinical practice. British Society of Gastroenterology. *Gut* 1999; **45**(Suppl. 4): IV1–IV11.

47 Lindor KD, Bru C, Jorgensen RA *et al.* The role of ultrasonography and automatic-needle biopsy in outpatient percutaneous liver biopsy. *Hepatology* 1996; **23**: 1079–1083.

48 Younossi ZM, Teran JC, Ganiats TG *et al.* Ultrasound-guided liver biopsy for parenchymal liver disease: an economic analysis. *Dig Dis Sci* 1998; **43**: 46–50.

49 Farrell RJ, Smiddy PF, Pilkington RM *et al.* Guided versus blind liver biopsy for chronic hepatitis C: clinical benefits and costs. *J Hepatol* 1999; **30**: 580–587.

50 Robles-Diaz G, Chavez M, Lopez M *et al.* Critical analysis of 1263 percutaneous hepatic biopsies carried out over a 12-year period (1970–1981) in the Salvador Zubiran National Institute of Nutrition. *Rev Gastroenterol Mex* 1985; **50**: 13–17.

51 McGill DB, Rakela J, Zinsmeister AR *et al.* A 21-year experience with major hemorrhage after percutaneous liver biopsy. *Gastroenterology* 1990; **99**: 1396–1400.

52 Maharaj B, Bhoora IG. Complications associated with percutaneous needle biopsy of the liver when one, two or three specimens are taken. *Postgrad Med J* 1992; **68**: 964–967.

53 Cadranel JF, Rufat P, Degos F. Practices of liver biopsy in France: results of a prospective nationwide survey. For the Group of Epidemiology of the French Association for the Study of the Liver (AFEF). *Hepatology* 2000; **32**: 477–481.

54 Piccinino F, Sagnelli E, Pasquale G *et al.* Complications following percutaneous liver biopsy. A multicentre retrospective study on 68,276 biopsies. *J Hepatol* 1986; **2**: 165–173.

55 Manolakopoulos S, Triantos C, Bethanis S *et al.* Ultrasound-guided liver biopsy in real life: comparison of same-day prebiopsy versus real-time ultrasound approach. *J Gastroenterol Hepatol* 2007; **22**: 1490–1493.

56 Al Knawy B, Shiffman M. Percutaneous liver biopsy in clinical practice. *Liver Int* 2007; **27**: 1166–1173.

57 Papini E, Pacella CM, Rossi Z *et al.* A randomized trial of ultrasound-guided anterior subcostal liver biopsy versus the conventional Menghini technique. *J Hepatol* 1991; **13**: 291–297.

58 Muir AJ, Trotter JF. A survey of current liver biopsy practice patterns. *J Clin Gastroenterol* 2002; **35**: 86–88.

59 Pasha T, Gabriel S, Therneau T *et al.* Cost-effectiveness of ultrasound-guided liver biopsy. *Hepatology* 1998; **27**: 1220–1226.

60 Riley TR, III. How often does ultrasound marking change the liver biopsy site? *Am J Gastroenterol* 1999; **94**: 3320–3322.

61 Caturelli E, Giacobbe A, Facciorusso D *et al.* Percutaneous biopsy in diffuse liver disease: increasing diagnostic yield and decreasing complication rate by routine ultrasound assessment of puncture site. *Am J Gastroenterol* 1996; **91**: 1318–1321.

62 Angtuaco TL, Lal SK, Banaad-Omiotek GD *et al.* Current liver biopsy practices for suspected parenchymal liver diseases in the United States: the evolving role of radiologists. *Am J Gastroenterol* 2002; **97**: 1468–1471.

63 Caturelli E, Solmi L, Anti M *et al.* Ultrasound guided fine needle biopsy of early hepatocellular carcinoma complicating liver cirrhosis: a multicentre study. *Gut* 2004; **53**: 1356–1362.

64 Bolondi L, Gaiani S, Celli N *et al.* Characterization of small nodules in cirrhosis by assessment of vascularity: the problem of hypovascular hepatocellular carcinoma. *Hepatology* 2005; **42**: 27–34.

65 Bruix J, Sherman D. Management of hepatocellular carcinoma. *Hepatology* 2005; **42**: 1208–1236.

66 Bruix J, Sherman M, Llovet JM *et al.* Clinical management of hepatocellular carcinoma. Conclusions of the Barcelona-2000 EASL conference. European Association for the Study of the Liver. *J Hepatol* 2001; **35**: 421–430.

67 Llovet JM, Fuster J, Bruix J. The Barcelona approach: diagnosis, staging, and treatment of hepatocellular carcinoma. *Liver Transpl* 2004; **10**: S115–120.

68 Llovet JM, Burroughs A, Bruix J. Hepatocellular carcinoma. *Lancet* 2003; **362**: 1907–1917.

69 Stigliano R, Marelli L, Yu D *et al.* Seeding following percutaneous diagnostic and therapeutic approaches for hepatocellular carcinoma. What is the risk and the outcome? Seeding risk for percutaneous approach of HCC. *Cancer Treat Rev* 2007; **33**: 437–447.

70 Silva MA, Hegab B, Hyde CJ *et al.* Needle track seeding following biopsy of liver lesions; a systematic review and meta-analysis. *Gut* 2008; **57**: 1592–1596.

71 Sawyerr AM, McCormick PA, Tennyson GS *et al.* A comparison of transjugular and plugged-percutaneous liver biopsy in patients with impaired coagulation. *J Hepatol* 1993; **17**: 81–85.

72 Sherman M, Goodman ZD, Sullivan S *et al.* Liver biopsy in cirrhotic patients. *Am J Gastroenterol* 2007; **102**: 789–793.

73 Forssell P, Bonkowsky H, Anderson P *et al.* Intrahepatic hematoma after aspiration liver biopsy. A prospective randomized trial using two different needles. *Dig Dis Sci* 1981; **26**: 631–635.

74 Schlichting P, Holund B, Poulsen H. Liver biopsy in chronic aggressive hepatitis. Diagnostic reproducibility in relation to size of specimen. *Scand J Gastroenterol* 1983; **18**: 27–32.

75 Holund B, Poulsen H, Schlichting P. Reproducibility of liver biopsy diagnosis in relation to the size of the specimen. *Scand J Gastroenterol* 1980; **15**: 329–335.

76 Cholongitas E, Senzolo M, Standish R *et al.* A systematic review of the quality of liver biopsy specimens. *Am J Clin Pathol* 2006; **125**: 710–721.

77 Persico M, Palmentieri B, Vecchione R *et al.* Diagnosis of chronic liver disease: reproducibility and validation of liver biopsy. *Am J Gastroenterol* 2002; **97**: 491–492.

78 Siddique I, El Naga HA, Madda JP *et al.* Sampling variability on percutaneous liver biopsy in patients with chronic hepatitis C virus infection. *Scand J Gastroenterol* 2003; **38**: 427–432.

79 Rousselet MC, Michalak S, Dupre F *et al*. Sources of variability in histological scoring of chronic viral hepatitis. *Hepatology* 2005; **41**: 257–264.

80 Kalambokis G, Manousou P, Vibhakom S *et al*. Transjugular liver biopsy –indications, adequacy, quality of specimens, and complications – a systematic review. *J Hepatol* 2007; **47**: 284–294.

81 Blasco A, Forns X, Carrion JA *et al*. Hepatic venous pressure gradient identifies patients at risk of severe hepatitis C recurrence after liver transplantation. *Hepatology* 2006; **43**: 492–499.

82 Cholongitas E, Quaglia A, Samonakis D *et al*. Transjugular liver biopsy: how good it is for accurate histological interpretation? *Gut* 2006; **55**: 1789–1794.

83 Miraglia R, Luka A, Gruttadauria S *et al*. Contribution of transjugular liver biopsy in patients with the clinical presentation of acute liver failure. *Cardiovasc Intervent Radiol* 2006; **29**: 1008–1010.

84 Donaldson B, Gopinath R, Wanless I *et al*. The role of transjugular liver biopsy in fulminant liver failure: relation to other prognostic indicators. *Hepatology* 1993; **18**: 1370–1376.

85 Dawson M, McCarthy P, Walsh M *et al*. Transjugular liver biopsy is a safe and effective intervention to guide management for patients with a congenital bleeding disorder infected with hepatitis C. *Intern Med J* 2005; **35**: 556–559.

86 Shin JL, Teitel J, Swain MG *et al*. A Canadian multicenter retrospective study evaluating transjugular liver biopsy in patients with congenital bleeding disorders and hepatitis C: is it safe and useful? *Am J Hematol* 2005; **78**: 85–93.

87 Burroughs AK, Dagher L. Liver biopsy. In: Classen M, Tytgat G, Lightdale C, eds. *Gastrointestinal Endoscopy*. Thieme, New York, 2002: 252–259.

88 Burroughs AK, Groszmann R, Bosch J *et al*. Assessment of therapeutic benefit of antiviral therapy in chronic hepatitis C: is hepatic venous pressure gradient a better end point? *Gut* 2002; **50**: 425–427.

89 Gamble P, Colapinto RF, Stronell RD *et al*. Transjugular liver biopsy: a review of 461 biopsies. *Radiology* 1985; **157**: 589–593.

90 Lebrec D, Goldfarb G, Degott C *et al*. Transvenous liver biopsy: an experience based on 1000 hepatic tissue samplings with this procedure. *Gastroenterology* 1982; **83**: 338–340.

91 Bull HJ, Gilmore IT, Bradley RD *et al*. Experience with transjugular liver biopsy. *Gut* 1983; **24**: 1057–1060.

92 Bruzzi JF, O'Connell MJ, Thakore H *et al*. Transjugular liver biopsy: assessment of safety and efficacy of the Quick-Core biopsy needle. *Abdom Imaging* 2002; **27**: 711–715.

93 Papatheodoridis GV, Patch D, Watkinson A *et al*. Transjugular liver biopsy in the 1990s: a 2-year audit. *Aliment Pharmacol Ther* 1999; **13**: 603–608.

94 Guido M, Rugge M. Liver biopsy sampling in chronic viral hepatitis. *Semin Liver Dis* 2004; **24**: 89–97.

95 Vibhakorn S, Cholongitas E, Kalambokis G *et al*. A comparison of four- versus three-pass transjugular biopsy using a 19-G Tru-Cut needle and a randomized study using a cassette to prevent biopsy fragmentation. *Cardiovasc Intervent Radiol* 2008; **32**: 508–513.

96 Demetris AJ, Ruppert K. Pathologist's perspective on liver needle biopsy size? *J Hepatol* 2003; **39**: 275–277.

97 Smith TP, Presson TL, Heneghan MA *et al*. Transjugular biopsy of the liver in pediatric and adult patients using an 18-gauge automated core biopsy needle: a retrospective review of 410 consecutive procedures. *AJR Am J Roentgenol* 2003; **180**: 167–172.

98 Cholongitas E, Quaglia A, Samonakis D *et al*. Transjugular liver biopsy in patients with diffuse liver disease: comparison of 3 cores with 1 or 2 cores for accurate hstological interpretation. *Liver Int* 2007; **27**: 646–653.

99 Groszmann RJ, Garcia-Tsao G, Bosch J *et al*. Beta-blockers to prevent gastroesophageal varices in patients with cirrhosis. *N Engl J Med* 2005; **353**: 2254–2261.

100 Samonakis DN, Cholongitas E, Thalheimer U *et al*. Hepatic venous pressure gradient to assess fibrosis and its progression after liver transplantation for HCV cirrhosis. *Liver Transpl* 2007; **13**: 1305–1311.

101 Imamura H, Kawasaki S, Bandai Y *et al*. Comparison between wedge and needle biopsies for evaluating the degree of cirrhosis. *J Hepatol* 1993; **17**: 215–219.

102 DeWitt J, LeBlanc J, McHenry L *et al*. Endoscopic ultrasound-guided fine needle aspiration cytology of solid liver lesions: a large single-center experience. *Am J Gastroenterol* 2003; **98**: 1976–1981.

103 Afdhal NH, Nunes D. Evaluation of liver fibrosis: a concise review. *Am J Gastroenterol* 2004; **99**: 1160–1174.

104 Pinzani M. Non-invasive evaluation of hepatic fibrosis: don't count your chickens before they're hatched. *Gut* 2006; **55**: 310–312.

105 Rockey DC, Bissell DM. Noninvasive measures of liver fibrosis. *Hepatology* 2006; **43**: S113–120.

106 Koda M, Matunaga Y, Kawakami M *et al*. Fibroindex, a practical index for predicting significant fibrosis in patients with chronic hepatitis C. *Hepatology* 2007; **45**: 297–306.

107 Wai CT, Greenson JK, Fontana RJ *et al*. A simple noninvasive index can predict both significant fibrosis and cirrhosis in patients with chronic hepatitis C. *Hepatology* 2003; **38**: 518–526.

108 Imbert-Bismut F, Ratziu V, Pieroni L *et al*. Biochemical markers of liver fibrosis in patients with hepatitis C virus infection: a prospective study. *Lancet* 2001; **357**: 1069–1075.

109 Naveau S, Poynard T, Benattar C *et al*. Alpha-2-macroglobulin and hepatic fibrosis. Diagnostic interest. *Dig Dis Sci* 1994; **39**: 2426–2432.

110 Sebastiani G, Alberti A. Non invasive fibrosis biomarkers reduce but not substitute the need for liver biopsy. *World J Gastroenterol* 2006; **12**: 3682–3694.

111 Castera L, Vergniol J, Foucher J *et al*. Prospective comparison of transient elastography, Fibrotest, APRI, and liver biopsy for the assessment of fibrosis in chronic hepatitis C. *Gastroenterology* 2005; **128**: 343–350.

112 Sebastiani G, Vario A, Guido M *et al*. Stepwise combination algorithms of non-invasive markers to diagnose significant fibrosis in chronic hepatitis C. *J Hepatol* 2006; **44**: 686–693.

113 Friedrich-Rust M, Ong MF, Martens S *et al*. Performance of transient elastography for the staging of liver fibrosis: a meta-analysis. *Gastroenterology* 2008; **134**: 960–974.

114 Afdhal NH. Diagnosing fibrosis in hepatitis C: is the pendulum swinging from biopsy to blood tests? *Hepatology* 2003; **37**: 972–974.

115 Fraquelli M, Rigamonti C, Casazza G *et al*. Reproducibility of transient elastography in the evaluation of liver fibrosis in patients with chronic liver disease. *Gut* 2007; **56**: 968–973.

116 Cales P, Oberti F, Michalak S *et al.* A novel panel of blood markers to assess the degree of liver fibrosis. *Hepatology* 2005; **42**: 1373–1381.

117 Rigamonti C, Donato MF, Fraquelli M *et al.* Transient elastography predicts fibrosis progression in patients with recurrent hepatitis C after liver transplantation. *Gut* 2008; **57**: 821–827.

118 Corpechot C, El NA, Poujol-Robert A *et al.* Assessment of biliary fibrosis by transient elastography in patients with PBC and PSC. *Hepatology* 2006; **43**: 1118–1124.

47 Drug induced liver disease: Mechanisms and diagnosis

Raúl J Andrade[1] *and M Isabel Lucena*[2]

[1] Liver Unit, Gastroenterology Service, "Virgen de la Victoria" University Hospital and School of Medicine, Centro de Investigación Biomédica en Red de Enfermedades Hepáticas y Digestivas (CIBEREHD), Málaga, Spain
[2] Clinical Pharmacology Service, "Virgen de la Victoria" University Hospital and School of Medicine, Centro de Investigación Biomédica en Red de Enfermedades Hepáticas y Digestivas (CIBEREHD), Málaga, Spain

Introduction

The liver is central to the biotransformation of virtually all drugs and foreign substances and, hence, an adverse hepatic reaction is a potential complication of nearly every medication that is prescribed. The list of drugs capable of inducing liver damage increases from year to year [1–5], and in the last decades this also included several herbal remedies [6–10], and dietary supplements [11, 12]. Indeed, drug-induced liver disease (DILI) is an increasing health problem, accounting for >50% of cases of acute liver failure in Western countries [13], and for the 4–10% of cases of jaundiced patients taken as a whole, admitted to a general hospital [14–16]. Moreover, a recent study suggests that roughly 1% of medical inpatients develop DILI during the course of hospitalization [17].

The overall frequency of DILI was assessed in a community-based study performed in France over a three-year period, which found an annual incidence of 14 cases per 100,000 inhabitants [18]. To be included as true cases in this study the patients had to have symptoms, so this latter figure is probably an underestimation of the actual number of cases that occurred. In addition, this figure was 16 times as high as the number notified to the French network of pharmacovigilance, revealing the main drawback of spontaneous reporting systems, which is under-reporting.

The frequency of DILI associated with specific drugs is unknown. At best, scattered data for the numerator (total number of affected subjects) are available for some medications, but information on the denominator is derived mainly from prescribing data (as a surrogate for data on number of persons and time of exposure); however, this does not accurately reflect the population exposed. Nevertheless, the frequency of unpredictable hepatotoxicity associated with the use of a given medication is suggested to be around 1 per 10,000 to 1 per 100,000 exposed individuals [19, 20]. In two large databases of DILI cases prospectively recorded, the Spanish and American Registries of hepatotoxicity, which are not restricted to specific agents and can be regarded as representative of clinical practice, antibacterial agents, non-steroidal anti-inflammatory drugs and central nervous system agents were reported to rank as the main compounds incriminated in DILI [21, 22]. In both databases, amoxicillin-clavulanate was the single agent most frequently responsible for DILI.

An important currently unresolved difficulty is that the diagnosis of DILI is not standardized, relying largely on the circumstantial evidence of exposure to a drug or herbal product and its relationship to the start of symptoms, the effect of discontinuation of the suspected toxic substance on outcome, and the exclusion of other causes of liver disease (see below). The rare occurrence of DILI, together with the lack of specific diagnosis have an important impact in terms of epidemiological data concerning the problem and is a barrier for progress in the understanding of the mechanisms involved.

Mechanisms

Hepatotoxicity directly related to the dose of a compound is the hallmark of *intrinsic* "dose-dependent" type A adverse drug reactions. Acetaminophen (paracetamol) is in practical terms the only marketed drug whose capacity of producing liver injury is closely related to the total dose consumed. On the contrary, *idiosyncratic* DILI, which represents the majority of DILI in clinical practice, is typically

Supported partly by research grants from the Agencia Española del Medicamento, Fondo de Investigacion Sanitaria FIS PI 07/0980 and EC07/90910 and Boehringer-Ingelheim, Barcelona.

Evidence-Based Gastroenterology and Hepatology, 3rd edition.
J. McDonald, A.K. Burroughs, B. Feagan, and M.B. Fennerty. © 2010
Blackwell Publishing Ltd

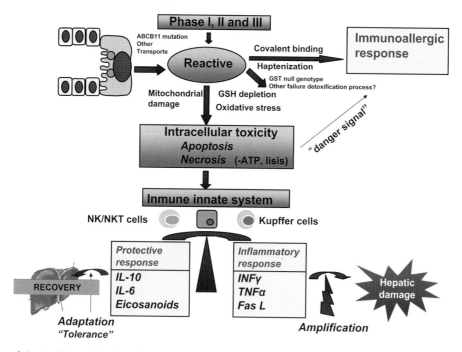

Figure 47.1 Pathways of chemical injury in the liver (upstream mechanisms) and their modulation by the immune system (downstream mechanism). GSH: Glutathione; GST: glutathione-S-transferase.

a non-predictable (not based on the pharmacology of the drug) type B adverse drug reaction. Idiosyncratic reactions cannot be usually predicted from preclinical studies. They are classified as immunoallergic (hypersensitivity features present), or metabolic, although this is more an arbitrary division and overlap between categories can occur. The classical concept of idiosyncratic DILI includes the lack of a clear dose relationship. That said, it has been recently re-emphasized that even in allergic adverse drug reactions, a dose threshold is required, as these reactions are very rare when the dose of any drug is less than 10 mg per day [23]. Actually, 77% out of 598 cases of idiosyncratic DILI included in a Swedish database occurred in patients taking drugs at daily dose of at least 50 mg (higher doses), 14.2% at doses of 11–49 mg (intermediate doses), and only 9% at doses equal or less than 10 mg (lower doses) [24]. Furthermore, it has also been pointed out that most drugs, that either have been withdrawn from the market, or have received a black box warning due to hepatotoxicity were prescribed at daily doses greater than 50 mg/day [25].

A recent definition states that idiosyncratic reactions are toxic responses determined by individual susceptibility to (host) factors that increase the penetrance and expressivity of the intrinsic toxicity of a drug (or a drug metabolite) [26]. Indeed, development of DILI is a complex, multi-step process in which the toxic potential of the drug, genetic and acquired factors, as well as individual deficiencies in the adaptive processes, that limit the extent of the injury, determine the susceptibility to the rare occurrence of idiosyn-

cratic hepatotoxicity (see Figure 47.1) [27]. Thus, most patients tolerate the drug without adverse liver effects or there is a background of mild, and often transient, asymptomatic liver injury (i.e. statins, isoniazid), indicating an adaptation to the drug and further tolerance. Therefore, the combination of susceptibility factors coupled with drugs that (due to variation in handling between different phases of drug metabolism, detoxification, and transport) reach a threshold for exposure to drug or toxic metabolites, enhances the risk of idiosyncratic hepatotoxicity.

Several mechanisms and pathways may be involved in DILI. Most frequently, damage is initiated through the formation of reactive drug metabolites that can be directly toxic or induce immune reactions [28, 29]. In other instances drugs can impair mitochondrial function, which may decrease fat oxidation (causing fat accumulation) and/or energy production leading to cell death [30, 31]. Also parent drugs or reactive drug metabolites, either through direct toxicity or immune reactions, may open the mitochondrial permeability transition pore, which subsequently results in necrosis or apoptosis [32]. A unifying hypothesis that involves underlying genetic or acquired mitochondrial abnormalities as a major determinant of susceptibility for a number of drugs that target mitochondria and cause DILI has been proposed [26]. The mitochondrial hypothesis requires gradually accumulating and initially silent mitochondrial injury in heteroplasmic cells, which then reaches a critical threshold and abruptly triggers liver injury. This is consistent with the fact that, typically, idiosyncratic DILI is delayed (by weeks or months). New animal models (e.g. the Sod2+/– mouse) provide supporting evidence for this concept [26]. However, genetic analyses of DILI patient samples are ultimately needed to provide evidence for this proof-of-concept [26].

In drug-induced immune-mediated hepatic injury, the drug reactive metabolites trigger an adaptive immune response directed against the drug-modified liver components, resulting in acute or chronic liver damage. Advances in the understanding of the pathogenesis of hepatotoxicity are hampered by the fact that no satisfactory animal models for idiosyncratic DILI have been developed. Recent evidence in experimental acetaminophen hepatotoxicity clearly indicates that the balance between the pro-and anti-inflammatory mediators determines the susceptibility and severity of liver injury [33]. Conceivably, these insights could be extrapolated to idiosyncratic DILI in humans, particularly the role of the innate immune system and cell-death pathways.

Risk factors

Most of the risk factors that have been identified are the ones which influence drug disposition and metabolism. Incomplete information in case reports has precluded analyses of drug-related, environmental risk factors and clinical presentation profiles, which, however, can be obtained in large cohorts of patients with DILI [21, 22, 34–37]. Known risk factors are, nevertheless, poorly predictive of hepatotoxicity, and in many instances of DILI no risk factor can be identified [38].

Environmental factors

There are several *environmental factors* that appear to operate in determining individual susceptibility.

Age
Elderly patients are more vulnerable to DILI. In particular, increased age is a susceptibility factor for developing hepatotoxicity to antituberculous drugs [39]. Older age has also been implicated in amoxicillin-clavulanate induced cholestasis [40, 41]. In contrast, valproic acid and erythromycin hepatotoxicity are more common in childhood [42]. Older age, rather than being a predisposing factor to DILI, seems to have an impact on the phenotypic expression of toxic liver damage, strongly favoring the appearance of a cholestatic pattern of injury [21, 43].

Gender
Women are more susceptible than men to most forms of DILI [18, 44–46]. For instance, autoimmune hepatitis triggered by drugs is seen almost exclusively in women [47],

and diclofenac hepatotoxicity has been reported more frequently in women with osteoarthritis [42].

However, new epidemiological data have challenged this traditional belief, showing a similar sex distribution in DILI cases [21, 48], with a higher prevalence of female gender only at younger ages [43]. Yet, female gender is considered to be a risk factor for developing fulminant liver failure [21], and female sex accounted for 76% of patients presenting with drug-induced acute liver failure in the USA who were transplanted [49]. Similarly to age, gender may influence the clinical presentation of DILI as women are over represented in the hepatocellular type of injury [43].

Chronic alcohol consumption
A history of alcohol intake was considered to be a general risk factor for idiosyncratic DILI, and as such scores 1 + point in the standard clinical scale for assignation of causality developed by experts, the CIOMS (Council for International Organizations of Medical Sciences) or RUCAM (Roussel Uclaf Causality Assessment Method) scale [50]. However, for most of the drugs capable of inducing hepatotoxicity there is no evidence for a role of alcohol in potentiating toxicity. In practical terms, chronic alcohol intake increases the risk of developing liver fibrosis during methotrexate therapy, enhances acetaminophen hepatotoxicity by inducing cytochrome P-450 (CYP) 2E1 (with generation of higher levels of the reactive metabolite and depletion of glutathione stores), as well as susceptibility to liver damage from isoniazid, halothane and cocaine [42].

Concomitant drugs
These are capable of modulating the hepatotoxic potential of other drugs through CYP or hepatic transport system induction, inhibition or substrate competition. In addition, concomitant medication with hepatotoxic potential may further increase the risk [51]. Concurrent use of anticonvulsants which induce drug metabolism greatly increases the risk of hepatotoxicity due to valproate [42]. The concurrent use of isoniazid and rifampicin, a potent microsomal inducer, enhances the risk of isoniazid hepatotoxicity [52].

Underlying disease states
Controversy exists as to whether pre-existing liver disease is a susceptible factor for the development of hepatotoxicity. The presence of chronic hepatitis B, hepatitis C infection or co-infection with human immunodeficiency virus (HIV) increases the risk of isoniazid hepatotoxicity or elevated transaminases on HAART (highly active antiretroviral therapy) [53]. The increased susceptibility exhibited by HIV patients suggests a role for cytokine imbalance [54]. Rifampicin is more hepatotoxic when used for control of itching in patients with primary biliary cirrhosis [55].

Obesity, diabetes mellitus type 2 and insulin resistance are known risk factors for steato-hepatitis, and have also been shown, along with psoriasis, to increase the risk of developing liver fibrosis during methotrexate therapy [56].

Genetic risk factors

Idiosyncratic hepatotoxicity is not predictable based either on the pharmacology of the drug or the dose administered, even when confounding variables such as environmental factors are taken into account. On the other hand, recurrence of liver injury with re-exposure to the drug often occurs under different clinical circumstances, indicating that susceptibility to hepatotoxicity could depend principally on host genetic factors [57]. Association studies have sought for single nucleotide polymorphisms (SNPs) in candidate genes, which are those presumably involved in drug bioactivation/detoxification processes as well in the immune response (see Table 47.1).

The reactive metabolite hypothesis states that most DILI instances would result from the production of reactive metabolites [20, 28, 29, 58, 59], which accumulate within the hepatocyte to levels that exceed a critical threshold. Once this threshold is crossed the damage is initiated. In liver, CYPs are more abundant in the centrilobular (zone 3) than periportal regions. Therefore, centrilobular necrosis, which represents one typical histological feature of serious acute drug-induced liver injury, may indeed indicate that drug metabolizing enzymes have a major role in pathogenesis. Only anecdotal reports suggest a role of CYP 450 polymorphisms in hepatotoxicity. For example, CYP2D6 deficiency is associated with perhexiline hepatotoxicity [60], and may occur in up to 10% of Europeans [61]. CYP 2C19 deficiency was suggested to be associated with Atrium (a phenobarbitone containing combination preparation) liver injury [62]. However, 60 patients with DILI caused by drugs known to be substrates of *CYP2C9* and *CYP2C19*, showed a similar prevalence of allelic variants to those in other European populations, and there were no patients exhibiting very low enzyme activity with *CYP2C9* *3/*3 and *CYP2C19* *3/*3 genotype [60]. These data suggest that CYP2C9 and CYP2C19 genetic polymorphisms might not be a predictable potential risk factor for DILI. Indeed, variant genotypes of CYP, associated with lower enzyme activity could not account for higher susceptibility to DILI, as an intact or even enhanced enzyme activity (determined by environmental rather than genetic factors) seems to be required for the formation of reactive metabolites.

An alternative possibility is that reactive metabolites may not undergo detoxification, either because they are poor substrates, or because of failure of detoxification enzyme function (due to genetic polymorphisms). Phase II enzymes are known to be polymorphically expressed. The major Phase II genes implicated in hepatotoxicity are N-acetyltransferase 2 (*NAT2*) and the glutathione S-transferases M and T (*GSMT* and *GSTT*).

In Chinese patients on antituberculosis therapy, carriers of *NAT2* genotypes which are associated with slow acetylation, had four-fold risk of developing isoniazid-induced hepatotoxicity [63]. Regular monitoring of serum aminotransferase was thus suggested in slow *NAT2* acetylators receiving isoniazid treatment [64]. The same authors showed that subjects with *CYP2E1 c1/c1, were* 2.5 times more likely to develop hepatotoxicity when compared with the other genotypes. The odds ratio for hepatotoxicity increased to 7.4 when *CYP2E1 c1/c1* was combined with slow acetylator status [65].

Oxidative stress induced by the reactive metabolites or reactive oxygen species generated by drugs, may be the final common pathway underlying DILI. Individual vulnerability to a drug might then not be closely related to the rate of parent drug metabolism, but related to deficiencies in the detoxification process, or in drug transporters which ultimately determine the level of exposure to the reactive metabolite. In this regard, glutathione S-transferase (GST), a major phase II family of conjugation enzymes, prevents the binding of reactive metabolites to cellular proteins and modulates the by-products of oxidative stress, catalyzing the conjugation of electrophilic moieties to glutathione [66].

The importance of GST as a general detoxification mechanism in DILI is underlined by the fact that it acts for a variety of metabolites derived from aflatoxin, acetaminophen, benzo(a)pyrene, bromobenzene, or felbamate, and other substances [67–72]. In humans, the activity of the cytosolic GSTs M1 (μ) and T1 (θ) are polymorphically expressed due to complete *GSTM1* and *GSTT1* gene deletions, that occur in homozygosity (null genotypes) in 50%, and 10–25% of Caucasian subjects respectively [73]. A significant association with *GSTM1-GSTT1* null genotype was found in Japanese patients with troglitazone induced DILI [74], and in a cohort of French [75], but not British patients [76], with tacrine-induced DILI. An association with GSTM1 (but not *GSTT1*) null genotype, was also identified in Indian patients with antituberculosis drug-induced hepatotoxicity (52% vs 24% in controls, p < 0.05) [77], and in Chinese patients with antituberculosis drug-induced hepatotoxicity, (2.23 fold-increased risk) [78]. Taken together, and consistent with studies in animal models, these findings point to a role for these enzyme activities as a general protective mechanism against hepatotoxicity. This hypothesis was tested in a study involving 154 patients with a diagnosis of DILI due to an array of medications. Carriers of double *GSTT1-M1* null genotypes were 2.70 times more likely to develop hepatotoxicity, when compared with non-carriers. The odds ratio for DILI patients receiving antibacterials, and NSAIDs were 3.52 and 5.61 respectively. Patients with amoxicillin-clavulanate hepatotoxicity had a 2.81-fold increased risk. There was a

Table 47.1 Genetic factors associated with idiosyncratic hepatotoxicity.

Genotype associated	Drug	Reported consequence for DILI susceptibility	Reference
Cytochrome P450			
CYP2E1 c1/c1	Antituberculosis	Increased DILI incidence	Huang et al., 2003
CYP2C9 *2, *3	Diclofenac	No association	Aithal et al., 2000
CYP2C9/2C19 *2, *3	Various drugs induced DILI and substrate of this CYP	No association	Pachkoria, 2007
Phase II conjugation enzymes			
NAT2 slow acetylator variants	Antituberculosis	Risk factor for DILI	Huang et al., 2002
GSTM1 null	Antituberculosis	Risk factor for DILI	Huang et al., 2007
GSTT1-GSTM1 double null	Troglitazone	Risk factor for DILI	Watanabe et al., 2003
GSTT1-GSTM1 double null	Tacrine	Risk factor for DILI	Simon, 2000
GSTT1-GSTM1 double null	Various	Risk factor for DILI	Lucena et al., 2008
MnSOD T/C or C/C	Antitituberculosis	Risk factor for DILI	Huang et al., 2007
UGT2B7*2 allele	Diclofenac	Increased DILI incidence	Daly et al., 2007 Goekkurt et al., 2007
Transporter genes			
ABCB11 (BSEP) T1331C	Various (n = 32)	Increased incidence of cholestatic injury	Lang et al., 2007
ABCB11 (BSEP) T1331C	Various (n = 188)	Increased incidence of hepatocellular injury	Andrade et al., 2008
ABCC2 C-24T	Diclofenac	Cellular accumulation of metabolite acylglucoronide	Daly, 2007
ABCC2 C-24T G1249A, T3563A, G4581A	Various	No association with DILI	Lucena et al., 2008
Immune response			
HLA-DRB1*1501-DRB5*0101-DQB1*0602 haplotype	Amoxicillin-clavulanate	Increased risk in cholestatic/mixed hepatotoxicity	Hautekeete et al., 1999
HLA-DRB1*1501-DRB5*0101-DQA1*0102-DQB1*0602	Amoxicillin-clavulanate	Increased risk in cholestatic/mixed damage	O'Donohue et al., 2000
HLA DRB1*0701 DQB1*0201 DQA1*0102	Antituberculosis	Increased risk of DILI	Sharma et al., 2002
HLA DRB1*15 DQB1*06	Various	Increased incidence of cholestatic/mixed hepatotoxicity	Andrade et al., 2004
HLA DRB1*07 and HLA DQB1*02	Various	Protective in cholestatic/mixed hepatotoxicity	Andrade et al., 2004
HLA DRB1*0701	Ximelagatran	Increased incidence of elevated ALT	Kindmark et al., 2008
IL-10 −627 AA/AC + IL4 −590 TT/CT	Diclofenac	Increase DILI incidence	Aithal et al., 2004
IL-10 −1082G/A, −819 C/T, −592 C/A	Various	No association with DILI Low and intermediate IL-10 haplotype associated with the worst DILI outcome.	Patchkoria et al., 2008

statistically significant predominance of women in the combined null genotype (p < 0.001) [79].

The Manganese Superoxide Dismutase (MnSOD) is also a critical determinant of cellular defence against toxic insult to the liver. A study including 115 subjects with DILI (63 with antituberculosis hepatotoxicity) showed that those with a variant *C* allele (genotype *T/C* or *C/C*) of *MnSOD* had an increased risk of hepatotoxicity compared to those with *MnSOD T/T* genotype, considering all drugs together (adjusted OR: 2.44), but also in the sub-category of anti-tuberculosis drugs (adjusted OR: 2.47) [78].

The functions of ATP-Binding-Cassette (ABC) transporters, which determine the excretion or accumulation of certain reactive metabolites, make them obvious candidate genes in the identification of susceptible individuals to develop DILI. In a study a single nucleotide polymorphism in exon 13 of *ABCB11*, 1331T > C (V444A), which is associated with decreased hepatic BSEP expression, was significantly more frequent in drug-induced cholestasis than in hepatocellular injury, or in the control population [80]. In contrast, carriers of the *ABCB11*, 1331T > C polymorphism were found to have a two-fold increased risk of developing toxic hepatocellular damage in a cohort of 188 Spanish DILI patients [81].

With the availability of increasing information on new polymorphisms and their functional significance, it is currently feasible in some cases to perform genotyping for different polymorphisms concomitantly. A study involving 24 patients with diclofenac-induced liver injury showed that simultaneous possession of variant of UDP-glucuronosyl-transferase (that mediates the glucuronoconjugation of diclofenac to a paradoxically reactive metabolite acyl-glucuronide) the *UGT2B7*2* allele (associated with increased activity), and the *ABCC2* (that transports the glucuronide to the biliary canaliculus), *C-24T* variant (associated with reduced activity) was more common in DILI patients compared with controls. Haplotype distributions for *CYP2C8* (which plays a role in the metabolism of diclofenac to 5-hydroxydiclofenac) were also significantly different in patients with hepatotoxicity [36]. Interestingly, in this study, 21% of the community control population was positive for both the "at-risk" *UGT2B7* and *ABCC2* genotypes [36]. It is clear that the incidence of serious hepatotoxicity is much lower than these figures. Indeed, genetic polymorphisms of drug metabolism, although increasing the risk of DILI, do not explain why all patients with a given polymorphism do not develop DILI when treated with the relevant drug.

Immunological factors

Once hepatic cells become stressed by the toxic insult, the response of the innate and acquired immune system (downstream events), appear to determine whether liver injury subsides or progresses to clinical disease (see Figure 47.1) [27].

Variations in the production of immunoregulatory cytokines (genetic polymorphisms) such as IL-10 and IL-4 have also been reported to contribute to the susceptibility to diclofenac hepatotoxicity [82]. The observed polymorphisms, resulting in low *IL-10* and high *IL-4* gene transcription, could favour a Th-2 mediated antibody response to neoantigenic stimulation associated with disease susceptibility.

As the increased susceptibility related to these downstream events may be less drug-specific than those involved in the accumulation of reactive metabolites, it might be possible to group cases of DILI associated with a heterogeneous group of drugs. In a cohort of 146 patients with DILI the analysis of three polymorphisms: −1082G/A, −819C/T, and −592C/A in the *IL-10* gene promoter, did not reveal any association with the predisposition to develop hepatotoxicity. However, the low IL-10 producing haplotype was more prevalent in DILI patients coupled with the absence of peripheral blood eosinophilia [83]. All cases with serious DILI outcome carried low or intermediate IL-10 producing haplotypes and had normal or low eosinophil counts. [83] Indeed, low IL-10 producing haplotype, leading to a reduced or absent rise in peripheral eosinophil count, could be a marker of an unfavorable outcome of DILI, supporting the concept of accelerated Th1 T-cytotoxic response.

HLA genotyping

Major histocompatibility complex molecules (i.e. class I and II HLA molecules) participate in antigen presentation to immunocompetent cells and in the regulation of the immune response. Significant association has been reported between *DRB1*1501-DRB5*0101-DQB1*0602* haplotype and cholestatic hepatitis related to amoxicillin-clavulanate [84]. Also a genome-wide association study using 866,399 markers in 51 cases of flucloxacillin DILI and 282 controls matched for sex and ancestry showed an association peak in the major histocompatibility complex (MHC) region with the strongest association (P = 8.7 × 10(−33)) seen for rs2395029[G], and other SNPs all of which are a part of an extended MHC 57.1 haplotype present in <4% of Europeans, which is associated to hypersensitivity to abacavir [85]. However, even in cases of DILI with no evidence of allergy, such as those induced by ximelagatran (hepatocellular type, delayed in latency, no eosinophilia), using a wide genome screen approach, a strong genetic association between elevated alaninoaminotransferases (ALT) and the HLA class-II alleles *DRB1*07* and *DQA1*02* was also recently shown, suggesting a possible immune pathogenesis. Consistent with this hypothesis, immunological studies suggest that ximelagatran may have the ability to act as a contact sensitizer, and hence be able to stimulate an adaptive immune response [86].

A large cohort of cases with drug-induced liver disease due to variety of agents with a wide range of manifestations may be suitable in the evaluation of the effect of genetic factors on the phenotype expression of hepatotoxicity [87]. The *HLA DRB1*15* and *DQB1*06* alleles of the class II HLA system participate in increased susceptibility to the development of a cholestatic/mixed pattern in drug-induced liver injury, thus providing indirect evidence about the immunoallergic nature of this specific pattern of damage and explaining, at least in part, why a given drug may cause different patterns of liver damage [87].

Diagnostic approach and tools for causality assessment

The phenotypic expressions of DILI may present in several ways (clinical and pathological) that resemble known forms of acute and chronic liver disease; the severity ranges from sub-clinical elevations in liver enzyme concentrations to acute liver failure. Mainly, drugs tend to induce acute hepatitis, cholestasis or a mixed condition (see Table 47.2) [47].

Liver histology (although not very specific and, at best, "compatible with") is still the ideal tool for defining the pattern of liver damage. However, since a liver biopsy specimen is often not available, the pattern of drug-related liver injury is, from a practical standpoint, classified according to laboratory data [88, 89]. The classification scheme was proposed by CIOMS [88] and recently updated by the Food and Drug Administration Drug Hepatotoxicity Committee (see Table 47.3) [89].

The acute hepatocellular (cytotoxic, cytolytic) type of liver injury is the most common expression of hepatotoxicity and it is observed with many drugs (see Table 47.4) [21, 22]. Patients with acute hepatocellular injury related to drugs are at risk of acute liver failure. The presence of combined increases in ALT and bilirubin levels in DILI reflects a substantial loss in hepatocellular function and potential for liver failure [90]. **B4** These parameters are considered a specific indicator of severe hepatotoxic potential of a drug. In patients with acute drug-induced hepatitis the presence of jaundice is the most significant predictor of mortality/liver transplantation. The observation by Hyman Zimmerman, known as "Hy's rule" [47], predicts a mean mortality (or its surrogate marker, liver transplantation) of 10% (range 5–50%) for jaundiced patients with acute toxic hepatocellular damage. Hy's rule has been validated in large case series from Spain and Sweden in which analysis of pooled data showed that other variables such older age,

Table 47.2 Key clinical aspects in drug-induced liver disease.

DILI clinical issue	Key point	To be remembered
Presentation	• DILI may resemble any acute and chronic liver disease. • Acute hepatocellular presentation predominates.	• Hypersensitivity features occur in less than a quarter of patients.
Prognosis	• Female sex, hepatocellular damage and high bilirubin levels on presentation are risk factors for the development of fulminant hepatic failure. • Cholestatic/mixed damage is more prone to chronicity.	• Classification of damage by biochemical criteria is useful to stratify prognosis.
Diagnosis	• Relies largely on exclusion of other causes of liver injury. • Rules for assigning causality in DILI do not substitute clinical judgment. • The "signature" (consistent clinical, pathologic and latency presentation) for a given drug may be variable.	• CIOMS/RUCAM scale provides a framework to guide diagnosis in DILI, and adds consistency and reproducibility to clinical judgment. • Complexity of CIOMS/RUCAM scale precludes its implementation in routine clinical practice.

Table 47.3 The classification of the type of liver damage according to the Council for International Organizations of Medical Sciences (*J Hepatol* 1990, **11**: 272) and recently updated by the Food and Drug Administration Drug Hepatotoxicity Committee (www.fda.gov/cder/livertox/presentations2005).

Hepatocellular: Increase >3N ALT or when R ≥ 5
Cholestatic: Increase >2N AP or when R ≤ 2
Mixed: Increase >2N ALT and AP or 2 < R > 5

$$R = \frac{ALTxN}{APxN}$$

N: Upper limit of normal; BC: Conjugated bilirubin; BT: Total bilirubin; ALT: Alanin-aminotransferase; AP: Alkaline phosphatase.

Table 47.4 Drugs and compounds predominantly associated with hepatocellular or cholestatic damage.

Hepatocelullar damage	Cholestatic damage
Acarbose	Amoxicillin clavulanic acid
Allopurinol	Azathioprine
Amiodarone	Captopril, enalapril, fosinopril
Amoxicillin, Ampicillin	Benoxaprofen
Anti-HIV:	Bupropion
(didanosine, zidovudine, protease inhibitors)	Carbamazepine
Non-steroidal anti-inflammatory drugs	Carbimazole
(ibuprofen, diclofenac, piroxicam,indometacin)	Cloxacillin, dicloxacillin
Asparaginase	Clindamycin
Bentazepam	Ciprofloxacin, norfloxacin
Bromfenac	Contraceptive steroids
Chlormethiazole	Cyproheptadine
Cocaine, Ecstasy and amphetamine derivatives	Diazepam, Nitrazepam
Diphenytoin	Erythromycins
Disulfiram	Estrogens
Ebrotidine	Gold compounds,penicillamine
Fluoxetine, paroxetine	Herbal remedies:
Flutamide	(Chaparral leaf (*Larrea tridentate*), Glycyrrhizin, Greater celandine
Halothane	(*Chelidonium majus*))
Herbal remedies	Irbesartan
((Chaso and Onshido, Herbalife®	Lipid lowering drugs:
Germander (*Teucrium chamaedrys*), senna Pennyroyal oil, kava-kava (*Piper*	(atorvastatin, fluvastatin)
Methysticum), *Camellia sinnensis* (green tea), Chinese herbal medicines))	Macrolide antibiotics
Leflunomide	Mirtazapine
Lipid lowering drugs:	Penicillin G
(lovastatin, pravastatin)	Phenotiazines (chlorpromazine)
Isoniazid	Raloxifen
Ketoconazole	Rofecoxib, Celecoxib
Mebendazole, albendazole, pentamidine	Rosiglitazone, pioglitazone
Mesalazine	Sulfamethoxazole-trimethoprim
Methotrexate	Sulfonylureas:
Minocycline	(Glibenclamide,Chlorpropamide)
Nitrofurantoin	Sulindac
Nefazodone	Terbinafine
Omeprazole	Tamoxifen
Pemoline	Tetracycline
Pyrazinamide	Ticlopidine, Clopidogrel
Risperidone	Thiabendazole
Ritodrine	Tricyclic antidepressants:
Sulfasalazine	(Amitriptyline, Imipramine)
Telithromycin	
Terbinafine	
Tetracycline	
Tolcapone	
Topiramate	
Trazodone	
Troglitazone	
Trovafloxacin	
Valproic acid	
Venlafaxine	
Verapamil	
Vitamin A	
Ximelagatran	

female gender and AST levels were independently associated with a poor outcome [21, 38]. **B4** Further analysis of the Swedish database, has found that there was also a significant linear relationship between daily dose and the outcome of death/liver transplantation (2%, 9.4% and 13.2% in <10, 11–49, and >50 mg/day groups respectively, p = 0.03) [24]. **B4** On the contrary, it has recently been suggested that eosinophilia accompanying DILI may be associated with a better short-term prognosis [91, 92]. Actually, none of the patients included in the Spanish Registry with idiosyncratic DILI who died, evolved to liver failure, or required a liver transplantation had eosinophilia, whereas this feature was found in the 23% of the patients with milder outcomes [21]. **B4** Of note is that the height of transaminases in acute hepatocellular DILI lacks prognosis significance. Indeed, a decrease in liver enzymes after drug withdrawal in patients with severe DILI may reflect rather than a clinical improvement, a limited hepatic reserve associated with impending liver failure [90]. Moreover, if acute injury is superimposed on underlying liver disease, monitoring liver function tests may be difficult to interpret. For example, if advanced cirrhosis is present, the severity of liver injury may be underestimated by the height of the serum ALT measurements [93].

Acute cholestatic injury is caused by many drugs, including anabolic and contraceptive steroids, which characteristically produce DILI with minimal or absent accompanying inflammation. Other medications, which include amoxicillin-clavulanate, macrolide antibiotics and phenothiazine neuroleptics, typically cause variable degrees of portal inflammation and hepatocyte necrosis, in addition to marked cholestasis, which is predominantly centrilobular (see Table 47.4) [42, 47].

In mixed hepatic injury, the clinical and biological picture is intermediate between the hepatocellular and the cholestatic patterns, and features of either type may predominate. By definition, the ALT/AP ratio is between 2 and 5 (see Table 47.3). When faced clinically with a mixed hepatitis picture, the gastroenterologist should always suspect and seek a potentially hepatotoxic medication, since this type of injury is far more characteristic of drug-induced hepatotoxicity than of viral hepatitis [47]. Almost all drugs that produce cholestatic injury are also capable of inducing a mixed pattern.

Drug-induced acute cholestatic and mixed lesions progress less frequently to acute liver failure than the hepatocellular type. However, their resolution is generally slower, with a higher likelihood towards chronicity in one study (9% vs 4% respectively; p < 0.031) [94]. In contrast, in the hepatocellular pattern with jaundice at presentation, the severity of chronic lesions was greater (higher incidence of cirrhosis and chronic hepatitis) [94, 95]. Cardiovascular and central nervous system drugs are the main groups leading to chronic liver damage [94]. Of the

whole population included in the Spanish Registry, 5.6% of patients had biochemical evidence of chronicity [94], a figure similar to that reported in the Swedish population (6%), even though the majority of the patients included in this latter study were identified in an outpatient basis and had mild to moderate DILI [96]. A higher prevalence of chronicity (14%) has been reported in the analysis of the first 300 patients enrolled in the cooperative group Drug Induced Liver Injury Network in USA [22]. Further studies on the natural history of DILI are ongoing.

The diagnosis of DILI remains a challenge because, except for the very rare circumstance in which an unintentional positive re-challenge may confirm the putative involvement of a drug, the evidence that is usually collected is often circumstantial. It is often based on subjective impressions from previous experiences, and can lead to inaccurate diagnosis [97]. At present, the diagnosis of DILI is complex and not standardized, and is made with varying levels of confidence, relying largely on exclusion of other causes of liver disease and identification of a signature pattern of disease manifestations, in relation to starting and stopping of the suspected drug or herbal medication [98]. The process is time-consuming and delays clinical diagnosis; at least until other possible causes of liver disease have been excluded. It has been considered as the Achilles heel in the field of hepatotoxicity. Confounding features include multiple drugs prescribed, lack of information on doses consumed, as well as the stop and start dates [99]. A careful "step-by-step" approach is outlined in Figure 47.2 [100].

This issue has important implications not only for practicing clinicians, but also for conducting research into the risk factors, mechanisms and natural history of DILI, and from a medico-legal and drug regulation/development standpoint [101]. The use of causality assessment methods does add some consistency to the diagnostic process, by translating the suspicion into a quantitative score and by providing a framework that emphasizes the features that merit attention in cases of suspected hepatic adverse reaction (see Table 47.2) [102].

A controversial issue is the role of liver biopsy in the diagnosis of DILI. Indeed, since there are no histological findings specific for toxic damage, liver biopsy should not be performed routinely for this indication [103]. Furthermore, a liver biopsy specimen which is often taken several days after the clinical presentation of the symptoms, when the pathological features are beginning to wane, may generate perplexity and confusion in cases in which chronological sequence criteria are critical and when exclusion of alternative causes appear to incriminate the drug [104]. Currently, a reasonable approach for performing a liver biopsy in patients with suspected DILI is restricted to some specific situations: (1) the patient may have an underlying liver disease and, hence, it is difficult to ascribe the picture to the candidate drug or to a

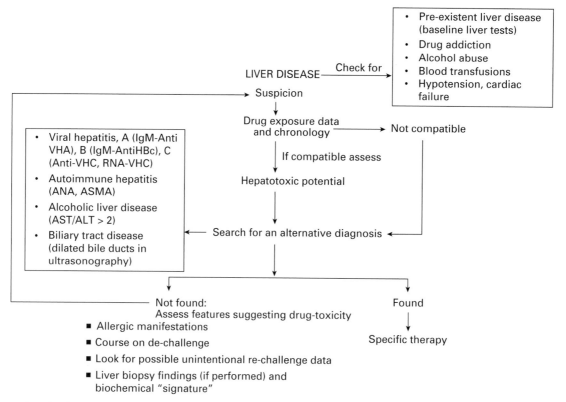

Figure 47.2 Algorithm for step-by-step approach to a suspected case of drug-induced liver disease.

recrudescence of the disease [104]; (2) to characterize the pattern of injury with those drugs that had not been previously incriminated in hepatotoxicity [1, 3, 105]; and (3) for identifying more severe or residual lesions (e.g. fibrosis) which could have prognostic significance. For instance, in some chronic variants of hepatotoxicity, clinical and laboratory features poorly reflect the severity of the liver injury [105], and a liver biopsy may clarify its true magnitude. Furthermore, severe bile duct injury during cholestatic hepatitis has been shown to be predictive of clinical evolution into chronic cholestasis [106], and, in a retrospective study, the presence of fibrosis in the index liver biopsy was related to the development of chronic liver disease [107].

Prompt recognition of potentially hepatotoxic drugs as the cause of liver injury is the most important aspect in the management of hepatotoxicity. It is of paramount importance as immediate stoppage appears to decrease the risk of progression to acute liver failure or chronic liver injury [94, 95]. The fact that the diagnosis of hepatotoxicity still relies upon careful history taking (completeness of data and accuracy) and a correct interpretation of the patient's clinical manifestations and laboratory data, should not be underestimated. An approach to diagnosis following clinical judgment, that closely depends on physician's skill, and that is not standardized, results in categories of causation that can be defined as drug-related (e.g. acetaminophen

over dosage, cases of positive re-challenge), clearly non-drug related (an alternative explanation found, negative de-challenge) or possibly drug-related (temporal sequence, possible competing cause, de-challenge positive) [104]. This last judgment in which subjectivity prevails and in which there is no strong argument for confirming or ruling out drug causality represents the majority of situations in clinical practice. Consequently, agreement among physicians who evaluate a given case of drug-suspected hepatotoxicity may differ strongly, and indeed has been shown to lead to inaccurate diagnosis [97].

To ascertain the putative role of a drug on the basis of quantitative criteria, clinical and laboratory data are assessed with probabilistic approaches (based on Bayesian statistics) and algorithms or clinical scales. The qualities usually required for a diagnosis scale are reproducibility and validity. Reproducibility ensures an identical result regardless of who the user is, and when the scale is used. Validity means the method is able to distinguish between cases where the drug is responsible and cases where it is not [104]. It is worth noting that none of the things that are currently measured have proven to be reliable in assessing causality for drug-induced liver injury. Therefore, more convincing evidence of validity is difficult to obtain in the absence of a unanimously accepted "gold standard" defining "truth" (see Table 47.2).

The first method developed in the area of DILI and, at present, the most prominent adjudication system in use by experts/researchers/sanitary authorities is CIOMS or RUCAM (Roussel Uclaf Causality Assessment Method) scale, which provides a standardized scoring system, in which the limits and content of most criteria were decided by consensus, among experts, on the basis of organ-oriented characteristics [50]. The parameters are outlined in Table 47.5. The time to onset and course criteria vary according to whether cases present with hepatocellular or cholestatic/mixed liver injury, since the latter may occur after a longer post-cessation interval and resolve much more slowly. The CIOMS/RUCAM scale provides a scoring system for seven axes in the decision strategy in which the answers correspond to weighted numeric values that are summed to give a total score. The scores are translated into categories of suspicion: definite or highly probable (score >8), probable (score 6–8), possible (score 3–5), unlikely (score 1–2) and excluded (score (</= 0). This method was originally validated using cases of drug-induced liver disease with known positive re-challenge (the major type of evidence recognized as demonstrating the role of a drug), and the system performed well when these cases were assessed, based on data prior to re-challenge, or when concomitant drugs were included [98]. This tool has the advantage of providing a framework that emphasizes topics that need to be addressed in cases of suspected hepatic adverse reaction, in order to improve the consistency of judgments. The major drawback is its complexity. It requires training and is less efficient when a user is unfamiliar with the format. The scale may seem cumbersome and while reading across the page, care needs to be taken not to misunderstand the questions, otherwise careless errors can be made [102]. Hence, it is not generally used by practicing physicians, who presumably find it confusing and difficult to apply.

A simpler but also organ-specific method, the Clinical Diagnostic Scale (CDS) (also called the M&V scale), was developed and tested by Maria and Victorino from Portugal [108]. In contrast with the CIOMS/RUCAM scale, the M&V scale includes questions that apply only to immune-allergic hepatitis. Furthermore, there are differences in the periods allowed for the end of treatment and the onset of liver injury and for the disappearance of liver abnormalities after withdrawal of treatment, as well as different criteria to define drug injury. The CDS/M&V scale is classified using five ratings: >17, relationship definite; 14–17, probable; 10–13, possible; 6–9, unlikely; <6 excluded. The CDS/M&V scale was validated using real and fictitious cases of immunoallergic drug-induced liver injury immunological mechanism (high percentages of positive immunological tests in cases classified as definite or probable), and was compared with the external standard or experts' classification.

The merits of the CIOMS/RUCAM scale and the CDS/M&V scale were compared in a population of 215 patients reported to a Registry [109]. Causality in this population was verified by three experts as drug-induced (185), or as non-drug caused (30 cases). Complete agreement between the CDS/M&V scale and the CIOMS/RUCAM scale was obtained in only 42 cases (18%). The CDS/M&V scale, classified only about one-third of the cases as probable or definite, and tended to underestimate the probability of causality. It was not unexpected, due to the arbitrary weights given to relevant assessment criteria, that the performance of the M&V scale was poor in drug injury with long latency periods (i.e. amoxycillin/clavulanic acid), evolution to chronicity after withdrawal (cholestatic pattern), or death (due to the lack of de-challenge data). On the contrary, the best agreement between scales was found for idiosyncratic immunologic DILI cases.

The need for more accurate and simple tools in drug hepatotoxicity has lead investigators to evaluate the performance of the Naranjo Adverse Drug Reactions Probability Scale (NADRPS), which is not liver specific but valuable in the overall evaluation of adverse drug reactions [110]. The attractive aspect of the Naranjo scale is its simplicity (see Table 47.5). The NADRPS involves ten "yes", "no" or "unknown or non-applicable" questions. The adverse drug reaction is assigned to a probability category, on the basis of the total score as "definite" ≥ 9, "likely" = 5–8, "possible" = 1–4, "unlikely" ≤ 0. In comparison with the CIOMS scale assessing a cohort of 225 cases of suspected DILI, the Naranjo scale had a low sensitivity and negative predictive value and it was neither reproducible nor valid for evaluating drug hepatotoxicity, and thus its use for this purpose is not recommended [111]. Indeed, the Naranjo algorithm was designed for evaluation of adverse drug reactions related to pharmacological actions of the drugs, and hence has questions such as "drug concentrations and monitoring", "dose relationship", "placebo response", which are clearly not relevant to idiosyncratic DILI.

However, limitations of the CIOMS/RUCAM scale have also been highlighted [90, 99, 112], such as the poor definition of the components needing to be answered, poor diagnostic capability when two drugs are given with the same temporal sequence, and the arbitrary weighting and selection of important validation criteria, such as the cutoff age point, known relevant risk factors and better estimates of temporal chronology. All of these are taken into consideration for each case under evaluation (see Table 47.5). Indeed, a recent report has shown a low reliability of the RUCAM instrument, and, moreover, poor agreement among experts in the analysis of 40 well-defined DILI cases [113]. Each case was adjudicated by three reviewers, each working independently. After an interval of at least four months,

Table 47.5 Scores for individual axes of most commonly used diagnostic scales.

CIOMS/RUCAM		Maria & Victorino/CDS		Naranjo	
Axis	**Score**	**Axis**	**Score**	**Axis**	**Score**
Chronological criteria		**Chronological criteria**		Previous reports on ADR	+1 to 0
(according to type of liver damage: hepatocellular or cholestatic/mixed)				Onset of the ADR after drug administration	+2 to −1
Time to onset of the event		From drug intake until onset event			
Suggestive	+2	4 days to 8 weeks	+3		
Compatible	+1	Less than 4 days or more than 8 weeks	+1	Improvement of ADR after drug withdrawal or antagonist	+1 to 0
From drug withdrawal until onset event		From drug withdrawal until onset event			
Compatible	+1	0 to 7 days	+3	Positive rechallenge	+2 to −1
Course of the reaction		8 to 15 days	0		
Highly suggestive	+3	More than 15 days	−3	Presence of alternative causes	+2 to −1
Suggestive	+2	Normalization of laboratory values			
Compatible	+1	Less than 6 mo (cholestatic) or 2 mo (hepatocellular)	+3	Positive rechallenge with placebo	+1 to −1
Against the role of the drug	−2				
Inconclusive or not available	0	More than 6 mo or 2 mo	0		
Risk factors				Toxic drug levels in biological fluids	+1 to 0
Age(≥50 y)	+1 to 0	**Other causes**			
Alcohol or	+1 to 0	Complete exclusion	+3		
Pregnancy (cholestatic)	+1 to 0	Partial exclusion	0	Reaction dosed-related	+1 to 0
		Possible alternative causes	−1		
		Probable alternative causes	−3	Previous reaction to the same or related drugs	+1 to 0
Concomitant drug(s)		**Extrahepatic manifestations**			
Absence	0	4 or more	+3		
Time to onset incompatible	0	2 or 3	+2	ADR confirmed by any objective evidence	+1 to 0
Compatible but unknown reaction	−1	1	+1		
Compatible and known reaction	−2	None	0		
Role proved in this case	−3				
None or information not available	0				
Exclusion non drug-related causes		**Rechallenge**			
Rule out all causes	+2	Positive	+3		
6 causes excluded	+1	Negative or not performed	0		
4 or 5 causes excluded	0				
<4 causes excluded	−2				
Probable hepatic etiology	−3				
Previous information on hepatotoxicity		**Known Reaction**			
Reaction known	+2	Yes	+2		
Reaction published but unlabelled	+1	No (drugs marketed < 5 y)	0		
Reaction labelled in the SPC	0	No (drugs marketed > 5 y)	−3		
Rechallenge					
Positive	+3				
Compatible	+1				
Negative	−2				
Not available or not interpretable	0				

CIOMS: Council for International Organizations of Medical Sciences; RUCAM: Roussel Uclaf Causality Assessment Method; CDS: Clinical Diagnostic Scale; SPC: Summary Product Characteristic; ADR: adverse drug reaction.

With CIOMS/RUCAM, score ≤ 0, diagnosis of excluded; 1–2 unlikely; 3–5, possible; 6–8 probable; >8 highly probable or definite.

With Maria & Vitorino/CDS, score > 17, definite; 14–17, probable; 10–13, possible; 6–9, unlikely; <6, drug hepatotoxicity excluded.

With Naranjo Adverse Drug Reaction Probability scale, score ≥ 9 diagnosis of definite; 5–8, likely; 1–4 possible; ≤0, doubtful.

cases were re-adjudicated by the same reviewers. Test-retest differences ranged from −7 to +8 with complete agreement in only 26% of cases. On average, the maximum absolute difference among the three reviewers was 3.1 on the first occasion and 2.7 on the second, although much of this variability could be attributed to differences between the enrolling investigator and the external reviewers. Under the best-case scenario, the test-retest reliability among the site principal investigators was only 0.65, while the inter-rater reliability among the external reviewers, was unacceptably low at 0.46. The authors concluded that the mediocre reliability of the RUCAM is problematic for future studies of DILI [113].

It would be important, nevertheless, to accommodate all relevant information into an ideal scoring system and to eliminate low impact items. This is now feasible with the use of large datasets of cases. Clinicians attribute a crucial value to the presence of clinical signs of hypersensitivity, which is not a domain in the scale. Besides, when liver biopsy findings are available, they should be taken into account for the evaluation of alternative causes, and also to reach a definitive diagnosis if an eosinophilic hepatic infiltrate, centrozonal damage (highest content of cyto-chrome P450), granulomas and microesteatosis are evident. Furthermore, assessment of known genetic risk factors for hepatotoxicity could be further evaluated. Indeed, a com-puterized scale that could integrate in a dynamic way all available knowledge with regard to the given drug and its signature in a particular patient population would be of great value. A modified RUCAM/CIOMS instrument termed DWW-J (Digestive Disease Week-Japan) has been proposed [115]. In this approach, the indirect evidence of immunoallergy such as eosinophilia, or a positive *in vitro* lymphocyte stimulation test, were weighted; no case in which the temporal criteria did not fall within the accepted limits was excluded, and the domain regarding concomi-tant drugs was deleted [114]. The performance of the DWW-J scale was then evaluated in 127 DILI cases and 46 controls with 423 putative drugs. As compared with CIOMS the modified scale showed a higher sensitivity but a poorer specificity [115].

International consensus is needed to agree upon common definitions, diagnostic criteria, terminologies and instruments to assess the causality in DILI and it is now feasible by the concerted actions of several investigators working in this area [21, 22, 35, 37]. Hopefully, a new instrument will be developed to improve the consistency, accuracy and objectiveness in causality assessment in hepatotoxicity. Such a goal, will allow better planning and interpretation of genetic studies and this, in turn, will enhance knowledge and research into the mechanism underlying DILI.

References

1 Andrade RJ, Lucena MI, Martín-Vivaldi R *et al.* Acute liver injury associated with the use of ebrotidine, a new H₂-receptor antagonist. *J Hepatol* 1999; **31**: 641–646.

2 Herrine SK, Choudary C. Severe hepatotoxicity associated with troglitazone. *Ann Intern Med* 1999; **130**: 163–164.

3 Lucena MI, Andrade RJ, Rodrigo L *et al.* Trovafloxacin-induced acute hepatitis. *Clin Infect Dis* 2000; **30**: 400–401.

4 Lee WM, Larrey D, Olsson R *et al.* Hepatic findings in long-term clinical trials of ximelagatran. *Drug Saf* 2005; **28**: 351–370.

5 Brinker A, Wassel R, Lyndly J *et al.* Telithromycin-associated hepatotoxicity: clinical spectrum and causality assessment of 42 cases. *Hepatology* 2008; **49**: 250–257.

6 Benninger J, Schneider HT, Schuppan D *et al.* Acute hepatitis induced by greater celandine (*Chelidonium majus*). *Gastroenterology* 1999; **117**: 1234–1237.

7 Stickél F, Baumuller HM, Seitz KH *et al.* Hepatitis induced by kava (*Piper methysticum rhizoma*). *J Hepatol* 2003; **9**: 62–67.

8 Adachi M, Saito H, Kobayashi H *et al.* Hepatic injury in 12 patients taking the herbal weight loss aids Chaso or onshido. *Ann Intern Med* 2003; **139**: 488–492.

9 Neff GW, Reddy KR, Durazo FA *et al.* Severe hepatotoxicity associated with the use of weight loss diet supplements contain-ing ma huang or usnic acid. *J Hepatol* 2004; **41**: 1062–1064.

10 Bonkovsky HL. Hepatotoxicity associated with supplements containing Chinese green tea (*Camellia sinensis*). *Ann Intern Med* 2006; **144**: 68–71.

11 Elinav E, Pinsker G, Safadi R *et al.* Association between con-sumption of Herbalife® nutritional supplements and acute hepatotoxicity. *J Hepatol* 2007; **47**: 514–520.

12 Schoepfer AM, Engel A, Fattinger K *et al.* Herbal does not mean innocuous: 10 cases of severe hepatotoxicity associated with dietary supplements from Herbalife® products. *J Hepatol* 2007; **47**: 521–526.

13 Ostapowicz G, Fontana RJ, Schiødt FV *et al.* Results of a pro-spective study of acute liver failure at 17 tertiary care centers in the United States. *Ann Intern Med* 2002; **137**: 947–954.

14 Whitehead MW, Hainsworth I, Kingham JGC. The causes of obvious jaundice in South West Wales: 2000. *Gut* 2001; **48**: 409–413.

15 Björnsson E, Ismael S, Nejdet S *et al.* Severe jaundice in Sweden in the new millennium: causes, investigations, treatment and prognosis. *Scand J Gastroenterol* 2003; **38**: 86–94.

16 Vuppalanchi R, Liangpunsakul S, Chalasani N. Etiology of new-onset jaundice: how often is it caused by idiosyncratic drug-induced liver injury in the United States? *Am J Gastroenterol* 2007; **102**: 558–556

17 Meier Y, Cavallaro M, Roos M *et al.* Incidence of drug-induced liver injury in medical inpatients. *Eur J Clin Pharmacol* 2005; **61**: 135–143.

18 Sgro C, Clinard F, Ouazir K *et al.* Incidence of drug-induced hepatic injuries:a French population-based study. *Hepatology* 2003; **36**: 451–455.

19 Larrey D. Drug-induced liver diseases. *J Hepatol* 2000; **32**: 77–88.

20 Park BK, Kitteringham NR, Maggs JL *et al*. The role of metabolic activation in drug-induced hepatotoxicity. *Annu Rev Pharmacol Toxicol* 2005; **45**: 177–202.

21 Andrade RJ, Lucena MI, Fernández MC *et al*. Drug-induced liver injury: an analysis of 461 incidences submitted to the Spanish Registry over a 10-year period. *Gastroenterology* 2005; **129**: 512–521.

22 Chalasani N, Fontana R, Bonkovsky MD, Watkin PB *et al*. Causes, clinical features, and outcomes from a prospective study of drug-induced liver injury in the United States. *Gastroenterolology* 2008; **135**: 1924–1934.

23 Seguin B, Utrecht J. The danger hypothesis applied to idiosyncratic drug reactions. *Curr Opin Allergy Clin Immunol* 2003; **3**: 35–42.

24 Lammert C, Einarsson S, Saha C. Relationship between daily dose of oral medications and idiosyncratic drug-induced liver injury: search for signals. *Hepatology* 2008; **47**: 2003–2009.

25 Uetrecht J. Idiosyncratic drug reactions: current understanding. *Annu Rev Pharmacol Toxicol* 2007; **47**: 513–539.

26 Boelsterli UA, Lim PLK. Mitochondrial abnormalities. A link to idiosyncratic drug hepatotoxicity? *Toxicol Appl Pharmacol* 2007; **220**: 92–107.

27 Kaplowitz N. Idiosyncratic drug hepatotoxicity. *Nature Rev Drug Discovery* 2005; **4**: 489–499.

28 Walgren JL, Mitchell MD, Thompson DC. Role of metabolism in drug-induced idiosyncratic hepatotoxicity. *Crit Rev Toxicol* 2005; **35**: 325–361.

29 Pessayre D. Role of reactive metabolites in drug-induced hepatitis. *J Hepatol* 1995; **23**(Suppl. 1): 16–24.

30 Berson A, De Beco V, Letteron P *et al*. Steatohepatitis-inducing drugs cause mitochondrial dysfunction and lipid peroxidation in rat hepatocytes. *Gastroenterology* 1998; **114**: 764–774.

31 Pessayre D, Berson A, Fromenty B *et al*. Mitochondria in steatohepatitis. *Semin Liver Dis* 2001; **21**: 57–69.

32 Pessayre D, Haouzi D, Fau D *et al*. Withdrawal of life support, altruistic suicide, fratricidal killing and euthanasia by lymphocytes: different forms of drug-induced hepatic apoptosis. *J Hepatol* 1999; **131**(4): 760–770.

33 Liu ZX, Govindarajan S, Kaplowitz N. Innate immune system plays a critical role in determining the progression and severity of acetaminophen hepatotoxicity. *Gastroenterology* 2004; **127**: 1760–1774.

34 Hoofnagle JH. Drug-induced liver injury network (DILIN). *Hepatology* 2004; **40**: 773.

35 Daly AK, Aithal GP, Leathart JBS *et al*. Genetic susceptibility to diclofenac-induced hepatotoxicity: contribution of UGT2B7, CYP2C8, and ABCC2 genotypes. *Gastroenterology* 2007; **132**: 272–281.

36 Molokhia M, McKeigue P. EUDRAGENE: European collaboration to establish a case-control DNA collection for studying the genetic basis of adverse drug reactions. *Pharmacogenomics* 2006; **7**: 633–638.

37 Björnsoon E, Olsson R. Outcome and prognostic markers in severe drug-induced liver disease. *Hepatology* 2005; **42**: 481–489.

38 DeLeve LD. Risk factors for drug-induced liver disease. In: Kaplowitz N & DeLeve LD, eds. *Drug-Induced Liver Disease*, Informa Healthcare, New York, 2007: 291–305.

39 Gronhangen RC, Hellstrom PE, Froseth B. Predisposing factors in hepatitis induced by isoniazid, refampin treatment of tuberculosis. *Am Rev Respir Dis* 1978; **118**: 161–166.

40 Garcia Rodriguez LA, Stricker BH, Zimmermann HI. Risk of acute liver injury associated with the combination of amoxicllin and clavulanic acid. *Arch Intern Med* 1996; **156**: 1327–1332.

41 Hussaini SH, O'Brien CS, Despott EJ *et al*. Antibiotic therapy: a major cause of drug-induced jaundice in southwest England. *Eur J Gastroenterol Hepatol* 2007; **19**: 15–20.

42 Kaplowitz N, Deleve LD. *Drug-induced Liver Disease*. Informa-Healthcare, New York, 2007.

43 Lucena MI, Andrade RJ, Kaplowitz N *et al*. Phenotypic characterization of idiosyncratic drug-induced liver injury: the influence of age and gender. *Hepatology* 2009; **49**(6): 2001–2009.

44 Fris H, Andreasen PB. Drug-induced hepatic injury: an analysis of 1100 cases reported to the Danish Committee on Adverse Drug Reactions between 1978 and 1987. *J Intern Med* 1992; **232**: 133–138.

45 Watkins PB, Seef LB. Drug-induced liver injury: summary of a single topic clinical research conference. *Hepatology* 2006; **43**: 618–631.

46 De Valle MB, Av Klinteberg V, Alem N *et al*. Drug-induced liver injury in a Swedish University hospital out-patient hepatology clinic. *Aliment Pharmacol Ther* 2006; **24**: 1187–1195.

47 Zimmerman HJ. *Hepatotoxicity. The Adverse Effects of Drugs and Other Chemicals on the Liver*, 2nd edn. Lippincott Williams & Wilkins, Philadelphia, 1999.

48 Ibáñez L, Pérez E, Vidal X *et al*. Prospective surveillance of acute serious liver disease unrelated to infectious, obstructive, or metabolic diseases: epidemiological and clinical features, and exposure to drugs. *J Hepatol* 2002; **37**: 592–600.

49 Russo MW, Galanko JA, Shrestha R *et al*. Liver transplantation for acute liver failure from drug induced liver injury in the United States. *Liver Transpl* 2004; **10**: 1018–1023.

50 Danan G, Bénichou C. Causality assessment of adverse reactions to drugs I. A novel method based on the conclusions of international consensus meetings: application to drug-induced liver injuries. *J Clin Epidemiol* 1993; **46**: 1323–1330.

51 De Abajo FJ, Montero D, Madurga M *et al*. Acute and clinically relevant drug-induced liver injury: a population based case-control study. *Br J Clin Pharmacol* 2004; **58**: 71–80.

52 Pessayre D, Pentata M, Degott C *et al*. Isoniazid rifampicin fulminant hepatitis: a possible consequence of enhancement of isoniazid hepatotoxicity by enzyme induction. *Gastroenterology* 1977; **42**: 284–289.

53 Bonfanti P, Landonio S, Ricci E *et al*. Risk factors for hepatotoxicity in patients treated with highly active antiretroviral therapy. *J Adquir Immune Defic Syndr* 2001; **27**: 316–318.

54 Kaplowitz N. Drug-induced liver injury. *Clin Infect Dis* 2004; **38**(Suppl. 2): S44–S48.

55 Lewis JH. The rational use of potentially hepatotoxic medications in patients with underlying liver disease. *Expert Opin Drug Saf* 2002; **1**: 159–172.

56 Rosenberg P, Urwitz H, Johansson A *et al*. Psoriasis patients with diabetes mellitus type 2 are at high risk of developing liver fibrosis during methotrexate treatment. *J Hepatol* 2007; **46**: 1111–1118.

57 Aithal GP. *Genetic basis of idiosyncratic hepatotoxicity.* In: Andrade RJ, ed. *Hepatotoxicity.* Permanyer Publications, Barcelona, 2007: 39–55.

58 Gillette JR. Keynote address: man, mice, microsomes, metabolites, and mathematics 40 years after the revolution. *Drug Metab Rev* 1995; **27**: 1–44.

59 Williams DP, Kitteringham NR, Naisbitt DJ *et al.* Are chemically reactive metabolites responsible for adverse reactions to drugs? *Curr Drug Metab* 2002; **3**: 351–366.

60 Pachkoria K, Lucena MI, Ruiz-Cabello F *et al.* Genetic polymorphisms of CYP2C9 and CYP2C19 are not related to drug-induced idiosyncratic liver injury. *Br J Pharmacol* 2007; **150**: 808–815.

61 Morgan MY, Reshef R, Shah RR *et al.* Impaired oxidation of debrisoquine in patients with perhexiline liver injury. *Gut* 1984; **25**: 1057–1064.

62 Alvan G, Bechtel P, Iselius L *et al.* Hydroxylation polymorphisms of debrisoquine and mephenytoin in European populations. *Eur J Clin Pharmacol* 1990; **39**: 533–537.

63 Huang YS, Chern HD, Su WJ *et al.* Polymorphism of the N-acetyltransferase 2 gene as a susceptibility risk factor for antituberculosis drug-induced hepatitis. *Hepatology* 2002; **35**: 883–889.

64 Sharma SK, Balamurugan A, Saha PK *et al.* Evaluation of clinical and immunogenetic risk factors for the development of hepatotoxicity during antitubercular treatment. *Am J Respir Crit Care Med* 2002; **166**: 916–919.

65 Huang YS, Chern HD, Su WJ *et al.* Cytochrome P450 2E1 genotype and the susceptibility to antituberculosis drug-induced hepatitis. *Hepatology* 2003; **37**: 924–930.

66 Hayes JD, Flanagan JU, Jowsey IR. Glutathione transferases. *Annu Rev Pharmacol Toxicol* 2005; **45**: 51–88.

67 Gum SI, Jo SJ, Ahn SH *et al.* The potent protective effect of wild ginseng (Panax ginseng C.A. Meyer) against benzo (alpha) pyrene-induced toxicity through metabolic regulation of CYP1A1 and GSTs. *J Ethnopharmacol* 2007; **112**: 568–576.

68 Tanaka K, Kiyosawa N, Watanabe K *et al.* Characterization of resistance to bromobenzene-induced hepatotoxicity by microarray. *J Toxicol Sci* 2007; **32**: 129–134.

69 Morishita K, Mizukawa Y, Kasahara T *et al.* Gene expression profile in liver of differing ages of rats after single oral administration of acetaminophen. *J Toxicol Sci* 2006; **31**: 491–507.

70 Chan K, Han XD, Kan YW. An important function of Nrf2 in combating oxidative stress: detoxification of acetaminophen. *Proc Natl Acad Sci USA* 2001; **98**: 4611–4616.

71 Eaton DL, Bammler TK, Kelly EJ. Interindividual differences in response to chemoprotection against aflatoxin-induced hepatocarcinogenesis: implications for human biotransformation enzyme polymorphisms. *Adv Exp Med Biol* 2001; **500**: 559–576.

72 Dieckhaus CM, Roller SG, Santos WL *et al.* Role of glutathione S-transferases A1-1, M1-1, and P1-1 in the detoxification of 2-phenylpropenal, a reactive felbamate metabolite. *Chem Res Toxicol* 2001; **14**: 511–516.

73 Lo HW, Ali-Osman F. Genetic polymorphism and function of glutathione S-transferases in tumor drug resistance. *Curr Opin Pharmacol* 2007; **7**: 367–374.

74 Watanabe I, Tomita A, Shimizu M *et al.* A study to survey susceptible genetic factors responsible for troglitazone-associated hepatotoxicity in Japanese patients with type 2 diabetes mellitus. *Clin Pharmacol Ther* 2003; **73**: 435–455.

75 Simon T, Becquemont L, Mary-Krause M *et al.* Combined glutathione-S-transferase M1 and T1 genetic polymorphism and tacrine hepatotoxicity. *Clin Pharmacol Ther* 2000; **67**: 432–437.

76 De Sousa M, Pirmohamed M, Kitteringham NR *et al.* No association between tacrine transaminitis and the glutathione transferase theta genotype in patients with Alzheimer's disease. *Pharmacogenetics* 1998; **8**: 353–355.

77 Roy B, Chowdhury A, Kundu S *et al.* Increased risk of antituberculosis drug-inducedhepatotoxicity in individuals with glutathione S-transferase M1 null mutation. *J Gastroenterol Hepatol* 2001; **16**: 1033–1037.

78 Huang YS, Su WJ, Huang YH *et al.* Genetic polymorphisms of manganese superoxide dismutase, NAD(P)H: quinone oxidoreductase, glutathione S-transferase M1 and T1 and the susceptibility to drug-induced liver injury. *J Hepatol* 2007; **47**: 128–134.

79 Lucena MI, Andrade RJ, Martínez C *et al.* Glutathione-S-transferase M1 and T1 null genotypes as susceptibility factor for idiosyncratic drug-induced liver injury. *Hepatology* 2008; **48**: 588–596.

80 Lang C, Meier Y, Stieger B *et al.* Mutations and polymorphisms in the bile salt export pump and the multidrug resistance protein 3 associated with drug-induced liver injury. *Pharmacogenet Genomics* 2007; **17**: 47–60.

81 Andrade RJ, Crespo E, Ulzurrun E *et al.* Polymorphic bile salt export pump transporter is a major determinant of hepatocellular drug-induced liver injury. *Hepatology* 2008; **48**: 468A (abstract).

82 Aithal GP, Ramsay L, Daly AK *et al.* Hepatic adducts, circulating antibodies, and cytokine polymorphisms in patients with diclofenac hepatotoxicity. *Hepatology* 2004; **39**: 1430–1440.

83 Pachkoria K, Lucena MI, Crespo E *et al.* Analysis of IL-10, IL-4 and TNF-alpha polymorphisms in drug-induced liver injury (DILI) and its outcome. *J Hepatol* 2008; **49**: 107–114.

84 Hautekeete ML, Horsmans Y, Van Waeyenberge C *et al.* HLA association of amoxicillin-clavulanate–induced hepatitis. *Gastroenterology* 1999; **117**: 1181–1186.

85 Daly A K, Donaldson P T, Bhatnagar P *et al.* HLA-B*5701 genotype is a major determinant of drug-induced liver injury due to flucloxacillin. *Nat Genet* 2009; **41**: 816–819.

86 Kindmark A, Jawaid A, Harbron CG *et al.* Genome-wide pharmacogenetic investigation of a hepatic adverse event without clinical signs of immunopathology suggests an underlying immune pathogenesis. *Pharmacogenomics J* 2008; **8**: 186–195.

87 Andrade RJ, Lucena MI, Alonso A *et al.* HLA class II genotype influences the type of liver injury in drug-induced idiosyncratic liver disease. *Hepatology* 2004; **39**: 1603–1612.

88 Benichou C. Criteria of drug-induced liver disorders. Report of an International Consensus Meeting. *J Hepatol* 1990; **11**: 272–276.

89 Navarro V. Hepatic adverse event nomenclature www.fda. gov/cder/livertox/presentations2005/Vic_Navarro.ppt (accessed on 21 August 2007).

90 Navarro VJ, Senior JR. Drug-related hepatotoxicity. *N Engl J Med* 2006; **354**: 731–739.

91 Björnsson E, Nordlinder H, Olsson R. Clinical characteristics and prognostic markers in disulfiram-induced liver injury. *J Hepatol* 2006; **44**: 791–797.

92 Björnsson E, Kalaitzakis E, Olsson R. The impact of eosinophilia and hepatic necrosis on prognosis in patients with drug-induced liver injury. *Aliment Pharmacol Ther* 2007; **25**: 1411–1421.

93 Russo MW, Watkins PB. Are patients with elevated liver tests at increased risk of drug-induced liver injury? *Gastroenterology* 2004; **126**: 1477–1480.

94 Andrade RJ, Lucena MI, Kaplowitz N *et al*. Outcome of acute idiosyncratic drug-induced liver injury: Long-term follow-up in a hepatotoxicity registry. *Hepatology* 2006; **44**: 1581–1588.

95 Björnsson E, Davidsdottir L. The long-term follow-up after idiosyncratic drug-induced liver injury with jaundice. *J Hepatol* 2009; **50**: 511–517.

96 Björnsson E, Kalaitzakis E, av Klinteberg V *et al*. Long-term follow-up in patients with mild to moderate drug-induced liver injury. *Aliment Pharmacol Ther* 2007; **26**: 79–85.

97 Aithal GP, Rawlins MD, Day CP. Accuracy of hepatic adverse drug reaction reporting in one English health region. *BMJ* 1999; **319**: 1541.

98 Kaplowitz N. Causality assessment versus guilt-by-association in drug hepatotoxicity. *Hepatology* 2001; **33**: 308–310.

99 Lee WM, Senior JR. Recognizing drug-induced liver injury: current problems, possible solutions. *Toxicol Pathol* 2005; **33**: 155–164.

100 Andrade RJ, Camargo R, Lucena MI *et al*. Causality assessment in drug-induced hepatotoxicity. *Expert Opin Drug Saf* 2004; **3**: 329–344.

101 Kaplowitz N. Drug-induced liver disorders: implications for drug development and regulation. *Drug Saf* 2001; **24**: 483–490.

102 Andrade RJ, Robles M, Fernandez-Castañer A *et al*. Assessment of drug-induced hepatotoxicity in clinical practice: a challenge for gastroenterologists. *World J Gastroenterol* 2007; **13**: 329–340.

103 Bianchi L. Liver biopsy in elevated liver function tests? An old question revisited. *J Hepatol* 2001; **35**: 290–294.

104 Lucena MI, Andrade RJ, Camargo R, García-Cortés M. Causality assessment. In: Kaplowitz N & DeLeve LD, eds. *Drug-Induced Liver Disease*, Informa Healthcare, New York, 2007: 325–344.

105 Andrade RJ, Lucena MI, Alcantara R *et al*. Bentazepam-associated chronic liver disease. *Lancet* 1994; **343**: 860.

106 Degott C, Feldmann G, Larrey D *et al*. Drug-induced prolonged cholestasis in adults: a histological semiquantitative study demonstrating progressive ductopenia. *Hepatology* 1992; **15**: 244–251

107 Aithal PG, Day CP. The natural history of histologically proved drug induced liver disease. *Gut* 1999; **44**: 731–735.

108 Maria V, Victorino R. Development and validation of a clinical scale for the diagnosis of drug-induced hepatitis. *Hepatology* 1997; **26**: 664–669.

109 Lucena MI, Camargo R, Andrade RJ *et al*. Comparison of two clinical scales for causality assessment in hepatotoxicity. *Hepatology* 2001; **33**: 123–130.

110 Naranjo CA, Busto U, Sellers EM *et al*. A method for estimating the probability of adverse drug reactions. *Clin Pharmacol Ther* 1981; **30**: 239–245.

111 Garcia-Cortés M, Lucena MI, Pachkoria K *et al*. Evaluation of Naranjo adverse drug reactions probability scale in causality assessment of drug-induced liver injury. *Alim Pharmacol Ther* 2008; **27**: 780–789.

112 Lee WM. Assessing causality in drug-induced liver injury. *J Hepatol* 2000; **33**: 1003–1005.

113 Rochon J, Protiva P, Seeff LB *et al*. Reliability of the Roussel Uclaf Causality Assessment Method for assessing causality in drug-Induced liver injury. *Hepatology* 2008; **48**: 1175–1183.

114 Takikawa H, Takamori Y, Kumagi T *et al*. Assessment of 287 Japanese cases of drug induced liver injury by the diagnostic scale of the International Consensus Meeting. *Hepatol Res* 2003; **27**: 192–195.

115 Watanabe M, Shibuya A. Validity study of a new diagnostic scale for drug-induced liver injury in Japan-comparison with two previous scales. *Hepatol Res* 2004; **30**: 148–154.

Index